D0540377

Scott-Brown's

Diseases of the Ear, Nose and Throat

Volume 1
Basic Sciences

Titles of other volumes

Volume 2 The Ear
Volume 3 The Nose and Sinuses
Volume 4 The Pharynx and Larynx

Scott-Brown's

Diseases of the Ear, Nose and Throat

Fourth Edition

Volume I

Basic Sciences

Editors

John Ballantyne, FRCS, HON FRCS (I)

Consultant Ear, Nose and Throat Surgeon,
The Royal Free Hospital and King Edward VII Hospital for Officers, London;
Civilian Consultant in Otolaryngology to the Army

John Groves MB, BS, FRCS

Consultant Ear, Nose and Throat Surgeon
The Royal Free Hospital, London

Butterworths

London Boston
Sydney Wellington Durban Toronto

United Kingdom London — **Butterworth & Co (Publishers) Ltd**
88 Kingsway, WC2B 6AB

Australia Sydney — **Butterworths Pty Ltd**
586 Pacific Highway, Chatswood, NSW 2067
Also at Melbourne, Brisbane, Adelaide and Perth

Canada Toronto — **Butterworth & Co (Canada) Ltd**
2265 Midland Avenue, Scarborough, Ontario, M1P 4S1

New Zealand Wellington — **Butterworths of New Zealand Ltd**
T & W Young Building, 77–85 Customhouse Quay, 1, CPO Box 472

South Africa Durban — **Butterworth & Co (South Africa) (Pty) Ltd**
152–154 Gale Street

USA Boston — **Butterworth (Publishers) Inc**
10 Tower Office Park, Woburn, Massachusetts 01801

First edition 1952
Second edition 1965
Reprinted 1967
Reprinted 1968
Third edition 1971
Reprinted 1977
Fourth edition 1979

ISBN 0 407 00147 6 Individual volume
ISBN 0 407 00143 3 Set of four volumes

British Library Cataloguing in Publication Data

Scott-Brown, Walter Graham
Scott-Brown's diseases of the ear, nose and throat. – 4th ed.
Vol. 1: Basic sciences
1. Otolaryngology
I. Ballantyne, John II. Groves, John
616.2'1 RF46 79-41008

ISBN 0-407-00147-6
ISBN 0-407-00143-3 Set of 4 vols

Phototypeset in Great Britain by
Filmtype Services Limited, Scarborough
Printed and bound by William Clowes & Sons Ltd, Beccles and London

Introduction to the Fourth Edition

Some eight years after the last edition of this work appeared it may now seem to the practising clinician that the present decade has been a relatively quiet one in the history of our specialty. In fact, there has been a steady growth in the scientific foundations upon which an increasing amount of our practice is built, and it is therefore not surprising that the first volume, *Basic Sciences*, has now been considerably enlarged.

There has also been a steady expansion of clinical knowledge, and in planning this new edition we quickly became aware that no single volume from the last edition could stand without revision.

Sadly, the list of authors has been depleted by deaths and retirements of old friends and colleagues, whose contributions to British otolaryngology will never be forgotten. We thank sincerely all our colleagues, both old and new who have spared no effort in preparing their manuscripts for this new presentation. The connoisseur will notice that a number of distinguished contributors from overseas have again been invited; we hope that this broadening of outlook will be welcomed by readers, and it is in keeping with the concepts of Mr W G Scott-Brown who originated the text nearly 30 years ago and who continues to flourish and to practice.

In some parts of the work, notably in Volume 2 (*The Ear*), advances in academic research have out-paced our ability to classify neatly a plethora of theories, facts (and sometimes fancies) for clinical application. Retaining the clinical approach as far as possible has compelled us, therefore, to commission chapters (for example in the field of sensorineural deafness) which overlap one another very considerably in content, while differing widely in emphasis. We hope that the reader will bear with this, and that the overall presentation will form a wider basis for learning than could be achieved by a more rigidly structured approach.

As far as we could we have used metric and SI units of measurement, even though a sense of humour is needed to accept some of the numerical absurdities which result. We are increasingly aware, too, that the SI system has brought upon us a hybrid and irrational system, heavily be-spattered with eponymously named units, at a time when eponyms are discouraged in the basic scientific disciplines. We are confident that the present generation will continue to honour Eustachius, Morgagni, Paget, Pott, Rosenmüller, and a hundred and one other great names, however the winds of pseudo-change may blow.

It is a great pleasure to thank and acknowledge all those who have helped so much in the preparation of this edition. We are grateful to those many colleagues who have lent us illustrations; to our registrars who have read proofs, criticized, advised and encouraged; and to those artists who have drawn new illustrations. Among the latter we thank especially Mr Frank Price for his unfailing generosity and technical skills. Equally we thank Mr Cedric Gilson and the Photographic Department of the Royal Free Hospital for their tremendous and willing efforts to provide so many of the new photographs.

Finally our gratitude goes to our publishers, Butterworths, who have done so much to lighten our editorial tasks.

London, 1979
John Ballantyne
John Groves

Introduction to the Third Edition

A radical new departure is made in the presentation of this work in four separately available volumes. This has been done for two main reasons. First, there is a real need, we feel, to recognize the diverse requirements of different readers – the newcomer to the specialty who needs a compact presentation of the special anatomy, physiology and radiology (for preparation for the DLO Part I and Primary FRCS examinations), and the specialist who is more interested in, say, the ear than in the throat. Secondly, advances are more numerous and more rapid in some sub-divisions of the specialty than in others so that it will be advantageous in the future to revise one volume at a time. The reduction in bulk of the individual volumes results, we hope, in easier handling and more pleasant reading.

A consequence of this change in format and policy is that page and chapter cross-references between different volumes cannot be given, nor is it practicable any longer to compile the symptom index featured in the last edition. To offset the former disadvantage some overlapping of subject material has been deliberately introduced wherever it was felt that too frequent referral to another volume would otherwise be necessary. Each volume has its own Table of Contents and Index, the latter compiled on the basis of noun-entries only.

The text throughout has been comprehensively revised. As a matter of general editorial policy, for this and for any subsequent editions which may appear under our direction, we have invited contributions only from those of our colleagues who are still actively engaged in hospital, university or college practice; and it has been our pleasure to welcome several new contributors. By including several new chapters, we have been able to remedy some of the omissions from earlier editions (for example, 'Congenital Diseases of the Larynx'), and also to give due emphasis to such topics as 'Acoustic Trauma' and 'Acoustic Neuroma', each of which now demands a separate chapter. The weights and liquid measures of all drugs, as well as the measures of distance, are all given in the metric system.

We are grateful to all the authors for submitting their work on schedule so that the production can be uniformly up-to-date. We warmly appreciate the efforts and enthusiasm of the Publisher's Editorial Staff, and the kind help we have received from colleagues, artists, and many friends too numerous to be named. It has been a tremendous encouragement to have the continuing interest of Mr W G Scott-Brown, CVO, MD, FRCS, who has read and contributed substantially to the editing of a large part of this edition. We wish to thank him for the honour of his invitation to join in the editorship of this standard textbook, which was established solely by him in the First Edition of 1952. Although he has now handed over completely the pleasant duties of joint Editorship to us and our successors, it remains his book and it retains his name.

London, 1971
John Ballantyne
John Groves

Introduction to the Second Edition

The objects set out in the Introduction to the First Edition have been the guiding principles in the present work. In order to make this new edition authoritative and contemporary in outlook, I asked two of my colleagues to join me as co-editors and I have been most fortunate in having the help and inspiration of John Ballantyne and John Groves. We have together re-cast the main sections, sub-sections and chapters and have given more emphasis to those departments of the specialty which have undergone the greatest changes. We have also made great efforts to have all contributions written and despatched to the printer within one year of starting the project, in order that all the articles shall be finished at the same time and be up-to-date when published. This object has been achieved thanks to the cooperation of our contributors.

It will be seen that the sections on physiology have been extended and improved and the chapters on the ear have been considerably altered and enlarged to include the many fresh ideas and techniques associated with both infective and non-infective ear conditions. The sections on endoscopy have been re-arranged to make the subject as practical as possible for our specialty. It is hoped that the necessary curtailment has not given rise to any major omissions. Neoplasms of the larynx and pharynx have been separated and new chapters on voice and speech have been introduced.

The index has been completely revised, and an innovation in a textbook of this size is an additional index – a symptom index – which is complete for the whole work at the end of each volume. It is hoped that this may be particularly useful to candidates for higher examinations and to general practitioners looking for causes of particular symptoms.

It is a pleasure to acknowledge the generous help which has been given by all the contributors, a number of them new to this book, and to artists and friends, for their kindly and stimulating interest. It is not possible here to record individual acknowledgments, but a special word of thanks must be made to the Editorial Staff of the Publishers.

London, 1965
W G Scott-Brown

Introduction to the First Edition

This work has been compiled with the object of presenting a textbook on Diseases of the Ear, Nose and Throat which would include most of the subject matter required by students and post-graduates with sufficient detail for those taking the higher specialized qualifications. It should also be a suitable reference book for general practice.

To achieve this it was decided to ask a number of teachers, examiners and other well-recognized authorities in the specialty to contribute articles on this general plan while leaving them free to put forward their own views of the particular subject in their own way. This has in some cases meant the presentation of individual preferences, classifications or theories, but as far as possible these have been integrated with the more usual views to give a balanced appreciation of the subject. It is hoped that this individuality of articles will give a more stimulating approach to the subject in spite of some overlapping of subject matter and differences of opinion.

Each section is prefaced by its anatomy and physiology as an essential basis to the understanding of the subject, and also to include in a concise manner the material necessary for the examinee. Methods of examination on the other hand have been cut to a minimum as they can only be learnt by the practical examination of patients. After considerable deliberation it was decided to include a chapter on plastic surgery of the nose and ear which should set out what can be done rather than entering into details of technique which are largely the province of the plastic surgeon.

My thanks are due in the first place to all the contributors who have lightened the editorial burden: they have all been most cooperative and have given freely of their time, knowledge and, in many cases, helpful criticism. Acknowledgement is made in the text for opinions and illustrations used.

I must particularly thank the Publisher's team, all of whom have been not only helpful but also encouraging during the many unavoidable delays and difficulties in the production of a new work.

London, 1952
W G Scott-Brown

Colour plates in this volume

Contributors to this volume

John Ballantyne, FRCS, HON FRCS (I)
Consultant Ear, Nose and Throat Surgeon, The Royal Free Hospital and King Edward VII Hospital for Officers, London; Civilian Consultant in Otolaryngology to the Army

A J Benson, MSC, MB, CHB
Senior Medical Officer (Research), Head, Vestibular Physiology Section, Royal Air Force Institute of Aviation Medicine, Farnborough, Hants

B J Bickford, MB, BS, FRCS
Formerly Consultant Cardiothoracic Surgeon, Broadgreen Hospital, Liverpool and Royal Liverpool Children's Hospital, Liverpool

L H Capel, MD, FRCP
Physician, London Chest Hospital, Rhinitis Clinic, Royal National Throat, Nose and Ear Hospital; Allergy Clinic, St Mary's Hospital, London

Peter Clifford, MB, MCH, FRCS
Consultant Head and Neck Surgeon, The Royal Marsden Hospital, London and Surrey and King's College Hospital, London

Ellis Douek, FRCS
Consultant Ear, Nose and Throat Surgeon, Guy's Hospital, London

C C Evans, MD, FRCP
Consultant Physician, Royal Liverpool and Broadgreen Hospitals, Liverpool

A J Fourcin, PHD
Professor of Experimental Phonetics, University of London

D B Fry, PHD
Emeritus Professor of Experimental Phonetics, University of London

R A Green, MA, MB, BCHIR (CANTAB), FFARCS
Consultant Anaesthetist, The Royal Free Hospital and St George's Hospital, London

John Groves, MB, BS, FRCS
Consultant Ear, Nose and Throat Surgeon, The Royal Free Hospital, London

W J Hamilton, MD, DSC, FRCS, FRCOG, FRSE
Formerly Emeritus Professor of Anatomy, University of London

R J Harrison, MD, DSC, MD
Formerly Professor of Anatomy, University of Cambridge

P W Head, OBE, QHS (ROYAL NAVY) MB, BS, FRCS (ENG), DLO
Consultant Otorhinolaryngologist, Royal Naval Hospital, Haslar, Gosport: Consultant Adviser on Otorhinolaryngology to MDG (Naval)

Bridget T Hill, PHD, CCHEM, FRIC, FIBIOL
Head, Laboratory of Cellular Chemotherapy, Imperial Cancer Research Fund, London

Paul Noone, MA, BM, BCH, MRCPATH
District Superintendent Radiographer, The Royal Free Hospital, London

P F King, OBE, FRCS (ED), DLO
Royal Air Force Consultant Adviser in Otorhinolaryngology and Reader in Clinical Aviation Medicine, Institute of Aviation Medicine, RAF Farnborough

R F McNab Jones, FRCS
Surgeon in Charge, Ear, Nose and Throat Department, St Bartholomew's Hospital; Surgeon, Royal National Throat Nose and Ear Hospital, London

Paul Noone, MA, BM, BCH, MRCPATH
Consultant Medical Microbiologist, The Royal Free Hospital, London

J E Pettit, MD, FRCPA, MRCPATH
Associate Professor of Haematology, University of Otago Medical School, Dunedin, New Zealand

L A Price, MB, BS, MRCP
Senior Lecturer in Medicine, Institute of Cancer Research and Honorary Consultant Physician, Royal Marsden Hospital, London

D B L Skeggs, MA, BM, BCH, FRCT, DMRT
Director of Radiotherapy, The Royal Free Hospital, London; Honorary Consultant Radiotherapist, Royal Northern Hospital, London

P M Stell, CHM, FRCS
Professor of Otorhinolaryngology, University of Liverpool

William B Young, MBE, FRCR, FRCSE
Honorary Consultant, The Royal Free Hospital, London; Consultant Radiologist, The Wellington Hospital, London

Contents

I Anatomy of the ear
John Ballantyne

Descriptive and applied anatomy of the human ear

External ear

The external ear consists of two parts, the auricle (or pinna) and the external auditory canal (or meatus).

The auricle

The auricle consists of a single irregularly-shaped thin plate of yellow fibrocartilage about 0.5–1 mm in thickness, covered with skin (*Figure 1.1*) and connected with the surrounding parts by ligaments and muscles.

The concha is the well of the ear. The helix forms the outer rim of the auricle; it begins at the concha and ends at the lobule. The tragus is a small lid that overlaps the concha anteriorly.

The cartilage is continuous with that of the external auditory canal and it extends throughout the entire auricle, except in the lobule and the part between the tragus and the helix. The absence of cartilage in this latter situation (the incisura terminalis) is utilized in one type of endaural incision (p. 46), which can be made without cutting through cartilage.

The skin is covered with fine hairs which are furnished with sebaceous glands. It is firmly adherent on the anterior surface, looser on the posterior surface. Hence in any infection, the swelling is more noticeable in the lax tissues behind the auricle.

The fact that the auricle is formed of a single sheet of cartilage is also important surgically, for if the perichondrium is stripped up by haemorrhage or suppuration, the whole cartilage may necrose.

The abundant blood supply of the auricle is derived from small branches of the external carotid artery, the posterior surface being supplied by the posterior auricular artery, the anterior surface by the anterior temporal artery.

Owing to the relatively little depth of tissue between the skin and the cartilage, these vessels lie in a very exposed position, and the ear is therefore unusually subject to frostbite.

The veins of the auricle enter the superficial temporal and posterior auricular veins. The former vein joins the posterior facial vein and drains into the internal jugular vein, whilst the latter drains into the external jugular vein. Posteriorly communicating branches enter the emissary vein which leads intracranially into the lateral venous sinus.

The nerve supply of the auricle is derived from the second and third cervical spinal nerves, and from the trigeminal nerve. The great auricular nerve (C2, 3) supplies the skin of the lower third of the lateral (anterior) surface and lower two-thirds of the medial (posterior) surface; the auriculo-temporal (fifth cranial) nerve supplies the rest of the lateral (anterior) surface; and the lesser occipital nerve (C2) the rest of the medial (posterior) surface.

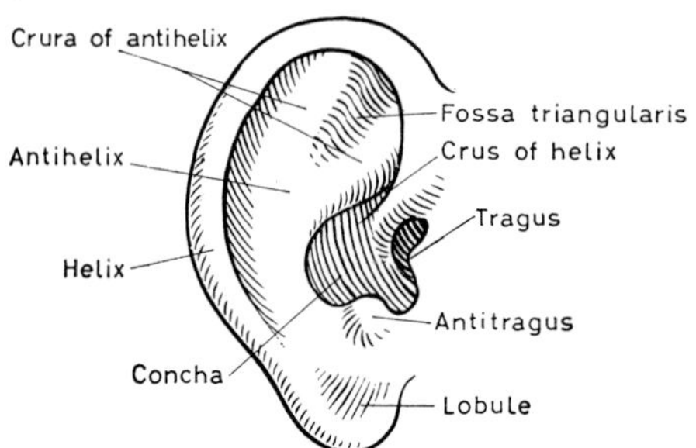

Figure 1.1 The auricle

The presence of two fissures in the cartilage, the fissures of Santorini, enables the vessels and nerves to pass through from one surface to the other.

The lymphatic drainage from the posterior surface is to the glands at the mastoid tip; from the tragus and from the upper part of the anterior surface to the parotid glands; and from the inferior part to glands beneath the ear.

The external auditory canal

The external auditory canal is about 2.5 cm in length in the adult, from the bottom of the concha to the tympanic membrane, which separates it from the tympanic cavity at its medial end.

It runs a tortuous S-shaped course, its general direction being inwards and slightly upwards and backwards in the outer cartilaginous part; inwards and slightly downwards and forwards in the inner bony part. The canal is straightened, therefore, by lifting the mobile auricle upwards and backwards and pulling it slightly outwards.

The curvature of the external canal serves as a protection to the tympanic membrane.

In newborn and young infants, the tympanic membrane lies in an almost horizontal position. Since it marks the inner boundary of the external auditory canal and since there is no bony canal as yet developed from the annulus tympanicus, the external canal is more or less collapsed upon the surface of the drumhead. In order to expose the tympanic membrane in these very young children, the manipulation of the external ear is therefore almost exactly opposite to that in the adult, for it is necessary to pull the auricle downwards and backwards.

The cartilaginous portion of the canal forms its outer one-third. The cartilage is continuous with that of the auricle and it is deficient superiorly. Superficially, this deficiency is continuous with the space between the tragus and the crus of the helix; more deeply it is filled with fibrous tissue which also binds the medial border of the cartilage to the lateral border of the bony tympanic plate.

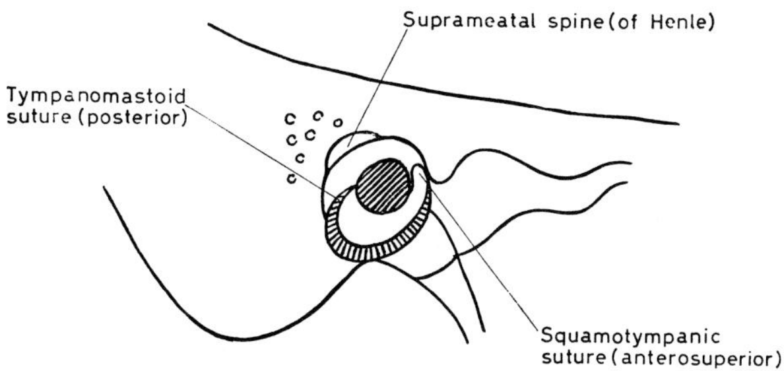

Figure 1.2 The endomeatal sutures

The bony portion of the canal forms its inner two-thirds, and is formed by the tympanic and squamous portions of the temporal bone. Its postero-superior portion is formed by a part of the squama, the remainder by the tympanic plate.

Prominent bony spines may project from the free outer border of the tympanic plate at the squamotympanic and tympanomastoid sutures (*Figure 1.2*). The presence of these endomeatal sutures and spines may make it difficult to separate an intact cuff of skin from the bony canal.

Two constrictions occur in the external auditory canal: (i) at the junction of the cartilaginous and bony portions; and (ii) at the isthmus. This is the narrowest part of the canal and is situated about 5 mm (approximately 0.2 in) from the tympanic membrane.

The tympanic membrane closes the canal obliquely, and its obliquity is such that the anterior wall and floor are slightly longer than the posterior wall and roof.

From the isthmus, the floor of the canal dips steeply downwards and forwards to form the anterior recess. It may be difficult to remove debris from this recess, or to strip the outer epidermal layer from the skin of this region in tympanoplastic procedures.

The skin of the external auditory canal is continuous with that of the auricle. It lines the whole of the canal and extends over the outer surface of the tympanic membrane. In the words of Eldon Perry (1957) 'the external auditory canal is the only skin-lined *cul-de-sac* in the human body'.

The skin of the outer one-third is about 1–1.5 mm thick and it is closely adherent to the cartilage. This portion of the skin is provided with hairs, sebaceous glands and ceruminous glands.

The hairs and sebaceous glands are identical with those in other parts of the body. Tiny, short vellus hairs line the whole of the cartilaginous portion of the canal, but large terminal hairs, the tragi, occur only in adult males, in whom they form a secondary sexual characteristic. The sebaceous, or oil glands, are abundant in the canal, and almost all of them open into the lumina of the hair follicles.

The ceruminous glands lie in the deeper portion of the dermis, and it has been estimated that the average human ear contains between 1000 and 2000 of these glands.

They are simple coiled tubular glands, the secretory cells being cuboidal and surrounded by an outer myo-epithelium (*Figure 1.3*). This myo-epithelium is flattened and contains smooth muscle, and its contraction compresses the lumen of the tubule, with expulsion of the contents.

When it reaches the epidermis, the duct empties either into the lumen of a hair follicle or on to the free epidermal surface.

When examined microscopically (Perry), the secretory product of the ceruminous glands appears on the wall of the canal at the orifices of the ceruminous ducts as tiny, white, watery droplets. If allowed to remain undisturbed, it slowly dries to form a sticky semi-solid. If removed and kept for a number of days, it gradually darkens in colour.

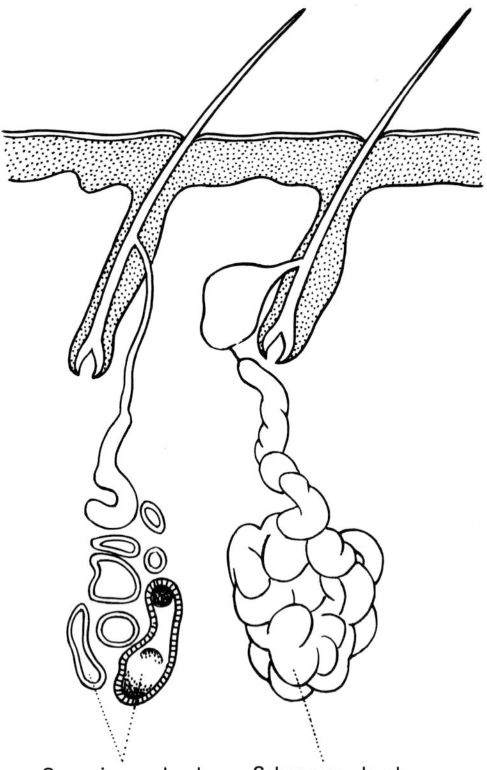

Figure 1.3 The skin of the external auditory canal. (After Lim, 1976)

The large lumen of the ceruminous gland serves as a reservoir until some stimulus causes the pre-formed secretion to be delivered to the skin surface. Apart from being slightly smaller, the ceruminous glands are identical in every respect histologically with the apocrine sweat glands in the human axilla and they have, indeed, been referred to as 'the apocrine sweat glands of the ear canal'. They also react to exactly the same stimuli as the apocrine sweat glands, these stimuli including smooth-muscle stimulants, especially such adrenergic drugs as adrenaline (epinephrine) and noradrenaline; strong emotional stimuli, such as fear, anxiety and pain, due to release of endogenous adrenergic mediators; and mechanical manipulation. In some subjects, vigorous chewing may cause enough distortion of the canal to produce this effect.

Wax (cerumen) is a mixture of the secretory products of the sebaceous and ceruminous glands. There are two main types of wax in humans: the 'wet' type, found in Caucasians and Negroes, both of whom have well-developed modified apocrine glands; and the 'dry' type, found in Orientals, in whom the ceruminous glands are sparse.

Wax contains a high concentration of lipid, most of it contributed by the sebaceous glands, and this lipid accounts for the hydrophobic properties of wax which are considered to be a part of the physical protective mechanism of canal skin. It has been suggested that wax also possesses antibacterial properties, and its consistent absence from infected ear canals has been presented as supporting evidence. Furthermore, the recent discovery of lysozyme and immunoglobulins in wax has raised the possibility that enzymatic and immunological defence systems may exist in the external auditory canal. Although their source is uncertain, it is known that sweat glands secrete immunoglobulins, and sweat glands are but modified apocrine glands (Lim, 1976).

In the inner bony portion of the external auditory canal, the skin is much thinner, being only about 0.1 mm thick. It is firmly adherent to the periosteum and is closely adherent to the sutures between the tympanic plate and the squama. It contains no glands or hairs. Self-cleansing of the ear canal is effected by migration of the skin covering the tympanic membrane and deep external canal, and Alberti (1964) has shown that the usual pattern of migration is centrifugal, from the umbo, at an overall rate equivalent to that of the growth of a finger nail, i.e. at the rate of about 0.05 mm per day.

Relations of the external auditory canal

Anteriorly, the canal is related deeply to the glenoid fossa of the temporo-mandibular joint (this is a useful landmark in entering the middle-ear cavity in congenital atresia of the external auditory meatus with middle-ear deformities) and the inner two-thirds of the head of the mandible; more superficially, the superficial temporal vessels, the auriculo-temporal nerve, the upper part of the parotid salivary gland and the pre-auricular 'lymph gland'. Posteriorly, it is related to the mastoid air-cells, and deeply to the vertical portion of the facial nerve. The mastoid antrum lies posteromedial and superomedial to the sloping squamous portion of the deep bony canal. Above it, lies the middle cranial fossa; below it, the parotid gland.

The blood supply of the external ear is derived anteriorly from the auriculo-temporal branch of the superficial temporal artery, and posteriorly from branches of the post-auricular division of the external carotid artery.

The nerve supply of the external auditory canal includes: (i) auriculo-temporal nerve (V), anterior half; (ii) auricular (Arnold's, Alderman's) nerve (X), posterior half.

Tympanic membrane

The tympanic membrane is an elliptical disc stretched obliquely across the medial end of the external auditory canal. It is about 10 mm high and 8 mm from front to back. It is set in such a way that the roof and posterior wall of the external auditory canal are shorter than the floor and anterior wall (*see Plate 4a, facing page 222*).

The membrane (or drumhead) is convex towards the tympanic cavity, and the point of maximum convexity is called the umbo (the Latin word for the knob on the centre of a warrior's shield).

The tympanic membrane has three layers: (1) An outer epithelial layer, which is continuous with the epithelium of the external auditory canal. This layer consists of only two layers of cells. (2) A middle fibrous layer, in the pars tensa but not so much in the pars flaccida. This layer contains a spider's web arrangement of radial and circular fibres, the former being inserted peripherally into the fibrous tympanic annulus and being lateral to the latter which contains parabolic and transverse fibres in addition to circular fibres. (3) An inner mucosal layer.

The handle of the malleus gives origin to the radial fibres of the fibrous layer and is covered medially with the mucosal layer. Its short process projects laterally (*Figure 1.4*).

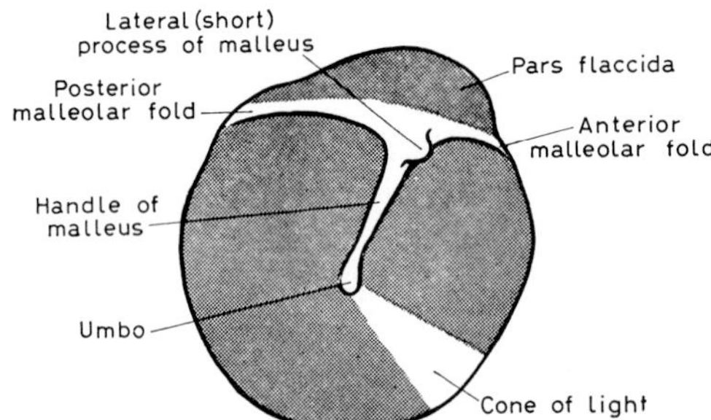

Figure 1.4 The right tympanic membrane (otoscopic appearance)

The greater part of the membrane is formed by the pars tensa, which is thickened peripherally into a fibrocartilaginous annulus. This thickened circumference fits into the grooved tympanic sulcus, which is a ring-like groove in the tympanic ring of the temporal bone; and the thickening itself allows the surgeon to dislocate the membrane out of the sulcus without tearing it.

The tympanic ring is an incomplete circle deficient above, and the fibrous layer is absent in the small part of the membrane which occupies the notch of Rivinus, where the ring is deficient. This pars flaccida, or Shrapnell's membrane, is attached above to the squama.

The fibrous annulus is carried from the anterior and posterior extremities of the notch of Rivinus to the lateral process of the malleus, thus forming the anterior and posterior boundaries of the pars flaccida, and raising up slight ridges of the mucous membrane called the anterior and posterior malleolar folds. The annulus is inserted into the tympanic sulcus.

The *vascular supply* of the tympanic membrane is derived partly from internal sources and partly from external sources.

Internally, the membrane is supplied by: (a) The arteria nutrica malleo-incudei, a twig from the middle meningeal artery, which supplies Shrapnell's membrane. (b) The vascular circle at the periphery, formed by: (i) the anterior tympanic artery, a branch of the internal maxillary artery, which enters the middle ear via the petrotympanic fissure, along the exit of the chorda tympani; (ii) the posterior tympanic artery, a branch of the stylomastoid artery, entering the middle ear with the chorda tympani; (iii) a tubal twig, from the ascending pharyngeal anastomosis.

Externally, the membrane is supplied by the *arteria manubrii*, whose origin is uncertain.

This artery lies behind the malleus in the upper part of its course, but directly on it further down. It divides into two branches which re-unite to form an elliptical loop. Branches from this loop radiate and anastomose with vessels coming from the tympanic vascular ring described above.

The *nerve supply* of the tympanic membrane is derived: (a) internally, from the tympanic plexus (IX); (b) externally, from (i) the auriculo-temporal nerve (V), in its anterior half, (ii) the auricular (Arnold's, Alderman's) nerve (X), in its posterior half.

The auricular branch of the vagus nerve passes from the fossa of the jugular bulb to the vertical portion of the bony facial canal, emerges with the facial nerve from the stylomastoid foramen and then curves laterally and upwards on the anterior surface of the mastoid process to supply the posterior halves of the external auditory canal and tympanic membrane.

A single injection of local anaesthetic solution into the soft tissues on the anterior aspect of the mastoid process and tympanic plate gives perfectly adequate analgesia for myringotomy, for example for fluid (non-suppurative) collections in the middle ear.

The patterns of the vascular and nervous supplies of the tympanic membrane are more or less parallel. The middle of the posterior half is relatively free of supply from either system, thus affording the surgeon a favourable site for paracentesis.

Middle-ear cleft

The middle-ear cleft consists of the eustachian tube, the tympanic (middle-ear) cavity, the aditus ad antrum, the mastoid antrum and the pneumatic system of the temporal bone (*Figure 1.5*).

The whole cleft is lined by a continuous layer of epithelium, which is respiratory in type in the eustachian tube and antero-inferior part of the tympanic cavity; this is a columnar epithelium, ciliated in parts. Above and behind this level the epithelium is flattened.

The eustachian (pharyngo-tympanic) tube

The eustachian tube is named after Bartolomeus Eustachius (1520–74), who at one time held the Chair of Anatomy at Rome. His book on the ear, *Epistola de Auditus Organis*, appeared in 1562 and is probably the earliest work to deal exclusively with the ear. The structure which is now known as the eustachian tube was known to the Greeks and mentioned by Aristotle, but Eustachius was one of the first to describe its structure, course and relations with accuracy. He divided it into bony and cartilaginous parts, the latter being lined with a mucous membrane similar to that of the nasal cavity, but he did not hazard an opinion as to its function.

The eustachian tube (auditory tube, pharyngotympanic tube) is about 3.75 cm long in the average adult.

It is directed upwards, backwards and outwards from its lower opening in the lateral wall of the nasopharynx towards its upper opening in the anterior wall of the tympanic cavity. The lower opening lies behind and on a level with the posterior end of the inferior turbinate (*Figure 1.6*).

The tube is more horizontal and relatively wider and shorter in the infant and young child than in the adult.

The upper one-third of the eustachian tube is a bony extension of the middle-ear cavity which takes a descending diagonal course at an angle of 40 degrees from the horizontal. It is widest at its entrance into the tympanic cavity, narrowest at its lower end (the isthmus) where the tube is flattened and has a diameter of only about 2 mm. The bony portion lies below the canal for the tensor tympani muscle (*Figure 1.7*), between the tympanic plate and the petrous portion of the temporal bone. It is only surgically accessible through the floor of the middle cranial fossa. Pneumatic (air) cells (the peritubal cells) may surround this part of the tube and are usually extensions of cells arising in the middle-ear cavity and following along the course of the tube. The internal carotid artery, passing through the carotid canal, lies medial to it.

The lower two-thirds of the tube form a narrow, slit-like fibrocartilaginous passage which passes downwards, forwards and medially towards the nasopharyngeal orifice from the isthmus where it makes an angle of about 160 degrees with the bony portion. When seen in cross-section, the cartilaginous part looks somewhat like a shepherd's crook, the cartilage being confined to the upper and medial parts of the tube, the remainder being composed of membrane.

Three muscles lie in close proximity to the tube: (a) The tensor tympani muscle lies along the roof of the bony tube in its own bony canal, from which its fibres take origin.

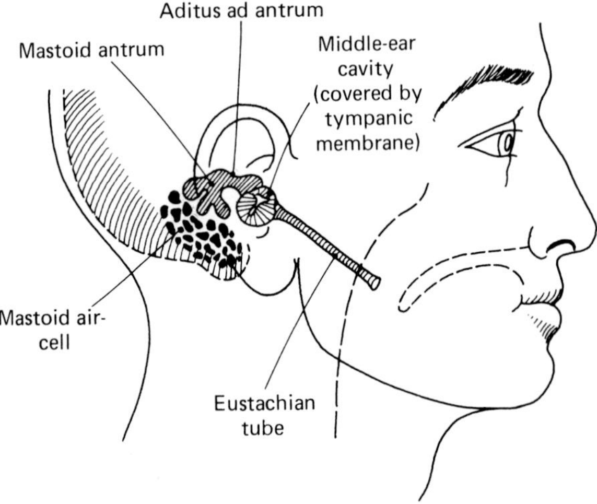

Figure 1.5 The right middle-ear cleft (schematic diagram)

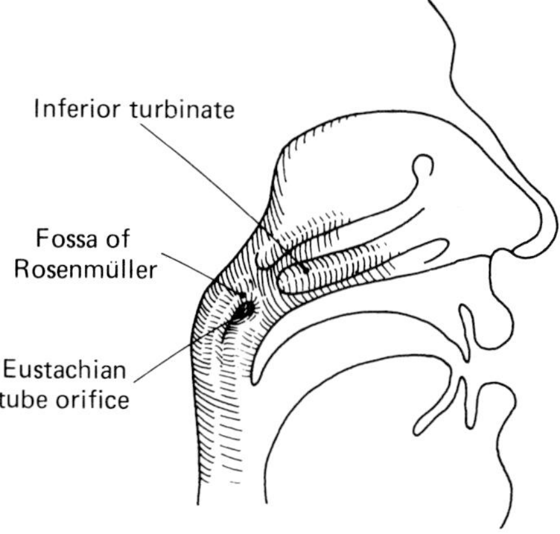

Figure 1.6 The lower orifice of the eustachian tube

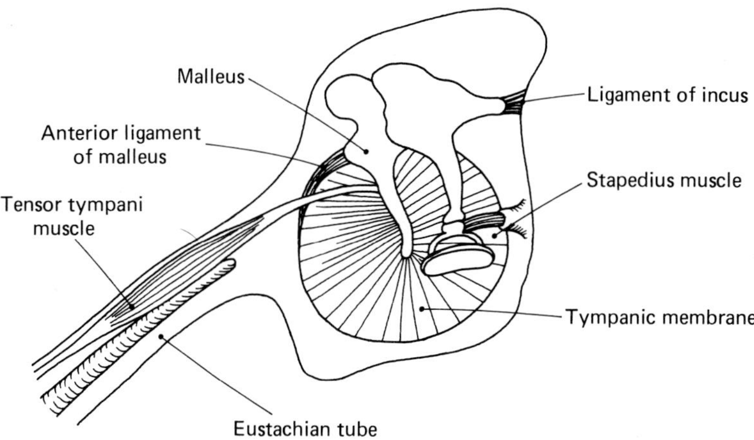

Figure 1.7 The inner (medial) aspect of the right eustachian tube and middle-ear cavity

(b) The levator palati muscle arises from the base of the petrosa and passes under the floor of the tube. It is inserted directly into the soft palate and meets its fellow of the opposite side. (c) The tensor palati muscle is the only one which has any function in opening the tube (*Figure 1.8*).

It arises from the bony wall of the scaphoid fossa, the spine of the sphenoid and along the whole length of the border of the short superolateral limb of the tubal cartilage. It passes like a pulley around the pterygoid hamulus and then meets fibres from the opposite side in an aponeurosis, forming a part of the soft palate. The tube is normally closed at rest but it is opened on swallowing or yawning by the combined action of the tensor palati muscle and the sphincter of the nasopharyngeal isthmus.

The lumen of the eustachian tube is lined with ciliated columnar epithelium. No glands occur in the bony tube, but seromucinous glands occur towards its pharyngeal end.

Gerlach described a tubal tonsil near the pharyngeal end of the tube, but in his own

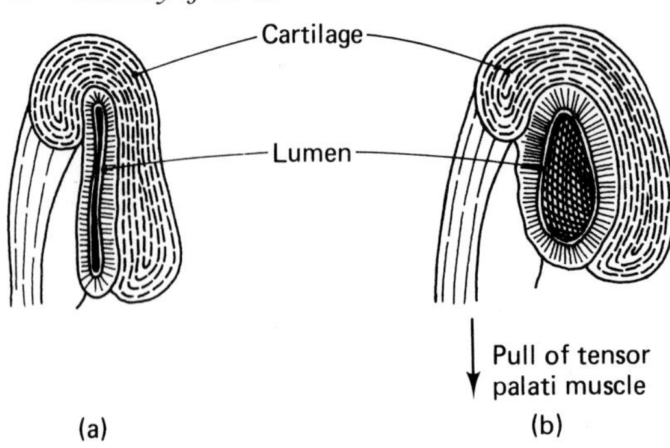

Figure 1.8 The cartilaginous portion of the right eustachian tube (schematic diagram): (a) tube closed; (b) tube open, demonstrating the pull of the tensor palati muscle

illustrations an infection was present in every case. Eggston and Wolff (1947) described 47 specimens, only one of which showed a tubal tonsil; and in this single case, it was found in a six-month-old infant with a heavy bilateral otitis media. It would appear, therefore, that this so-called tonsil is, in fact, a collection of lymphocytes rather than an organized nodule. However, the fossa of Rosenmüller (*Figure 1.6*), which lies behind the nasopharyngeal orifice, is normally packed with small but well-organized lymph nodules.

The *blood supply* of the eustachian tube is derived from: (i) the *ramus meningeus accessorius*, a branch of the middle meningeal artery which passes outside the skull; (ii) the artery of the pterygoid canal, or vidian artery, a branch of the internal maxillary artery; and (iii) a branch from the ascending pharyngeal artery.

The *nerve supply* of the tube is derived from the tympanic plexus and the sphenopalatine ganglion.

The middle-ear (tympanic) cavity

The middle-ear (tympanic) cavity lies between the external and inner ears. It has the form of a biconcave disc, and measures about 15 mm (rather more than 0.5 in) from above downwards, 13 mm (about 0.5 in) from behind forwards. It is very narrow in its transverse diameter, measuring about 6 mm across in its upper part, 4 mm in its lower part, and only 2 mm at its narrowest part, in the centre.

The cavity has lateral and medial walls, a roof and a floor, and anterior and posterior walls.

The *lateral wall* consists mainly of the tympanic membrane, and partly of bone above and below the membrane. Accordingly the cavity is divided into three parts: (a) the mesotympanum, medial to the tympanic membrane; (b) the epitympanum (attic), medial to the bone of the horizontal part of the squama (the outer attic wall), above the tympanic membrane; (c) the hypotympanum, below the drumhead.

The *medial wall* separates the middle ear from the inner ear and it is readily distinguished by the presence of the promontory, a smooth rounded bony projection covering the basal turn of the cochlea (*Figure 1.9a*).

The fenestra ovale (oval window), lies above and slightly behind the promontory. The niche of the oval window measures 2.5 mm by 1.2 mm and has a depth of 3 mm. It opens into the vestibule of the inner ear and is closed in life by the footplate of the stapes and its annular ligament.

The fenestra rotunda (round window) lies below and behind the promontory. Its

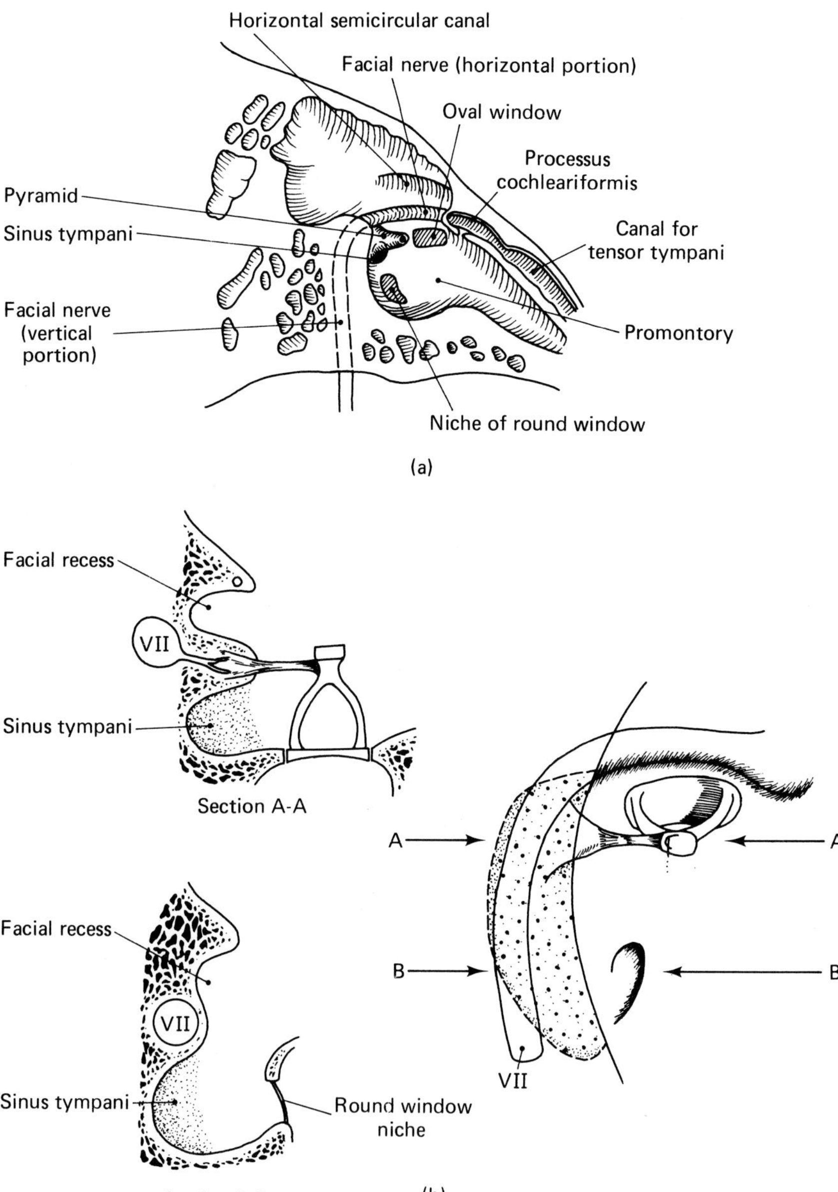

Figure 1.9 (a) The medial wall of the middle-ear cavity: (b) the sinus tympani and the facial recess. The correct anatomical description of the sinus tympani is that it starts above at the oval window niche; it occupies a groove deep to the descending portion of the facial nerve and to the pyramid and passes behind the round window niche to the hypotympanum. The facial recess is a term not yet accepted by anatomists: it is an alternative name for the suprapyramidal recess (Sheehy and Patterson, 1967). The facial recess may be entered from the mastoid by opening up small cells usually present between the fossa incudis, the deeper posterior bony canal and the descending portion of the facial nerve. (From Thorburn, 1967, reproduced by courtesy of the Editor of *Proceedings of the Royal Society of Medicine*)

niche measures 1.5 mm by 1.2 mm and it faces posteriorly. It opens into the scala tympani of the basal turn of cochlea and is closed in life by the secondary tympanic membrane, which is well protected by the promontory, lying at a depth of 2 mm within its niche.

The niches of the two labyrinthine windows communicate, at their posterior extremity, with a deep recess, the *sinus tympani* (*Figure 1.9b*). Lateral to the sinus, and separated from it by the facial canal and pyramid, is the *facial recess*. This latter recess is bounded laterally by the postero-superior part of the tympanic annulus and superiorly by the short process of the incus.

The facial recess leads from the postero-superior portion of the tympanic cavity into the aditus and antrum; and it can be approached surgically from the mastoid antrum (posterior tympanotomy) thus exposing an area which is otherwise very difficult of access.

Just above the oval window is the horizontal tympanic portion of the facial nerve, lying within the bony fallopian canal which may not uncommonly be deficient, especially on its inferior aspect.

The horizontal semicircular canal also lies in the medial wall of the tympanic cavity, above the facial nerve.

The *roof of the middle-ear cavity* separates it from the middle cranial fossa. It is known as the tegmen tympani and is formed partly by the petrous portion of the temporal bone and partly by the squama. It is normally a thin plate of bone, and the petrosquamous suture may persist throughout life. In some cases blood vessels pass through it, thus providing a pre-formed pathway for infection to spread from the middle ear to the middle cranial fossa.

The *floor of the tympanic cavity* is also a thin plate of bone, separating the cavity from the jugular bulb. Occasionally the floor may be defective, and when a dehiscence is present the jugular bulb encroaches on the cavity, and the bulb may be injured in surgical procedures on the middle ear. It is in this part of the bulb that the glomus jugulare (jugular body) is situated.

The *anterior wall* is narrow because the lateral and medial walls converge anteriorly. It presents four openings which are, from above downwards: (1) The small orifice of the canal of Huguier, through which the chorda tympani escapes from the middle ear. (2) The canal for the tensor tympani muscle. (3) The tympanic orifice of the eustachian tube. The septum between the tubal orifice and the canal for the tensor tympani is prolonged backwards along the medial wall of the cavity as a shelf of bone called the processus cochleariformis (and its end is moulded) to form a pulley round which the tensor tympani tendon turns abruptly in a lateral direction to be inserted into the handle of the malleus, just below its neck (*Figure 1.7*). Below the opening of the eustachian tube is a plate of bone which separates the tympanic cavity from the carotid canal. (4) The glaserian fissure, containing the tympanic artery and the anterior ligament of the malleus.

The *posterior wall* presents (towards its upper end) an opening (the aditus ad antrum) which leads backwards from the epitympanum into the mastoid antrum.

Below this lies the pyramid, a small, hollow conical projection through which emerges the tendon of the stapedius muscle, which passes forwards to be inserted into the neck of the stapes. The pyramid is perforated on its summit, and the aperture leads into a canal which curves backwards and then downwards until it opens into the lower part of the fallopian canal.

Lateral to the pyramid, and separated from it by the facial recess, is the opening through which the chorda tympani nerve enters the middle ear; deep to it, between the windows and a little behind them, is the sinus tympani. The relationship of the vertical portion of the facial nerve to the posterior wall is seen in *Figure 1.9b*.

The anatomy of the facial nerve is discussed in more detail on p. 39.

The contents of the middle-ear cavity

Besides air, which fills the cavity, the middle ear contains: (1) the auditory ossicles; (2) two muscles; (3) the chorda tympani nerve; and (4) the tympanic plexus of nerves.

The *auditory ossicles* derive their names from the blacksmith's forge. They are (a) the malleus (or hammer); (b) the incus (or anvil), and (c) the stapes (or stirrup) (*Figures 1.4* and *1.7*).

The malleus is the largest of the ossicles. It is about 7.5–8 mm in length. It has a head and a neck; anterior and lateral (short) processes; and a handle. The head is in the attic and articulates with the body of the incus. The anterior ligament of the malleus is attached to its anterior process. The handle of the malleus, directed downwards and slightly backwards, is firmly attached to the middle fibrous layer of the tympanic membrane. The malleus is suspended by an anterior ligament; a superior ligament attached to the tegmen tympani; and a lateral ligament between its lateral process and the margins of the notch of Rivinus.

The incus measures about 6 mm × 6 mm. It resembles a bicuspid tooth, and its body articulates with the head of the malleus. This lies in the attic, as also does the short process, to which the ligament of the incus is attached. The long process of the incus descends behind the handle of the malleus and parallel to it. At its lower end there is a very small medially-directed lenticular process, which articulates with the head of the stapes. The length of the long process is rather more than one-half of that of the handle of the malleus.

The stapes is the smallest bone in the body. It has a head and a neck; anterior and posterior crura; and a footplate which is held in the oval window by the annular ligament. The stapedius tendon is inserted into the posterior surface of the neck.

The superior margin of the footplate is convex, whereas the inferior margin is relatively straight, occasionally concave, thus giving the base a reniform outline.

The anterior crus is usually more slender and straighter than the posterior crus.

The *intratympanic muscles* are mainly striated muscles but many may contain some non-striated fibres. They are (a) the tensor tympani muscle and (b) the stapedius muscle (*Figure 1.7*).

The tensor tympani is a tiny though relatively long bipennate muscle which runs for 12 mm above the eustachian tube. It arises mainly or wholly from the bony tunnel above the osseous part of the tube and passes backwards and laterally through this tunnel.

In the middle-ear cavity, its tendon turns at right angles around the processus cochleariformis and passes laterally, to be inserted into the medial surface of the malleus, just below its neck. It is innervated by a branch of the fifth cranial nerve.

The stapedius is a relatively short, bulky muscle. It occupies the pyramid and the canal which curves downwards from it. Its tendon enters the tympanic cavity through the aperture on the summit of the pyramid and is inserted into the back of the neck of the stapes. It is supplied by a branch of the seventh cranial nerve, and its contraction pulls the stapes posteriorly and slightly outwards, around a pivot at the posterior end of the footplate. The actions of the intratympanic muscles are controlled reflexly, and it is thought that they protect the inner ear against the harmful effects of loud noise.

The *chorda tympani nerve* is the chief nerve of taste. It is a branch of the facial nerve and it arises in the fallopian canal at a variable distance above the stylomastoid foramen. Ascending in a narrow tunnel, it enters the middle-ear cavity through its posterior wall, lateral to the pyramid.

Within the middle ear itself it passes forwards, medial to the malleus and lateral to the incus (*Figure 1.10*) outside the mucous membrane, and therefore (correctly speaking) outside the cavity itself.

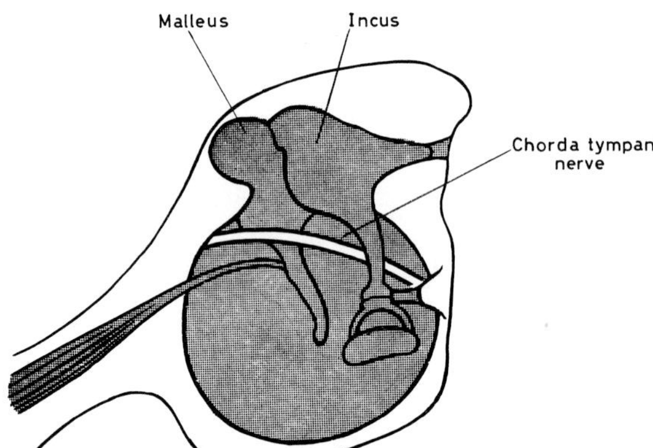

Figure 1.10 The right chorda tympani nerve, showing the course within the middle-ear cavity, viewed from the inner (medial) aspect of the cavity

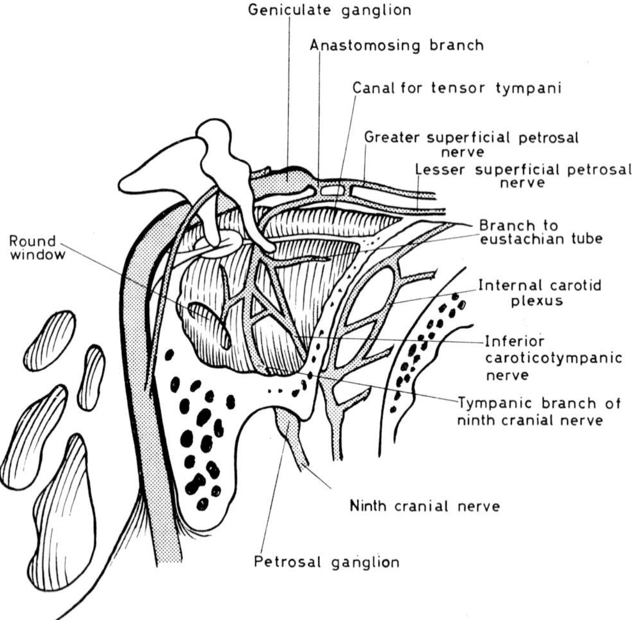

Figure 1.11 The right tympanic plexus

It escapes from the tympanic cavity through the canal of Huguier (*see* p. 12) at the uppermost part of the anterior wall of the cavity. It is carried herein to the medial end of the squamotympanic fissure, whence it passes downwards and forwards to join the lingual nerve through which its sensory fibres are distributed to the mucous membrane of the anterior two-thirds of the tongue.

The chorda tympani also contains parasympathetic secretory fibres which are relayed to the submandibular and sublingual salivary glands through the submandibular ganglion.

The *tympanic plexus* of nerves is derived from the tympanic nerve. This is a very slender nerve which arises from the glossopharyngeal (ninth cranial) nerve, immediately below the skull.

It enters a small hole between the carotid canal and the jugular fossa and ascends through a narrow canal into the tympanic cavity (*Figure 1.11*).

On the medial wall of the middle ear, under the mucous membrane, it breaks up to form the tympanic plexus, whose sensory fibres supply the mucous membrane of the eustachian tube, the middle-ear cavity, the mastoid antrum and the mastoid air-cells.

The plexus is joined by two minute caroticotympanic nerves, which arise in the carotid canal from the sympathetic plexus around the internal carotid artery.

It also sends a root to the lesser superficial petrosal nerve, where secretory (parasympathetic) fibres are sent on the first stage of their course to the parotid gland.

The mucous membrane of the middle-ear cavity

A thin, delicate mucous membrane lines the whole of the middle-ear cavity and is reflected on to the ossicles and the tendons of the tensor tympani and stapedius muscles. It is continuous with the mucous membrane of the eustachian tube and the mastoid antrum.

In general it consists of a single non-ciliated cuboidal epithelium, two or three cells deep, without a basement membrane, but in parts the cells may be of the simple or ciliated columnar type, especially near the entrance of the eustachian tube and in the hypotympanum.

As one follows the cuboidal cells back into the mastoid antrum and peri-antral cells, they become reduced to a single row of flattened squamous cells.

Compartments and folds of the middle ear

The mucous membrane is thrown into a series of folds by the intratympanic structures; they are of importance surgically because they divide the middle ear into compartments and they carry blood vessels to the ossicular chain.

The ossicular chain, with its ligaments, the tendons of the tensor tympani and stapedius muscles, and the chorda tympani nerve are described by Proctor (1964) as the viscera of the tympanic cavity. The mucosal folds he considers as its mesenteries.

The attic, or epitympanum, is almost completely separated from the mesotympanum by the ossicles and their folds, except for two small but constant openings which Proctor calls the isthmus tympani anticus and the isthmus tympani posticus (*Figure 1.12a*).

The transversely-placed superior malleolar fold normally divides the attic into a smaller anterior compartment (the anterior malleolar space), which lies above the tensor tympani fold which may prevent cholesteatoma from reaching the anterior mesotympanum from the attic; and a larger posterior compartment. The posterior

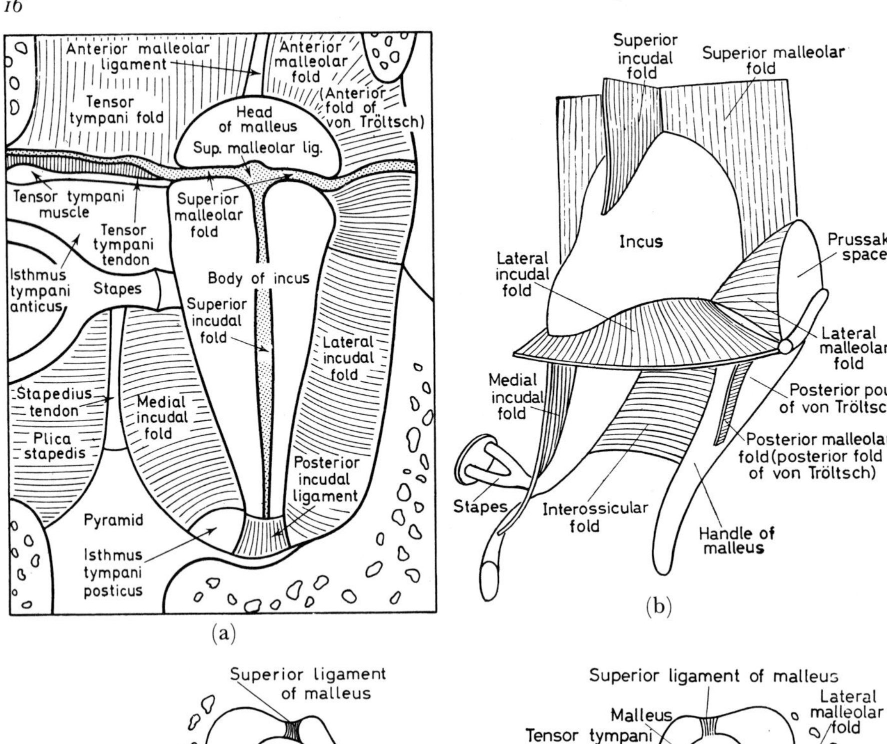

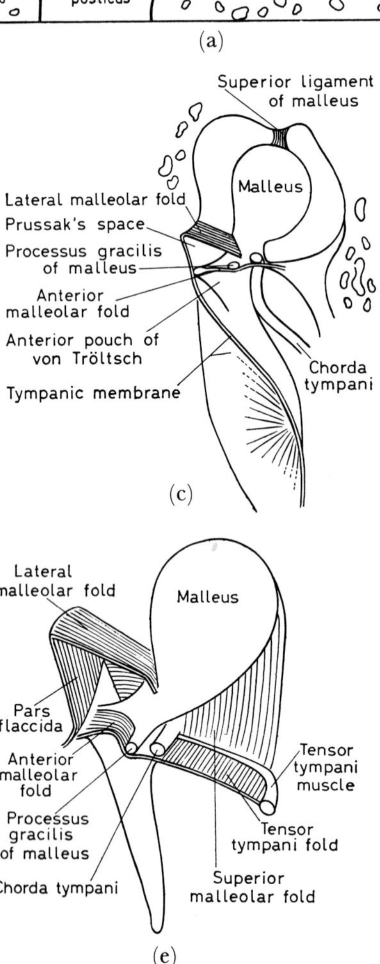

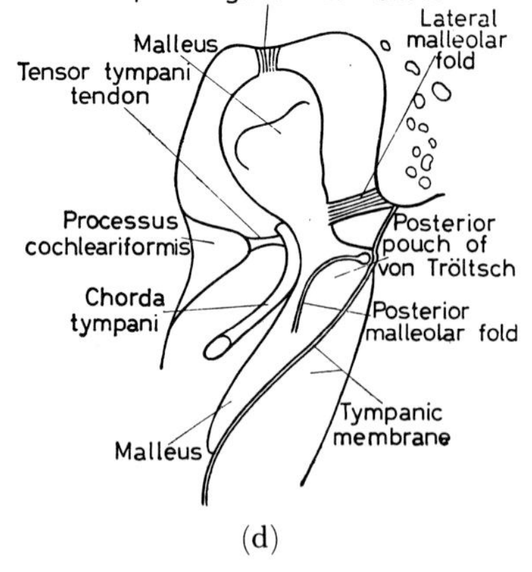

Figure 1.12 The compartments and folds of the middle ear (after Proctor): (a) the attic folds; (b) postero-superior and lateral view of right middle ear; (c) the anterior pouch of von Tröltsch, anterior aspect; (d) the posterior pouch of von Tröltsch, posterior aspect; (e) Prussak's space, showing the posterior two-thirds of the space, seen from behind

compartment is further subdivided by the superior incudal fold into the superior incudal space (lateral to the fold) and the medial incudal space (medial to the fold). The entrance into Prussak's space is usually located between the lateral malleolar fold and the lateral incudal fold. This latter fold may arrest the passage of keratin, through a postero-superior marginal perforation, into the attic.

Beneath the floor of the attic, in the upper part of the mesotympanum, there are three components: the inferior incudal space; the anterior pouch of von Tröltsch; and the posterior pouch of von Tröltsch.

The inferior incudal space (*Figure 1.12b*) is limited: superiorly, by the lateral incudal fold; medially, by the medial incudal fold; laterally, by the posterior malleolar fold (posterior fold of von Tröltsch); and anteriorly, by the interossicular fold, which lies between the long process of the incus and the upper two-thirds of the handle of the malleus.

The anterior pouch of von Tröltsch (*Figure 1.12c*) lies between the anterior malleolar fold (*Figure 12e*) and that portion of the drumhead anterior to the handle of the malleus.

The posterior pouch of von Tröltsch (*Figure 1.12d*) lies between the posterior malleolar fold and that portion of the tympanic membrane posterior to the handle of the malleus.

The chorda tympani nerve usually lies in the free margin of the posterior malleolar fold.

Prussak's space (*Figure 1.12e*) is a small space lying between the neck of the malleus internally and Shrapnell's membrane (the membrana flaccida) externally.

It is bounded below by the short (lateral) process of the malleus, and above by fibres of the lateral malleolar fold, which fan out from the neck of the malleus to be inserted along the entire rim of the notch of Rivinus.

A cholesteatoma may extend from Prussak's space, under the lateral incudal fold, into the posterior mesotympanum.

However, the mucosal folds may limit infection to one or several of the compartments in the middle ear; and if disease is thus limited it may be possible to control it in the affected compartment while preserving the integrity and function of adjacent structures.

The mucosal folds and their remnants are often considered as residues of inflammation or as adhesions. It must be emphasized, therefore, that they occur in fairly constant anatomical positions which can be explained by the embryological development of the middle ear.

The vascular supply of the middle-ear cavity

The arterial supply is derived from numerous sources. The arteries to the tympanic cavity are small and they travel through dense bone.

The superior region is supplied by three branches of the middle meningeal artery. These are the superficial petrosal and superior tympanic arteries, and the ramus nutricia incudomallei.

The inferior region is supplied by the inferior tympanic artery, a branch of the ascending pharyngeal artery.

The anterior region is supplied by: (a) the anterior tympanic artery, a branch of the internal maxillary artery which enters the middle ear through the petro-tympanic fissure, along the exit of the chorda tympani nerve; (b) the ramus-tympanici, a fine branch of the internal carotid artery.

The posterior region is supplied by the posterior tympanic artery, a branch of the mastoid artery. This latter vessel is a branch of the stylomastoid artery, itself derived from the posterior auricular artery, and it gives off the mastoid artery in the fallopian canal.

The ossicles are supplied as follows. The malleus and incus are at least partly supplied by the ramus nutricia incudomallei, a branch of the middle meningeal artery. The malleus also receives a branch from the anterior tympanic artery. The incus, according to Nager and Nager (1953), is also supplied by the incudal artery, another branch of the anterior tympanic artery. This latter artery enters the middle ear through the petro-tympanic fissure, and its incudal branch usually enters the incus on the lateral side of its body. Inside the body of the incus, the artery forms a vascular network which gives rise to branches supplying the short and long processes.

Brownlie Smith (1962) questions whether the vessel running down the long process supplies the very tip of the long process, with the lenticular process. There is some evidence that, while the incus is supplied mainly by the incudal artery, the tip of the long process with the lenticular process is supplied, at least in part, by vessels which come up from the head of the stapes around the capsule of the incudostapedial joint. This vascular network around the joint is supplied by branches of the superior and inferior tympanic arteries.

In some work carried out in St. Louis, Alberti (1964) described in great detail the blood supply of the incudostapedial joint and the lenticular process. According to this author, the blood supply of these structures is derived from three different groups of vessels which anastomose in this region; they are vessels which pass in the mucosa covering the stapedius tendon; vessels which climb up the stapes crura; and vessels which descend down the incus (*Figure 1.13*).

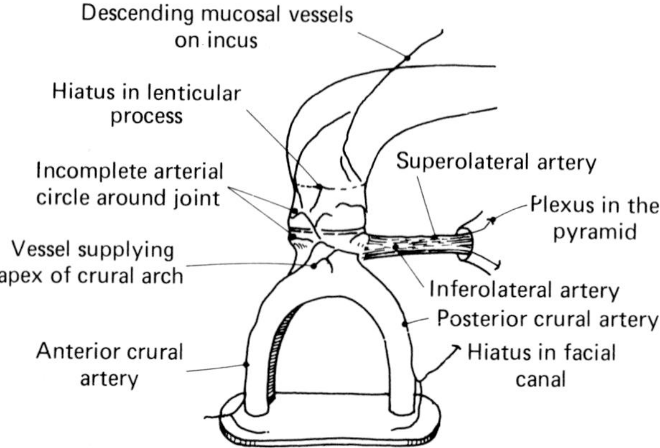

Figure 1.13 The blood supply of the incudostapedial joint and stapes (after Alberti)

Two constant and several inconstant mucosal vessels are found passing along the stapedius tendon. These are: (1) a small vessel on the superolateral surface of the tendon; and (2) a larger vessel on the inferolateral surface, both of them arising from the plexus surrounding the facial nerve within the fallopian canal.

The vessels which ascend the stapedial crura are: (1) the anterior stapedial artery, which is a branch of the conjoined superior and inferior tympanic arteries; and (2) the posterior crural artery, which is a branch of the superior petrosal artery.

According to Nager and Nager, the blood supply of the long process is derived from two sources: the incudal artery, referred to above; and a branch of the posterior tympanic artery which descends in the mucosa covering the long process. Alberti found two inconstant groups of mucosal vessels passing down the incus, one on the lateral side and one on the medial side.

The stapes is supplied by two groups of vessels: the first, which is concerned mainly with supplying the footplate and crura, is derived from the anterior tympanic artery anteriorly and the plexus surrounding the facial nerve posteriorly; the second group which supplies the apex of the crura, the head and neck of the stapes, the incudostapedial joint and a variable portion of the lower end of the incus, arises from the plexus which surrounds the facial nerve and emerges into the tympanum near the pyramid where the vessels anastomose with each other before passing along the stapedius tendon. Both groups of stapedial vessels anastomose on the neck of the stapes, the conjoined vessels then passing over the incudostapedial joint, to supply it by means of incomplete proximal and distal arterial circles.

At a variable distance from the incudostapedial joint, either on the lenticular process, or on the long process proper, vessels which pass from the stapes anastomose with those which descend the incus.

If a wire or plastic prosthesis is crimped too tightly over the incus, it may obstruct some of the mucosal vessels and thus interfere with the blood supply of the mucosa, and possibly of the ossicle itself; but wire, by its own natural resilience, is likely to be less harmful in this respect than other less yielding materials.

The intratympanic muscles are supplied as follows: (a) the tensor tympani, by the ramus musculus tensor tympani, and a branch of the nutrient artery of the malleus and incus, both arising from the middle meningeal; (b) the stapedius, by the ramus musculus stapedius, a branch of the stylomastoid artery.

The venous drainage is of relatively greater significance than the arterial supply, for the veins are much larger; they often lie within the operative field of the otological surgeon; and they are not infrequently subjected to pathological changes.

The middle ear and its contents drain into the sigmoid sinus and the jugular bulb; and into the middle meningeal (and internal jugular) veins.

The nerve supply of the middle-ear cavity

The sensory nerve supply is derived from the glossopharyngeal (ninth cranial) nerve, through the tympanic plexus (*see* p. 15).

The tensor tympani muscle is supplied by the mandibular nerve (a branch of the trigeminal, or fifth cranial, nerve), by way of the otic ganglion; it also receives a twig from the tympanic plexus.

The stapedius muscle is supplied by a branch of the facial (seventh cranial) nerve.

Aditus ad antrum

The aditus ad antrum leads backwards from the upper attic space of the epitympanum into the mastoid antrum. The bony prominence of the horizontal semicircular canal lies between its medial wall and its floor; and the short process of the incus lies on its floor. The facial nerve lies on a plane below and deep to the opening of the aditus from the attic.

Mastoid antrum

The mastoid antrum is an air-chamber situated in the temporal bone and is lined with a simple epithelium with a single row of flattened squamous cells. This mucosa is continuous, anteriorly with that of the tympanic cavity, through the aditus ad antrum; posteriorly with that of the mastoid air-cells, through several openings.

In the average adult, the mastoid antrum measures about 14 mm from front to back; 9 mm from top to bottom; and about 7 mm from side to side. Its anterior wall receives the posterior opening of the aditus ad antrum. Its medial wall is related to the posterior and horizontal semicircular canals. It is formed by the petrous portion of the temporal bone. Its roof, the tegmen antri, separates the antrum from the temporal lobe and its meningeal coverings, in the middle cranial fossa. Its lateral wall is formed by the squamous portion of the temporal bone. The suprameatal (Macewen's) triangle forms its bony surface marking, the antrum lying about 15 mm (just over 0.5 in) deep to the bone in the adult; in children it is much more superficial.

Its posterior wall and floor are formed by the mastoid portion of the temporal bone. It is through this part of the antrum that it communicates, by several openings, with the mastoid air-cells.

Mastoid process

The mastoid process lies behind the tympanic portion of the temporal bone and, on a deeper level, the styloid process.

The word 'mastoid' is derived from the two Greek words mastos (a breast) and eidos (resemblance). There is no actual process at birth; for the mastoid portion of the temporal bone is flat at first and the stylomastoid foramen, through which the facial nerve emerges, lies immediately behind the tympanic ring (*see Figure 1.41*). Later, when the lateral part of the mastoid portion grows downwards and forwards to form the process, the stylomastoid foramen comes to lie on the under-surface of the temporal bone.

According to Alexander (1917), the development of the mastoid process is dependent entirely on the development of the sternomastoid muscle. Hence its development does not really begin until the end of the first year of life when the infant begins to walk and to hold its head erect. It does not form a definite elevation until the end of the second year and achieves its definitive size only at puberty.

During the period of development of the mastoid process, the bone is normally filled with marrow, except in the antrum and the peri-antral cells; but the majority

(80 per cent) of mastoids become honeycombed with air spaces. The cellular type of mastoid is therefore regarded as normal in the adult. In some persons, however, marrow persists within the bony structure of the mastoid (diploeic type); and in others air-cells and marrow spaces are wholly or almost absent (the acellular, sclerotic or 'ivory' type) (*Figure 1.14*).

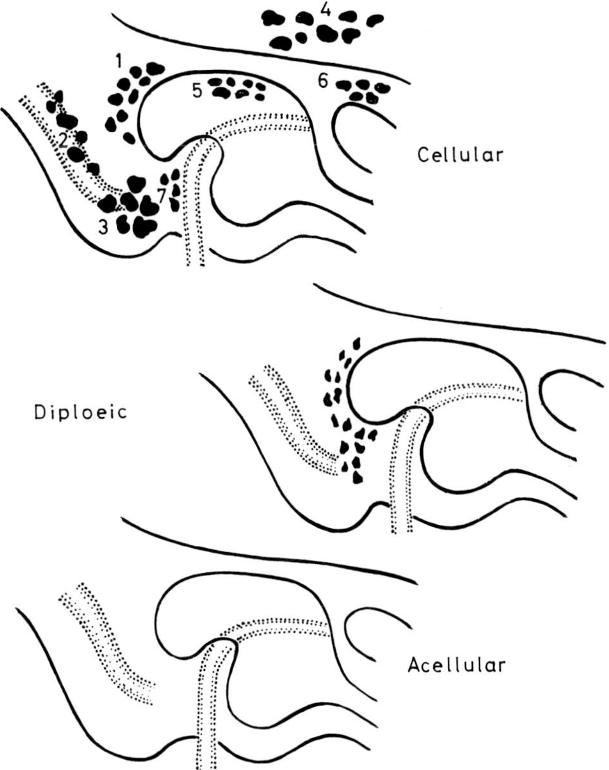

Figure 1.14 The three mastoid types. (1) Peri-antral cells. (2) Perisinus cells. (3) Tip cells. (4) Petrosal cells. (5) Peri-labyrinthine cells. (6) Zygomatic cells. (7) Retrofacial cells

The process of pneumatization, whereby the mastoid process becomes filled with air spaces, is closely associated with the descent and development of the process.

Pneumatic system of the temporal bone

'Pneumatization may be defined as the process of air-space formation within the temporal bone' (Eggston and Wolff, 1947), and the air-cells which occur within the mastoid form but a part of a much more extensive pneumatic system which may invade wide areas of the temporal bone.

Within the mastoid itself, the mastoid antrum is the only air-cell that is constantly present; but cells may also occur in close proximity to the antrum (the peri-antral cells); the sigmoid sinus (the perisinus cells); and at the tip (the tip cells). Superficial tip cells lie superficial to the posterior belly of the digastric muscle, deep tip cells deep to it. Between them is the digastric ridge which points directly to the stylomastoid foramen and provides a surgical guide to the facial nerve.

They may also be found in the body and apex of the petrosa, those at the apex including cells under the gasserian (trigeminal) ganglion, and around the carotid artery and the bony eustachian tube; and in close relationship to the labyrinth (the perilabyrinthine cells) within the petrosa; these perilabyrinthine cells may occur about the arch of the superior semicircular canal (supralabyrinthine); beneath the labyrinth (infralabyrinthine); or behind it (retrolabyrinthine cells).

Zygomatic cells may extend forwards into the zygoma.

In the fetal temporal bone the potential air spaces are filled either with mesenchyme or with haemopoietic bone-marrow, and the process of pneumatization begins with the resorption of mesenchyme early in the third fetal month. The potential air spaces do not contain air until the child is born, but the process of pneumatization is greatly hastened after birth.

It is not until air enters the middle ear at birth, permitting the loose embryonic connective tissue to condense and thin, that pneumatization accelerates, continuing throughout infancy and early childhood. In the petrous apex, pneumatization may continue into early adult life.

Resorption of mesenchyme progresses rapidly during the first two months of infancy. It is practically complete in the middle ear by the sixth month, and in the mastoid antrum by the first birthday. From this time onwards, pneumatization of the mastoid is solely a matter of resorption of the haemopoietic marrow in the diploeic bone.

Pneumatization of the petrous apex begins later than in the mastoid, about the third or fourth year, but in some cases of well-pneumatized mastoid the apex may contain marrow throughout life.

Radiological evidence of pneumatization in the mastoid is not usually present until about the third year of childhood (Law, 1913) and it continues until puberty, when its definitive size is attained. The two mastoids are essentially similar so that when there are, for example, large pneumatic cells on one side, there will also be large pneumatic cells on the other.

It has already been said that the pneumatic temporal bone is regarded as the normal, but this, of course, allows no chance for individual variation and affords no explanation for the many temporal bones with marked diploeic characteristics, especially at the petrous apex.

However, the fact remains that the majority of mastoids are of the cellular type and one must therefore ask oneself why some are not.

Albrecht (1930) believed that most of the damage done to the mesenchyme was due to bleeding from suffocation or birth injury, and he also mentioned the presence of infected meconium.

Wittmaack (1931) believed that deficient pneumatization resulted from infantile otitis media which interfered with the normal absorption of diplöe.

Tumarkin (1959) believes that 'frustration of pneumatization' results from failure of aeration of the middle-ear cleft, due to blockage of the eustachian tube. This occurs particularly in upper respiratory 'catarrh'.

Diamant and Dahlberg (1945) contend that dense bone is congenital and is a normal variant.

Relations of the middle-ear cleft

The many complications of inflammatory and neoplastic diseases of the middle-ear cleft result mainly from direct spread of the pathological process to surrounding structures. A knowledge of its relations is therefore of the utmost importance.

The external auditory canal is separated from the middle-ear cavity by the tympanic membrane.

The inner ear (or labyrinth) is separated from the cavity by its medial wall, which has been described.

The temporal lobe of the brain, in the middle cranial fossa, is separated from the tympanic cavity by the thin tegmen tympani, which is formed partly by the petrous and partly by the squamous portion of the temporal bone; it is separated from the mastoid antrum by the tegmen antri.

The carotid canal, containing the internal carotid artery, is separated from the lower part of the tympanic cavity, anteriorly, by a plate of bone which merges with the floor of the cavity.

The jugular bulb is closely related to the bony floor of the cavity, which may be deficient in part. There is no reliable surface landmark to the location of the sigmoid sinus.

The ninth, tenth and eleventh cranial nerves emerge from the skull through the jugular foramen, alongside and just medial to the jugular bulb, and may be involved in glomus tumours arising from the dome of the bulb.

The ganglion of the fifth cranial nerve lies in a shallow depression on the anterior surface of the petrous apex, between two layers of dura.

The sixth cranial nerve, the motor nerve to the lateral rectus muscle of the eye, comes into close proximity with the middle-ear cleft, as it runs along the posterior surface of the petrous apex, in the posterior cranial fossa, on its way to Dorello's canal; this canal is formed by the petroclinoid ligament, which stretches from the tip of the apex to the posterior clinoid process of the sphenoid bone.

The fifth and sixth cranial nerves may be involved in suppuration within the apex, to produce Gradenigo's syndrome, pain behind the eye, diplopia and aural discharge.

The seventh cranial (facial) nerve is closely related to the middle-ear cavity in its horizontal and vertical tympanic portions. Its bony covering (the fallopian canal) may be very thin, or totally deficient in parts, the nerve being covered only by the tympanic mucoperiosteum in as many as 10 per cent or more of temporal bones.

The internal auditory canal

This is a short canal, nearly 1 cm in length, lined by dura; it passes into the petrous in a lateral direction. It is closed at its lateral end (or fundus) by a plate of bone presenting numerous apertures (*Figure 1.15*). The auditory nerve, the facial nerve and the internal auditory artery and vein pass along the canal.

The vertical plate of bone separates the fundus of the internal auditory canal from the internal ear. On the medial aspect, the plate is divided by a transverse crest into a small upper and a larger lower area. Anteriorly, above the crest, is the opening of the facial canal. Behind this and separated from it by a vertical ridge (Bill's bar) is the

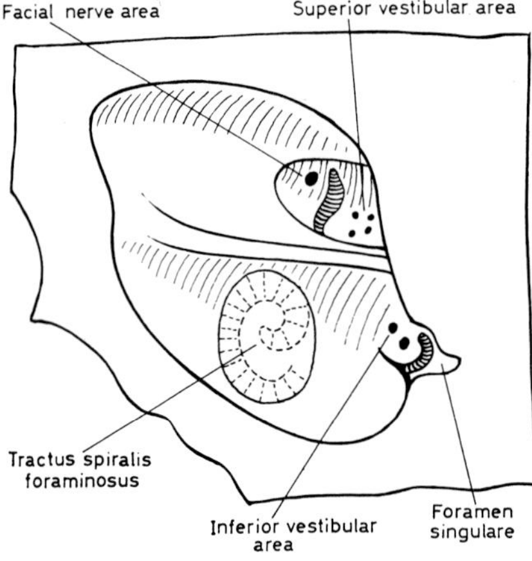

Figure 1.15 The right internal auditory canal

superior vestibular area. It shows a small depression containing numerous openings for the passage of filaments of the vestibular nerve to the utricle, saccule and superior and lateral semicircular ducts.

Below the transverse crest, anteriorly, is found the cochlear area, which presents a spirally-arranged series of foramina (the tractus spiralis foraminosus) and a central canal. The foramina and the canal transmit the nerve filaments to the cochlea.

The inferior vestibular area lies behind the cochlear area and, through its foramina, nerves pass to the saccule.

Behind the inferior vestibular area and slightly below it is the foramen singulare through which passes the nerve to the posterior semicircular duct.

The inner ear

The inner ear lies in the temporal bone. It is called the labyrinth (literally, a 'structure of winding passages') and consists of two parts: (i) the osseous periotic labyrinth; and (ii) the membranous otic labyrinth.

The osseous labyrinth

This consists of cavities in the petrous part of the temporal bones. There are three main parts: the vestibule; three bony semicircular canals; and the bony cochlea (*Figure 1.16*).

The vestibule

This is a small ovoid bony chamber, about 5 mm in length. It is placed between the medial wall of the middle ear and the outer part of the internal auditory canal.

The fenestra ovale (vestibuli), in the lateral wall of the vestibule, is separated from the middle ear by the footplate of the stapes and its annular ligament. Just within the oval window lies a relatively spacious portion of the vestibule, known as the perilymphatic cistern.

A small aperture in the posterior part of the medial wall of the vestibule leads into

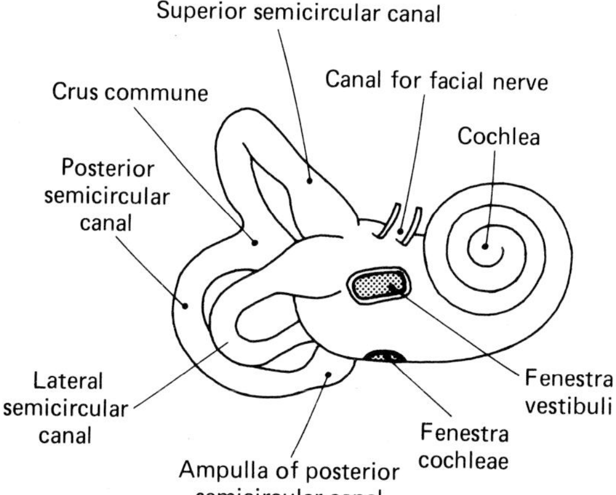

Figure 1.16 The right bony labyrinth

the aqueduct of the vestibule, a small canal which passes backwards to the posterior surface of the petrous bone, where it opens under the dura.

The three bony semicircular canals

These open into the posterior part of the vestibule by five round apertures, the two vertical canals (the superior and posterior canals) joining posteriorly to form the *crus commune* (*Figure 1.17*). Each canal forms considerably more than half a circle, and the diameter of their lumina is slightly more than 1 mm.

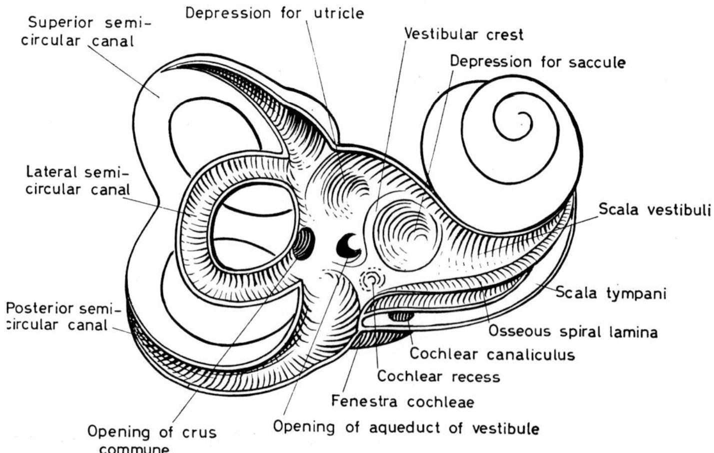

Figure 1.17 Interior of the right bony labyrinth, viewed from lateral aspect

The superior semicircular canal lies almost transverse to the long axis of the petrous. Its highest point lies beneath the arcuate eminence, on the anterior surface of the petrous.

The posterior semicircular canal lies in a plane parallel to the posterior surface of the petrous.

The horizontal semicircular canal lies in the angle between the superior and posterior canals. It makes a bulge on the medial walls of the attic, aditus and antrum.

The two horizontal canals lie in exactly the same plane, which, in the anatomical position of the head, slopes downwards and backwards at an angle of 30 degrees to the horizontal.

The bony cochlea

The bony cochlea lies in front of the vestibule and resembles a snail shell in shape. Its base is directed towards the bottom of the internal auditory canal, and its long axis runs outwards, slightly forwards and slightly downwards from base to apex. It coils for $2\frac{3}{4}$ turns, a distance of about 35 mm (Wrightson, quoted by Eggston and Wolff, 1947) around a central bony axis known as the modiolus, which forms the inner wall of the bony canal of the cochlea, which is wound spirally round it (*Figure 1.18*). The

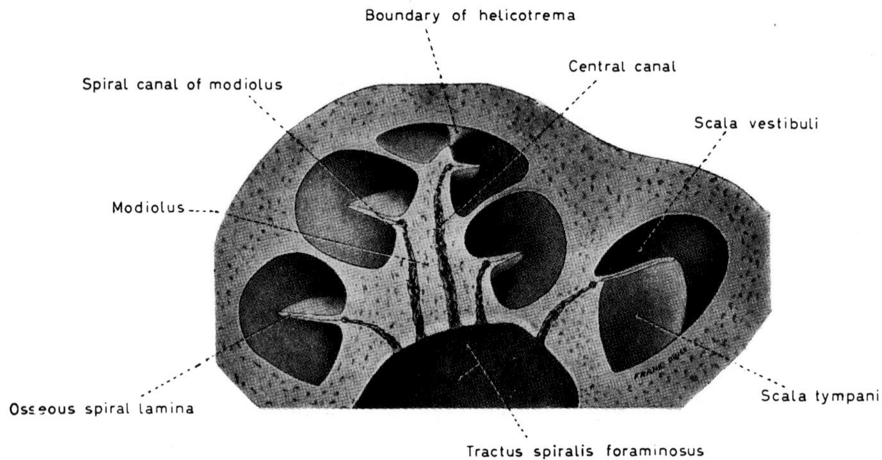

Figure 1.18 Section through the bony cochlea

bony canal is about 3 mm in diameter in its first turn, which produces the bulge of the promontory on the medial wall of the middle-ear cavity, but narrows progressively towards its apex.

The modiolus is thick at the base, but rapidly tapers towards its apex.

The osseous spiral lamina projects from the modiolus into the bony canal and forms a sheet of bone which winds spirally round the modiolus 'like the thread of a screw' (Cunningham, 1959).

The modiolus is traversed by numerous minute canals and one more conspicuous than the others runs lengthwise in the centre. The spiral lamina is also tunnelled by small canals in communication with those in the modiolus, whilst one – the spiral canal of the modiolus – winds spirally around the modiolus in the attached margin of the spiral lamina. All these channels convey filaments from the cochlear nerve to the duct of the cochlea; and the spiral canal lodges the spiral ganglion, which is the ganglion of the cochlear nerve.

The osseous labyrinth is lined throughout with a delicate endosteum, and contains perilymph fluid, in which the membranous labyrinth is situated.

The membranous labyrinth

This is a continuous series of communicating sacs and ducts within the bony labyrinth. The otic labyrinth may be divided into: the pars superior or vestibular labyrinth; the endolymphatic sac and duct; and the pars inferior or cochlea. It consists of: the saccule and utricle, in the bony vestibule; the three membranous semicircular ducts, in the bony canals; and the ductus cochlearis (scala media), in the bony cochlea (*Figure 1.21*). The membranous labyrinth contains endolymph fluid.

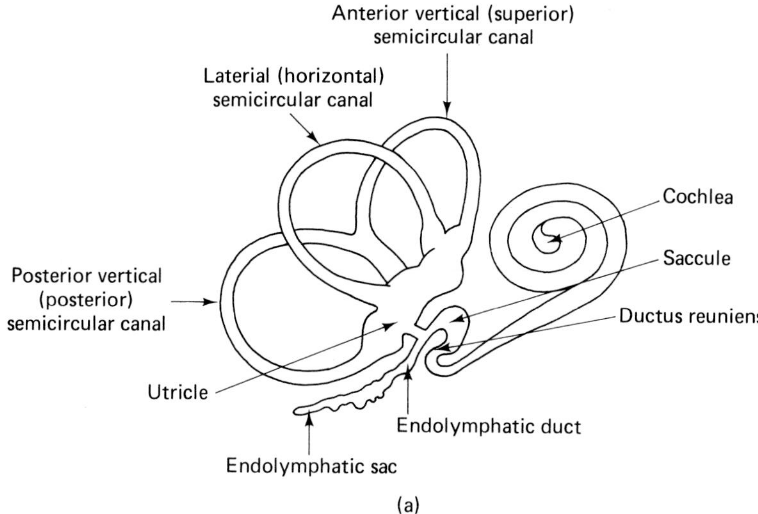

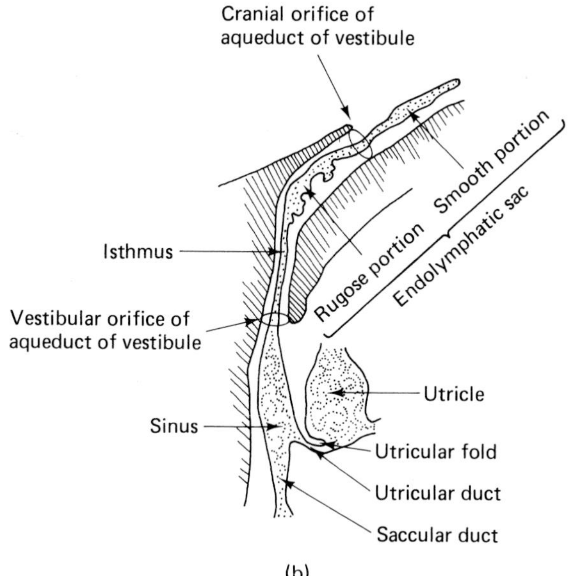

Figure 1.19 (a) The right membranous labyrinth; (b) the endolymphatic duct (after Bast and Anson)

The saccule and utricle

The utricle occupies a depression on the upper wall of the vestibule; the saccule is smaller and lies in a depression below and in front of the utricle (*Figure 1.17*). These two sacs communicate indirectly by means of a slender membranous tube called the endolymphatic duct (*Figure 1.19a*); this duct occupies the bony aqueduct of the vestibule and divides into two branches (the utricular duct and saccular duct) which separate to open respectively into the utricle and the saccule.

The endolymphatic duct has an initial dilatation, known as the sinus (*Figure 1.19b*), before it narrows to enter the bony aqueduct. The aqueduct enlarges beyond the isthmus of the duct; and in this expanded portion, the duct is surrounded by vascular connective tissue and lined by a rugose membrane which forms the proximal part of the endolymphatic sac. The relatively smooth distal part of the sac is contained within the dura mater covering the posterior surface of the petrous pyramid, where it ends close to the sigmoid sinus.

The utricular duct, on leaving the utricle, curves at an acute angle to form a valve-like fold over the orifice of the duct. This utriculo-endolymphatic 'valve' is so constructed that it allows inflow but not outflow of endolymph.

A short, narrow tube, called the ductus reuniens, connects the saccule with the duct of the cochlea.

The three membranous semicircular ducts

These open into the posterior part of the utricle by five separate openings, and are set at right angles to one another, like the three faces of a cube. Hence they represent the three planes of space.

At one or other end, each of the semicircular ducts dilates into an ampulla, which completely fills a corresponding dilatation of its bony canal. The long axis of each ampulla measures about 2 mm.

Elsewhere, however, the membranous ducts (with a diameter of only 0.4×0.2 mm) are considerably narrower than the bony canals (with a diameter of slightly more than 1 mm), and the ducts are attached to the outer walls of the canals by delicate fibrous strands.

The vestibular receptor organs (*Figure 1.20a*)

A special sensory epithelium, the *crista*, is found in each ampulla, and each is supplied by a branch of the vestibular division of the eighth cranial nerve.

In the utricle and saccule, there is also a patch of specialized epithelium, the *macula*. That of the utricle is in a horizontal plane, that of the saccule in a vertical plane. The latter can often be clearly seen during the performance of a stapedectomy operation, after removal of the stapedial footplate.

The epithelium of these receptor organs contains three basic structures: sensory cells containing hairs on their free surface; supporting cells; and a gelatinous substance lying on the hairs and composed mainly of mucopolysaccharides which are thought to be secreted by the supporting cells.

The vestibular cells (*Figure 1.20b*) are of two types: the Type 1 cell, which is rounded and flask-shaped, and surrounded by a nerve chalice; and the Type 2 cell, which is cylindrical and has no chalice.

In the ampullary cristae, there are relatively more Type 1 cells on the summit of the crista, relatively more Type 2 cells on its sides. The hairs do not jut freely into the

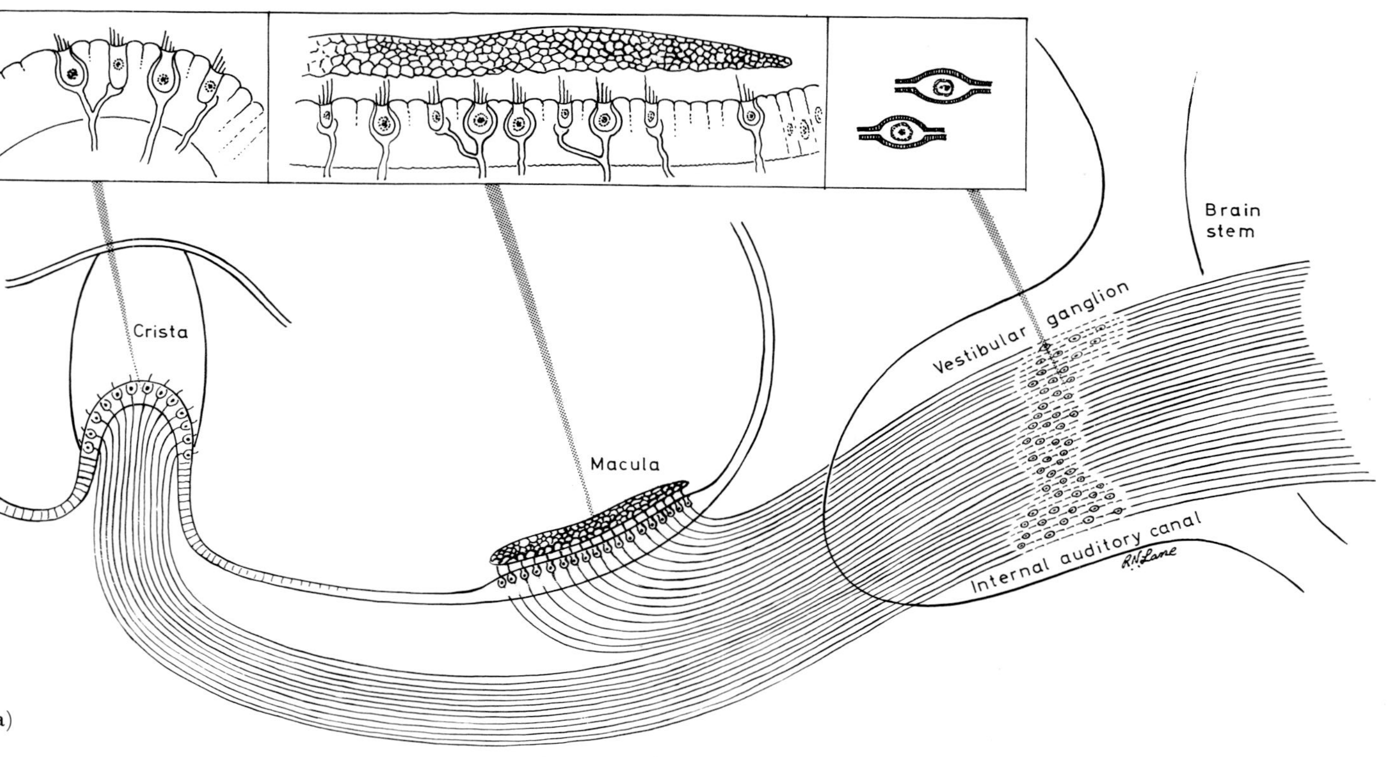

Figure 1.20 (a) Plan of the vestibular receptor organ

Kinocilium

Stereocilia

1

2

I

II

(b)

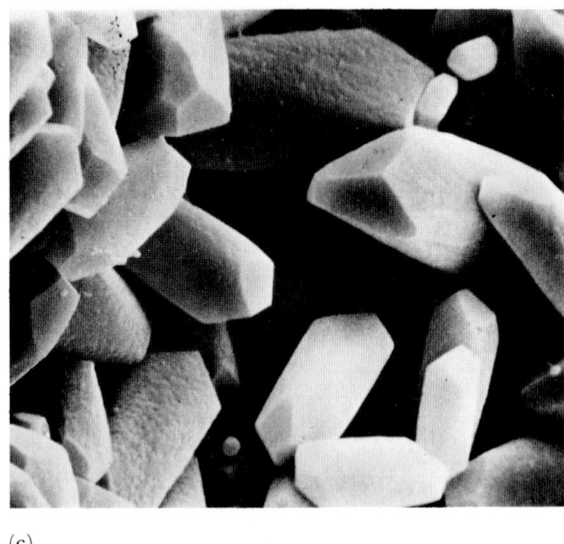

(c)

Figure 1.20 (b) the vestibular sensory cells (after Engström); (c) statoconia (by courtesy of H. Lindeman)

endolymph but into a gelatinous substance, dome-shaped in the ampullae, where it is known as the cupula; flattened in the utricular and saccular maculae, where a number of crystals (the statoconia) are embedded in it (*Figure 1.20c*). This latter is called the statoconial membrane.

Sensory hairs protrude from the surface of each sensory cell. These consist of one kinocilium and many stereocilia; and the kinocilium is longer than the stereocilia, which gradually decrease in length as the distance from the kinocilium increases.

The stimulus to the vestibular sensory cells is generally considered to be a shearing motion of the cupulae and statoconial membranes on the epithelial surfaces of the cristae and maculae. This mechanical stimulus probably acts primarily on the hairs of the sensory cells. Secondarily, this mechanical energy is converted into action potentials in the sensory nerve fibres innervating the cells.

Flock and Wersäll (1963) showed that stimulation of the hairs in a direction away from the stereocilia towards the kinocilium produced depolarization of the sensory cell, with a resultant increase in the frequency of nerve impulses; whilst stimulation in the opposite direction produced hyperpolarization, with a reduction in the frequency of nerve impulses.

Lindeman (1969) has shown that, in the ampullary cristae, the cells are all polarized in one direction. In the utricular and saccular maculae, however, there is an arbitrary line which divides them into two areas, the sensory cells being polarized in the utricle towards the dividing line, in the saccule away from it. Furthermore, he found that on the crista of the horizontal semicircular duct all sensory cells are morphologically polarized towards the utricle, on the cristae of the two vertical canals away from it.

The scala media (ductus cochlearis)

In axial section (*Figure 1.21*), this is roughly triangular in shape. The base of the triangle is formed by the basilar membrane which stretches from the free border of the osseous spiral lamina, via the tympanic lip of the spiral limbus, to the spiral ligament. This ligament is composed of a thickening of the endosteal lining of the outer wall of the bony canal of the cochlea, and it supports the cells of the outer sulcus. Continuous with these are the cells of the stria vascularis, which contains numerous capillaries and forms the outer wall of the scala media. The third side of the triangle is formed by

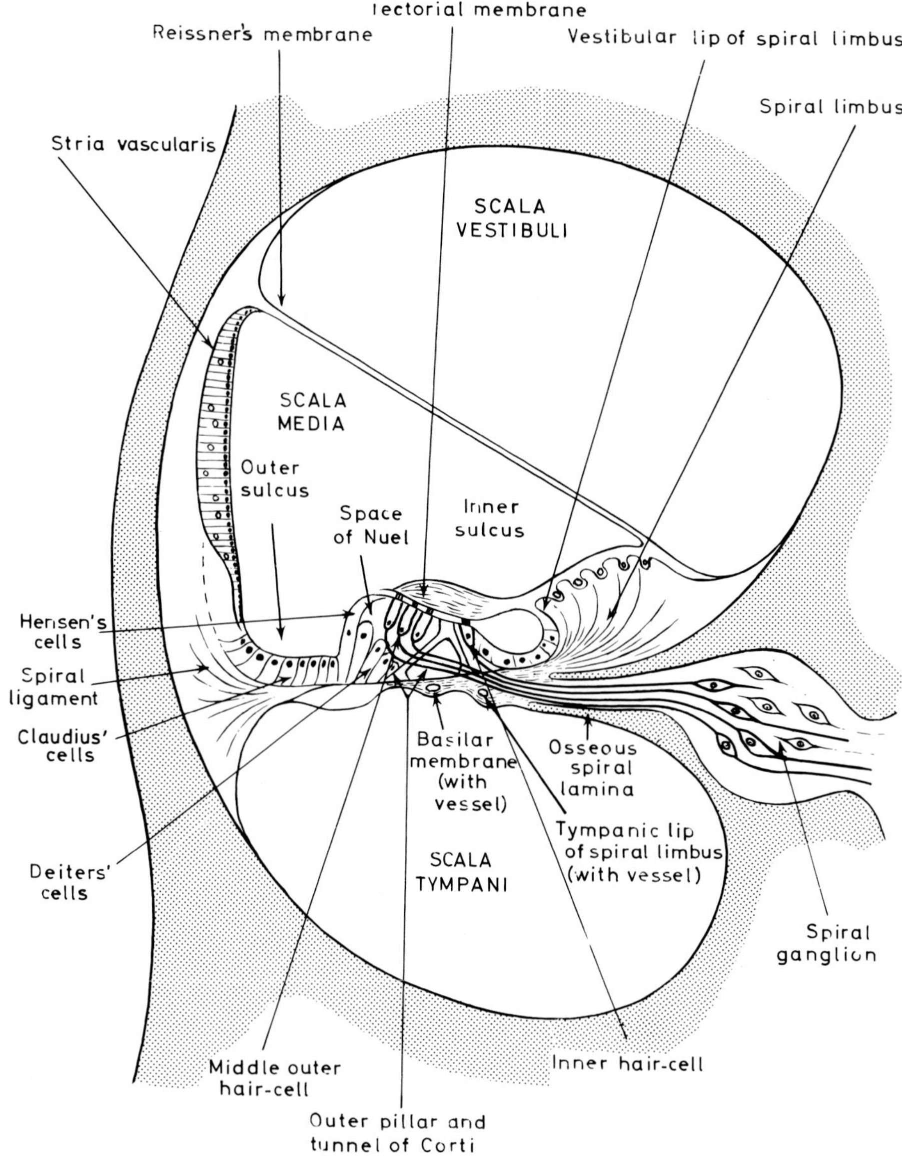

Figure 1.21 The scala media (axial section of cochlea)

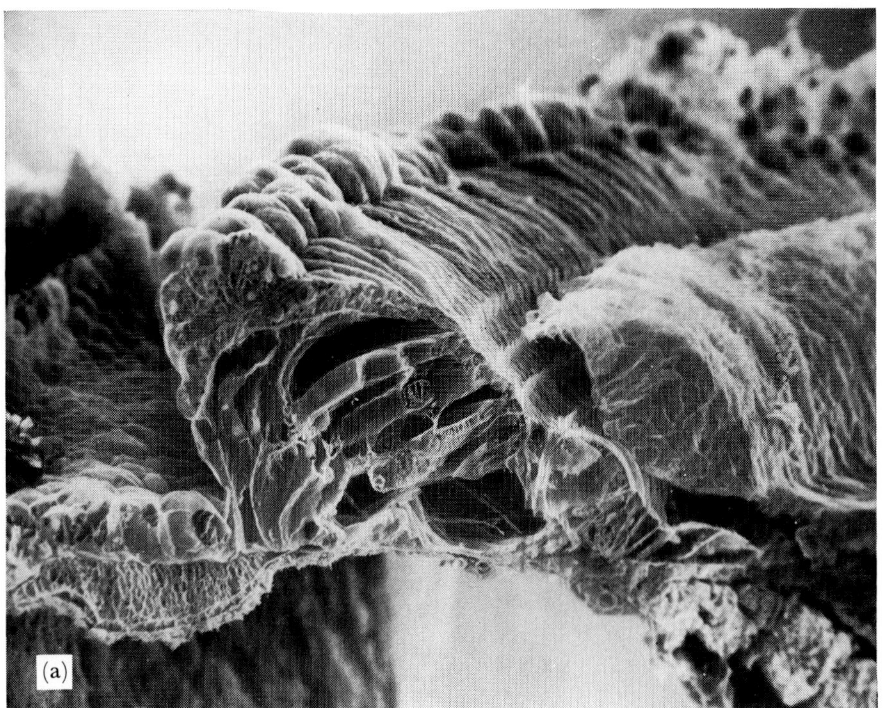

Rows of hairs

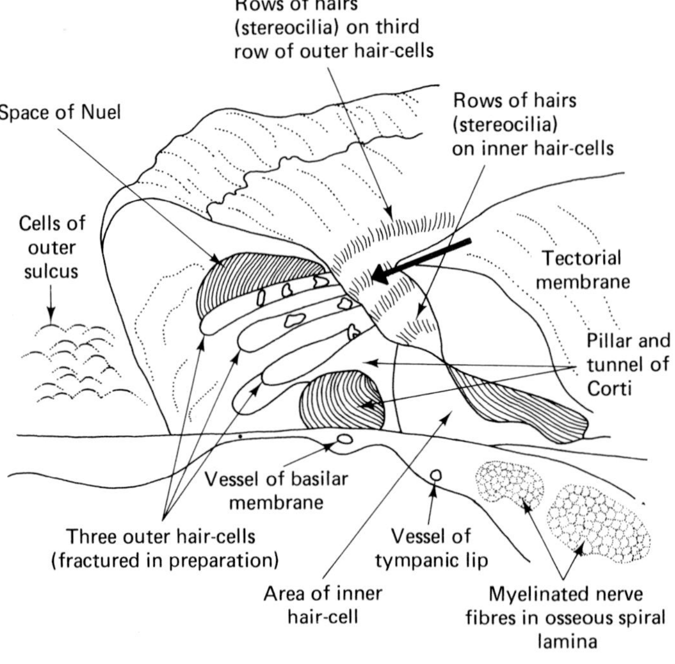

(b)

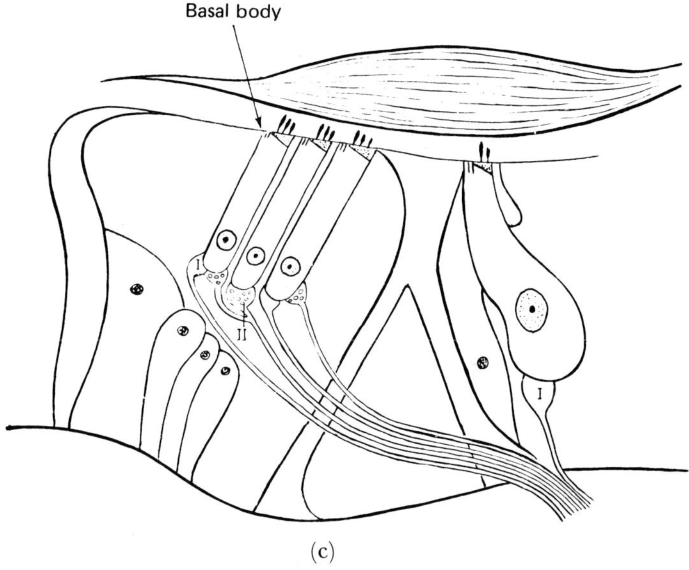

(c)

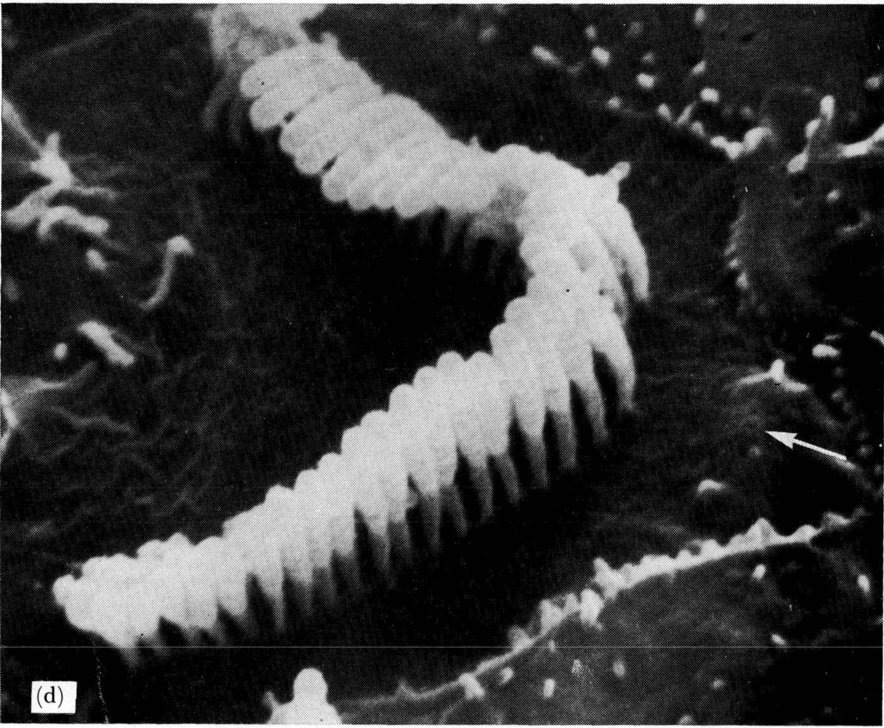

Figure 1.22 (a) Scanning electron micrograph of organ of Corti (× 590) (Reproduced by courtesy of Göran Bredberg); (b) diagrammatic representation of (a). The solid arrow shows the position of stereocilia on one second-row outer hair-cell which is seen in (d); (c) The inner and outer hair-cells of the organ of Corti; (d) the hairs of one outer hair-cell of the second row. The arrow points to the basal body (× 26000)

Reissner's membrane, which stretches diagonally from the spiral limbus to the outer bony wall of the cochlea.

The scala vestibuli and scala tympani

The scala media ends as a blind sac and separates the bony canal of the cochlea into two passages. The upper chamber of perilymph is the scala vestibuli, which is closed by the footplate of the stapes; it communicates functionally with the middle ear through the oval window. The lower one is the scala tympani, which is closed by the secondary tympanic membrane; it communicates functionally with the middle ear through the round window. These two chambers communicate with one another, at the apex of the modiolus, through the helicotrema [Latin *helix* (snail) + *trema* (hole); hole in the snail shell].

The scala tympani is also in connection with the subarachnoid space, by way of the cochlear aqueduct in the cochlear canaliculus (*see Figure 1.17*). The aqueduct contains a reticular network of connective tissue known as the periotic duct.

The cochlear receptor organ

The organ of Corti is the sense organ of hearing and it is set upon the basilar membrane throughout the whole length of the membranous cochlea. As in the vestibular receptor organs, there are three main structures: sensory cells with hairs; supporting cells; and the overlying gelatinous tectorial membrane.

The hair-cells are disposed in a single row of inner hair-cells, astride the inner rod (or pillar) of Corti; and three or four rows of outer hair-cells, outside the outer pillar and supported externally by the cells of Hensen (*Figure 1.21*). There are approximately 17 000 hair-cells in each organ of Corti, about 4500 in the inner, 12 500 in the outer rows. Minute hairs 4 μm long and 0.1 μm thick, project from the free surfaces of the hair-cells into the tectorial membrane, which is attached externally to the spiral limbus.

The space between the pillars is the tunnel of Corti, which contains the 'cortilymph' (Engström, 1960).

The inner hair-cells (*Figure 1.22c*) are bulbous in shape, thus resembling the Type 1 cells of the vestibular labyrinth; and the hairs are arranged in two rows in the form of a double V, with their apices directed away from the modiolus. The outer hair-cells are columnar in shape, like the Type 2 vestibular cells; and the hairs are arranged in three rows in the form of a wide triple W, with their apices also directed away from the modiolus. The kinocilium of the vestibular cells is represented in the cochlear hair-cells by a simple basal body (*Figure 1.22d*).

Innervation and central connections (the eighth cranial nerve)

The eighth cranial nerve has two distinct divisions, subserving respectively the functions of equilibration and hearing.

The vestibular nerve

The fibres of this nerve ramify around the hair-cells of the vestibular receptor organs. There are two types (*Figure 1.20b*): Type I fibres, which are probably afferent and include the nerve chalices around the Type 1 cells; and Type II fibres, which are richly granular and probably efferent.

Within the epithelium there is a plexus of very fine unmyelinated fibres, each of which appears to make contact with the chalices of the Type 1 cells, with a large number of Type 2 cells and with thicker intraepithelial fibres.

From this plexus, proximal to the epithelium, myelinated neurones pass, through two main subdivisions of the vestibular nerve, to the large bipolar cells of the vestibular ganglion. The upper branch innervates the cristae of the superior vertical and lateral semicircular canals, the macula of the utricle and a small portion of the macula of the saccule (*Figure 1.23*); the lower branch innervates the major portion of the macula of the saccule and the posterior vertical canal.

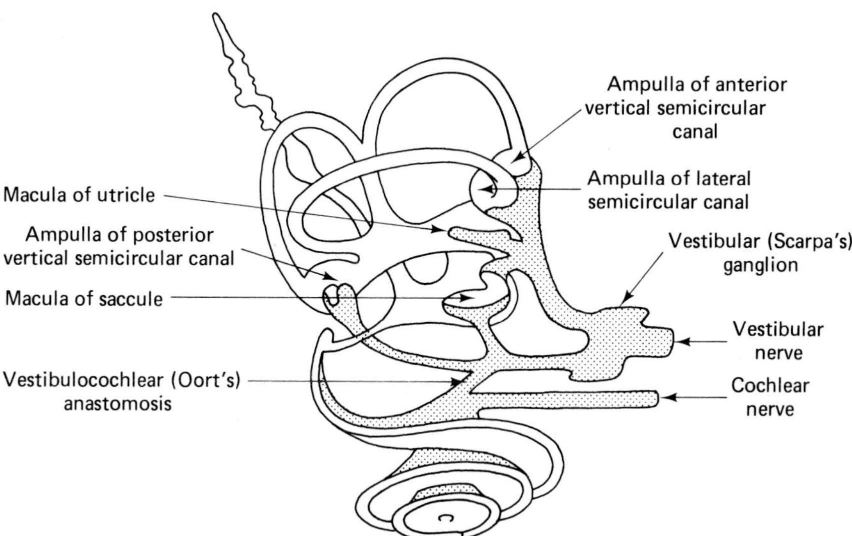

Figure 1.23 The vestibular nerve (after Lindeman)

Situated in the internal auditory canal, the vestibular (Scarpa's) ganglion is usually depicted as having separate superior and inferior portions, but Ballantyne and Engström (1969) found that the ganglion cells formed (in higher mammals) but one oblique ganglion, scattered ganglion cells being seen only rarely at a distance from the main body of the ganglion.

Central connections of the vestibular nerve

In travelling the length of the internal auditory canal, most of the vestibular nerve runs above the cochlear nerve. As the dendrites leaving the vestibular ganglion enter the lower border of the pons, the nerve lies above and medial to the cochlear nerve. The fibres from the three semicircular ducts come together as they pass backwards in the medulla. Most of the fibres of the vestibular nerve terminate in the vestibular nuclei in the pons and medulla, close to the floor of the fourth ventricle.

The vestibular nuclei

There are four nuclei on each side (*Figure 1.24*): (1) The lateral vestibular nucleus, in the lateral part of the medulla, and dominated by impulses from the utricular macula; (2) the superior vestibular nucleus, above the lateral nucleus, in the angle of the fourth ventricle; (3) the medial nucleus, which receives afferent fibres from the

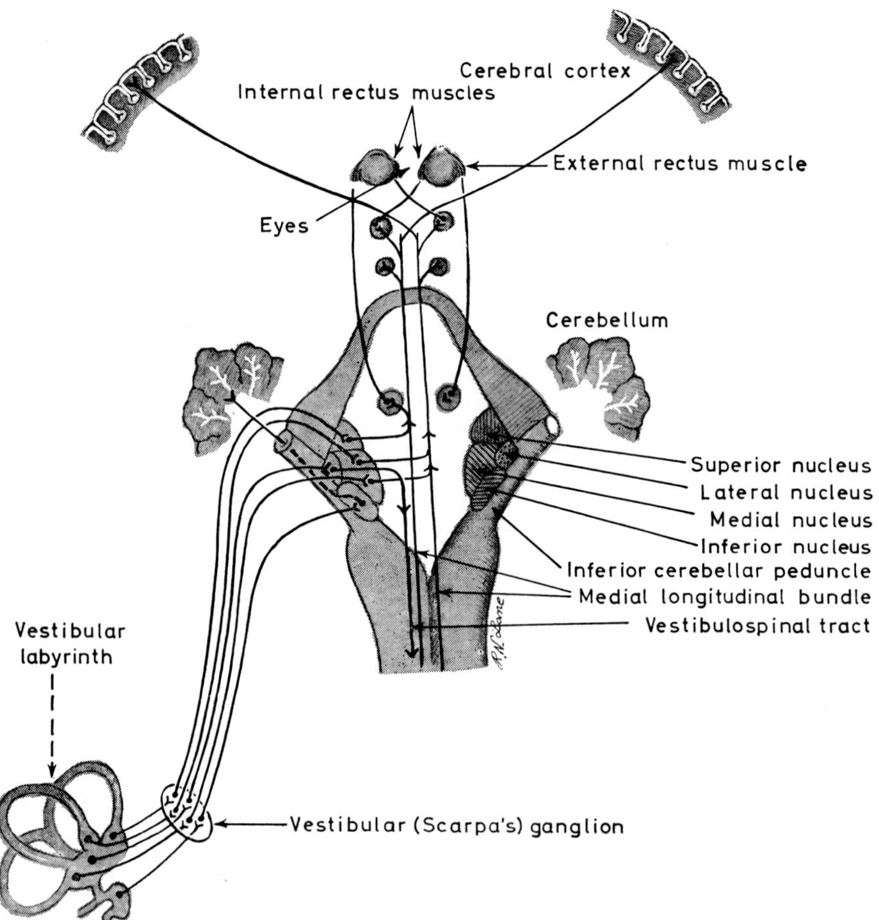

Figure 1.24 The central connections of the vestibular nerve

cristae of the semicircular canals; (4) the inferior nucleus, which receives afferent fibres from the cristae and from the saccular macula. The superior and medial nuclei also receive afferents from the cerebellum.

Secondary central pathways

Efferent fibres from the vestibular nuclei pass to: (1) The vestibulospinal tract, and thence to the spinal cord, from the lateral nucleus. This nucleus is responsible for myotatic reflexes and reflex muscle tone. (2) The medial longitudinal bundle, which receives ascending fibres from the superior nucleus and a few from the medial nucleus. This nucleus exerts its influence upon the extrinsic muscles of the eye, through the nuclei of the third, fourth and sixth cranial nerves. The medial longitudinal bundle is the foremost ascending projection in the vestibular apparatus. (3) The cerebellum, from the inferior nucleus.

In the central vestibular pathways, there are both crossed and uncrossed fibres. The reticular substance in the brain stem receives fibres both from the nuclei themselves and from higher cortical centres, the latter exerting an influence upon the nuclei. Hence the reticular substance plays an important part in the regulation of activity within the vestibular system.

The cochlear (acoustic) nerve

The terminal fibres of this nerve end in contact with the hair-cells. As in the vestibular epithelium, there are two types of nerve fibres (*Figure 1.22c*): Type I fibres which are sparsely granulated and probably afferent; and Type II fibres, which are richly granulated and probably efferent.

These fibres pass through the osseous spiral lamina to the bipolar cells of the spiral ganglion, the cells of this ganglion being generally smaller than those of the vestibular ganglion. They are located in a long bony canal (Rosenthal's canal), which winds spirally from base to apex of the cochlea. The neurones peripheral to the ganglion cells are distributed to the organ of Corti, most of them taking a direct radial course.

The nerve fibres pierce the basilar membrane through the habenula perforata, or foramina nervosa. These foramina are situated in the tympanic lip of the spiral limbus and are minute canals, 1–3 μm wide and 1–2 μm long, arranged in a continuous spiral row beneath the inner hair-cells. Proximal to the habenula perforata the fibres are myelinated; distal to it, they are unmyelinated.

Some of the fibres pass directly to the inner hair-cells, each fibre supplying several hair-cells and each hair-cell being innervated by several fibres.

The remaining fibres pass between the inner pillars of Corti, most of them taking a direct radial course across the tunnel to the outer hair-cells. Below these cells, the fibres turn in a spiral direction, three groups of spiral fibres being thus formed, one beneath each row of outer hair-cells. Each of the radial fibres travels for approximately one-quarter to one-third of a turn of the cochlea. Hence most of these nerve fibres innervate many outer hair-cells, and most of the outer hair-cells are innervated by many fibres.

Apart from 25 000 or more afferent fibres, there are also about 500 efferent (centrifugal) fibres which originate in the superior olivary nucleus and pass to the hair-cells. These fibres form the olivocochlear bundle of Rasmussen (1960), which joins the cochlear nerve by way of the vestibulocochlear (Oort's) anastomosis (*Figure 1.23*).

The efferent fibres lose their myelin sheaths as they perforate the habenula perforata with the afferent fibres, and they form two bundles of spiral nerve fibres: an inner spiral bundle, beneath the inner hair-cells; and a spiral tunnel bundle, in the tunnel of Corti, most of the fibres of the latter bundle turning towards the outer hair-cells.

Spoendlin (1969) found, in experiments with cats, that most of the afferent neurones ended at the inner hair-cells; only a minority, crossing the tunnel of Corti in its lower part, were associated with the outer hair-cells. He believes that most of the radial fibres crossing the tunnel belong to the efferent innervation of the organ of Corti.

Central connections of the cochlear nerve

The thousands of dendrites leaving the spiral ganglion become entwined together like the strands of a rope. After leaving the internal auditory canal, the cochlear nerve enters the brain stem at the upper border of the medulla, just below the lower border of the pons and close to the inferior cerebellar peduncle (*Figure 1.25a*).

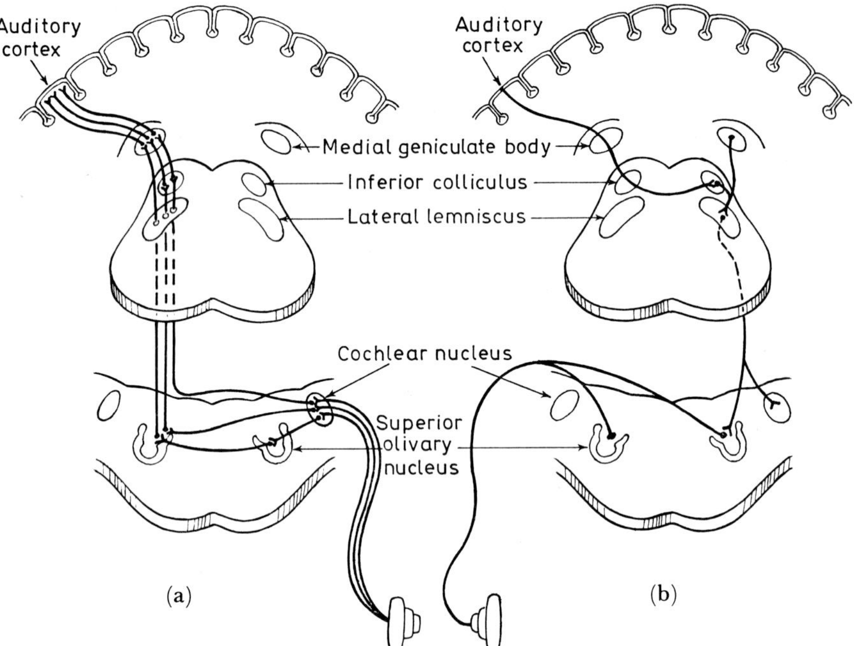

Figure 1.25 The central connections of the cochlear nerve: (a) afferent fibres; (b) efferent fibres

Lying lateral and inferior to the entrance of the vestibular nerve as they enter the brain stem, the afferent fibres of the cochlear nerve terminate in the cochlear nucleus of the same side. From this nucleus, most of them cross the midline, some of the fibres entering the lateral lemniscus of the opposite side directly, others after relaying through the heterolateral superior olivary nucleus. All of these fibres in the lateral lemniscus terminate in either the inferior colliculus or the medial geniculate body (the primary auditory centres).

A few of the afferent fibres may terminate in the superior olivary nucleus of the same side, and thence in the homolateral lateral lemniscus to the inferior colliculus and medial geniculate body of that side.

There is an interconnection between the inferior colliculi of the two sides.

After leaving the medial geniculate body the fibres pass to the higher auditory centres in the temporal lobe.

The efferent fibres (*Figure 1.25b*) originate in the superior olivary nucleus, about one-fifth of them being homolateral, the remainder heterolateral, in origin. These efferent fibres appear to be linked, at brain stem level, with the cochlear nuclei; and to be under the control, by descending fibres, of the cerebral cortex. The significance of these efferent fibres is not yet understood.

The facial (seventh cranial nerve)

The nerve enters the temporal bone through the internal auditory meatus together with the auditory nerve, nervus intermedius, and the internal auditory artery and veins, all these structures being sheathed in a prolongation of the subarachnoid space with its meninges.

At the lateral extremity of the internal auditory meatus the nerve continues, with the nervus intermedius, into the bony fallopian canal, which runs above the labyrinth, separated from the middle cranial fossa by a very thin layer of bone.

The tympanic (or horizontal) portion of the nerve begins where the nerve now turns posteriorly from the geniculate ganglion into the medial wall of the middle ear, where it stands out clearly in its bony canal just above the promontory and the niche of the oval window, and below the horizontal semicircular canal. The anterior end of this portion of the facial canal is marked by the processus cochleariformis with the emerging tensor tympani tendon, and from this point the nerve slopes downwards at an angle of 30 degrees from the horizontal as it proceeds backwards.

The mastoid (or vertical) portion of the facial nerve begins at the pyramidal eminence for the stapedius muscle and tendon, where the nerve makes its second turn, downwards, towards the stylomastoid foramen. This pyramidal turn carries the nerve just posterior to the tympanic cavity, at the posterior extremity of the sulcus tympanicus. This portion of the nerve lies at great depth, rarely less than 1.8 cm from the outer mastoid surface in the adult.

As long as the short process of the incus is in its normal position, the surgeon need not worry about the facial nerve while taking down the facial 'bridge' (of the outer attic wall) in radical mastoid surgery, for the nerve always lies deep to the incus.

The tympanomastoid suture, in the posterior bony wall of the external auditory canal, is the surgical landmark of the vertical portion of the facial nerve, the nerve lying directly medial, sometimes a little posterior but never anterior, to this plane.

The nerve emerges from the stylomastoid foramen. The posterior belly of the digastric muscle is attached to the digastric groove, on the inner surface of the mastoid tip, between the superficial and deep tip cells of the mastoid process. This groove is the surgeon's infallible guide to the facial nerve, at the point where it emerges from the foramen, at the anterior end of the groove.

From the stylomastoid foramen the nerve turns forward, passes lateral to the base of the styloid process, and enters the parotid gland. Within the gland subdivision begins, usually first into upper and lower branches, and then again into the six peripheral branches. These branches run forwards in the plane between the superficial part of the parotid gland, and the ramus of the mandible and masseter muscle.

The facial nerve contains:

(1) Motor fibres, to the muscles of facial expression, and the buccinator, stapedius, digastric and stylohyoid muscles.

(2) Secretomotor parasympathetic fibres, to the lacrimal and nasal glands, and to the submandibular and sublingual salivary glands.
(3) Taste fibres, from the taste-buds of the palate and the anterior two-thirds of the tongue.

In addition, some evidence suggests that there may be cutaneous sensory fibres from a small area of the external ear, accounting for the distribution of the vesication in herpes oticus.

The motor fibres have their cell bodies in the facial nucleus in the pons. The nucleus receives pyramidal fibres from the contralateral motor cortex and a smaller number from the homolateral side. In addition, fibres from the spinal tract of the trigeminal nerve and fibres from the corpus trapezoideum play upon the facial nucleus. The motor fibres sweep around the nucleus of the sixth cranial nerve and emerge from the brain stem at the lower border of the pons. Crossing the cerebello-pontine angle in a lateral and forward direction, the nerve is closely related to the two divisions of the auditory nerve, the nervus intermedius and posteriorly the anterior inferior cerebellar artery.

The parasympathetic nerve fibres originate in the superior salivary nucleus and leave the brain stem in the nervus intermedius. At the geniculate ganglion these fibres mingle with those of the motor nerve trunk. Those destined to innervate the submandibular and sublingual glands continue in the facial nerve as far as the chorda tympani. They finally reach the submandibular ganglion by way of the chorda and the lingual nerve. Parasympathetic motor fibres for the lacrimal gland leave the geniculate ganglion in the greater superficial petrosal nerve, and reach their destination by way of the vidian nerve, the maxillary nerve, and its zygomatic branch. The secretomotor fibres for the nasal mucosa leave the facial nerve by the same route.

The taste fibres from the anterior two-thirds of the tongue travel in the lingual nerve, and then join the facial nerve by way of the chorda tympani. After ascending the facial nerve, the taste fibres have their cell bodies in the geniculate ganglion. From the palate taste fibres first follow the palatine nerves, and then pass through the sphenopalatine ganglion, vidian nerve and greater superficial petrosal nerve to reach the geniculate ganglion. The central axons of all these taste neurones continue in the nervus intermedius to the brain stem. Their final destination is the tractus solitarius.

The branches of the facial nerve from above downwards are:

(1) The greater superficial petrosal nerve, at the geniculate ganglion.
(2) The nerve to stapedius, which passes upwards and forwards, from the commencement of the vertical segment of the facial nerve.
(3) There is much variation in the exact level of origin of the chorda tympani which may be anywhere from 1 to 2 mm below the nerve to stapedius, to the stylomastoid foramen or even lower. Furthermore, the chorda may spring from the front, lateral, or posterior aspect of the nerve trunk. These variables can create difficulties in operations on the nerve if the chorda is used as a landmark for the main trunk.
(4) Below the stylomastoid foramen are the branches to the stylohyoid and digastric

muscles and the post-auricular branch to the occipitofrontalis and external auricular muscles.

(5) The final fanwise branching of the nerve in the face has six main subdivisions: (a) temporal; (b) upper zygomatic; (c) lower zygomatic; (d) buccal; (e) mandibular; (f) cervical. These form a complex branching and anastomosing network in which extensive interconnections with the finer branches of the trigeminal nerve are found. There are also many small branches which cross the midline and innervate a limited muscular field on the opposite side of the face.

Within the confined space of the fallopian canal special attention to the blood supply of the nerve is necessary; a detailed account is given by Blunt (1954). The stylomastoid artery, a branch of the occipital artery, enters the foramen and runs upwards anterior and slightly medial to the nerve, sending short branches at intervals around and into it. At the geniculate ganglion the petrosal branch of the middle meningeal artery enters the canal and runs distally to anastomose with the stylomastoid artery. Within the internal auditory meatus the nerve is supplied by the internal auditory artery and in the posterior cranial fossa by the anterior inferior cerebellar artery. The veins form a plexus around the nerve, from which efferent vessels run obliquely, first between the sheath and the nerve and then through the sheath to lie on its outer surface. Apart from small veins accompanying the chorda tympani, the venous drainage leaves the canal mainly at the stylomastoid foramen and at the genu. Sympathetic nervous control of vasomotor tonus is presumed to be effective through the cervical sympathetic fibres distributed around the branches of the external carotid artery.

Microscopic studies indicate that, like other peripheral nerves, the facial contains medullated axons of varying size, and presumably of varying conductivity speeds.

It seems possible that the larger fibres which have the faster conduction rates, are concerned with voluntary movement, while the smaller diameter 'slow' fibres may be responsible for emotional and reflex movements. The question of maintenance of facial 'tonus' is a little obscure, since muscle spindles – the essential stretch receptors – have apparently not been demonstrated in the facial muscles.

Each medullated nerve fibre branches near its termination into fibrils distributed to the motor end-plates of its own motor unit. In the face, motor units have a comparatively small number of muscle fibres, so that the patterns of muscular activity which are possible are correspondingly large in number, and refined in detail and complexity.

Throughout the fallopian canal the nerve (and its two infrageniculate branches) are enclosed in a fibrous sheath. As exposed during surgical procedures this sheath consists from without inwards of:

(1) A tough, shiny, grey periosteal layer.
(2) A vascular plane of arteries and venous plexus, embedded in loose connective tissue.
(3) A firm fibrous layer perforated by the vessels and on its deep surface in contact with the perineural connective tissues.

Although a clear plane of dissection is found between the sheath and the nerve, this plane is crossed by innumerable connective tissue strands which require careful division and separation if a length of the nerve is to be uncovered.

At the internal auditory meatus the sheath blends with the dural coverings of the nerve, while at the stylomastoid foramen it fuses with the periosteum and with the adjacent fascial layers covering the digastric muscle, the parotid gland and carotid vessels.

The sheath is easily recognized under the dissecting microscope and it is a valuable barrier against mechanical injury and infection. It should be opened only if there are proper surgical indications for doing so.

The blood supply of the labyrinth

The arterial blood supply of the labyrinth is derived principally from the labyrinthine (internal auditory) artery (*Plate 1a, facing page 46*).

This artery usually arises from the anterior inferior cerebellar artery, which is one of the major branches of the midline basilar artery, formed by the confluence of the paired vertebral arteries; occasionally, however, it may arise directly from the basilar, or even the vertebral, artery.

The labyrinthine artery passes down the internal auditory canal and divides into the anterior vestibular artery and the common cochlear artery, the latter soon dividing into two terminal branches, the vestibulocochlear artery and the cochlear artery.

The anterior vestibular artery supplies the vestibular nerve, much of the utricle and parts of the semicircular ducts.

Upon arrival at the modiolus, in the region of the basal turn of the cochlea, the vestibulocochlear artery divides into its terminal vestibular and cochlear branches, which take opposite directions. The vestibular branch supplies the saccule, the greater part of the semicircular canals, and the basal end of the cochlea; the cochlear branch, running a spiral course around the modiolus, ends by anastomosing with the cochlear artery. The vestibular and cochlear branches both supply capillary areas in the spiral ganglion, the osseous spiral lamina, the limbus, and the spiral ligament.

In the internal auditory canal, the cochlear artery runs a spiral course around the acoustic nerve. In the cochlea, it runs a serpentine course around the modiolus, as the spiral modiolar artery, which is an end-artery (*Plate 2, facing page 46*). Arterioles leave this artery, to run centrifugally and to radiate over both the scala vestibuli and the osseous spiral lamina. They end in spiral capillary systems in the lamina and the external wall of the cochlea.

In the latter situation, it is the stria vascularis which has excited most interest because of its apparent role both in the formation and absorption of endolymph and as the source of electrical potentials. The stria consists of a network of capillaries which appear to be composed of endothelial cells only.

The capillaries from the external wall of the cochlea are drained into collecting venules which radiate centripetally, to empty into veins which run spirally, like the artery, around the modiolus (*Plate 2, facing page 46*).

In this region of the external wall, there is a preponderance of arteries in the scala vestibuli, and of veins in the scala tympani.

The whole of the apical region of the cochlea is drained by the anterior spiral vein (*Plate 1b, facing page 46*). A small part of the middle turn and all the basal turn are drained by the posterior spiral vein. These two branches of the spiral vein join with the anterior and posterior branches of the vestibular vein, in the region of the basal turn, to form the vein of the cochlear aqueduct – the principal vein of the cochlea – which runs in a separate channel close to the aqueduct of the cochlea, and empties into the jugular bulb.

The vestibular labyrinth is drained: from the anterior part by the anterior vestibular vein, which becomes the labyrinthine vein and accompanies the artery of the same name, usually ending in the superior petrosal sinus; from the posterior part by the vein of the vestibular aqueduct which passes alongside the endolymphatic duct to the sigmoid sinus.

This description of the vascular supply of the cochlea is based on the work of Axelsson (1968).

The anatomical basis of referred otalgia

It is a *sine qua non* that the ear must be very carefully examined in any patient who complains of earache. And indeed, in the majority of such patients, the cause of this symptom is to be found in the ear itself. However, one is confronted from time to time with a patient whose main (or only) complaint is of earache, sometimes continuous, sometimes intermittent and not uncommonly neuralgic in quality. In such cases the pain may be referred to the ear from remote or related structures whose sensory nerve supply also sends branches to the ear.

The rather complex sensory nerve supply of the ear has been described in the relevant parts of 'Descriptive Anatomy of the Ear' (*see* pp. 2, 5, 7 and 19), but it can perhaps be best summarized pictorially (*Figures 1.26* and *1.27*).

The sensory nerve supply of the ear is derived from branches of the second and third cervical spinal nerves and from branches of the fifth, ninth and tenth cranial nerves.

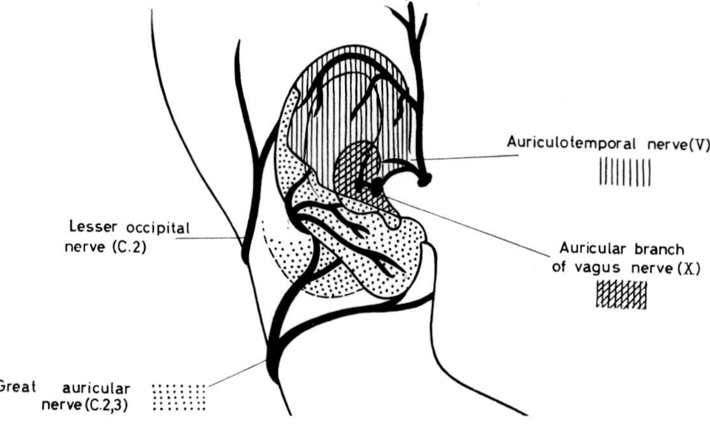

Figure 1.26 Sensory nerve supply of the lateral aspect of the ear

The great auricular nerve is derived from the second and third cervical spinal nerves and supplies the skin of the lower third of the lateral (anterior) surface of the auricle, and the skin over the mastoid process.

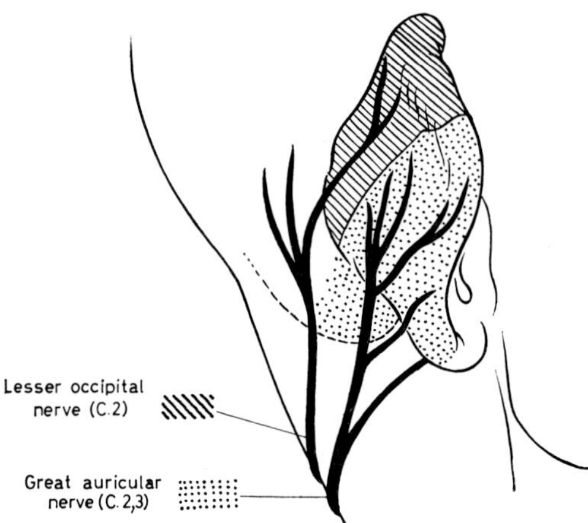

Figure 1.27 Sensory nerve supply of the medial aspect of the ear

The lesser occipital nerve is derived from the second cervical spinal nerve and supplies the skin of approximately the upper one-third of the medial (posterior) surface of the auricle.

The auricular branch of the auriculotemporal nerve is a terminal branch of the lowest, mandibular division of the trigeminal (fifth cranial) nerve. It supplies approximately the upper two-thirds of the lateral (anterior) surface of the auricle, and the anterior halves of the external auditory canal and tympanic membrane.

The tympanic plexus is derived from the tympanic branch of the glossopharyngeal (ninth cranial) nerve, and it supplies the mucous membrane of the whole middle-ear cleft. The auricular branch of the vagus (tenth cranial) nerve supplies a small part of the auricle and roughly the posterior half of the external auditory meatus and tympanic membrane.

This nerve is alternatively known as Arnold's nerve, or the 'Alderman's nerve', the latter nickname originating from the fact that aldermen attending banquets in bygone days were purported to have stimulated their pre-prandial appetites by stimulation of this branch of the vagus by the introduction into the ear of spirit! This is also the nerve that so often makes a patient cough when instruments are introduced, and indeed there is even a case on record of a death from syringeing, presumably due to vagal stimulation.

Referred otalgia, then, may be referred via the second and third cervical spinal nerves, as in lesions of the upper cervical discs, arthritis of the cervical spine, 'fibrositis' of the upper part of the sternomastoid muscle or herpetic lesions; via the fifth cranial nerve as in lesions of the nose and paranasal sinuses, especially in infections or neoplasms of the maxillary or sphenoidal sinus, and in pressure on the middle turbinate from high deviation or swelling of the septum; in lesions of the nasopharynx, such as ulceration, neoplasm or acute inflammatory lesions, or after adenoidectomy; and in lesions of the teeth and jaws, such as dental caries, apical abscess and impaction of the molar teeth (particularly in the lower jaw), malocclusion (including overclosure of the jaws, as in Costen's syndrome) and arthritis of the temporo-mandibular joint; in lesions of the salivary glands and ducts, due either to an acute inflammatory lesion or to the presence of calculi; and in sphenopalatine neuralgia.

The oropharynx, laryngopharynx and base of the tongue receive their sensory nerve supply from the ninth and tenth cranial nerves and a wide variety of lesions arising within this territory may cause referred otalgia. In the oropharynx, acute pharyngitis and tonsillitis, peritonsillar abscess (quinsy) and abscesses in the parapharyngeal and retropharyngeal spaces may cause earache, whilst this is also a common complaint after tonsillectomy. Ulceration (especially tuberculous) and neoplasia in these areas may also cause otalgia, whilst less common causes include primary glossopharyngeal neuralgia and elongation of the styloid process, the latter causing pressure on this nerve as it winds round the process. Rarely, the vagus may be stimulated by oesophageal disease.

Finally, there is a doubtful sensory division of the seventh cranial nerve, which has been held responsible for the earache of herpes zoster oticus, including the Ramsay Hunt syndrome.

Tonsillitis and tonsillectomy, dental lesions and ulcerations and neoplasms of the upper digestive tract are the most common causes of referred otalgia, but the full investigation of an obscure case may demand a thorough examination of all those anatomical areas which come within the very widespread area of distribution of all those sensory nerves whose branches supply the ear.

Anatomical principles of temporal bone surgery

The several parts of the middle-ear cleft and the labyrinth may be approached surgically in a variety of ways.

Incisions

Endomeatal

Although it has been used for many different purposes in the past (for instance, as an approach to the middle-ear cavity for 'tympanosympathectomy' by Lempert, and for the eradication of limited attic disease by Tumarkin), the endomeatal incision has been much more widely adopted since it was used by Rosen for mobilization of the stapes. It provides by far the most satisfactory approach to the mesotympanum (permeatal tympanotomy), for such operative procedures as removal or mobilization of the stapes; destruction of the labyrinth through the oval window (Cawthorne); removal of 'glue' from the middle-ear cleft in cases of exudative otitis media, and for the exact diagnosis and, where feasible, the surgical correction of certain derangements of the ossicular system due to congenital or traumatic causes.

Used for these purposes, the standard incision is made (in the erect 'anatomical' position of the head) from 12 o'clock, through the skin and periosteum of the posterior deep meatal wall, to 6 o'clock, coming outwards in the middle of its course to a distance of at least 6 mm from the posterior attachment of the tympanic annulus in its sulcus (*Figure 1.28a*).

A variety of other endomeatal incisions may be employed for the purpose of removing exostoses from the external canal; for reducing bony humps from the anterior deep meatal wall, where an unusually deep anterior recess adds to the difficulty of exposing the anterior edge of an anterior perforation, as in myringoplasty; or for the fashioning of free or pedicled skin flaps for tympanoplastic procedures.

Endaural

The endaural incision may be regarded as an extension of the endomeatal incision, and indeed a major part of the endaural incision is endomeatal. This endomeatal part of the incision (*Figure 1.28b*) is made just internal (medial) to the junction of the bony and cartilaginous meatus and it is made through the skin and periosteum on to the

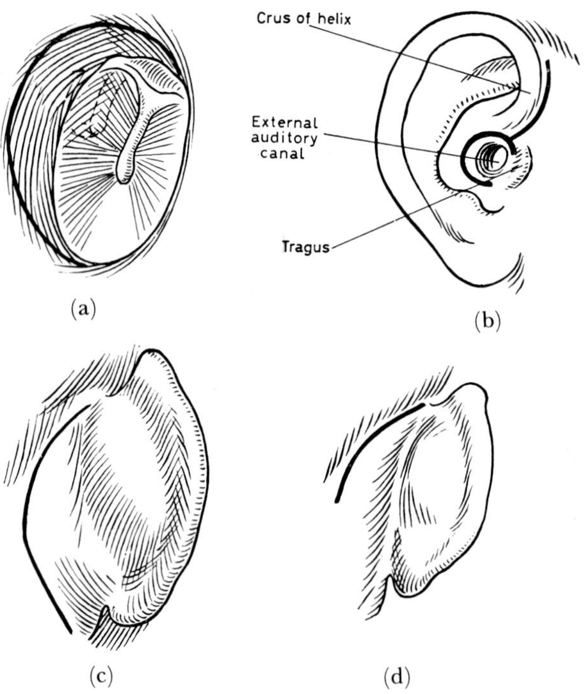

Figure 1.28 Incisions for temporal bone surgery: (a) endomeatal incision; (b) endaural incision; (c) post-aural incision, in adults and older children, (d) post-aural incision, in infants and very young children

bone itself. The incision usually extends (in the right ear) from the 3 o'clock position anteriorly, through 12 o'clock down to 6 o'clock posteriorly. Hereafter, a cuff of skin may be reflected (dissected) off the bony meatal wall to the tympanic annulus and the notch of Rivinus (*see* endomeatal sutures and spines, p. 3).

The second, or superficial part of the endaural incision passes outwards through the incisura terminalis and upwards between the tragus and crus of the helix from the 12 o'clock position of the endomeatal incision to the point where the anterior part of the helix leaves the side of the head (*Figure 1.28b*). Hence cartilage is avoided and the risk of perichondritis or cartilage necrosis is thereby greatly reduced.

The endaural incision was popularized by Lempert in his one-stage operation for fenestration of the horizontal semicircular canal, and later for destruction of the labyrinth through this canal in cases of Menière's disease; it is also very widely

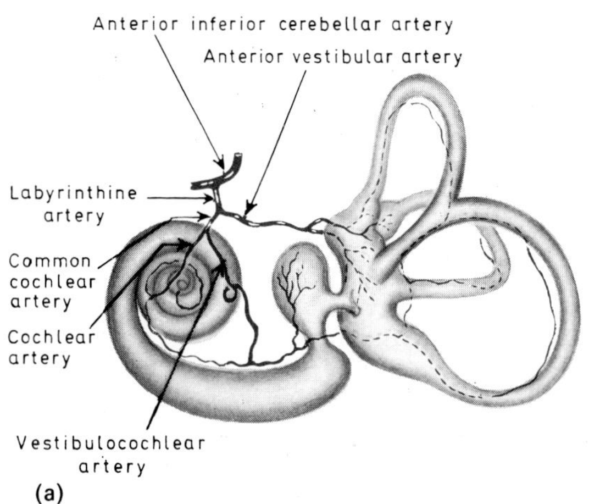

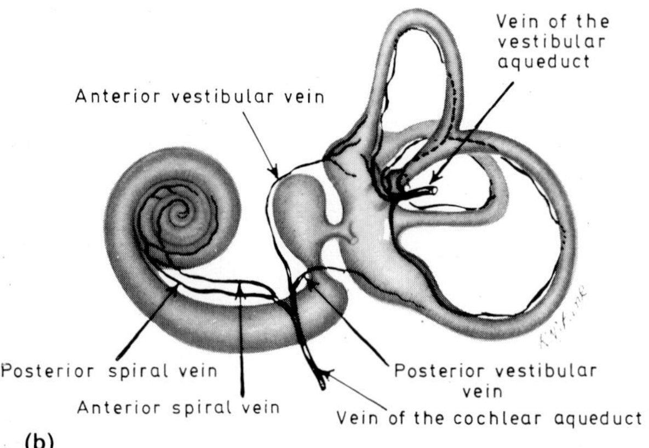

Plate 1 Vascular supply of the inner ear (after Axelsson): (a) arteries; (b) veins

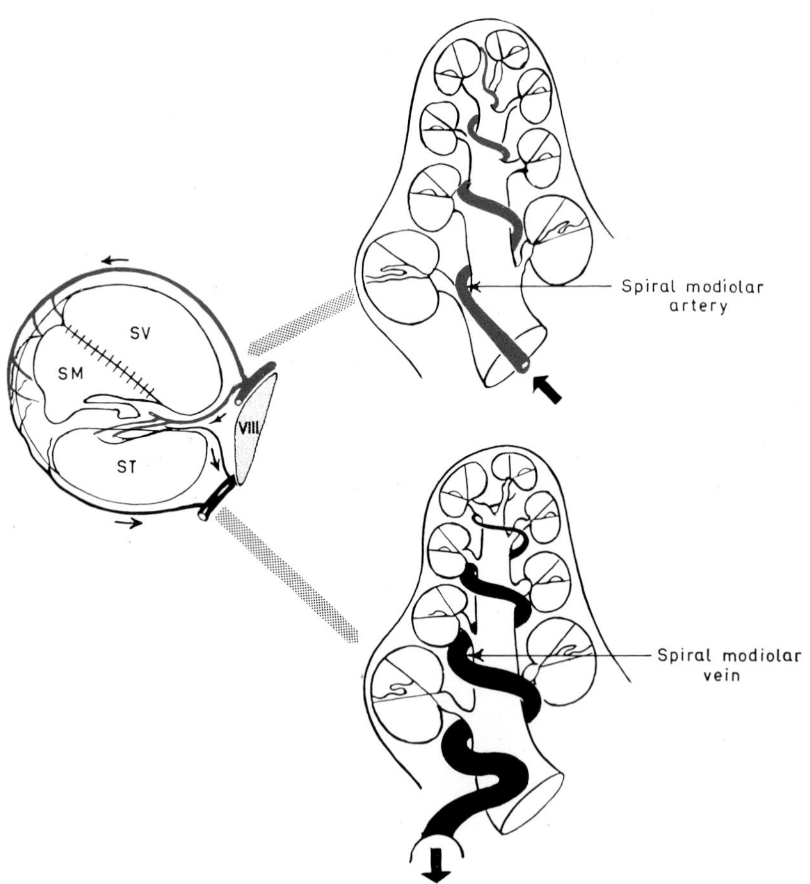

Plate 2 Cochlear vasculature (after Axelsson)

employed in all forms of radical mastoid surgery, with or without plastic reconstruction of the sound-conducting apparatus.

It is used particularly for operations on the hypocellular mastoid or when the operative procedure is directed mainly to the tympanic cavity (including the epitympanum), the aditus and the antrum. It may also provide freer access to the deep external auditory canal when it is grossly narrowed.

Post-aural

The post-aural incision (*Figure 1.28c*) is made, in the adult, from just above the point where the ear leaves the side of the head, to the tip of the mastoid process, curving backwards between these points, usually about 1 cm or so behind the attachment of the auricle in the middle of its course.

If the incision is made in, or too near to, the post-aural sulcus, meatal stenosis is likely to result; and in an infant the incision must be modified, to avoid damage to the superficially-placed facial nerve (*Figure 1.28d*).

The post-aural incision allows complete exposure of the entire mastoid cellular system, right down to the tip cells, and is to be preferred to the endaural incision in the conservative (cortical or Schwartze) operation for acute mastoiditis. It is also usually employed in the re-opening of an old mastoidectomy cavity and for exploration of the vertical part of the facial nerve.

It should be emphasized that these three standard incisions can be extended and combined into a wide variety of combinations and permutations. For example, the endaural or post-aural incision can be extended upwards into a superior incision for the purpose of exposing the temporalis muscle; this muscle is used in muscle-plasty operations for obliteration of the mastoid 'bowl', and its fascia is often employed (either from its superficial or its deep surface) for tympanoplastic repair. Furthermore the endaural incision can be modified for the excision of a congenital pre-auricular sinus or cyst, and a combined endaural–post-aural incision used when the sinus extends backwards and downwards towards the mastoid tip.

Permeatal tympanotomy and atticotomy

This provides the most direct approach to the middle-ear cavity, either through the endomeatal incision or through the extended endomeatal approach of the endaural incision.

After separation of the skin and periosteum from the bone of the posterior deep meatal wall, the tympanic annulus is dislocated out of its sulcus (preferably at its postero-superior angle in the first instance). Forward reflection of the resultant small tympanomeatal flap allows exposure of the posterior half of the mesotympanum (*Figure 1.29*).

The chorda tympani nerve, lying superficial to the long process of the incus, is the first structure to come into view; most of the long process, with its lenticular process, is easily seen in most cases, together with the incudostapedial joint, and the stapedius tendon passing forwards to be inserted into the neck of the stapes. Sometimes the crura and footplate of the stapes may be partially visualized, and the round window niche is seen to lie below and behind the bony bulge of the promontory. Part of the horizontal portion of the bony facial (fallopian) canal may also be seen.

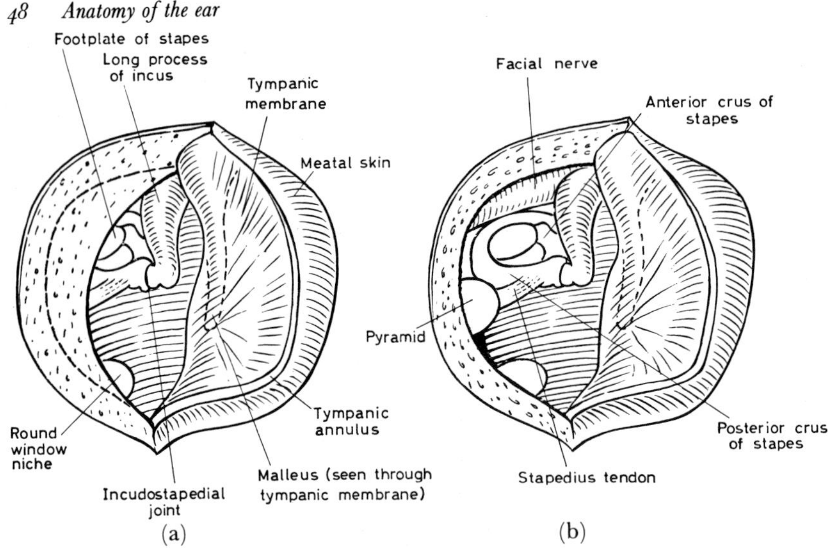

Figure 1.29 Permeatal tympanotomy: (a) initial exposure of posterior half of mesotympanum. The dotted line indicates the area of bone that has to be removed to expose the pyramid, stapedius tendon and footplate of stapes; (b) exposure of pyramid, stapes and labyrinthine windows

However, the origin of the stapedius tendon through the bony pyramid can usually be seen only after removal of bone from the postero-superior angle of the deep meatus; this also allows better exposure of the facial canal and the footplate area. Removal of the bone of the outer attic wall will also permit a limited exposure of the attic.

Bony surface landmarks

After making the endaural or the post-aural incision, periosteum is reflected from those areas of the temporal bone behind, above and sometimes in front of the bony external

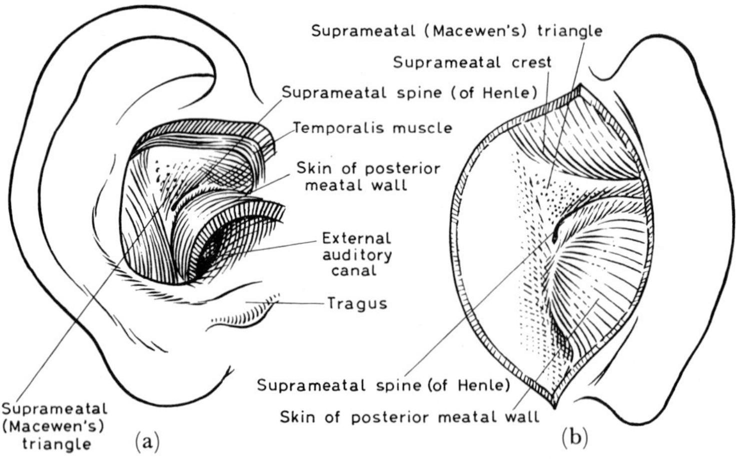

Figure 1.30 The spine of Henle and Macewen's triangle: (a) endaural incision; (b) post-aural incision

canal. This exposes two bony landmarks of particular surgical importance (*Figure 1.30*).

The suprameatal spine (spine of Henle) usually marks the postero-superior angle of the external auditory canal.

The suprameatal triangle (Macewen's triangle) forms a shallow roughened depression immediately behind the spine.

Its boundaries are formed by the suprameatal crest, above; the orifice of the bony external canal, in front; and a vertical line which is tangential below to the posterior margin of the meatus and cuts the suprameatal crest above.

In the average adult, the antrum lies about 1.5 cm deep to the triangle.

The bone over the infant's antrum is cribriform, so that an otitis media is actually subperiosteal, and early oedema and redness of the skin occur over this area. The mastoid process does not begin to appear until the second year of life, and the osseous meatus begins to develop at about the same time by the lateral growth of the early incomplete ring of the tympanic bone.

It should be emphasized that there is no reliable surface marking for the sigmoid sinus, whose position is extremely variable and may rarely be found immediately behind the posterior wall of the bony meatus, especially near the floor.

Surgical approach to the mastoid antrum

The mastoid antrum is often the first part of the middle-ear cleft to be exposed in the surgical treatment of diseases of the cleft, other than those which are strictly limited to the tympanic cavity itself.

Whilst the post-aural incision is to be preferred in cases of acute mastoiditis (now relatively rare) and is still used by many surgeons for all extratympanic surgical procedures, the endaural incision gives a more direct 'head-on' approach to the 'key area' of the attic, aditus and antrum (*Figure 1.31*).

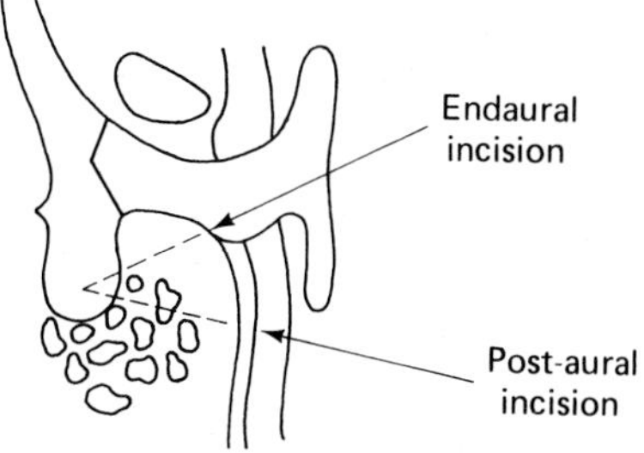

Figure 1.31 Surgical approaches to the mastoid antrum (schematic horizontal section through the external auditory canal and middle-ear cleft, as seen from above)

When the post-aural incision is used, the antrum is approached through Macewen's triangle. With the endaural incision, it is approached partly through this triangle, and partly by the more direct approach through the sloping postero-superior wall of the bony external auditory canal.

Surgical exenteration of the mastoid air-cell system

After the antrum has been fully exposed, the entire air-cell system is exenterated. In the cellular mastoid, this exenteration will extend downwards to the very tip of the mastoid, and forwards into the zygomatic process, when zygomatic cells are present; such a clearance of the cells will reveal further bony landmarks (*Figure 1.32*). In the hypocellular and acellular mastoid some of these landmarks will be less clearly defined.

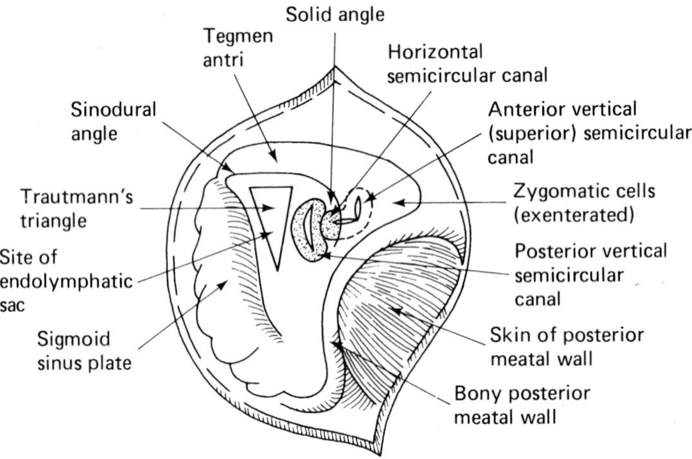

Figure 1.32 The solid angle, the sinodural angle and Trautmann's triangle

The bony plate of the sigmoid sinus presents as a smooth rounded plate of bone after all the cells have been removed. It is extremely variable in position.

The bony tegmen antri covers the temporal lobe of the brain, in the middle cranial fossa. It may be extremely thin.

The sinodural angle is the angle between the tegmen antri and the sigmoid sinus (and posterior cranial fossa).

The solid angle is formed by the solid bone in the angle formed by the three semicircular canals, medial to the antrum.

Trautmann's triangle is a part of the bony plate of the posterior cranial fossa, behind the antrum. It is bounded by the sigmoid sinus, the bony labyrinth and the superior petrosal sinus, which runs along the upper border of the petrous temporal bone and ends in the transverse sinus at the point where it is continuous with the sigmoid sinus.

Exposure of the attic and aditus ad antrum

Proceeding from the position just described, let us imagine that all the skin covering the mastoid and squamous portions of the temporal bone has been removed; that the bony external canal has been denuded of its cutaneous lining; and that the tympanic

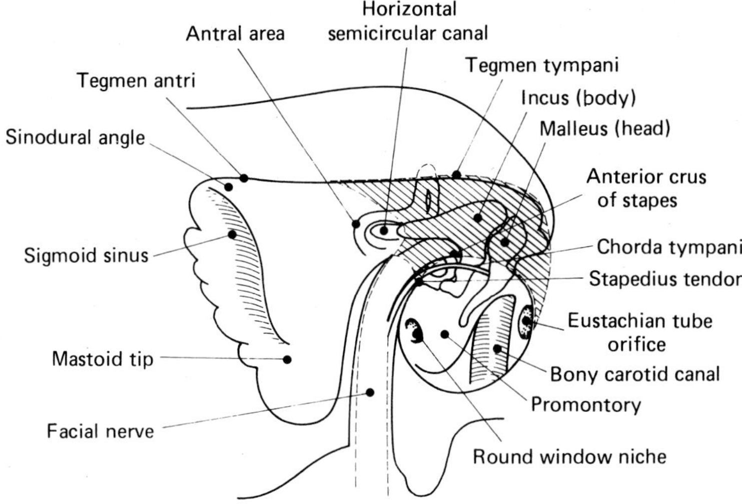

Figure 1.33 Surgical exposure of the normal middle-ear cleft. (The striped area represents the outer wall of the attic and aditus ad antrum)

membrane has been removed. We are now left with a temporal bone in which the ossicles remain in their normal position (*Figure 1.33*).

The handle of the malleus, together with its short (lateral) process and a part of its neck, are seen; so also is a part of the long process of the incus, together with its lenticular process, the incudostapedial joint, the stapedius tendon, a limited amount of the crura and a part of the footplate. Above the footplate, the lower border of the bony facial canal may be visualized, and the chorda tympani nerve is seen to pass between the long process of the incus and the neck of the malleus. The bony bulge of the promontory is clearly discerned and below and behind it is the niche of the round window. The upper tympanic orifice of the eustachian tube is seen anteriorly.

But the head of the malleus (and the remainder of its neck), the body and short process of the incus (with a part of the long process) and the incudomalleolar joint are still hidden from view by the bony bridge which remains between the mesotympanum in front and the mastoid antrum behind. This bridge is formed by the outer walls of the attic and aditus, represented by the striped outline in *Figure 1.33*.

Remove the bridge and still we are unable to see much of the horizontal portion of the bony facial canal and the bony bulge of the horizontal semicircular canal, both of them lying in the medial wall of the attic and aditus.

Remove the malleus and incus, however, and we are left with the entire middle-ear cleft (apart from the eustachian tube) in a state which resembles very closely a complete radical mastoidectomy (*Figure 1.34a*). In the operation for fenestration of the horizontal semicircular canal, the canal is exposed by removing the incus, with the head and neck of the malleus. The posterior end of the canal can be adequately exposed, usually through a post-aural incision, without removing even the incus; this route is employed for ultrasonic destruction of the vestibular labyrinth in certain cases of Menière's disease.

The semicircular canals are clearly seen, and below the horizontal canal is the horizontal portion of the fallopian canal. Emerging just below the anterior end of the facial canal, close to the level of the geniculate ganglion, is the tendon of the tensor tympani muscle, passing laterally from its exit from the cochleariform process to the neck of the malleus. This tendon may be very prominent, when it is easily confused by the unwary with nerve fibres. The bony carotid canal may be seen between the eustachian orifice and the promontory.

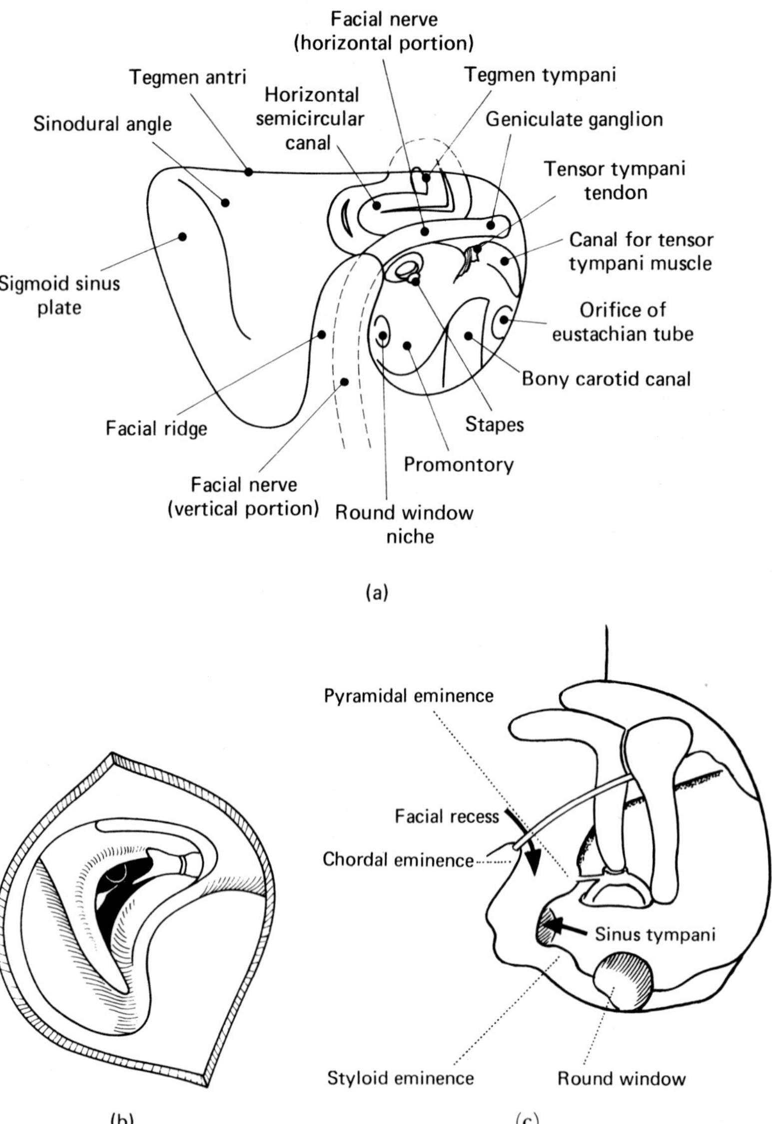

Figure 1.34 (a) The surgical anatomy of the complete radical mastoid cavity; (b) exposure of the facial recess; (c) the facial recess and sinus tympani (after Proctor)

Exposure of the facial recess (posterior tympanotomy)

It has been demonstrated recently that disease can often be removed from all parts of the middle-ear cleft without removing the 'bridge' of the postero-superior bony canal wall. This is done by combining a permeatal approach (lateral tympanotomy) with an approach through the mastoid antrum (posterior tympanotomy).

In posterior tympanotomy, an initial cortical mastoidectomy is carried forwards sufficiently far to expose the incus and head of malleus (*Figure 1.34b*). The 'facial triangle' is then dissected, by removing the bone which lies between the posterior part of the tympanic annulus and the vertical portion of the facial nerve, up to the bend between the horizontal and vertical portions. This brings the surgeon into the facial recess (*Figure 1.34b*), lateral to the vertical portion of the nerve, and permits him to visualize the stapes and sinus tympani, in the posterior reaches of the mesotympanum.

Exposure of the endolymphatic sac

The endolymphatic sac, whose exposure may be indicated in some cases of Menière's disease, can be reached through an extended cortical mastoidectomy. The sac is situated half-way between the sigmoid sinus and the midpoint of the bony posterior semicircular canal (*Figure 1.32*).

Exposure of the internal auditory canal

Provided that they have not extended below the jugular bulb, tumours of the eighth cranial nerve and cerebello-pontine angle may be removed by way of a cortical mastoidectomy and translabyrinthine approach (*Figure 1.35a*). All air-cells from the sinodural angle and over the sigmoid sinus must be exenterated.

The tympanic portion of the facial nerve is skeletonized and kept in view throughout the procedure. The bony labyrinth is removed; in order that an adequate exposure of the internal auditory canal may be obtained; this must include the whole of the superior semicircular canal.

The internal acoustic meatus may also be approached through the posterior cranial fossa (sub-occipital approach, *Figure 1.35b*) or through the middle cranial fossa (*Figure 1.35c*).

(a)

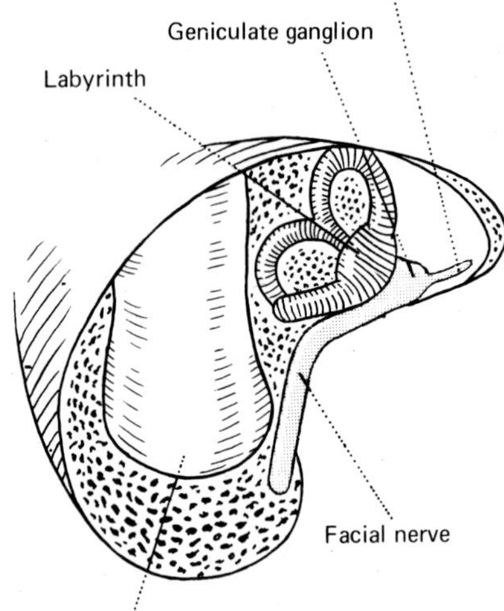

Gtr. superficial petrosal nerve
Geniculate ganglion
Labyrinth
Facial nerve
Sigmoid sinus

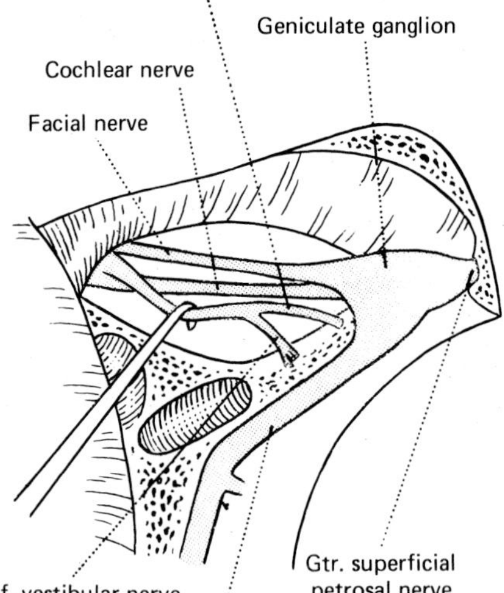

Sup. vestibular nerve
Geniculate ganglion
Cochlear nerve
Facial nerve
Inf. vestibular nerve
Gtr. superficial petrosal nerve
Facial nerve

(b)

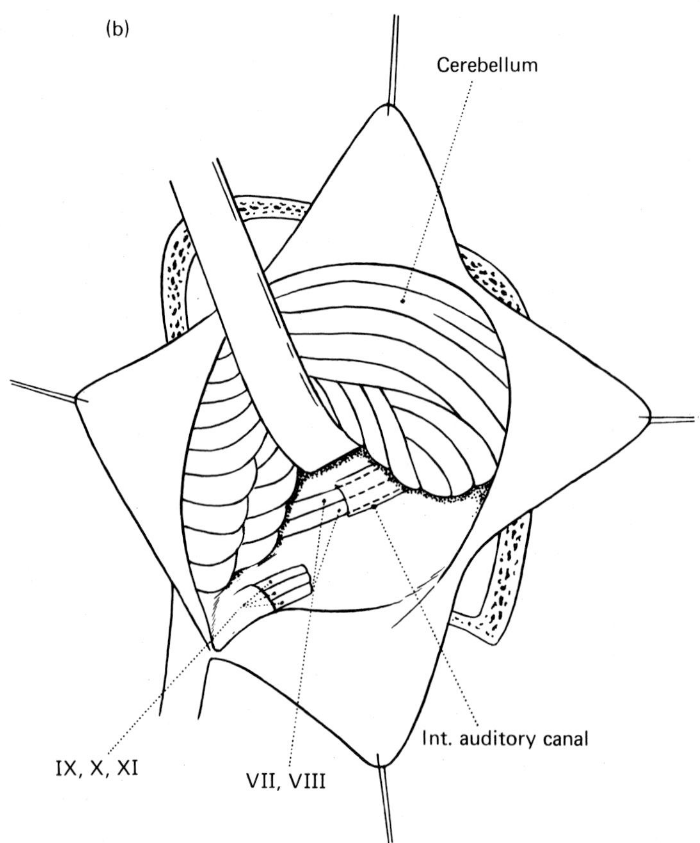

Cerebellum
Int. auditory canal
IX, X, XI
VII, VIII

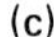
(c)

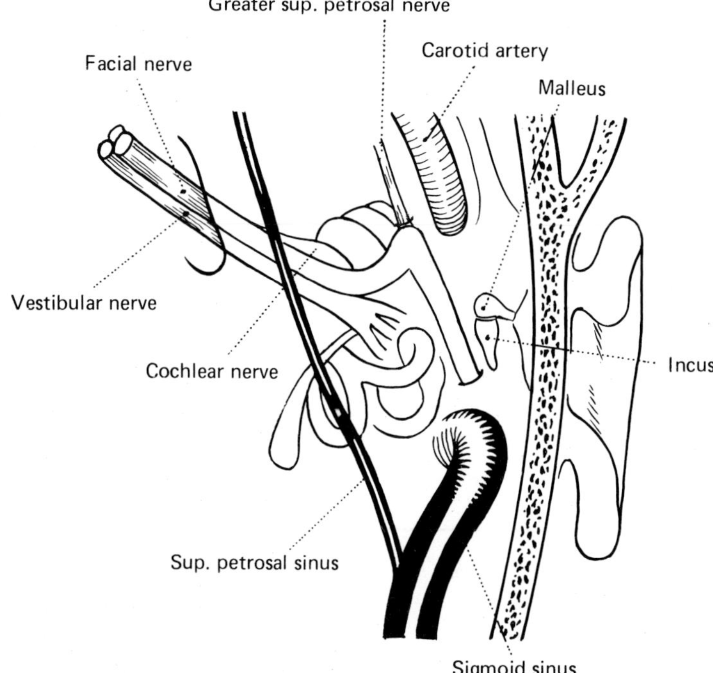

Figure 1.35 Surgical approach to the internal auditory canal: (a) translabyrinthine approach: *Left* Initial stage *Right* Disposition of nerves after removal of labyrinth and posterior wall of internal auditory canal; (b) posterior fossa approach; (c) Middle fossa approach (after Fisch)

Development of the human ear

The ear is the first organ of special sense to become differentiated in man, for the inner ear reaches full adult size and configuration by midterm. The external and middle ear, however, are not completely formed at birth.

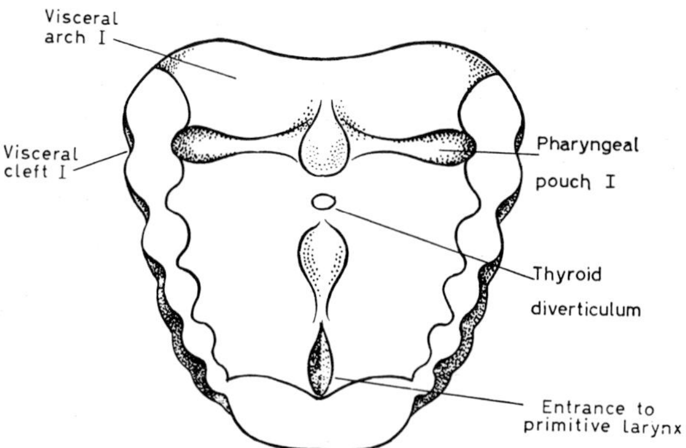

Figure 1.36 The primitive visceral arches and clefts

During the early stages of fetal development, a series of six visceral arches appears on the lateral aspect of the head. These mesenchymal arches form ridges in the overlying ectoderm and corresponding projections in the entoderm of the pharynx.

The ridges become separated from one another by a series of furrows where ectoderm and entoderm come into contact with one another. The ectodermal furrows form the visceral clefts. The entodermal furrows form the pharyngeal pouches.

The external ear

The auricle

The auricle arises from the outer part of the first visceral cleft, where six cartilaginous tubercles appear towards the end of the first fetal month; three on the first (mandibular) arch; three on the second (hyoid) arch (*Figure 1.37*).

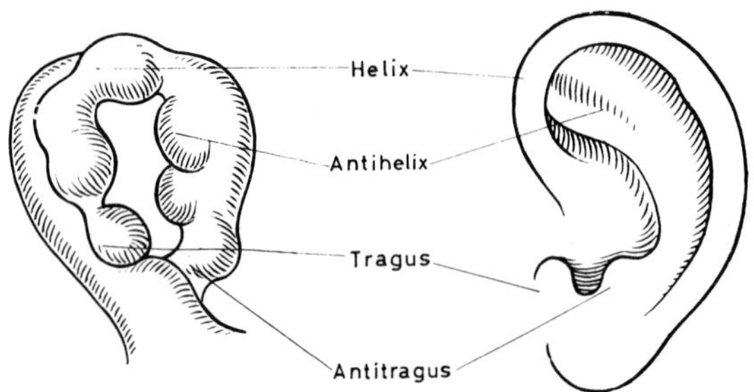

Figure 1.37 Development of the auricle

Many investigators believe that the auricle is developed from the growth and fusion of these tubercles, the tragus coming from the most ventral one on the mandibular arch; the antitragus from the most ventral one on the hyoid arch; and the helix from the fusion of the remainder.

However, a second school of thought holds that the tubercles are of minor importance, disappearing after a certain stage of their development has been attained.

In any case, the tubercles are clearly evident in the third month of fetal life, when rapid changes occur. According to Evans, it is at this time that the greater number of malformations are produced.

The external auditory canal

The external auditory canal is formed from the ectoderm of the first visceral cleft (*Figure 1.38*).

The primary external auditory canal is a funnel-shaped tube from which the cartilaginous meatus and a small portion of the bony canal are formed. From this tube a solid core of epithelium extends inwards, but this core eventually hollows out

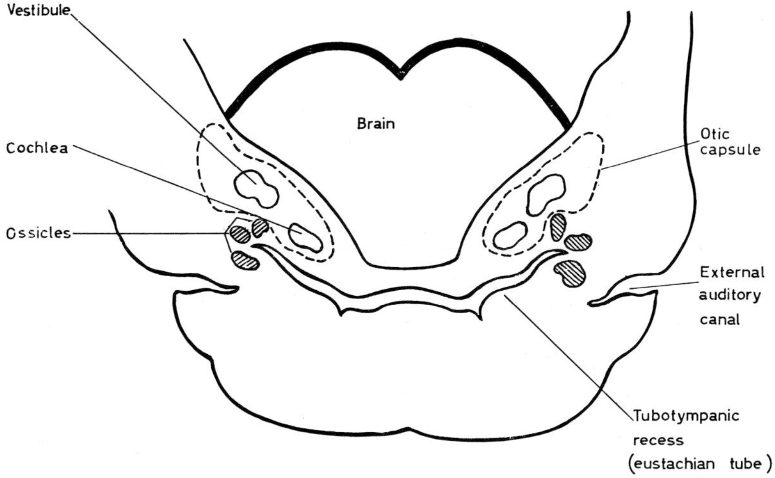

Figure 1.38 Development of the ear (human embryo, eight weeks)

to form the inner portion of the canal (the so-called secondary meatus), the blind end of which forms the outer epidermal layer of the tympanic membrane.

Most of the bony canal is derived from the os tympanicum which develops, first of all in the floor of the first visceral cleft, as an incomplete circle deficient above. At birth it is still an open ring. After birth, however, it grows outwards, along the floor and sides of the external auditory canal, to form the tympanic plate; some time elapses before this incomplete ring can form a complete external canal. Thus a gaping fissure (the glaserian fissure) leads to the middle-ear cavity, and through this fissure haemorrhage and infection may pass readily from the middle ear, to cause sagging of the superior canal wall.

Furthermore, the anterior and posterior portions grow more rapidly than the rest and this leaves a foramen in the floor of the canal. This is the foramen of Huschke, which may be present throughout life.

The tympanic membrane

The tympanic membrane has three layers: (1) an outer epithelial layer, from the ectoderm of the visceral cleft; (2) a middle fibrous layer, from the mesoderm between the first visceral cleft and the tubotympanic recess; (3) an inner mucosal layer, from a part of the recess.

The middle-ear cleft

The middle-ear cleft is developed from the entoderm of the tubotympanic recess, which is pushed out from the first pharyngeal pouch to approach the surface between the first and second visceral arches (*Figure 1.38*).

Towards the end of the second fetal month, the eustachian tube is clearly seen as a relatively direct extension from the primitive pharynx, but at this stage the middle ear is only a potential cavity, being solidly filled with mesenchyme in which the ossicles are embedded. The mastoid antrum appears during the sixth or seventh month, as a dorsal expansion of the middle-ear cavity, but the mastoid air-cells do not begin to form until the end of fetal life.

The ossicles may all be defined in the eighth fetal week, embedded in a solid mesenchyme.

In the embryo of six weeks, there appears in the region of the lower jaw a sizeable bar of cartilage which extends superolaterally to the region of the ear. This is Meckel's cartilage, which is formed from the mesoderm of the first visceral arch (*Figure 1.39*). At

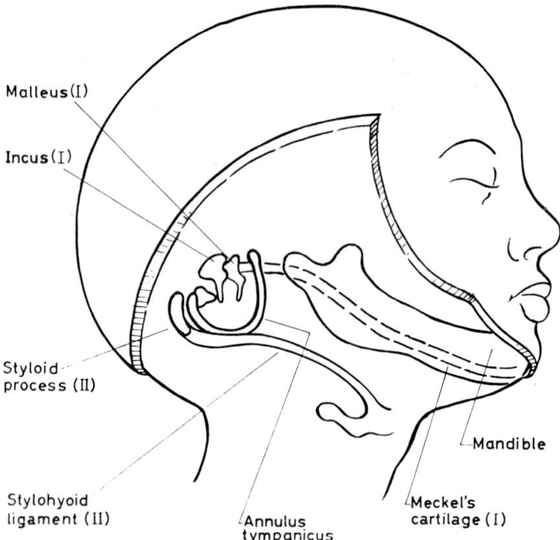

Figure 1.39 Development of the ossicles

its aural end it bears two swellings, one of which is conventionally thought to form the malleus, the other the incus. Broman states that, even at this early date, the malleo-incudal joint is present. Hough (1964), on the other hand, believes that the malleus and incus arise from separate specific mesenchymal cells and not from Meckel's cartilage.

The hyoid bar is formed in the mesoderm of the second visceral arch and from it come the head, neck and crura of the stapes; the styloid process; and the stylohyoid ligament. Hanson, Anson and Bast (1959) believe that a part of the long process of the incus as well as the greater part of the stapes is developed from second arch tissue, and this view is in keeping with Alberti's work (1964) on the blood supply of these areas (*see* p. 18).

Cauldwell and Anson (1942) stated that the stapes is derived from two sources, the footplate coming in part from the otic capsule (*see* p. 63). This occurs as early as the third month. By the end of this month, the stapes assumes its definitive form and by this time the annular ligament has formed. On the basis of meticulous reconstructions, Bast and Anson (1949) consider that the footplate of the stapes is derived either exclusively from the lateral wall of the otic capsule or from a dual origin, in part from the capsule and in part from the second arch cartilage (Bowden, 1977). In the light of surgical experience with congenital ossicular lesions, Pracy (1977) favours the view that the footplate is composed of two layers, an inner endosteal 'wafer' and an outer second arch 'wafer'.

By the end of the fifth month a thin layer of perichondrium exists between the footplate of the stapes and the labyrinth. The ultimate size of the stapes is attained at the end of the seventh fetal month (Broman).

Development of the mucosal folds

Between the third and seventh fetal months, the gelatinous tissue of the middle-ear cleft is gradually absorbed. At the same time the primitive tympanic cavity develops by the growth, into the cleft, of an endodermal-lined fluid pouch extending from the eustachian tube. Four primary sacs then bud out (*Figure 1.40*). They are the saccus anticus, the saccus medius, the saccus superior and the saccus posterior.

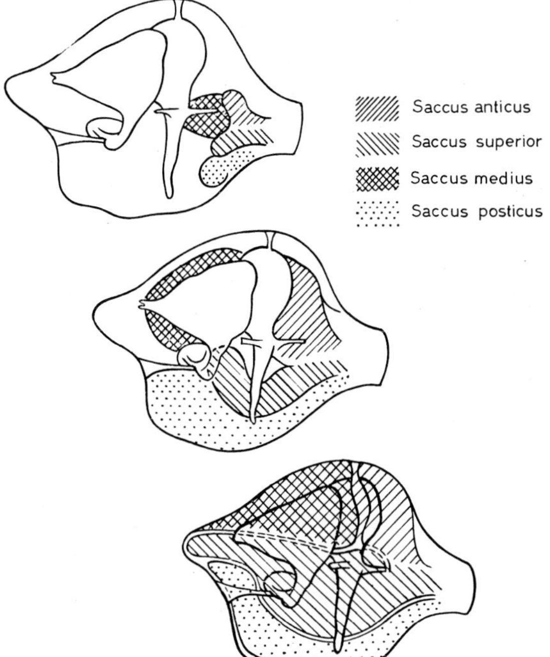

Figure 1.40 Development of the mucosal folds of the middle ear (after Proctor)

Where these pouches contact each other, mucosal folds are formed. Between the mucosal layers of the folds are remnants of the mesoderm, including the blood vessels which supply the 'viscera' of the tympanic cavity.

The saccus anticus, the smallest, forms the anterior pouch of von Tröltsch.

The saccus medius forms the attic. It breaks up into three saccules – anterior, medial and posterior. The posterior saccule eventually pneumatizes that portion of the mastoid air-cell system which is derived from the pars petrosa of the temporal bone.

The saccus superior forms the posterior pouch of von Tröltsch and the inferior incudal space. Eventually it pneumatizes that portion of the mastoid which is derived from the pars squamosa.

The saccus posticus extends along the hypotympanum to form the round window niche, the sinus tympani and the greater portion of the oval window niche.

The temporal bone

The temporal bone is derived from four distinct morphological elements: the os tympanicum; the styloid process; the squama; and the petromastoid (*Figure 1.41*).

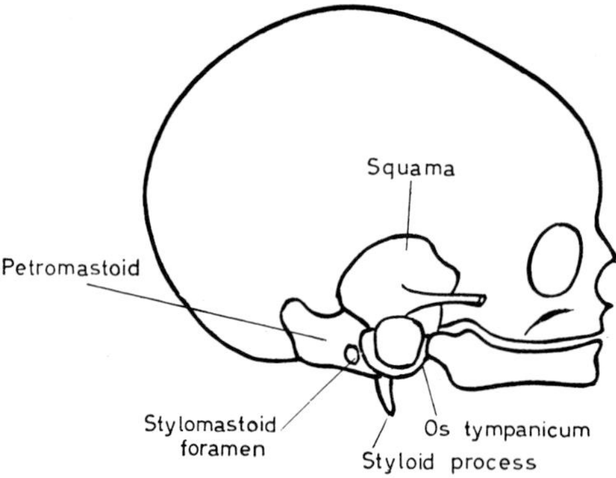

Figure 1.41 Development of the temporal bone

The os tympanicum and its subsequent fate have been described with the development of the external auditory canal. The styloid process is developed from the cranial end of the cartilage of the second visceral arch.

The squama is ossified in membrane and is developed to help in the protection of the brain. The postero-inferior portion of the squama grows downwards behind the tympanic ring to form the lateral wall of the mastoid antrum. The petromastoid is pre-formed in cartilage as a protective capsule for the membranous labyrinth.

The tubotympanic recess lies at first on the inferolateral aspect of the petrosa, but as the latter enlarges, the recess comes to lie anterolaterally. A cartilaginous flange grows downwards and outwards from the lateral part of the petrosa across the recess and above Meckel's cartilage, to form the tegmen tympani. This process also grows downwards to form the lateral wall of the eustachian tube. In this way the tympanic cavity and proximal part of the tube are included in the petrous portion of the temporal bone.

A second flange grows outwards below the recess to form the jugular plate.

The petrous of the adult is frequently spoken of as the petrous pyramid but it never truly develops the shape of a perfect pyramid, and the apex may be defined as that portion of the petrosa anteromedial to the cochlea. According to Profant (1931), the apex does not develop before the seventh fetal month.

At birth, the annulus tympanicus is beneath the skull, lying in an almost horizontal plane. By the third month of infancy, as a result of the upward and lateral rotation of the petrous bone, it appears on the inferolateral aspect of the skull. It is this somewhat horizontal position of the tympanic membrane in early infancy that makes paracentesis a difficult and hazardous procedure for the uninitiated. Gradually the annulus assumes its verticolateral position.

The mastoid portion of the temporal bone is at first flat, and the stylomastoid foramen, through which the facial nerve emerges, lies immediately behind the tympanic ring. As air-cells develop, the lateral part of the mastoid portion grows downwards and forwards to form the mastoid process. Hence the stylomastoid foramen comes to lie on the under-surface of the bone. This descent is accompanied by an increase in the length of the facial nerve canal. The mastoid process does not form a definite elevation until the end of the second year of life.

The mastoid process begins to develop during the second year of life, by downward extension of the squamous portion to conceal partially the petrous portion, and of the petrous portion to form the mastoid tip.

These two parts of the mastoid process may fuse imperfectly, leaving a more or less distinct petrosquamous suture line in the lateral surface.

Within the mastoid process cells grow from the antrum, which is well defined and pneumatized by the seventh month, to the mastoid tip; and laterally and radially in the squamous portion. A well-marked septum, known as Körner's septum, may persist between the cell tracts. This septum is a remnant of the petro-squamous suture, and the surgeon may fail to discover the deeper system of cells in the petrous portion of the mastoid process if he is misled by this septum.

As the process develops, the thin incomplete ring of the infant's tympanic portion grows laterally and inferiorly to form the osseous external auditory canal, with two suture lines: (i) a well-marked deep tympano-squamous suture in the antero-superior meatal wall; and (ii) a shallower, less distinct tympanomastoid suture in the posterior meatal wall (*see* p. 3).

The lateral growth of the tympanic portion and mastoid process causes the lateral surface of the temporal bone to assume a vertical position in the adult.

At the same time, the stylomastoid foramen and facial nerve come to lie quite deeply at the lateral surface of the mastoid process, well protected from the usual vertical post-aural incision.

Since there is no mastoid process at birth, the facial nerve in the infant emerges from the stylomastoid foramen on to the lateral surface of the skull where it can be cut by the usual vertical post-aural incision; therefore, an incision for a post-aural subperiosteal abscess in an infant must be made in a more horizontal plane. The mastoid antrum lies above the tympanic ring in the infant, about 2 mm deep to the bony surface.

The inner ear

The inner ear is developed from ectoderm in the region of the hindbrain. A thickening of the ectoderm, the auditory (otic) placode, becomes invaginated to form the auditory (otic) vesicle (*Figure 1.42*).

This is detached from the surface and, carrying a layer of mesoderm around it, it sinks into the mass of mesoderm which is the rudiment of the petrous bone. As it sinks into the petrous mass, the vesicle draws a tail behind it which is the rudiment of the ductus endolymphaticus. The saccus endolymphaticus develops as an expansion of the distal end of the ductus endolymphaticus.

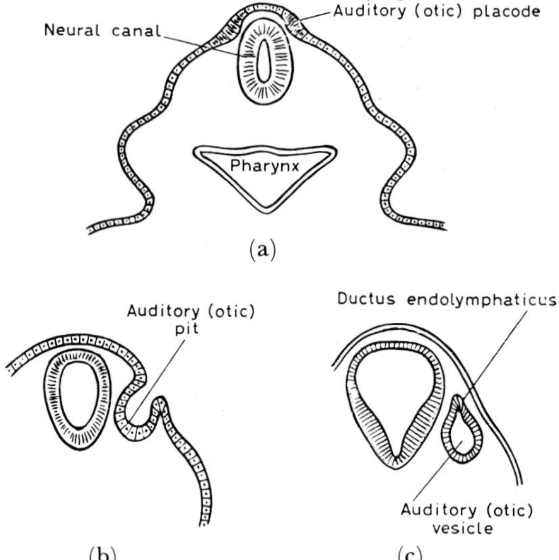

Figure 1.42 Development of the inner ear

The membranous labyrinth is formed from the otic vesicle (*Figure 1.43*) and it is the first part of the ear mechanism to make its appearance (Gray). By the sixth week of embryonic life, the three semicircular canals are well-formed, the ampullated expansions being clearly defined and the crus commune established.

At this stage, the dependent portion of the vesicle has not only elongated as the cochlear pouch, but has begun to assume its snail-shell coil.

At the end of the first month, the human inner ear exhibits only an endolymphatic space. The perilymphatic spaces have not yet developed although the end-organs are beginning to differentiate.

The first perilymphatic space to form is that just within the oval window, in the vestibule, the cisterna perilymphatica. In the human embryo, this occurs in the latter

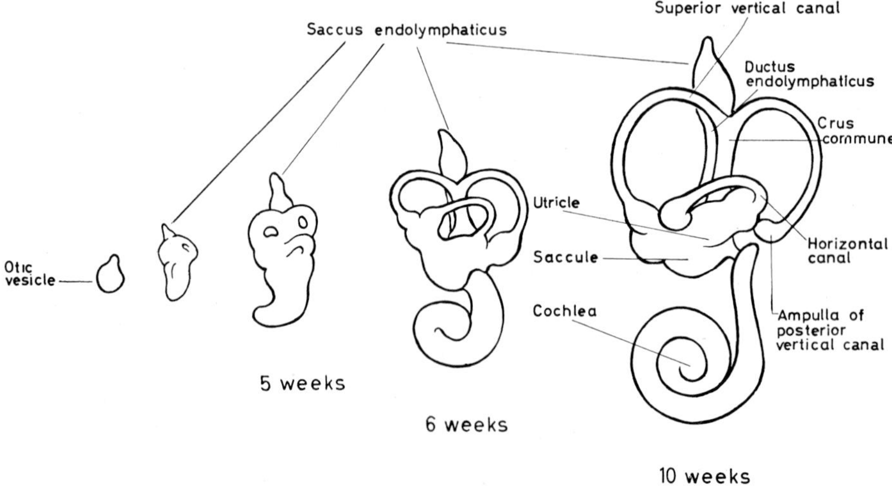

Figure 1.43 Development of the membranous labyrinth

part of the third fetal month and it is done by a process of 'dedifferentiation of tissue' (Streeter, 1918, 1922).

The second perilymphatic space begins to form just within the round window. This is the scala tympani.

Following the appearance of this scala, the scala vestibuli forms as an extension of the cisterna perilymphatica in the basal portion of the cochlea.

The aqueductus cochleae develops relatively late as an 'out-pouching' from the subarachnoid spaces (along the glossopharyngeal nerve, towards the scala tympani).

The neuro-epithelial structures of the membranous labyrinth are basically similar in type, but they become modified in form in accordance with their final respective functions. Each of the sensory end-organs consists of hair-cells, supporting cells and an overlying gelatinous substance in which the hairs are embedded. They are the maculae of the utricle and saccule, the ampullary cristae of the semicircular canals, and the organ of Corti.

The formation of the vestibular end-organs advances more rapidly than that of the cochlear end-organs, hairs or vibrissae appearing sooner on the vestibular end-organ than on the cochlear end-organ.

The maculae develop from the utricular and saccular epithelia at the points where the nerves enter their walls. This begins at the seventh week, and by the twelfth week the hair-cells and supporting cells can be differentiated. Between the fourteenth and sixteenth weeks, otoconia have appeared in the gelatinous layer.

The ampullary cristae also form at the points where the nerve fibres enter the ampullae of the semicircular canals. They begin to develop at the same time as the maculae but, instead of remaining flat, they become elevated into a ridge covered by a gelatinous cupula.

The epithelium of the cochlear duct begins to differentiate in the basal turn at about eight weeks, and is followed by the middle and apical turns. The organ of Corti and tectorial membrane are recognizable in the basal turns by the twelfth week, and at four months the cochlea is almost in its adult form. Alexander (1917) showed the organ of Corti formed by the fifth fetal month of human life.

The hair-cells and supporting cells of the organ of Corti can be differentiated by the twelfth week, and the gelatinous tectorial membrane is seen to lie on their free surface. The tunnel of Corti can be recognized by the fifteenth week.

'The inner ear is the only organ that reaches full adult size and complete differentiation by mid-term, even before the tiny fetus has become a viable premature infant' (Shambaugh, 1959, after Anson and Bast). But 'The more recently-acquired cochlear end-organ not only is the last in the labyrinth to differentiate, but also is less stable (and more subject to developmental anomalies and acquired disease) than the older vestibular region'.

The otic capsule

The otic capsule develops in the mesoderm which surrounds the membranous labyrinth. The mesoderm changes to 'precartilage' and later to true cartilage, and at the end of the second fetal month, the membranous labyrinth is embedded in a cartilaginous ear capsule. This in turn becomes dedifferentiated, and in the fifth fetal month ossification of the otic capsule occurs by a process of incrustation (Bast, 1930)

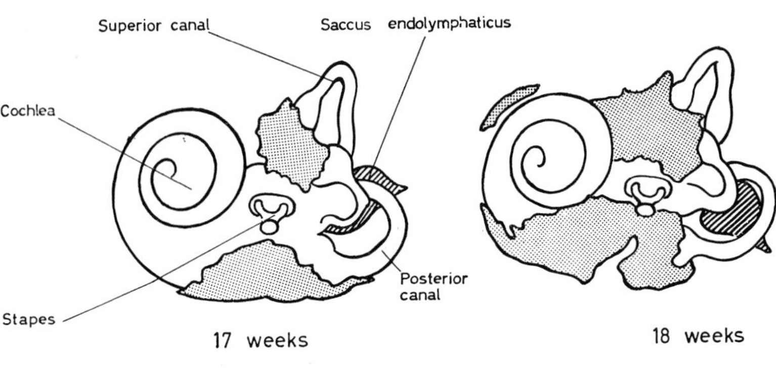

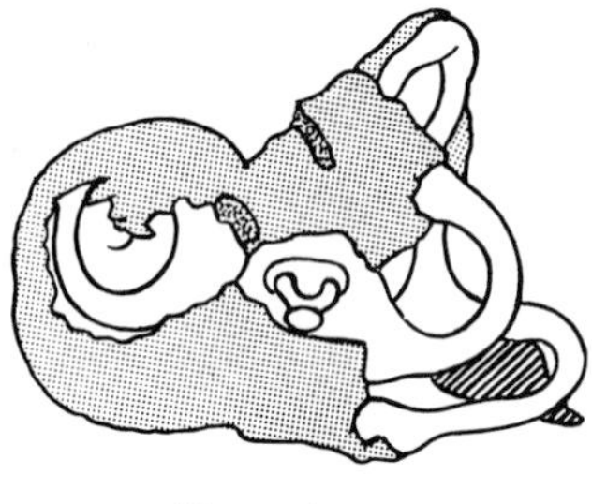

Figure 1.44 Ossification of the otic capsule (after Bast)

(*Figure 1.44*). From this time onwards, the otic capsule is known as the *petrosa*, forming one of the four component parts of the temporal bone.

The petrosa gradually becomes encased with dermal or membranous bone so that at birth three distinct layers of bone are discernible: an outer layer of periosteal bone (which is lamellar in type), presenting all the usual characteristics of bone elsewhere in the body; an inner layer of endosteal bone (also of lamellar type), lining the contours of the labyrinth and relatively thin; and, between these two, and peculiar to this region in the adult, enchondral bone, which is characterized by the presence of so-called 'cartilage rest' cells, or globuli interossei.

The fissula ante fenestram consists of an irregular ribbon of connective tissue that extends through the bony otic capsule from the vestibule (just anterior to the oval window) to the tympanic cavity (near the processus cochleariformis) (Shambaugh, 1959).

The auditory nerve

The rudiment of the eighth cranial nerve appears in the fourth week as the auditory ganglion, which lies between the auditory vesicle and the wall of the hindbrain. At first it is fused with the ganglion of the seventh cranial nerve (acousticofacial ganglion) but later the two separate. The cells of the ganglion are mainly derived from those of the neural crest but probably some come from the neurectoderm of the auditory vesicle. The auditory ganglion divides into a vestibular and a cochlear part, each associated with the corresponding division of the eighth cranial nerve.

By the seventh week, the cochlear nerve is laid down and has its main characteristics, including its twisting fibres; the spiral ganglion is recognized at the eighth week, and the spiral ganglion and cochlear nerve have linked up with their sensory end-organ by the twelfth week.

References

Alberti, P. W. R. M. (1963). *Laryngoscope*, **73**, 605

Alberti, P. W. R. M. (1964). *Journal of Laryngology*, **78**, 808

Albrecht, W. (1930). *Acta otolaryngologica*, **14**, 221

Alexander, G. (1917). *Diseases of the Ear in Childhood*, 2nd edn. Philadelphia; Lippincott

Axelsson, A. (1968). *Acta otolaryngologica*, Suppl. 243

Ballantyne, J. C. and Engström, H. (1969). *Journal of Laryngology*, **83**, 19

Bast, T. H. (1930). *Contributive Embryology*, **21**, 53

Bast, T. H. and Anson, B. J. (1949). *The Temporal Bone and the Ear*. Springfield, Ill.; Thomas

Blunt, M. J. (1954). *Journal of Anatomy*, **88**, 520

Bowden, Ruth E. M. (1977). *Proceedings of the Royal Society of Medicine*, **70**, 807

Cauldwell, E. W. and Anson, B. J. (1942). *Archives of Otolaryngology*, **36**, 891

Compere, W. E. Jnr. (1958). *Transactions of the American Academy of Ophthalmology and Otolaryngology*, **62**, 444

Compere, W. E. Jnr. (1964). *Journal of Laryngology*, **78**, 649

Cunningham's Manual of Practical Anatomy (1959). Ed. by J. C. Brash, 12th edn. Vol. III. London; Oxford University Press

Diamant, M. and Dahlberg, C. (1945). *Hereditas*, **31**, 520

Diamant, M. and Dahlberg, C. (1952). *Practical Oto-rhinolaryngology* (Suppl. 1), **14**, 1

Eggston, A. A. and Wolff, D. (1947). *Histopathology of the Ear, Nose and Throat*. Baltimore; Williams and Wilkins

Engström, H. (1960). *Acta Morphologica Neerl-Scandinavica*, **3**, 195

Flock, A. and Wersäll, J. (1963). *Journal of Ultrastructural Research*, **8**, 193

Gray's Anatomy (1958). Ed. by T. B. Johnston, D. V. Davies and F. Davies, 32nd edn. London; Longmans

Hamilton, W. J. and Harrison, R. J. (1952). In *Diseases of the Ear, Nose and Throat*. Ed. by W. G. Scott-Brown, 1st edn. London; Butterworths

Hanson, J. R., Anson, B. J. and Bast, T. H. (1959). *Manchester Quarterly Bulletin, Northwest University Medical School*, **33**, 358

Hough, J. (1964). Summer Meeting, Section of Otology, *Royal Society of Medicine*, 26th June

Law, F. (1913). *Annals of Otology, Rhinology and Laryngology, St. Louis*, **22**, 635

Lim, D. (1976). *Laryngoscope*, **86**, 1164

Lindeman, H. (1969). *Advances in Anatomy, Embryology and Cell Biology*. New York; Springer-Verlag

Nager, G. T. and Nager, M. (1953). *Annals of Otology, Rhinology and Laryngology, St. Louis*, **62**, 923

Owen, G. R. (1951). *Transactions of the American Otological Society*, 189

Owen, G. R. and Compere, W. E. Jnr. (1959). In *Surgery of the Ear*. Ed. by G. E. Shambaugh, Jnr. Philadelphia; Saunders

Perry, Eldon T. (1957). *The Human Ear Canal*. Springfield, Ill.; Thomas

Pracy, R. (1977). *Proceedings of the Royal Society of Medicine*, **70**, 823

Proctor, B. (1964). *Journal of Laryngology*, **78**, 631

Profant, H. (1931). *Archives of Otolaryngology*, **13**, 347

Shambaugh, G. E. Jnr. (1959). *Surgery of the Ear*. Philadelphia; Saunders

Sheehy, J. L. and Patterson, M. E. (1967). *Laryngoscope*, **77**, 330

Smith, A. Brownlie (1958). *Journal of Laryngology*, **72**, 330

Smith, A. Brownlie (1962). *Journal of Laryngology*, **76**, 140, 403

Spoendlin, H. (1969). *Acta Otolaryngologica*, **67**, 239

Streeter, G. L. (1917). *American Journal of Anatomy*, **21**, 299

Streeter, G. L. (1918). *Contributive Embryology Carnegie Inst.*, **7**, 1

Streeter, G. L. (1922). *Contributive Embryology Carnegie Inst.*, **14**, 111

Tumarkin, A. I. (1959). *Journal of Laryngology*, **73**, 34

Witmaack, K. (1931). *Archives der Ohren, Nasen und Kehlk Heilkunde*, **129**, 207

2 Physiology of hearing

John Groves

Introduction

Whether or not man has a monopoly of language, his versatility in communication is pre-eminent, yet his ears are no more efficient than those of many lower species. In man it is by virtue of his intellectual capacity that hearing becomes the vital basis for the acquisition of speech and language, and these skills in their turn are the most important tools of constructive thought. For man, the ear is the main portal through which his mind and faculties are developed and trained. When we try to evaluate the significance of hearing we might also remember its place in art. Through this most exquisite of the senses men have created and developed the wordless language of music, which speaks directly to the intellectual, aesthetic, and emotional structure of human personality.

The actual experience of hearing, the appreciation of sound in all its qualities, is a function of the auditory areas of the temporal lobes of the brain. The use made by the animal of what it hears depends upon the development and training of the neighbouring psycho-auditory areas. In this field the term *psycho-acoustics* is sometimes used to embrace the study of what a person hears, what he can discriminate, how his hearing can be measured, and so on. It must be remembered that in these matters it is the overall functions of hearing which are under scrutiny – the performance of the whole auditory apparatus from the ear to the mind. The ear itself can be regarded as a device for detecting acoustical information, and for encoding this information for transmission by the auditory nerve. In traversing the central nervous system with its many synaptic connections, the coded acoustical information is processed, correlated with the pattern of impulses from the opposite ear, and finally presented to the cerebral cortex in a form which informs the hearer of pitch, loudness and location of the sound source.

An account is given of some of the salient facts of auditory physiology, not because a final coherent theory of hearing can be built upon them, but because they are facts which concern the otologist and which must all be given their proper place and value in future research and theories.

The physical nature of sound

Strictly speaking, sound is a sensation – a phenomenon existing only in the auditory perceptive apparatus of the hearer. The physicist, however, studies the external physical disturbances which can result in auditory stimulation. In this restricted sense the term 'sound' may properly be used, provided that whenever necessary the context is made to show that sound waves or energy, and not the sensation of sound, is under discussion. 'Acoustics' is definable as the study of sound, dealing with vibratory motion perceptible through the organ of hearing.

The external physical disturbances of sound have two essential vehicles, the *sound source* which liberates energy in a characteristic manner, and the *medium* through which the energy is transmitted to the hearer.

Sound sources

The human larynx, tuning forks and musical instruments, have in common the property of converting mechanical energy applied to them into a characteristic vibratory energy. This vibratory energy can travel as sound waves in any suitable medium. When a tuning fork is struck a quantity of energy is stored in it by the bending of its molecules, against the natural stiffness (elasticity) of the steel of which it is made. Almost instantly the prongs spring apart again with a momentum which carries the system beyond the resting point and bends the prongs of the fork in the opposite direction. At the limit of outward movement all momentum has been lost and the elasticity of the outwardly bent steel causes the prongs to swing towards each other again. This cycle is repeated again and again. The energy initially stored, however, is steadily dissipated as heat due to friction between the molecules of the fork and as sound energy imparted by the vibrating prongs to the surrounding air. The excursions of the prongs therefore decrease steadily in amplitude until eventually the fork comes to rest and is silent. Although the *amplitude* of vibration falls steadily from its initial maximum, the rate or *frequency* of the vibrations remains constant throughout and is expressed as the number of completed cycles (double vibrations)/s. This frequency is characteristic of the individual tuning fork, and is determined by its design. The factors influencing the frequency include the mass of the vibrating parts, and the elasticity (or stiffness) of the metal of which the fork is made. Tuning forks can be constructed to vibrate at frequencies ranging from 16 Hz to over 8000 Hz. Since the frequency of vibration determines the pitch, and doubling the pitch of a musical note raises it by exactly one octave, this range spans nine octaves.

Many of the percussion type of musical instruments function in a manner strictly similar to that of the tuning fork. In other percussion instruments, such as the drum with its stretched membrane, and the piano with stretched strings, the *linear* elasticity of the vibrator is utilized, and in these cases the frequency of vibration is determined by the mass, elasticity, length and degree of tightness or tension of the membrane or string.

The human vocal cords, closely applied to each other in phonation, represent another type of sound source. In this case a steady flow of expired air delivered through the glottis sets up a steady state of vibration in the free margins of the cords. The frequency is determined by the mass and elasticity of the vibrating parts and in this example also by the length and tension of the cords. The last two factors are variable and are controlled by the tonic contraction of the intrinsic laryngeal muscles. The vibrations of the cords impose themselves upon the expiratory air column so that at all levels above the glottis, through the pharynx and mouth, sound energy flows freely.

Similar mechanisms are utilized in the design of reed instruments such as the oboe (double reed), clarinet (single reed) and harmonica. Again we have elastic vibrators set in motion by a flow of air. In the brass instruments the principles are the same, the players' lips in controlled tension performing the vibratory function.

It should be noted at this stage in the discussion that, in contrast to the tuning fork and percussion instruments which commence vibration at a maximum amplitude and more or less rapidly subside to rest, the larynx and the wind instruments can maintain a steady amplitude which can continue indefinitely. The amplitude will depend on the velocity of the air current which actuates the vibratory elements, and can be varied at the will of the speaker or player.

A like contrast can be made between strings vibrating momentarily from being struck or plucked, and strings vibrating at sustained, controlled amplitude as when played upon with a bow.

All of the above examples are natural sound sources in that the characteristic sound patterns they liberate are created by them from the physical energy applied. The chief property of all natural sound sources is that in greater or lesser degree they are tuned by the relationships between their physical properties of mass (inertia) elasticity, length, tension and so on, so that when activated they will vibrate at a predetermined or *resonance* frequency.

Natural sources differ radically from reproducers such as loudspeakers or telephones. The latter are 'slave' devices driven by variations of electrical current and designed to vibrate as closely as possible in imitation of whatever variation of electrical current may be applied to them. Reproducers, therefore, have built-in detuning or *damping*, a physical concept which has great significance in the study of auditory physiology. Resonances in such follower or 'slave' devices should ideally be absent, or kept to low relative intensity levels, and if possible confined to frequencies outside the range of signal frequencies to be handled.

Media in sound transmission

A sound source vibrating in a complete vacuum cannot be heard. Sound energy can travel only by vibrations transmitted in a gaseous, liquid or solid medium. The physical changes occurring in the medium are summarized as an alternating condensation and rarefaction of its constituent molecules impressed upon them by the vibrating sound source and following faithfully its frequency and amplitude. The vibratory pattern of changes in the medium travels as a sound wave with diminishing amplitude until, eventually, through dissipation as heat, the energy can carry no further and silence reigns. Whatever the nature of the sound, and whatever the medium may be, it is the *energy* which flows through the medium, while the molecules of the medium itself, oscillating back and forth in alternating condensation and rarefaction, retain their overall position in space unchanged.

The important physical attributes of a sound-transmitting medium are its density

(D) and its elasticity (E). The velocity at which a sound wave travels is proportional to the square root of the ratio between elasticity and density $\left(\text{velocity} \propto \sqrt{\frac{E}{D}}\right)$. It will be obvious, therefore, that the speed of sound must differ very greatly as between one medium and another, and under varying conditions of temperature and barometric pressure. The speed of sound in air at sea level is about 330 m/s or 1120 km/h. (Note: higher speeds are *supersonic*. The term *ultrasonic* refers to vibratory energy with a frequency higher than the audible range. The terms are sometimes, unfortunately, confused.)

Sound waves

While it is essential always to retain a clear mental picture of the propagation of sound energy from molecule to molecule in periodic vibration along the axis of propagation, it is also essential to understand how this form of energy flow can be graphically represented in the conventional wave diagram used by physicists.

The simplest type of sound wave is that which consists of only one frequency and which is constant in amplitude. If a graph is plotted to indicate the displacement of a single vibrating particle in the sound medium from its normal resting position, against the time axis, we obtain a curve commencing at zero at the beginning of the cycle. During the first half of the cycle the particle is displaced to a maximum in one direction, and then returns to the resting position. During the second half of the cycle the particle continues to move, past the zero point, and swings to a maximum in the opposite direction. As the cycle is completed the particle returns to its starting point, zero. Its successive displacements, measured and plotted with respect to time, have drawn for us a sine wave, a representation of a pure tone (a sound consisting of only one given frequency). Mathematicians call this a sine wave because it is the curve

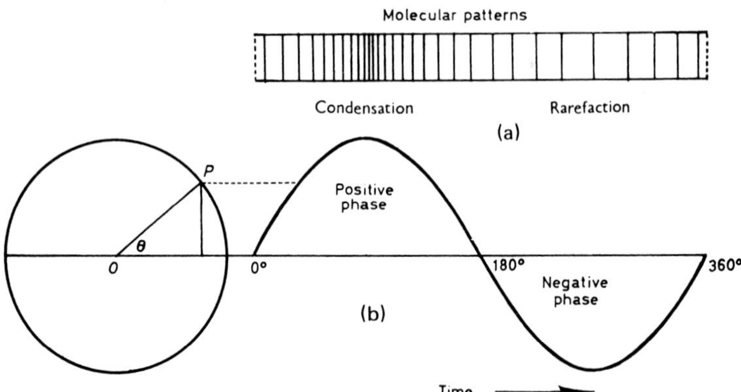

Figure 2.1 Basic concept of a sinusoidal sound wave: (a) the longitudinal condensation-rarefaction sequence in the molecules at a given point in a sound-conducting medium during a complete cycle; (b) the derivation of the sine wave as a projection of the angular displacement with respect to time of the point P moving at constant velocity in a circle. The form of the curve is a function of sin θ (or cos θ)

obtained when the sine (or cosine) of the angular displacement of a point moving in a circle at uniform velocity is plotted graphically with respect to time (*Figure 2.1*). This mathematical point must be made in order to show the meaning of the expression *phase angle*. Any given moment during the cycle of vibration can be identified by reference to its projection upon the circle diagram. Thus at zero time (commencement of the cycle) the phase angle is zero. At maximum positive (peak) displacement of the particle the phase angle is 90 degrees. As displacement passes through zero towards negative values the phase angle is 180 degrees and at maximum negative displacement it is 270 degrees. Finally, at completion of the cycle the phase angle is 360 degrees.

Two or more sound waves are said to be *in phase* if, at a given point in space, their phase angle is the same. Their peaks and troughs are additive and the amplitude of vibration is equal to the sum of the amplitudes of the individual waves. Sound waves are in opposite phase if their phase angles differ by 180 degrees. In this condition the peaks and troughs cancel each other, and the sound waves are abolished. For all other phase angle differences the resultant of two sound waves will be an algebraic summation at a level somewhere between the 'in' and 'opposite' extremes just described.

Dimensions of sound energy

Frequency

This has already been defined as the number of complete vibrations or cycles/s (Hz). It confers upon a sound its apparent musical *pitch*. In most conditions pitch and frequency have a constant and predictable relationship, but we shall see later that pitch can appear to alter with high levels of sound intensity even though the frequency remains unchanged. The audible range of frequency extends in humans from 16 to about 20 000 Hz. Vibrations at lower frequencies than the audible range are called *subsonic*, and those above the audible range are classed as *ultrasonic*.

Wavelength

As with all forms of wave motion, wavelength is measured from the commencement of one cycle to the commencement of the next. Wavelength and frequency are simply related, by the formula:

$$\underset{\text{(Hz)}}{\text{frequency}} = \frac{\text{velocity (cm/s)}}{\text{wavelength (cm)}}$$

The velocity (and therefore the wavelength) depend (see above) on the particular medium under consideration. In air the wavelength of a sound wave will be about 10.5 m for a frequency of 32 Hz. Sounds of higher frequency have progressively shorter wavelengths, for example 32.5 cm for 1000 Hz and 2.5 cm for 13 000 Hz.

Intensity

Although apparent loudness depends on the intensity of a sound the terms represent different phenomena. Intensity is the quantitative objective measure of sound energy. In a given medium it will be proportional to the amplitude and frequency of the waves, or to the velocity of the individual particles as they vibrate back and forth, or to the pressure exerted by the particles upon neighbouring objects, or to the rate of energy flow in ergs/s, that is, watts. These various modes of expressing the intensity of a sound each have their particular uses, and they can be expressed as peak (or maximum) values measured instantaneously at their maxima during the cycle. More usually they are expressed as 'root mean square' (rms) values, a mathematical way of stating 'average' energy for each completed cycle. Thus sound intensity can be expressed, as is usual in clinical work, as *sound pressure*, in dynes/cm^2 (peak or rms), or as *particle velocity*, in cm/s (peak or rms), or as *power*, in watts.

Sound ratios

Because the sounds in which we are interested biologically range over such a vast span it is not always convenient to express sound intensity in the absolute terms defined above. Instead, a logarithmic scale is used, and this has the additional advantage of conforming to the proportional scales of increment which are most clearly apparent to the ear as equivalent changes in loudness. Just as the ear detects pitch as a doubling of frequency for each octave up the scale (a logarithmic function) so it estimates loudness increments on a logarithmic basis.

The sound intensity to be defined is expressed as the logarithm of the ratio between it and another reference sound intensity. The figure thus obtained is the ratio between the two sounds in bels. A more convenient unit for most purposes is the decibel and the formula becomes:

$$\text{dB} = 10 \log \frac{J_1}{J_2}$$

where J_1, J_2, are the intensities (in watts) of the two sounds, or

$$\text{dB} = 20 \log \frac{P_1}{P_2}$$

where P_1, P_2, are the pressures of the two sounds (in dynes/cm^2).

We are able to express in decibels the ratio between the intensities of widely different sound levels with great convenience and clarity. Thus a sound level ten times greater than the reference level is 10 dB greater. A ratio of 100 times is represented by 20 dB, 1000 by 30 dB, and so on through the scale. A ratio of one million times is 60 dB, and 130 dB indicates a ratio of 10 to the thirteenth power.

Any two sounds can be compared in intensity on the decibel scale – for example, the signal-to-noise ratio for an electronic amplifier may be specified as being 'not less than 70 dB'. This means that the ratio of the desired amplified signal to unwanted spurious electronic 'noise' in the output of the instrument is not less than 10 000 000:1.

If desired, a specified reference sound level can be used to which all other sound levels can be related. A commonly used reference level is that of 0.0002 dynes/cm^2, an intensity which is very close to the normal threshold of hearing of the human ear at 1 000 Hz.

Propagation of sound waves

From a point source sound waves radiate in a spherical manner equal in intensity in every direction. They obey the inverse square law in that the intensity at any point is inversely proportional to the square of the distance from the sound source. These conditions obtain only in a so-called *free field*, that is, one in which there are no physical boundaries to the medium in which the sound energy is travelling.

If the medium is bounded in any way a great variety of effects are produced according to the ways in which the sound waves are reflected, absorbed and diffracted (scattered). A wave-front which strikes a soft irregular surface will be largely absorbed and dissipated, while hard dense surfaces reflect sound waves very readily. These properties are freely manipulated in the acoustical treatment of rooms and halls, to control or eliminate echoes and reverberation, and to achieve an optimum spread of undistorted sound to all parts of an auditorium.

It is of more than passing interest to otologists to consider the effect caused by an obstruction in the path of a sound wave-front. Sounds of low frequency having wavelengths far greater than the physical dimensions of the obstruction are hardly affected and the wave-front reforms perfectly beyond the obstacle. High-frequency sounds, however, behave differently. Beyond the obstacle the broken wave-front does not reform and a sound 'shadow' is cast. As will be shown later such effects are important in connection with binaural ability to localize sound sources.

In an enclosed space interaction between an incident sound wave and its own reflection can result in so-called *standing waves*. In these conditions tests of hearing, for example with the live voice, can be misleading, because sound intensity will be maximal at each antinode of the standing wave, and negligible near each node.

Sound at an interface between media

As mentioned above, a sound wave, on arriving at the boundary of its supporting medium, may be reflected or absorbed by the material of which the boundary is constructed. For example, if the medium is air and the boundary is water, 99.9 per cent of the sound energy is reflected. This effect is governed by the specific acoustic resistances of the medium and the boundary. If the values for these factors are known for both air and water the ratio of sound energy reflected to sound energy absorbed can be calculated*.

When the values of acoustic resistance (or impedance) of two media, such as air and water, are widely different, as in the example given above, we speak of *impedance mismatching*, and most of the sound energy is reflected. When the impedances are similar, or approximated by an intervening mechanical device, we speak of *impedance matching*, and a high proportion of sound is absorbed at the interface and propagated in the new medium.

The concept of acoustic impedance need not be limited to simple homogeneous media. Any mechanical system capable of periodic vibration has an acoustic impedance which can be calculated from a knowledge of its physical dimensions of mass, elasticity and frictional resistance to vibration†. Similarly, a cavity, whether it contains air or liquid, has an acoustic impedance value which can be measured, or can be calculated from its dimensions, shape, volume, etc., and indicates in what ratio sound energy will be accepted by it from an adjacent specified medium. Alteration of any of the relevant physical characteristics of a vibrating system will change its impedance. If matching between two systems is thereby improved, sound transmission is increased, while if mismatching results, sound transmission will be impaired.

Changes in the mass of a vibrating sound system alter the transmission of high frequencies more than low ones, while changes in stiffness have their greatest effects in the lower frequency range. *Figure 2.2* shows how stiffness, mass and friction may be correlated in their effects upon the overall impedance of the ear. Changes in mass or

*The *specific acoustic resistance of air*,

$$R_1 = \sqrt{(d \times S)} = 41.5 \text{ ohms/cm}^2$$

where d is the density and S the bulk modulus of elasticity of air.

Calculated from the same formula, the *specific acoustic resistance of sea water*, R_2, is 161 000 ohms/cm^2. The ratio, r, between the two acoustic resistances $= \frac{R_1}{R_2} = \frac{161\ 000}{41.5} = 3880$ is substituted in the following formula for the actual energy *transmission* ratio, T.

$$T = \frac{4r}{(r+1)^2} = 0.001$$

This result tells us that 0.1 per cent of sound energy will continue in the new medium, water, while 99.9 per cent is reflected. The ratio is 1000:1, or 30 dB. This is close to the value found experimentally for the transmission loss in the ear if the middle-ear transformer mechanism is destroyed.

†The acoustic impedance of a vibrating system having mass, stiffness (elasticity) and frictional resistance is calculated from the formula:

$$I = \sqrt{\left(r^2 \times \left(mf - \frac{s}{f}\right)^2\right)}$$

where I is the impedance, r the frictional resistance, m the mass, s the stiffness and f the frequency.

From this it is evident that high values for f will exaggerate the effect of changes in mass, while low frequency values will emphasize the effect of changes in stiffness. Changes in r (frictional resistance) are not frequency dependent. Johansen (1948) gives a most lucid account of some otological applications of these principles.

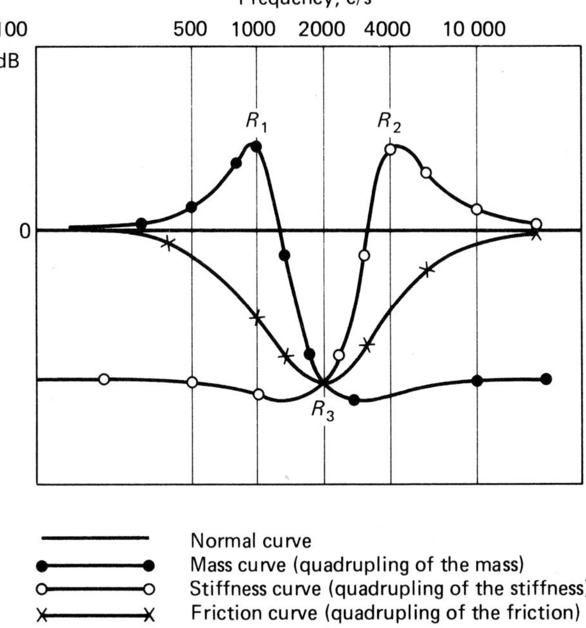

Figure 2.2 Theoretical (calculated) threshold value curves for the ear (after Johansen, 1948). The horizontal line represents normal hearing threshold. Quadrupling the mass of the vibrating parts gives the *mass* curve, with impaired transmission for higher frequencies and the resonance point R_1 shifted towards the base. Quadrupling the stiffness gives the *stiffness* curve with impaired transmission for lower frequencies, and the resonance R_2 shifted towards the treble. Quadrupling the friction has equal effects on bass and treble frequencies on either side of the resonance point R_3.

stiffness also impose alterations in phase upon the signal being conducted in an acoustical system.

Complex sounds

In his everyday work with sound the otologist must beware of the notion of sine waves or pure tones. In nature they hardly exist, and they are very difficult to produce artificially, completely free from harmonic distortion and 'electronic noise'. Furthermore, it is the everyday complex sounds which patients want to hear.

Harmonics

The individual tone quality of a musical instrument, which distinguishes it from pure-tone generators (audiometer, tuning fork) depends upon the mixture of overtones or harmonics with the fundamental frequency. For example, the violin produces a different pattern from the mouth-organ, both as to the number and intensity of the harmonics generated. These overtones have frequencies which represent simple multiples or ratios of the fundamental frequency and the many different sine waves present are summated algebraically into an elaborate wave-form (*Figure 2.3*).

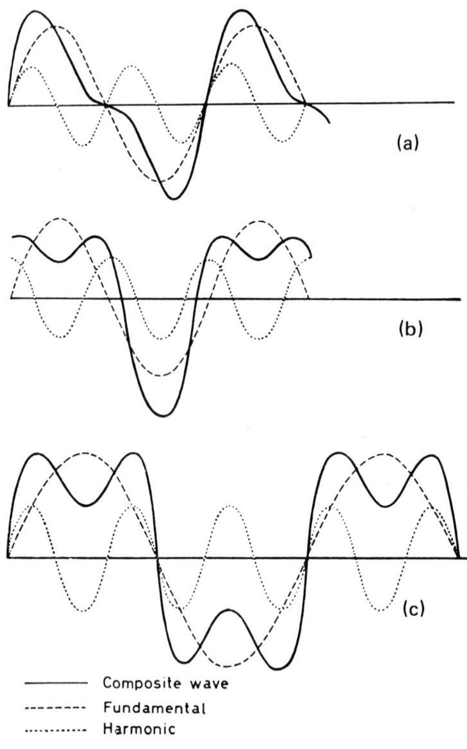

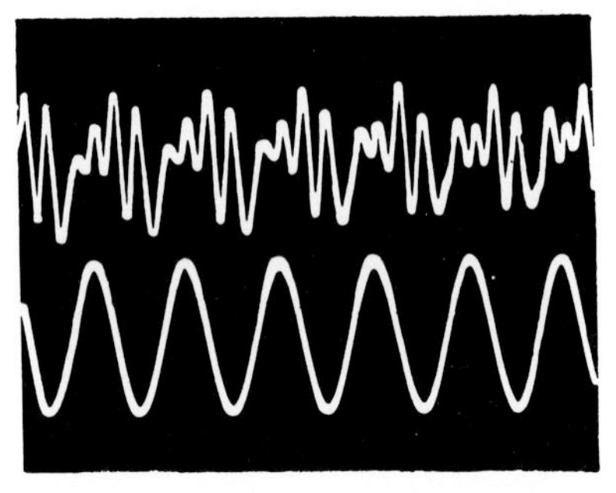

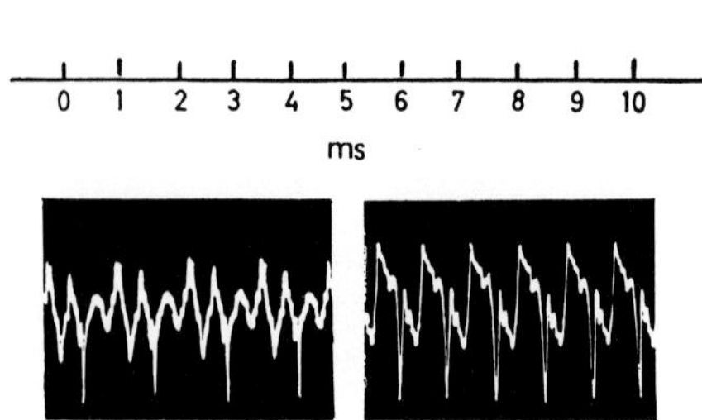

Figure 2.3 The synthesis of compound sound waves from their constituent sine waves.

(a) Fundamental tone with second harmonic of half amplitude.

(b) Fundamental tone with second harmonic, but in different phase.

(c) Fundamental tone with third harmonic at half amplitude.

((a), (b) and (c) reproduced from Wilson, 1957, *The Gramophone Handbook*, by courtesy of Methuen)

(d) Oscillogram of violin note with pure tone below for comparison (600 Hz).

(e) Oscillogram of harmonica. This is rich in tone colour and varies quite a lot according to the frequency played.

((d) and (e) reproduced by courtesy of Wharfedale Wireless Works Ltd. and Mr. G. A. Briggs)

Harmonic distortion is the spurious generation of *unwanted* multiples or sub-multiples of the fundamental. It occurs in electronic and acoustical devices, and these require careful design to keep such distortion within acceptable limits. The normal ear has this defect also, as is shown later.

Noise

In the realms of physics noise is not necessarily a loud sound or a sound which annoys the hearer. Rather it is defined as superfluous, unwanted or random sound energy, unrelated to the sounds being measured, amplified or otherwise studied. Noise is usually (but not necessarily) an aperiodic sequence of vibrations. A 50 Hz 'hum' due to alternating current electricity mains supply, and the high-pitched hiss due to thermal agitation of the molecules in an electrical resistor, are examples of electronic noise. It is possible electronically to produce sound which contains all the frequencies from the lowest to the highest limits of audibility. By analogy with white light this is known as 'white' noise.

Transients

So far we have considered mainly sounds of sustained intensity, but a large part of our auditory experience comprises brief, sudden, complex noises known as 'transients'. Obvious examples are the percussion instruments (drums, cymbals) but speech is full of these components, and so is everyday domestic life; *Figure 2.4* shows wave-forms of some of these sounds. It should be noted how great is the initial amplitude and how rapidly the sound decays. In experimental work with the ear isolated click sounds produced by the discharge of an electrical condenser are widely used.

Speech

Obviously speech is the most complex and vital of all sounds, including a great number of different harmonics, transients and noises. It is analysed in detail elsewhere, and is not discussed further here.

Beats

When two tones of dissimilar frequencies are sounded simultaneously their sound pressures are additive whenever the wave-peaks coincide. This condition occurs with a frequency equal to the difference in frequency between the two tones. Thus a 50 cycle beat results with tones of 250 and 300 Hz. The beat effect is clearly audible at slower rates, such as will result when the tones differ only by a few Hz.

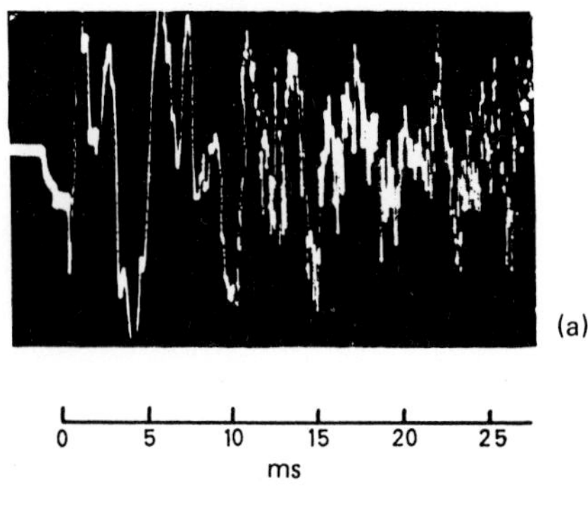

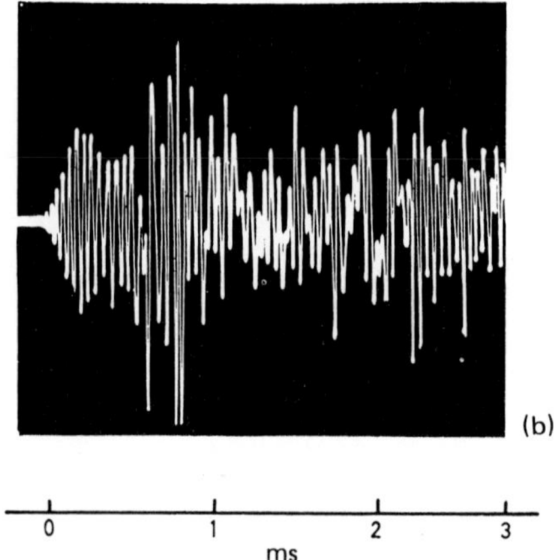

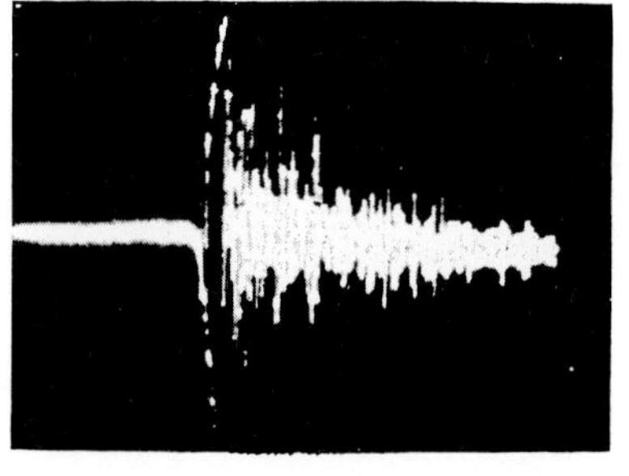

Figure 2.4 Oscillograms of some familiar transients. (Reproduced by courtesy of Wharfedale Wireless Works Ltd. and Mr. G. A. Briggs.) (a) Snare drum. The transient attack here is very sharp. The uneven wave-form shows that this is a noise rather than a musical note. (b) Cymbal. The harmonics here go as high as 25 000 Hz and the starting transients are very sudden and clear. (c) Handclap. This is obviously a noise with rapid starting and decay transients

Fourrier's analysis

The apparent chaos of the world of sound wave-forms resolves itself most beautifully into the orderliness of the perfect sine wave. Fourrier showed mathematically that any wave-form, however complex, can be analysed and broken down into a number of constituent sine waves each with a definite frequency and amplitude. It has usually been assumed that such a frequency analysis is performed in the inner ear, but recent researches suggest that other mechanisms operate for the perception of transients and complex sounds (Tonndorf, 1962).

Electronic techniques

Electronic devices permit the accurate representation of sound wave patterns by variations in the flow of electrons in an electrical circuit. With the aid of these devices sound wave patterns can be manipulated in practically any way desired – they can be measured, amplified, filtered, reproduced and even photographed. All of these techniques have relevance to otological practice and research, and the principles of the fundamental devices should be understood.

Transducers

To convert sound waves into equivalent variations of electron flow a microphone is necessary. A flexible elastic membrane in the path of the sound wave is set into sympathetic vibration and mechanically excites the sensitive element to which it is attached. Being suitably damped, this membrane can vibrate at any frequency required, and with amplitude proportional to that of the incident sound wave. The sensitive element may consist of a cartridge of carbon granules, a magnetic vibrator within a coil of wire, a piezo-electric crystal (whose mechanical distortion sets up electrical currents), or the two plates of an electrical condenser. Whatever the particular type of microphone, it will, when connected to a suitable circuit, generate an electric signal whose wave-form, as a complex alternating current, is a replica of the sound pattern impinging upon the instrument.

To convert electrical energy back into sound waves an earphone or a loudspeaker is required. In either case the fluctuations in electron flow are made to set up equivalent fluctuations in a strong magnetic field by being passed through a suitably designed coil of wire. These changes in the magnetic field are made to cause appropriate vibrations in a metallic diaphragm (earphone) or in a larger movable cone (loudspeaker) which, in turn, 'drives' the surrounding air medium. The electrical and mechanical design are such as to give maximum damping, and the system responds more or less accurately to all wave-forms imposed upon it by the electronic signal.

Other examples of transducers could be cited, but it is sufficient to understand that their role is the conversion of one form of vibratory energy into another. Transduction as a function of the cochlea is considered later in this chapter.

Amplifiers

Electronic wave-forms representing acoustical energy can be increased in amplitude by means of valve or transistor amplifiers. A simple one-stage valve amplifier is shown in *Figure 2.5*.

This is a basic triode circuit in which the voltage fluctuations of the signal are applied to the grid of the valve. The valve itself has a high tension voltage across it so that electrons flow in a steady stream from the heated cathode to the anode. The grid potential with respect to earth controls the rate of flow of current through the valve, and when the grid voltage fluctuates with the applied signal the electron flow from cathode to anode is made to vary similarly. These changes in the current passing

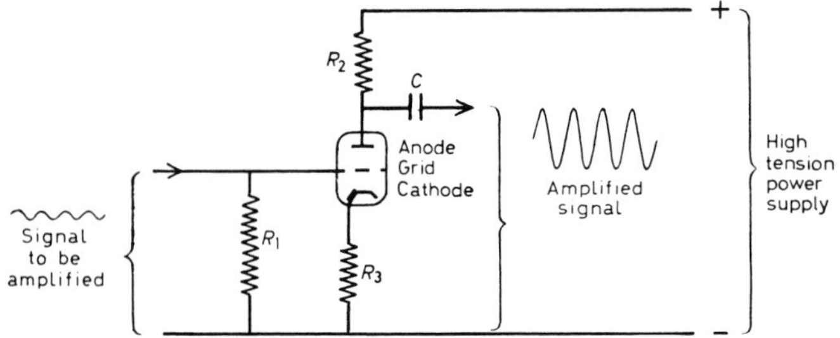

Figure 2.5 Theoretical circuit diagram of a triode valve amplifier

through the valve have identical wave-form to the applied signal, but their amplitude is enormously greater, the necessary energy for the increase being derived from the high tension supply to the valve. The amplified signal is available at the anode load resistor R_2, and can be tapped off (being alternating current) through a capacitor C, independently of the unwanted high tension potential of the anode.

The amplification is expressed as a ratio, and a triode circuit can be so designed, by the values assigned to R_1, R_2, R_3, and to the high tension voltage to give any desired amplification or gain from unity to over 100.

Multi-stage amplifiers consist of this basic circuit repeated twice, three times, or more, the amplified signal from stage one being applied to the grid of the next stage and so on. Practical limitations to the amount of amplification which can be used are imposed by the 'noise' generated in the various components, and amplified to unmanageable levels in the succeeding stages of the amplifier. In many applications transistors have replaced the thermionic valve. They perform the same functions as valves but have the advantages of being very much smaller and more reliable in terms of their long working life. Transistors also require much smaller power supplies for their working voltage and, since they operate 'cold', no separate heater current supplies are needed.

Just as mechanical and acoustical systems must be matched with respect to their acoustical impedances, so electronic circuits require impedance matching if signals are to pass from one to another without decrement. If, for example, a microphone with a low output impedance is to transfer its signal to an amplifier with a high input impedance, the two are easily matched by means of a transformer whose primary and secondary windings are in the required ratio. Similar transformers are used to match the high impedance of the output stage of an amplifier to the low impedance of the 'speech' coil of its loudspeaker.

Direct analogy can be made between these electronic matching arrangements, and the impedance matching effects achieved by mechanical means in the handling of sound waves passing from one system to another. These concepts are essential to the evaluation of the mechanisms of sound propagation in the ear.

Filters

Often it is necessary to amplify and reproduce a part of a sound signal free from unwanted frequencies which may be unavoidably present in the original sound source. Filter circuits can be designed which will attenuate to negligible levels an unwanted band of frequencies, while passing on the desired signal virtually undiminished. These effects are obtained by design techniques which make use of the selective impedances of capacitors and inductors, which vary according to signal frequency. These are the electrical analogues of stiffness and mass which, as pointed out above, influence impedance in a mechano-acoustical system selectively according to frequency.

In electronic equipment bass-boost, bass-cut, top-boost and top-cut networks can be arranged to increase or attenuate a given range of frequencies exactly as desired. The range of frequencies allowed to pass on from such networks can be a very narrow band spanning as little as half an octave, a broad band of, say, four octaves (for example, 500–4000 Hz, as in many hearing aids) or, indeed, any desired range envisaged in the filter circuit design.

Oscillators

The electronics engineer can manipulate capacitances and inductances in other ways, producing a resonating or tuned circuit. The tuning may be sharply peaked (confined to a narrow frequency band) or fairly broad. Under suitable conditions, with an energy source applied across a valve or transistor, electron flow can be made to oscillate at any required frequency and with any desired wave-form. Such an oscillator or signal generator, combined with the necessary measured amplification and attenuation circuits, forms the basis of an audiometer.

Frequency response curves

It will be realized at this stage in the discussion that any system, mechanical or electrical, which conducts sound waves or their electronic equivalents may – either by accident or design – favour certain frequencies at the expense of others. The manner in which a system handles sounds can be plotted as a frequency response curve, which immediately reveals this major aspect of the fidelity of the system. Frequency is

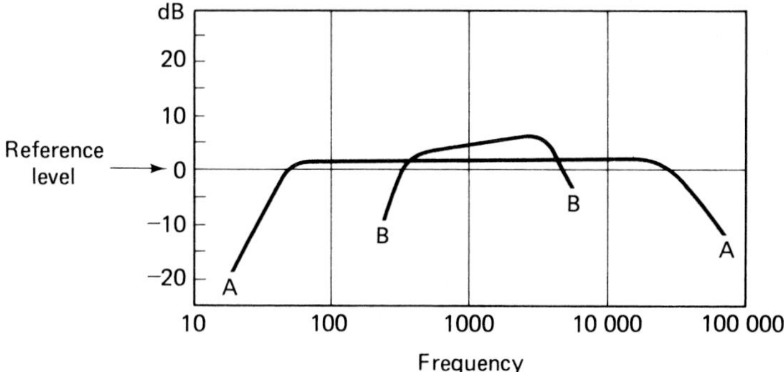

Figure 2.6 Examples of frequency response curves. (A) high-fidelity amplifier, showing good 'linear' response over almost the whole audible range of frequencies. (B) hypothetical hearing aid, with restricted response curve and steep cut-off in both bass and treble

plotted horizontally against intensity in dB on the vertical scale: 0 dB is an arbitrary reference level. Positive values represent increased transmission or amplification and negative values diminished transmission or attenuation (*Figure 2.6*).

The perfect system would show a completely linear response throughout the audible range of frequencies. In practice, most devices, despite damping, will have one or more resonance points on the graph where peaks will appear, and most devices also will show a more or less steep cut-off in the lowest range of frequencies. Some frequency response curves for hearing aids are given in Volume 2.

It will be noted that if a curve deviates from the linear it will have a slope whose steepness is expressed in 'decibels per octave'. This is a useful term in defining the behaviour of filter circuits and frequency selective systems in general.

The performance of the ear

Before considering the details of the hearing mechanism it is necessary to state in physical terms what is known regarding the overall ability of the auditory apparatus.

Perception of frequency as pitch

The range of pitch audible to the human ear extends from about 16 Hz to between 15 000 and 20 000 Hz. The upper tone limit is higher in children and young adults than it is in older people. *Pitch discrimination*, that is, the ability to distinguish between two sounds of almost identical pitch, varies from one individual to another, and at different intensity levels. The musical octave is subdivisible into 12 equal semi-tones, but a person with a 'good ear' can detect many discrete changes in pitch between each semi-tone and the next above or below it. In the vicinity of 1000 Hz the ear can detect a change in frequency of as little as 3 or 4 Hz. The smallest change in frequency the ear can detect under given conditions is known as the *difference limen for frequency*.

A few unusual people are unable to recognize pitch as a property of sound and are said to be *tone deaf*; the cause is not known. At the opposite extreme is another small group of individuals who have *absolute pitch*. These latter not only enjoy perception of pitch in the normal way but can also identify the pitch of a sound without the aid of another reference tone of known pitch.

Perception of intensity as loudness

The sensitivity of the ear is greatest in the frequency range 2000–3000 Hz. In this frequency band it is able to detect a sound pressure of about 0.0002 dynes/cm^2. The threshold of sensitivity is progressively higher, both up and down the frequency scale from this point, and can be plotted graphically (*Figure 2.7*). At its most sensitive the ear has a threshold some 15–30 dB higher than the intensity of ubiquitous ambient sound energy generated by random molecular movement – known as Brownian movement. Evidently nature's limit to the threshold sensitivity of the ear is well adjusted to the limit beyond which increased acuity would become a liability.

The ear performs smoothly with sounds of increasing intensity and can recognize as discrete changes in loudness extremely small changes in intensity. The smallest detectable change is called the *intensity difference limen.* This varies according to frequency and intensity of the signal and is altered in certain pathological conditions.

With increasing intensity the limit is reached above which sound energy causes discomfort or pain. At 1000 Hz this level is around 130 dB above threshold, but at both higher and lower frequencies the limit of tolerance is lower. The curves for threshold of sensitivity and loudness tolerance, both plotted with respect to frequency, are superimposed in *Figure 2.7.*

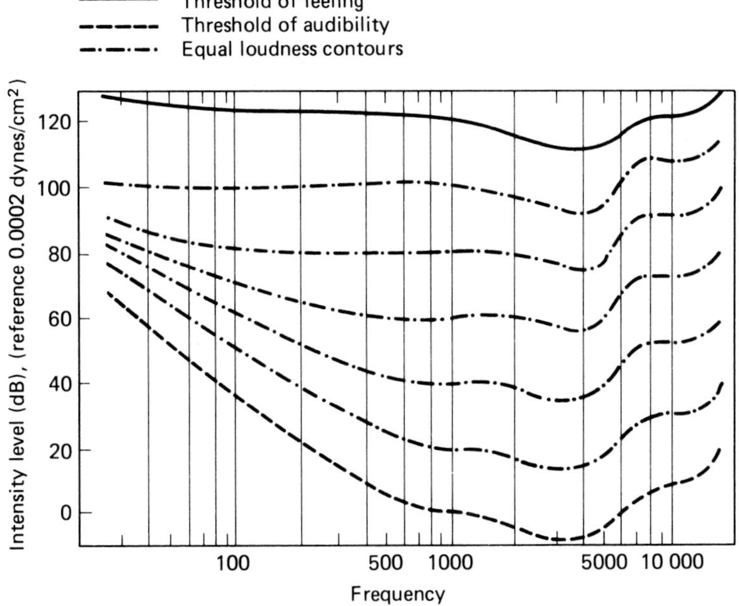

Figure 2.7 Equal loudness curves for the human ear (after Fletcher and Munson, 1933)

Most people find it difficult to compare subjectively, with respect to loudness, sounds of different frequency. This has been studied and recorded in detail by Fletcher and Munson (1933) whose *equal loudness contours* are represented by the broken lines in *Figure 2.7.* These curves join points on the graph at different frequencies of identical (apparent) loudness.

Binaural hearing effects

There are numerous hearing functions which appear to depend upon adequate bilateral hearing.

(1) Absolute threshold – with two good ears the sensitivity is in the region of 3–4 dB better than for either ear alone.

(2) Location of a sound source – the stereophonic effect – depends upon correlation in the central nervous system between different sound patterns at the two ears. This is discussed in greater detail on p. 115.

(3) Ability to pick out and follow a particular sound sequence while rejecting or ignoring unwanted sounds. Although this a faculty largely dependent upon cerebral processes, the necessary sound data require good binaural hearing for their detection and processing.

These and other aspects of binaural hearing appear to indicate that a pair of ears not only perceives the necessary frequencies and intensities but is also able to inform the central nervous system of *phase differences* between the two sides.

The physiology of sound conduction

The sound conducting mechanism extends from the pinna to the organ of Corti. Each part of it forms a link in the acoustical chain which overall is designed to carry out the following functions.

(1) *Collection and transmission of sound energy*, involving impedance matching at every stage, and particularly in the major matter of matching between the external air and cochlear fluids (*Figure 2.8*).

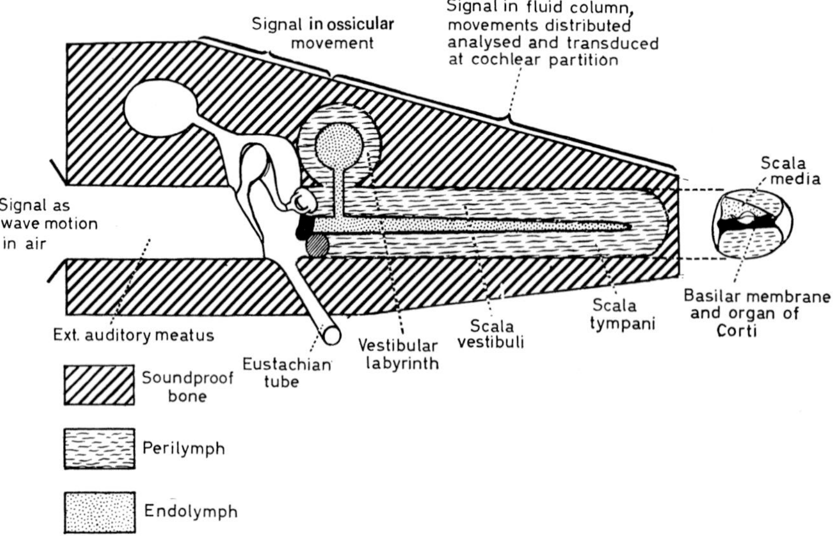

Figure 2.8 Scheme of the sound conducting apparatus, omitting the intratympanic muscles

(2) *Protection of inner ear from excessively loud sounds* – a function carried out by the tympanic muscles without sacrificing sensitivity for low intensity sound levels.

Physiology of the external ear

The *pinna* functions as a sound collector, intercepting sound energy and deflecting it into the auditory canal. In many animals the pinna can be rotated so as to achieve optimum sound interception by alignment with the direction of the sound source. In man the external auricular muscles have lost this function and the pinna itself has no useful range of movement. Nevertheless, it still has value in sound collection, and its effect can be augmented by the cupped hand behind the ear.

The *external auditory meatus*, by virtue of its tortuous shape, its vibrissae and the wax it secretes, affords considerable protection against physical violence and the entry of foreign material. In the remote depths of the meatus the tympanic membrane is almost immune to direct injury.

The acoustic functions of the external meatus appear to be very simple – namely to permit air-borne sound waves to reach the tympanic membrane. A conductive hearing loss results if the meatus is totally occluded due to any cause, but a severe degree of narrowing, less than complete occlusion, does not significantly affect hearing. The frequency response curve for the meatus is not perfectly linear. If the sound pressure in the deep meatus is measured and compared with the pressure immediately outside the meatus, a linear relationship is evident for the lower and

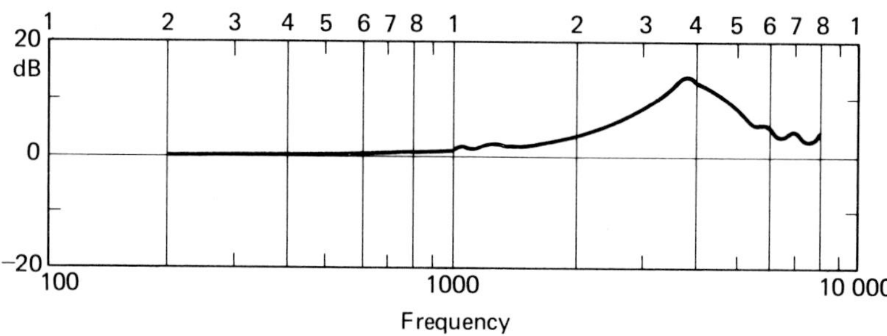

Figure 2.9 Resonance of the external auditory meatus, showing the peak at the characteristic frequency just below 4000 Hz. (Reproduced from *Physiological Acoustics* by Wever and Lawrence, by permission of Princeton University Press – after Wiener and Ross)

middle frequencies, but at around 4000 Hz a resonance, peaking to some 12 dB above the signal intensity, is found. At this frequency the sound wavelength is four times the length of the auditory canal (*Figure 2.9*). These are the conditions required for resonance to occur in any tube which, like the ear canal, is closed at one end.

Physiology of the middle ear

An understanding of the physiology of the middle ear must begin from the oval and round windows of the labyrinth. In order that vibratory movements may take place at the cochlear partition in response to sound energy it is essential that the two windows are free to vibrate reciprocally, that is, in opposite phase. This cannot occur if both windows are exposed to the same wave-front under the same functional conditions, and in this situation no to-and-fro movement of the cochlear fluids could result. In the intact ear sound energy is applied *preferentially* through the tympanic membrane and ossicular chain to the *oval* window. Only a very small fraction of the total energy reaches the round window by air conduction across the middle-ear cavity, and this in-phase pressure is far too weak to interfere significantly with the reciprocal pressure on the round window reaching it by the cochlear fluid and oval window route. The intact tympanic membrane thus 'protects' the round window while 'feeding' the ossicular chain and oval window.

There was formerly controversy over the mechanisms outlined above, it being held by some that the 'aerotympanic route' to the round window was the important route. Current views, however, almost unanimously affirm that the round window functions as a 'relieving point' and does not lie in the direct sound pathway to the cochlea. Its mobility, however, is as essential to normal hearing as that of any other part of the vibrating system.

The tympanic membrane

Many workers have studied the dynamics of the tympanic membrane, notably Dahmann and Békésy. From their researches we know that the drum membrane vibrates in a manner quite different from that of a simple stretched elastic membrane. Methods for observing and measuring the movements of the membrane resulting from a change in pressure in the meatus include the attachment of small mirrors or the sprinkling of fine particles of silver upon the surface of the drumhead. Measurement of their displacement can then be made by observation of the deflection of a beam of light.

Békésy used an electrical probe to measure the linear displacement of the membrane. This method has the advantage of allowing normal vibrations to be measured, uninfluenced by the loading effects due to the weight of optical reflecting devices. A fine metallic probe acts as one plate of a condenser, and its tip is fixed very close to the membrane without actually touching it. The membrane itself serves as the other plate. An alternating current applied across the two 'plates' will flow through this capacitative arrangement whose electrical impedance will vary with any change

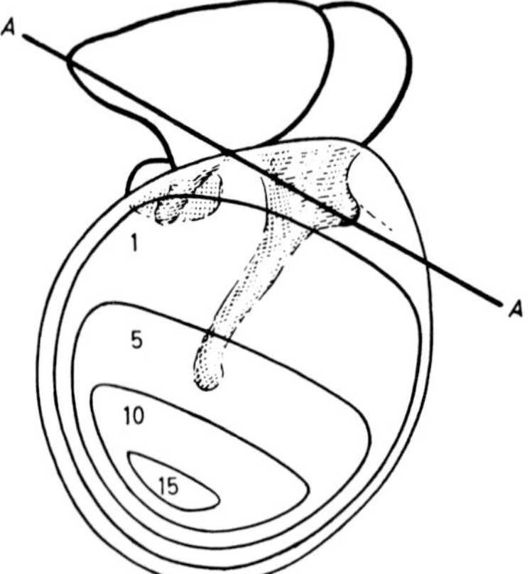

Figure 2.10 Vibration of the tympanic membrane (after Lawrence, 1962). Below 2400 Hz the whole membrane vibrates in the same phase with a pattern shown by the equal amplitude lines. The combined mass of the head of the malleus and the body of the incus lies above the axis of rotation, A-A, counterbalancing the structures below that level

in the distance separating the probe from the drumhead. Displacements of the membrane can thus be directly measured from the alternating current which flows in the circuit. Békésy used this method to plot the movements in each portion of the membrane, and *Figure 2.10* summarizes his findings. The area of maximum displacement is seen near the lower margin. As might be supposed from this finding, the central part of the membrane in fact vibrates as a sheet suspended from a curvilinear axis near its upper edge. The central part of the membrane vibrates more or less uniformly at frequencies up to 2400 Hz. For tones of higher frequency Békésy found that the vibration of the malleus handle lags behind that of the membrane.

The ossicular chain

The mode of vibration of the various elements of the ossicular chain can be deduced from their dimensions and from the arrangements of their ligamentous supports and joint surfaces. Actual vibrations can be measured by means of mirrors attached to the ossicles, by means of stroboscopic light observations, and by cinematography. Naturally, most of the relevant observations have been made on the fresh cadaver ear.

The *malleus and incus* vibrate as a combined unit, rocking on a linear axis which runs from the anterior ligament of the malleus to the attachment of the short process of the incus in the fossa incudis (*Figure 2.10*). When reciprocating movements of the conducting system take place the mass of the body of the incus and the head and neck of the malleus, lying above this axis, serve to balance the mass of the drumhead, malleus handle, long process of incus and stapes lying below it.

The *stapes* is often imagined to move in and out in the oval window niche with the simple movement of a piston. Békésy showed that the matter is more complex than this (*Figure 2.11*). With sounds of moderate intensity the anterior end of the footplate

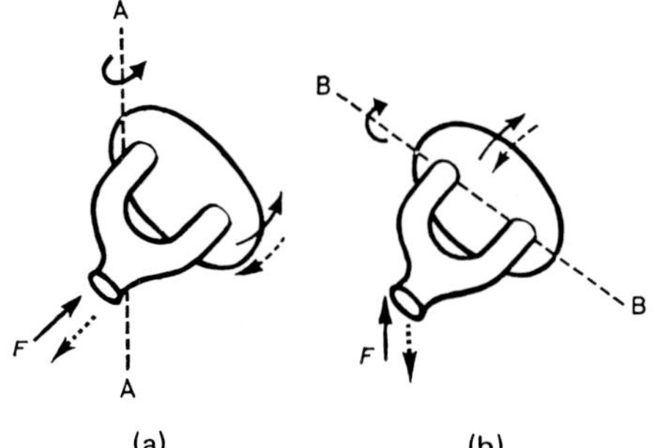

Figure 2.11 Vibratory motion of the stapes (after Békésy, 1960): (a) normal mode of vibration through the axis A-A; (b) mode of vibration at high sound intensities through the axis B-B

oscillates with a greater amplitude than the posterior end. In other words, a rocking movement occurs about a transverse axis near the posterior end. This mode of vibration is probably determined by the fact that the fibres of the annular ligament are longer at the anterior end than those at the posterior end. With high sound levels the mode of action changes and a side-to-side rocking movement is seen about an axis running longitudinally through the length of the footplate. The volume displacement of the inner-ear fluids will be proportionately less in the second vibratory mode than in the first, and presumably these alternative stapedial mechanisms constitute a protective arrangement for minimizing too violent stimulation of the inner ear. It may be that the controlling mechanism for this arrangement operates through the intratympanic muscles which will be discussed in more detail later.

Cochlear fluids

The cochlear fluids must be recognized as an essential part of the sound conducting mechanism, as indeed are the *basilar membrane* and all vibrating structures within the cochlea. Since the details of their physiology have such a profound bearing on the study of sound perception, they are fully discussed later (p. 105) but at this stage it is sufficient to appreciate the mechanical presence of the twin fluid columns of scala vestibuli and scala tympani, separated by the elastic cochlear partition and terminated by the round window membrane. This vibratory system of fluids and membranes provides the mechanical loading on the inner surface of the stapes footplate. Its acoustic impedance is the essential component in the conducting mechanism to which the external ear is matched, and we must now consider how this matching is achieved by the middle-ear apparatus.

The transformer mechanism of the middle ear

It has already been explained (p. 74) that the specific acoustic resistances of air and water respectively are mismatched to a degree which appears to involve a loss in sound energy transfer from the one medium to the other of 1000 to 1, or 30 dB. In the intact middle ear a considerable degree of impedance matching is brought about, so that, while the amplitude is greatly reduced at the oval window as compared with amplitude at the tympanic membrane, the force of the vibrations at the oval window is increased in the same proportion. This desirable effect depends on:

(1) *The ossicular chain lever ratio* – The malleus and incus jointly act as a lever, pivoting upon the axis of rotation. The malleolar arm is longer than the incudal arm in the ratio of 1.3:1. This ratio varies among different species of animal, but can be directly measured. That the expected lever ratios are in fact operative in the presence of sound energy has been shown experimentally by Wever and

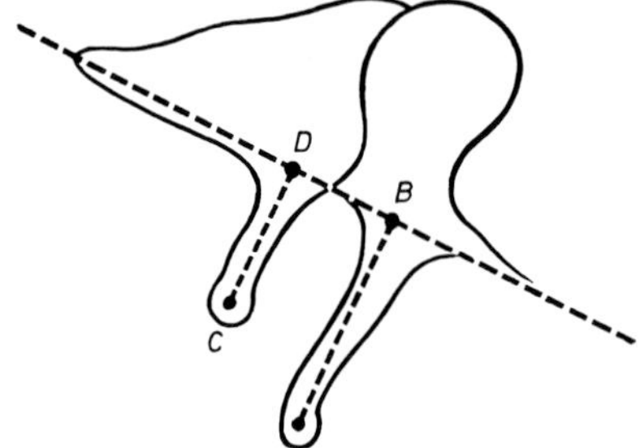

Figure 2.12 The lever ratio of the human ossicular chain. The effective lever arms *AB* and *CD* are in the ratio 1·3 to 1·0

Lawrence (1954). They applied a vibrating probe at various points on the malleus and incus and were able to calculate the effective lever ratios at each point, using the round window cochlear microphonic as their index of sound conduction.

(2) *The areal ratio of the tympanic membrane and oval window* – There is an hydraulic effect between these two structures increasing the force of the vibrations at the oval window. If it is assumed that the sound energy accepted by the tympanic membrane reaches the oval window undiminished, the increase in force will be in the same ratio as the ratio between the effective areas of the membrane and the oval window. (It should be realized that the effective area of the tympanic membrane is appreciably less than its total area since it is fixed all around the periphery.) On the basis of the equal displacement contours of Békésy (*see Figure 2.10*) and measurements of volume displacement in the cadaver ear, Wever and Lawrence deduce that the effective area for the tympanic membrane is two-thirds of the anatomical area. If the area of the oval window is measured an effective areal ratio between these two structures of 14:1 is obtained.

The overall ratio for the middle ear is the product of the ossicular chain lever ratio and the areal ratio between the tympanic membrane and the oval window. This gives an approximate figure of 18.3. By definition the impedance transformation ratio is the square of this figure and is therefore 336. We have already seen that the ratio of acoustic impedance of air and water is 3880 so it becomes evident that the impedance matching due to the middle ear, although very substantial, is theoretically, at least, less than ideally required.

Further consideration, however, shows that the impedance of the inner-ear conductive apparatus is substantially different from that of an unbounded volume of sea water. The elastic structures of the round window and the cochlear partition have a complex and important effect, and *Table 2.1* (from Wever and Lawrence) shows that the calculated impedances for the inner ear as a whole vary greatly with

Table 2.1 Calculated impedance of the inner ear at various audio-frequencies. (The acoustic impedance of an unbounded volume of sea water is 161 000 mechanical ohms/cm²)

Frequency (Hz)	*Inner-ear impedance* (ohms/cm²)
100	1 580 000
200	1 510 000
300	1 090 000
500	585 000
700	330 000
1000	169 000
1500	117 000
1600	121 000

(Reproduced from *Physiological Acoustics*, by Wever and Lawrence, by permission of Princeton University Press.)

frequency. It is obvious that where one middle-ear mechanism must 'match into' so wide a range of inner-ear impedances a working compromise is necessary.

Békésy measured the pressure transformation ratio in human cadaver ears by finding the sound pressure required at the inner surface of the footplate to cancel a known sound pressure at the surface of the tympanic membrane. His results showed a ratio ranging from 12:1 to 19:1 (22–24 dB) at frequencies up to 2400 Hz.

Direct measurements were made by Wever and Lawrence of the loss of sensitivity due to removal of the middle-ear transformer mechanism in the cat's ear. They first found the sound pressure needed to evoke a standard cochlear microphonic response at the round window with the middle ear intact. They then removed the tympanic membrane and ossicular chain but left the footplate undisturbed. Sound energy was then applied directly to the oval window by way of a tube cemented to its margins. The greater intensity required to evoke the same cochlear microphonic potential was measured. The differences between the two sound levels, expressed in dB and plotted against frequency, are shown in *Figure 2.13*. The losses shown are those due to loss of

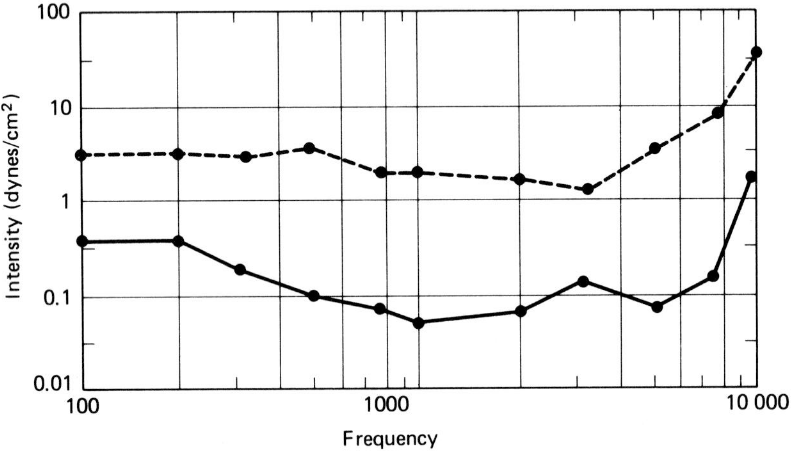

Figure 2.13 The mechanical transformer action of the middle ear. The continuous curve indicates the performance of the intact ear. The interrupted curve shows the greater sound intensity required to evoke the same round window microphonic voltage when the sound is applied directly to the oval window. The difference between the two curves represents the transmission loss due to removal of the transformer mechanism. (Reproduced from *Physiological Acoustics*, by Wever and Lawrence, by permission of Princeton University Press)

the transformer mechanism only, since the principle of preferential application of sound energy to the oval window was maintained in the conditions of this experiment. The average transmission loss calculated from the graph is around 30 dB, a figure comparable to the loss in the human ear after fenestration operations and some tympanoplastic procedures. This value of 30 dB is close to the theoretical figure of 25 dB for the human ear, as calculated from the transformation ratio 18:1 (the product of the areal and lever ratios discussed above).

Disorders of middle-ear function

Total loss of the middle-ear mechanism

This disorder which leaves the two mobile windows equally exposed to sound waves, results clinically in a hearing loss of some 40–60 dB. It has been argued that in this condition the cochlear fluids are able to vibrate effectively, although at greatly reduced amplitude, because of the depth of the round window niche and the oblique angle at which the round window membrane is set. Such factors, however, are not significant for the wavelengths with which we are concerned in auditory physiology, except possibly at the highest frequencies. Békésy investigated the simultaneous sound pressure levels at the two windows in a cadaver preparation lacking the tympanic membrane, malleus and incus. His so-called reciprocal technique gave measurements directly from the inner-ear side of the two windows, thus excluding any effects due to inner-ear mechanisms. He concluded that in such a condition there is only a negligible pressure and phase difference at the two windows, except at the higher frequencies. Békésy suggests that residual hearing in complete loss of the middle ear is probably attributable to yielding of the inner-ear contents. Of course, the bony walls do not yield significantly but, it is argued, blood vessels and capillaries can yield by expression of their contents beyond the labyrinth confines. Békésy points out that this possibility is greater in the vestibular labyrinth than in the scala tympani so that positive sound pressures acting equally at both windows press the basilar membrane towards the scala vestibuli (*see Figure 2.14a*). Békésy's view appears to be

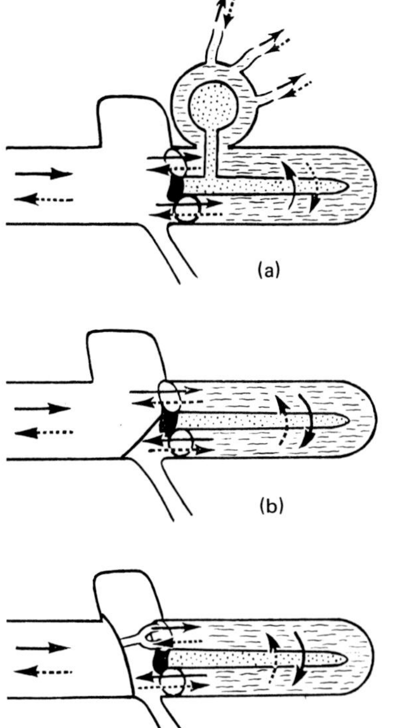

Figure 2.14 Common derangements of the conducting mechanism. In each illustration the direction of displacement during the compression phase of an incident sound wave is represented by the continuous arrows, and during the rarefaction phase by the interrupted arrows. (a) Total loss of the tympanic membrane and ossicular sound pathway. Displacement of the basilar membrane can only occur by virtue of the yielding of the vascular contents of the labyrinth. This yielding is greater on the vestibular side, so that the basilar membrane moves in that direction during compression. (In (b) and (c) below, and in the normal ear, the opposite displacement occurs towards the scala tympani)

(b) Round window baffle effect. The shielding of the round window permits free reciprocal movement of the cochlear fluids, with selective application of sound energy to one window only. The transformer mechanism is lost

(c) Columellar mechanism. The tympanic membrane, applied directly to the stapes, conserves the areal ratio and the selective route for sound to one window only. The loss of the lever ratio (1·3 to 1) is the only deficiency

confirmed by his observation that there is an apparent change of phase in perception of sounds in such an ear (consistent with the reversed direction of basilar membrane displacement) and that this phase change reverts to normal if an effective 'eardrum–round window' prosthesis is inserted.

Békésy repeated his measurements of sound pressure differences at the two windows, referred to above, after removal of the incus and stapes, but with the tympanic membrane left intact. In this condition of the cadaver ear his results indicated an additional hearing loss of 1–5 dB, as compared with the effect of removing the membrane as well as the ossicles. The otologist will recognize here an equivalent condition to dislocation of the ossicular chain behind an intact drumhead, in which he is accustomed to a hearing loss of some 40–60 dB.

The round window baffle effect

In an ear lacking drumhead, malleus and incus, remarkably good hearing is preserved if a membrane encloses the lower part of the tympanum so that the round window is protected from direct sound energy (*see Figure 2.14b*). In this condition there is no transformer mechanism, but the principle of preferential sound conduction to the oval window is maintained. Reciprocal movement of the two windows is facilitated. Instead of the loss of 40–60 dB due to the loss of the middle ear, we have theoretically only the loss due to the transformer device, namely 25 dB. It is by no means unusual to find hearing of this comparatively good standard after a Type 4 tympanoplasty. After radical mastoidectomy a spontaneously formed membrane may give the same effect, while the classic Lempert fenestration operation reproduces the same conditions, albeit with a new 'oval' window. Some workers have attributed the success of the fenestration technique to other factors, such as resonance effects in the bony cavity, mobilization of the cochlear fluids, and so forth, but the essential conditions are, of course, the creation of a mobile substitute for the oval window exposed to direct sound vibrations, and the establishment of the round window baffle effect.

The columellar effect

If the drumhead should be adherent to the head of the stapes, so bypassing the malleus and incus (*see Figure 2.14c*), the portion of the transmission ratio due to the areal ratio of the membrane and oval window remains effective although the ossicular chain lever ratio (1.3:1) is lost. It is unimportant if the malleus and incus are damaged or destroyed in this condition – indeed, the stapes superstructure itself can be lost and a plastic rod substituted – provided that good mechanical linkage between the oval window and the drumhead is established. The arrangement imitates the single ossicle, or columella, of lower vertebrates, and it provides in ideal circumstances hearing approaching normal levels.

It should be appreciated that such disorders of the conducting apparatus as are described above will result in changes in the physical characteristics of the vibrating structures. Mass and elasticity changes will have frequency-selective effects, while changes in frictional resistance will affect all frequencies equally. The otologist must therefore expect not only alterations in threshold sensitivity of the ear, but also changes in frequency response, and phase distortion with its effects on binaural directional hearing.

Perforation of the tympanic membrane

A small hole in the drumhead has no appreciable effect on sound conduction provided that the rest of the conducting apparatus is normal. Larger losses of the membrane represent a diminution of the areal ratio as well as permitting direct access of sound waves to the round window. The sound transformation is diminished and the preferential conduction of energy to one window only is disturbed. The degree of hearing loss will depend on the extent to which each of these mechanisms is impaired.

Stapes fixation

Reduced mobility of the stapes due to disease results in increased stiffness and increased frictional resistance at the oval window. According to the severity of the condition, the transformer mechanism will be impaired. At 30 dB hearing loss the transformer effect is lost altogether. Provided that some portion of the annular ligament remains flexible reciprocal cochlear fluid movement can still take place, but now the aerotympanic route and the round window membrane become the principal avenues for sound conduction. When total fixation occurs involving the whole of the annular ligament as well as the footplate, reciprocal vibration of the cochlear fluid columns is gravely limited even though the round window membrane remains normal. Residual hearing for air-conducted sound probably now depends upon the compressibility of the inner-ear blood vessels mentioned earlier in another connection.

Effects of static pressure changes

Optimum performance of the middle-ear mechanism requires equal pressures on the outer and inner surfaces of the tympanic membrane. The external air pressure in the meatus is balanced in the middle ear by the intermittent opening of the eustachian tube by reflex muscular action (*see* Chapter 1, p. 9). This balance can be disturbed by eustachian-tube obstruction, by rapid changes in the atmospheric pressure (*see* Chapters 6, and 7) and experimentally by means of pressure changes applied by a closely fitting tube in the meatus. Experimental observations show that a loss of some 5 or 6 dB for frequencies below 1000 Hz results from pressure changes of 10 cm of water, whether these changes are in the positive or the negative sense.

Békésy states that these findings indicate that any change in static pressure increases the tension of the fibres of the drumhead, and so increases its acoustic impedance for all frequencies below its resonance frequency (800–1500 Hz). The hearing for higher frequencies (above about 1800 Hz) appears not to be appreciably altered by static pressure variations.

Tympanic muscle reflexes

The stapedius and tensor tympani muscles act directly upon the ossicular chain. They cause alterations in tension and stiffness, as well as movement of the structures to which they are attached. If the incudostapedial joint is disrupted, the stapes can be seen to rock backwards and outwards when the stapedius muscle contracts. The tensor tympani not only increases the tension in the fibres of the tympanic membrane, but also draws the malleus slightly medially and forwards, a movement which can be seen and measured under magnification.

Some normal persons can voluntarily contract the tensor tympani, and in many people the contraction of the intratympanic muscles is audible to the subject. It is easily demonstrable that sound is the effective stimulus causing reflex contraction of these muscles. The reflex arc is from the cochlea, through the cochlear nuclei and superior olivary body to the motor nuclei of the fifth and seventh cranial nerves. The reflex is consensual, that is, bilateral regardless of whether the sound stimulus is applied to one or both ears. In addition to the motor nerve supply from the facial nerve (to stapedius) and the trigeminal nerve (to tensor tympani) it has been shown that fibres from the tympanic plexus of nerves reach the tensor tympani muscle and innervate it (Lawrence, 1962). It is not yet known whether these fibres are motor or sensory.

The reflex activity of the intra-aural muscles can be studied by direct (optical) observation in animals, and in the human ear when a perforation of the drumhead exposes the stapedius tendon and stapes to view. Variations in the position of the tympanic membrane caused by the muscle reflexes can be measured, if the external meatus is closed, by the resulting changes of static pressure in the outer ear. This type of investigation, known as tympanomanometry, has the advantage of being suitable for the intact living human ear, and has been used notably by Mendelson (1961), and by Weiss and his colleagues (1962). Another technique suitable for use in human subjects as well as in animals, is the measurement of changes in the acoustic impedance of the ear caused by the muscle reflex (Metz, 1951, and others). This change in impedance is thought to result chiefly from the increase in stiffness of the middle-ear mechanism which occurs when the tympanic muscle reflex is brought into play. In the cadaver the muscle actions have been studied by observation of the effect of attaching weights to the tendons. In experimental animals the effect of such manoeuvres upon the transmission characteristics of the middle ear can be investigated by measurement of the round window microphonic potentials.

The chief questions to be answered in connection with the tympanic muscle reflexes are:

(1) What are the characteristics of effective stimuli which will result in reflex activity?
(2) How do the muscles respond to reflex excitation, in terms of latency time, adaptation to continued stimulation, combinations of more than one stimulus, and so on?
(3) What are the effects of reflex muscle activity on the sound transmission characteristics of the conducting mechanism?

Stimulus

The stimulus has been found by all workers to be sound of high intensity. For example. Weiss and his colleagues found by tympanomanometry in human subjects an average threshold for excitation of the reflex of 92 dB above normal sensation threshold, regardless of the frequency employed. Moller (1961) claims that the threshold is lower for noise than it is for pure-tone stimuli. He also found that ipsilateral stimuli have a lower threshold than contralateral stimuli, and that bilateral stimuli have the lowest threshold of all. The question is still further complicated because the rate of onset of the stimuli is also relevant, and for the lower frequencies the threshold of the stapedius reflex is lower than that for the tensor.

The responses of the tympanic muscles

The *latency time* of the reflex has been measured by many workers and in numerous experimental animals. Perlman and Case (1939) found a figure of 10 ms for the human stapedius, a finding confirmed by Fisch and Schulthess (1963). For the combined muscle action in man Metz (1951) observed a latency which became progressively shorter as the stimulus intensity was raised, and Kato made a similar observation for the cat.

Strength of contraction

In response to the onset of stimulation a maximum contraction is quickly reached, but if stimulation continues the muscle response falls to a lower sustained level. That this is due to a process of adaptation and not to fatigue is shown by the fact that if the stimulus is interrupted and then immediately resumed, the muscle contraction is repeated at full initial strength. The strength of contraction increases as the strength of the stimulating sound is increased and is greater for stimuli of low frequency than for higher tones. The reflex can be abolished by exposure to very strong stimuli (for example, 140 dB at 1000 Hz for 20 s) and Perlman states that this is due to fatigue, not in the muscle but presumably in the neural circuit of the reflex arc.

Summation of stimuli occurs when two tones of equal contraction-inducing power are applied simultaneously to produce twice the power of muscle contraction. This results only if both the stimuli are above the reflex threshold. Perlman (1960) has given a lucid account of these matters, and the reader is advised to study his paper for more details. Jepsen (1963) should also be consulted.

Effects upon sound transmission

All the experimental work indicates that contraction of the tympanic muscles restricts the vibrations of the ossicular chain, tenses the tympanic membrane, and reduces the sensitivity of the ear (as measured by the cochlear potentials in animals and subjectively in man). Weiss and his colleagues deduced from tympanomanometric studies that in man reflex displacement of the drumhead is the resultant of the opposing pressures of the two muscles. They conclude that the membrane is displaced laterally by the stapedius and medially by the tensor, and obtained evidence in support of this from patients suffering from stapes fixation due to otosclerosis. Their paper should be consulted for further details of this important work, but it is of interest to note here that in a fairly large series they found that 5 per cent of human subjects had no reflex demonstrable by their most sensitive technique, using stimuli up to 115 dB above hearing threshold.

Many workers have believed that in man only the stapedius muscle is active in response to sound stimuli. Certainly the stapedius has a shorter latency time and develops a stronger contraction than the tensor in animal investigations.

The effect of the muscle reflex upon the performance of the ear, as stated above, is a reduction in transmission, and this is due to an increase in stiffness of the vibrating parts. As theoretically expected, this attenuation is frequency-selective for the lower tones. In experimental work on the guinea-pig the effect is limited to frequencies below about 1200 Hz, and at higher frequencies Wiggers (1937) found that the reflex actually caused a small increase in sensitivity. This enhancement of sensitivity in the middle frequency range has also been observed in the cat.

The physiological role of the tympanic muscle reflex

There can be very little doubt that this reflex mechanism serves to protect the cochlea from excessive stimulation by loud noise. Since the reflex comes into play at sound levels of 70–90 dB above threshold, becomes increasingly more effective with increasingly loud stimuli, and is most effective as an attenuator for the more damaging lower frequencies, the device seems well adapted to this purpose. Experiments have shown that animals in whom the reflex has been abolished by nerve or tendon section develop the inner-ear lesions of acoustic trauma much more readily than intact controls. The mechanism has its limitations, however. The latency time implies that no protection is offered against sound of explosively sudden onset, while the partial relaxation of the muscles during adaptation to longer stimuli reduces to some extent the cover given. Hilding (1961) has shown that acoustic trauma due to sudden loud sounds (gunfire) can be prevented in animals by the prior excitation of the tympanic muscle reflex with a short tone of 1000 Hz at 100 dB. Loss of the stapedius reflex in humans with facial paralysis results in hyperacusis or phonophobia, and the effect of stapedius tendon section at stapedectomy presumably raises a hazard of acoustic trauma for patients who have noisy occupations.

Tumarkin (1945) has objected to the protection theory on the grounds that excessively loud sustained noise could hardly occur in nature, and is merely a byproduct of modern life.

Another function put forward for the tympanic muscle reflex is that it selectively *augments* auditory function at low and moderate sound levels. Simmons and Beatty (1962) have used 'chronically implanted' electrodes in the cat to investigate this problem and they claim that 'the minor amplitude modulations of auditory input which are produced by the middle-ear acoustic reflex at moderate and low sound intensities in the cat may contribute significantly to signal analysis or attention mechanisms of the auditory system'. At high sound levels the attenuation of the masking effect of low-frequency noise by the muscle reflex may well be valuable in making more intelligible the wanted middle and high frequencies. As we have already seen, the latter are not influenced by the reflex, and in the cat and guinea-pig are actually enhanced by it.

Lastly, the middle-ear muscles have a very simple and obvious function, namely to provide stability of suspension for the ossicular chain. The tendons, possibly supported by a resting tonus of their muscle fibres, appear to maintain ossicular alignment in a way which becomes only too obvious to the surgeon when he has divided them.

Hearing by bone conduction

The otologist's chief interest in the phenomenon of hearing by bone conduction lies in its value as an index of cochlear function. In everyday experience there are three main ways in which hearing is brought about by bone-conducted sound. These are:

(1) The sound vibrations of the skull caused by the subject's own voice.
(2) Skull vibrations due to 'free-field' sound energy. The whole head vibrates with ambient sound pressures in the same way that the tympanic membrane itself does. This mode of hearing, bypassing the normal meatal route, imposes a

practical limit to the amount of attenuation of, and protection from, injurious loud noise which can be achieved with ear-muffs or plugs.

(3) Skull vibrations caused by direct application of a vibrating body to the head, as in tuning-fork tests.

None of these sources of bone-conducted sound is particularly useful physiologically, and the auditory apparatus has evolved so as to achieve maximum sensitivity to air-conducted sound while these unwanted bone-conducted sources are attenuated as much as possible. The mammalian ear has developed as we know it primarily as an adaptation to terrestrial instead of aquatic life, and in the process the physical construction of the ear and its orientation in the skull have evolved in favour of air-borne sound reception, with minimum interference from sounds generated within or conducted through the head.

It has been shown conclusively that the manner of stimulation of the sense organ is the same for both air- and bone-conducted sounds – the final common mechanism is the vibration of the basilar membrane which results from oscillatory movements of the cochlear fluids. As to the way in which these fluid oscillations are brought about by skull vibrations there are three main theories which require attention.

(1) The *translatory*, or inertial, mechanism. When the head vibrates as a whole the ossicular chain, because of its inertia, lags behind the general vibration of the skull. The stapedial footplate therefore oscillates with respect to the oval window, and the inner-ear mechanism performs just as it does for air-borne sound.

(2) The *compressional* mechanism. This theory supposes that when the skull vibrates the bony capsule of the labyrinth is alternately compressed and decompressed by fluctuating twisting forces in the surrounding bone. In each cycle, therefore, the labyrinthine fluids are first squeezed and then relaxed. Because the oval window is many times less yielding than the round window this alternate compression and decompression of the fluids will be compensated mainly at the more compliant round window, and the basilar membrane will vibrate accordingly. Theoretically, if this mode of bone conduction is operative, rigidity, even fixation, of the oval window should actually enhance the efficiency of the arrangement with regard to displacement of the basilar membrane.

(3) The *effect of the mandible*. This heavy bone lags behind the vibrations of the skull so that the head of the mandible causes vibrations of the cartilaginous meatus. These vibrations of the meatus are then transmitted by the normal air-conduction route to the cochlea. This theory is supported by the fact that occlusion of the meatus by light pressure on the tragus enhances the loudness of a bone-conducted sound, whereas an occlusion in the deep bony meatus has no effect.

Much evidence has accrued in support of each of the above theories, and it seems probable that all play a part in bone conduction. The effect of a pathological condition of the ear upon bone-conduction thresholds will depend upon the extent to which one or more of these mechanisms may be impaired or enhanced.

Experimental studies by Békésy (1960), Bàràny (1938), and Kirikae (1959) show how the skull vibrates in response to acoustic energy. It is found that in the lower frequency range the skull vibrates as a whole without deformation. Such a mode of

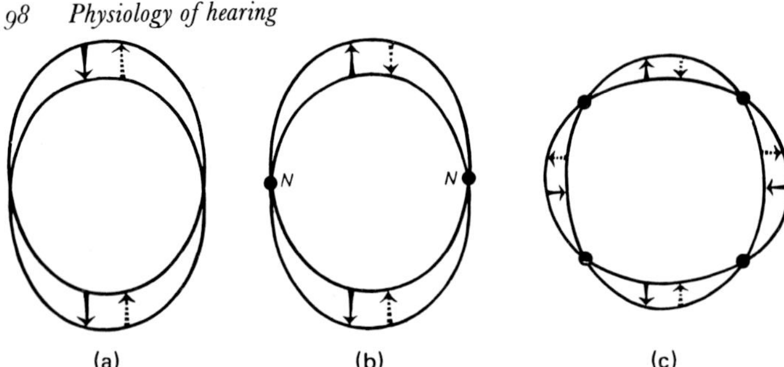

Figure 2.15 Simplified patterns of vibration of the skull in response to sound energy at various frequencies: (a) at frequencies below 800 Hz the head moves as a whole in following the applied vibration to and fro; (b) at the resonance frequency of the skull (800–1200 Hz) bending occurs in the skull walls at the nodal points *N*, *N*. Opposite poles of the skull now move alternately towards and away from each other in the positive and negative phases of the applied vibration; (c) above the resonance frequency additional nodal points appear, and more numerous but smaller vibrating segments of the skull wall are found. Twisting and compressional forces develop in the bones, including, of course, the labyrinthine capsule

vibration requires an inertial mechanism for hearing by bone conduction. At higher frequencies – 800 Hz and above – it is found that bending occurs in the bones of the skull, and nodal (that is, stationary) points appear (*Figure 2.15*) as the frequency rises. In this condition the frontal and occipital regions move alternately towards and away from each other, while the temporal regions do likewise but in opposite phase. It is this mode of vibration which results in the compressional mode of labyrinthine stimulation. We thus have evidence that the translatory (inertial) mechanism is important for bone conduction of lower frequencies, and the compressional mechanism for the higher range.

Certain aspects of bone conduction are not readily explained, however, by the simple mechanisms just described. Discrepancies encountered in the Weber, Bing and Gelle tests, and the shape of the so-called Carhart notch due to stapes fixation, all require more detailed study. Allen and Fernandez (1960) state that 'alteration of the conduction mechanism causes an alteration of the inner-ear vibratory mechanism which changes the intensity and phase of vibrations delivered to the cochlea. It is the change of phase which primarily determines lateralization of the Weber. Also changes in the conduction mechanism can prevent the escape of energy from the vestibular compartment through the ossicular chain. This improves the bone-conduction threshold mainly around the resonance frequency of the conduction mechanism.' The reader will find further discussion in the works of Bàràny (1938), Békésy (1960), Carhart (1950), Kirikae (1959), Wever and Lawrence (1954) and Zwislocki (1953).

Cochlear function

There are two essential processes in the cochlea, namely *transmission* and *transduction*. The former accounts for the transference of acoustic energy from the oval window to the hair-cells, while the latter is the process by which this sound energy pattern is converted at the organ of Corti into action potentials in the auditory nerve. These processes must be performed in such a way as to account for all the known phenomena of hearing in terms of pitch, loudness, phase discrimination, and so on. Theories of hearing have been increasing in complexity, sophistication, and numbers, over the past 100 years. With the compilation of more and more experimental data the many gaps in knowledge are being filled, but the casual or non-specialist student of the subject finds increasing difficulty in following the seemingly endless arguments and discrepancies which appear in disciplines and terminologies more and more removed from the domain of ordinary clinical life. The almost total inadequacy of present-day management of inner-ear diseases must surely be the otologist's incentive to keep up with scientific work in this field.

Before the principles of transmission and transduction in the cochlea are discussed some account is given of cochlear metabolism, including electrical activity.

Chemistry of the cochlear fluids

Microchemical analysis of inner-ear fluids has provided data of value in recent times. The most striking discovery has been that while perilymph has a composition much like that of other extracellular fluids, the endolymph has a remarkably high potassium concentration and a low sodium content, similar to that of intracellular fluids. *Table 2.2* [taken from Vosteen's (1963) monograph] summarizes the present available data for the composition of the relevant fluids. It is supposed that the high level of potassium is 'pumped' into the endolymph from the blood by the activity of the stria vascularis, although other mechanisms have been suggested.

At present the physiological role played by the unique composition of the endolymph remains obscure. The high K/low Na ratio appears to lead to the following important conclusions:

(1) The walls of the scala media present a barrier to the passage of electrolyte ions.

(2) The positive endolymphatic potential (*see below*) cannot be due to electrolyte concentrations because these would result in a negative and not a positive voltage.

(3) The hair-cells and non-medullated nerve fibres of the organ of Corti cannot be bathed in endolymph. This follows from the neurophysiological fact that nerve action potentials cannot arise in the presence of a high potassium concentration outside the polarized membrane of nerve cells. We are led by this to the facts that the fluid in the tunnel of Corti (cortilymph) cannot be endolymph, and that an impermeable barrier separates the upper surfaces of the hair-cells from the scala media. Lawrence (1960), however, presents contrary arguments to the effect that the cortilymph *is* endolymph, although he admits that the problem of how the nerve fibres could function in a high potassium concentration remains unsolved.

The problem of the so-called cortilymph has received much attention. On electron microscopic evidence, Engström (quoted by Vosteen) believes that the tunnel is completely closed in every direction, and that the cortilymph is an intra-epithelial accumulation of intracellular fluid. Other evidence indicates that the cortilymph is chemically similar to perilymph and that it is probably derived from the scala

Table 2.2 Composition of inner ear fluids (data from Vosteen, 1963)

Substance or measure	*Blood serum*	*CSF*	*Perilymph*	*Endolymph*	*Author*
Man					
Sodium, mEq/l	141	141	135–150	13–16	Rauch
Potassium, mEq/l	5	2.5	7–8	140–160	Rauch
Chlorine, mEq/l	101	126	135	120–130	Rauch
Magnesium, mg/100 ml	2	2	2		Rauch
Protein, total	7000	10–25	70–100	20–30	Rauch
CO_2, mEq/l	27	18	10	20	Rauch
Phosphor Anorg., mg/100 ml	2	1	1–3	0.8–1.3	Rauch
pH	7.35	7.35	7.2	7.5	Rauch
Cat					
Sodium, mEq/l	155	162	164	66	Citron, Exley, *et al.*
Potassium, mEq/l	6.7	5.9	6.0	117.0	Citron, Exley, *et al.*
Chlorine, mEq/1		150 152	150 158	151 151	Citron, Exley, *et al.*, Ledoux
Protein, mg/100 g		31 25	268 142	118	Ledoux, Citron, Exley, *et al.*
Non-protein nitrogen, mg/100 g		20	21		Citron, Exley, *et al.*
Co_2, vol/100 ml (stp)		43.2	32.0	31.5	Ledoux
pH		7.45	7.87	7.82	Ledoux
Refractory index, 22 °C		1.33435	1.33495	1.33455	Ledoux
Osmotic pressure		1.017	1.046	1.058	Aldred, *et al.*

tympani. Schuknecht and Seifi (1963) demonstrated in the cat the presence of minute openings in the osseous spiral lamina which lead from the scala tympani to the habenula perforata and organ of Corti. Von Ilberg (1968) demonstrated, in guinea-pigs, that particles of thorium dioxide injected into the perilymphatic space could be subsequently found in certain situations which suggested that the cortilymph space communicates freely with the scala tympani; and he concluded that cortilymph might in fact be identical with perilymph. Engström himself does not necessarily subscribe to this view but, whatever the composition of this fluid in Corti's tunnel, Axelsson (1968) believes that nearby vessels, which he described, in the basilar membrane and tympanic lip may be of some importance in its formation and absorption. Being much nearer to the organ of Corti than is the stria vascularis, he suggests that they may also be concerned in supplying oxygen to the organ, although this has been widely believed to be a function of the stria (*see below*).

Origin, circulation and absorption of the perilymph

The similar chemical compositions of the perilymph and of the cerebrospinal fluid (CSF), and the existence of the aqueduct of the cochlea which joins the subarachnoid and perilymphatic spaces, have suggested that perilymph is indeed CSF. The embarrassing and unending flow of perilymph which has occasionally occurred from the vestibule during stapedectomy operations indicates that in these conditions at least a free flow of CSF may occur from the subarachnoid space to the labyrinth. However, although perilymph is chemically similar to CSF, detailed analysis shows differences in the concentrations of amino-acids as well as in the protein fractions as revealed by immune electrophoresis. Experimental evidence suggests, however, that in the intact ear the perilymph is produced within the labyrinth, probably as a direct blood filtrate from the vessels of the spiral ligament. Work by Axelsson (1968) suggests formation in the scala vestibuli and absorption in the scala tympani.

Origin, circulation and absorption of the endolymph

Endolymph is thought by some authorities to be secreted by the stria vascularis or by the adjacent tissues of the outer sulcus. The evidence is circumstantial and is based upon:

(1) The extremely rich blood supply of the stria.
(2) The presence of glandular ducts shown histologically in the region of the outer sulcus.
(3) The very strong activity of oxidative enzymes, indicating a high metabolic rate in the vicinity of these ducts (Vosteen).
(4) Marked similarities of electron-microscopic detail between the tissues of the stria which face the scala media and those of glandular structures in other parts of the body.

The special composition of the endolymph with its high potassium and low sodium content indicates that this fluid is produced by an active secretory energy-consuming process, and the region of the stria vascularis is well adapted to the purpose. Whether the ducts of the outer sulcus might also be concerned with re-absorption or with pressure regulation in the scala media remains uncertain.

The 'classic' route of re-absorption is the endolymphatic duct and sac, although this is not universally agreed. The fact that the sac was experimentally destroyed in cats without apparent changes in the scala media or in the hearing (Lindsay *et al.*, 1952) suggested that other routes must exist. Later work, however, (Kimura, 1967; Schuknecht *et al.*, 1968) demonstrated labyrinthine hydrops and atrophy of the organ of Corti after destruction of the saccus. Biochemical analysis (Fernandez, 1967) reveals differences between the cochlear and saccus endolymphs which are compatible with a re-absorptive process in the latter organ.

Naftalin and Harrison (1958) suggested that endolymph is derived from perilymph across Reissner's membrane, and is re-absorbed by the stria vascularis. They account for the reversed electrolyte concentration by suggesting that the stria vascularis is selective, leaving potassium in the endolymph at a raised concentration. This point is re-inforced by analogy with similar ionic adjustments by the renal tubules, and the possible influence of aldosterone upon these processes in the ear is raised.

Work supporting the theory of Naftalin and Harrison has been published by Lawrence *et al.* (1961) based upon the electron-microscopical structure of Reissner's membrane and upon the effects of localized injuries of Reissner's membrane on cochlear function.

To summarize, it remains still uncertain whether the perilymph or the stria vascularis is the origin of the endolymph, and whether the circulation is radial (across the scala media), longitudinal towards the saccus, or a combination of both routes. That two separate systems, cochlear and vestibular, may exist (perhaps demarcated by the utriculo-endolymphatic valve) remains a real possibility (Seymour, 1954).

Oxygen distribution and utilization in the cochlea

It is probable that the organ of Corti has no direct blood supply and depends for its metabolic activities upon diffusion of oxygen from the stria vascularis across the scala media. It is generally believed that this arrangement is necessary for the acoustic insulation of the hair-cells from inevitable noise arising in blood vessels.

Energy-producing metabolic processes depend upon the function of specific intracellular enzymes, and the distribution of these enzymes in the cochlea has been well described by Vosteen. From such histochemical studies deductions are possible regarding the rates and types of carbohydrate metabolism and oxygen utilization in different parts of the organ of Corti and stria vascularis.

Misrahy *et al.* (1958) showed convincingly that oxygen reaches the hair-cells from the scala media. They injected into the scala media a mixture of glucose and the enzyme glucose-oxidase, thus rendering the endolymph oxygen-deficient. Immediately the cochlear microphonics disappeared. By making such injections at localized points of the cochlea, and selecting appropriate test frequencies Misrahy showed that the effect of such oxygen deprivation was localized to the injected turn.

In other experiments Misrahy showed with a recording electrode introduced into the scala media that there is a gradient of oxygen tension which is highest (44–70 mmHg) near the stria vascularis, and lowest near the organ of Corti (16–25 mmHg). Vosteen comments that on this basis the oxygen tension would be nearing the critical level in some parts of the organ of Corti – that is, the level (3–4 mmHg) below which all oxidative metabolism ceases.

It would appear from these facts that the high metabolic rate of the organ of Corti is maintained by oxygen supplies which are only just adequate. Many experiments show that cochlear function is severely and rapidly depressed by lowered oxygen tension in the bloodstream, or by obstruction of the arteries or veins of the cochlea.

The effects of sound stimulation upon the oxygen tension in the scala media are of great interest. Misrahy showed that after a brief increase the oxygen tension falls rapidly and markedly. Yoshioka (quoted by Vosteen) found that the blood supply of the stria vascularis is affected by intense sound stimuli. It appears, therefore, that such stimuli will tend to reduce the oxygen supply to the organ of Corti at a time when its metabolic activity and oxygen needs are greatest. In such circumstances the sensory cells must be vulnerable, and these observations have obvious interest in connection with the pathogenesis of noise deafness.

Electrical potentials in the cochlea

The study of electrical phenomena in the inner ear is of prime importance in all matters relating to the physiology and pathology of hearing. Two main types of potential have been identified, the steady or resting state potentials, and the superimposed a.c. voltage fluctuations due to acoustic stimulation.

The *resting potentials* were discovered and measured by the insertion of exploring micro-electrodes into various parts of the cochlea under microscopic observation. The most striking finding is a *positive* potential of some 80 mV in the scala media (with reference to scala tympani) known as *endolymphatic potential* or EP.

Insertion of the electrode into a hair-cell reveals a *negative* potential of about 80 mV so that there is an overall potential difference between the scala media and the interior of the hair-cells of 160 mV. In physiological work generally this is a strikingly high voltage difference to find across a cell membrane.

A small positive potential of some 5 mV is also noted in the scala vestibuli. *Figure 2.16* shows the distribution of these resting potentials.

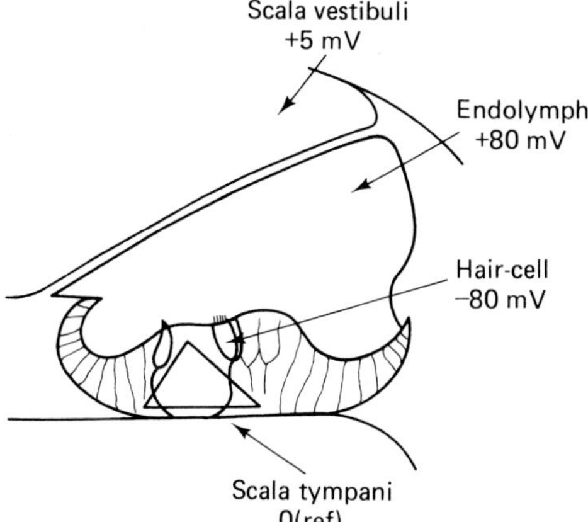

Figure 2.16 The electrical polarization (d.c. potentials) within the cochlea

The EP is not due to the differences in electrolyte composition of the various scalae, since these would lead to a negative and not a positive electrical potential. Tasaki and Spyropoulos (1959) showed that the EP was highest directly over the stria vascularis, and was present even in guinea-pigs with complete congenital absence of the organ of Corti. It appears likely that in addition to its other functions, the stria vascularis is responsible for the maintenance of EP. Vosteen has suggested that EP may be a by-product of the potassium 'pump'.

The *electrical responses* of the cochlea to acoustic stimulation were first described by Wever and Bray. These responses can be detected from any part of the cochlea or auditory nerve, and appear at the very conveniently accessible round window. They have been measured and studied extensively in animals and in man. As an indication of sound transmission in the conducting apparatus they have been the essential basis of much of the experimental work from which our knowledge of middle-ear function has been built up. (Their application to clinical work is discussed in Chapter 1, Vol 2.) It is accepted that the microphonic potentials follow with linear fidelity the waveform and amplitude of the acoustic stimulus from the lowest intensity levels that can

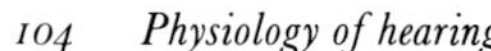

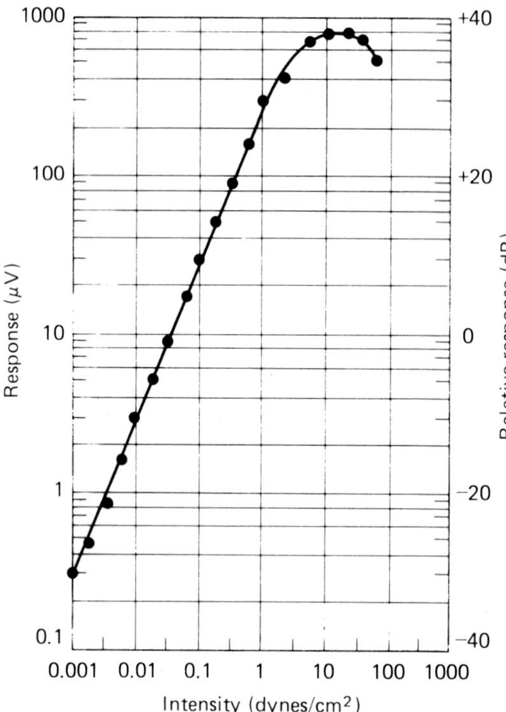

Figure 2.17 Cochlear microphonic potentials (in the cat) showing a linear relationship between intensity of stimulus at 1000 Hz (abscissa) and cochlear response (ordinate). Note the onset of distortion at stimulus levels just above 1 dyne/cm^2. (Reproduced from Wever, 1949, *Theory of Hearing*, by courtesy of John Wiley)

be measured (well below sensation threshold) up to levels of around 1 dyne/cm^2. Beyond this point distortion sets in and the response curve (*Figure 2.17*) rolls off and begins to fall. Frequency response is accurate throughout the audible range and beyond. There is no latent period between the stimulus and the microphonic and adaptation and fatigue are not observed. It has been found that the microphonic potentials are a composite of several electrical activities. These are:

(1) The auditory nerve *action potential*, or AP, which consists of an aggregate of the action potentials of the individual nerve fibres. These potentials are similar to those of other nerves – namely, a spike discharge preceded by a latent period and followed by a refractory period. The AP component of the microphonics is large when the electrode is near the modiolus or the nerve trunk, but is relatively small when recorded from the scalae or round window.

(2) The *cochlear microphonic*, or CM. This is the main component and confers upon the cochlear potentials the characteristics described above. It has two elements, CM1, which is oxygen dependent and is abolished by oxygen lack or by death of the individual, and CM2, about 10 per cent of the whole, which can still be elicited for several hours after total oxygen deprivation or death.

The origin of CM is conclusively shown to be the physical stimulation of the hair-cells and, by use of differential recording electrodes above and below a given point on the basilar membrane, its place of origin along the cochlea has been shown to be determined by the stimulus frequency. When the hair-cells have degenerated from streptomycin poisoning, or are congenitally absent, CM is absent too. It has been suggested that CM is generated at the hair-cell–tectorial membrane area by a purely piezo-electrical effect due to deformation by sound vibrations of the hairs or hair-cell bodies. Davis (1957, 1958) considers this improbable and suggests that the physical disturbances at this point act by varying the electrical resistance of the cell membrane. We have already seen that there is a potential of some 160 mV across this membrane, so that relatively large currents may flow when the resistance of the membrane is altered. This action would be similar to that of a thermionic valve, and the energy developed in the microphonic potentials would be derived not from the acoustic signal which triggers them, but through the biological 'high tension' voltage supply maintained in the resting state. Such a theory for the transduction of acoustic to electrical energy is a very attractive one, first because it provides a situation where amplification as well as transduction can occur, and secondly because of the obvious facility with which such electrical processes could stimulate the nerve endings of the auditory nerve. Naftalin (1968) offers an important and extended discussion of the biophysical problems of transduction in the cochlea and his paper should be studied in the original.

(3) *Summation potentials*, or SP. This last type of cochlear potential, like CM, results from acoustic stimulation, and consists of a change in EP which may be in the positive or the negative sense (SP+ and SP−). Unlike CM it does not follow the actual instantaneous values of the sound stimulus, but is proportional to the r.m.s. (root mean square) acoustic pressure. In more technical terms it is a rectified and 'detected' version of the sound signal – a representation of the wave-form's envelope, not of the individual waves themselves.

SP becomes most conspicuous at higher sound levels, beyond the point at which distortion begins in CM. It is thought to originate in the hair-cell–reticular lamina area, like CM, but is probably the product of a different mode of differential vibration between the organ of Corti and the tectorial membrane from that which produces CM. Davis suggests that SP is mainly produced by the inner hair-cells, which are regarded as effective for higher sound intensities, in contrast with CM, produced in the much more sensitive outer hair-cell system.

Cochlear hydrodynamics

There is a basic assumption underlying present-day theories of hearing, and which has been relied upon throughout this chapter, that the cochlear fluids vibrate instantaneously from window to window. These movements are those of a fluid column vibrating back and forth without significant compression and rarefaction of its constituent molecules. This means that a sound wave, as such, does not travel through the cochlear fluids. This conception is supported by powerful physical arguments, but the reader should bear in mind that an assumption lacking direct experimental proof is being made. Opposite views have been put forward to the effect that actual waves may be propagated in the fluid medium, and in this, as in so many other auditory questions, the last word may still be unwritten.

Accepting the usual and most likely view of the mode of the fluid vibrations, we must now consider how the cochlear partition is caused to vibrate. It is on this point that most of the discussions regarding the mode of action of the inner ear have centred. At the present time Békésy's extensive researches are generally considered to give the most valid account. He used models of the cochlea, and also made direct observations under magnification of the basilar membrane in motion. This work has shown that in response to acoustic vibrations applied to either of the scalae, a so-called travelling wave appears. This wave begins from the basal end of the basilar membrane and moves towards the apex. It increases in amplitude as it moves until a maximum is reached. Beyond this the amplitude falls rapidly and there is an alteration in the phase of the vibrations. In the surrounding fluids eddy currents appear immediately beyond the point of maximum amplitude.

It has been repeatedly observed that the form of the travelling wave is independent of frequency, but that the region of maximum displacement of the basilar membrane varies according to the frequency. High-pitched sounds cause a 'short' travelling

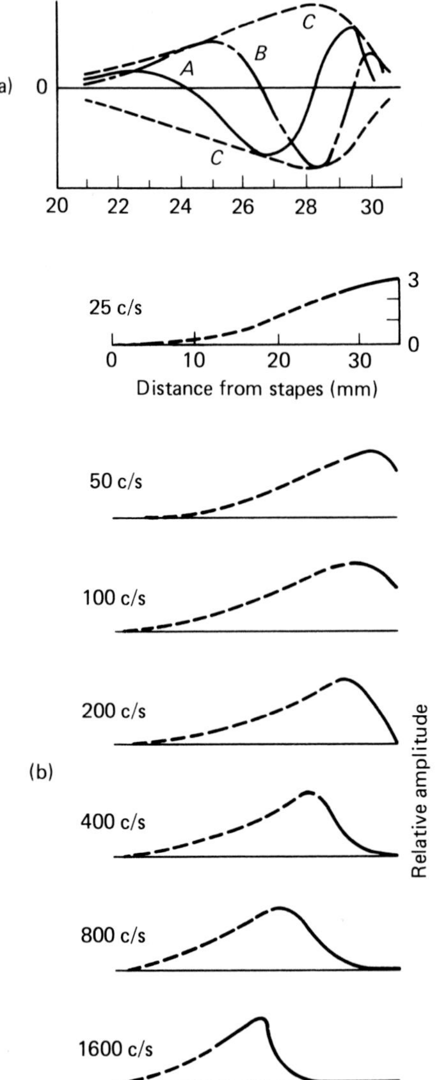

Figure 2.18 The travelling wave concept.

(a) Detail of the form of vibration of the cochlear partition (for 200 Hz [c/s] at two different moments, A and B within a cycle. The broken lines, *C*, *C*, show the displacement 'envelope' for one whole cycle (after Békésy, 1960)

(b) Travelling wave envelopes indicating the loci of maximum displacement at different frequencies (for clarity only one half of each envelope is shown) (after Békésy, 1960)

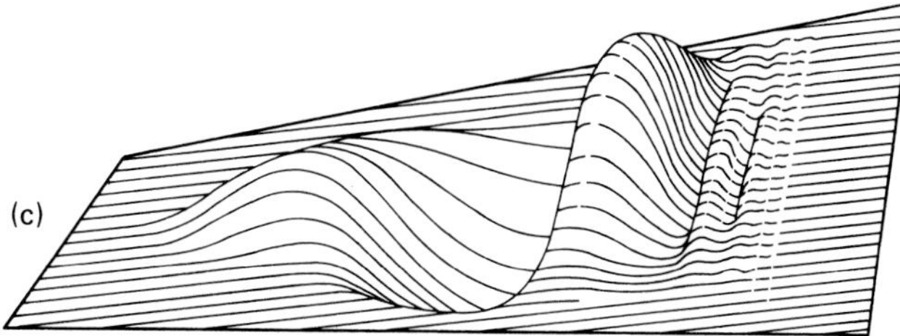

(c) Pictorial display (after Tonndorf, 1962) showing how the fixed margins of the basilar membrane necessitate a transverse deformation as well as a longitudinal one. At the point of maximum displacement longitudinal and transverse curvatures are equal. On the stapedial or proximal side of the maximum displacement transverse curvature predominates, and on the distal side the longitudinal curvature is the more marked

wave which does not extend beyond the basal turn. Middle and low frequency stimuli have their maxima progressively nearer the apex as the frequency is lowered (*Figure 2.18*).

Theories of hearing

The facts given above render improbable both of the classic theories of hearing. In their original forms these theories (of Helmholtz and Rutherford) appeared to be mutually exclusive and contradictory. It will be shown below that in modified versions they probably supplement each other in a way that their originators did not anticipate.

Helmholtz suggested that frequency analysis by the ear was due to the fact that each pitch would cause resonant vibration of its own particular 'place' on the basilar membrane. It was postulated, with some support from anatomical observations, that the length, mass and tension of the combined basilar membrane and organ of Corti varied progressively from the base to the apex of the cochlea so as to form a series of tuned resonators. Unfortunately for this hypothesis the basilar membrane far from meets all the physical requirements of a series of highly tuned resonators. In fact, damping, not resonance, is the more conspicuous property of this complex system. Another objection, stressed by several workers, is that the known ability of the ear to distinguish accurately very small shifts of frequency would require that the fibres of the basilar membrane should be under strong tension across the membrane while preserving independence of action (very loose coupling) in the longitudinal direction. The evidence is against this. In particular, the observation that a probe applied perpendicularly to the membrane causes a circular indentation implies very strongly that the tension is the same in all directions.

It is now generally accepted that along the basilar membrane there is a significant gradation of the length of its constituent fibres, of the mass of the vibrating parts and, possibly the most important, of their stiffness. These factors can account for the comparatively 'flat' or damped response curve of the travelling wave, but not for the sharply tuned system proposed by Helmholtz.

Rutherford's 'telephone' hypothesis of cochlear action suggested that the basilar membrane vibrates uniformly in all its parts and that its amplitude represents the intensity of the signal. Meanwhile, he postulated, the frequency of the signal is represented by the rate of the firing of the auditory nerve fibres. Such an hypothesis reduces the complexity of the auditory nerve to that of a mere piece of wire and relegates to the central nervous system all problems relating to frequency analysis. Such a view has never been acceptable in the light of what is known of neurophysiology. The refractory period of nervous action would in itself limit the upper frequency of the system to less than 1000 Hz.

A great variety of theories bearing their author's names have attempted to overcome the difficulties inherent in Rutherford's and Helmholtz's hypotheses. In general they have not withstood the test of time and newer discoveries, but the interested reader will find them reviewed by Wever (1949), and will appreciate what efforts of penetration and intellect have, down the years, been applied to this thorny problem.

Wever himself appears to have been the first to put forward the so-called *volley theory* of hearing, and because this theory meets many of the facts and has steadily received confirmation from subsequent experimental findings, it must be described here in some detail. The theory states that the place principle accounts for perception of high frequencies (above 5000 Hz) which stimulate the hair-cells in the basal turn only. Low frequencies (below 400 Hz) stimulate the entire organ of Corti, and are represented in the auditory nerve by nerve fibre responses which are directly synchronous with the applied signal wave-form (in Hz). Between 400 and 5000 Hz groups of fibres fire asynchronously so that, despite the limitation of the frequency capacity of each individual fibre, the frequency of the signal is presented to the CNS by sequential firing in pairs, trios or quartets of fibres. There is presumed to be a gradual transition from one mode of action to the next, as signal frequency is raised or lowered. *Figure 2.19* indicates how the volley principle might operate for a tone of intermediate frequency.

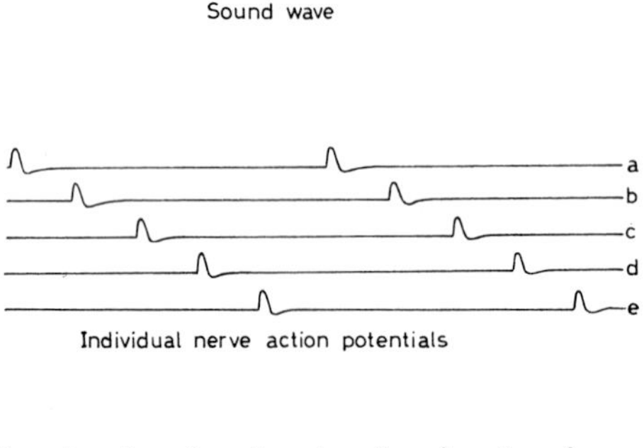

Figure 2.19 The 'volley theory' (after Wever, 1949). Above is a sine wave trace representing a tone of intermediate frequency. Each nerve fibre, (a) to (e), responds in turn with a spike potential, to every fifth cycle. The brain receives from the combined activity of these five neurones a synchronous relay of spike potentials representing the original frequency

It will be evident that such a theory of cochlear action would fit satisfactorily the travelling wave principle for the basilar membrane. It will also be evident that if the frequency dimension is transduced in terms of the rate of nerve fibre discharges, the dimension of loudness must presumably be transduced by a mechanism which controls the numbers of active nerve fibres. Schuknecht (1958) summarized the possible variables in a pattern of neuronal activity as follows:

(1) Frequency of impulses in a single fibre (below 1000 Hz).
(2) Time relation between impulses in the various fibres.
(3) Selectivity as to which fibres are being activated.
(4) The number of fibres activated.

The volley theory is supported by direct recordings of action potentials in the auditory nerve, and its individual fibres. Recordings of the cochlear microphonics along the cochlear spiral also re-inforce the idea that high frequencies are transduced only in the basal turn. An important contribution to the volley theory has emerged from the study of the effects of partial section of the auditory nerve (Guild, Dandy). It seems that whatever part of the nerve is divided by a cut commencing from its periphery the result is always a high-tone deafness. The fibres from the basal turn are arranged spatially from the modiolus around the outer aspect of the nerve trunk. The lower frequencies, which the volley theory maintains are subserved by larger areas of the basilar membrane and more of the nerve fibres, would understandably be far less vulnerable to a partial nerve trunk lesion of this kind.

Another sphere of research, namely the study of stimulation deafness, indicates very strongly the operation of the place principle for the higher frequencies. After acoustic trauma electrical, audiological and histological studies show clearly selectivity of injurious sounds, according to their frequencies, for certain places along the organ of Corti.

Further considerations

The reader will find much interest in the extended treatment of the volley theory, and the travelling wave, in the writings of Wever (1949), Békésy (1960), Lawrence (1960, 1962), Davis (1957, 1958) and others. At this point we must move on to consider the implications of these matters in terms of the mechano-electrical processes at the organ of Corti.

As has already been pointed out, one of the chief objections to a process of frequency analysis by place is the fact that the basilar membrane is not sharply tuned. Indeed, direct observation of the travelling wave shows that the membrane vibrates over wide areas, and its area of maximum displacement is fairly diffuse. This must mean that the area over which the hair-cells are stimulated is correspondingly wide. Such a broad zone of stimulation cannot easily account for the known ability of the ear in terms of pitch discrimination.

In theoretical terms some authors suggest that frequency discrimination is based not upon the broad localization of the maximum displacement, but upon sensory detection of its mathematical derivatives, for example the slope of the displacement curve or the rate of change of the slope. This merely suggests what happens without indicating how it is done. Searches have been made for mechanisms which might permit a 'sharpening' of pitch discrimination, and at least two interesting possibilities are open.

From a study of the lie of the fibrils in the tectorial membrane Békésy deduced that their oblique orientation from the fixed to the unattached margin would result, during acoustic stimulation, in three different modes of pressure on the underlying hairs near the maximum displacement of the travelling wave. Immediately proximal to the point of peak displacement a radial shearing action would occur. At the point of peak displacement the pressures would be perpendicular to the plane of action. Finally, just distal to the point of peak displacement a longitudinal shearing force would be present. That these modes of action have different stimulation values was shown by an experiment in which a microprobe was used to vibrate the tectorial membrane in various directions relative to the hair-cells. Each mode produces a different intensity of CM response. From these ideas it can be argued that the central nervous system receives sufficient data from which it can 'select' the indicated frequency while suppressing the adjacent ones. A neurophysiological process termed 'funnelling' (*see below*) provides a possible central mechanism for this process.

Another possibility is that the summation potential, which is probably evoked by a longitudinal shift of the tectorial membrane, particularly over the inner hair-cells, is sufficiently localized in relationship to the basilar membrane displacement to be the actual triggering stimulus which determines frequency discrimination. Yet another differentiating factor arises from the architectural differences in the inner and outer parts of the organ of Corti. The structure of this complex is such that the outer hair-cells are subjected to a different pattern of pressures from the inner hair-cells and are stimulated by much lower sound intensities than the latter. There is here a possible mechanism for the analysis of loudness, and possibly also an explanation of loudness recruitment in end-organ lesions.

Innervation of the hair-cells

In man there are about 17 000 hair-cells in each cochlea and the auditory nerve contains some 25 000 fibres. These fibres flow outward from the spiral ganglion in an orderly arrangement to the organ of Corti. As they are followed peripherally they lose their medullary sheaths and divide into branches. Some of the branches terminate on the bases of inner hair-cells, while others cross the floor of the tunnel of Corti and, coursing up and down the basilar membrane, terminate upon outer hair-cells. Each fibre therefore reaches several hair-cells, and each hair-cell receives branches from many fibres. Different types of nerve endings have been described upon the hair-cells, but at present very little is known of how they may differ functionally. Perhaps the most remarkable work in this connection was the tracing of the efferent cochlear fibres (*see below*) to the hair-cells by Kimura and Wersall (1962), who suggested that the larger nerve endings are the efferent terminations of the olivocochlear bundle of Rasmussen, while the smaller endings are those of afferent fibres.

A more detailed account of the innervation pattern of the hair-cells is given in Chapter 1, and it will be appreciated that the complexities of overlapping as between groups of hair-cells and groups of fibres must provide a matrix or computer mechanism for peripheral analysis along the basilar membrane. If the reader recalls the (oversimplified) account of cochlear action outlined in the previous few pages, the differential vibration patterns to which the travelling wave exposes the hair-cells along the cochlear axis, and the differential vibration patterns across the cochlea as between inner and outer hair-cells, and if he then visualizes the possibilities of neuronal summation among branches of 17 000 individual nerve fibres, each 'receiving' from a number of hair-cells, he may appreciate, even without fully understanding its mechanism, that here is a transducer with a capacity for analysis fully adequate for its task.

Action potentials in the auditory nerve

Each individual nerve fibre obeys the all-or-none principle, responding with a spike potential if the stimulus rises above threshold. The size of the action potential depends on the state of the nerve at the moment of stimulation, and cannot be varied in any way by varying the stimulus. The action potentials of individual auditory nerve fibres have been studied by many workers, notably Tasaki (1957) and Kiang *et al.* (1962). It has been shown that each fibre has an optimum frequency of sound stimulus for which its threshold is lowest. As the stimulus frequency is moved away from this optimum the threshold intensity rises until, beyond certain frequency ranges, the fibre will not fire at any intensity. Thus each fibre has an optimum stimulus frequency, and a limited response 'area' above and below it (*Figure 2.20*). The discharge rate for a single fibre is related to stimulus intensity, and extends over a dynamic range from threshold to a maximum of some 25 dB above.

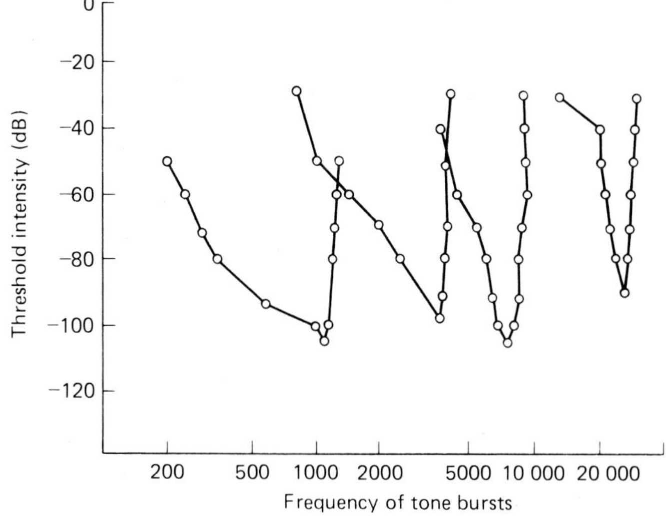

Figure 2.20 'Response areas' of individual auditory nerve fibres (after Kiang *et al.*, 1962). Representative response areas or tuning curves for four different auditory nerve fibres. Each curve is obtained by setting the intensity of tone bursts and measuring the frequency range for which spike responses are obtained. The limits of this frequency range for a number of intensities are represented by points joined to produce a 'curve'. The abscissa of the lowest point of each curve is defined as the characteristic frequency of that unit

Although the discharge rate of single neurons is rather irregular, the volley theory is supported by the observation that the rate of firing in groups of fibres corresponds to the stimulus frequency up to about 1500 Hz. The orderly localization of frequency along the basilar membrane correlates in a re-assuring way with the spatial arrangement of the individual fibres in the nerve trunk as identified by their optimum stimulus frequencies.

The action potentials for the whole nerve trunk indicate that higher sound intensities to some extent cause activity of increasing numbers of fibres, but the problem of intensity-coding still appears to cause misgivings among authorities who regard the classic difficulties of frequency-coding as virtually solved.

The efferent cochlear system

Experimental stimulation of the efferent cochlear fibres in the floor of the fourth ventricle has been shown to increase the threshold for afferent nerve potentials resulting from acoustic stimulation of the ear. Other work indicates that the efferent nerve endings upon the hair-cells liberate acetylcholine, and that acetylcholine esterase disappears from the organ of Corti after section and degeneration of the efferent tracts. Further data will doubtless have major significance for the physiology of hearing, for it appears that in this efferent system we have a kind of negative feedback arrangement linked at brain stem level with the cochlear nuclei and under control from cortical levels by descending fibres. The possibilities for the regulation of the sensitivity of the sense-organ complex are numerous, both by reflex and through conscious channels (variations in attentiveness 'listening', and so on). It may be that in the reflex activity of the efferent fibres a servomechanism responds to stimulus–intensity changes, holding the afferent fibre activity within limits which the spatial and temporal coding system can handle. The efferent cochlear system should prove a very fruitful field of study over the next few years.

Recruitment

Loudness recruitment due to inner-ear disease has received various explanations in pathophysiological terms, but concrete evidence regarding its causes is lacking. It must be remembered that the recruitment effect is a continuous function over the whole intensity range of the deafened ear, and is characterized by reduced intensity limen. Tumarkin (1954) has suggested that selective loss of the more sensitive outer hair-cells causes the observed threshold impairment, while the comparatively normal inner hair-cells 'take over' at normal outputs for higher sound intensities. Such a mechanism does not easily account for over-recruitment, or the reduction of difference limen. It appears feasible that the efferent cochlear nerves might repay study in this connection. If, indeed, a feedback mechanism exists as suggested above, regulating within certain broad limits the response patterns for the afferent fibres according to changes in signal intensity, it would be easy to understand how functional impairment of this mechanism could result in recruitment, over-recruitment, and difference limen changes.

Masking

The masking of a tone by a louder sound of approximately similar frequency is called *ipsilateral direct masking*. This mechanism is independent of the central nervous system, and electrical studies show that the signal tone and the masking sound are both represented in the cochlear microphonic. Therefore, the masking process must occur by interaction of the two sounds at the transduction stage of the hair-cell–neurone complex. Presumably the nerve fibres required for the signal frequency are pre-empted by the masking sound, but the precise mechanism is not clear.

The investigations of Fletcher and Munson (1937), and more recently of Hood, have defined the optimum characteristics for a masking sound – a narrow band of filtered white noise centred on the frequency of the test tone.

Remote masking

Remote masking is the term used to describe changes in threshold of a tone caused by a masking sound in a different frequency range. To achieve the same degree of masking, a higher intensity of masking sound is required than is necessary for direct masking.

Transcranial masking

This is due to acoustical leakage of a masking sound around the head to the opposite ear.

Central masking

Central masking results from the intermingling of the central connections of the two ears. Presumably final common neural pathways are pre-empted by the masking sound from one ear, to the exclusion of the masked tone from the other.

Distortion in the ear

There are several forms of sound distortion to which the ear, in common with other acoustic devices, is subject. These are:

(1) *Frequency distortion* – the 'preferential' transmission of certain frequencies as compared with others.
(2) *Phase distortion* – changes in the phase relationships of the constituent frequencies of a complex sound.
(3) *Amplitude distortion* – non-linear variations in the responses caused by changes in signal intensity. In its worst form this distortion is observed at the highest intensities where the response curve begins to 'roll off' due to gross overloading.

Amplitude distortion is perhaps the most important of the above. It results in the generation of spurious harmonic and so-called combination tones. Combination tones occur if the ear is stimulated with two or more tones simultaneously, whereupon additional frequencies corresponding to both the sums and the differences of the signal frequencies are heard by the subject, and are detectable in the cochlear microphonic potentials. Another remarkable phenomenon at high intensity levels is the apparent change in pitch of a tone when its intensity is increased.

These distortions in hearing function have been extensively studied since they would appear to offer clues concerning the physiology of hearing. Wever and Lawrence (1954) discuss them in detail and conclude that, within the physiological range of the ear, distortion of all kinds is virtually absent in the conducting mechanism which functions throughout with remarkable linearity. From the sustained purity of the signal as traced acoustically from the ossicular chain and from the round window itself, they argue convincingly that both the combination tones and harmonic distortion present in the microphonic response must originate in the electromechanical events at the organ of Corti. Without going into further details here, it should be noted that their view represents a departure from earlier theories, which held that the middle-ear mechanism was the main source of overtones, combination tones, and other distortion processes.

Central processes of hearing

In the brain stem acoustic stimulation of the ear results in neuronal activity which can be followed by exploring electrodes. It has been shown that there is a close correlation between the plan of the cochlear nucleus and of the cochlea. In traversing the nucleus an electrode can plot a sequence of stimuli of varying frequency, which corresponds with the sequence along the basilar membrane. The cochlea is said to be *unrolled* in the cochlear nucleus. It is at this level that some degree of 'funnelling' (with sharpening of pitch perception) is thought to occur. Electrode studies have shown that when a given group of neurones in the cochlear nucleus is activated by a sound stimulus of appropriate frequency at the ear, resting activity is inhibited in the adjacent neurones.

In ascending the brain stem the second- and third-order neurones undergo partial decussation, and interaction of stimuli from the two ears becomes possible. Neuronal circuits subserving the tympanic muscle reflexes and others linking with the efferent cochlear system add to the complexities of the region.

Cortical activity in audition

Information on the physiology of the auditory cortex in man is based upon direct stimulation of the auditory areas during operations under local anaesthesia (Penfield and Rasmussen, 1950) supplemented by fragmentary details of the effects of known pathological lesions. Recently, techniques for the direct recording of brain activity through the intact skull in response to sensory stimulation of hearing, have become available in the form of electric response audiometry (Chapter 2, Volume 2). Animal experiments, such as those of Neff (1958) and of Roberts (1960), have shown by direct recording from the surface of the brain that the spread of auditory activity is much wider than was previously thought, and involves temporal lobe, insula, suprasylvian areas, anterior lateral gyri, and part of the motor area.

In terms of sound analysis, the main facts which have so far emerged are that pitch recognition, and the learning of conditioned reflexes to sound stimuli can occur after ablation of the auditory cortex. Localization of a sound source, however, and sound pattern discrimination are affected by cortical lesions. In man stimulation of the cortex causes various complex auditory hallucinations and recalls auditory memories. Spatial projections in terms of frequency are not clearly definable.

Localization of a sound source

Monaurally, a fair estimate of the position of a sound source in relation to the hearer can be made if the subject can alter the position of his head while the signal continues. This facility is complex and must be based upon at least two different sound patterns received, and at cortical levels the ability to remember the first while comparing it with the second. A judgment, perhaps based upon experience of similar situations, is then made.

Of greater physiological interest is the mechanism of binaural localization of a sound source. In the study of this phenomenon it is necessary to consider the following.

The available sound clues

Physical measurements in a free sound field show that at the position of the two ears of a dummy head there are interaural differences in respect of sound intensity, phase, and time of onset of the stimulus. Interaural intensity differences are greater for higher frequencies because of the sound 'shadow' effects of the head. Differences in phase angle at the two ears depend upon the wavelength (and therefore frequency) of the signal. The difference in time of arrival of the stimulus at the two ears depends on the different distances between each ear and the sound source, but for a low frequency pure-tone stimulus the phase difference, expressed as time, is the same as the time difference. Detailed measurements (Nordlund, 1962) show that the interaural intensity differences are irregular in relation to changes in position of the sound source, whereas phase and time differences have a constant and predictable linear relationship to the angular position of the sound source.

Utilization of localizing clues

By means of binaural testing with earphones, and in free-field conditions, Nordlund found that:

(1) Interaural phase differences are useful clues only below 1400 Hz. Since intensity differences are negligible at lower frequencies, the phase differences must form the basis for sound localization in this range.

(2) Interaural intensity differences are the basis for sound location for frequencies above 1400 Hz. Because of the irregular relationships between the angular location of the sound and the intensity differences, accurate localization for high frequencies can only be achieved if the head can be moved to scan the sound field and centre itself in the balance position where the intensities at the two ears become equal.

(3) Time differences are probably important for localization of complex sounds, and particularly for transients.

A degree of accuracy of localization ranging from 5 to 17 degrees is achieved in experimental conditions.

Neurological mechanisms

The neurological mechanisms involved in binaural sound localization have been reviewed by Rosenzweig (1961). The necessary interaction between the neuronal response patterns from the two ears has been sought at all levels. It would appear that the lowest level at which this could occur is at the superior olivary nuclei. Numerous ablation experiments indicate that the auditory cortex is essential, but it appears possible that after removal of only one hemisphere sound localization can still be achieved.

Clinical assessment of sound localizing ability may become a useful tool. Lesions of the conducting mechanism which result in a phase alteration (for example, the fenestration operation) have a measurable effect on sound localization, and a system of audiometric investigation as planned by Nordlund may eventually help in the topognosis of neurological, as well as ear, disorders.

Throughout this chapter the reader will, it is hoped, be aware of omissions and inconsistencies. For example, the all-important question regarding the final conversion of acoustic energy into nervous impulses has not been discussed. Whether this takes place through direct electrical stimulation of nerve endings or through chemical mediation (for example, by liberation of acetylcholine) is far from being decided. Even the generally accepted views concerning the mechanisms of sound conduction and sound transformation regularly come under fire. Other difficulties are not lacking. The code form through which the ear presents acoustical data to the brain is still imperfectly understood. When once this code is known, in terms of the precise spatial and temporal activities of the auditory nerve, we can expect to have a clarification of how the cochlea functions, based upon precise knowledge of what it does. Similarly, when the full encoded pattern which reaches the cochlear nuclei from the ear is understood the study of the central mechanisms of sound perception will be made easier.

References

Allen, G. W. and Fernandez, C. (1960). *Annals of Otology, Rhinology and Laryngology*, **69,** 5

Axelsson, A. (1968). *Acta otolaryngologica, Stockholm*, Suppl. 243

Bàràny, E. (1938). *Acta otolaryngologica*, Suppl. 26

Békésy, G. von (1960). *Experiments in Hearing.* New York; McGraw-Hill

Carhart, R. (1950). *Archives of Otolaryngology*, **51,**

798
Davis, H. (1957). *Physiological Reviews*, **37**, 1
Davis, H. (1958). *Laryngoscope*, **68**, 349
Fernandez, C. (1967). *Archives of Otology*, **86**, 222
Fisch, V. and Schulthess, G. V. (1963). *Acta otolaryngologica, Stockholm*, **56**, 287
Fletcher, H. and Munson, W. A. (1933). *Journal of the Acoustical Society of America*, **5**, 82
Fletcher, H. and Munson, W. A. (1937). *Journal of the Acoustical Society of America*, **9**, 1
Hilding, D. A. (1961). *Transactions of the American Academy of Ophthalmic Otology*, **65**, 297
Ilberg, von (1968). *Archiv fur Klinische und experimentelle Ohren, Nasen und Kelhkunde Heilkunde*, **192**, 163
Johansen, H. (1948). *Acta otolaryngologica, Stockholm*, Suppl. **74**, 65
Jepsen, O. (1963). In *Modern Developments in Audiology* (Ed. by J. Jerger). New York; Academic Press
Kiang, N. Y-S., Watanabe, T., Thomas, E. C. and Clark, L. F. (1962). *Transactions of the American Otological Society*, **50**, 264
Kimura, R. S. (1967). *Annals of Otology*, **76**, 664
Kimura, R. S. and Wersall, J. (1962). *Acta otolaryngologica, Stockholm*, **55**, 11
Kirikae, I. (1959). *Acta otolaryngologica, Stockholm*, Suppl. 145
Lawrence, M. (1960). *Annals of Otology*, **69**, 480
Lawrence, M. (1962). *Annals of Otology*, **71**, 705
Lawrence, M., Wolsk, D. and Litton, W. (1961). *Transactions of the American Otological Society*, **49**, 92
Lindsay, J. R., Schuknecht, H. F., Neff, W. D. and Kimura, R. S. (1952). *Annals of Otology*, **61**, 697
Mendelson, E. S. (1961). *Journal of the Acoustical Society of America*, **33**, 146
Metz, O. (1951). *Acta otolaryngologica, Stockholm*, **39**, 397
Misrahy, G. A., Shinabarger, E. W. and Arnold, J. E. (1958). *Journal of the Acoustical Society of America*, **30**, 701
Misrahy, G. A., de Jonge, B. R., Shinabarger, E. W. and Arnold, J. E. (1958). *Journal of the Acoustical Society of America*, **30**, 705
Misrahy, G. A. Hildreth, K. M. Shinabarger, E. W. Clark, L. C. and Rice, E. A. (1958). *Journal of the Acoustical Society of America*, **30**, 247
Moller, A. (1961). *Annals of Otology*, **70**, 735
Naftalin, L. (1968). In *Progress in Biophysics and Molecular Biology*. Oxford and New York; Pergamon Press
Naftalin, L. and Harrison, M. S. (1958). *Journal of Laryngology*, **72**, 118
Neff, W. D. (1958). *Laryngoscope*, **68**, 413
Nordlund, B. (1962a). *Acta otolaryngologica, Stockholm*, **55**, 405
Nordlund, B. (1962b). *Acta otolaryngologica, Stockholm*, **54**, 75
Penfield, W. and Rasmussen, T. (1950). *The Cerebral Cortex of Man*. New York; Macmillan
Perlman, H. B. (1960). *Archives of Otololaryngology*, **72**, 201
Perlman, H. B. and Case, T. J. (1939). *Annals of Otology*, **48**, 663
Roberts, L. (1960). *Annals of Otology*, **69**, 830
Rosenzweig, M. R. (1961). *Psychology Bulletin*, **58**, 376
Schuknecht, H. F. (1958). *Laryngoscope*, **68**, 429
Schuknecht, H. F. and Seifi, A. E. (1963). *Annals of Otology*, **72**, 687
Schuknecht, H. F., Northrop, C. and Igarashi, M. (1968). *Acta otolaryngologica, Stockholm*, **65**, 479
Seymour, J. C. (1954). *Journal of Laryngology*, **68**, 689
Simmons, F. B. and Beatty, D. L. (1962). *Science*, **138**, 590
Tasaki, I. (1957). *Annual Review of Physiology*, **19**, 417
Tasaki, I. and Spyropoulos, C. S. (1959). *Journal of Neurophysiology*, **2**, 149
Tonndorf, J. (1962). *Journal of the Acoustical Society of America*, **34**, 1337
Tumarkin, A. (1945). *Journal of Laryngology*, **60**, 337
Tumarkin, A. (1950). *Journal of Laryngology*, **64**, 178
Tumarkin, A. (1954). *Journal of Laryngology*, **68**, 411
Vosteen, K. H. (1963). *Translations of the Beltone Institute for Hearing Research*, No. 16
Weiss, H. S., Mundie, J. R., Cashin, L. J. and Shinabarger, E. W. (1962). *Acta otolaryngologica, Stockholm*, **55**, 505
Wersall, R. (1958). *Acta otolaryngologica, Stockholm*, Suppl. 139
Wever, E. G. (1949). *Theory of Hearing*. New York; John Wiley
Wever, E. G. and Lawrence, M. (1954). *Physiological Acoustics*. Princeton University Press
Wiggers, H. C. (1937). *American Journal of Physiology*, **120**, 771
Zwislocki, J. (1953a). *Journal of the Acoustical Society of America*, **25**, 986
Zwislocki, J. (1953b). *Journal of the Acoustical Society of America*, **25**, 752

3 Physiology of equilibration

John Groves

Maintenance of equilibrium depends upon coordinated interaction of many senses. Sight, touch, and proprioception are all of high importance, but the vestibular apparatus is perhaps the most vital. Its normal function is so unobtrusive that it might well be termed a 'sixth sense', and yet its derangement is so dramatic and incapacitating an event that activities essential to life may become impossible.

The human infant acquires postural control and locomotory coordination almost painfully slowly, by comparison with many quadrupeds which follow the herd within minutes of birth. His *acquired* skill in equilibration, however, later transcends native instinct. Not only may he sit on a horse – he can learn to ride a bicycle, sail the seas, ski, skate, fly an aeroplane, or pilot a space-craft in weightlessness.

Perfect equilibration may be defined as reflex control of bodily posture in relation to environment, reflex control of muscular coordination in relation to movement, and accurate cortical awareness which is essential for voluntary purposive regulation of activity. The neurological systems involved in these processes are all so closely interrelated that they must be considered together, although it is the vestibular apparatus which happens to be the otologist's chief concern.

Sensory systems in equilibration

Light touch and pressure receptors in the skin detect bodily contact with the environment. The most important areas of skin are on the soles of the feet, the hands, and the buttocks. Changing sensations reflect the interplay of gravity, body-attitude, weight and movement, and are an essential source of data in walking, 'feeling one's way' (especially in the dark), flying 'by the seat of one's pants' (as in aviation, equitation, cycling, motoring, etc.).

Proprioception, the function of the stretch receptors of tendon and muscle, and of the organs of joint sensation, provides data regarding the instantaneous mechanical disposition of the musculo-skeletal system, as it relates to the force of gravity acting upon it. In the stationary condition, these sensory data are the principal basis of posture, maintained by antigravity tonus in the muscles subjected to stretch by the body's weight. All movements are a co-ordinated adjustment of posture superimposed upon this constantly appropriate static relationship to gravity.

The cutaneous and proprioceptive sensory systems depend upon the integrity of the peripheral sensory nerves, the posterior spinal roots, the long tracts of the spinal cord, their medullary relay stations, and their secondary neuronal connections with the cerebellum and midbrain. Their importance for maintenance of posture, and for balance in movement, has been demonstrated in nerve section experiments, but is sufficiently obvious to the clinician in peripheral neuritis, tabes dorsalis, and spinal lesions to require no description here.

Vision plays the most immediately obvious part in continuous monitoring of the environment. Known verticals and horizontals, and all familiar objects provide instantaneous data of the subject's position in space. Distances, speeds of linear and angular movement, changes of direction, can all be estimated, with experience, and the data thus acquired by the central nervous system can be integrated with those received by other sensory systems to form a correct assessment on which posture, and movement both reflex and voluntary, are based. Acute loss of sight gravely impairs balance during more complex locomotory activities, though some, but not all, of these may be re-learned in time through re-education of the remaining senses.

Vestibular sensation, subserved by the receptor mechanisms of the vestibular labyrinths, detects two distinct modalities – *orientation* with respect to the pull of gravity and *acceleration*, both angular and linear.

All of these sensory systems are closely linked in the central nervous system. In the brain stem vestibular second-order neurones in the medial longitudinal bundle ascend to the oculomotor nuclei, providing a short reflex pathway for co-ordination of head and eye movements. Descending (vestibulospinal) extrapyramidal tracts play upon the anterior horn cells and thereby continuously regulate somatic muscular tonus. The reticular formation also receives an important contribution from the vestibular system. Other connections reach the cerebellum and thalamus, and from the latter fibres relay to the temporal lobe cortex. Vestibular areas in the temporal lobe and pre-occipital region of both cat and man have been identified by numerous workers. Penfield (1957) stimulated the superior temporal gyrus at brain operations under local analgesia and noted the patients' descriptions of vertiginous sensations. Computer-averaged cortical responses to rotation are reported by Spiegel, Szekely and Moffet (1968), and Milojevic and St. Laurent (1966) describe vestibular areas in the cat located in the suprasylvian and ectosylvian gyri.

An account of vestibular physiology *must* begin with this survey of equilibration, and the central nervous system, because much of the basic research, both past and present, observes the effect upon posture, gait, and eye movements (including nystagmus) of a given intervention or stimulus at the vestibular end-organ. We may review cochlear function in isolation from the CNS mainly because of the ready availability of the cochlear microphonic at the round window. No such convenience exists for monitoring peripherally the effects of stimulating the vestibular labyrinth. This unfortunate fact, due to anatomical arrangement, may seem paradoxical if one recalls that both of these sensory organs have evolved from the lateral line of fishes, are basically responsive to mechanical disturbances of hair-cells, and have the same anatomical and biophysical environment.

Physiology of the vestibular labyrinth

Historical

In the nineteenth century the classical observations of the pioneers Flourens (1830), Menière (1861), and Ewald (1892) established positively that the semicircular canals are concerned with the maintenance of equilibrium, and that their destruction or derangement results in vertigo and nystagmus.

Ewald's contribution was crucial in that he demonstrated that displacement of the labyrinthine fluids in the pigeon's semicircular canal, either towards, or away from, the ampulla results in a reflex movement of the head and eyes in the plane of the canal and in the direction of the endolymph current.

Major contributions have followed at an increasing pace, emerging from many new disciplines. Bárány (1907) showed that endolymph flow, with consequent nystagmus, could result from warming or cooling the external auditory meatus. This so-called caloric vestibular response has been developed, notably by Hallpike and colleagues, not only as a physiological research tool, but as a valuable clinical test (*see* Volume 2). Bárány also investigated vestibular function by observing post-rotational vertigo and nystagmus. His simple rotating chair was the predecessor of today's sophisticated servocontrolled devices employed for precise study of pre-rotational vestibular activity. Magnus (1924) described the tonic labyrinthine reflexes in the decerebrate cat, and showed that they were abolished by eighth nerve section or by selective destruction of the otolith organ.

Adrian (1943) recorded nerve discharge activity in the vestibular nuclei of cats during stimulation of the labyrinth. He was able to define gravity receptors for posture and linear acceleration, and rotation receptors for turning movements.

Recording of eighth nerve action potentials (Lowenstein and Sand, 1940) by micro-electrodes placed upon single nerve fibres provided the first direct indication of vestibular responses to experimental stimuli. Neurosurgery has provided data regarding cortical representation of vestibular activity (Penfield, 1957). More recently electron microscopy has clarified the functional anatomy of the inner ear (*see* Chapter 1), whilst microchemical analysis of tissue fluids, and the use of radioactive tracers have led to better knowledge of essential metabolic processes.

The study of vestibular function in conditions of zero-gravity (which was essential for manned exploration of space) has resulted in major contributions to this branch of physiology.

Labyrinthine fluids

The perilymph and endolymph are common to the vestibular and cochlear labyrinth and the reader is referred to p. 34. *Vestibular endolymph* requires further comment. Like the cochlear endolymph, it contains high potassium and low sodium concentrations. Its production, circulation, and re-absorption are as yet uncertain. The so-called vestibular 'dark cells', found near the cristae and maculae and described by Dohlman (1964, 1965) and Hamilton (1965) have structural features suggestive of a secretory function (Nakai and Hilding, 1968). Dohlman (1967) however, suggested their function might be the selective re-absorption of sodium from the endolymph.

Circulation of the endolymph, as stated on p. 121, remains a controversial topic. Dyes, pigments, isotopes, or labelled enzymes injected into the scala media or semicircular canals have been found by many workers to accumulate in the saccus endolymphaticus. Similarly, parenterally-administered isotopes have been traced through the cochlear and vestibular secretory tissues, and the endolymph, to the saccus. Surgical destruction of the saccus results in hydrops of the labyrinth. Kimura, Lundquist and Wersäll (1964) regarded the ultrastructure of the saccus as suggestive of a secretory function, whereas Adlington (1968) reached an opposite conclusion. There is therefore considerable weight of evidence to suggest that endolymph is produced, and re-absorbed at several different sites. The 'radial' and 'longitudinal' theories of circulation still have their protagonists, but as Lundquist (1967) suggests these concepts need not be mutually exclusive. Both processes may be active, with a slow longitudinal flow towards the saccus where substances of high molecular weight and cellular debris may be absorbed and phagocytosed.

The role, if any, of the utriculo-endolymphatic valve (Bast, 1928), in controlling circulation of endolymph has been debated by Secretan (1944) and Seymour (1954), but remains undecided.

Functional anatomy of the vestibular sense organs

The detailed morphology is described in Chapter 1, but it is necessary here to note the following points.

The cupulae, overlying the cristae of all three ampullae are composed of a jelly-like substance, very similar to that of the tectorial membrane, and composed of sulphomucopolysaccharides. Each cupula at its free border makes a close seal with the roof of the ampulla and the hairs of the hair-cells are embedded in its substance. The cupula is displaced towards or away from the utricle by movement of the endolymph in one or other direction, and in these conditions has the physical characteristics of a heavily-damped pendulum.

The macula of the utricle lying flat in an almost horizontal plane is covered by its otolithic membrane. This consists of a gelatinous matrix similar to that of the cupula, but contains innumerable crystals of calcite (statoconia) ranging in size from 0.5 μm to about 30 μm (in the guinea-pig). The hairs of the utricular macular hair-cells are embedded in this statoconial membrane.

The macula of the saccule lies on the medial wall of the saccule in a vertical plane, and is covered by a statoconial membrane like that of the macula utriculi.

Functional polarization of the vestibular sense organs

Each hair-cell has 50–110 stereocilia, and one kinocilium which lies at the periphery of the bundle of stereocilia. This asymmetrical arrangement coincides with a functional polarization of the cell. Displacement of the hairs is believed to alter the electrical state of the cell. Displacement towards the kinocilium results in depolarization, while the opposite movement away from the kinocilium, is accompanied by hyperpolarization (*Figure 3.1*).

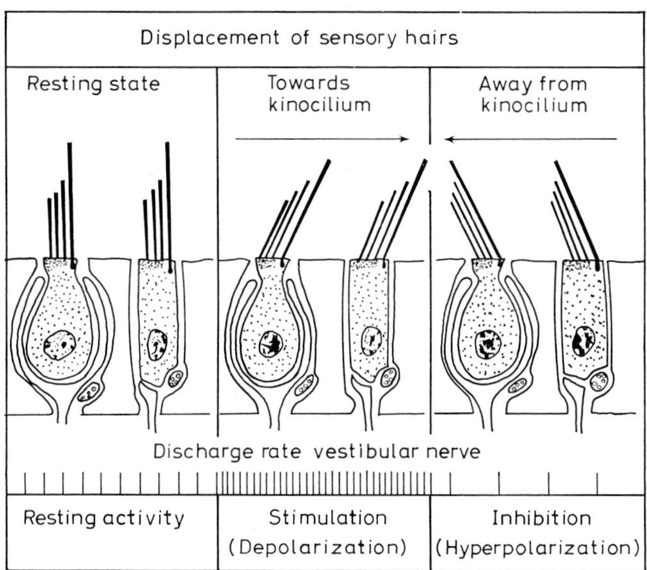

Figure 3.1 Schematic illustration of the relation between hair-cell orientation and the pattern of stimulation of the innervating nerve fibres in the mammalian crista. (From Wersäll, Gleisner and Lundquist, 1967, reproduced by courtesy of Messrs J. & A. Churchill)

Lindeman (1969) describes the polarization patterns for each of the sensory regions of the vestibular apparatus. On the crista of the lateral canal, all of the hair-cells have their kinocilia on the utricular side. On the other two cristae the kinocilia are all orientated away from the utricle.

The maculae can be divided into two areas by an arbitrary curved line, with opposite polarization on each side. On the macula utriculi the cells have their kinocilia towards this line, whilst on the macula sacculi they are orientated away from it (*Figure 3.2*). As the figure indicates the arrangement is such that in the macula utriculi there are sensory cells orientated spatially in every direction in the plane of the organ.

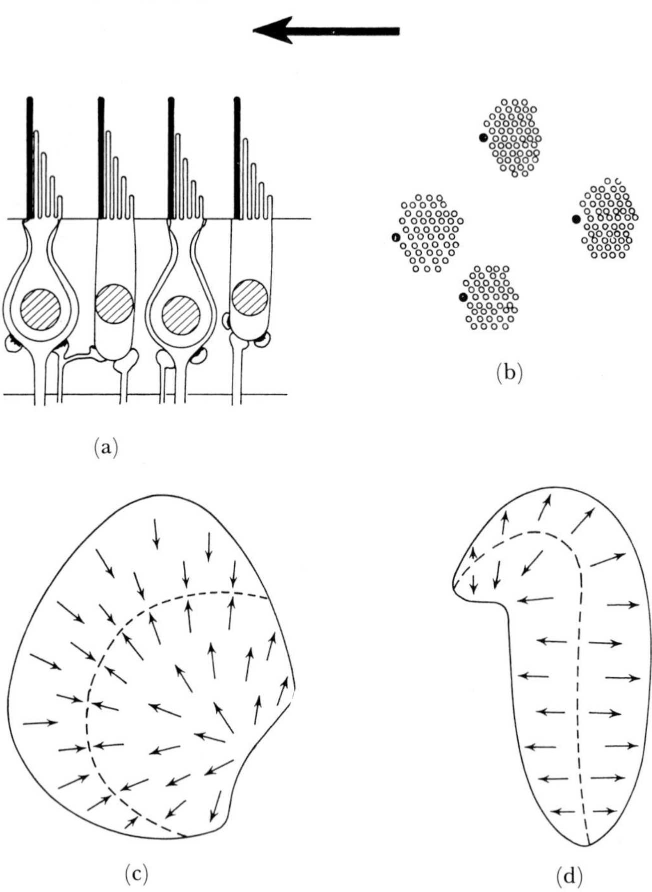

Figure 3.2 Diagram illustrating the morphological polarization of the sensory cells (above) and the polarization pattern of the maculae in man (below). The morphological polarization (arrow) of a sensory cell is determined by the position of the kinocilium in relation to the stereocilia: (a) a section perpendicular to the epithelium; (b) section parallel to the epithelial surface. Note increasing length of the stereocilia towards the kinocilium. The macula utriculi (c) as well as the macula sacculi (d) are divided by an arbitrary curved line into two areas – pars externa and pars interna – with opposite morphological polarization. On the macula utriculi the sensory cells are polarized towards the dividing line, on the macula sacculi away from the dividing line. (From Lindeman, 1969, reproduced by courtesy of the Editor of *Journal of Laryngology and Otology*)

Electrical polarization of the vestibular sense organs

Numerous workers have carried out micro-electrode studies of animal labyrinths, and of the lateral line organs of certain fishes. By analogy with the confirmed electrical conditions in the cochlea it is expected that a positive d.c. endolymph potential and a negative intracellular potential would be present. Confirmatory evidence is at present lacking; Smith and her colleagues were unable to confirm Trincker's reports of high positive potentials in the endolymph and cupula, and although they observed negative values of 30–70 mV in the cells of the cristae they were unable to tell whether these were sensory or supporting cells.

Vestibular nerve action potentials

In many different animals it has proved possible to record individual nerve fibre action potentials in the various branches of the vestibular nerve. In the 'resting' state these sensory fibres have a spontaneous discharge rate of 10–20/s whether they arise from cristae or maculae.

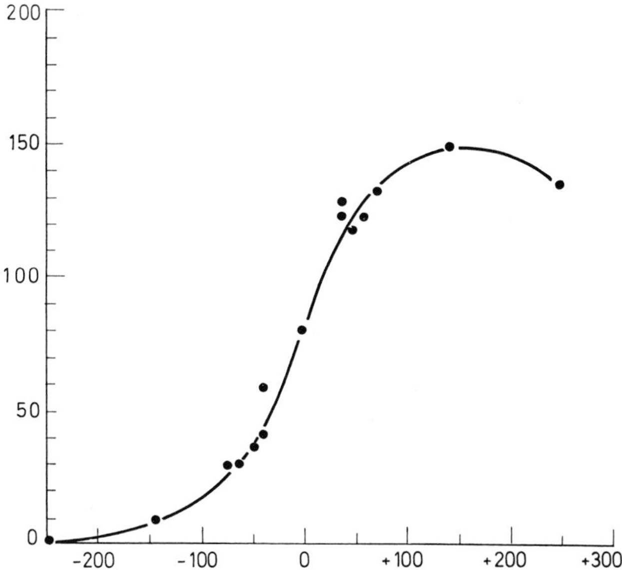

Figure 3.3 Characteristic curve of action potential frequency plotted against impulse stimuli, using a three-unit preparation of the horizontal semicircular canal of the ray. Abscissa: stimulus strength (rotational velocity (deg/s) at 'stop'). Ordinate: response frequency (action potentials/s). (The mechanical impulses are produced by sudden stopping of steady speed rotations.) (From Groen, Lowenstein and Vendrik, 1952, reproduced by courtesy of the Editor of *Journal of Physiology*)

The cause of this resting activity is not known as it is difficult if not impossible, certainly for the maculae, to eliminate completely any possibility of external stimuli in a laboratory animal preparation. The effect however, is that the labyrinth at rest, or more accurately, in the normal, neutral, position of the head is 'biased' to a point in the middle of its sensory range (*see Figure 3.3*) so that functional response to stimulation can be bi-directional (increase or decrease of activity) in each afferent nerve fibre.

Mechanisms of the vestibular sensory organs

Semicircular canals

Ewald's experiment has already been mentioned in which he stimulated the lateral canal by changing the pressure inside it. A surgical opening was made, and a cannula, attached to a pump, fixed into it. A sudden positive pressure caused head and eye movements to the contralateral side. A negative pressure caused the opposite reaction. The conclusion that movement of the endolymph stimulated the crista ampullaris has remained the accepted basis of physiology to the present day. During angular acceleration or deceleration the endolymph, due to its inertia, lags behind and thereby exerts pressure within the ampulla. As soon as acceleration or deceleration ceases and a constant velocity of rotation is attained, the endolymph ceases to move relative to its surroundings and stimulation ends. The semicircular canals are therefore sensitive only to *changes* of *angular* velocity. (Linear acceleration, rotational velocity, centrifugal force, and spatial orientation are all detected by the otolith organ.)

Later workers made the cupula and its movements visible by injecting opaque materials such as Indian ink into the endolymph. It was then realized, and more recently confirmed by ultra-microscopy, that the cupula reaches the roof of the ampulla and therefore seals effectively its lumen. Furthermore the cupula was seen to move in either direction with any displacement of the endolymph (*Figure 3.4*).

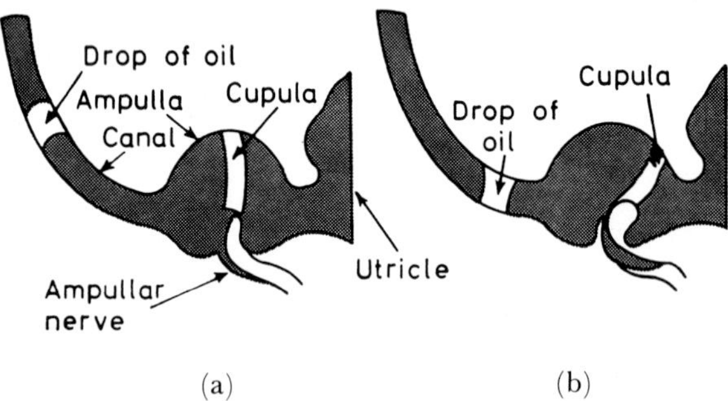

Figure 3.4 The ampulla and semicircular canal in the living state before and during angular acceleration. The cupula, situated on the top of the crista, traverses the entire lumen of the ampulla; (a) the cupula in its normal position; (b) the cupula during angular acceleration. Note the shift of position of the oil droplet in the endolymph during acceleration. (From Dohlman, 1935, reproduced by courtesy of the Editor of *Proceedings of the Royal Society of Medicine*)

Such cupular displacements occur in the intact animal as shown by nystagmus during angular acceleration, whilst in experimental animals the vestibular nerve action potentials show corresponding increase or decrease in discharge rates as compared with the resting state. Lowenstein demonstrated these changes with measured deceleration stimuli (*see Figure 3.3*). The graph illustrates proportional changes in nervous discharge rates from the horizontal canal crista in both directions of stimulation (ampullopetal and ampullofugal) with the resting discharge rate poised in the middle of the straightest part of the response curve.

These findings correlate perfectly with the observed functional and morphological polarization of the hair-cells described above, and the correlation is confirmed by the fact that on stimulation of the superior and posterior canals by rotational accelerations in the appropriate planes the converse results are obtained. Ampullopetal (i.e. towards the utricle) displacement of the cupula in these canals *reduces* the nerve discharge rates and ampullofugal displacement increases it.

The threshold of effective stimulus intensity for the canals (in man) is an acceleration (or deceleration) of about 0.2–0.5 degrees/s^2. The figure varies somewhat according to the duration of stimulus, shorter stimulation times requiring greater acceleration to achieve threshold.

Caloric stimulation gives similar and compatible results in man and animals, confirming yet again that displacement of the endolymph is the effective stimulus. This basic physical mechanism is interestingly endorsed by the recent observation that caloric vestibular reactions (which depend upon thermally induced changes in specific gravity of the endolymph) are abolished in the condition of weightlessness (zero-gravity).

It was once supposed that the displacement of endolymph in the canals whether induced by angular acceleration, or by caloric stimulation, was a continuous or 'streaming' flow, and that the nystagmus after stimulation persisted until the momentum of the endolymph was dissipated. The realization that the cupula closely seals the ampulla shows that this old idea is erroneous, and it is currently thought that the after-nystagmus is due mainly to the (comparatively) slow return of the damped cupula to its resting position when the endolymph pressure upon it (due to acceleration) ceases.

Correlation of responses between the several semicircular canals is obviously of a highly complex kind. In each labyrinth, a rotational stimulus exactly in the plane of any canal will be maximal, and in either direction, whilst the other two canals will remain at rest. Angular acceleration in any intermediate plane will result in simultaneous activity of two or even three canals, and the intensity of response in each will be in vectorial proportion based upon the angles between the functional axes of the canals and the plane of movement.

In the intact animal an exact mirror image of these events simultaneously occurs in the opposite labyrinth. Each ampullopetal stimulus on one side is matched in the other ear by an equal ampullofugal displacement in the functionally paired canal. (In this 'push-pull' arrangement the lateral canals form one pair whilst each posterior canal is parallel to and therefore paired with the superior canal of the opposite side.)

The utricle

The hair-cells of the macula utriculi are stimulated, as shown by changes in the appropriate nerve action potentials, by the effect of gravitational pull upon the otolith (statoconial membrane). The calcite of which the statoconia are composed has a specific gravity of 2.93–2.95. The pressure thus exerted on the nearly horizontal macula when the head is stationary stimulates a resting discharge the rate of which will be different for every different orientation of the head. This variation can occur in respect not only of overall discharge rate but also of the differential discharge patterns amongst the individual nerve fibres, as a consequence of the morphological polarization pattern of the hair-cells described above. For example, when the head is tilted so that the recording ear is undermost, the discharge rate increases in proportion to the angle of tilt.

These static labyrinthine responses were postulated in detail by Magnus in his studies of reflex postural behaviour. He observed reflex adjustments of postural tone in the decerebrate cat for each different position of the head, even when the neck righting reflexes were eliminated. He showed that these static labyrinthine reflexes were abolished by destruction of the otolith or by eighth nerve section.

Being, thus, a sensory receptor responding to the pull of gravity, the otolith organ must also respond to linear acceleration and to centrifugal force. The gravitational forces generated by these stimuli must act upon the otolith organ in summation with the influence of environmental gravity, in respect of both intensity and direction. These expectations have been confirmed experimentally.

The saccule

The function of the saccule remains an enigma. It is phylogenetically related more closely to hearing than to equilibration, and in many lower animals a microphonic type of response to sound stimuli below 800 Hz has been demonstrated. The macula sacculi and its statoconial membrane are structurally almost replicas of those of the utricle, and these structures lie in a vertical plane which one might regard as 'strategically' complementary to that of the utricle. The afferent fibres terminate in the vestibular nuclei. Despite all this anatomical compatibility with an equilibratory function, no very firm experimental evidence has been found in mammals. Lowenstein (1956) stated that positional responses exactly like those of the utricle were detectable in the posterior third only of the elasmo-branch macula sacculi. Other work shows that the macula sacculi may also be concerned with low frequency vibration. Its functions may indeed be very different in different orders of the vertebrate kingdom, and experimental findings must be regarded with corresponding caution and reserve.

Transduction in the vestibular sense organs

As described for the cochlea (p. 103) there is a fundamental question as to how a mechanical stimulus results in a nerve action potential. In the vestibular sense organs the mechanical stimuli, as we have seen, are, in the *ampullary* displacement and deformation of the *cupula*, in the *utricle* a variable pressure (due to gravity) upon the *macula* by the statoconial membrane. In every plane except the truly horizontal, the membrane must also tend to slip downwards, creating a shearing effect.

It is believed, as noted earlier, that stimulation occurs in association with a change in the degree of electrical polarization between the structures outside and the interior of the hair-cell. The mechanism for such an electrical change is not known.

Actual bending or shearing forces upon the hairs may be responsible, though some authorities consider a kind of 'piezo-electrical' effect in the deflected cupula is a distinct possibility. Analogous theories for tectorial membrane function in the cochlea (Naftalin, 1968) are of interest in this connection. The specific directionality of the responses to stimulation do point, however, towards a cellular, rather than an extracellular source of electrical changes. The respective roles of the stereocilia and the kinocilium are discussed by Lowenstein (1967) but no firm conclusions have been reached.

A similar uncertainty prevails as to whether the afferent nerve terminals upon the hair-cells are stimulated directly by the electrical changes, or by the liberation of a chemical transmitter-substance from the hair-cells.

Efferent vestibular nerve fibres, arising from the region of the lateral vestibular nuclei, travel outwards in the vestibular nerve and its branches to all of the vestibular sense organs. Their function is at present unknown. It has been suggested that they may regulate the sensitivity and the resting discharge activity of the hair-cells, and if this is so they must play some part in the processes of transduction.

Integrated functional activity of the vestibular system

Through their CNS connections the labyrinths serve to maintain equilibrium, and in particular the posture of the head and eyes. Consequently, during movement the gaze can be stabilized upon any required external object by an automatic adjustment of extra-ocular muscle tonus. If the movement continues and the object passes out of visual range, the eyes flick rapidly back to fix upon another point. This process continuously repeated therefore causes alternating slow and fast eye movements, or nystagmus. In this example we have *optokinetic* nystagmus. The slow movement is purely reflex at brainstem level, whilst the quick (corrective) movement depends upon cerebral cortical adjustment. Pure optokinetic nystagmus, uninfluenced by vestibular stimulation, is observed when the subject is at rest and his environment moves (e.g. in 'railway nystagmus'), or in clinical testing as described in Volume 2.

Vestibular nystagmus displays the same slow–quick characteristics. It occurs during angular acceleration or deceleration and also for a brief period following such stimuli ('after-nystagmus').

Since nystagmus of both these types is mediated through the oculomotor and abducens nuclei, the reticular formation, and the complex cortical control of both, they may augment or inhibit one another in algebraical summation. Vestibular nystagmus, for example, can be markedly influenced by preventing fixation of the gaze (as by blindfolding), or by cortical activity (as by conversation or the performance of mental arithmetic).

In man the capacity to register and respond posturally to labyrinthine stimulation is normally perfectly adequate for everyday conditions. It is common knowledge, however, that some have a better sense of balance than others, which seems to be an intrinsic physical attribute. The finest skaters, ballet dancers and acrobats might well be termed 'vestibular athletes'. Pilots, too, and especially astronauts, must possess better than average vestibular aptitude before selection for training. Their training programmes, however, include systematic augmentation of this aptitude, which is shown to be capable of considerable development. So-called habituation to repeated vestibular stimulation can be demonstrated in flying personnel as a diminished nystagmic response to rotation tests, and similar findings have been noted in other vestibular athletes. To some extent at least habituation may depend upon a trained ability consciously to suppress after-nystagmus as long as the eyes remain open. In a fast pirouette the skater or dancer fixes the gaze on the same distant point for as long as possible during each rotation, and returns to it at the earliest possible instant in the next successive turn.

Singleton (1967) demonstrated that previously induced habituation (to caloric stimulation) in cats was abolished by ablation of the cerebellar nodulus. His experiments support the view that the nodulus exerts an inhibitory effect on vestibular centres and on the oculo-vestibular reflex arc.

Motion sickness results from excessive stimulation of the labyrinths. Nausea and vomiting occur, from activity of the dorsal nucleus of the vagus, together with a fall of blood pressure and bradycardia.

It has long been recognized that deaf persons may be more tolerant of conditions which cause motion-sickness (James, 1882). Several workers have since reported that labyrinthine-defective subjects remained well under a variety of stimuli which cause sickness in normal controls. Kennedy and his colleagues (1968) reviewed the literature and described an experiment which showed immunity to sea-sickness in extreme storm conditions at sea.

Why some people should be abnormally prone to motion-sickness is not understood, though for the average 'occasional sailor' habituation will usually restore well-being during a prolonged voyage.

Effects of labyrinth destruction

Unilateral labyrinth destruction

Loss of one labyrinth results in:

Skew deviation of the eyes towards the side of the lesion.
Spontaneous nystagmus towards the opposite side.
Flexion of the neck and rotation of the occiput towards the side of the lesion.
Increased extensor tonus in the limbs of the opposite side.

In addition there are spontaneous movements – the body turns or rolls, there is head nystagmus, and a falling towards the operated side.

A patient will prefer to lie with the affected ear uppermost because the severity of the nystagmus and vertigo is aggravated if he tries to look towards the normal side.

These reactions are due to imbalance, amounting to total unilateral loss, of the normal sensory input between the two sides of the vestibular system.

In long-term experiments, and in the human patient, compensation takes place over a period of a few weeks and the overt symptoms and signs disappear. Compensation is thought to be due to adaptation in the regulating activities of the brain stem. Vestibular function tests (*see* Volume 2) reveal a permanent preponderance of induced nystagmus towards the intact ear.

Bilateral labyrinth destruction

Bilateral labyrinth destruction results in a severe loss of tone in all of the postural muscles. There is no nystagmus or true vertigo, but there is a severe degree of imbalance and ataxia. Without the aid of sight, the animal cannot stand. Underwater disorientation is complete, and the animal (or human) subject is as likely to swim downward as upward. These disabilities are permanent.

References

Adlington, P. (1968). *Journal of Laryngology*, **82,** 101

Adrian, E. D. (1943). *Journal of Physiology*, **101,** 389

Bárány, R. (1907). *Physiologie und Pathologie des Bogenganapparates beim Mehschen.* Vienna; Deuticke

Bast, T. H. (1928). *Anatomy Record*, **40,** 61

Dohlman, G. F. (1935). *Proceedings of the Royal Society of Medicine*, **28,** 137

Dohlman, G. F. (1964). *Annals of Otology*, **73,** 708

Dohlman, G. F. (1965). *Acta otolaryngologica, Stockholm*, **59,** 275

Dohlman, G. F. (1967). In *Myotatic, Kinaesthetic and Vestibular Mechanisms*, pp. 138, 143. London; Churchill

Ewald, J. R. (1892). *Physiologische Untersuchungen uber das Endorgan des Nervus Octavus.* Wiesbaden; Bergmann

Flourens, M. J. P. (1830). *Mémoires Académie Royale des Sciences, Paris*, **9,** 455

Groen, J. J., Lowenstein, O. and Vendrik, A. J. H. (1952). *Journal of Physiology*, **117,** 329

Hamilton, D. W. (1965). *Journal of Morphology*, **116,** 339

James, W. (1882). *American Journal of Otology*, **4,** 239

Kennedy, R. S., Graybiel, A., McDonough, R. C. and Beckwith, Fr. D. (1968). *Acta otolaryngologica, Stockholm*, **66,** 533

Kimura, R., Lundquist, P-G. and Wersäll, J. (1964). *Acta otolaryngologica, Stockholm*, **57,** 517

Lindeman, H. H. (1969). *Journal of Laryngology*, **83,** 9

Lowenstein, O. (1956). *British medical Bulletin*, **12,** 110, 114

Lowenstein, O. (1967). In *Myotatic, Kinaesthetic and Vestibular Mechanisms*, p. 121. London; Churchill

Lowenstein, O. and Sand, A. (1940). *Proceedings of the Royal Society*, Series B, **129,** 256

Lundquist, P-G. (1967). In *Myotatic, Kinaesthetic and Vestibular Mechanisms*, p. 147. London; Churchill

Magnus, R. (1924). *Korpestellung.* Berlin; Springer

Menière, P. (1861). *Gazette medical, Paris*, **16,** 29

Milojevic, B. and St. Laurent, J. (1966). *Aerospace Medicine*, **37,** 709

Naftalin, L. (1968). 'Acoustic Transmission in the Peripheral Hearing Apparatus', In *Progress in Biophysics and Molecular Biology.* Oxford; Pergamon Press

Nakai, Y. and Hilding, D. (1968). *Acta otolaryngologica, Stockholm*, **66,** 120

Penfield, W. (1957). *Annals of Otology*, **66,** 691

Secretan, J. P. (1944). *Acta otolaryngologica, Stockholm*, **32,** 117

Seymour, J. C. (1954). *Journal of Laryngology*, **68,** 689

Singleton, G. T. (1967). *Laryngoscope, St. Louis*, **77,** 1579

Spiegal, E. A., Szekely, E. G. and Moffet, R. (1968). *Acta otolaryngologica, Stockholm*, **66,** 81

Wersäll, J., Gleisner, L. and Lundquist, P-G. (1967). In *Myotatic, Kinaesthetic and Vestibular Mechanisms*, p. 109. London; Churchill

4 Anatomy of the nose, nasal cavity and paranasal sinuses

W J Hamilton and R J Harrison

Embryology

An understanding of the development of the nose, mouth, palate, air sinuses, pharynx and oesophagus requires a knowledge of the formation and fate of the primitive foregut. This, in turn, presupposes a grasp of the arrangement of the original yolk sac vesicle and an appreciation of the significance of the folding of the embryonic head.

In its early stages the embryo is a bilaminar disc of ectoderm and endoderm between which a layer of mesoderm later develops on each side of, and in front of, the notochordal–prochordal plate complex (*Figure 4.1*). It is to this mesoderm that the term 'paraxial' is applied. This is the arrangement of embryonic tissues immediately prior to the formation of the head fold – an event which directly conditions a number of important results.

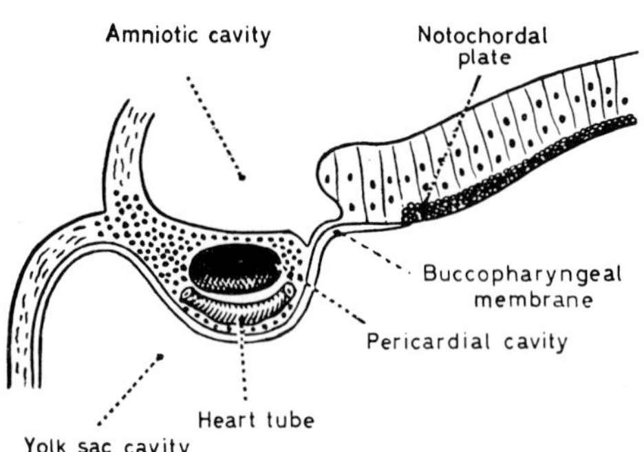

Figure 4.1 A diagrammatic longitudinal midline section through the cranial half of the embryonic disc in a pre-somite human embryo to show the relationships of the pericardial cavity and the buccopharyngeal membrane before the formation of the head fold

(1) Head-folding brings the cardiogenic region, the future septum transversum and cranial mesoderm, from their original anterior positions so that they then lie on the ventral embryonic aspect and are thereafter ventral to the foregut. This is a radical and fundamental change in the arrangement of structures which were originally anterior to the prochordal plate (*Figure 4.2*).

(2) The foregut extends forwards as an endodermal diverticulum, the closed anterior extremity of which lies in part immediately adjacent to the surface ectoderm and

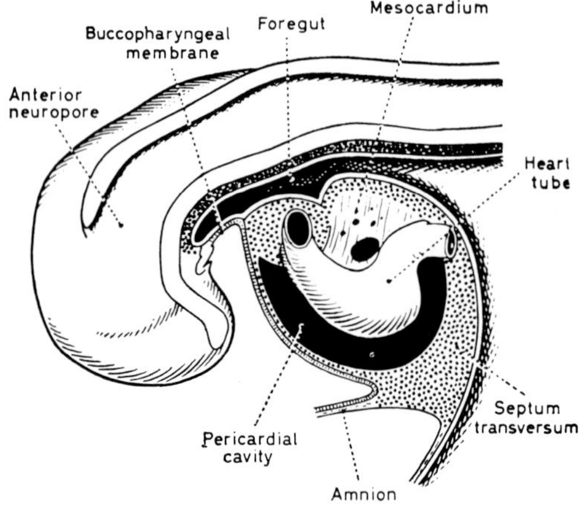

Figure 4.2 A diagrammatic longitudinal midline section through the cranial half of the embryonic disc of a 14-somite embryo to show the rotation of the heart tube resulting from the formation of the head fold

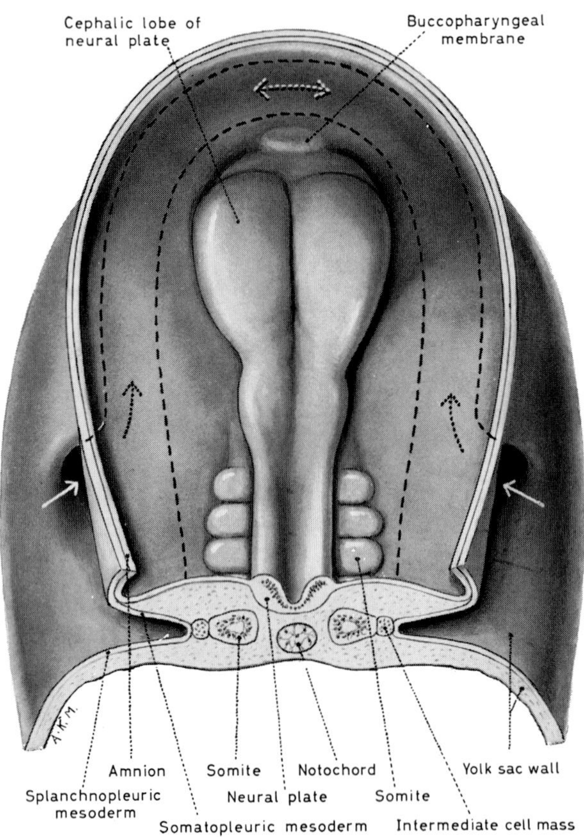

Figure 4.3 A schematic representation of the cranial part of a somite embryo to show the relationships of the intra-embryonic coelom, the development of the neural plate and the continuity between the intra-embryonic coelom and the extra-embryonic coelom

with it forms the buccopharyngeal membrane. It is this diverticulum which is now properly spoken of as the 'primitive foregut'.

(3) The paraxial mesoderm on each side of the notochordal process is present as thickened longitudinal masses which become subdivided into somites. Intermediate cell masses of mesoderm lie between somitic and lateral plate mesoderm, the latter subsequently splitting to enclose the intra-embryonic coelom. Cranial to the somite region only the lateral plate mesoderm of each side extends forwards to fuse cranially in the midline and thus, by its splitting, surrounds the pericardial cavity and leads to the development and function of the coelomic ducts (*Figure 4.3*). With the possible exception of 'somites' for the extrinsic eye muscles, no somites are found in the mesoderm cranial to the notochord, nor are there intermediate cell masses. The diffuse, unsegmented mesoderm does exist, however, as far forwards as the cephalic extremity of the embryonic disc. It is this mesoderm (branchial) which condenses cranially as the forerunner of the branchial arch components (*Figure 4.3*), and also surrounds the more caudal derivatives of the foregut proper.

Although the above account implies a sequence of events described separately, many are occurring synchronously. All are vital both to the development of the fundamental pattern displayed in the foregut region and to an understanding of the subsequent morphogenetic changes.

The foregut can be divided, descriptively, into cranial and caudal portions. The former gives origin to the endodermal part of the mouth, most of the pharynx, and the endodermal epithelium of the respiratory system. The caudal portion gives origin to the oesophagus, stomach and the duodenum as far as the entrance of the bile duct.

Development of nasal cavity

The external nose

Epithelial thickenings, known as nasal placodes, are the first indication of the development of the nose. These appear on the infralateral side of the head region above the stomatodaeum in embryos of 5–6 mm C.R. length, which is 28–30 days ovulation age (Streeter, 1945). Initially the placodes are convex but with the proliferation of the surrounding mesenchyme, accompanying the formation of the medial and lateral nasal folds, the placodes soon come to lie in depressions which ultimately deepen sufficiently to form the olfactory pits. The medial nasal folds fuse to form a central elevated part known as the frontonasal process. With further growth of the nasal folds each olfactory, or nasal, pit becomes deeper, forming a nasal sac (*Figure 4.4*) (Streeter, 1948).

As the nasal folds develop, the maxillary processes grow forwards from the mandibular region. This state of affairs can be seen in embryos 9–12 mm C.R. length (*Figure 4.5*).

The maxillary process grows medially underneath the developing eye and eventually comes into contact with the lateral nasal process. With further growth, the

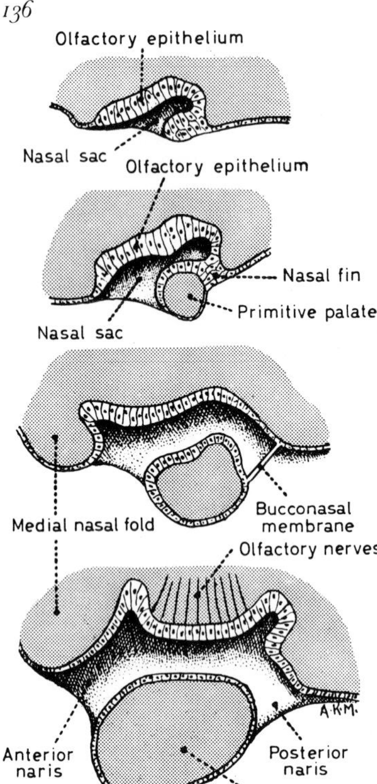

Figure 4.4 Schemes to show the development of the nasal sac, nasal cavity and primitive palate (based on Streeter)

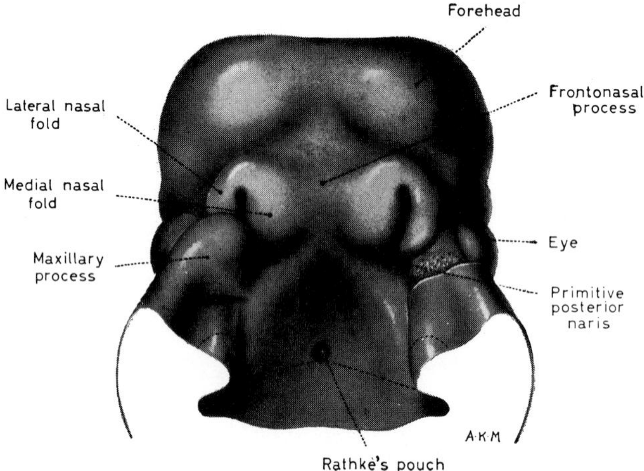

Figure 4.5 A drawing of the roof of the stomatodaeum of a 12 mm human embryo to show the development of the primitive anterior and posterior nares by the approximation of the maxillary processes to the lateral and medial nasal folds. Part of the left maxillary process has been removed. The previous site of attachment of the buccopharyngeal membrane is represented by the interrupted line. The maxillary palatal processes are just appearing. (Reproduced by courtesy of Professors Hamilton, Boyd and Mossman)

maxillary process spreads medially so that the olfactory pit now becomes the primitive nasal cavity. Eventually the maxillary process comes to overlap the lower part of the frontonasal process (*Figures 4.6* and *4.7*). When this state has become established the tissues for the development of the upper lip and the alveolar process of the maxilla are formed. The lateral nasal processes approach each other so that the frontonasal process is depressed to form the primitive nasal septum (*Figure 4.7*). After the overgrowth of the maxillary mesoderm, the free lower surface of the fronto-nasal process forms the primitive palate. The nasal cavities at this stage of development consist of two narrow channels which open anteriorly at the external nares. Posteriorly, however, each cavity is still closed by the thinned-out posterior wall of the original nasal sac, forming a temporary bucconasal membrane behind the primitive palate (*Figure 4.4*).

It will be seen that the tissues of the upper lip are derived entirely from the maxillary process. As the fronto-nasal process is developed from the region which is

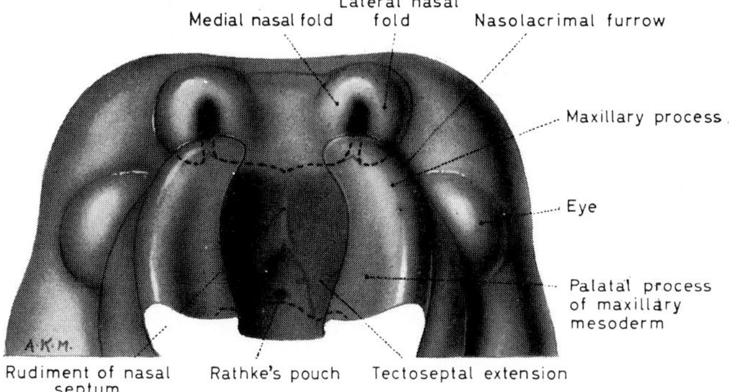

Figure 4.6 The roof of the stomatodaeum of a 12.5 mm human embryo. The interrupted line indicates the extent of the lateral and medial nasal folds and the frontonasal process. (Reproduced by courtesy of Professors Hamilton, Boyd and Mossman)

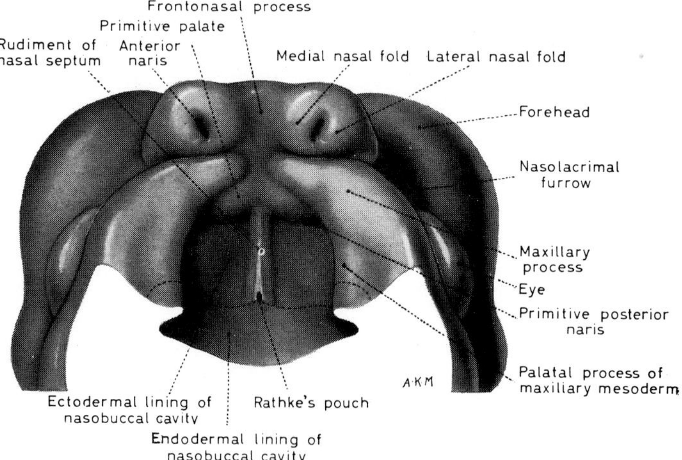

Figure 4.7 The roof of the stomatodaeum of a 13.5 mm human embryo. (Reproduced by courtesy of Professors Hamilton, Boyd and Mossman)

supplied by the ophthalmic division of the trigeminal nerve, that part of the nose which develops from the fronto-nasal process derives a nerve supply from the anterior ethmoidal nerve, a branch of the ophthalmic nerve. At the line of contact between the maxillary process and the lateral nasal process, the ectoderm enclosed sinks in and forms the nasolacrimal duct.

The above description of the development of the medial portion of the upper lip is based on the work of Frazer (1931) and Boyd (1933), confirmed by Streeter (1948).

In embryos of 12–14 mm C.R. length the bucconasal membranes rupture and continuity is established on each side between the corresponding nasal sac and the roof of the mouth (*Figure 4.4*). The regions of continuity are the primitive posterior nares, and they lie behind and above the primitive palate. Many embryologists, however (*see* Warbrick, 1960, for review), believe the mesoderm of the central part of the upper lip to be of fronto-nasal origin.

The nasal cavity and palate

At first the primitive nasal cavity is a single chamber roofed by stomatodaeal ectoderm anterior to the line of attachment of the now ruptured buccopharyngeal membrane, and by foregut endoderm posterior to that line.

The upper and anterior part of the front-nasal process forms the primitive nasal septum. The lower surface of the fronto-nasal process remains to form the primitive palate, above and lateral to which are the posterior nares (*Figure 4.7*). Extending from the site of Rathke's pouch to the level of the posterior edge of the frontonasal process, a median ridge develops on the inferior surface of the roof of the buccal cavity (*Figure 4.7*). This ridge is formed by an extension of mesoderm, deep to the ectodermal lining, from the maxillary process of each side, the so-called tectoseptal expansion. This expansion becomes continuous with the mesodermal tissue of the frontal process to form the definitive nasal septum.

This septum gradually grows backwards and downwards as a distinct midline elevation with a free edge reaching as far as where Rathke's pouch projects from the roof of the buccal cavity.

As the nasal septum develops, each mass of maxillary mesoderm provides a medially-directed extension – the palatal process (*Figure 4.7*). It extends medially with a free edge below and behind the primitive posterior nares and level with the primitive palate. The tongue lies below the primitive palate in front but, more posteriorly, it projects temporarily between the maxillary palatal processes and the enlarging nasal cavities (*Figure 4.8*). The free edges of the maxillary palatal processes subsequently fuse, first with the posterior margin of the primitive palate, and then progressively, from before backward, with each other in the middle line and also eventually with the lower free edge of the nasal septum (*Figure 4.9*). The stomatodaeum and olfactory pits are thus subdivided into an upper pair of nasal cavities and a lower cavity, the definitive mouth. This obviously constitutes the embryological basis for the separation of the respiratory and alimentary systems in the nasal region; the former now bypasses the mouth and each system can perform its own specific function without impediment. The tongue is now rapidly depressed from the nasal cavities by the progressive fusion of the maxillary palatal processes with the primitive palate and with each other. This fusion also results in a posterior migration

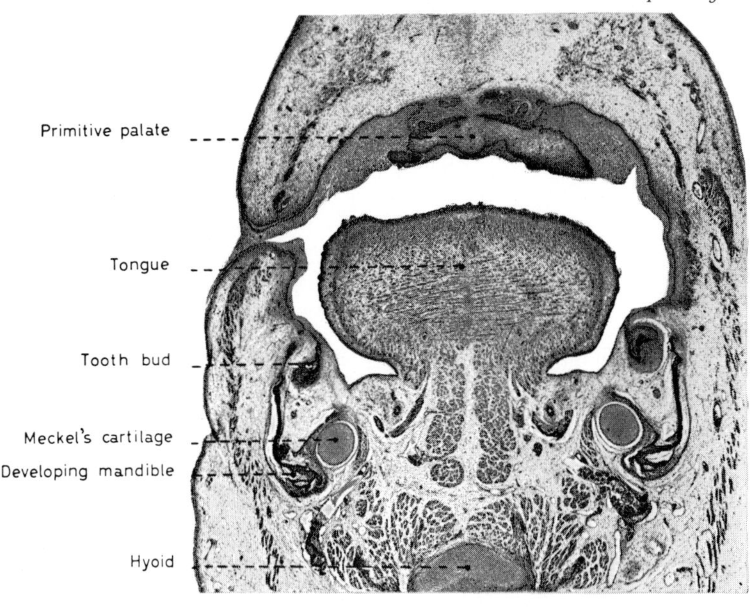

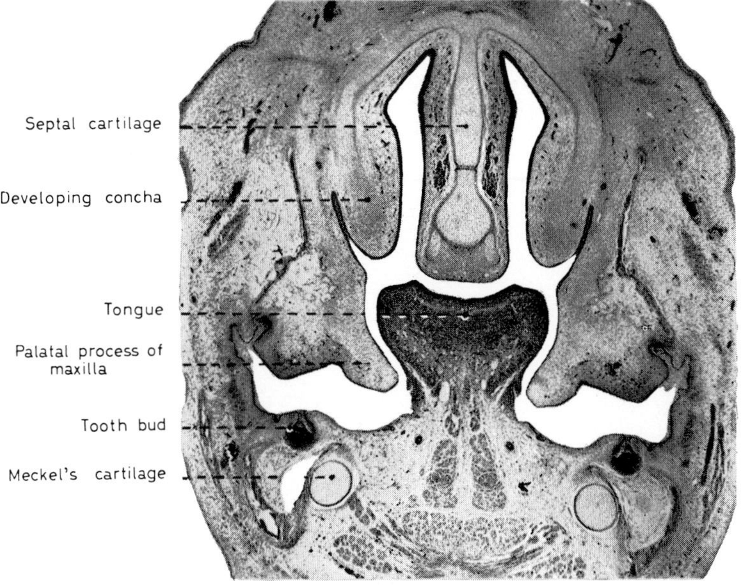

Figure 4.8 Photographs of two sections through the developing palate of a 20 mm human embryo. The upper section shows the anterior part of the primitive palate; the lower section passes through the posterior part of the palate and shows the palatal processes on each side of the tongue

of the posterior nares so that they eventually lie on each side of the posterior free edge of the adult nasal septum.

In later development membranous ossification from the premaxillae extends into the primitive palate, and from the maxillae and palatine bones into the maxillary

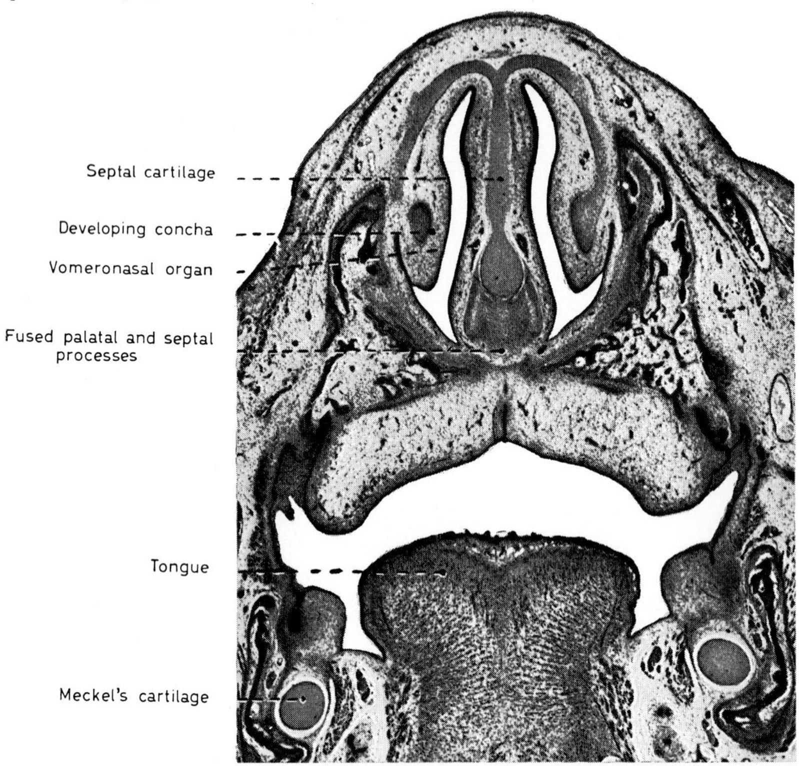

Figure 4.9 Photograph of a section through the palate of a 48 mm human embryo. The palatal processes have fused with each other and with the septal process

palatal processes. The posterior portions of the latter, however, do not become ossified; they extend beyond the nasal septum and fuse to form the *soft palate* and *uvula*. A small opening, the naso-palatine canal, persists for a time in the middle line between the primitive palate and the maxillary palatal processes. Eventually epithelial fusion obliterates the naso-palatine canal. Its position is represented throughout life, however, in the hard palate by a foramen known as the *incisive canal*.

Anomalous fusion, or lack of fusion, of the maxillary palatal processes with each other or with the posterior margin of the primitive palate results in some form of *cleft palate*. Cleft palate is frequently associated with *hare-lip*. In this condition there has been an apparent failure of fusion between the maxillary process of one (unilateral hare-lip) or both (bilateral hare-lip) sides with the fronto-nasal process. Hare-lip may, however, be due to an initial abnormality in the establishment of the primitive palate (Töndury, 1950; Warbrick, 1960). If both maxillary processes fail to reach the middle line the lower margin of the nasal septum appears in the palatal cleft as a free edge. If only one process fails to reach the middle line then only one nasal cavity communicates through the palatal cleft with the mouth (*see* Holdsworth, 1963, for details).

The paranasal sinuses

During the development and growth of the palate, and more locally of the frontonasal process, the primitive nasal cavity extends upwards. On its lateral surface a series of ectodermal elevations appear. These fuse to form three main elevations, into which mesenchyme migrates and later differentiates into osteogenic tissue. The three elevations become the superior, middle and inferior turbinates (conchae). The superior turbinate is derived from the embryonic maxilloturbinate, the other two from the ethmoturbinates. Occasionally a supreme turbinate develops above the superior concha. A small anterior elevation called the nasoturbinate is rudimentary in man, and in the adult becomes the agger nasi.

The paranasal sinuses in the adult are air-containing spaces communicating with the nasal cavity. They develop late in fetal life or in the early post-natal period. There are four sinuses on each side – maxillary, sphenoidal, frontal and ethmoidal. The maxillary sinus appears first and is initially represented as a depression in the nasal wall below the middle turbinate. The depression rapidly becomes a groove, grows laterally and invades the body of the maxilla. The sinus grows in spurts associated with eruption of the molar teeth and reaches its full size after the time of eruption of the permanent dentition. The sphenoidal sinus appears before birth; it is a small but definite cavity at birth. After five years it has invaded the pre-sphenoid bone and there are successive periods of rapid growth at about the age of ten years and later at puberty. The frontal and ethmoidal sinuses are represented merely by epithelial diverticula at birth. The frontal sinus develops as an upgrowth from the diverticulum that is to form the anterior ethmoidal sinus. Growth begins at about the sixth month of intra-uterine life, but the developing sinus only invades the frontal bone within the first year after birth. The sinus grows steadily for about ten years, but shows a more rapid growth at puberty. The ethmoidal sinuses develop from grooves between the embryonic ethmoturbinates and are present as little diverticula during the last month of fetal life.

The sinuses continue to grow and alter in shape until the age that general growth in bone ceases. There is some evidence that the epithelium of the invading mucous membrane of the sinuses is capable of influencing the destruction of bone. Occasionally the sinuses enlarge excessively and their walls may press on branches of the trigeminal nerve in the vicinity.

Anatomy of nose and nasal cavity

The supporting framework of the external nose consists of a bony part and a number of paired and unpaired cartilages. The bones consist of the anterior part of the body of the maxilla with its frontal process, the nasal spine of the frontal bone and the nasal bones. The nasal bones articulate with the medial surface of the frontal process of the maxilla and superiorly with the medial part of the nasal notch of the frontal bone. They rest superiorly on the anterior surface of the nasal spine of the frontal bone and articulate inferiorly in the middle, by means of a small crest, with the lower part of the perpendicular plate of the ethmoid bone. Their free lower borders are attached to the upper lateral cartilages of the nose. Hence the bony aperture to the external nose is bounded by the projecting free lower borders of the nasal bones above, by the anterior edges of the maxillae on each side, and by the fusion of the bodies of the maxillae (pre-maxillae) below. A small median projecting spine, the anterior nasal spine of the maxilla, is present on the anterior aspect of the lower border of the aperture. The bony part of the nasal septum does not project into the external nose and thus the anterior nasal aperture in the prepared skull is a single pear-shaped opening.

The flexible framework is basically a single central septal cartilage, two upper and two lower nasal cartilages, and the two smaller alar cartilages (*Figure 4.10*). The septal

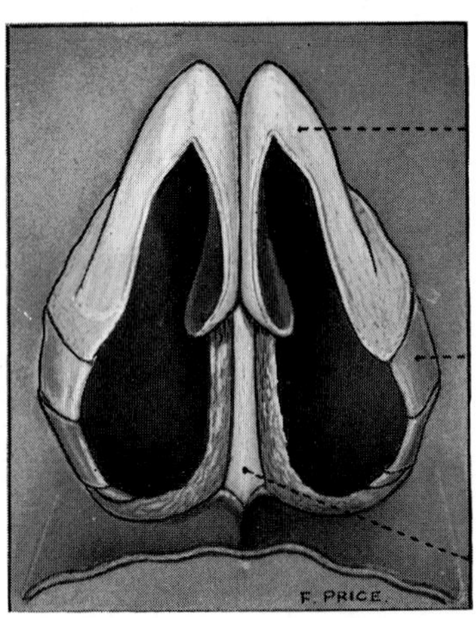

Figure 4.10 The cartilages of the nose seen from below

cartilage is somewhat quadrilateral in shape (*Figure 4.16*). It is attached to the perpendicular plate of the ethmoid bone postero-superiorly, to the internasal crest and suture superiorly, to the anterior border of the vomer posteriorly, and to the nasal crest of the maxillae and the anterior nasal spine inferiorly. To the antero-superior border of the septal cartilage are attached the two upper nasal cartilages. Of these latter, the upper part is continuous with the septal cartilage, whereas the lower part is relatively free, there being only a perichondrial attachment. The lower nasal cartilage is loosely attached by its medial septal process to the lower inferior part of the septal cartilage.

The posterior border of the septal cartilage is often elongated in the form of a narrow process, so that it fits in between the vertical plate of the ethmoid bone and the anterior border of the vomer. This process is frequently well-marked in children. A narrow prolongation of cartilage, the subvomerine cartilage, which may be part of, or distinct from, the septal cartilage, passes backwards parallel to the postero-inferior surface of the septal cartilage. It forms the support for the lower part of Jacobson's organ.

The upper nasal cartilage is triangular in shape (*Figure 4.11*) and, in addition to being attached to the septal cartilage as described above, is attached to the anterior edge of the nasal bone and the frontal process of the maxilla. Inferiorly, it is connected to the lower nasal cartilage by fibrous tissue. The lower nasal cartilage is thin and is bent round the external aperture to form a medially-placed septal process which is attached by fibrous tissue to the septal cartilage and to the process of the opposite side (*Figure 4.10*). Posteriorly the lower cartilage is connected with the frontal process of

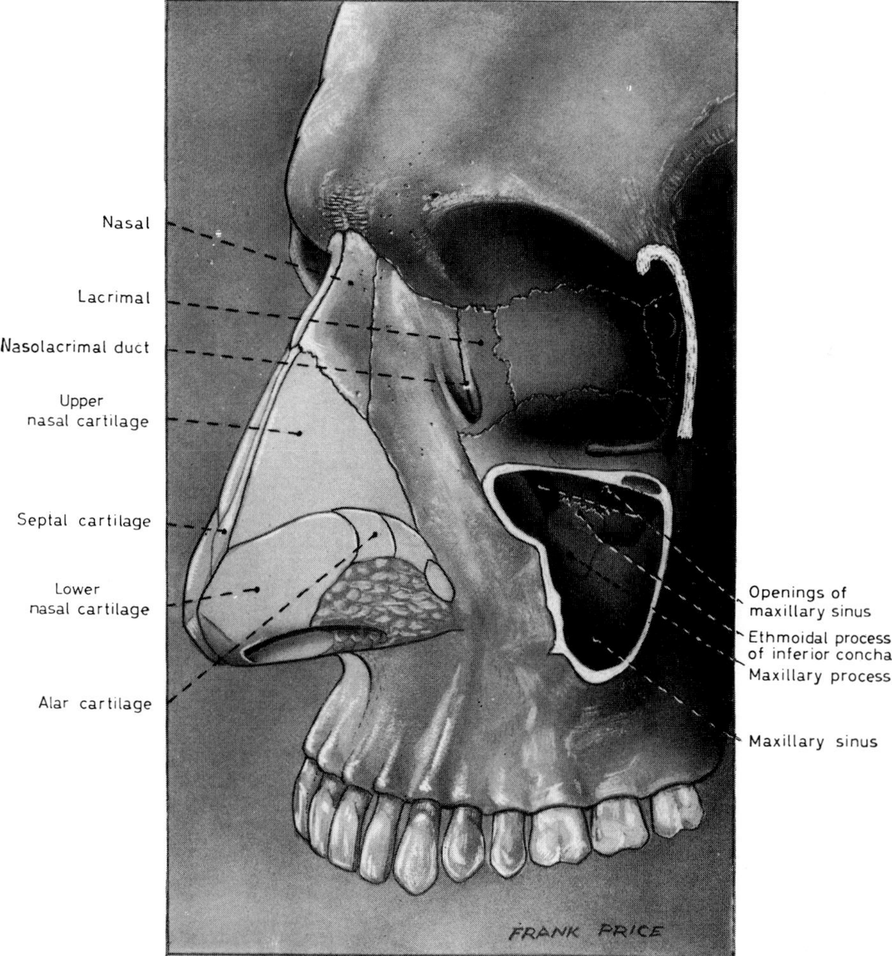

Figure 4.11 The cartilages of the nose. The maxillary sinus has been opened to show the medial wall

the maxilla by a strong fibrous membrane in which are several small alar cartilages. The contours of the alae of the nose derive their rounded appearance from the wedge of fibrous fatty tissue which is adherent to the lower edges of the alar cartilages (*Figures 4.10* and *4.11*).

The lower cartilage is relatively loosely attached and thus the lower part of the nasal septum and the tip of the nose are movable (septum mobile nasi) upon the more firmly attached septal cartilage. At the apex of the nose the two lower nasal cartilages end at a small notch, and here also the two cartilages are relatively loosely attached (*Figure 4.11*). The muscles bringing about the movement of the alae and the lower part of the septum are the procerus; the nasalis, consisting of a transverse part (compressor naris) and an alar part (dilator naris); and the depressor septi. The muscles are either attached to the cartilages or, as in the compressor naris, pass across the nose from the maxilla to a central aponeurosis. Their action is as their names indicate, but they are seldom well-developed in man; all are innervated by the upper buccal branches of the facial nerve.

It should be noted that the skin over the lower part of the nose is thicker and more securely attached to the cartilages than is the skin on the upper part. A large number of sebaceous glands are present in the skin of the alae. The skin is supplied through the infratrochlear branch and the anterior ethmoidal branch of the ophthalmic nerve, and also from the infra-orbital branch of the maxillary nerve. The blood supply is from the facial artery to the alae and lower part of the septum, and from the external nasal branch of the ophthalmic artery and the infra-orbital branch of the maxillary artery to the lateral surface and septum. The arterial and nerve supply from the ophthalmic artery and nerve indicate the developmental origin of the external nose.

The bony structure of the nasal cavity

The nasal cavity is divided into right and left halves by the median nasal septum. Each cavity extends from the nares (nostrils) anteriorly to the posterior nasal apertures or choanae posteriorly where it communicates with the nasopharynx.

Owing to the deficiency of the bony septum anteriorly, the nasal cavity in the prepared skull presents a single anterior opening. The cavity is wide below at the floor and narrows above to the roof. Each half of the cavity has a roof, a floor and a lateral and a medial wall. The medial walls are formed by the two sides of the septum. Each half of the cavity communicates with the maxillary, sphenoidal, frontal and ethmoidal sinuses of the same side.

The roof has a sloping anterior (frontonasal) portion, a more horizontal central part and a sloping posterior (sphenoidal) portion (*Figure 4.12*). The front part is made by the nasal bones and the under-surface of the nasal spine of the frontal bone. The central part is made by the cribriform plate of the ethmoid bone. The posterior sloping part of the roof is made by the under-surface of the body of the sphenoid bone, which is partially covered over by the alae of the vomer, the sphenoidal process of the palatine, and the vaginal process of the medial pterygoid plate (*Figure 4.13*).

The floor is concave from side to side and is slightly concave from before backwards (*Figure 4.14*). The anterior three-quarters is formed by the junction of the palatine processes of the two maxillae and the posterior quarter by the union of the horizontal plates of the two palatine bones (*Figure 4.13*). Anteriorly, close to the base of the septum, is the incisive fossa. In the roof of the fossa are two lateral incisive canals and two median incisive foramina. The latter transmit the long sphenopalatine nerves. The lateral incisive canals represent the site of the embryonic communication between the nasal and buccal cavities and thus define the line of union on the palate of the pre-maxilla with the maxilla.

The anterior nasal aperture has already been described (p. 14). The posterior nasal apertures are separated by the posterior free edge of the vomer; the alae of the latter spread laterally at their junction with the body of the sphenoid bone above, and thus help to form part of the roof. The vaginal process of the medial pterygoid plate passes medially to meet the ala of the vomer and so forms part of the roof (*Figure 4.13*). The remainder of the roof is formed by the body of the sphenoid bone; the floor of the aperture is formed by the free edge of the horizontal plate of the palatine bone.

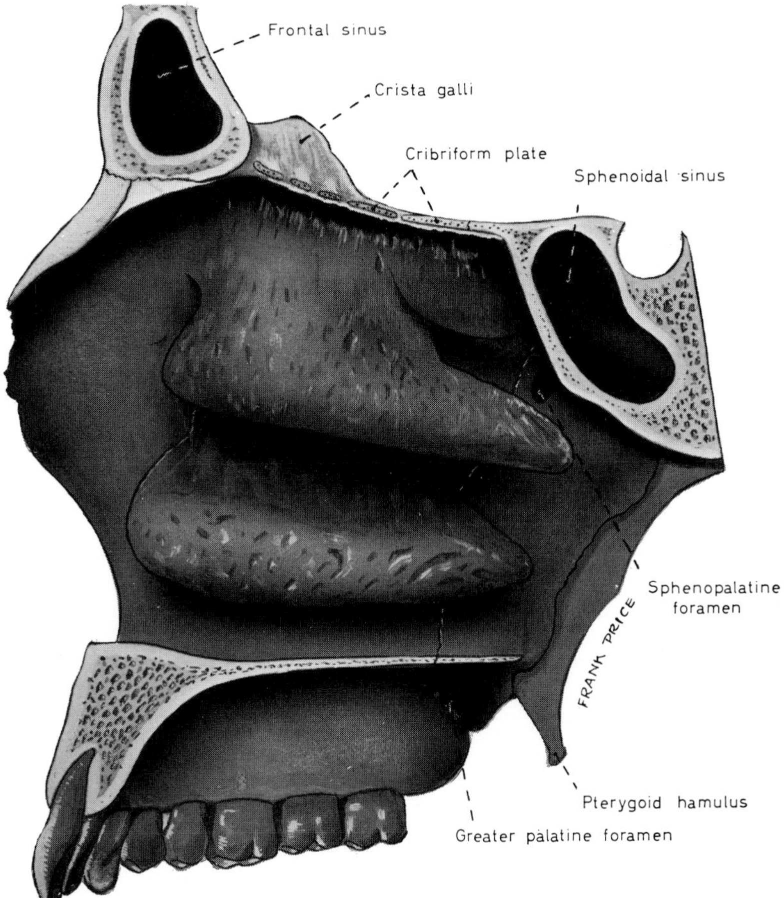

Figure 4.12 The appearances of the lateral bony wall of the nasal cavity with the conchae in position

The lateral wall of each nasal fossa is composed of a number of bones and presents a complicated form owing to the presence of three scroll-like projections (*Figure 4.12*), the superior, middle and inferior turbinate bones. The description of this wall is given with the turbinates in position, and after their partial removal to display the lateral walls of the meatuses.

Anteriorly, the wall is formed by the inner aspect of the nasal bone, the frontal process and anterior part of the body of the maxilla, and it is overlapped by the anterior end of the inferior turbinate. The upper middle part of the wall is formed by the medial surface of the ethmoidal labyrinth, with the superior turbinate projecting from its postero-superior part, and the middle turbinate from its anterior and middle surfaces (*Figure 4.14*).

The superior turbinate is the smallest of the turbinates and may be reduced to only a small ridge about 1.25 cm below the cribriform plate. Above and behind the superior turbinate is a small depression, the spheno-ethmoidal recess, into which opens the sphenoidal sinus.

The middle turbinate is large and its anterior part extends forward to articulate

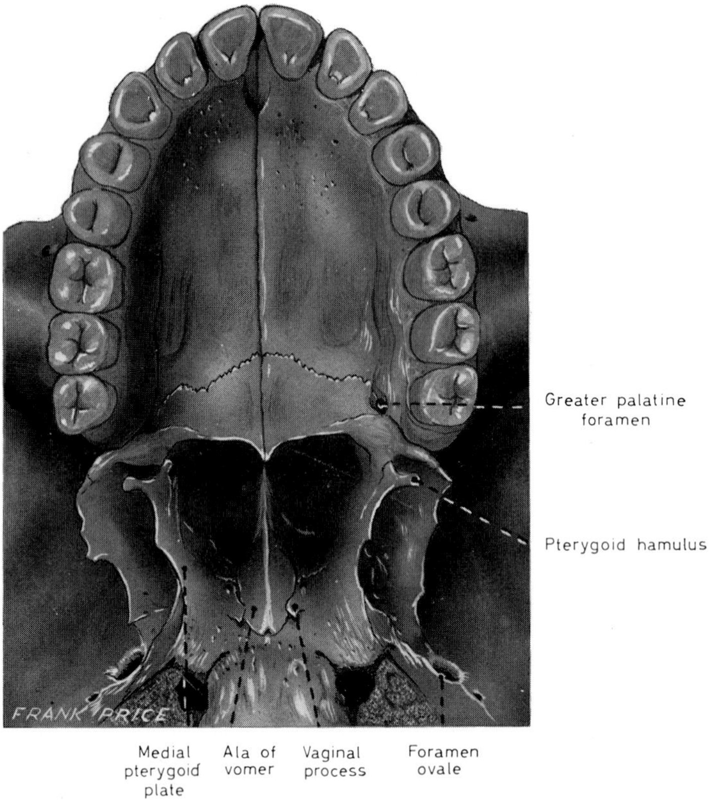

Figure 4.13 The palate and posterior nasal apertures seen from below

with the ethmoidal crest on the frontal process of the maxilla. The posterior edge extends as far back as the medial surface of the perpendicular plate of the palate. The free edge is turned down and inwards and curves from the anterior to the posterior attachments. Below the middle turbinate in the middle part of the lateral wall is a gap partially closed by a number of bones. Of these, the largest is the inferior turbinate, and it extends, as already indicated, from the body of the maxilla to the ethmoidal crest on the perpendicular plate of the palatine. Below the turbinate the middle part of the lateral wall is formed by the body of the maxilla. The posterior part of the lateral wall is formed by the perpendicular plate of the palatine and the inner surface of the medial pterygoid plate. In the upper part of the perpendicular plate, and between it and the sphenoid, is the sphenopalatine foramen. It should be realized that the inferior turbinate is a separate entity, whereas the superior and middle turbinates are projections from the ethmoidal labyrinth.

The spaces overhung by the turbinates are called the meatuses (*Figure 4.15*). Removal of the three turbinates at their attachments reveals the structure of the lateral wall of each meatus (*Figure 4.14*). The small superior meatus shows an opening which leads into the posterior ethmoidal sinus. Immediately below the attachment of the middle turbinate is a swelling, varying in size, known as the bulla ethmoidalis. This bulla is produced by the bulging out of part of the middle ethmoidal sinus; the opening of this sinus lies on or above the bulla ethmoidalis. Below the bulla the long

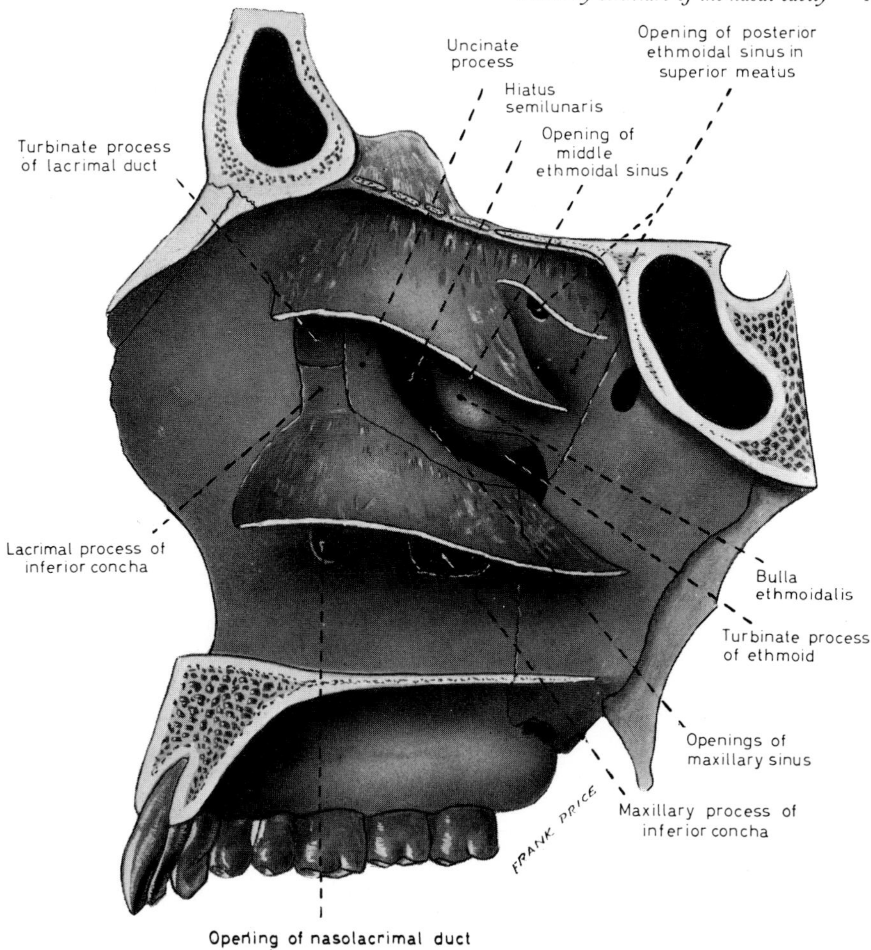

Figure 4.14 The lateral bony wall of the nasal cavity; the turbinates are cut short at their attachments to display the three meatuses

curved uncinate process of the ethmoid projects downwards and backwards from the anterior extremity of the ethmoidal labyrinth to articulate with the ethmoidal process of the inferior turbinate; this process partially closes the opening in the maxilla which leads into the maxillary sinus (antrum of Highmore). The uncinate process articulates in front with the ethmoidal process of the lacrimal bone and with the lacrimal process of the inferior turbinate as far back as the ethmoidal process. The postero-superior surface of the uncinate process has a free edge which forms the lower boundary of a curved fissure, the hiatus semilunaris. The upper boundary of the hiatus is formed by the bulla ethmoidalis. The descending process of the lacrimal bone and the lacrimal process of the inferior turbinate together form the medial bony wall of the nasolacrimal duct. From the middle of the superior border of the inferior turbinate the maxillary process passes downwards and further closes the opening of the maxillary sinus by articulating with the maxilla and the maxillary process of the palatine.

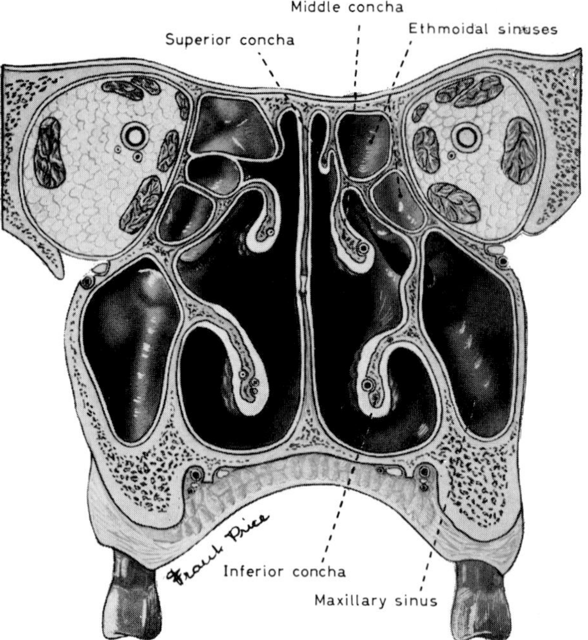

Figure 4.15 A coronal section through the conchae, ethmoidal and maxillary sinuses

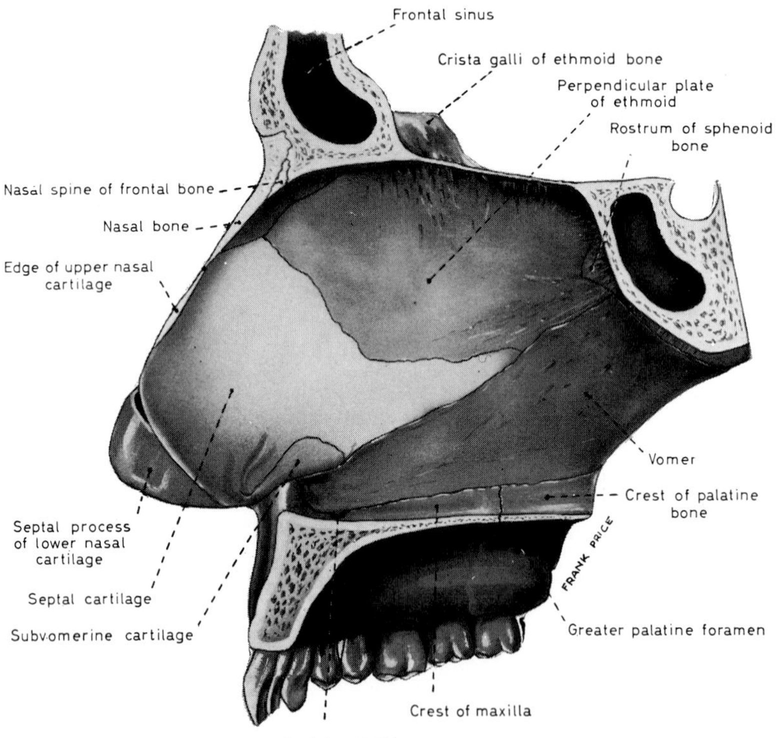

Figure 4.16 The cartilaginous and bony septum of the nose

Superiorly, the hiatus is continuous with the infundibulum, into which the anterior ethmoidal sinuses open, and which may, in 50 per cent of subjects, communicate with the frontal sinus. The latter sinus, however, may drain separately into the anterior part of the meatus. The opening of the maxillary sinus is found in the posterior part of the hiatus semilunaris. The bony wall of the meatus may be deficient below the hiatus semilunaris, but the deficiency is usually closed by mucous membrane.

The inferior meatus is the largest of the three meatuses and, in its deepest part, near the anterior end, is the opening of the nasolacrimal duct. Sometimes the lower edge of the inferior turbinate descends vertically for a varying distance before turning abruptly backwards. More frequently, the two portions continue without any marked irregularity.

The central septum (*Figure 4.16*) is formed by the perpendicular plate of the ethmoid above and anteriorly, and by the vomer below and behind. The perpendicular plate articulates with the nasal spine of the frontal bone above and is attached behind to the cribriform plate. Posteriorly, the perpendicular plate articulates with the body of the sphenoid bone. The upper end of the vomer is thickened to form two alae which spread out on the under-surface of the sphenoid and are held in place by the vaginal processes of the medial pterygoid plates (*Figure 4.13*). The rostrum of the sphenoid bone, a small anteriorly directed wedge of bone projecting from the body of the sphenoid bone, fits in between the postero-inferior edge of the ethmoid bone and the antero-superior angle of the vomer. Inferiorly, the vomer articulates with the nasal crest, the latter being a slight ridge at the junction of the horizontal plates of the two maxillae and palatine bones. The septum is often deflected at the vomero-ethmoidal suture, causing disparity in the size of the two halves of the nasal cavity. Ridges of bone may occasionally be found projecting from one or both sides of the septum.

The cavity in the recent state

Each half of the nasal cavity in the recent state can be divided into four parts, the vestibule, the atrium, the olfactory and the respiratory regions (*Figure 4.17*). The vestibule is the expanded portion within the anterior aperture of the nose. It is bounded laterally by the ala of the nose and the lateral nasal cartilages and medially by the lower part of the septum. The vestibule can be further subdivided into a lower part lined with skin and containing sebaceous glands and long strong hairs, the vibrissae, and an upper part, also lined by skin, but which is smooth. It is limited above and posteriorly by the elevated limen nasi which corresponds to the margin of the lower nasal cartilage. The upper region extends into the atrium, which is marked by a depression on the lateral wall anterior to the upper end of the middle turbinate. The atrium is defined above by a ridge of mucous membrane, the agger nasi, which runs from the upper end of the middle turbinate above the atrium and then downwards towards the vestibule. The agger nasi is most marked in the newborn; it represents the nasoturbinate bone which is found in many mammals. The groove above the agger nasi leads up to the olfactory region and is called the sulcus olfactorius nasi.

The olfactory region consists of the upper part of the nasal cavity and is related to the superior turbinate and the upper part of the septum. The cribriform plate of the

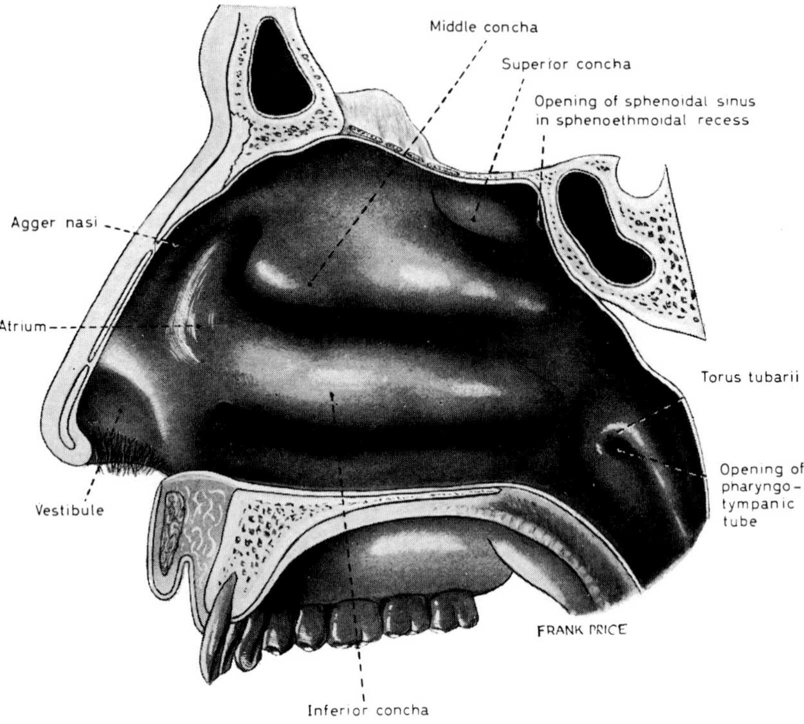

Figure 4.17 The lateral wall of the nasal cavity in the recent state

ethmoid bone forms its roof. The remainder of the nasal cavity forms the respiratory portion.

The mucous membrane of the nasal cavity is inseparably applied to the periosteum or perichondrium. It is thick and vascular, being most developed over the turbinates, the septum and on the floor, whereas that of the sinuses is relatively thin. The epithelium varies in structure; in the lower respiratory part of the cavity, except in the pre-turbinate area, it is ciliated columnar in type.

Numerous goblet cells are present in the epithelium beneath which is an almost continuous layer of mucous and serous glands. In addition, there are aggregations of lymphoid tissue. By contrast, in the upper olfactory region, and in the vomeronasal organ (*see below*), olfactory epithelium is present. This consists essentially of biopolar nerve cells and supporting cells with oval nuclei. Beneath the olfactory epithelium is a layer of serous, tubular, branched nasal glands. The epithelium of this region has a distinct yellow colour in man, as opposed to the brown coloration present in some animals.

A small depression may be present at the lower edge of the septal cartilage, over the incisive canal, marking the position of the original canal that connected the buccal cavity with the nasal cavity in the embryo. A small opening may lead backwards into a blind pouch, placed in the septum close to this depression. The pouch represents the vomeronasal organ (Jacobson) (*Figure 4.16*), which is well developed in some animals, but is vestigial in man. The pouch is backed by a slip of cartilage, the subvomerine cartilage, placed in the lower part of the septum. The organ is an accessory olfactory area, and is supplied by twigs from the olfactory nerve. In the human embryo, up to the eighth week, the epithelium in the vomeronasal organ is relatively better developed, but it soon undergoes retrogressive changes. A patent naso-palatine canal has been reported in the adult; air or dye-stuff could be sucked from the nasal cavity into the mouth.

Blood vessels and nerves

The nasal cavity derives its blood supply from several sources (*Plate 3, facing page 206*). The anterior and posterior ethmoidal branches from the ophthalmic artery enter the nasal cavity through the anterior and posterior foramina in the cribriform plate of the ethmoid bone. The anterior ethmoidal artery supplies the septum and upper part of the lateral wall, and it sends a terminal branch on to the dorsum of the nose between the nasal bone and the upper nasal cartilage. The spheno-palatine branch of the maxillary artery enters the nasal cavity by the spheno-palatine foramen. It gives off a large septal branch which passes downwards and anastomoses with the terminal branches of the greater palatine artery and the labial branch of the facial artery. It also gives off a number of lateral nasal branches, which ramify over the turbinates and in the meatuses. The greater palatine artery descends through the greater palatine canal to emerge on the oral surface of the palate through the greater palatine foramen. It runs forward in a groove on the palatal surface of the maxilla to the incisive canal. Branches pass through this canal to anastomose with the septal branches of the spheno-palatine artery. In the greater palatine canal a number of branches penetrate the perpendicular plate of the palatine bone and anastomose on the lateral wall with the lateral nasal branches of the spheno-palatine artery. The superior labial branch of the facial artery ascends through the upper lip and gives off both septal and alar branches.

In the mucous membrane of the nose the arrangement of the blood vessels is said by Swindle (1935, 1937) to consist of a superficial venous plexus and a deeper arteriolar system, arranged parallel to the long axis of the nose. The venous plexus is especially marked over the lower turbinates and the lower part of the septum. It has been shown by Harper (1947) that the main arteries occupy an interosseous position and branches pass from these arteries to form a fine subepithelial plexus. From this plexus the blood passes into irregularly arranged cavernous spaces which resemble those found in erectile tissue. The cavernous tissue appears early in development, being present in embryos of 44 mm and being well developed at the 150-mm stage (Boyd and Harper, 1946). Arterio-venous anastomoses are also described in the nasal mucosa; these may play an important part in the control of the erectile tissue.

The venous plexus drains to the neighbouring large veins, the spheno-palatine vein and the anterior facial vein, and from the ethmoidal to the ophthalmic veins, and there are communications with the cerebral veins through the cribriform plate. A communicating vein may pass through the foramen caecum, which lies between the crista galli and the frontal crest, and when this foramen is patent, this vein opens into the superior sagittal sinus.

The nerve supply of the mucous membrane is derived from the anterior ethmoidal branch of the nasociliary nerve, the anterior superior dental branch of the maxillary nerve, the nerve of the pterygoid canal, the long spheno-palatine nerve, the greater palatine nerve and nasal branches from the spheno-palatine ganglion (*Plate 3, facing page 206*). With the exception of the nasociliary nerve, all the branches supplying the nasal cavity are derived from the maxillary nerve. These nerves carry the tactile and protopathic sensory fibres, and also those secretomotor fibres supplying the nasal glands. The olfactory nerves pass through the foramina in the cribriform plate of the ethmoid in a series of bundles, each of which is enclosed in a tube of pia and arachnoid. The meninges thus have a close relationship with the mucosa at this point. The olfactory fibres immediately enter the under-surface of the olfactory bulb, in which they ramify and form synapses. In rabbits, experimental investigation of the flow of particulate matter from the cerebrospinal fluid has shown that fine Indian ink particles can pass along the sheaths of the olfactory nerve bundles to reach the connective tissue stroma and lymphatic plexuses of the nasal mucosa (Field and Brierley, 1948). It is possible that there may be a retrograde flow of material from the nasal mucosa to the cerebrospinal fluid.

The lymphatic drainage from the anterior part of the nasal cavity is to the submandibular glands through the lymph vessels of the skin of the nose. The posterior portion of the cavity drains to the upper deep cervical glands and to those at the back of the pharynx. Further discussion of the lymphatic drainage of the nasal cavity and the paranasal sinuses is to be found in an article by Dixon and Hoerr (1944).

The paranasal sinuses

The paranasal sinuses are, on each side, maxillary, frontal, sphenoidal and ethmoidal.

Maxillary sinus

The maxillary sinus is the largest of the paranasal sinuses; it is a pyramidal cavity extending into the body of the maxilla (*Figures 4.15* and *4.18*). The pyramidal space lies with its apex directed laterally and with its base towards the nasal cavity. The apex sometimes extends into the zygomatic process of the maxilla, or even into the zygomatic bone. The floor of the sinus is made by the alveolar process of the maxilla, and in the adult the level of the floor is about 1.0 to 1.2 cm below that of the nasal cavity, whereas in the edentulous skull the level of the floor rises above that of the nasal cavity. The roof is formed by the orbital surface of the maxilla and is ridged by the canal of the infra-orbital nerve. The anterior wall is fairly thick and is formed by the anterior part of the body of the maxilla. The medial wall, however, is thin, being composed of the nasal surface of the maxilla, the descending part of the lacrimal bone, the uncinate process of the ethmoid, the maxillary process of the inferior concha, and the perpendicular plate of the palatine bone. The opening of the sinus (*Figure 4.18*) is a small slit between the inferior turbinate, its maxillary process, the uncinate process of the ethmoid bone and the perpendicular plate of the palatine bone. In the prepared skull, the opening of the sinus is double, but in the recent state the posterior opening is usually closed by mucoperiosteum. The opening to the sinus is found in the posterior part of the hiatus semilunaris in the middle meatus. There is occasionally, however, in

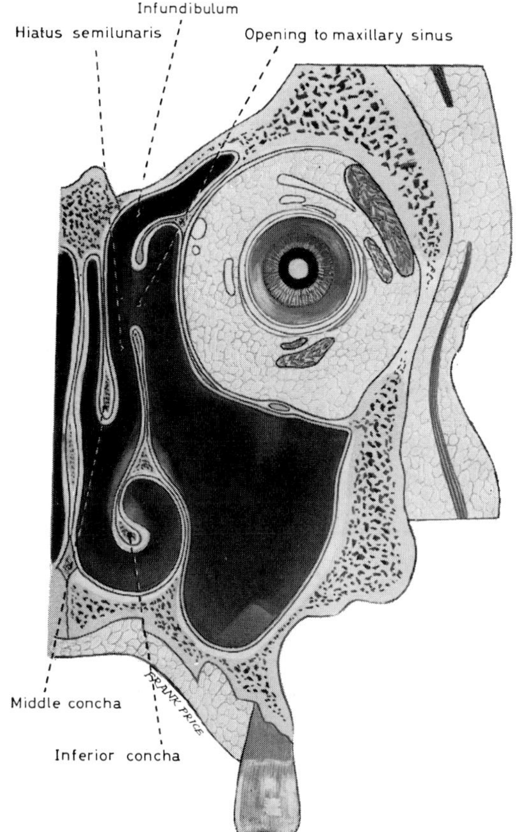

Figure 4.18 A coronal section through the maxillary sinus

the recent state, an accessory opening placed posteriorly. The following average dimensions of the adult sinus have been given: height, opposite first molar tooth, 3.5 cm; breadth, 2.5 cm; depth, 3.2 cm (Turner, 1901). A large sinus in the adult may hold 30 ml (1 fl. oz).

The lower part of the sinus may be subdivided by incomplete bony septa lying between the roots of the teeth. The number of teeth in relation to the floor of the sinus varies with age and with the size of the sinus; occasionally, all the teeth of the upper jaw from the canine to the third molar are found to be in relation with the floor. The posterior wall is often ridged by the projection of the alveolar canals which convey the posterior superior dental nerves and vessels to the teeth. The mucoperiosteum is frequently raised into a series of folds and ridges. The two sinuses are usually equal in size, but are not necessarily so; rarely, one sinus is completely absent.

The mucous membrane of the maxillary sinus is supplied by branches from the posterior superior dental branch of the maxillary nerve. The blood supply is from the posterior superior dental artery and from the spheno-palatine artery.

Frontal sinus

The two frontal sinuses are found in the frontal bone above and deep to the superciliary ridges (*see Figures 4.12* and *4.14*). A prominent superciliary ridge is not necessarily associated with a large frontal sinus. The two sinuses are usually unequal in size and each has the shape of an irregular pyramid with its apex directed upwards. They are separated by a thin septum of bone, which is seldom in the midline, and may occasionally be deficient. The septum may be placed obliquely, occasionally separating the sinuses almost in the coronal plane. The sinuses of men are generally larger than those of women, but there is great individual variation. A small accessory sinus may be found interposed between the lower parts of the two main sinuses. Frequently the sinuses extend backwards into the substance of the orbital plate of the frontal bone and they may extend as far back as the optic foramen.

The anterior wall is formed of diploic bone, and is the thickest of the walls, varying from 1 to 5 mm in thickness. The posterior wall is thinner, but is composed of more compact bone. The floor slopes medially downwards and backwards towards the opening of the fronto-nasal duct. The duct runs down through the front of the ethmoidal labyrinth and enters either the ethmoidal infundibulum (in 50 per cent of subjects), or else opens independently into the anterior end of the middle meatus. The following dimensions of the sinus have been given: height, 3 cm; breadth, 2.5 cm; and depth, 2 cm. The sinuses are fairly well developed at the age of 7 years, but they continue to increase in size until after puberty. The nerve supply of the sinus is from the supra-orbital nerve, but there are also branches direct from the nasociliary nerve. The blood supply is from the supra-orbital and anterior ethmoidal arteries.

Sphenoidal sinus

The body of the sphenoid bone is hollowed out by the ingrowth of the two sphenoidal sinuses from the nasal cavity (*see Figures 4.12* and *4.14*). Occasionally the sinuses spread laterally to invade the greater and lesser wings and the medial and lateral pterygoid plates of the sphenoid and occasionally even into the basilar part of the occipital bone. The sinuses are separated by a septum which is seldom in the midline and is sometimes deficient. Further partial septa may be present in the upper part of the sinuses: a well-marked lateral recess may be present. The irregularities in the shape of the sinuses are probably due to the developing sinuses coming successively into contact with the several independent centres of ossification of the sphenoid bone. Anteriorly the sinuses are covered by the thin sphenoidal turbinates (bones of Bertin) which were originally associated with the cartilaginous nasal capsule. These bones are at first free elements, but they fuse imperceptibly with the rest of the body of the sphenoid at about the tenth year or later. The sphenoidal turbinates fit over the anterior part of the sinus and are attached to the back of the ethmoid bone. A foramen in the centre of each turbinate allows the sinus of each side to communicate with the nasal cavity at the spheno-ethmoidal recess. Average measurements of the size of the adult sinus have been given as: height 2 cm; breadth, 1.8 cm; and depth, 2 cm; at birth the sinus is about 4 mm in height and 2 mm across. The sinus has many important relations which may cause elevations in its walls. Laterally, it is related to the optic nerve and to the cavernous sinus and its contents; superiorly, it is related to the under-surface of the frontal lobes and to the olfactory tracts. The pituitary gland lies above and posteriorly.

The nerve supply of the sinus is from the posterior ethmoidal branch of the nasociliary nerve and the blood supply is derived from branches of the spheno-palatine artery.

Ethmoidal sinuses

These sinuses consist of thin-walled cavities varying in size and number (3–18) and constitute the ethmoidal labyrinth. The labyrinth is suspended on each side from the edges of the cribriform plate of the ethmoid bone (*see Figure 4.15*). It rests inferiorly on the maxilla and is attached to the front of the sphenoidal concha. The posterior part of the labyrinth is separated from the maxilla by the perpendicular plate of the palatine. The orbital plate of the ethmoid bone forms the medial wall of the orbit, but it ceases to cover the labyrinth anteriorly, being replaced by the lacrimal bone which articulates with the frontal process of the maxilla anteriorly.

The sinuses contained within the labyrinth are arranged in three main groups, separated by thin-walled septa of bone. The sinuses of the three groups do not communicate with one another, neither do the sinuses of one group communicate with each other except by their ducts. The groups are referred to as the anterior, middle and posterior ethmoidal sinuses. The sinuses of each group open into the nasal cavity either through a common channel, one for each group, or else by independent openings. These three groups of sinuses may not be confined to the ethmoidal labyrinth; frequently they pass beyond into the maxilla below, the sphenoid bone behind and the frontal bone above.

The posterior ethmoidal sinuses open into the superior meatus below the superior turbinate. One or more of the posterior ethmoidal sinuses may communicate with the sphenoidal sinus. The posterior ethmoidal sinus is supplied by the posterior ethmoidal nerve and by the short spheno-palatine branches of the spheno-palatine ganglion. The blood supply is from branches of the spheno-palatine artery.

The middle ethmoidal sinuses open either immediately above or on the bulla ethmoidalis. The latter is a bony rounded projection into the middle meatus, lying above the hiatus semilunaris. It is partially formed by the bulging out of the middle ethmoidal sinuses. The middle group is sometimes included with the anterior.

The anterior ethmoidal sinuses open into the infundibulum, a curved tunnel which passes upwards in the anterior part of the ethmoidal labyrinth from the anterior end of the middle meatus. In 50 per cent of subjects it continues as the fronto-nasal duct to the frontal sinus, but the latter sinus may open independently into the middle meatus.

The anterior and middle ethmoidal sinuses derive their nerve supply from the anterior ethmoidal branch of the nasociliary nerve. The blood supply is from the branches of the spheno-palatine artery, but there are also additional twigs from the anterior ethmoidal artery.

The mucous membrane

The mucous membrane lining the paranasal sinuses is continuous with that of the nasal cavity through their openings. It is, however, thinner than that of the nasal cavity and it is closely applied to the periosteum. Numerous goblet cells are present and the mucus is swept into the nasal cavity by the ciliated columnar epithelium. The blood supply is relatively poor, which accounts for the pale yellow colour of the lining mucous membrane in the living subject. Cilia are not uniformly distributed over the sinuses, but are always found near the openings.

References

Boyd, J. D. (1933). *Journal of Anatomy, London*, **67**, 409

Boyd, J. D. and Harper, W. F. (1946). *Journal of Anatomy, London*, **80**, 231

Dixon, F. W. and Hoerr, N. B. (1944). *Laryngoscope*, **54**, 165

Field, E. J. and Brierley, J. B. (1948). *British Medical Journal*, **1**, 1167

Frazer, J. E. (1931). *A Manual of Embryology*. London; Baillière, Tindall & Cox

Harper, W. F. (1947). *Journal of Anatomy, London*, **81**, 392

Holdsworth, W. G. (1963). *Cleft Lip and Palate*, 3rd edn. London; Heinemann

Streeter, G. L. (1945). *Contributions to Embryology at the Carnegie Institution*, **31**, 27

Streeter, G. L. (1948). *Contributions to Embryology at the Carnegie Institution*, **32**, 133

Swindle, P. F. (1935). *Annals of Otology, Rhinology and Laryngology, St. Louis*, **44**, 913

Swindle, P. F. (1937). *Annals of Otology, Rhinology and Laryngology, St. Louis*, **46**, 600

Töndury, G. (1950). *Acta Anatomica*, **11**, 300

Turner, A. L. (1901). *Accessory Sinuses of the Nose*. London; Churchill

Warbrick, J. G. (1960). *Journal of Anatomy, London*, **94**, 351

5 Physiology of the nose and paranasal sinuses

Ellis Douek

Functions of the nose

The nose is an exposed organ subject to frequent and widespread ailments. Together with the sinuses it has, in the past, been particularly prone to serious and chronic bacterial infection. Today, although it is still open to viral infection, a major part of nasal disease is either the result of injudicious and often self-inflicted medication or to contrived changes in the environment. The most important of these are central heating and air-conditioning; but the combination of a mild allergy to house dust with the excessive dryness of a centrally-heated interior, and compounded by addiction to nasal decongestants, produces changes now very commonly seen. The treatment offered to patients, especially surgical treatment, is usually based on mechanical considerations and many failures result from overlooking the functional aspects of the nose and its lining.

The primary functions of the nose may be classified as follows:

(1) the respiratory channel;
(2) air-conditioning of the air stream;
(3) filtration;
(4) olfaction;
(5) vocal resonance;
(6) speech;
(7) nasal reflex functions.

Respiratory channel

The nasal passages constitute the uppermost part of the conducting passages along which the ventilation of the pulmonary alveolar surface is maintained. They serve as a natural airway, distinct from the buccal cavity, enabling respiration to proceed during mastication.

Respiratory air currents

The tidal air drawn in and forced out through the nose in the inspiratory and expiratory phases of normal respiration appears to traverse, in the main, fairly well-defined pathways through the nasal passages.

The course of these air currents has been determined: (1) by drawing air charged with ammonia vapour through the nose of a cadaver in which pieces of litmus paper had been placed; (2) by direct observation and cinematography of the path of smoke through a head divided sagittally with the septum replaced by a glass plate; and (3) by inserting moistened strips of litmus paper in the nose of a subject and studying the effect of inhaling the fumes of hydrochloric acid.

Inspiratory air currents

The pathway of inspired air through the nasal cavity is determined by the following factors: (1) the downward direction of the anterior nares; (2) the smallness of the inlet to the nasal cavity compared with the size of the posterior outlet; (3) the shape of the nasal cavity; and (4) the 'streamlining' of the anterior ends and surfaces of the turbinates, which causes them to exercise a minimal resistance to the inflow of air.

As a consequence of these anatomical features, the inspired air entering through the anterior naris is directed upwards in a narrow stream medial to the middle turbinate and then downwards and backwards in high, vaulted or parabolic curves. The stream fans out somewhat as it traverses the posterior choana. The main current passes close to the septum and the cold, dry, contaminated, inspired air does not enter the recessed meatuses (*Figure 5.1*).

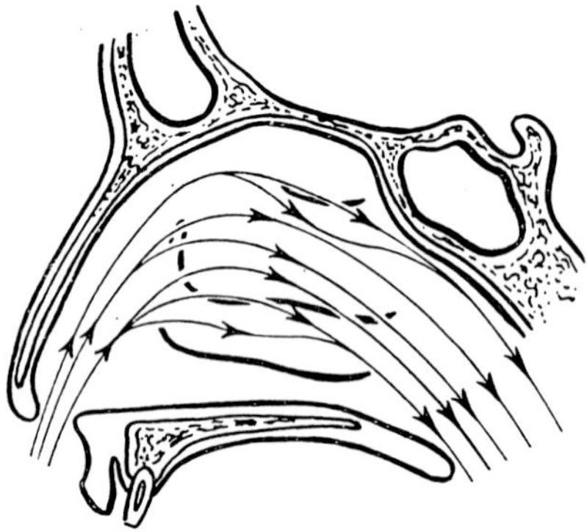

Figure 5.1 Diagram of inspiratory air currents

The relative rigidity of the fibrous and cartilaginous framework of the alae nasi prevents their collapse under the negative pressure of inspiration, which varies from −6 mm of water in normal inspiration to −200 mm of water in a maximal inspiratory effort.

Expiratory air currents (*Figure 5.2*)

In expiration the air enters the choana from the nasopharynx and follows much the same route as do the inspiratory air currents. Anteriorly, on meeting the constriction at the upper limit of the vestibule, the air current divides. A portion passes out through the nostril, and the remainder forms a large, central eddy, whirling back through the inferior meatus and rising to join the main stream from the nasopharynx. Part of this central eddy passes under the middle turbinate.

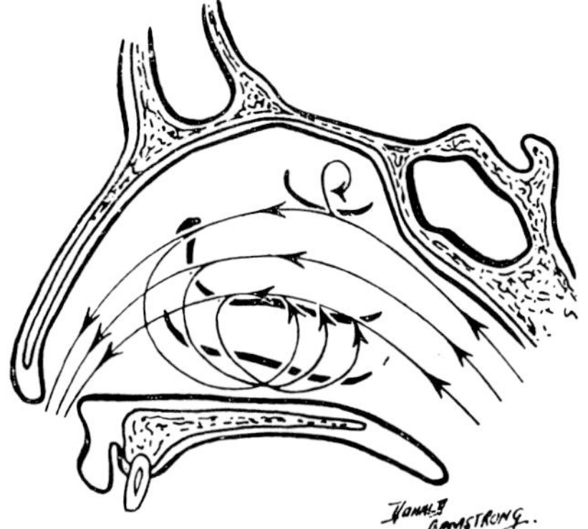

Figure 5.2 Diagram of expiratory air currents

Resistance and obstruction to air currents

It seems clear that except in forced respiration the respiratory air currents are restricted to the central part of the nasal chambers. Air currents do not pass through the lower part of the nasal cavities, nor does any considerable volume pass up into the relatively small olfactory area of the human nose. Narrowing of the nasal cavity in the region of the middle meatus constitutes therefore an important obstruction to the free passage of air. Septal deviations, spurs, polypi, mucosal hyperplasia and other causes of obstruction disturb the respiratory air currents. The air stream is thus diverted on to mucosal areas not adapted for heating and humidification. This may result in imperfect conditioning of the air and also produces local changes in the mucosa with reduction in resistance to bacterial invasion. A valvular function has been attributed to the inferior turbinate: the engorgement and depletion of its mucosa controls the passage of air through the nose.

The intranasal pressure varies from about -6 mm to $+6$ mm of water with the inspiratory and expiratory phases of normal respiration. The magnitude of these pressure fluctuations is dependent on the relative size of nostril and choana. The resistance to the flow of air through the nasal passages has been studied quantitatively. In normal noses the resistance is low. Shrinking of the mucosa with drugs reduces this frictional resistance markedly. With partial nasal obstruction the resistance may be nearly doubled.

Nasal component in airway resistance

The tidal air drawn in during inspiration meets with a frictional resistance to that air flow. This frictional resistance is partly between the molecules of the inspired air stream and partly between the moving mass of air and the walls of the conducting respiratory passages, that is, the nasal chambers, pharynx, larynx, the tracheo-bronchial tree and the intrapulmonary air-passages.

The air-flow resistance between a moving gas and the duct along which it is flowing, varies directly with the density of the gas, its velocity of flow and the length of the duct. The resistance varies also inversely with the fourth power of the diameter of the tube. Therefore small changes in the diameter of the channel along which a gas is flowing will bring about large changes in the resistance.

The nasal chambers contribute a notable portion of the total airway resistance. This nasal component in resistance to flow varies in different species. In man it probably provides 30 per cent of the total resistance. When the width of the nasal air channel is reduced by septal deviations, polypi or mucosal swelling due to allergy, inflammation or reflex vasodilatation to emotional stress, the resistance to air flow may become markedly increased.

The work performed in overcoming airway resistance in drawing air into the lungs is one of the elements of the total work done by the muscles of respiration. The contribution of the nasal passages to air-flow resistance may be of definite clinical importance since an increase in this resistance in pathological states of the nose is the main cause of symptoms.

Air-conditioning

Inspired air is both heated and moistened during its passage through the nose. It is assumed that this is beneficial in some way, probably in the protection of the alveolar epithelium and the lower reaches of the tracheo–bronchial tree. On the other hand, no absolute evidence has been produced regarding the effects of oral and nasal breathing. Tracheostomized patients have often been studied from that point of view and the reports have generally been reassuring. The recordings of Ingelstedt (1970) and Ingelstedt and Toremalm (1960, 1961) have demonstrated the difference in temperature and moisture between nasal and mouth breathing and although the question still remains open the clinician has no doubt of the value of normal nasal respiration. He has a definite experience of increased catarrhal problems which include the ears and larynx and an increased incidence of sinus problems. Most of all he knows that reassuring the patient about the most unpleasant subjective pharyngo–laryngeal and aural sensations associated with nasal obstruction will quickly end the latter's confidence.

Moisture appears to be of critical importance because dehydration will deplete the mucous blanket which protects the cilia. Drying of the cilia may be particularly destructive and nasal function grossly impaired.

Heating

Heating is closely bound up with moisture because of ordinary physical laws and it also has a similar place in the physiology of the transfer of gases. In this way, just as heat and moisture are taken up from warm vascularized nasal mucosa during inspiration, the saturated heated expired air gives up both water and heat to the relatively cooler, drier nasal lining.

The amount of heat lost through the nose will depend on the degree of dilatation of mucosal arterioles and of the sinusoids. Also important is the environmental temperature, and it has been calculated that in Arctic conditions about half the total heat and water is recovered by the nose while in temperate climates it would be about one-third (Cole, 1953). In general, the amount of heat and water lost from the respiratory tract amounts to 10–20 per cent of the total body loss. During violent exertion there is a tendency to breathe through the mouth so that less heat is taken up and more given off than during ordinary nasal breathing. This loss of heat should be considered in association with the increased muscular and metabolic activities involved with exercise. In dogs a good deal of heat is eliminated by panting although in humans this can result in carbon dioxide loss and alkalosis.

According to Negus (1958) the reason for warming inspired air is mainly to allow a greater amount of water vapour to be carried. To some extent it has a role in the regulation of body temperature but he could find no significant evidence that it was necessary in order to protect the respiratory system from cold air.

Moistening

The protection of the pulmonary alveolar epithelium from the effects of dust and other foreign particles in the inspired air is dependent largely on the continuous activity of the ciliated epithelium of the respiratory passages. Adequate saturation of the inspired air with water vapour is essential to the maintenance of the efficient functioning and the integrity of the ciliated epithelium. Absence of moisture, even for a few minutes, results in cessation of ciliary beating and in degeneration of the cilia. One barrier to the invasion of the mucosa by pathogenic bacteria is thus removed.

Moisture is also essential for the proper cleansing of the pharyngeal mucosa and for the protection from drying of the lining of the pulmonary alveoli. The exchange of respiratory gases between alveolar air and the blood in the pulmonary capillaries takes place through the film of moisture on the alveolar surface.

The almost complete saturation of the inspired air is effected with remarkable efficiency in the nasal cavities. Variations in the environmental temperature and humidity in different geographical regions and with different seasons of the year are of great importance in relation to the ability of the nasal mucous membrane to achieve saturation of the inspired air.

Failure of this humidifying function results in drying of the mucosa of the pharynx, larynx, trachea and bronchi. Drying of the larynx and of the tracheo-bronchial tree results in accumulation of strings of ropy mucus and inspissated secretions. This is followed by hyperplasia and reduced resistance to infection.

The origin of the moisture appears to be from two sources:

Secretion

There are two groups of glands in the nasal mucosa – large anterior groups and smaller lateral glands. The cells are either mucous- or serous-producing but the quantity of fluid produced is not known. Generally speaking it is unlikely that enough moisture is produced in this way to explain the complete saturation of the inspired air which reaches the alveoli.

Transudation

This is the passage of fluid through or between cells. It is the main method of humidification of inspired air, as atropinization can virtually abolish secretion without affecting saturation of inspired air. A great many factors are involved and many of them are imperfectly known. Nevertheless, the following are known to have an important place:

(1) *Hydrostatic pressure* – this is the simple process of ultrafiltration resulting from a difference of pressure between two sides of a membrane. This difference is provided by the circulation. The pressure in the tissue spaces is about 20 mmH_2O which is enough to cause transudation by a filter action.
(2) *Osmotic pressure* – this must work in the opposite direction to hydrostatic pressure.
(3) *The nature of the cell membranes and the intercellular cement substance* – little is known of the relationship between this and the transference of water but there is a considerable biochemical and hormonal influence.

Filtration

This aspect of nasal function, namely the cleansing of the inspired air from noxious particles, micro-organisms, etc. has recently been given renewed importance. The increasing pollution of the environment and the extraordinarily exposed nature of the nasal mucosa has placed upon it considerable stress, and at the same time aroused interest in its mechanisms.

Movement of particles

The particles which enter the nose are suspended in the air and the manner of their deposition depends on a number of factors:

(1) *Mass and density of the particles* – the greater the mass and density, the greater the effects of gravity and the more rapidly deposition will take place.

(2) *Air flow and shape of the particles* – the larger the size of the airway, the greater the velocity of flow, the less likely it is to be deposited early. Air resistance will be greater on a large irregular particle and be more likely to slow it down. On the other hand, the inertia of a heavy particle travelling at a greater velocity will not allow it to follow the air flow in a turbulent system and it is more likely to be deposited on the lateral walls.

The velocity of the air flow itself is less at the beginning of inspiration, accelerating and also increasing turbulence. The major part of the particulate matter is deposited in the anterior part of the nose but further amounts are deposited around the conchae and along bends in the septum as well as in the pharynx.

(3) *Diffusion*– although small particles can be removed by diffusion this probably happens very little at the flow-rates existing in the nose. Nevertheless, it is possible that some gases are removed in this way.

The nasal lining

The walls of the nasal chambers and accessory sinuses are lined almost entirely by a pseudostratified, columnar, ciliated epithelium. Only the olfactory area and the pre-turbinal region are non-ciliated. Human nasal cilia are delicate, tapering filaments, approximately 7 μm long and 0.3 μm thick, projecting from the free border of each cell. The free end of each cilium is curved slightly in the direction of the ciliary beat.

Electron microscopy has revealed that there are small slender projections under 1 μm in length called microvilli scattered between the main cilia. Each ciliated cell has approximately 250 cilia and 150 microvillous processes. The cilia have the usual ultrastructure of nine peripheral double filaments and two central filaments.

Ciliary movement is described as consisting of a 'forward' or effective stroke followed by a 'backward' or recovery stroke. The effective stroke is much more rapid than is the recovery stroke; it occupies only one-fifth of the time of one cycle. Moreover, the effective stroke constitutes the propulsive phase, the cilium remains rigid and the movement is vigorous. The recovery stroke is less rapid and less vigorous, and the cilium is relatively limp (*Figure 5.3*).

The cilia of the nasal mucosa beat at a frequency of 10–15 beats/s at the normal nasal temperature of 30°C. This produces a streaming movement of the overlying mucus which has been estimated at 0.25–0.75 cm/min. This movement is not equally rapid in all parts of the nose. As a general rule, it is more rapid in the posterior two-thirds of the nasal chambers than in the anterior third, and more active in the protected meatal recesses than on the exposed surfaces of the turbinates and the septum. The mucous covering of the non-ciliated pre-turbinal region is drawn back by the traction exerted by the cilia immediately behind this area. The clinically significant fact has been established experimentally that, provided the normal functional efficiency of the ciliated epithelium is maintained, the entire mucous blanket of the nose can be propelled into the pharynx every 20–30 min. The mucous covering of the paranasal sinuses is cleared in less than 10 min. Impairment of ciliary action or decreased secretion of mucus predisposes to penetration by bacteria into the nasal mucous membrane.

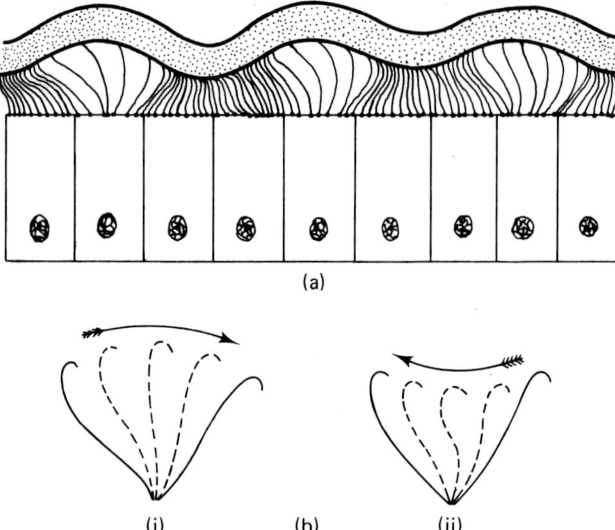

Figure 5.3 (a) Diagram of ciliated cells with overlying mucous blanket. Mucous blanket consists of outer layer of viscid mucus resting on a thin layer of serous fluid. (b) Diagram of ciliary action: (i) propulsive stroke of a single cilium: (ii) recovery stroke

The ciliary pathways

The pathways along which the cilia of the nose direct the mucus from the paranasal sinuses and the nasal chambers have been revealed by the researches of Lowndes Yates (1924), Hilding (1932) and others. The pattern of mucus clearance is shown in *Figure 5.4* and is summarized below.

From middle and inferior meatuses: main antral stream

The mucus from the mucosa of the anterior part of the lateral wall passes backwards through the middle and inferior meatuses. In the middle meatus it is joined by mucus from the sinuses opening into this recess. Mucus from the antrum streams back chiefly along the upper portion of the middle meatus to its posterior end. From here this main stream passes laterally and downwards, anterior to the pharyngeal ostium of the pharyngo–tympanic tube. The main stream continues down just behind the posterior pillar of the fauces. A portion is directed anterior to the posterior pillar into the recess between the tonsil and the posterior pillar. The main stream is joined by streams from the superior meatus and the sphenoidal sinus.

From the superior meatus

From the superior meatus, including mucus from the posterior ethmoidal cells, the stream passes into the nasopharynx and divides into two portions. The larger anterior stream extends down in front of the eustachian opening and joins the main antral

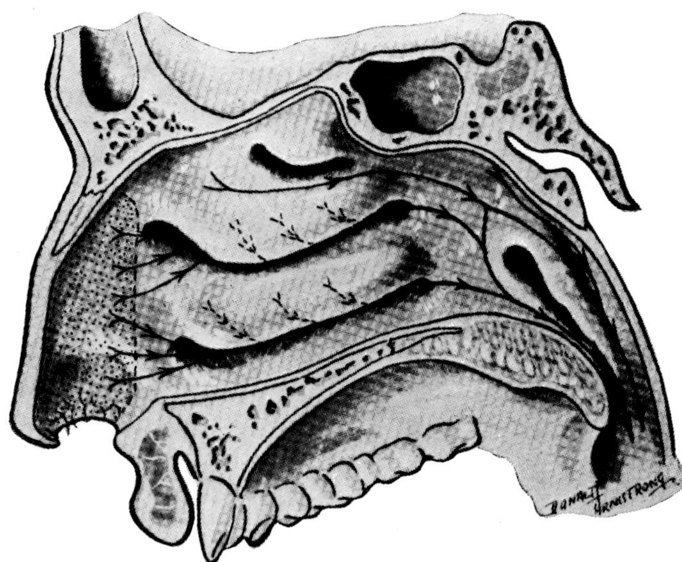

Figure 5.4 Pathways of clearance of mucus from lateral wall of nose

stream. The smaller posterior portion passes behind the eustachian orifice and downwards through the fossa of Rosenmüller, and then curves forward to join the main stream.

From the sphenoidal sinus

From the ostium of the sphenoidal sinus mucus passes down to the top of the nasal choana and then backwards on the roof of the nasopharynx, spreading in a fanwise manner into a series of streams, which pass outwards and join the main antral stream just below the lower margin of the palate.

These combined streams pass down posterior to the posterior pillar to the level of the dorsum of the tongue. A small part is conveyed across the tongue to the glosso–epiglottic pouch. the larger part continues down to the piriform sinus. From here the mucus is swallowed.

Factors influencing ciliary activity

The protection of the respiratory epithelium rests to an important extent on ciliary activity. The effects on the frequency and speed of ciliary beating, of drying, temperature, pH changes, and of various solutions introduced into the nose are, therefore, of definite clinical importance. This subject has been extensively investigated, particularly by Proetz (1953) on excised human sinus mucosa and by Negus (1934).

Drying

Adequate moisture is essential for the maintenance of the integrity and normal functional activity of the cilia. Drying of slight degree causes cessation of ciliary activity; prompt moistening restores normal activity. Drying for a few minutes leads to destruction of cilia. The sensitivity of cilia to lack of moisture underlies the importance of conditions in which excessive drying may occur in the nose. These conditions fall into three main groups: (1) prolonged breathing of excessively dry air, (2) inadequate secretion by mucosal glands, and (3) deviation of the inspired air stream by septal deflections, spurs or polypi. The deviated inspiratory air current is concentrated upon a restricted area of mucosa in excess of the local capacity to saturate the air. Excessive local evaporation results, with greatly increased viscosity of the nasal mucus. For efficient ciliary action a film of moisture and a mucous blanket of suitable viscosity is essential. Thus, local stasis of the mucous blanket and cessation of ciliary activity result.

Temperature

The optimal range of temperature for ciliary activity studied in excised human nasal mucosa is 28–33 °C (Proetz). The normal human nasal temperature has been recorded as about 32 °C.

Fall of temperature depresses the frequency of ciliary motion, and at about 7–10 °C all activity ceases. Warming to normal nasal temperature restores activity.

Rise in temperature results in depression of activity at 35 °C and in coagulation and irreversible arrest at 43–45 °C.

Saline solutions

The action of varying concentrations of sodium chloride on ciliary motion has been investigated on excised human sinus mucosa.

With isotonic saline solution (0.9 per cent sodium chloride solution) cilia remain active for prolonged periods.

Hypertonic saline solutions inhibit ciliary activity. All activity ceases in 4.5–5 per cent saline solution; activity returns when the mucosa is replaced in normal saline solution.

With hypotonic saline solution (0.3–0.2 per cent saline solution) all ciliary motion ceases. The ciliary mechanism is permanently damaged.

Changes in pH

Cilia are readily paralysed by acid solutions. If the pH is reduced to 6.4 or less, ciliary action is arrested (Negus, 1934). A rise in the pH is better tolerated. Ciliary activity is increased in dilute alkaline solutions. Cilia will function actively for prolonged periods in saline solutions of pH 8.5. The effect of dilute acids and alkalis is reversible; neutralization restores normal ciliary action.

The reaction of normal human nasal secretions is disputed. Determinations of the pH of collected secretions are vitiated by the disturbance of acid–base balance that occurs as a result of the evolution of carbon dioxide on exposure to air. The development of the glass electrode has made it feasible to record the pH of nasal secretions *in situ* with ease and precision. Parkinson's (1945) measurements gave an average pH value of 7.0, but Fabricant (1945) claims that the reaction in the clinically normal nose is on the acid side of neutrality and fluctuates in the majority of cases over a pH range from 5.5 to 6.5. Nasal pH is affected by temperature changes; rise of temperature tends to lower and cold to increase the pH. Inflammatory and allergic conditions of the nose and paranasal sinuses are associated with changes in the hydrogen-ion concentration of the nasal mucus. Correlation of the culturable bacterial content of the nose with characteristic changes in the pH in various types of nasal infections has been investigated. During acute rhinitis and the active phase of allergic rhinitis the nasal secretions tend to become alkaline in reaction (pH 8.0). The reaction returns to normal as the condition subsides. Fabricant has stressed the special clinical significance of these changes and the need for considering changes of reaction in the treatment of upper respiratory infections. Nasal solutions which restore the nasal pH to normal are recommended. Proetz has demonstrated in cases of chronic sinusitis that the cilia are functioning actively even when bathed in pus.

Drugs

The effects on ciliary action of drugs used intranasally are summarized below.

Adrenaline (1:10 000) causes reversible inhibition of ciliated cells when they are exposed to it for 20 min. Higher concentrations produce more rapid effects; immediate and irreversible cessation of ciliary motion is produced by 1:1000 adrenaline solution.

Ephedrine sulphate (0.5 per cent solution) does not affect ciliary action. Even with 2 per cent ephedrine, ciliary activity is not markedly depressed.

Cocaine (2.5 per cent solution) has little immediate action in the majority of experiments. Continuous application for 1 h stops ciliary activity. Five per cent solution causes arrest of ciliary motion in 2–3 min; the cilia cannot be resuscitated. Ten per cent solution produces immediate and complete ciliary paralysis.

2-Aminoheptane in isotonic solutions in varying concentrations from 0.5 to 4 per cent, does not produce impairment of ciliary action.

Amphetamine, although a volatile vasoconstrictor, is without appreciable action on cilia when inhaled. Direct application to the mucous membrane of a 1 per cent solution decreases the frequency of the ciliary beating, and more concentrated solutions (3 per cent) cause complete inhibition of the movements.

Acetylcholine causes an increase in the rate of ciliary beating.

Ether and chloroform, in high concentrations in the inspired air, have no effect on the nasal cilia in the living animal. Both liquids, however, on direct application cause immediate ciliary paralysis.

Regulation of ciliary action

Ciliary motion is an inherent property of ciliated cells. The cilia beat in orderly succession and the activity passes smoothly from cell to cell. The mechanism of ciliary movement and of the coordination of the rhythmic regulated activity of the cells of a ciliated epithelium is not clear.

The movements of cilia are probably the result of shortening of the longitudinally disposed contractile structures visualized as the peripheral filaments by the electron microscope. The effective stroke may be due to initial shortening of these contractile filaments on one side and the recovery stroke by the subsequent contraction of the contractile elements within the cilium on the opposite side.

Ciliary action is independent of the nervous system; excised portions of ciliated mucosa show sustained normal ciliary activity. Cilia were regarded as being spontaneously in constant action. Lucas (1935) questioned the validity of this conclusion. The normal ciliary activity had been studied by observing the rate of passage of particles across the ciliated surface, and these particles acted as stimuli.

Using a reflection method, Lucas claimed that unstimulated cilia were completely quiescent.

The rate of ciliary activity can be influenced by the extrinsic autonomic nerve supply. The precise effects are uncertain. In amphibian buccal mucosa sympathetic stimulation has been said to cause acceleration of ciliary movement. Greater speed of effective phase and greater amplitude of movement of the cilia accompany the increased frequency. This response is contrary to the inhibitory effect of high concentrations of adrenaline on human sinus mucosa, mentioned above. Stimulation of the parasympathetic fibres has an inhibitory effect. Lucas, on the other hand, adduced evidence that the cilio–accelerator fibres are in the cranial parasympathetic system and that sympathetic stimulation has no effect. Since these results are all based on experimental investigations of amphibian buccal mucosa, it is not certain how far they are applicable to human nasal mucous membrane.

Apart from its direct physical effect on deposed particles, the nasal secretion contains bactericidal compounds (e.g. lysozyme or muramidase) and immunoglobulins of which IgA is the most important. Hughes and Johnson (1973) described a circadian rhythm in which the highest concentration of IgA was during the night and the lowest in the afternoon. There was also a seasonal and individual difference.

By far the most important aspect of this nasal protective function is the filtration effected by the film of mucus which covers the surface of the nasal mucosa. This mucous blanket forms a continuous protective covering. The physical properties and chemical composition of the mucous layer are not known exactly, because of the difficulty of collecting it from the normal nose in any appreciable quantity. The secretions of the mucosal glands and goblet cells are diluted by a watery transudate passing through the lining epithelial layer and by the secretion of the lacrimal glands. The approximate composition is water, 96 per cent, inorganic salts, 1–2 per cent, and mucin, 2.5–3 per cent. It is extremely thin, elastic, highly viscous, and has a fair degree of tensile strength. The maintenance of the normal tenacity and viscosity of the nasal mucus is essential for the efficient functioning of the mucociliary apparatus. Small changes in mucin content produce relatively large changes in viscosity. Increased or decreased viscosity interferes with ciliary propulsion.

The mucous blanket consists of two layers. An outer layer of viscous mucus rests upon a thin layer of serous fluid which facilitates the movements of the cilia. The ends of the cilia are in contact with the overlying film of mucus. Ease of vibration of the cilia and of movement of the overlying mucous layer is thus ensured (*Figure 5.3*).

Finely divided particulate matter, dust, soot, pollens and micro-organisms are filtered out of the inspired air by adhering to the mucous film. Two factors are held responsible for the adhesion of foreign matter to the sticky mucus; these are direct impaction of the particles on to the surface of the mucus, and attraction by electrostatic surface charges (Proetz). The efficiency of this filtration is such that the posterior part of the nasal chambers contains very few bacteria and the sinuses are normally bacteriologically sterile.

Olfaction

The role of olfaction in the lower animals is of considerable and well-documented importance. Its role in the human is of much less note and it was often stated in the past that its sole physiological function was in the reflex secretion of digestive juices. Research in animals has demonstrated such an extensive range of functions, however, that it bears reassessing in man. The discovery of pheromones and their use in agriculture has particularly demanded a review of smell in man. This is because their place as sex attractants, territorial markers and aggression induction is so subtle that it is not possible to positively deny it in man. Despite this revival of interest over the last decade it has not been possible to investigate olfaction in comparable detail in man so that most of what is described here relates to animal work.

The basic functions of olfaction are related to (1) food intake, (2) reproduction, and (3) communication.

These will be discussed first and the review of the mechanisms involved will follow. (The application of olfactory problems to human pathology will be dealt with in Volume 3.)

1. Olfaction and food intake

All animals have to eat and this process involves two basic aspects. In the first instance the right food has to be selected and, indeed, the definition of a food must be a substance which is recognizable by the central nervous system to be of nutritive value. Not only has it to be selected but it should be taken in the right quantities by the mouth. The second aspect is the metabolic one where the ingested food is broken down to the body's requirements. One of the results of these metabolic changes is the regulation of the first part of the intake by a feedback effect.

The mechanisms responsible for this recognition are mainly the chemical senses of taste and smell, although visual and tactile clues also have a place. The sense of taste itself only provides biochemical information in the form of four modalities: salt, sweet, sour and bitter, and it is the sense of smell which provides the main elements of flavour which is what we mean by recognition. An interesting aspect of the relationship between olfaction and natural foods is that it is not the actual substance of nutritive value which provides the olfactory stimulus; it is not the fat, carbohydrate or protein which is odoriferous but rather the impurities that go with them. Nevertheless, there is enough behavioural information (von Bekesy, 1964) as well as experimental work (Leveteau and MacLeod, 1968) to confirm our natural belief that the sense of smell is primordial in seeking out foods. The place of innate responses as opposed to learned responses in food selection has not been fully determined in either man or animals, but the place of smell in adjusting food intake according to palatability has been shown beyond doubt (Le Magnen, 1956 a and b, 1960).

It is probable that simple innate responses are modified by experience and that this contributes through palatability and preferences to the intake of food. The regulation of this intake then depends on hunger and its metabolic signals (Le Magnen and Tallon, 1968).

The neurophysiology of this mechanism has been extensively studied (Anand and Pillai, 1976; Oomura *et al.*, 1967; Larue and Le Magnen, 1968). The primary role falls on the lateral and ventromedial hypothalamic centres. These respond directly to metabolites and to afferents from the alimentary tract and mouth. Implanted electrodes in these centres have recorded typical arousal responses to olfactory stimuli in the lateral hypothalamic centre though less consistently in the ventromedial hypothalamic centres.

2. Reproduction

It has been long suspected that smell plays a role in the biological processes of reproduction but it is only with the discovery of pheromones that its place has been fully accepted. Previously it was discussed in the emotional language of perfumery and prejudice.

The name pheromone was first used to describe sex attractants in insects but odorous chemicals of this type have been found in other animals including mammals.

There is a similarity between hormones and pheromones in that they are both formed by glands and that they affect behaviour, development and reproduction of individuals. The difference is in the fact that pheromones are produced by one individual and affect another.

Le Magnen (1952) showed that adult rats discriminate between the sexes by olfaction and that males can differentiate between receptive and quiescent females. Since then numerous examples of the place of olfaction in sexual behaviour have been found.

Bruce (1970) classified these responses into three types:

(a) *releaser pheromones* – which produce an immediate reversible response, e.g. by recognition;
(b) *primer pheromones* – which are slow to develop, requiring prolonged stimulation, and act through the anterior pituitary. Examples are the control of oestrus which male mammals exert on females; and
(c) *imprinting pheromones* – stimulation at a critical period during development may result in a permanent modification of behaviour in the adult.

3. Communication

Pheromones have a communication role in that they appear to act in methods of territorial marking as well as in indicating fear or stress.

Electrophysiology of olfactory impulses

The electrical responses to olfactory stimuli have been extensively studied. Recordings can be made from the receptor surface itself up to the cerebral cortex. They will be discussed in the following order:

(1) the electro-olfactogram (EOG),
(2) the olfactory bulb and its projections,
(3) the higher centres.

1. The electro-olfactogram

The electrical impulse discharge along the afferent nerve fibre of a sense organ results from a local depolarization effect at the receptor cell. In other words, the receptor cell generates a potential which gives rise to the nerve impulse.

In 1954 Ottoson was able to record a slow potential in response to an olfactory stimulus from the rabbit. The fact that the response was unchanged by blocking nerve conduction with cocaine confirmed the suggestion that the potentials came from the receptors themselves. Later work on the frog (Ottoson, 1956) allowed him to apply controlled odorous stimuli on the olfactory epithelium and to record simultaneously from the mucosa, the nerve fibre and the bulb. This led to his giving the name electro-olfactogram (EOG) to the monophasic negative potential evoked by odours in the sensory region of the nasal mucosa.

The characteristics of the electro-olfactogram

The electrical response of the sensory epithelium to a puff of odorous air is a slow, negative, monophasic potential. It rises steeply and then falls exponentially back towards the base line.

The *amplitude* of the response increases with increasing volume of stimulating odorized air up to a maximum. This may be due to an increasing number of receptors activated, possibly with different sensitivity. Furthermore, the amplitude of the response is also a function of the concentration of the odorant.

The EOG has a *latent period* which varies from 200 to 400 ms for butanol. This is unlikely to be the true latent period as some time is taken by the stimulating particles to cross the layer of mucus on the surface of the epithelium. Also, in the technical process of stimulation there may be an air front free of particles pushed ahead of the odorized air. This means that the true latency may be nearer 100 ms.

The *rising phase* of the potential rises faster with increasing strength of stimulus. On the other hand, the time it takes to reach its peak remains constant despite differences in strength.

The *falling phase* of the potential is exponential and has a time constant of 0.9–1.4 s and the decay is a logarithmic function of the concentration and it is different for different substances.

Superimposed on the EOG are often seen oscillations with a frequency of 15–25/s. It is not clear what they represent but they are likely to be intermittent synchronous activity in groups of receptors or even in groups of nerve fibres.

The problem of how stimuli give rise to neuronal codes which enable the recognition of one from the other still remains to be elucidated. What is clear is that it must be formed into a spatial and temporal pattern of activation among the 50 000 fibres of the olfactory nerve. As each channel conveys purely quantitative information, quality must be closely associated with intensity.

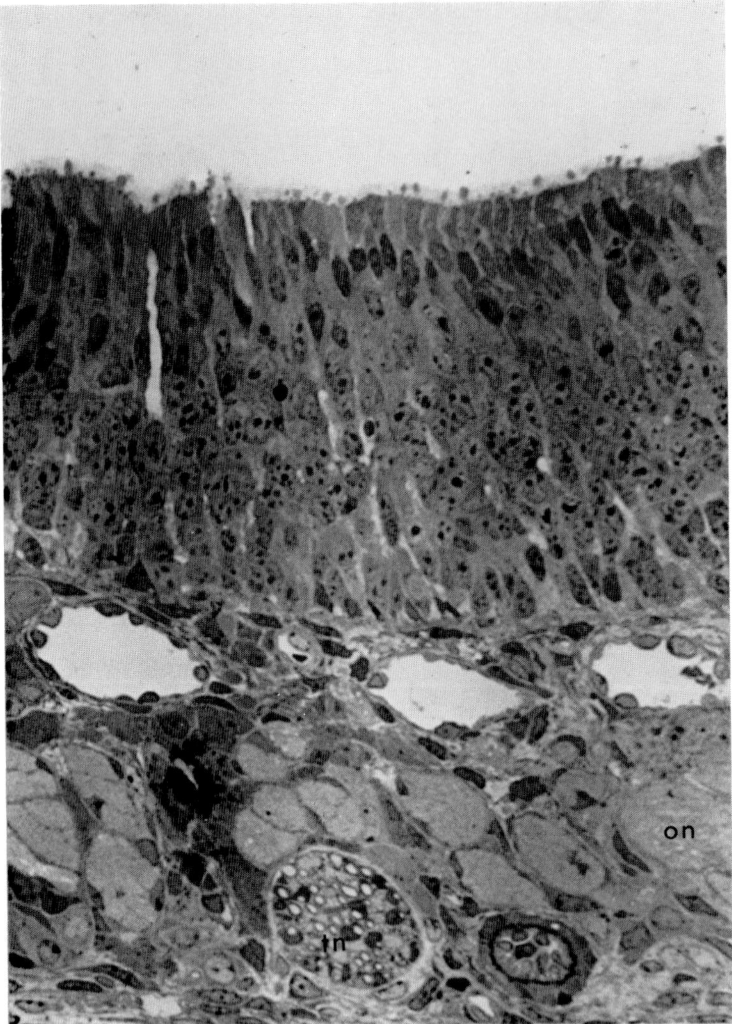

Figure 5.5 Light micrograph of a vertical section through the olfactory mucosa of a mouse, showing the sensory epithelium with nerve terminals at the surface, and, deeper, a zone of blood vessels, olfactory nerve bundles (on) and trigeminal nerve fasciculus (tn). Resin section, stained with toluidine blue. Magnification (× 800)

2. The olfactory bulb

Each glomerulus receives 26 000 olfactory fibres (Allison and Warwick, 1949) and appears to act as an integrating device. Leveteau and MacLeod (1965) recorded the summated synaptic potentials of these structures and found a negative slow potential starting 50 ms after the onset of the corresponding EOG and following a similar time course.

A glomerulus responds selectively to chemicals in an all-or-nothing manner (Leveteau and MacLeod, 1966 and 1969) whatever the stimulus intensity.

At the level of the mitral cells, where the second order neurons represent the convergence of ascending and descending influence the final message transmitted to the higher centres is elaborated. Døving (1964, 1966 b, c) was able to analyse single unit activity in the bulb of a frog, stimulated by different chemicals. He found three different types of responses: (1) inhibition – 80 per cent of the tests; (2) excitation – 10 per cent of the tests; and (3) lack of response – 10 per cent of the tests.

These responses were remarkably consistent for each unit and for the different chemicals and indeed some units appeared specific in the sense that they were inhibited by all except one chemical. The actual pattern of firing of the neurons was characteristic of the units themselves and independent of the stimulus whereas the frequency of firing was on the contrary related to the stimulus (Døving and Hyvarinen, 1969). Computer analysis of these response patterns in the frog showed unexpected agreement with psychophysical measurements in man, but it should be stressed that this applies to the level of the initial cells and second order neurons and not to the glomerular level.

The lateral olfactory tract is the bulb's projection to the forebrain. It makes direct ipsilateral connections during its course with all parts of the anterior olfactory nucleus, the olfactory tubercle, pre-pyriform cortex and periamygdaloid cortex, as well as the cortical nucleus of the amygdaloid complex.

There are also centrifugal fibres from all the ipsilateral olfactory areas of the brain and from the contralateral anterior olfactory nucleus.

3. The higher centres

These include the anterior olfactory nucleus which seems to be the real origin of the efferent impulses to the opposite bulb and to the ipsilateral forebrain through the anterior commissure.

The primary olfactory cortex lies at the rostral side of the telencephalon just behind the insertion of the olfactory tract, and includes the olfactory tubercle, the pre-pyriform and periamygdaloid areas.

Biedenbach and Stephens (1969, a, b) have carried out electrophysiological studies of this area and found that incoming olfactory potentials cause single-synapse excitations of the superficial neurons followed by inhibition. This reflex inhibition results from stimulation of the deeper cells.

The primary cortex has secondary projections but these are multiplexed as there are a hundred times as many fibres as those coming in from the mitral cells. They are projected to:

(1) *The thalamus* – which receives also a direct taste input in the same area. From there fibres travel to the fronto–lateral and orbito–frontal area of the neocortex. In this manner the olfactory pathway is similar to other sensory pathways.

(2) *The hypothalamus* – where they terminate in the lateral pre-optic nucleus and in lateral and peri-infundibular nuclei and the nuclei gemini. There is an important aspect here in that the hypothalamus is only two synapses away from the peripheral olfactory input (Kandel, 1964). This is quite different from other

sensory systems which are connected only indirectly and may be relevant to the role of olfaction in nutrition and reproduction.

(3) *The entorhinal and amygdaloid projections.*

(4) *Centrifugal fibres to the olfactory bulb* – it is through these fibres that negative potentials appear in both bulbs with unilateral stimulation of the pre-pyriform cortex. Most of the work done in this area has been in fish (Døving and Gemme, 1965, 1966) and despite the differences with mammals they have shown the manner in which third-order neurons control those of the second order. The former may themselves respond to stimuli which are not olfactory. By and large, these centrifugal fibres provide a negative feedback system from one bulb to the other as well as from the higher centres.

Odour discrimination

The question of exactly how odours are recognized from one another has not been resolved. There is evidence that receptors are selectively sensitive (O'Connell and Mozell, 1969; Gesteland *et al.*, 1965). On the other hand, it is possible that a spatio–temporal analysis of the odorant across the olfactory mucosa can also occur. Such a double system could provide a code based on a very large number of possible permutations.

The psychophysics of smell

Although electrophysiological studies in animals have given considerable information, the study of the senses requires human subjects who can take part in subjective experiments. This study of the relationship between the stimulus and the sensation is termed psychophysics. Here an attempt is made to put it in a mathematical form so that a system of scaling has to be devised. Subjects may be asked to estimate the strength of a stimulus by matching it with numbers (Stevens, 1966) and the judgments are averaged for groups of 10–20 subjects. Techniques of this type have shown that for a number of smells the following results (Stevens, 1957)

$$R = kS^b$$

when R is the perceived intensity, S the stimulus intensity, k is a constant referring to the intercept when the averages are plotted in double logarithmic coordinates, and b is also a constant referring to the slope. It can be expressed in logarithmic terms as

$$\log R = b(\log S) + \log k$$

Although these functions can apply to all senses b varies between them.

Adaptation, detection of odours and their classification have been studied using these techniques.

There seems to be a problem concerning adaptation and olfaction, because it is a well-known fact that sensitivity to a smell rapidly diminishes with duration of exposure. On the other hand, electrophysiological measurements (Ottoson, 1956) show the responses are maintained for a long time. Caine and Engen (1969) have studied the effect of intensity on adaptation using psychophysical measurements as well as the effect of the duration of the presentation. The longer the exposure the lower is the perceived intensity. This decrease is at first rapid and then slows down but does not appear to reach zero, so that it is unlikely that sensitivity can disappear completely. This would be more in keeping with the electrophysiological findings. Recovery from adaptation is rapid but it may depend on the nature of the odorant (Koster, 1968).

Theories of smell

The fact that there are an enormous number of olfactory theories still discussed shows that it has not yet been possible to develop a totally acceptable and comprehensive theory of smell. Nevertheless, a considerable amount of experimental evidence has been accumulated over the last two decades which gives a clearer picture of the situation and allows us to omit many theories which are only of historical interest.

It is necessary to separate the two questions of how stimulation takes place in the first instance from that of how the quality of an odour is decided.

Theories of stimulation

Vibration theories

If one considers that visual and auditory stimulation is the result of particular vibrations it is not surprising that olfactory vibrations have been suggested for many years.

More recently, Randebrock (1968) has modernized this theory by suggesting that olfactory perceptors are peptide chains vibrating in an α-helix. An odorant molecule forms a bond with the peptide thus modulating the vibration. At the other end of the helix the vibration is transmitted to the nerve.

Wright (1954, 1964, 1966) proposes a different theory. This implies that it is the molecular vibrations themselves which conform with vibrations on the sensitive surface. To conform the stimulant and receptor molecule must have near equal frequencies. Synchronous vibration would allow a closer approach and electronic bonding between them. Wright *et al.* (1967) have claimed that particular vibration frequencies allow the firing of only certain receptors and that these correspond to electrophysiological measurements in the bulb. These claims have not been accepted by Davies (1971).

Olfactory pigment theories

The role of the olfactory pigment (Briggs and Duncan, 1961, 1962) has been questioned. Some animals such as cows and dogs, have been found to have carotenes in the olfactory region and these workers suggest that as carotenoids can exist in numerous cis–trans forms and, indeed, the action of light on rhodopsins produces such changes, that the same effects can be produced by olfactory molecules. Little evidence has been shown in favour of this theory.

Rosenberg *et al.* (1968) have suggested that odorant molecules form a complex with certain olfactory pigments giving them an increased electrical conductivity.

Enzyme theories

These suggest that the activity of certain enzymes can be altered by adsorption of odorant molecules (Kistiakowski, 1950; Baradi and Bourne, 1951). Again, no valid evidence in favour of this theory has been produced.

Penetration and puncturing theory

This theory (Davies, 1953, a, b) is based on the manner in which, during excitation of a nerve axon, the excess of potassium ions inside the cell is able to escape across the lipid cell membrane while sodium enters the cell. During the resting phase the cell is able to pump ions back across its membrane against the gradient. It is this exchange of ions or 'puncturing' of the membrane that sets off the electrical discharge along the nerve. The cell membrane is like a bimolecular sandwich of protein and lipid. It is probably the proteins which provide the sodium pump and the lipid makes the membrane impermeable. According to Davies' theory the odorant molecule is able to penetrate the membrane of the olfactory receptor cell and diffuse through, leaving a hole. Through this hole leakage of ions occurs initiating the nerve impulse. Davies and Taylor (1957) and Davies (1962) were able to place this theory on a mathematical basis.

Theories of odour quality

Vibration theory

Wright (1965, 1967) suggested that odour quality is related to vibrations in the far infrared spectrum and although there has been some correlation between the musky odours in particular frequency bands, it has not been possible to develop this theory further for the time being.

Penetration and puncture theory

According to this theory adsorption and penetration of a molecule results in a hole in the membrane of the cell through which ions pass initiating the nervous impulse. The degree in which this flow will occur, however, may depend on the relative rate of diffusion of the penetrating molecule to that of membrane healing. It is also possible that the quality of healing varies from cell to cell. Different shapes of molecule presumably may also leave different sizes of hole. Davies refers to this as the 'hole sharpness factor' which he describes as

$$1 - t_{\mathrm{diff}}/t_{\mathrm{h}}$$

where t_{diff} is the time the odorant molecule takes to diffuse and t_{h} is the time the membrane takes to heal.

This factor, then, will depend on the size and shape of the molecule as well as on the quality of the membrane at this particular place.

Specific site theory

Amoore (1952, 1962, 1964) related the shape of odorant molecules to the shape of a specific site, a small but actual cavity, on the receptor cell. In the site an electron-seeking group has to be satisfied to initiate a response.

Obviously there cannot be an indefinite number of different sites and Amoore postulated that there must be a limited number of 'primary' odours to fit into a limited number of sites. By looking through the numerous smells of organic compounds it appeared that seven were very much more common than the others. The suggestion then is that they must be primary and the others composite. These odours were the following: ethereal, camphoraceous, musky, floral, minty, pungent and putrid.

The shape of the receptor site would be such as to accept odorant molecules of the appropriate size and shape. In further work Amoore (1961, 1967) showed that there was a statistical correlation between the profile of the molecules as represented by silhouette photographs of molecular models and the smell.

A number of objections can be made. The first is that the frequency-of-occurrence basis for the seven primary odours is the reports made by organic chemists. Thus, if there has been a lot of work done on substances with a musky smell by the perfumery industry, the figures will be weighted in favour of musk as a primary odour. Other objections are that there are many exceptions such as glycol which may fit sites but has no odour, and the vast ability to discriminate different odours which the nose has and which suggests more than seven primary odours.

On the other hand, the statistical correlation betweeen Amoore's silhouette photographs and odours gives correlation coefficients of between 0.45 and 0.66 which shows that they are definitely related.

In 1967 and 1968 Amoore had begun to carry out studies on persons with specific anosmia for certain odours.

At present the position is still uncertain but it does appear that there may be more than seven 'primary' odours. What constitutes a receptor is itself uncertain although one may speculate that it consists of a specific protein.

There is no doubt that an olfactory code has not yet been broken.

Sensitivity of the nose to smells

There appears at first to be a great variation of olfactory sensitivity between different individuals which to some extent seems to be due to training such as in the case of perfumes. There is also a considerable pathological element as in the case of rhinitis, not to speak of broad differences due to smoking.

There has also been a perpetual discussion regarding differences in olfaction between the sexes. In some cases there are definite differences in relation to the smell of certain musks between nubile women and men, but the rest of the differences are more anecdotal than scientifically demonstrated.

More important differences exist between humans and other species although they are not always meaningful. For instance, it is not of great import to suggest that certain insects may be able to smell a substance in minute quantities even though we may not be aware of it at all. It may well be that insects are unable to smell substances that are important to us. Nevertheless, differences between ourselves and other mammals are worth noting.

Using simple sniffing methods Neuhaus produced some average figures comparing thresholds between men and dogs. For instance,

	Man	*Dog*	
Butyric acid	7×10^9	9×10^3	molecules/cm^3

For like smells dogs can smell concentrations a million times lower than man. For other types of smell,

Man	*Dog*
$3^6 \times 10^8$	1×10^5

the difference is only a thousand times.

Many smells become different with dilution. In particular, certain musks and substances like indole and skatole which are intolerable in large concentrations are not only pleasant in high dilution but actually form the basis of many perfumes.

The sense of smell

Although a good deal of information has become available about various aspects of olfaction, about the behaviour of odorants and their chemistry, and about the electrophysiology of responses, we are as yet, far from understanding the basic mechanisms.

Vocal resonance

The voice is produced by the air-stream causing vibration of the vocal folds. This laryngeal tone is low pitched and is then transmitted to the pharynx, the mouth and the nose – three cavities.

The quality of the voice, its timbre, the richness of the tone, particularly in singing but also in speech, depends on its resonance through these cavities. Obstruction of the nasal cavity will suppress the overtones of the laryngeal voice and produce a distinctive impairment.

In such conditions the voice will be 'flat' or 'dead' and is referred to as 'nasal'. This type of problem is also known as rhinolalia clausa to distinguish it from the other type of 'nasal' condition, rhinolalia aperta. The latter is a defect of speech which means that the column of air rises through the nasopharynx into the non-obstructed nose in an uncontrolled manner. This occurs in cleft palate, paralysis, or shortening of the soft palate.

Speech

The role of the nose in speech production is distinctive from, though associated with, that in vocal resonance.

A number of sounds used in speech require the nose as a resonator. These could be consonants or vowels and the fine adjustments are produced by using the tongue and soft palate.

Consonants

To produce a nasal consonant the oral cavity is occluded by the mouth and at the same time the nose is opened to the air-stream by lowering the soft palate.

In this situation the pharyngeal and nasal cavities act as a single resonator. The oral cavity then acts as a secondary resonator whose size can be modified by the tongue. This allows a further distinction to be made between the different nasal consonants according to tongue position and lip movements.

Labials e.g. m
Dentals e.g. n
Palatals e.g. ng

In the nasal spectrum it is the lower formant, 200–300 Hz, that is nearer to the laryngeal tone which predominates.

Vowels

Vowel formants are not of primary importance in the nasals. The frequency of F1 is around 300–400 Hz, F2 500–1900 Hz and F3 1800–2600 Hz. Their role seems to be mainly transitional, influencing the pattern of the preceding and following vowels.

It appears that the relative impedance of the nose and mouth cavities affects the nasalization of vowels. If that of the nasal cavity is greater then the effect of the nose-resonator on the acoustic cavity is small. If, on the contrary, it is less then the nose has an important influence on the acoustic outcome.

The nasalized vowels have their intensity growing at 250 Hz and weakening again at 500 Hz, but there are other weak components between the vowel formants around 1000–2500 Hz.

Nasal reflexes

Vascular arrangements

The nasal mucosa has an abundant blood supply, mainly from the spheno-palatine branches of the maxillary artery and the anterior and posterior ethmoidal branches of the ophthalmic artery. Zuckerlandl (1900), Swingle (1935) and, more recently, Dawes and Prichard (1953) have described the detailed architecture of the nasal vascular bed.

The arterioles lie in the deeper part of the tunica propria and are arranged in parallel longitudinal rows. These arterioles supply periglandular and subepithelial capillary networks. The efferent vessels from this superficial capillary bed open into large sinusoidal venous spaces. The walls of these spaces are supported by abundant elastic tissue and by a marked development of circular and spirally arranged bundles of plain muscle. The ends of the sinusoids are furnished with sphincter muscles and Lucas (1935) has demonstrated these sphincters in sections of human nasal mucosa.

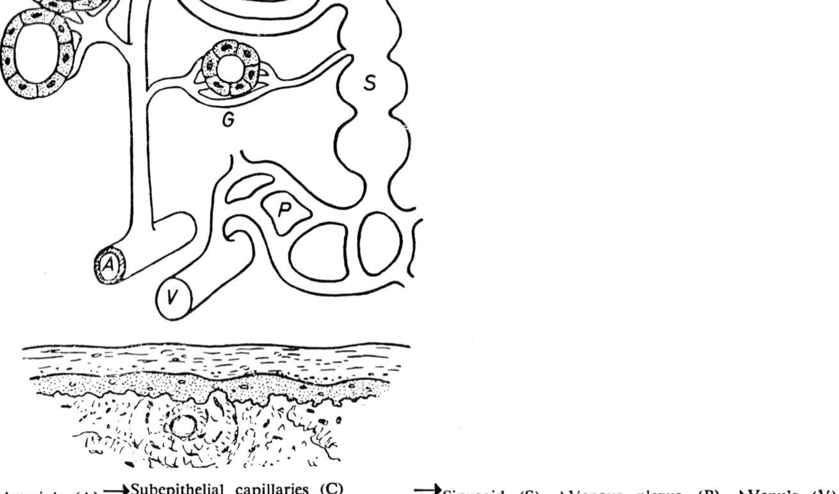

Figure 5.6 Simplified diagram of arrangement of blood vessels in the nasal mucous membrane

These sinusoids drain into a deeper venous plexus (*Figure 5.6*). This vascular organization constitutes a type of erectile cavernous tissue and is particularly well developed over the inferior turbinate, and the lower margin and posterior end of the middle turbinate. The corresponding parts of the septal mucosa are also highly vascular and erectile.

The existence of arterio–venous anastomoses in the nose had been claimed by Sucquet and by Harper; Dawes and Prichard (1953) at Oxford used microdissection techniques on neoprene-injected specimens and they provided for the first time detailed descriptions of the general pattern of distribution of nasal vessels in the common experimental animals. They also demonstrated unequivocally that arterio–venous anastomoses are present bypassing the periglandular capillary system.

The *vasomotor nerve supply* is derived from the autonomic nervous system. The *sympathetic* pre-ganglionic connector cells lie in the lateral horn of grey matter of the first and second thoracic segments of the spinal cord. Pre-ganglionic medullated axons emerge in the corresponding anterior nerve roots and pass through the mixed spinal nerves, their anterior primary rami and the white rami communicantes, to the corresponding ganglia of the sympathetic chain. Here they ascend in the cervical sympathetic chain, to end by synapsing around cells in the superior cervical ganglion. Post-ganglionic fibres pass from the superior cervical ganglion to the plexus around the internal carotid artery and then, in the deep petrosal nerve and the vidian nerve, to the spheno-palatine ganglion. They pass without relaying through the spheno-palatine ganglion, to be distributed in the palatine and naso-palatine branches of the ganglion to the nasal mucous membrane (*Figure 5.7*).

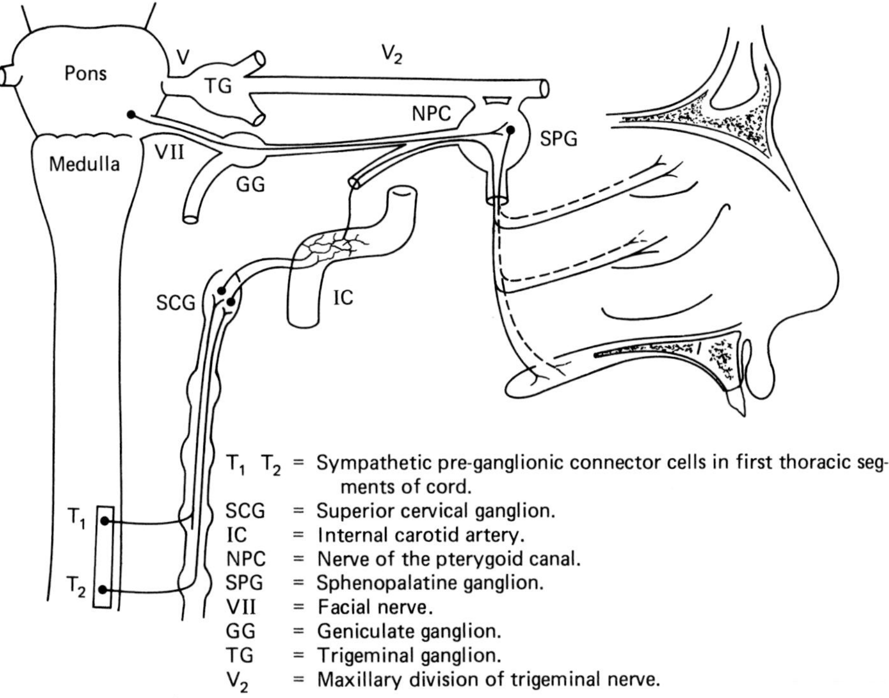

Figure 5.7 Diagram of automatic nerve supply of nasal mucous membrane

The *parasympathetic* supply is from pre-ganglionic cells in the superior secretory nucleus in the brain stem. The pre-ganglionic fibres emerge in the pars intermedia of the facial nerve to reach the geniculate ganglion. From this ganglion these fibres continue on, in the greater superficial petrosal nerve, to unite with the deep petrosal nerve composed of post-ganglionic sympathetic fibres from the internal carotid plexus, to form the nerve of the pterygoid canal (vidian nerve). These fibres then terminate in the spheno-palatine ganglion. Post-ganglionic parasympathetic fibres from the cells of this ganglion pass in the palatine, naso-palatine and pharyngeal branches to the mucosa of the nose and of the roof of the nasopharynx.

Experimental study of nasal vessels

The principles underlying some of the methods used in the experimental study of nasal blood vessels are shown in *Table 5.1*.

Table 5.1 Methods used in investigating nasal blood flow changes

(1) *Colour* of nasal mucosa (a) inspection
(b) photoelectric plethysmography (Hertzman)
(2) *Temperature* of nasal mucosa recorded by thermocouples (Mudd and Goldman, Ralston and Kerr, Richtner)
(3) *Volume* changes (a) intranasal balloon
(b) closed chamber technique (Tschalussow, Jackson)
(c) resistance to air flow

Indirect rhinometry
Hygrometric method (Zwaardemaker)
Rotating cylinder (Hellman)

Direct rhinometry
(a) Volume of nasal air flow
Movable vane or turbine in air-stream
(i) normal inspiration (Zwaardemaker, Undritz)
(ii) air sucked artificially through nasal chambers (Sternstein)
(b) Pressure in nose recorded by water manometer
(i) normal inspiration (Uddstromer, Spiers)
(ii) constant stream of air pumped into nose (van Dishoeck)
(iii) intermittent stream of air pumped into nose (Malcomson, Slome)
(c) Velocity of nasal air-stream (Blick, Zwaardemaker, Malan, Worms)

(4) *Pressure–Volume* recording
(5) Comparison of forced expiratory volume (1 s) through nose with forced expiratory volume (1 s) through mouth

These nasal vasomotor reactions can be studied by observations of the colour and temperature changes of the mucosa and its state of swelling or shrinkage. Temperature measurements are made by placing minute thermocouples in contact with the mucosa. Volume changes are followed by recording changes in the capacity of the nasal cavity from a rubber balloon in the nose connected to an optical recording system. Vasomotor changes may also be studied by recording with a water manometer the resistance to the inflow of air pumped into the nose under constant pressure. The temperature of the nasal mucosa depends on the amount of blood flowing through the superficial vessels. This is regulated by the tone of the arterioles. Rise of temperature indicates arteriolar dilatation; fall of temperature indicates arteriolar constriction. The colour of the mucosa is determined by the volume of blood in the capillaries and superficial venous spaces. This is dependent on the calibre of these superficial vessels. Constriction of the vessels causes pallor, whereas dilatation produces a red or bluish colour, depending on whether the blood flow is rapid or relatively stagnant. The colour of the normal nasal mucosa varies with age, type of complexion, temperature and humidity of inspired air, posture, exercise, body temperature and with menstruation and pregnancy.

Swelling of the nasal mucous membrane follows congestion of the cavernous tissue due to dilatation of the walls of the cavernous spaces, constriction of the deeper veins or dilatation of arterioles. Oedema of the mucous membrane also leads to swelling.

Four possible combinations of changes in mucosal temperature and volume have been recorded.

(1) Hyperaemia: rise of mucosal temperature (arteriolar dilatation) and swelling of the mucosa (congestion of the cavernous spaces).

(2) Ischaemia: fall in mucosal temperature (arteriolar constriction) and shrinkage of mucosa (collapse of cavernous spaces).
(3) Turgescence: fall in mucosal temperature (arteriolar constriction) and swelling of the mucosa (congestion of the cavernous spaces).
(4) Rise of mucosal temperature (arteriolar dilatation) and shrinkage of the mucosa (collapse of the cavernous spaces).

The superficial capillaries and deeper cavernous spaces may react independently to both nervous and pharmacological stimulation. The anatomical arrangement of the vascular bed is such that vasoconstriction of nasal vessels may be accompanied by constriction of the deep veins and thus by congestion of the cavernous tissue. Conversely, reflex arteriolar dilatation can be associated with emptying of the cavernous spaces, due to dilatation of the efferent veins.

Vasomotor responses

The relatively extensive vascular network of the nasal mucous membrane and the marked variations in its capacity and blood flow are related primarily to the functions of humidification and heating, and not to the nutritional needs of the mucosa. The responses of the nasal vascular bed to local stimulation and general bodily changes, and the participation of these vessels in the general reflex vasomotor reactions of the body, are of special clinical interest. The effects of stimulation and of section of the autonomic nerve supply of nasal vessels have been studied.

Stimulation of cervical sympathetic

The response to stimulation of the cervical sympathetic is an immediate and intense vasoconstriction. The threshold of stimulation for this response is remarkably low: mere handling of the sympathetic chain elicits a response. This may be correlated with the clinical fact that warming over the superior cervical ganglion may clear the airway in an occluded and congested nose. Increasing the strength of stimulation or the frequency of stimulation produces an increased degree of vasoconstriction. However, beyond a certain maximum, further increase in stimulation, as one would expect, produces no further increase in response. The vasoconstrictor effect of stimulation of these pre-ganglionic fibres is abolished by blocking synaptic transmission at the superior cervical ganglion.

This sympathetic innervation maintains a constant tonic vasoconstrictor action. Section of the cervical sympathetic chain (Horner's syndrome) is followed by nasal vasodilatation due to loss of the sympathetic vasoconstrictor tone.

Stimulation of parasympathetic

In experimental animals, stimulation of the trunk of the facial nerve central to the geniculate ganglion or of the greater superficial petrosal nerve causes dilatation of the nasal blood vessels.

Stimulation of the nerve of the pterygoid canal produces two types of response depending on the parameters of the stimuli employed. Weak stimulation causes vasodilation; stronger stimuli cause vasoconstriction. This diphasic response is explained by the fact that the nerve of the pterygoid canal contains both thick medullated pre-ganglionic parasympathetic vasodilator fibres and thin non-medullated post-ganglionic sympathetic vasoconstrictor fibres. These two groups of fibres have different excitation thresholds associated with the different fibre diameters.

Nasal vasomotor tone following operations on the autonomic nervous system

Clinical studies have confirmed that section of the cervical sympathetic is followed by hyperaemia, swelling of the nasal mucosa and hypersecretion. This effect is also produced by procaine block of the cervical sympathetic. Persistent nasal obstruction and congestion also develop after superior cervical ganglionectomy.

Interruption of the parasympathetic innervation of the nasal vascular bed was present in the cases described by Gardner and Stowell (1947) of resection of the greater superficial petrosal nerve. This operation resulted in a shrunken pale mucous membrane with excessive drying and crusting in the nose. Marked nasal vasoconstriction and drying has also been described in cases of geniculate herpes and of section of the trunk of the facial nerve.

Factors affecting nasal blood flow

The physiological and pharmacological responses of the blood vessels of the nasal mucous membrane are important in the consideration of the pathology and treatment of many nasal conditions.

The vasomotor mechanism of the nose is readily affected by nervous factors including both local and general reflex effects, and by hormonal and chemical factors.

Local factors

Temperature and humidity

Changes in the temperature and humidity of the inspired air result rapidly in vasodilatation or vasoconstriction. The mucosal blood flow is thus automatically adjusted to changes in climatic conditions. A fall in the temperature of the inspired air is compensated for by arteriolar dilatation and, consequently, an appropriately increased blood flow. This increased blood flow raises and maintains the mucosal temperature and increases the temperature gradient between the mucosal surface and the external environment. The mucosa acts, therefore, as a more efficient radiator, and adequate heating of the colder inspired air to body temperature in the nose is ensured. When nasal air currents are in abeyance, as in total laryngectomy, the nasal blood flow gradually becomes markedly reduced.

Vasoconstrictor and vasodilator drugs

The effects on the nasal mucosa of vasoconstrictor and vasodilator drugs have been carefully studied.

Sympathomimetic drugs applied locally produce a rapid vasoconstriction with blanching and shrinkage of the nasal mucous membrane. This local ischaemia may persist for 1–3 h.

The factors determining the choice of these vasoconstrictor compounds are (1) vasoconstrictor potency, (2) duration of effect, (3) toxicity and systemic side-effects, (4) local astringent and irritative effect, (5) secondary vasodilatation, (6) pH of solution, and (7) action on ciliary activity.

Adrenaline has a powerful vasoconstrictor effect. It can be used to produce a bloodless field in nasal operations. It is unstable except in acid solutions.

Ephedrine is less active but the effect is more prolonged. Local irritation and toxicity are less marked.

Neosynephrine hydrochloride is claimed to produce a more powerful and prolonged vasoconstriction.

2-Aminoheptane sulphate is an even more potent vasoconstrictor; 0.5 per cent solution is more than equivalent to 2 per cent solution of ephedrine.

Amphetamine is popularly used as a volatile decongestant.

Many of these sympathomimetic amines produce local irritation and a watery discharge. It is mainly due to this irritation that a secondary vasodilatation occurs after the vasoconstrictor action of the drug has passed off. Adrenaline and ephedrine are the worst offenders; propadrine, neosynephrine hydrochloride and 2-aminoheptane sulphate are claimed to cause minimal irritation and secondary vasodilatation.

These drugs are readily absorbed from the nasal mucosa. They may produce general systemic effects. Ephedrine, amphetamine and propadrine cause marked stimulation of the central nervous system. Adrenaline, noradrenaline and ephedrine produce circulatory effects, increasing the rate and especially the force of contraction and excitability of the heart. Neosynephrine hydrochloride, privine hydrochloride and 2-aminoheptane sulphate do not produce any significant side-effects.

When members of this group of drugs are administered systemically a similar though less intense nasal vasoconstriction results. Subcutaneous injection of 0.75 ml of 1:1000 adrenaline produces a pronounced drop in temperature of nasal mucosa and an increase in volume of the nasal cavities. This indicates constriction of the arterioles, accompanied by emptying of the cavernous vascular network.

Parasympathomimetic drugs, such as mecholyl, carbachol and neostigmine, produce congestion of the nasal mucosa with increased secretion.

The pharmacological reactions of the nasal vascular bed to these autonomic drugs are not significantly different in patients with vasomotor nasal disease.

Atropine, 0.1 per cent, causes capillary constriction and contraction of the cavernous tissue.

Cocaine produces marked contraction of the erectile spaces. The superficial capillaries are not significantly affected, except by high concentrations which cause slight contraction.

Inhalation of amyl nitrite causes transitory dilatation of the superficial vessels.

Histamine, which is widely distributed in all body tissues, has an action on the nasal mucous membrane which is of particular interest. This intracellular histamine appears to be present in a bound and inactive form. The main actions of histamine are marked dilatation and increased permeability of capillaries, dilatation of arterioles, fall of arteriolar blood pressure, contraction of plain muscle, such as the bronchiolar muscle, and increased secretion of various glands.

Intradermal injection of a histamine solution produces the characteristic triple response, which consists of the following.

(1) The red reaction: a maximal dilatation of the capillaries by a direct action on the capillary wall.
(2) Flare: dilatation of the surrounding arterioles giving a diffuse, irregular, flushed area. This is due to a local axon reflex, nerve impulses initiated by histamine being transmitted antidromically along an axon branching to the neighbouring arterioles.
(3) Wheal: an area of oedema corresponding to the area of capillary dilatation. The capillary paralysis is associated with increased permeability of the vessel wall. A protein-rich oedema fluid is filtered from the blood plasma into the extracellular tissue spaces.

Tissue injury results in the local liberation of histamine or a histamine-like substance. There is substantial evidence that histamine is the essential causative agent in anaphylactic shock and allergic states. In anaphylaxis, the initial interaction between antigen and antibody occurs within the body cells. This intracellular reaction results in injury to the cell, which leads to the liberation of histamine-like substances. Antihistamine drugs have been shown to be of definite therapeutic value in those conditions characterized by vascular phenomena in the nasal mucous membrane. The great majority of patients with hay fever are markedly benefited. In perennial rhinitis the benefit from antihistamine drugs is definite but not nearly so dramatic as in hay fever.

Compression of jugular veins and the common carotid artery. Congestion of nasal mucosa follows compression of the jugular veins. This may be a factor accounting for postural nasal obstruction when in the lateral horizontal position. Compression of the common carotid artery causes shrinkage of the mucous membrane, but this effect is only temporary, due to the opening up of an effective collateral circulation.

Trauma and infection

Local trauma and infection lead to the marked vascular changes characteristic of inflammation.

General factors

The calibre of the nasal vessels is affected by endocrine and nervous factors.

Endocrine

In hyperthyroidism intranasal temperature is raised. In hypothyroidism it falls below normal and the mucosa is pale and boggy. Cone (1933) concludes that these changes associated with abnormal metabolic rates are due to variations in sympathetic vasoconstrictor tone, as evidenced by the changes in colour, volume and temperature of the turbinates.

The secretions of the adrenal medulla and cortex and the sex hormones have effects on the nasal vascular bed. The relations between the nasal mucosa and menstruation and pregnancy are well known.

Emotional stress

Emotional states readily affect the degree of congestion or depletion of the nasal mucous membrane. The vasomotor and secretory reactions of the nasal mucous

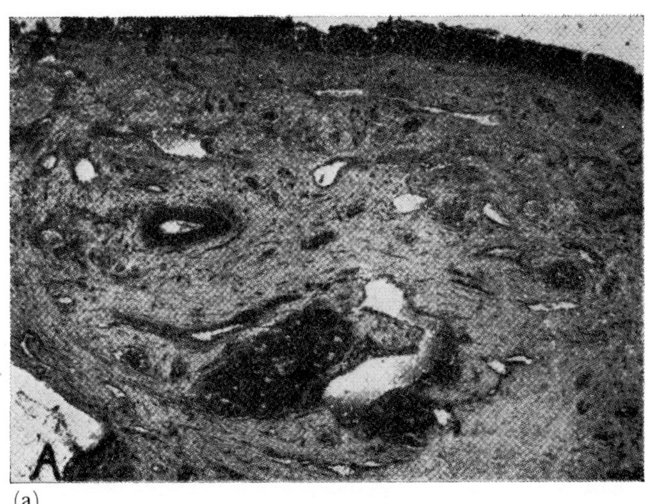

(a)

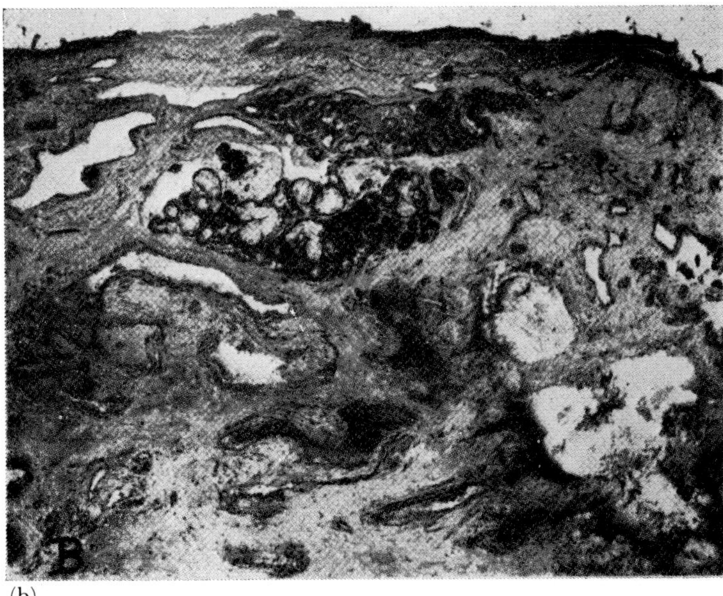

(b)

Figure 5.8 Effect of emotional stress on nasal mucous membrane: (a) section of biopsy from left lower turbinate during control period of relative relaxation and security; (b) section of biopsy from right lower turbinate 1 h later, during period of resentment and frustration; section shows oedema with marked vascular and lymphatic engorgement

membrane to emotional stress have been subjected to detailed experimental investigation by Holmes and his colleagues (1950). Two different patterns of response may be produced.

Fear and terror result in vasoconstriction and shrinking of the mucous membrane – a 'sympathetic' type of response.

Emotional situations causing resentment, humiliation, frustration and anxiety lead to a different pattern of reaction. This response is characterized by marked vascular engorgement, swelling of the erectile tissues of the turbinates and nasal septum, obstruction of the nasal airway and increased volume of nasal secretions (*Figure 5.8*).

This is a 'parasympathetic' type of response probably mediated through the greater superficial petrosal nerves. Nasal pain is often associated with this mucosal swelling. The pain may extend to the orbital, supra-orbital, zygomatic and temporal regions. Hyperaemic nasal mucosa has been demonstrated to have a lowered pain threshold.

A most convincing demonstration of the hyperaemia, lymphatic engorgement and hypersecretion in emotional states of frustration and rage, was provided by comparing the histological sections of a biopsy of the inferior turbinate of a subject during a period of intense emotional conflict, with sections of a similar biopsy from the same subject during a control period of relaxation and security.

These emotional responses may, when they are maintained for long periods, give rise to irreversible tissue changes. They may thus form the initial mechanism leading to the establishment of chronic nasal vasomotor disease.

The common syndrome of hyperaemia and swelling of the nasal mucous membrane, nasal obstruction, hypersecretion and pain, may be produced by a number of other stimuli, such as irritant fumes and dusts, inhalation of pollens and substances to which the subject is sensitized, cooling of the body surface, menstruation and pregnancy.

General vasomotor reflexes

The nasal vessels may be involved in the general sympathetic vasomotor responses of the body; indeed, they appear to reflect most sensitively any changes in peripheral vasomotor tone. Afferent impulses from the baroreceptors in the carotid sinus and aortic area reflexly inhibit the medullary vasomotor centre, thus adjusting the peripheral vascular bed to maintain the constancy of the arterial blood pressure. The reflex response to a rise of arterial blood pressure is peripheral vasodilatation, due to decreased sympathetic tone. A fall of arterial blood pressure results in peripheral vasoconstriction. Painful stimulation of peripheral cutaneous areas produces constriction of the nasal vessels. In exercise also these vessels are constricted.

Photoelectric plethysmography has been adapted to study vascular activity in the mucosa of the nasal septum. In the normal resting man spontaneous fluctuations of vasomotor tone may be present. Auditory and psychic stimulation, deep breathing, breath-holding and the cold pressor test all produce marked vasoconstrictor effects in the nasal mucosa. Similar vascular reactions occur more or less uniformly in the skin, especially in the exposed regions.

The nasal vessels may also react in other generalized sympathetic vasomotor responses in the body. Painful stimulation of peripheral cutaneous areas results in nasal vasoconstriction.

Asphyxia is associated with nasal vasoconstriction (Tatum, 1923). This effect is prevented by section of the cervical sympathetic and is therefore reflex in origin. Overventilation, on the other hand, produces dilatation of nasal vessels. This response is not affected by sympathectomy. These effects would appear to subserve a useful function, an adaptive reflex mechanism, reducing nasal resistance when the respiratory need is increased, and increasing resistance when respiration is depressed.

Vascular responses to cutaneous thermal stimulation

The participation of the vascular bed of the human nasal mucosa in the reflex vasomotor reactions of the body, especially to thermal stimulation of the skin, is of particular interest. These reflex responses have been subjected to experimental study by Spiesman (1935), and by Mudd, Goldman and Grant (1921), and have been re-investigated more recently by Ralston and Kerr (1945).

Effects of general cutaneous cooling

The effect of exposure to a cold environment is a sudden initial fall in nasal temperature and shrinkage of the mucosa, followed by a gradual swelling of the

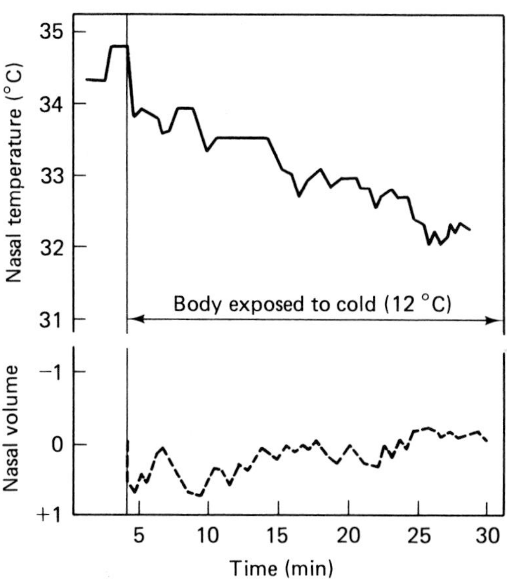

Figure 5.9 Vascular responses of nasal mucosa to cutaneous thermal stimulation. Effect of prolonged generalized cooling of the body. Progressive fall of temperature of nasal mucosa and initial decrease in volume of nasal cavity due to swelling of nasal mucosa. (Ralston and Kerr, 1945)

mucosa while the nasal temperature continues to decline. Reflex arteriolar constriction is accompanied by initial emptying and later distension of the vascular sinuses (*Figure 5.9*).

Effects of general cutaneous warming

Raised environmental temperature causes swelling and hyperaemia of the nasal mucosa.

The degree of vasomotor response depends on the rate of change of temperature. Rapid changes of temperature readily elicit reflex vasomotor responses in the nasal mucous membrane. Gradual and prolonged variations in environmental temperature have a relatively slight effect on the vascularity of the nasal mucous membrane. This is a result of the phenomenon of adaptation of the cutaneous thermal receptors. This reflex has a low threshold of stimulation; reflex vasoconstriction in the nose may occur with only slight cooling, such as may be caused by unwrapping a patient in a cool room, before any reflex vasoconstriction of skin vessels is demonstrable.

Effects of local cooling and warming

Local cutaneous cooling of the feet produces a pronounced initial drop in nasal temperature due to reflex vasoconstriction, succeeded by incomplete recovery. Although the cold stimulus is still being applied, the temperature stabilizes at a level below the original control temperature.

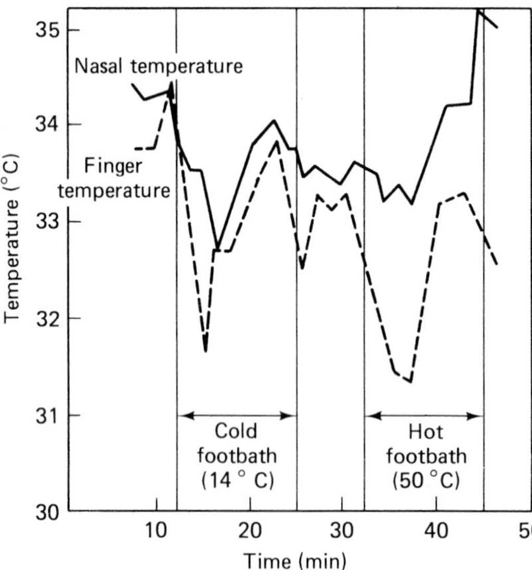

Figure 5.10 Vascular responses of nasal mucosa to cutaneous thermal stimulation. Effect of local cooling and heating on temperature of nasal mucosa and skin. Nasal temperature = ——; finger temperature = – – –. Cold footbath causes initial pronounced fall of nasal temperature with some recovery while cold stimulus is still being applied. Hot footbath causes slight drop of nasal temperature followed by rise to above normal level. (Ralston and Kerr, 1945)

Local cutaneous warming elicits a transitory vasoconstriction with decline in nasal temperature, followed by a steady rise to above the normal temperature (*Figure 5.10*).

Effects of cooling of a local area in a warm environment

Chilling of the feet in subjects exposed to a high environmental temperature brings about a marked drop in nasal temperature, associated with shrinkage of the mucous membrane. Then follow a rapid recovery to normal, and finally an elevated temperature and swelling of the mucosa. This experimental finding would appear to provide substantiation for the belief that exposure of a warm subject to a cold draught causes hyperaemia of the nasal mucosa.

No significant differences in response of nasal mucosa to thermal stimulation or to adrenaline can be demonstrated between normal individuals and hypersensitive subjects, including those with increased susceptibility to colds and sufferers from allergic rhinitis. Spiesman and his colleagues claimed that the initial ischaemic reflex response to cutaneous cooling is temporarily inhibited before and during a cold. In the active phase of allergic cases, the response becomes a reflex vasodilatation.

Clinical studies of neurectomy for chronic vasomotor rhinitis

Experimental studies of the innervation of the nasal blood vessels and the neural control of nasal blood capacity and flow, have provided a basis for proposals to treat certain forms of chronic vasomotor rhinitis by neurectomy. In these cases the underlying lesion is believed to be due to parasympathetic overactivity. Malcomson (1959) treated a few of these patients with some success, by section of the nerve of the pterygoid canal. The nerve was approached by a submucous route along the septum with mobilization of the mucosa of the nasopharynx and lateral wall of the nose at the upper part of the medial pterygoid plate. The 'vidian' nerve was then divided in the region of the pterygo–palatine foramen. Golding-Wood (1961) devised an operation for exposure of this nerve by a transantral route. The maxillary antrum was opened as in the Caldwell–Luc operation and a section of the posterior antral wall was removed. The region of the spheno-palatine fossa was thus exposed and dissected under direct vision. The nerve of the pterygoid canal was exposed and destroyed by electrocoagulation in the canal. In a series of 40 cases of severe vasomotor rhinitis, resistant to treatment and subjected to 'vidian' neurectomy, Golding-Wood claimed immediate relief in 90 per cent without any evidence of relapse, in some cases for up to four years.

Reflexes initiated from the nose

The nasal mucous membrane is the specific receptive field for a large variety of reflex responses affecting particularly the alimentary, cardiovascular and respiratory systems.

These reflexes may be broadly divided into two groups: (1) olfactory and (2) trigeminal, according to the receptors and afferent nerves involved. The olfactory group of reflexes follows stimulation of olfactory receptors and influences chiefly the secretions of the salivary, gastric and pancreatic glands. These conditioned reflexes are considered in the sections on olfaction and salivary secretion.

The second group includes reflex responses to excitation of receptors by touch, pressure, temperature, pain or chemical irritants. Trigeminal neurones form the afferent limb of these reflex arcs. These nasal reflexes include, among others, reflex changes in pulmonary ventilation, changes in laryngeal and bronchial muscle, and changes in heart-rate and blood vessels.

Nasal reflexes have been studied by Nadel and Comroe (1961), Nadel and Widdicombe (1962), Tomori and Widdicombe (1969), Corbett, Kerr and Prys-Roberts (1969) and Angell James and de Burgh Daly (1969).

Angell James and de Burgh Daly (1969) have carried out a careful analysis of the reflex cardiovascular and reflex respiratory effects following stimulation of the nasal mucosa in man, and analysed the mechanisms of these reflex responses. Irritation of the nasal mucous membrane may cause reflex sneezing or apnoea.

Reflex sneezing

Vascular engorgement of the nasal mucosa and secretion of nasal glands may trigger off this respiratory reflex. The vasodilatation and secretion may be reflexly produced, for example, by excitation of cutaneous thermal receptors by cold. In experimental animals Malcomson has shown that vasodilatation and secretion by stimulation of nasal parasympathetic innervation can cause sneezing. In man sudden intense illumination of the retina may also cause a sneeze reflex.

The reflex response in sneezing consists of a preliminary inspiration which may be either a single slow deep inspiration or a series of sharp inspiratory efforts, followed after a short pause by a sudden forcible expiratory movement. The soft palate remains depressed and the high velocity of air is forcibly expelled through the mouth and the nose.

The reflex cessation of breathing or sneezing on irritation of the nasal mucosa contrasts with the reflex effects of stimulation of the laryngeal and tracheo–bronchial mucous membranes. Stimulation of the larynx causes a cough reflex with bronchoconstriction and bradycardia. The receptors for laryngeal and tracheo–bronchial reflexes have been investigated by Widdicombe (1954) who identified three functionally distinct types of mechanoreceptors. The cough reflex in response to mechanical stimulation is most easily elicited from the larynx and the region of the bifurcation of the trachea. Chemical stimulation by irritant gases causes coughing by stimulation of receptors in the depths of the lungs.

The respiratory reflex response to stimulation of the respiratory mucosa contrasts with that of stimulating the cutaneous body surface. Stimulation of the mucosa lining the nose causes a protective reflex apnoea or an expiratory sneeze, and stimulation of the laryngeal and tracheal mucosa causes coughing. These represent attempts to exclude the irritant by preventing it entering the air-passages or to expel it by sneezing or coughing. In contrast stimulation of the skin surface causes an inspiratory gasp or increasing breathing.

Respiratory and cardiovascular effects of nasal irritation

In man very low concentrations of chemical irritants may cause increased breathing.

(1) Mild chemical irritants, e.g. cigarette smoke or ammonia vapour, cause depression of breathing with bronchial constriction accompanied by bradycardia and a rise of blood pressure.

(2) Other irritant fumes such as sulphur dioxide can cause either rapid shallow respiration or slow deep breathing with tachycardia. Strong irritants cause arrest of breathing.
(3) Introduction of cold water into the nose causes cessation of breathing and a rise of blood pressure. Reflex vagal cardiac arrest may be caused by immersion of the head in water permitting water to flow into the nose.
(4) Stimulation of the nasal mucosa with electrical pulses has been demonstrated to produce an increase in heart-rate. On the other hand stimulation of cutaneous fibres of the trigeminal nerve has been reported as causing slowing of the heart-rate and a decline of blood pressure.
(5) In experimental animals chemical irritation of the nasal mucosa by tobacco smoke, ether, chloroform or ammonia results in apnoea, laryngeal spasm and bronchial constriction. These respiratory reflex changes are accompanied by bradycardia and variable effects on arterial blood pressure. These reflexes are mediated along afferent fibres of the trigeminal nerve innervating the nasal mucous membrane. Local anaesthesia of the nasal mucosa or section of the trigeminal nerve abolishes these responses. Stimulation of the central end of the trigeminal nerves will cause reflex slowing of the heart, hypertension, bronchial constriction and arrest of breathing. This reflex bradycardia and broncho-constriction are due chiefly to an increase of vagal activity and they are almost completely suppressed by atropine.

Phillips and Raghavan (1970) studied, in sheep, the effect of reflexes from the nasobuccal region on thermoregulation. An increase in the temperature of the inspired air, while the ambient temperature was kept constant, resulted in an increased rate of breathing. This hyperpnoea was attributed to stimulation of warm receptors in the upper respiratory tract. Similarly a reflex decrease in temperature of the inspired air from cold receptors in the upper respiratory tract caused a decrease in respiratory rate.

Vascular and respiratory effects of nasal irrigation

Angell James and de Burgh Daly explored experimentally the effects of irrigation of the nose with water or isotonic saline at varying temperatures on the respiratory rate and depth, heart-rate and blood pressure of dogs. The responses evoked were (1) depression or inhibition of breathing in the expiratory position, (2) bradycardia, (3) diminution of cardiac output, (4) selective peripheral vasoconstriction, and (5) hypertension or sometimes hypotension. The temperature of the irrigating solution was not a significant factor.

They demonstrated that this nasal stimulation produced a varying effect on the peripheral vascular resistance in different parts of the systemic circulatory bed. In general the vascular resistance was increased by arteriolar constriction in the cutaneous muscle, splanchnic and renal circulations, but not in the cerebral circulation. This effect is illustrated in *Figure 5.11*. The increase in peripheral vascular resistance is expressed as a percentage change from the control. The vascular resistance in the legs rose by 125 per cent composed of a 30–40 per cent increase in cutaneous vascular resistance and a 300–350 per cent increase in resistance in the muscle vessels. Constriction in the splanchnic circulation is reflected in a rise in

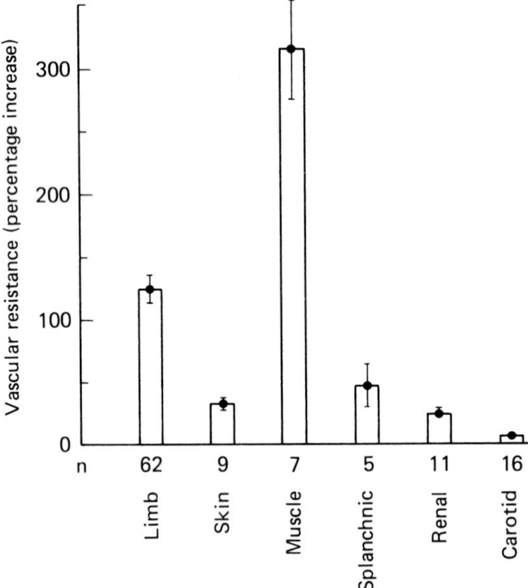

Figure 5.11 The effects of stimulation of the nasal mucous membrane on the vascular resistance (expressed as a percentage of the control value) in different vascular territories. (From Angell James and de Burgh Daly, 1969, reproduced by courtesy of the Editor of *Proceedings of the Royal Society of Medicine*)

resistance in that vascular territory of 50–60 per cent. The renal circulation shows a smaller increase of 10 per cent. These circulatory responses were due to vasomotor responses evoked reflexly from the nose, and were not secondary to changes in cardiac output or changes in pulmonary ventilation.

These effects were suppressed by ganglionic blocking drugs and also by adrenergic blocking agents. The afferent path of these reflex responses is in the sympathetic adrenergic vasomotor nerves.

The action on blood pressure of these nasal reflex responses is variable, depending on the effects on the cardiac output and on the peripheral vascular resistance. The arterial blood pressure is a product of the cardiac output and the peripheral resistance. The effect on blood pressure of these reflexes is therefore determined by the relative magnitudes of the hypertensive effect of peripheral vasoconstriction and the hypotensive action of the reduction of cardiac output resulting from the cardiac slowing.

Functional significance of these nasal reflexes

Another functional significance for these reflexes has been discussed by Angell James and de Burgh Daly. The respiratory air flow in its passage in and out through the nose in tidal ventilation might play a role in the maintenance of the normal rhythmic movements of inspiration and expiration similar to that of the Hering–Breuer pulmonary inflation reflex.

More definite irritation causes reflex apnoea, closure of the laryngeal sphincters and bronchoconstriction subserving a clearly protective function.

Angell James and de Burgh Daly have drawn attention to the special significance of these reflexes in diving mammals. Contact of water with the nasal mucosa causes apnoea with bradycardia and vasoconstriction. The continued apnoea during the diving results in progressive hypoxia and carbon dioxide retention and acidosis. These changes stimulate the arterial chemoreceptors and cause further reflex vasoconstriction.

Paranasal sinuses

Mucous membrane

The mucous membrane of the accessory nasal sinuses is directly continuous at the ostia of the sinuses with the mucous membrane of the nasal fossae. It consists of a pseudostratified, columnar, ciliated epithelium which rests on a tunica propria of loose connective tissue and elastic fibrils. The deeper part is inseparably blended with the periosteum of the bony sinus wall. The sinus mucosa thus resembles nasal respiratory mucous membrane, but is thinner and less vascular, and cavernous vascular spaces are not present. Goblet cells and glands are less numerous and found mainly close to the ostia.

Functions of the paranasal sinuses

Numerous functions have been attributed to the paranasal sinuses. None of these theories is based on any unequivocal evidence, and consequently there is no general agreement as to their specific functional role. The following 'functions' have been ascribed to these cavities.

Air-conditioning

They serve as supplementary chambers for conditioning the inspired air by heating and moistening. This function would necessitate a definite exchange of air between the nasal fossae and their accessory sinuses. The magnitude of this air exchange has been investigated by measuring simultaneously the pressure fluctuations in the nose and in the maxillary sinus. The normal respiratory excursions are accompanied by fluctuations in intranasal and intra-antral pressure which are of equal magnitude and practically simultaneous. Air exchange between the sinuses and the nasal cavities is dependent on these pressure variations. The volume of air exchanged in this sinus ventilation is approximately 0.1 per cent of the volume of the sinus with each respiratory cycle. The total replacement of the air in a sinus would take several hours. The air exchange with the paranasal sinuses forms, therefore, so insignificant a fraction of the total volume of the inspired air that the sinuses cannot be regarded as acting as additional humidifiers to any appreciable extent. Further, the sinus mucous membrane lacks the rich vascular bed and abundant glands of the nasal mucous membrane.

Vocal resonance

The sinuses may act as resonance chambers and affect the quality of the voice. The accessory nasal sinuses, which form a number of air-filled chambers with thin bony walls, have been regarded as sounding-boards for the primary tones produced at the vocal cords. Others claim that the position of the sinuses and of their ostia prevents them acting to any important extent as efficient resonators. Moreover, there is no correlation between resonance of voice and size of sinuses in lower animals.

Vestigial olfactory organs

In lower animals the sinuses contain complex olfactory organs and contribute a portion of the olfactory receptor surface.

Thermal insulators

The paranasal sinuses serve as temperature buffers, protecting the structures in the orbit and cranial fossae from the intranasal temperature variations. However, the largest sinuses are not interposed between the nose and any specially delicate tissues.

Formation secondary to bony re-adjustments

Proetz has suggested that the formation of the sinuses is secondary to the bony re-adjustments consequent upon the continued post-natal growth of the face. The frontal sinus, for example, is formed by the disproportionate growth of face and cranium, leading to a separation of the outer surface of the bone from the inner. Into the space so formed a diverticulum of nasal mucous membrane is drawn in.

Replacement of functionless bone

The origin of the sinuses has been attributed to replacement of functionless bone. The masticatory stresses in the upper jaw are transmitted from the alveolar processes to the skull by three vertical pillars or thickenings of bone in the maxilla. The functionally unstressed bone between these pillars undergoes re-absorption and the maxillary sinuses develop as invaginations of the nasal mucosa into this space. Similarly, it is suggested that the supra-orbital ridges are formed as a buttress for masticatory stresses, and the resulting remodelling and forward movement of the outer plate of the frontal bone give rise to the frontal sinus.

Aid to balance of head

It has been claimed that the sinuses aid in the balance of the head by reducing the weight of the bones of the face. However, even if the sinuses were replaced by bone, the resulting 1 per cent increase in weight could not be regarded as significant.

Ciliary action in clearance of mucus

The clearance of the mucous covering of the sinuses is carried out by ciliary propulsion. In the frontal and maxillary sinuses this transport has been demonstrated by Lucas (1935) to follow a spiral pathway towards the ostium. This ciliary action will maintain a constant direction of beat, that is, towards the natural ostium, even when an artificial antrostomy opening has been made.

Regeneration of the mucous membrane

Regeneration of the mucous membrane of the sinuses has been studied after various operations on experimental animals and in man. It has been definitely established that normal, functioning ciliated epithelium can be regenerated following operative removal of the complete lining of the maxillary sinus. This epithelial regeneration occurs mainly by growth from the margins of the operative opening into the sinus and, to a less extent, from islands of mucosa left behind.

Pain from the nasal and paranasal structures

Pain is one of the most important presenting symptoms in disease of the nasal passages and accessory nasal sinuses. An accurate description of pain should include its quality, intensity, duration and distribution and the reflex accompaniments, tenderness, muscular rigidity and autonomic effects. Such knowledge as is available about nasal pain is derived from two main sources: (1) clinical observations of the pain and its associated reactions, correlated with the exact site of the pathological lesions in the nose and sinuses; and (2) experimental investigations of the sensitivity to direct painful stimulation of the walls of the nose and sinuses in human subjects.

The nasal mucous membrane is sensitive to pain and to cold. It is unresponsive to touch and to warmth. Even light touch elicits pain of a surprising intensity and characteristically disagreeable quality. It is imperfectly localized and tends to be diffuse.

The nerves of the nasal mucous membrane terminate in an irregular plexiform arrangement of fine nerve endings. There is little reason for doubting that, as elsewhere in the body, these terminal ramifications constitute the peripheral receptive mechanism for pain.

Properties of pain receptors

Pain receptors in general react to extreme degrees of several kinds of injurious stimulation: thermal, barometric, chemical. Intensity of stimulation is signalled by the frequency of the discharge of nerve impulses from the receptors. Weak stimulation causes discharge of a train of impulses at a slow rate, and more intense stimulation causes a discharge at a higher frequency. With continuous stimulation at constant intensity, peripheral receptors show the phenomenon of adaptation. The rate of discharge of nerve impulses is initially high and then declines progressively to a steady rate. Pain receptors adapt very slowly. After the initial decline in the first few seconds the discharge is maintained. This is correlated with the protective function of pain. The train of impulses continues until the nocuous stimulating agent is removed.

The exciting stimulus in painful nasal affections may be the action of bacterial toxins or pressure arising from congestion and oedema of the mucosa. In the paranasal sinuses positive pressure may develop following occlusion of the sinus ostium. Sluder (1927) has described vacuum headache resulting from a negative pressure in a closed sinus. The effect of prolonged positive pressure within the maxillary sinus has been studied experimentally in man by inflating a balloon introduced into the sinus through a fistulous opening from the socket of an extracted upper molar. Pressures of 20 mmHg produced a sensation of fullness. Moderate pain was produced by pressure of 50–80 mmHg maintained for 2 h. There was associated engorgement of the turbinate, and anaesthetization of the turbinates abolished the pain. Pressures of 200 mmHg caused immediate pain.

Pathway of pain sensation

The pain sensibility from the nasal cavities is mediated by trigeminal neurones. The cell bodies of these fibres are located in the semilunar ganglion. The central axons of these cells enter the pons and synapse with cells of the sensory trigeminal nucleus. This consists of a main sensory nucleus in the pons and an elongated spinal nucleus extending through the medulla to the second cervical segment of the spinal cord. The

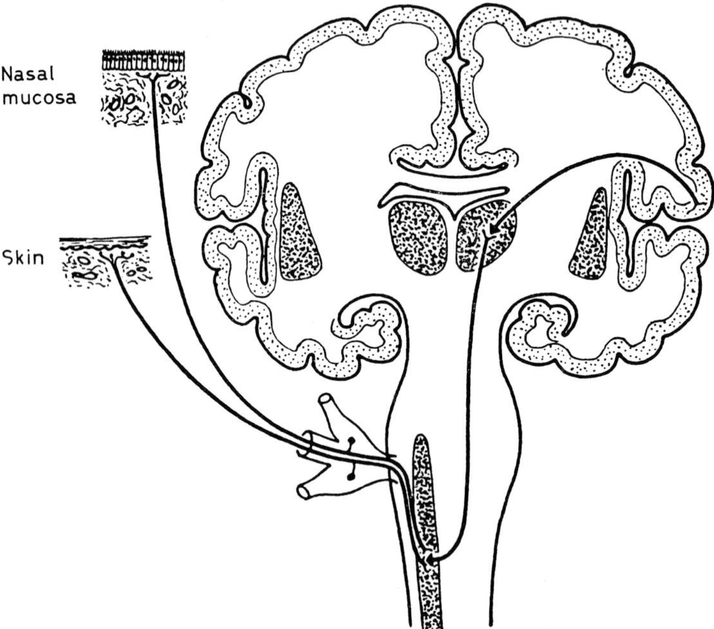

Figure 5.12 Diagram of pathway of pain (illustrating mechanism of referred pain)

fibres carrying pain impulses pass entirely to the spinal nucleus. Second-order neurones from this nucleus cross to the opposite side and ascend to relay in the postero-ventral nucleus of the thalamus. Third-order neurones are projected from the thalamus to the most inferior portion of the post-central gyrus of the cortex (*Figure 5.12*).

Distribution of pain

Pain may be experienced locally at the site of the lesion or it may be referred – chiefly to the peripheral distribution of the ophthalmic and maxillary divisions of the trigeminal nerve. The localization and main features of the headache commonly associated with disease of the accessory nasal sinuses are summarized below (*Table 5.2*). Headache diffusely localized over the frontal region along the distribution of the supra-orbital nerve with tenderness at the supra-orbital notch accompanies frontal sinus disease. In antral infections pain is felt over the maxillary region with local tenderness, and in the teeth. Acute abscess may cause also referred pain spreading over the entire area of trigeminal sensory innervation. Disease of the ethmoidal sinuses produces pain in the orbital region and over the vertex and parietal area of the skull. Acute sphenoidal sinusitis is typically associated with pain over the vertex and occipital region, accompanied by pain between and behind the eyes, in the upper jaw and teeth, and extending along the zygoma to the temple. In addition, earache and post-aural pain, simulating acute mastoiditis, and radiating pain with muscular stiffness in the back of the neck and shoulder, may occur.

Table 5.2 Distribution of referred pain from site of stimulation

Site of stimulation	*Local pain*	*Distribution of referred pain*	*Intensity in arbitrary units*
Nasal septum	Moderate	(1) Upper part – zygoma (2) Middle part – outer and inner canthus of eye	2–1
Turbinates	Sharp burning	(1) Inferior turbinate (a) anterior part – upper teeth (b) middle and posterior part – upper teeth, below eye and along zygoma (2) Middle turbinate – zygoma extending to ear and temple (3) Superior turbinate – inner canthus of eye, forehead and lateral wall of nose	4–6
Ostium of maxillary sinus	Intensely sharp and burning	Posterior nasopharynx, zygoma, temple and upper molar teeth	6–9
Frontonasal duct	Intense burning	Inner canthus, below eye, along zygoma, temple, angle of jaw and upper molar teeth	5–7
Sinuses			
Frontal	Moderate		1 plus–2 plus
Maxillary	Moderate		1 plus–2 plus
Sphenoidal	Moderate	Vertex of skull	1 plus–2 plus

This widespread referred pain is sometimes attended by vascular and secretory effects such as copious rhinorrhoea, profuse lacrimation and conjunctival hyperaemia. This syndrome constitutes the 'lower-half headache' or spheno-palatine neuralgia described by Sluder. It is attributed to irritation of the spheno-palatine ganglion or the nerve of the pterygoid canal as a result of extension of inflammation from the adjacent sphenoidal sinus. It may arise as a primary condition in the absence of intranasal suppuration. Sympathetic pathways are not involved in the afferent conduction of these 'pain' impulses. Paravertebral blocking of the cervical sympathetic does not prevent the pain nor modify its character or severity. Stimulation of the nasal mucosa still produced the same effect as before the injection of the sympathetic (Knight, 1948). Trigeminal sensory root section is followed by complete and lasting relief.

The character of the pain, its severity, time–duration curve and area of distribution depend largely on the nature and severity of the pathological condition. Pain from the nasal sinuses is generally of a dull, aching, non-pulsatile character. It is continuous rather than intermittent. In acute sinusitis, however, it may be of extreme severity and throbbing. It is less frequent at night and when lying down or resting. Pain from maxillary sinusitis may be relieved by lying down with the affected side uppermost. Increase in intensity of sinus pain is caused by shaking or lowering the head, by raising the venous pressure by coughing, straining or occluding the jugular veins, and by the vascular engorgement produced by emotion, alcohol or exposure to cold air.

Relative sensitivity of nasal structures

The sensitivity of the mucous membranes of the nasal cavities and paranasal sinuses has been investigated experimentally in man by McAuliffe, Goodell and Wolff (1945). The methods of painful stimulation employed were faradic, mechanical (by pressure with a probe) and chemical (by application of pledglets soaked in adrenaline solution). The mucosa of the ostium of the maxillary antrum was found to be most

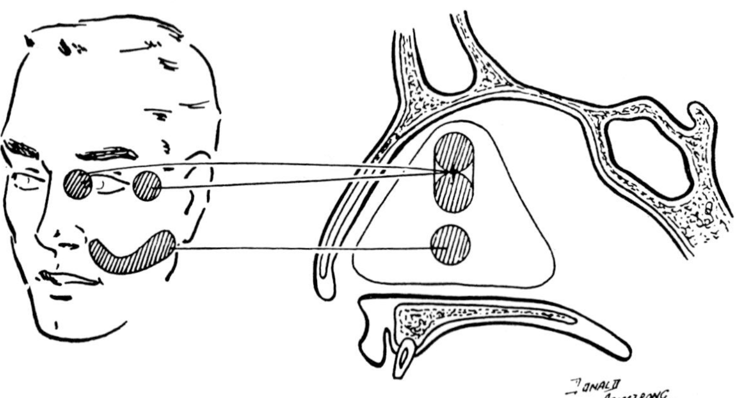

Figure 5.13 Diagram of areas of reference of pain from experimental stimulation of nasal septum. (After McAuliffe, G. W., Goodell, H. and Wolff, H. G.)

sensitive, followed in order of decreasing sensitivity by the fronto-nasal duct, turbinates, roof of the nasal cavity and septum of the nose. The mucosal lining of the maxillary and frontal sinuses were relatively insensitive, being approximately equal in sensitivity to the nasal septal region, in striking contrast with the marked sensitivity of the fronto-nasal duct and maxillary ostium. The experimentally induced pain was of a deep, diffuse, aching quality, continuous and generally referred to various areas in the peripheral distribution of the ophthalmic and maxillary divisions of the trigeminal nerve. This pain was accompanied in some cases by reflex lacrimation, photophobia, hyperalgesia and conjunctival injection or cutaneous erythema. The areas of reference from stimulation of various points are illustrated in *Figures 5.13, 5.14* and *5.15* and set out in *Table 5.2.*

Pain over the occiput and in the back of the neck could not be produced by excitation of any of the nasal or paranasal structures. Such pain is a not uncommon concomitant of sinus disease and is attributed by these workers to sustained reflex contraction of cervical and scalp muscles. This 'splinting' action of the muscles has been confirmed by electromyographic records.

In patients with section of the trigeminal nerve referred pain was not experienced on stimulation of the mucosa of the nose or of the sinuses.

Cutaneous hyperalgesia can be provoked by stimulation of the mucous membrane of the paranasal sinuses. It commonly and characteristically accompanies referred pain. Lewis (1942) stimulated the mucous membrane of the maxillary sinus with electrodes introduced through an antrostomy opening. Following stimulation after a latent period of 8 min, a little smarting was felt in the region of the malar process and lower eyelid. Hyperalgesia gradually developed, increasing in degree and extent until

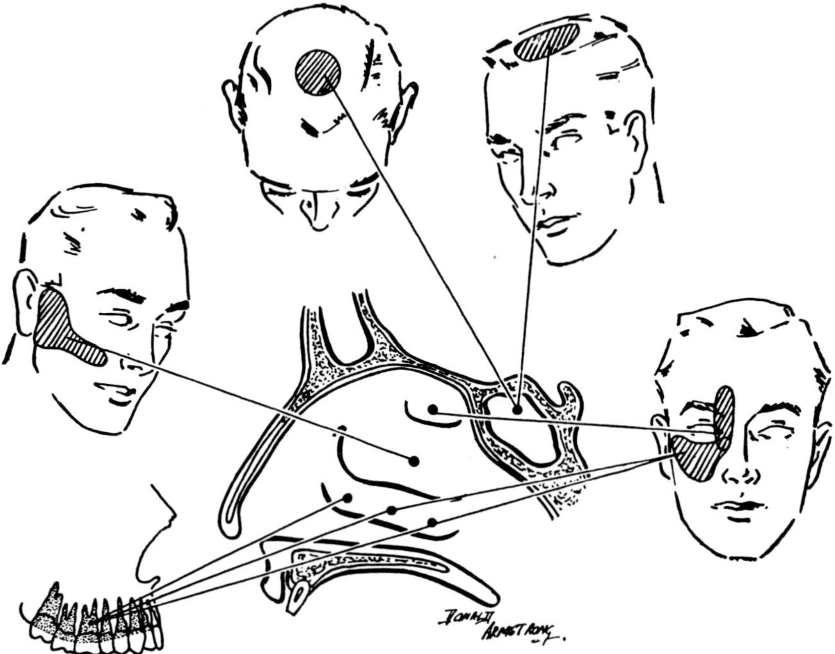

Figure 5.14 Diagram of areas of reference of pain from stimulation of the turbinates and the sphenoidal sinus. (After McAuliffe, G. W., Goodell, H. and Wolff, H. G.)

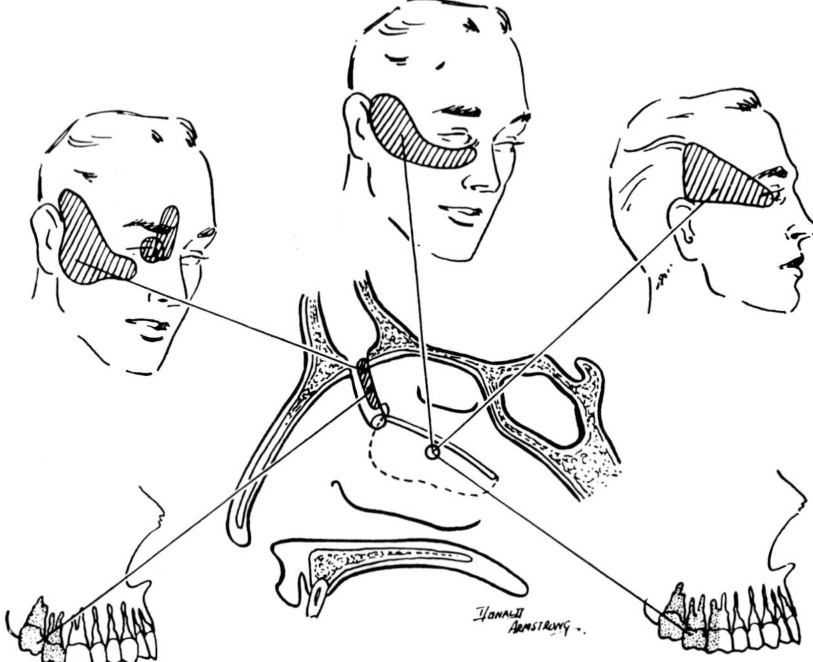

Figure 5.15 Diagram of areas of reference of pain from stimulation of frontal sinus, fronto-nasal duct and the ostium of the maxillary sinus. (After McAuliffe, G. W., Goodell, H. and Wolff, H. G.)

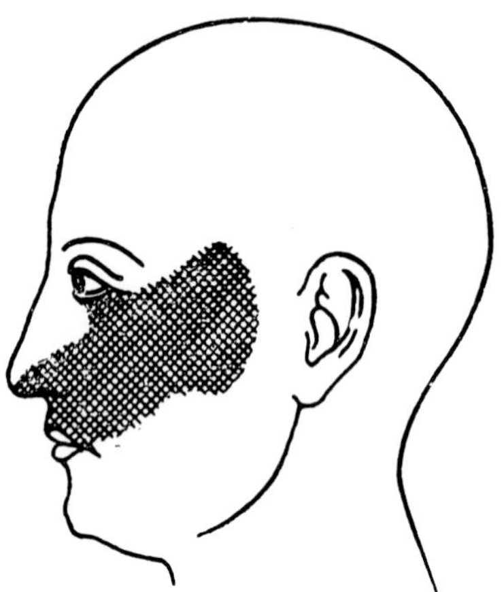

Figure 5.16 Diagram of area of hyperalgesia on experimental stimulation of mucous membrane of maxillary sinus (Lewis, 1942). (Reproduced by courtesy of *Clinical Science* and The Macmillan Co.)

the whole cutaneous area of the maxillary division of the trigeminal nerve was involved (*Figure 5.16*); a slight flush appeared on the cheek. An exactly similar distribution of hyperalgesia was set up by catarrh of the antrum in this subject.

Mechanism of referred pain

The mechanism underlying the reference of pain from one part of the body to another and the cause of the various associated reflex effects are not clearly understood.

Referred pain is a form of false localization arising from a central 'misinterpretation' by the cortical pain area. It is projected in the case of the nose to the cutaneous distribution of the fibres whose cells are located in the semilunar ganglion, through which the afferent pain impulses are entering the central nervous system.

One theory as to the mechanism of this false reference of pain is represented diagrammatically in *Figure 5.12*. Afferent fibres in the maxillary division of the trigeminal nerve from pain receptors in the nasal mucosa converge with afferent fibres in the same nerve from cutaneous pain endings, to end upon the same pool of sensory neurones in the sensory nucleus of the trigeminal nerve. Thus, these two pathways discharge along the same final neurones to a common cortical area. The cortical centre cannot distinguish the original peripheral source of the impulses reaching it by this single final pathway. Therefore, when the mucosa is stimulated, the afferent pain impulses, upon reaching the sensory cortex, are falsely localized. They are misinterpreted on the basis of previous experience as coming from the skin area from which impulses normally arrive at that point in the brain.

Sinclair, Weddell and Feindel (1948–9) have postulated, on the basis of their extensive investigations, that the essential anatomical factor concerned in the mechanism of referred pain and its associated phenomena is the branching of the peripheral axon. The afferent fibres conveying the impulses giving rise to the sensation of pain are branched, so that one limb innervates the site of the lesion and the other the area of reference of pain. For example, one limb of a branched peripheral trigeminal axon supplies the nasal mucosa while the other passes to the skin of the face. In this way pain impulses from the nasal mucosa must inevitably reach the same point in the central 'pain centre', leading to misinterpretation of their true area of origin.

This axonic branching mechanism also gives a reasonable interpretation of cutaneous hyperalgesia. Impulses from the axon branch supplying the nasal mucosa pass antidromically down the other branch. A stable chemical substance is liberated in this cutaneous area, which heightens the excitability of the cutaneous nerve terminals, producing hyperalgesia.

References

Adrian, E. D. (1956). *Journal of Laryngology*, **70,** 1

Blier, Z. (1930). *American Journal of Physiology*, **93,** 398

Cone, A. J. (1933). *Archives of Otolaryngology, Chicago*, **17,** 65

Corbett, J. L., Kerr, J. H. and Prys-Roberts, C. (1969). *Journal of Physiology, London*, **210,** 51P

Dawes, J. D. K. and Prichard, M. M. L. (1953). *Journal of Anatomy*, **87,** 311

van Dishoeck, H. A. E. (1936). *Acta Otolaryngologica, Stockholm*, **24,** 494

Fabricant, N. D. (1945). *Archives of Otolaryngology, Chicago*, **41,** 53

Fowler, E. P. (1943). *Archives of Otolaryngology, Chicago*, **37,** 710

Gardner, W. J. and Stowell, A. (1947). *Journal of Neurosurgery*, **4,** 105

Golding-Wood, P. H. (1961). *Journal of Laryngology*, **75,** 232

Grant, S. B., Mudd, S. and Goldman, A. (1920). *Journal of Experimental Medicine*, **32,** 87

Gray, J. (1928). *Ciliary Movement.* Cambridge University Press

Hertzman, A. B. and Dillon, J. B. (1939). *American Journal of Physiology*, **127,** 671

Hilding, A. C. (1932). *American Journal of Physiology*, **100,** 164

Holmes, T. H., Goodell, H., Wolf, S. and Wolff, H. H. (1950). *The Nose.* Springfield, Ill.; Thomas

Inglestedt, S. (1970). *Annals of Otology, Rhinology and Laryngology.* **79,** 475

Inglestedt, S. and Torelmalm, N. G. (1960). *Acta Otolaryngologica*, Supp. **158,** 1

Inglestedt, S. and Torelmalm, N. G. (1961). *Acta Physiologica, Scandinavica*, **51,** 1

Jackson, D. E. (1942). *Annals of Otology, Rhinology and Laryngology, St. Louis*, **51,** 973

James, J. E. Angell and Daly, M. de Burgh (1969). *Proceedings of the Royal Society of Medicine*, **62,** 1287

Knight, G. C. (1948). *Proceedings of the Royal Society of Medicine*, **41,** 587

Lewis, T. (1942). *Pain*. London; Macmillan

Lierle, D. M. and Moore, P. M. (1934). *Archives of Otolaryngology, Chicago*, **19,** 55

Lorenzo, H. J. (1951). *Journal of Biophysics and Biochemical Cytology*, **3,** 839

Lucas, A. M. (1935). *American Journal of Physiology*, **112,** 468

Malcomson, G. (1959). *Journal of Laryngology*, **73,** 73

McAuliffe, G. W., Goodell, H. and Wolff, H. G. (1945). *Research Publications of the Association of Nervous and Mental Diseases*, **23,** 185

Mudd, S., Goldman, A. and Grant, S. B. (1921). *Annals of Otology, Rhinology and Laryngology*, **30,** 1

Mullins, L. J. (1955). *American New York Academy of Sciences*, **62,** 247

Nadel, J. A. and Comroe, J. H. Jnr. (1961). *Journal of Applied Physiology*, **16,** 713

Nadel, J. A. and Widdicombe, J. G. (1962). *Journal of Applied Physiology*, **17,** 861

Negus, V. E. (1934). *Journal of Laryngology*, **49,** 571

Negus, V. E. (1954). *Annals of the Royal College of Surgeons*, **15,** 141

Negus, V. E. (1958). *Comparative Anatomy and Physiology of the Nose and Paranasal Sinuses*. Edinburgh and London; Livingstone

O'Neill, D. and Malcomson, K. (1954). *British medical Journal*, **1,** 554

Phillips, G. D. and Raghavan, G. V. (1970). *Journal of Physiology*, **208,** 2

Proetz, A. W. (1953). *Applied Physiology of the Nose* (2nd ed.). St. Louis; Mosby

Ralston, H. J. and Kerr, W. J. (1945). *American Journal of Physiology*, **144,** 305

Reading, P. and Malcomson, K. (1954). *British Medical Journal*, **1,** 552

Sinclair, D. C., Weddel, G. and Feindel, W. H. (1948–9). *Brain*, **71,** 7184

Slome, D. (1956). *Lectures on the Scientific Basis of Medicine*, **5,** 451

Sluder, C. (1927). *Nasal Neurology, Headaches and Eye Disorders*. St. Louis; Mosby

Spiesman, I. G. (1935). *American Journal of Physiology*, **115,** 181

Sternberg, H. (1925). *Zentralblatt fur Halsen, Nasen und Ohrenheilkunde*, **7,** 675

Sternstein, H. J. (1937). *Archives of Otolaryngology, Chicago*, **25,** 442

Swingle, P. E. (1935). *Annals of Otology, Rhinology and Laryngology, St. Louis*, **44,** 913

Tatum, A. L. (1923). *American Journal of Physiology*, **65,** 229

Tomori, Z. and Widdicombe, J. G. (1969). *Journal of Physiology, London*, **200,** 25

Tschalussow, M. A. (1913). *Pflüg. Arch. ges. Physiol.*, **151,** 523

Tschalussow, M. A. (1913). *Zentralblatte Biochemica Biophysica*, **15,** 338

Uddströmer, M. (1940). *Acta Otolaryngologica, Stockholm*, Suppl. 42

Undritz, W. (1930). *Acta Otolaryngologica, Stockholm*, **14,** 530

Wolff, H. G., Wolf, S., Goodell, H. and Holmes, T. H. (1949). *American Journal of Medical Science*, **218,** 16

Yates, A. L. (1924). *Journal of Laryngology*, **39,** 554

6 The ears and nasal sinuses in the aerospace environment

A J Benson and P F King

Otic barotrauma

The physiological changes which occur in the ears in the environment of aerospace are of importance to professional aviators and passengers alike, particularly as flight is now commonplace. That such changes occur with change of altitude, and hence of atmospheric pressure, has been known since man first took to the air. The celebrated balloonist J. A. C. Charles complained of severe pain in the right ear in his first flight in a hydrogen balloon in December 1783.

The development of aviation in this century gave a great impetus to the solution of problems arising from man entering a new environment. Despite the immense growth in aviation fostered by the opposing nations in the First World War, there appears to have been little interest in the mechanism of pressure change in the ears, though Sidney Scott (1919), a distinguished otologist of that time, recorded typical cases showing these effects.

The Second World War saw the use of air power on a wide scale by the warring nations, and this in turn led to great efforts to solve environmental problems. While Armstrong and Heim (1937) had described the sequence of events during pressure change in the ears, it was left to Dickson and his colleagues in the Royal Air Force to complete the ground work which gave an overall picture of otic barotrauma.

Definition and nomenclature

Unobstructed ventilation of the eustachian (auditory) tube will produce no changes, and hence no symptoms, in flight. The tube which becomes obstructed during pressure change will produce characteristic physiological changes in the ear(s) with signs and symptoms – and, in a proportion of cases, a chain of possible complications of relatively serious import.

The syndrome of total obstruction during pressure change is, or has been, known variously as aerotitis media (Armstrong and Heim, 1937), aviation pressure deafness (McGibbon, 1947), and otitic barotrauma (Dickson *et al.*, 1947 – but it is probably most accurately described as *otic barotrauma*. Collectively, the syndromes related to pressure changes are termed *dysbarism* (Hinchcliffe, 1972).

By definition, otic barotrauma is damage to the ears resulting from pressure. It is therefore likely to occur in any situation where a change of pressure is acting on the middle ear and tubal system. In this section we are concerned with such a mechanism in flight and in the decompression chamber, but it will also occur in diving, and in the clinical field when patients are treated in hyperbaric oxygen chambers (Morrison, 1972).

Boyle's law

Of first importance is a knowledge of the behaviour of gases when subjected to pressure, as this will govern the behaviour of gas in the tympanic cavity. This is exemplified by Boyle's Law which states that the pressure and the volume of an enclosed fixed mass of gas are inversely proportional.

In ascent from sea level through the atmosphere there is a progressive reduction in the atmospheric pressure, as shown in *Figure 6.1*. In round terms at 18 000 ft (5500 m)

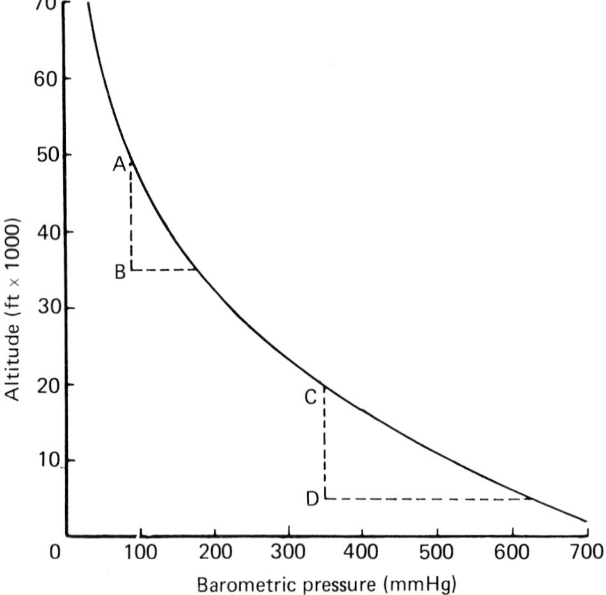

Figure 6.1 Relationship between altitude and barometric pressure. For any given rate of descent, the rate of pressure change increases as the altitude is reduced. A descent of 15000 ft is shown at AB and CD: in AB the pressure change is 91 mmHg, and in CD it is 283 mmHg

above sea level the pressure is half that at sea level, and this pressure is halved again at almost 34 000 ft (10 300 m). It will be appreciated that the change in differential pressure associated with a given change in altitude is much greater at relatively low altitudes than at great height.

In practical terms, this will mean that during ascent through the atmosphere from

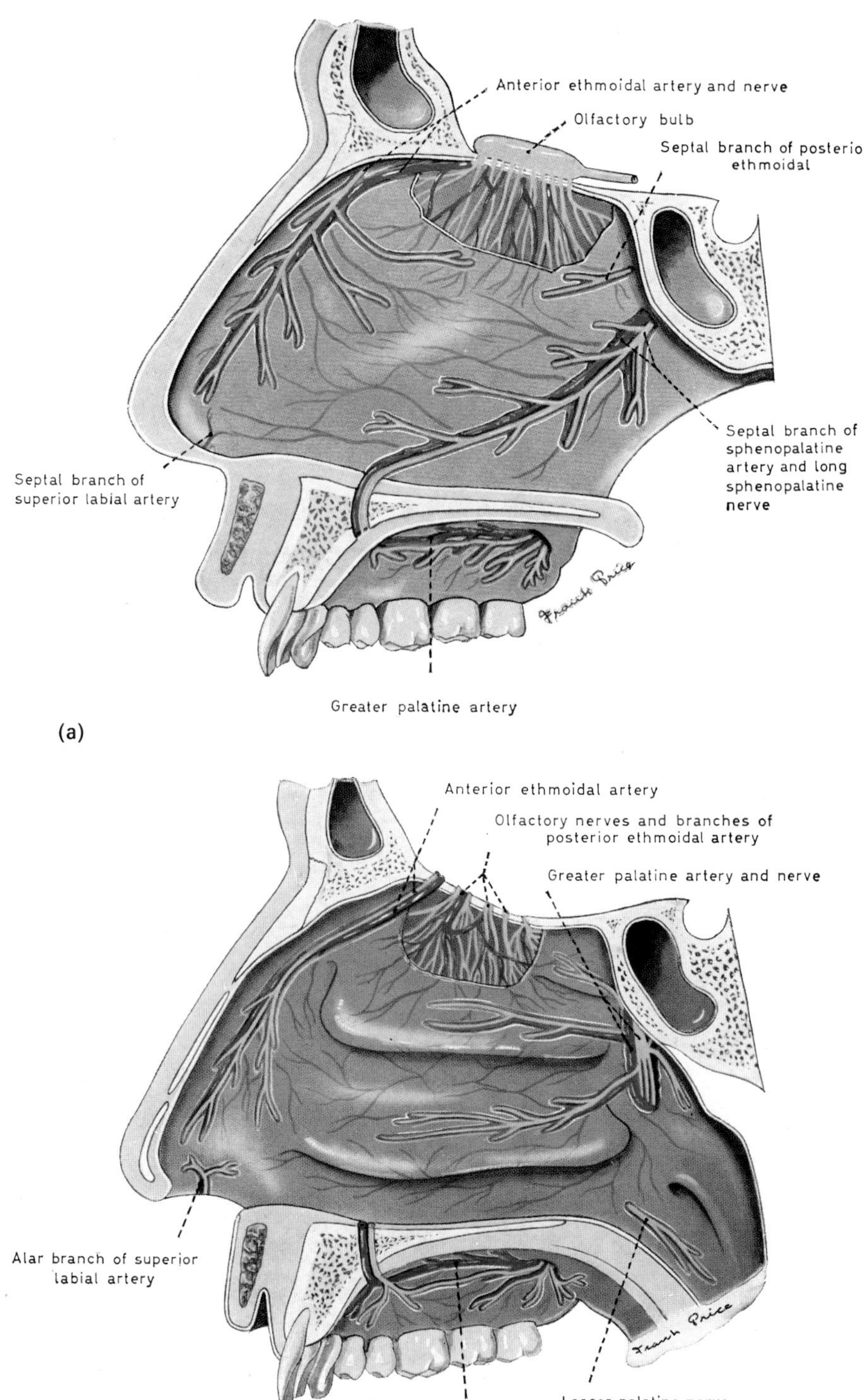

Plate 3 The blood vessels and nerves of: (a) the nasal septum; (b) the lateral wall of the nasal cavity

(*To face page* 206)

sea level, the atmospheric pressure will diminish, and as a result a given mass of gas contained within an elastic structure will expand. In the middle ear (*Figure 6.2*) the gaseous expansion will continue until it has pushed the tympanic membrane virtually to the natural limit of its excursion, an effect which can be studied with an otoscope in flight or during simulated flight in a decompression chamber. When the tympanic membrane has reached its limit there is an easy and involuntary escape of air along the eustachian tube, as described by Hartmann in 1879 and confirmed by Armstrong and Heim (1937). Movement of the membrane will only be impaired if it is restricted by scarring in the middle ear, or calcareous deposits in the tympanic membrane itself.

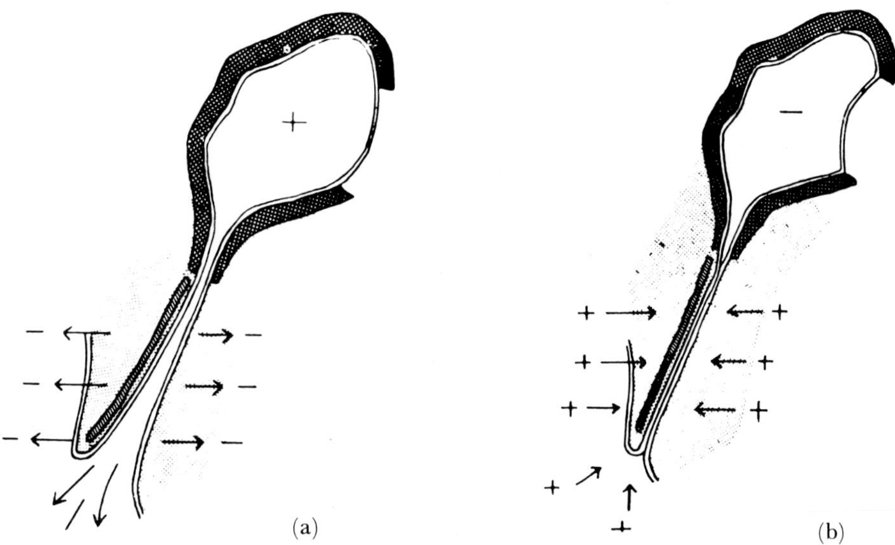

Figure 6.2 Diagrammatic representation of the middle ear during the ascent (a) and descent (b). With reducing environmental pressure on ascent, the air in the middle ear expands, bulges the tympanic membrane and passively opens the eustachian tube. In descent with increasing environmental pressure the tympanic membrane is forced inwards, and the soft parts of the eustachian tube are held in opposition

During descent from altitude the same physical laws apply, so that as the atmospheric pressure increases, the volume of gas in the middle ear decreases; but air does not normally enter the middle ear automatically, the eustachian tube must be opened and ventilation brought about by involuntary swallowing movements, which recur about every minute or so. Failure or delay in the mechanism will result in an increasing differential pressure acting on the soft, nasopharyngeal end of the tube. If this pressure closing the tube exerts a force greater than that which can be developed by the tubal dilator muscles, the tube will stay closed, and is said to be 'locked'. Thereafter the patho-physiological changes of barotrauma are inevitable. Armstrong and Heim (1937) have shown that a positive extra-tympanic pressure of 90 mmHg (12 kPa) will lock the tube, but this figure is variable and will depend on the intrinsic strength of the tubal dilator muscles.

Associated physiology of the eustachian tube

The detailed anatomy of the auditory tube has been given earlier, but a review of its function is essential to a clear picture of the mechanism of barotrauma.

The primary role of the auditory tube is to maintain the equality of air pressure across the tympanic membrane, which is necessitated by the absorption of gas through the mucous membrane in the middle ear, and the variations of ambient atmospheric pressure. This is achieved by opening the tube to permit the passage of gas along it.

It follows that in the resting phase the tube is closed, and this comes about from the combination of several factors such as the elasticity of the cartilaginous support, the venous pressure and the presence of a mucous blanket in the lumen of the tube. Quantitative data relating to some of these factors have not been determined, though Rundcrantz (1969) has shown that air volumes passing through the tube were much reduced during compression of the neck veins, or when the body was in a horizontal position compared to being in a position of elevation of 20 degrees (0.35 rad). Perlman (1967) has shown that relatively small pressure differences across the tube are needed for separation of the mucosal surface and breaking of the mucous film.

The muscular opening of the tube

The auditory tube is opened by swallowing, yawning and gaping movements – and in flight these actions are employed to initiate tubal opening.

The cartilaginous portion of the tube is cradled by muscles, but those concerned with the control of patency of the tube can be divided into two groups:

(a) Those muscles which by having an insertion into the walls of the tube exert a direct action.
(b) Those muscles which by anatomical association assist or influence tubal opening.

Of the muscles in the first group we should consider the tensor palati, levator palati, the salpingo-pharyngeus, and finally the tensor tympani muscle.

The *tensor palati muscle* is the most important of this group: it takes its origin from the wall of the scaphoid fossa, the spine of the sphenoid, and from the length of the antero–lateral aspect of the tubal cartilage. It passes round the pterygoid hamulus, joining the fibres of the opposing muscle from the other side in an aponeurosis forming part of the soft palate. McMyn (1940) believed that the tensor palati was the prime mover in opening the tube, and he considered that the other muscles in the supporting group acted synergistically. The view that the tensor palati is the *only* muscle involved in opening the tube was put forward by Rich (1920), and this view is supported by Macbeth (1960) on phylogenetic evidence in whales and porpoises, which have a well-developed levator palati muscle that appears to be the sole mechanism of opening the tube in these animals. Holmquist (1976) believes that both the tensor palati and the tensor tympani muscles act synergistically in relation to their action on the auditory tube, and as they have been shown to have a common embryological origin, and a common nerve supply from a branch of the 5th cranial nerve, this would not be surprising.

The role of the *tensor tympani muscle* in tubal opening is a relatively recent consideration. The muscle originates from the cartilaginous part of the tube and the adjoining part of the sphenoid bone, and from the walls of its own bony canal. Posteriorly it forms a tendon, which is angled at the processus cochleariformis to cross the tympanic cavity to the neck of the malleus. Its origin may well influence the opening of the tube (Ingelsted, Ivarsson and Jonson, 1967) and this is supported by the fact that the tube begins to open from the middle-ear end (Holmquist, 1976).

Proctor (1973) has given a full description of the other two muscles in this primary group – *levator palati* and *salpingo-pharyngeus*. The latter arises from the inferior part of the tubal cartilage near its pharyngeal end, and passes downwards to blend with palato-pharyngeus. The remaining muscle, the levator palati, arises from the under surface of the petrous bone, and from the medial lamina of the auditory tube. It

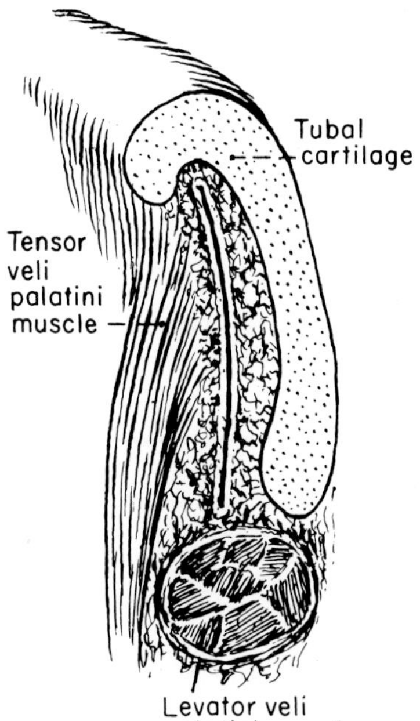

Figure 6.3 A diagram of a cross-section of the cartilaginous portion of the auditory tube, showing the relative positions of the tensor palati and levator palati muscles (after Holmquist, 1976)

gradually comes to lie on the inferior aspect of the tube, which it helps to support. Passing within the upper margin of the superior constrictor muscle, it spreads out into the soft palate – its fibres blending with those of its fellow from the other side. Its action is to elevate the soft palate at the beginning of swallowing. If one considers its action in association with the tensor palati muscle it is likely that the levator palati will support and hold the tubal cartilage to permit the tensor palati muscle to act on the curve of the tubal cartilage, and so open the lumen.

The muscles in the second, supporting, group which assist in the opening of the tube are the upper parts of the superior constrictor of the pharynx, and the sphincter of the nasopharyngeal isthmus, of which the palato–pharyngeus is a major contributor.

The passive state of the tube

In its natural state the auditory tube is collapsed – so that its closure is essentially a passive process. When the associated muscles relax, or when a static pressure is no longer acting to maintain tubal patency, the tubal lumen collapses. Aschan (1954) has shown that this passive closure starts at the nasopharyngeal end. It is an increasing pressure acting on the soft, nasopharyngeal end which compresses the collapsed tube, and will lead to barotrauma if the tube is not opened; this site of the obstruction was shown by McGibbon (1942).

It is also of importance that, following its opening, the tube should stay open long enough to permit the adequate passage of gas along its lumen. There is no agreement as to the length of time the tube stays open – and this varies between 0.1 and 0.9 s (Perlman, 1951; Aschan, 1955; Miller, 1965). This is of practical importance as Dickson and King (1954) have indicated that the *severity* of otic barotrauma sustained in flight is related to the rate of descent from altitude, and hence to the rate of pressure change. A slow opening time of the tube, from whatever cause, will therefore predispose to barotrauma. Other factors influencing the passage of gas along the tube will be the pressure difference across the tube, and the width and length of the narrowest part (Elner, Ingelstedt and Ivarsson, 1971).

Factors contributing to barotrauma

So far we have been concerned with the physical changes which occur in flight and the physiological mechanism which ventilates the middle ear. From the foregoing remarks it will be appreciated that any condition which either narrows the lumen of the tube by oedema, or increases the amount or viscosity of the mucus coating the tube, will predispose to barotrauma, either by reducing the rate of flow of gas along the tube, or by impairing the ability of the tube to open.

Such conditions are those that one would expect to play such a part, and include the effects of acute or chronic infection in the nose, particularly coryza, and also allergic and vasomotor rhinitis. To these should be added the long-term effects of malformation of the nasal skeleton, either congenital or traumatic in origin, together with gross malocclusion of the teeth and jaws.

Role of overpressure in the nasopharynx

We have seen that the eustachian tube will open passively in ascent, with the overpressure of gas contained in the middle ear. In descent, the tube will also open from overpressure of some degree applied at the nasal end of the tube, as in Valsalva's manoeuvre. This technique and Frenzel's manoeuvre are employed to assist in clearing the ears in flight or in the decompression chamber. A description of each of these techniques is given, as mention of them is omitted from many modern publications.

Valsalva's manoeuvre

This is performed when the subject attempts forcible expiration with the lips tightly closed and the nostrils occluded by digital compression of the nose. By this procedure the air pressure in the nasopharynx is raised to force air along the auditory tube to the middle ear. This technique was described originally by Antonio Valsalva in 1704, in his 'Tractus de Aure Humana' (Scott, Stevenson and Guthrie, 1949).

Although Valsalva's manoeuvre is commonly employed in flight to clear the ears, it can on occasion cause syncope. The raised intrathoracic pressure produced during the manoeuvre will result in an increase in central venous pressure and pooling of blood in the venous system. In addition, pulmonary stretch reflexes have a well recognized potential for inducing cardiac arrythmia. The combination of these two factors is believed to be responsible for the syncope which can occur (Duvoisin, Kruse and Saunders, 1962), and which could be disastrous if occurring in the pilot of a high performance aircraft.

Frenzel manoeuvre

Another mechanism to ventilate the middle ear was developed by Hermann Frenzel (1938, 1950). It consists of voluntarily closing the glottis and closing the mouth and the nose, while simultaneously contracting the muscles of the floor of the mouth and the superior pharyngeal constrictors. It is a technique which has to be taught and learned. Its advantage is that it can be performed in any phase of respiration and is independent of intrathoracic pressure. Chunn (1960) found that the mean tubal opening pressure when using the Frenzel manoeuvre was 6 mmHg (0.8 kPa), compared to a mean opening pressure of 33 mmHg (4.4 kPa) with the Valsalva technique. This can probably be explained by the use of the tensor palati muscle to open the tube in Frenzel's manoeuvre, whereas in Valsalva's manoeuvre no muscular opening of the tube occurs.

One further tubal opening technique worthy of description is the manoeuvre demonstrated by Toynbee in 1853, which opens the tube at ground level. It consists of swallowing with a closed nose. Initially, a small positive pressure develops in the nasopharynx, but is soon replaced by negative pressure (Thomson, 1958). It is useful in visually checking the patency of the tube.

Patho-physiology

Our knowledge of the patho-physiology of otic barotrauma owes much to the experimental work by Dickson, McGibbon and Campbell (1947) in which cats were decompressed to a pressure corresponding to an altitude of 20 000 ft (6100 m) and then recompressed. The histological changes seen were all vascular in nature, and included mucosal congestion, haemorrhage into the mucosa, oedema, seromucinous or haemorrhagic effusion and polymorph infiltration. These changes are shown in *Figure 6.4 a–d*. Such changes can be explained by the presence of a sub-ambient pressure in the middle ear. Such a negative pressure differential across the tympanic membrane is revealed by its invaginated appearance, while the varying degrees of congestion, the formation of solitary or multiple haemorrhagic bullae, blood or fluid in the middle ear or even rupture of the tympanic membrane, all accord with the proposed patho-physiological mechanism. The varied appearances of the tympanic membrane are shown in *Plate 4 a–h* (*facing page 222*).

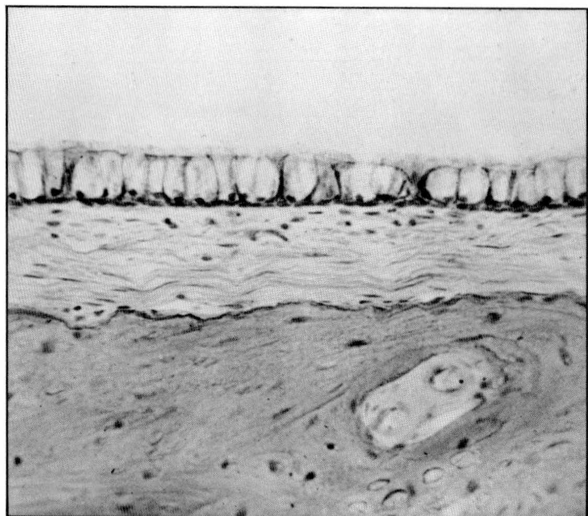

(a) Normal mucosa of middle ear

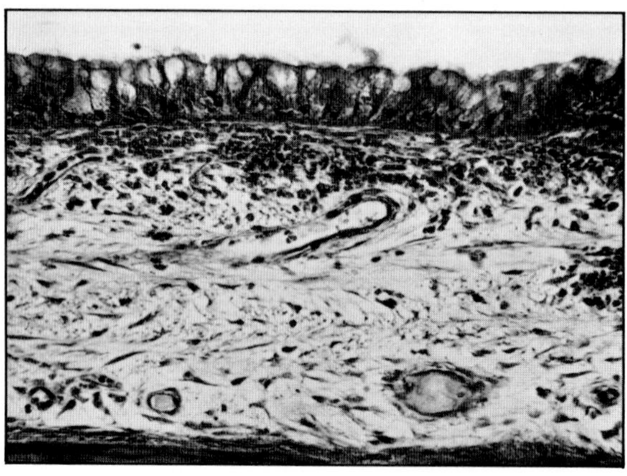

(b) Oedema of middle-ear mucosa, with sub-epithelial cellular infiltration

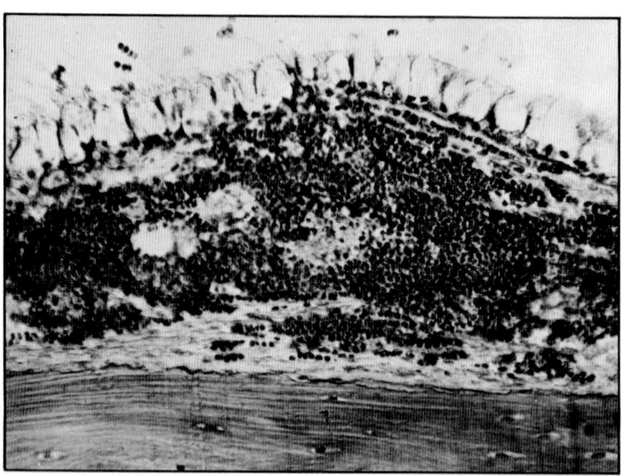

(c) Haemorrhage in middle-ear mucosa

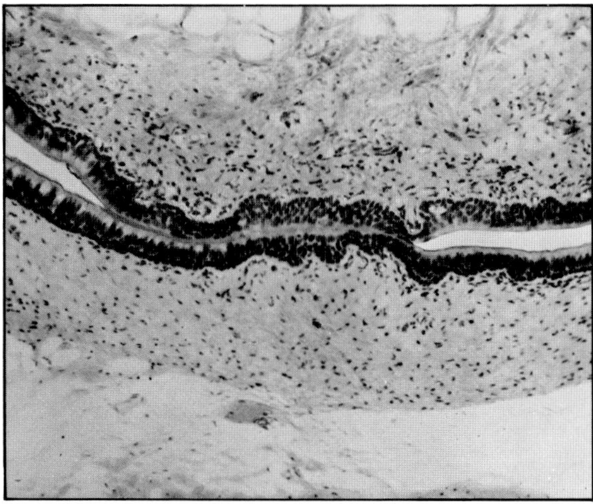

(d) Tubal obstruction

Figure 6.4 Histological preparations showing the tissue changes occurring in barotrauma induced experimentally in the ear

Range of middle-ear pressures

The production of these changes may be explained further by considering the effect of a loss of height through a known range.

If the middle ear should remain unopened in a descent from an altitude of say 10 000 ft (3050 m) above sea level, on reaching the ground (sea level) where the ambient pressure is 760 mmHg (101.3 kPa), the middle ear will contain air at a theoretical pressure of 522.6 mmHg (70 kPa) – there will thus be a pressure difference of some 237 mmHg (31 kPa).*

The absolute pressure within the blood vessels in the tympanic membrane is the sum of the ambient pressure (atmospheric pressure) plus the present blood pressure. If the capillary pressure is regarded as 20 mmHg (2.7 kPa) then the absolute pressure in the capillaries will be 780 (760 + 20) mmHg (103.9 kPa). The pressure of the tissue fluid surrounding the vessels is only 522.6 mmHg (70 kPa), and as a result the vessels become passively engorged.

Rupture of the tympanic membrane

As would be expected, the differential across the drumhead occurring during descent can be sufficiently great to rupture the tympanic membrane. The antero-inferior segment of the tympanic membrane (that portion sited close to the tympanic opening of the eustachian tube) is the site where tears commonly occur, but the membrane can tear anywhere, particularly if weakened by previous scarring. In acute barotrauma of rapid onset, with a fast rate of pressure change, the drumhead may be avulsed from the tympanic ring – the membranous remnants being wrapped round the handle of the malleus – leaving a wide open middle ear. Rupture of the drumhead due to barotrauma in flight was reported by King (1976) to have occurred in 38 of 897 ears with barotrauma.

* The actual pressure, assuming no venting of air into the middle ear, will be less because of the compliance of the tympanic membrane.

Rupture of the labyrinthine windows

The concept of rupture of the round or oval window membranes during barotraumatic change is relatively new. Goodhill (1971) drew attention to spontaneous rupture of the round window membrane following a rise in intracranial pressure from sudden coughing, sneezing or straining, and he believed that sudden middle-ear pressure change in flight might produce the same result. As long ago as 1933 Hughson and Crowe demonstrated that the round window membrane bulged outwards in the tympanic cavity during a rise of pressure in the cerebrospinal fluid.

In addition, increasing pressure acting on the drumhead and pushing it inwards will cause inward movement of the stapes at the oval window, though tearing of the annular ligament of the oval window is rare. Nevertheless, we have seen this occur in middle-aged aircrew.

Recent work by Tingley and MacDougall (1977) suggests that rupture of the round window membrane may be a cause of the symptoms of alternobaric vertigo in some instances.

However, there is a special risk for those who have had the operation of stapedectomy, and several cases of this nature occurring in flights have been reported. The possible fate of the stapedectomized ear in these circumstances has been investigated extensively by Rayman (1972). Tearing of one or both windows is associated with a sudden severe sensorineural hearing loss which may fluctuate, and there is sometimes, but not always, vertigo. Those who are to undergo, or who have had, stapedectomy should be warned of the possible hazard of flight to the hearing, and this places an additional responsibility on the surgeon. There is evidence to suggest that, of the variety of stapedial prostheses employed, a fat and wire assembly is the safest.

Delayed otic barotrauma

Otic barotrauma is normally associated with physiological changes at the time of the pressure change. However, there are occasions when the subject may experience symptoms (i.e. discomfort and deafness) several hours after the completion of a flight.

This delayed form of otic barotrauma occurs after long flights, when the breathing of 100 per cent oxygen has resulted in the middle ear containing a much raised tension of that gas. With occlusion of the tube, and an absence of active inflation of the middle ear (as would occur during sleep), the relatively rapid absorption of oxygen through the mucosa of the middle ear will result in the development of a significant pressure differential.

This phenomenon was reported originally by Comroe *et al.* (1945), and then investigated in some depth by Jones (1958, 1959) who found that in the absence of inflation, the rate of pressure change is doubled when the middle ear is filled with oxygen as opposed to being filled with air.

The signs of the condition are not so marked as in otic barotrauma of acute onset, and normally one would see only a marked invagination of the tympanic membrane – with, in some cases, a hint of fluid in the middle ear.

Chronic otic barotrauma

This is a clinical, rather than a physiological, condition in which one episode of barotrauma predisposes to another. Two factors are likely to be at work here:

(a) The original predisposing factor may itself be chronic.
(b) Oedema and interstitial bleeding in the tubal mucosa may result in a further decrease in the size of the tubal lumen, and so predispose to further attacks. It is likely that in both passengers and aircrew a return to flying was permitted before the tube had fully recovered, and so a further barotrauma was induced.

The role of pressurization and the pressure cabin

The adverse physiological effects of flight at high altitude are almost entirely due to the accompanying reduction of barometric pressure, so that the most logical way of securing satisfactory conditions for the occupants of high-flying aircraft is to provide within the aircraft an atmosphere that is at a pressure appropriate to bodily needs (*Figure 6.5*).

As the cabin pressure has to be greater than that of the surrounding atmosphere, the difference between the two pressures will be represented by a *differential* pressure tending to force the cabin walls outwards. It follows that the absolute pressure within the pressure cabin will be equal to the barometric pressure existing at a level below that at which the aircraft is flying. It is convenient to consider conditions *inside* the aircraft in terms of the altitude which is being simulated by pressurization. In pressure cabin aircraft, then, we have 'aircraft altitude' and 'cabin altitude'.

The effect of employing a pressure cabin is to reduce the range over which barometric pressure is acting, but it should be remembered that below 15 000 ft (4500 m) the rate of pressure increase will predispose to barotrauma, and this is an

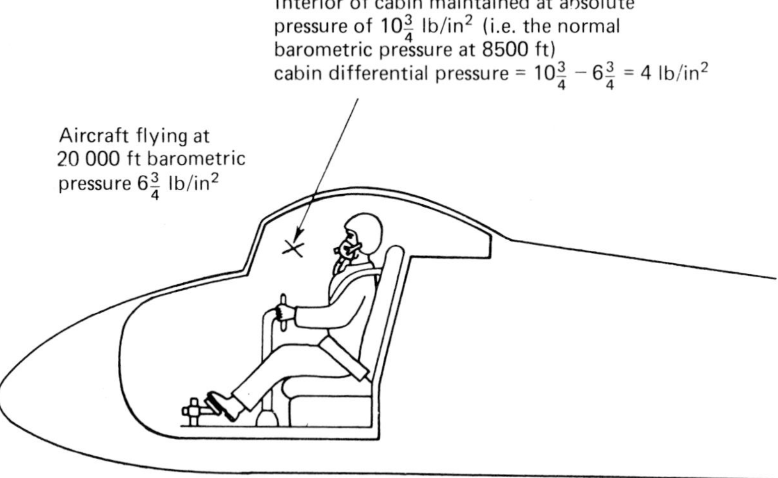

Figure 6.5 Pressure cabin aircraft in a situation where the aircraft altitude is 20 000 ft, and the cabin altitude is 8500 ft

important factor in deciding the rate at which pressurization should diminish when an aircraft is descending.

The practicalities of the situation have resulted in the concept of a high differential cabin and a low differential cabin. The high differential cabin is employed in transport aircraft in which the conveyance of passengers make it necessary to maintain a cabin altitude of 8000 ft (2440 m) even when the aircraft, like the supersonic transport, is flying at 60 000 ft (18 000 m). The maximum differential pressure involved is 430 mmHg (56.9 kPa). The low differential cabin is employed in military aircraft, when failure of the pressure cabin in combat must be accepted as an operational hazard. The risks of too great a pressure change on sudden decompression are minimized by employing a relatively low cabin differential pressure. Despite this, many military aircraft are provided with a high level of pressurization. Transport aircraft are commonly fitted with cabin pressure controllers, whose characteristics can be altered in flight. Although no variation can be made in the maximum permissible differential pressure, it is possible to select the altitude at which pressurization will start after take-off, and the rate of change of cabin pressure during ascent and descent.

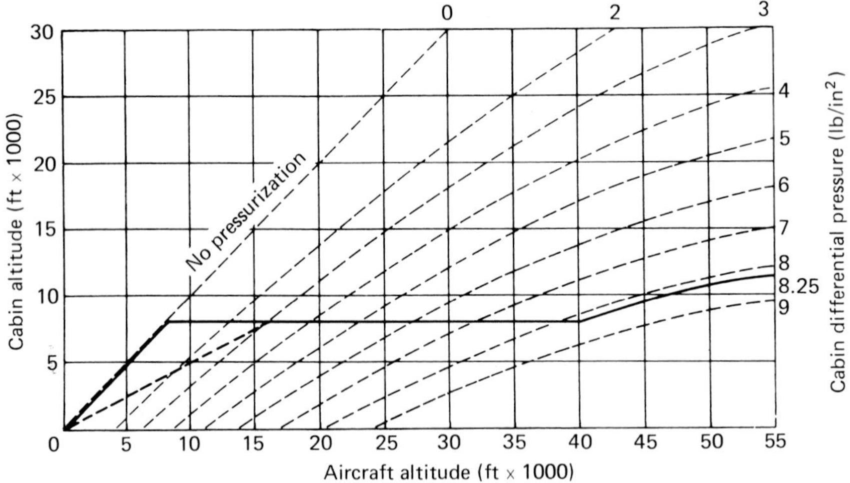

Figure 6.6 Graph illustrating, for a typical passenger aircraft, the relationship between aircraft altitude, cabin altitude, and cabin differential pressure

In the example shown in *Figure 6.6* (Brown, 1965) the alternative pattern, if adopted, would reduce the risk of barotrauma when carrying out a rapid descent below 8000 ft (2400 m), e.g. if the aircraft was descending at 1000 ft/min (5 m/s) below 8000 ft the rate of change of the cabin altitude would be 500 ft/min (2.5 m/s) – an effective reduction.

Sinus barotrauma

The paranasal sinuses also contain air, so, as with the ears, symptoms can arise when communication between the interior of the sinuses and the outside atmosphere fails to cope with changes in the surrounding atmospheric pressure.

The syndrome of pain developing in the frontal region or in the cheeks during or shortly after flight, sometimes associated with rhinorrhoea and epistaxis is commonly called *sinus barotrauma*, but it is also called aero-sinusitis, barotraumatic sinusitis, or dysbarism.

The frequency with which the condition occurs is difficult to assess. Campbell (1944) reported an incidence of sinus barotrauma to otic barotrauma as being one to 20; while Dickson and King (1954) gave an account of 328 patients suffering from barotrauma, of whom 250 suffered an otic lesion and 100 a sinus barotrauma (22 sustaining a combination of both lesions). King (1965) reporting a further series of 100 such cases found the frontal sinus to be involved in 70, the maxillary sinus in 19, the frontal and maxillary sinuses together in ten, and the ethmoid sinuses in only one.

Mechanism of production

The physical laws that apply to enclosed gas spaces of the ear also apply to gas-filled cavities of the sinuses (*Figure 6.7*); therefore, the production of physiological changes

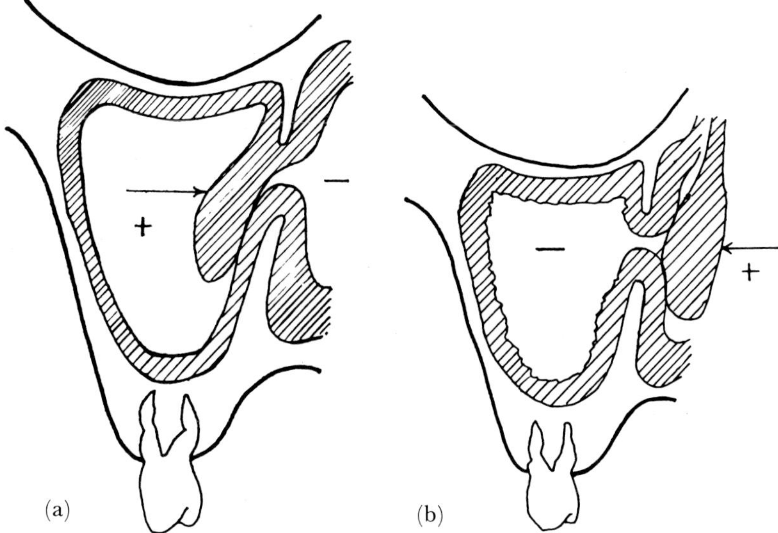

Figure 6.7 (a) Diagram indicating the mode of causation of antral barotrauma during ascent. The air in the sinus expands with decreasing environmental pressure and, in this instance, has forced a polyp into the ostium so blocking it. With continued ascent, an increasing differential is built up between the sinus and the environment. (b) The mode of causation of antral barotrauma in descent. With increasing environmental pressure, a polyp in the nasal fossa has been forced into the sinus ostium, so blocking it. With continued descent, and unrelieved obstruction, antral barotrauma will occur

within the sinuses during actual or simulated flight will hinge on the degree of patency of the ostium ventilating each sinus.

Occlusion of a sinus ostium may be due to a mucous plug, to oedema of the ostial mucosa, or to mechanical obstruction from such features as polypi, mucosal folds or neoplasm. Generally, the obstructing flap has a valvular action, so that air passes easily in one direction, but not in the other.

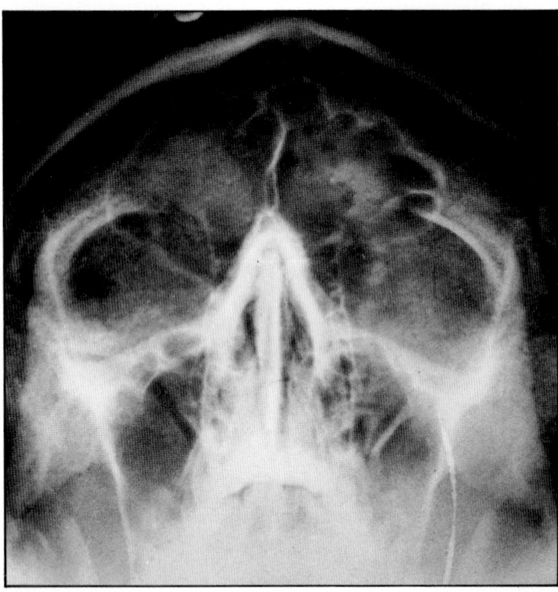

Figure 6.8 Right frontal sinus barotrauma. The right frontal sinus shows a pear-shaped swelling, the result of submucosal haemorrhage

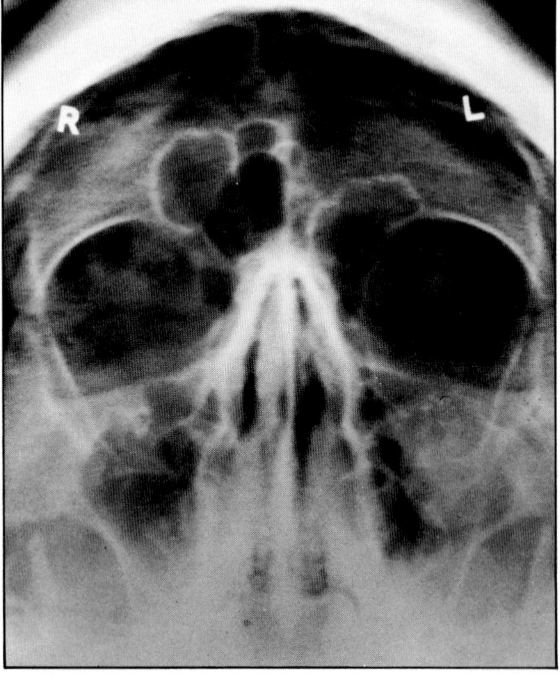

Figure 6.9 Left antral barotrauma. The left antrum shows a well-defined polypoid swelling, apparently arising from upper outer angle of the antrum. Lavage yielded blood clot on this side

Normally, the maximum difference in pressure between the substance of the mucosa and the air in a sinus equals the systolic blood pressure. For example, if the systolic figure is 130 mmHg (17.3 kPa) it follows that the absolute blood pressure (and hence the pressure within the mucosa) will be 130 + local barometric pressure (mmHg). During descent from altitude the absolute blood pressure increases steadily, and if there has been obstruction of a sinus ostium the air in the sinus will remain at a constant relatively low pressure. The pressure differential between the mucosa and the interior of the sinus will thus increase, so that the mucosa will become engorged. The change in pressure causes rupture of the mucosal vessels and produces a sub-epithelial haematoma, which may be large. These haematomata are demonstrable radiologically (*see Figures 6.8* and *6.9*) and may take up to two months or longer to resolve. The use of serial radiography in such a case can be a useful guide to the progress of treatment – though some of the radiological changes may remain despite treatment.

If there is obstruction of a sinus ostium before ascent, this will result in ischaemia of the mucosa during ascent. The change in the mucosa occurring in sinus barotrauma, and hence the signs and symptoms, will depend on the degree of pressure difference and the rate of change of pressure.

Many factors are responsible for the production of sinus barotrauma, and while each may be a specific cause, it is possible for several to be combined in any one instance. The factors may be listed as:

(1) *Developmental.* Valvular folds of mucous membrane, or pressure by a deviated nasal septum, septal spur, enlarged middle turbinal or ethmoid cells.
(2) *Traumatic.* Obstruction secondary to deformities resulting from old fractures of the nasal and facial bones.
(3) *Allergic.* Swelling of the mucous membrane, or polyposis resulting from nasal allergy or vasomotor rhinitis.
(4) *Infective.* Acute or chronic rhinitis (catarrhal or purulent), or acute or chronic sinusitis.
(5) *Neoplastic.* Obstruction from a simple or malignant tumour is possible, but barotrauma from this cause is rare.

The patho-physiological changes occurring in the affected sinus(es) give a well defined pattern of symptoms and signs. *Pain* is predominant, and it may or may not be localized to the affected sinus; it often originates above and behind the eyes, spreading to the temples and the vertex. It may also involve the face, and spread to the upper teeth. The pain is of sudden onset, and frequently severe, the severity being directly related to the rate of descent. Occasionally the pain may be severe enough to cause fainting, and there are recorded instances of this happening – disaster being averted by another pilot in the same aircraft. Discharge of straw-coloured fluid from the nose is not uncommon, and epistaxis can be heavy. These symptoms may be accompanied by the presence of free blood, or blood clot, in the nose, and tenderness over the affected sinus. In as many as 75 per cent of cases it will be possible to visualize the site and size of the submucosal haematoma by radiological means.

Unfortunately, radiological examination does not always distinguish between abnormalities which contribute to the barotrauma, and those which are the consequence of the unrelieved change in pressure (McGibbon, 1947).

Delayed sinus barotrauma

Delayed sinus barotrauma is relatively rare and occurs sometimes after the flight is completed. It is associated with long flights in which the breathing of high concentrations of oxygen has raised the tension of that gas in the sinuses. Occlusion of the sinus ostium will be followed by absorption of oxygen through the mucosa, with a consequent fall of pressure within that sinus. Frequently generalized headache develops after the onset of sinus pain, but this is variable in incidence and duration.

Management

Immediate treatment is directed to the relief of pain, and the ventilation of the affected sinus. The latter is relatively easily accomplished by the use of nasal decongestants and antihistamines. Auto-inflation is of no value. The ultimate aim of treatment will be to eradicate any causal pathology.

Surgical intervention may be required, but this is generally simple in nature and would include such procedures as submucous resection of the septum, antrostomy, ethmoidectomy, and intranasal enlargement of the fronto-nasal duct.

Pneumocoele

Pneumocoele of the antrum is included for completeness, as this appears to be aggravated by high altitude flying. So far, only two cases have been reported (Noyek and Zizmor, 1974; Zizmor *et al.*, 1975). A structural defect at the ostium causes a valvular effect which permits air to enter the antrum but prevents its escape. The symptoms in one case were aggravated by flight, and included a feeling of pressure in the cheek, worsened by sneezing. Valsalva's manoeuvre produced the appearance of a fluctuant swelling through a dehiscence in the inferolateral wall of the antrum. Radiological examination showed an expanded translucent antrum.

Dental barotrauma

Pain of dental origin in flight is probably commoner than is realized; Ashley (1977) reported that one in five of fighter pilots in the United States Forces suffered from pain of dental origin in flight, and this can be compared with a French Air Force survey in which over 6 per cent of flying personnel had suffered from this condition. Dickson *et al.* (1947) were more conservative in their view of the incidence, giving it as 1.3 per cent in 1000 men decompressed to 10 000 ft (3048 m), which they believed to concur with other collected data on the evidence of dental barotrauma in flight and during decompression.

Orban and Ritchey (1945) reviewed 250 cases in which dental pain occurred during decompression chamber runs. They made the point that it was important to differentiate this condition from maxillary sinus barotrauma. They showed that the syndrome occurred in the following teeth:

(a) Non-vital teeth.
(b) Partially-vital teeth.
(c) Vital teeth with early pulpitis.

In *non-vital teeth* the pulp may become necrotic, possibly following restoration or the use of irritant filling materials. Gas formation occurs in the autolysing pulp, and expansion of the gas on ascent can force infected material into the periapical tissue – so that it is likely that an apical abscess may develop within a day or two of flight.

In *partially-vital teeth* gas bubbles may be found in the pulp cornua under a deep cavity. The source and composition of the gas is not known, but severe pain may be experienced at altitudes up to 5000 ft (1500 m) in such teeth.

Dental pain in flight occurs most commonly in *vital teeth*, and typically will be experienced above 7000 ft (2000 m). Histological examination in such a case will show changes in the pulp, and the degree of pulpitis may have an influence on the severity of the symptoms. It will be seen from the foregoing that dental pain due to barotrauma would be expected to be rare where the cabin pressure is not at or near an equivalent altitude of 6000 ft (1800 m).

The detailed dental care is outside the scope of this work, but the prevention of pulpitis is important. Where possible flying should be stopped for 10–14 days after the completion of treatment for a suspect tooth.

In reaching a diagnosis it should be remembered that pain originating from the dental pulp is poorly localized cortically, so that all teeth on the affected side should be checked for their response to cold stimulation. Finally, pain of this nature is more likely to occur in a restored tooth than in an open cavity.

Pressure (alternobaric) vertigo

So far attention has been given to the traumatic effects of pressure change on the ear and sinuses, but it has long been recognized (Alt *et al.*, 1897) that changes in ambient pressure can also cause a transient disturbance of vestibular function in the absence of overt aural pathology. The occurrence of vertigo during ascent, or descent, was described by Wulfften Palthe (1922) and Armstrong and Heim (1937). However, the condition was not clearly recognized until Melvill Jones (1957) reported that 10 per cent of RAF pilots whom he had interviewed had experienced such symptoms. A later survey by Lundgren and Malm (1966) found an incidence of 17 per cent in flying personnel of the Royal Swedish Air Force. The disability is even more common (23 per cent) amongst divers (Lundgren, 1965) who commonly are exposed to greater and more rapid changes of pressure than aircrew.

Clinical features

The characteristic features of the syndrome, termed 'pressure vertigo' by Melvill Jones (1957) and 'alternobaric vertigo' by Lundgren (1965), is the occurrence of vertigo, of sudden onset, which coincides with the passive equilibrium of middle-ear pressure either during a rapid ascent or on voluntarily producing an overpressure in the middle ear by Valsalva's manoeuvre during descent or when on the ground. Typically, the vertigo is short lived, decaying in 5 s or less, though it can be of such an intensity that the associated nystagmus may prevent the pilot from being able to read aircraft instruments. Less commonly, the vertigo is weaker, there being only an illusory sensation of turning without impairment of vision, and it is more persistent, lasting for up to 1 min or even longer. There is considerable intersubject variability in the plane and direction of the vertigo, though it is usually of a consistent pattern in any one individual. There is no indication, however, from anamnestic reports that the middle-ear pressure change preferentially stimulates a particular group of semicircular canal receptors, as the illusory sensation of turning may be in pitch, yaw, roll, or about an oblique axis.

The case histories reported in the literature (Melvill Jones, 1957; Lundgren and Malm, 1966; Enders and Rodrigez-Lopez, 1970; Brown, 1971) accord with the authors' experience that pressure vertigo is more likely to trouble aircrew when there is difficulty in equilibrating middle-ear pressure, usually from congestion and inflammation of the nasal mucosa due to a common cold or other infection of the upper respiratory tract; such an association was noted in 70 per cent of cases. There are, however, a few individuals who suffer from pressure vertigo even in the absence of infection. Studies by Ingelstedt, Ivarsson and Tjernström (1974) suggest that those susceptible require a higher pressure differential between the middle ear and ambient than the norm to open the eustachian tube and vent gas to ambient. To date, however, passive forcing pressures and other measures of middle-ear mechanics have not been determined on aircrew suffering from pressure vertigo.

Pathophysiology

The mechanisms by which sensory receptors of the vestibular apparatus are stimulated by changes in middle-ear pressure is still a matter for conjecture. The dominant symptom – vertigo – strongly suggests that it is the ampullary receptors of the semicircular canals rather than the maculae that are stimulated. Furthermore, the transient nature of the disturbance accords with the theory proposed by Melvill Jones (1957), that the cupula is deflected when the overpressure in the middle ear is suddenly relieved on passive venting, or when middle-ear pressure is raised transiently above ambient by Valsalva's manoeuvre. Overpressure in the middle ear may not be transmitted equally to the fluid systems of the inner ear by the round and oval windows, for the stapes footplate might be moved against the pressure gradient by the outward displacement of the tympanic membrane. It is conceivable that with the sudden restoration of middle-ear pressure there is a movement of endolymph and perilymph which causes a displacement of the cupula of one or more of the semicircular canals of the ear involved. Unfortunately, little is known about the transient response of the hydrodynamic systems of the inner ear to large amplitude pressure changes, even in normal man, so it is difficult to explain why some individuals show an altered pattern of end-organ activity with such a stimulus and others do not.

The work of Ingelstedt, Ivarsson and Tjernström (1974) and Tjernström (1974)

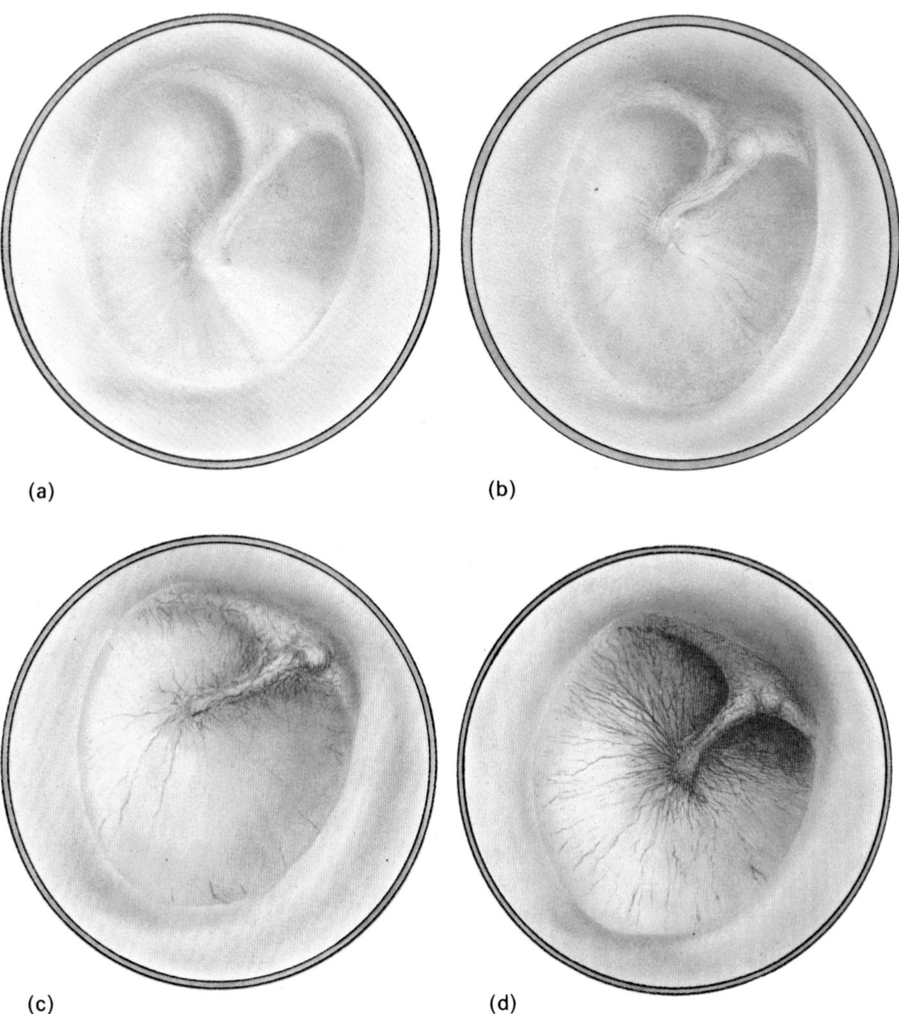

Plate 4 Appearance of the tympanic membrane in otic barotrauma: (a) normal right tympanic membrane; (b) tympanic membrane invaginated, with minimal congestion, during descent from altitude; (c) invagination of the tympanic membrane with congestion along the handle of the malleus; (d) attic congestion resulting from a relatively mild otic barotrauma; *(continued)*

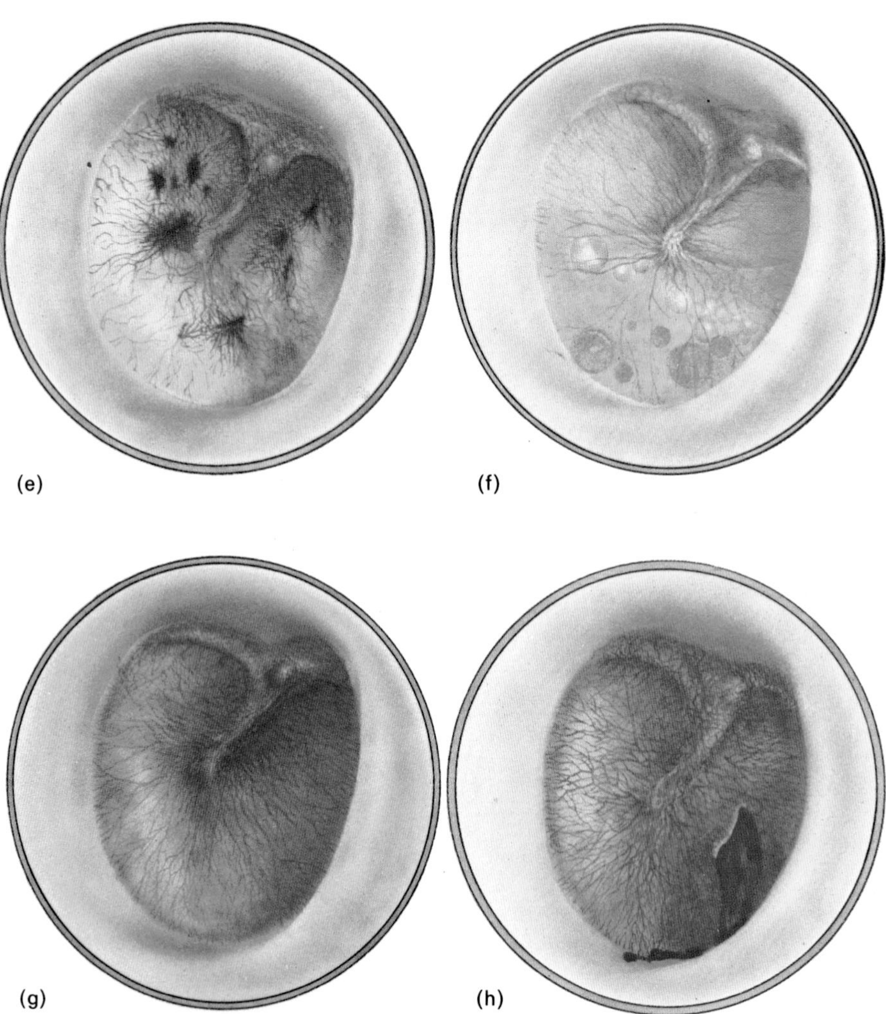

Plate 4 (*continued*) (e) scattered interstitial haemorrhages in tympanic membrane, these are usually residual in nature; (f) unresolved otic barotrauma with amber-coloured effusion in the middle ear. (The bubbles indicate attempts to ventilate the ear via the eustachian tube.); (g) marked congestion, with fresh haemorrhage into the middle ear; (h) rupture of the anterior portion of the tympanic membrane

has shown that 5 out of 79 otologically healthy subjects exposed to simulated ascents with a pressure change of 66 mmHg (8.8 kPa) in 25 s (equivalent to an ascent from ground level at approximately 5000 ft (1500 m)/min) developed vertigo when middle-ear pressure was allowed to equilibrate passively. Indirect measurement of middle-ear volume was used to identify the times of tubal opening. It was found that vertigo and concomitant nystagmus were not induced at the moment of tubal opening but rather that vestibular stimulation occurred when the relative overpressure in one ear was about 44 mmHg (5.9 kPa) or higher. However, not all subjects who had a high opening pressure developed vertigo. The additional requirement for the induction of symptoms was a definite asymmetry of the middle-ear pressures, caused by one ear equilibrating with low tubal opening pressures and the other needing a high opening pressure.

In a further series of experiments Tjernström (1974) demonstrated that vertigo and nystagmus could be induced in susceptible subjects by an overpressure in the middle ear when there was free communication of air between the middle ear and the external canal. He accordingly concluded that movement of the stapes against the pressure gradient, due to outward displacement of the tympanic membrane, was not an essential feature of the mechanism responsible for pressure vertigo, and that the transmission to the labyrinthine fluids of change in middle-ear pressure is more dependent upon the mobility of the membrane of the round window than movement of the stapes footplate. These results led Tjernström (1977) to propose that pressure vertigo might be due to a relative ischaemia of the sensory epithelium. He suggested that the overpressure in the middle ear is effectively transmitted to the fluid system of the inner ear because of the poor patency of the cochlear aqueduct when there is a rapid pressure change. The estimated pressure in capillaries of the inner ear is < 40 mmHg (5 kPa) above ambient, so if the fluids of the inner ear were pressurized to > 40 mmHg above ambient, by an overpressure in the middle ear, then circulatory insufficiency affecting structures within the inner ear is likely to ensue.

Although such a mechanism can not be refuted it must be pointed out that the vestibular reactions induced by the pressure change in the experimental studies of Ingelstedt and Tjernström are weak. The maximum slow-phase velocity of the nystagmus evoked (with eyes closed) was never greater than 5 degrees/s which, if occurring in flight, would be suppressed by fixation and would not cause blurring of vision nor be associated with the intense vertigo that are common features of the syndrome described by aircrew. Vascular insufficiency could well be responsible for the low grade and sometimes sustained vertigo that is reported by a minority of flying personnel with 'pressure vertigo', but in our opinion, it is unlikely to account for the severe yet brief disturbance of vestibular function that is often concomitant with equilibration of middle-ear pressure during ascent or active over-inflation (Valsalva's manoeuvre) during descent.

Management

The established association between the incidence of pressure vertigo and the impairment of middle-ear ventilation by upper respiratory tract infections implies that the most important prophylactic measure is the restriction of flying duties of aircrew when they are suffering from coryza or other conditions where there is congestion of the mucous membrane of the nasopharynx. Unfortunately, in some cases, it is the occurrence of pressure vertigo that first tells the aviator that he is developing a common cold.

On return to flying following an upper respiratory tract infection, susceptible aircrew should be advised to equilibrate middle-ear pressure frequently so as to minimize the development of high pressure differentials. The use of nasal decongestants may also be beneficial.

The repeated occurrence of vertigo associated with changes of middle-ear pressure, like any other form of persistent vertigo in aircrew, merits withdrawal from flying duties and investigation. If evidence of tubal dysfunction is not found the integrity of the round window membrane and the annular ligament of the oval window should be determined by tympanotomy. Tingley and MacDougal (1977) have described two aircrew with symptoms, not dissimilar to those of pressure vertigo, who were found to have a small defect in the round window membrane when this structure was visualized.

Air-sickness

Introduction

Air-sickness is a condition, characterized primarily by nausea, vomiting, pallor and sweating, that occurs when an aviator or passenger is exposed to certain patterns of aircraft motion. The syndrome and the development of the disability is indistinguishable from that induced by the motion of other aids to locomotion such as boats, motor vehicles, camels and elephants, or by fairground amusements like swings and roller coasters. Thus air-sickness, like sea-sickness, car-sickness and swing-sickness is just another form of *motion-sickness* or *kinetosis*. The term motion-sickness is, in some respects, a misnomer, for sickness carries the connotation of disease and obscures the fact that motion-sickness is a quite normal response of an individual, without organic or functional disorder, to motion with which he (or she) is unfamiliar and hence unadapted. Indeed, if the motion is severe and prolonged it is the absence, rather than the presence, of symptoms that is abnormal, for only those individuals without functioning labyrinths are truly immune (James, 1882).

Early in the history of powered flight it was found that sickness was induced by flight through turbulent air, tight turns, loops or other aerobatic manoeuvres, and clear descriptions of the natural history of the condition appeared shortly after the end of the First World War (Anderson, 1919; Head, 1920). However, the problem did not attract the attention of the scientific community until the Second World War when attempts were made to understand the mechanism of the condition and to develop prophylactic drugs. A further impetus to research was manned space-flight, where both Russian cosmonauts and, later, American astronauts reported that exposure to the weightless environment of orbital flight induced symptoms similar to those of the motion-sickness syndrome. There is not yet complete agreement that space-sickness is just another form of motion-sickness. However, the similarity of the signs and symptoms of space-sickness with those of terrestrial motion-sickness, the similarity of the time course of the development and decay of symptoms with continued exposure to the provocative environment, the relief of space-sickness by anti-motion drugs, and the identification of the cause of space-sickness within a general aetiological mechanism of motion-sickness, strongly suggest (and parsimony dictates) that space-sickness is just another form of motion-sickness (Benson, 1977).

Signs and symptoms

The cardinal symptom of motion-sickness is nausea; the cardinal signs are vomiting, pallor and sweating. Other signs and symptoms are frequently though more variably reported. In the early stages, a feeling of bodily warmth, increased salivation, eructation and flatulence are commonly associated with the development of nausea. An alteration of respiratory rhythm, with sighing and yawning, can be an early symptom, while hyperventilation may occur, particularly in those individuals who are anxious about either the cause or the consequences of the disability. Headache is another prodromal symptom, usually frontal in distribution, which may be accompanied by an ill-defined tinnitus, dizziness or 'light headedness'. In those with severe malaise, apathy and depression are not uncommon symptoms. They contribute to degradation of performance and may be of such severity that personal safety and survival are neglected.

Drowsiness is an important yet oft ignored symptom. Typically, feelings of lethargy and somnolence persist for many hours after withdrawal from provocative motion and nausea has abated. Indeed, in certain circumstances a desire to sleep may be the only symptom engendered by an unfamiliar motion stimulus, especially when the intensity of the stimulus is such that adaptation occurs without significant malaise (Graybiel and Knepton, 1976).

Natural history

Typically, the development of the motion-sickness syndrome follows an orderly sequence, the time scale being determined by the intensity of the provocative motion and by the susceptibility of the individual. But just as there are considerable individual differences in susceptibility so are there differences in the order in which particular symptoms and signs develop, or whether they appear at all in a particular individual. The earliest symptom is, commonly, a sensation of epigastric discomfort, best described as 'stomach awareness'. With continued exposure nausea increases in intensity and the cardinal autonomic signs appear, namely pallor and sweating. Vasoconstriction is most obvious in the face, in particular about the mouth. Sudomotor activity is usually confined to those areas of skin where thermal sweating rather than emotive sweating occurs and is accompanied by feelings of warmth. The afflicted individual seeks cool air and so may obtain symptomatic relief, but this is usually short lived. These symptoms commonly develop relatively slowly, but if the provocative motion continues there is rapid deterioration in well-being, the nausea becomes severe and culminates in vomiting or retching. Emesis often brings relief, but this may be short lived if the motion stimulus is severe or the individual is highly susceptible.

In fixed-wing aircraft prolonged exposure to provocative motion is, these days, relatively uncommon; even long distance transport or maritime reconnaissance flights are rarely longer than 10–12 h. The situation is different in space-flight, where the astronaut may be in an abnormal force environment for many days, even months. The clinical picture of the development of space-sickness is essentially the same as that already described, with the important exception that the provocative stimulus is not the motion of the vehicle *per se*, but movement of the astronaut within the vehicle. If the astronaut does not, or cannot, move his head then sickness is unlikely to occur. But if he does move about, and in particular makes rapid head movements, then the signs and symptoms of motion-sickness are likely to develop. Space-sickness has been reported within minutes of the pilot becoming established in orbit (Graybiel, Miller and Homick, 1974, 1975) and characteristically it is most severe during the first day in weightlessness. Symptoms become less as the flight progresses. Most astronauts have been able to make rapid head movements without discomfort after three days, and all but one have been symptom free after six days. Once this initial adaptation has occurred there has been no recurrence during the remainder of the flight (Berry, 1973). The time scale of adaptation to the abnormal force environment of space-flight is thus very similar to that described for sea-sickness (Groen, 1960) and for subjects living in a rotating room (Graybiel *et al.*, 1975) where sickness is also induced by head movement.

On return to earth, astronauts have observed that brisk movements of the head induced sensations of tumbling and vertigo similar to those experienced early in orbital flight. This phenomenon is akin to the *mal de débarquement* that sailors sometimes experience on return to land following a sea voyage in which they have had time to adapt to the motion of the ship. The disturbances occurring on return to a familiar environment after exposure to an atypical one are considered to be a manifestation of the adaptive process (Reason, 1970). This involves a modification of the processing of sensory information within the central nervous system and the establishment of new motor patterns appropriate to the atypical motion environment to which the individual has been exposed. But on return to a normal environment those sensory and motor patterns are no longer appropriate and will cause perceptual and equilibratory disturbances until the individual has readapted.

Space-flight is a good paradigm of adaptation to motion-sickness, but adaptation is a characteristic feature of man's response to prolonged or repeated exposure to provocative motion. In conventional flight it is manifest as a decreased susceptibility to air-sickness as the aviator gains experience. Individuals who adapt rapidly may report a regression of symptoms during a single flight, but more commonly the increase in tolerance to provocative manoeuvres is only achieved over the course of several flights. There is also a small proportion of the population (estimated at 5 per cent) who do not adapt and hence show no decrease in their susceptibility to motion-sickness with repeated exposure (Hemingway, 1946).

Aetiology

An adequate theory of the aetiology of motion-sickness, and hence air-sickness and space-sickness, should not only explain how the disability is produced by certain angular and linear accelerations, but should also account for the phenomenon of adaptation as well as the recurrence of symptoms when man returns to his normal environment after having adapted to an atypical one. Undoubtedly the vestibular apparatus plays a significant role in the genesis of motion-sickness because man, like other susceptible animals, does not get motion-sick unless he has a functional labyrinth (Money, 1970). The idea that motion-sickness is caused by vestibular 'overstimulation' *per se*, is, however, untenable. Quite strong and unfamiliar stimuli, like repeated stops of a rotating chair or the cyclical oscillation experienced on horseback, do not readily induce sickness, whereas much weaker stimuli, such as cross-coupled (Coriolis) accelerations (q.v.), can be highly provocative (Guedry, 1970). Furthermore, the vestibular 'overstimulation' theory does not account for the visually-induced forms of motion sickness (e.g. Simulator or Cinerama-sickness) nor does it attempt to explain adaptation or *mal de débarquement* phenomena.

'Neural mismatch theory'

The basic tenet of this theory is that in all situations where motion-sickness occurs, the information signalled by the eyes, the vestibular apparatus, and perhaps other

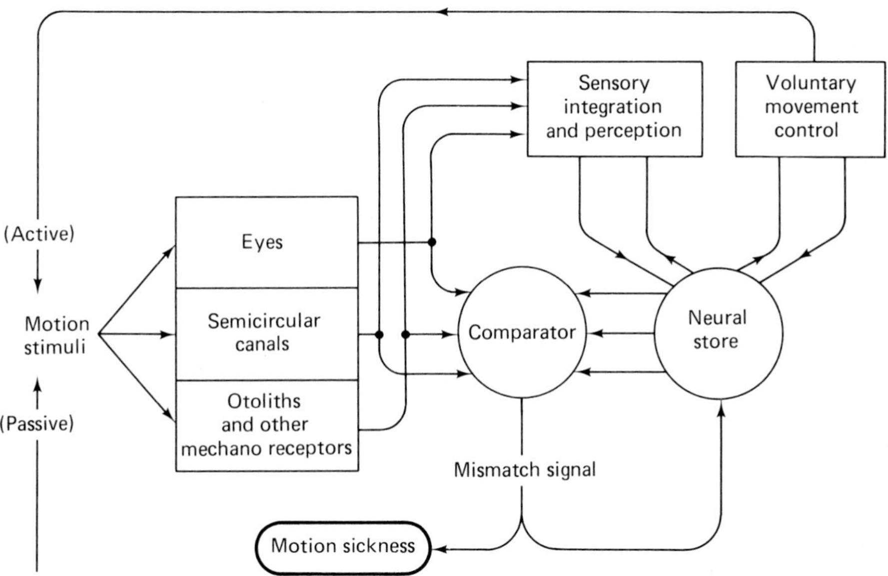

Figure 6.10 'Neural mismatch' model of motion-sickness

mechanoreceptors stimulated by forces acting on the body, is at variance with the inputs that are expected from past experience.

In functional terms the theory, as elaborated by Reason (1970) and by Reason and Brand (1975) proposes that within the central nervous system there is some form of store or memory which is linked to a comparator where signals from the sensory receptors and the neural store are correlated (*Figure 6.10*). If the signals from the receptors stimulated by the motion accord with the stored association, all is well. However, when the input signals do not agree with the expected (i.e. stored) information then, what may be termed an *error* or *mismatch* signal is generated. This mismatch signal has two effects. One is to modify the store so that a new association of cues is elaborated; in other words, the store is *rearranged*. The other effect is to initiate the sequence of neurovegetative and sensory responses which characterize the motion-sickness syndrome. Both of these responses are dependent upon the duration and intensity of the mismatch signal. A sustained, strong mismatch signal is likely to provoke sickness and concurrently a significant rearrangement of the store. Conversely, a weak mismatch signal, provided it is sustained, can allow rearrangement (i.e. adaptation) to occur without engendering disturbing nausea and vomiting, although certain features of the motion-sickness syndrome, in particular drowsiness and lethargy, may appear.

Table 6.1 Identification of type of motion cue mismatch in situations where motion-sickness is provoked

	Type of Motion Cue Mismatch	
	Visual (A)–Vestibular (B)	*Canal (A)–Otolith (B)*
Type 1 A and B simultaneously signal contradictory information	(a) Looking from side or rear window of aircraft (b) Inspection through binoculars of ground or aerial targets from moving aircraft	(a) Cross-coupled (Coriolis) stimulation head movement during rotation about another axis (b) Head movement in abnormal force environment which may be stable (e.g. hyper- or hypo-gravity) or fluctuating (e.g. during linear oscillation)
Type 2(a) A signals without expected B signal	(a) 'Simulator sickness'. Piloting of fixed base simulator with moving external visual display (V.F.A.)	(a) 'Space-sickness'. Head movement in weightless environment (b) Pressure (alternobaric) vertigo
Type 2(b) B signals without expected A signal	(b) Looking inside aircraft when exposed to motion	(a) Low frequency (< 0.5 Hz) linear oscillation (b) Rotation about non-vertical axis

Nature of the provocative stimulus

Two sensory systems are commonly involved in situations where motion-sickness occurs, namely the visual system and the vestibular system. The latter may be further divided into the angular acceleration receptor system of the semicircular canals and the linear acceleration (or force environment) receptor system of the utricular and saccular maculae (i.e. the otolith organs). Other receptors like cutaneous pressure receptors and stretch receptors in muscles and supporting tissues are stimulated by changes in the force environment, but in general they may be considered to act synergistically with the otoliths and need not, here, be considered separately.

Two main types of motion cue mismatch can be identified, according to the sensory systems involved; one is a *visual–vestibular* mismatch, the other a *canal–otolith* (or *intra-vestibular*) mismatch. Examples of the different types of mismatch that occur in aerospace flight and engender air or space-sickness are summarized in *Table 6.1*; characteristic features of each situation are described below.

Visual–vestibular mismatch

Type 1

In this category both the eyes and the vestibular receptors simultaneously signal motion, but of an unrelated or incompatible kind. Sensory cues in the two modalities do not accord with expectation based on prior experience and hence are in conflict. One example is the sickness suffered by an observer in a helicopter or light aircraft who attempts to see a target on the ground with the aid of binoculars. Relative movement of the visual aid and the observer's head generate certain visual motion cues, but these are unlikely to be correlated with vestibular cues that signal, in a modified form, the angular and linear accelerations of the head. Direct observation of the passing landscape from the side or rear windows of a vehicle which is changing direction or speed also causes sickness even when an optical device is not employed to exaggerate visual motion cues.

Type 2

In this category two types of conflict may be identified: (a) when there are visual motion cues without the expected vestibular cues, and conversely, (b) when the vestibular cues are not accompanied by the expected visual cues. The former is more important in relation to theories of motion-sickness than to sickness in the air, for it relates to simulator-sickness or other forms of motion-sickness induced by visual stimuli without there being any physical motion of the subject, and hence no stimulation of vestibular receptors. In fixed base simulators (i.e. those without motion systems) that are provided with a realistic visual display of the outside world, it is the experienced pilot who is more likely to suffer nausea than an individual with little or no experience of the changing force environment of flight (Miller and Goodson, 1960; Guedry, 1970). This difference presumably reflects the greater strength of the association between specific visual and vestibular cues that are established in the experienced aviator, and hence the more severe sensory mismatch when he is confronted by the absence of the expected vestibular motion cues in a fixed base simulator. It is noteworthy that motion-sickness rarely occurs when the simulator is given some motion, even though the physical characteristics of the motion are but a caricature of the real motion of the aircraft.

The type 2b visual vestibular mismatch, in which the vestibular receptors signal motion but the expected visual motion cues are absent, occurs when an individual looks at the visual scene within the moving vehicle. This type of mismatch features in all types of transportation devices where the passenger or operator has no view of the outside world. Motion of the vehicle is transduced by the inertial receptors of the vestibular apparatus but correlated visual information is absent because the visual scene, within the aircraft or ship, moves with the observer.

Intravestibular (semicircular canal–otolith) mismatch

Although the nature of the visual stimuli received by a person aboard a moving vehicle can significantly increase or decrease his liability to develop motion-sickness, it must be recognized that it can develop in many situations where there is no visual input. Indeed, in order to explain the highly provocative nature of certain types of motion it is necessary to identify several categories of intravestibular mismatch where the semicircular canals and otoliths signal conflicting or uncorrelated information.

When the head is moved, either voluntarily or passively, in a vehicle which itself is rotating or subject to an abnormal (i.e. other than 1 g) force environment then cues provided by the canals and otoliths will differ from those that are generated when the same head movement is made in a stable terrestrial (1 g) environment.

As with visual–vestibular conflict two types of intravestibular mismatch may be identified; Type 1 when both the semicircular canals and otoliths signal motion; and Type 2 when one of these receptor systems signal motion in the absence of the expected signal from the other.

Type 1

An angular movement of the head made in a vehicle which itself is turning engenders a cross-coupled (*syn.* Coriolis) stimulus to the semicircular canals, provided the plane of the head movement differs from the plane of rotation of the vehicle. If the head movement is made shortly after the beginning of a turn then the cross-coupled stimulus does not evoke any inappropriate sensation of angular motion (Guedry and Benson, 1978). But if vehicular rotation is sustained (i.e. more than 5 s) or the head movement is made during angular deceleration from a sustained turn, then the vestibular cue will be erroneous; the rotation signalled by the canals will accord neither with that of the imposed rotation nor with that of the head movement. In addition, the signal from the stimulated canals will persist after completion of the head movement, for the deflected cupulae will take 10 s, or more, to return to their neutral position. During the period the canals are generating inappropriate angular motion information, the otoliths provide correct information about the attitude and change of attitude of the head with respect to gravity; there is, therefore, a mismatch between the cues provided by the two groups of receptors. In susceptible individuals just one head movement (e.g. moving the head in roll from one shoulder to the other) can induce nausea and vomiting when rotating at, say, 30 rev/min on a Bárány chair. In flight such high angular rates are rarely achieved, but repeated head movements made in an aircraft which is turning can be highly provocative.

Cross-coupled stimulation is not the only cause of sensory mismatch associated with head movements for, when a head movement is made in an abnormal force environment, the otolithic cues about the change of orientation of the head relative to the force vector differ from those evoked by the same head movement when made in the normogravic (1 g) environment (Schöne, 1964). The semicircular canals, however, are little influenced by linear accelerations so in a wide variety of flight conditions, ranging from the zero gravity of orbital flight to the hypergravity experienced by astronauts during launch and re-entry, the canals correctly signal the angular movement of the head. Accordingly, in an atypical force environment, any head movement which alters the orientation of the head with respect to the force vector produces a mismatch between vertical canal and non-veridical otolith cues. This type of mismatch is not confined to space flight, for in modern high performance aircraft sustained accelerations of several g are produced by large radius turns of low (e.g. 3 degrees/s) angular velocity. Head movements made while executing such a manoeuvre will, of course, involve cross-coupled stimulation of the canals, but of only liminal intensity. Indeed, we would suggest that in most flight situations where head movements cause, or contribute to, motion-sickness, the principal aetiological factor is the atypical nature of otolithic rather than semicircular canal sensory information.

Type 2

As before, two types of mismatch can be identified: (a) when the canals signal rotation in the absence of the expected and correlated signal from the otoliths and (b) when movement is transduced by the otoliths but there is no accompanying signal from the canals.

Space-sickness can fall into category 2a, for in weightlessness slow regular movements of the head will be correctly sensed by the canals but there may be no change in the afferent discharge from the macular receptors. However, when the angular movement is rapid, the transient linear acceleration experienced by the otoliths may be as high as $5\,m/s^2$ so they will be stimulated, albeit in an atypical manner; sensory mismatch is Type 1 rather than Type 2 (Benson, 1977).

Pressure (or alternobaric) vertigo (*q.v.*) is a condition which may occasionally be accompanied by the motion-sickness syndrome. Overpressure in the middle ear stimulates the semicircular canals without apparent involvement of the otoliths. So a situation arises in which the canals erroneously signal rotation while the otoliths signal a stable head position. The mismatch is thus essentially the same as that which occurs when a clinical caloric test is performed and a semicircular canal is selectively stimulated. The patient may feel that he is rotating about a longitudinal (z) body axis, while gravireceptors tell him that he is lying on a couch and that there is no angular motion of his head with respect to gravity. The nausea, and rarely vomiting, that may disturb patients following irrigation in the caloric test is, in essence, another manifestation of an intravestibular mismatch and is not aetiologically different from motion-sickness.

Type 2b mismatch occurs when man is exposed to linear oscillation or sustained rotation about a non-vertical axis. The pilot of an aircraft executing a prolonged roll is continually reorientated with respect to gravity but once a steady rate of roll has been achieved there is no stimulus to the semicircular canals. Thus he receives strong otolithic cues about the continued rotation but no correlated signal from the canals, once the effect of the initial angular acceleration in roll has died away.

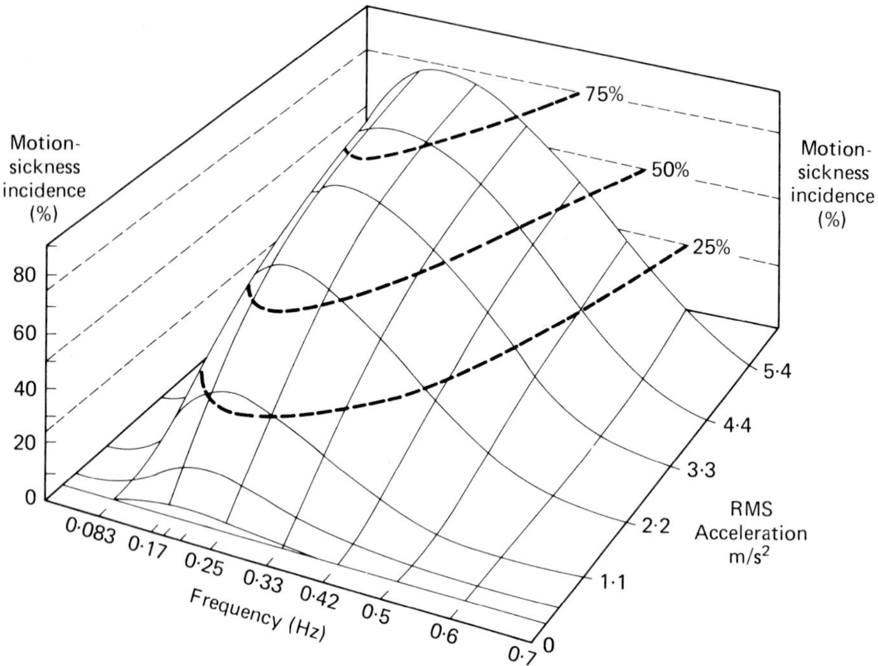

Figure 6.11 Motion-sickness incidence as a function of wave frequency and acceleration for 2 h exposures to vertical sinusoidal motions (from McCauley *et al.*, 1976)

Less potent but considerably more important as a cause of motion-sickness are the linear accelerations that are experienced in an aircraft flying through turbulent air. In such a motion environment there are regular, or irregular, changes in the magnitude and direction of the force vector without significant changes in angular velocity. In a number of experiments, carried out on swings (Fraser and Manning, 1950), vertical oscillators (O'Hanlon and McCauley, 1974; McCauley *et al.*, 1976) and modified lifts (Alexander *et al.**), it has been shown that the incidence of sickness bears an inverse relationship to the frequency of oscillation (*Figure 6.11*). This well-defined relationship between the frequency of the translational motion and sickness rate accords with observations made in flight; aircraft with a high natural frequency of oscillation (0.8–0.9 Hz) produce less sickness than those which respond at a lower frequency (0.4 Hz) to the perturbations produced by turbulent air (Kennedy *et al.*, 1972).

The reason why linear oscillation at 1 Hz does not produce sickness while oscillation at 0.1 Hz is highly provocative can probably be explained by the nature of the expected correlation of canal and otolith organ activity established during normal locomotor activities. The dominant frequencies reaching the head during walking, running, jumping, etc., lie in the range 0.5–10 Hz and it is in this frequency domain that the canals and the otoliths signal angular and linear velocity in a dynamic and not necessarily correlated manner. But at lower frequencies a change in the angular position of the head in the pitch (antero-posterior) and roll (lateral tilt)

* The Wesleyan University studies, carried out by Alexander, Cotzin, Hill, Klee, Ricciuti and Wendt, are conveniently summarized by Baker (1966).

axes will be signalled by the otoliths acting in their 'static', position sensing, rôle, and will normally be accompanied by a commensurate signal from the vertical semicircular canals. Thus, when the gravireceptors are stimulated by a slowly changing force vector there is an expectation that there will be a concomitant signal from the canals. If there is no stimulation of the canals, as during linear oscillation, there is a Type 2b mismatch and motion-sickness is likely to be induced.

Neural centres and pathways involved in motion-sickness

Neural mismatch is a useful concept with which to collate aetiological factors of motion-sickness, but it is now necessary to try and give neurophysiological and neuro-anatomical substance to the theory. Regrettably, the picture is far from complete, though certain elements are reasonably well understood from experimental work on animals (*Figure 6.12*). It is well established that the vestibular apparatus and the vestibular cerebellum (uvula and nodulus) are essential for the development of the motion-sickness syndrome and, by inference, the integrity of the vestibular nuclei is also mandatory. The activity of the vestibular nuclei is influenced not only by the vestibular input but also by visual, somato-sensory and cerebellar afferents (Duensing and Schaefer, 1959; Dichgans and Brandt, 1972; Henn, Young and Finley, 1974; Schaefer, Schott and Meyer, 1975), so the convergence necessary for the comparator to function can be identified at this level. However, it is perhaps more likely that the vestibular cerebellum functions both as comparator and neural store, and that it controls and mediates the process of adaptation.

The nature of the 'mismatch signal' and the means by which it initiates the sensory and autonomic responses of the motion-sickness syndrome are even more speculative. Whether by neural or humoral circuits it acts through the *Chemoreceptive Trigger Zone* and the *Vomiting Centre* of the brain stem to initiate the integrated motor response of vomiting (Wang and Chinn, 1954; Reason and Brand, 1975). Modification of the

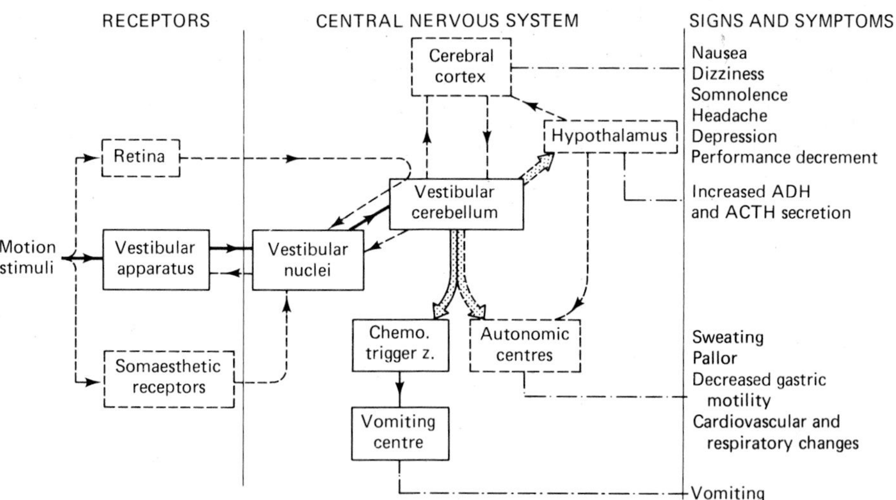

Figure 6.12 Structures involved in motion-sickness

activity of hypothalamic nuclei is reflected by the increased secretion of anterior pituitary hormones (ADH and ACTH) (Money and Wood, 1970) and may be responsible for the changes in vasomotor and sudomotor activity that are important features of the motion-sickness syndrome. But neither hypophysectomy nor partial destruction of the hypothalamus prevents vomiting in dogs exposed to provocative motion stimuli. Indeed, decerebrate dogs can be made motion-sick (Money, 1970).

The relatively slow development of the signs and symptoms of motion-sickness and their persistence after withdrawal of the causal motion is suggestive of the accumulation of some neuro-humoral agent (Pestov, 1967; Graybiel, 1969), though to date this has not been identified. Neither has understanding of the mediating system been enhanced by the study of the neuro-pharmacology of antimotion-sickness drugs (Lukomskaya and Nikol'skay, 1971; Wood, 1970; Wood and Graybiel, 1972; Graybiel *et al.*, 1975) where effectiveness does not appear to be related to the generic group (e.g. antihistamines, parasympatholytics). In general they are central sedatives, though the analeptic amphetamine is a notable exception.

Incidence of air- and space-sickness

Because of the very large inter-subject differences in susceptibility to motion-sickness and variations in the intensity, duration and nature of provocative motion, the incidence of air-sickness ranges from a fraction of 1 per cent of passengers in civil jet transport to 100 per cent in aircrew exposed to severe turbulence. Large jet transport aircraft usually fly at high altitudes in calm air and attempts are made to avoid severe weather systems, so the exposure to turbulence is confined to ascent and descent and few passengers are inconvenienced. Such considerations do not apply in military aviation, where high performance aircraft execute high rate turns and other provocative manoeuvres, while some operational duties require prolonged flight at low altitude, as in maritime reconnaissance. Such flights rarely cause sickness of the pilot, but other crew members, who have no control of the aircraft and often a poor view of external visual references, are more likely to become sick. For example, some 50 per cent of navigators of high performance aircraft suffer from air-sickness at some time during training, though the majority adapt and are rarely afflicted on operational duties. The severe turbulence experienced during 'hurricane penetration' flights caused symptoms in 90 per cent of experienced crew while all the men who had not flown in such conditions before were affected, a third reporting severe symptoms (Kennedy *et al.*, 1972).

Susceptibility to motion-sickness is very much influenced by the level of protective adaptation, gained largely by exposure to the provocative motion, so it is not surprising that air-sickness is seen most frequently during flying training. A survey of routine post-flight reports of RAF flying instructors (Dobie, 1974) revealed that 39 per cent of the student aircrew population were affected by air-sickness, and in 15 per cent of the students the disability was of sufficient severity to lead to disruption or abandonment of the training flight. Typically, air-sickness is most troublesome during initial training flights; thereafter the incidence falls as the student becomes adapted to motion of the aircraft but may rise again when aerobatic or high '*g*' manoeuvres first feature in the training programme (Tucker *et al.*, 1965).

The incidence of space-sickness is no less variable than that of air-sickness. Early

American experience in the small Mercury and Gemini vehicles, where sickness did not apparently occur, contrasted with the reports of early Russian cosmonauts who, like Titov, suffered 'unpleasant sensations resembling sea-sickness' on making head movements when established in orbital flight (Yemel'yanov, 1968). With the advent of the Apollo programme the picture changed and American astronauts began to report symptoms which are now categorized as space-sickness. In the 14 flights of the Apollo series 50 per cent of the astronauts had symptoms of varying severity. Similarly, in the spacious Skylab, five of the nine astronauts suffered from space-sickness, despite attempts to promote protective adaptation before space-flight by aerobatics and zero gravity parabolas in conventional aircraft, and despite the administration of anti-motion-sickness drugs once in orbit.

Factors influencing susceptibility

There are very considerable differences between individuals in their susceptibility to motion-sickness and hence air-sickness. Although the syndrome may be more readily provoked, in a particular individual, by one form of motion than another, there is considerable evidence to show that those who are prone to sickness in one motion environment are also likely to suffer when exposed to other types of provocative motion (Kennedy and Graybiel, 1962; Money, 1972). Space-sickness may, however, be an exception, for the limited data available reveal no apparent correlation between susceptibility to provocative stimuli in a terrestrial environment (including aircraft motion) and the occurrence of space-sickness.

The intensity and character of the motion-stimulus is, of course, the principal determinant of whether an individual develops sickness. Nevertheless, a number of factors concerning the physical and mental constitution of the individual have been identified as influencing susceptibility to motion-sickness.

Age

Motion-sickness is rare in infants below the age of two years, but with maturation susceptibility increases rapidly and is at a peak between the ages of 2 and 12 years. Over the next decade the incidence of sickness falls and this decline in susceptibility continues with increasing age, so that by the age of 50 years motion-sickness is quite rare (Reason and Brand, 1975). The reduction in susceptibility with age has been noted both for sea-sickness (Chinn, 1951) and air-sickness (Lederer and Kidera, 1954).

Sex

Females are more susceptible to motion-sickness than males of the same age (Reason, 1967). The reason for this sex difference, which has long been recognized and which applies to both children and adults, is not understood. It is most likely to be due to hormonal factors, as in women the incidence of motion-sickness reaches a peak during menstruation (Schwab, 1954) and susceptibility is increased during pregnancy.

Psychological factors

Nausea and vomiting are not uncommon symptoms of fear and anxiety, hence it is commonly assumed that anxiety increases susceptibility to motion-sickness. Yet despite the affirmation by a number of authors that motion-sickness is first and foremost a neurotic reaction there is little objective evidence to support this opinion (*see* Reason and Brand (1975) for a review of this topic). It must, however, be acknowledged that positive but weak correlations have been obtained between psychometric measures of neuroticism and susceptibility to motion-sickness. Likewise, it has been shown that introverts (as assessed by the Eysenck Personality Inventory) are more disturbed by a provocative stimulus and adapt more slowly than extraverts. Perceptual style is another dimension of personality which has been found to correlate with susceptibility (Barrett and Thornton, 1968; Kennedy, 1975), but the aetiological significance of this relationship, as with those mentioned above, is a matter for conjecture. Certainly they do not explain the wide inter-subject variation in susceptibility that exists in a group of men, or women, of similar ages and similar exposure to motion. Reason (1970) suggests that these differences are attributable to two other constitutional factors, namely receptivity and adaptability, which relate to the manner in which an individual processes sensory information.

Receptivity refers to the way in which the sensory stimuli are transduced, such that a given stimulus evokes a more powerful subjective experience in a person of high receptivity than in one of low receptivity. Hence, according to Reason's theory, a 'receptive' has a more intense mismatch signal and is therefore more likely to suffer from motion-sickness than the non-receptive when exposed to provocative motion. The term 'adaptability' describes the rate at which an individual adapts to an atypical motion environment, or, in more general terms, the rate of the sensory rearrangement. Those who are slow adaptors take longer to rearrange the neural store and attenuate the mismatch signal than those who are fast adaptors. Hence the slow adaptor is the more likely to suffer from motion-sickness. Although high receptivity and low adaptability both increase susceptibility, this does not mean that slow adaptors are also receptives (or vice versa) for it has been shown that these two factors are essentially unrelated (Reason and Graybiel, 1972).

Although the concepts of receptivity and adaptability can explain the way in which an individual will respond on first exposure to unfamiliar motion, his response on subsequent exposure to the motion will depend upon the extent to which he has been able to retain the adaptation acquired during previous exposures. Anamnestic reports and laboratory experiments have shown that the retention of adaptation (i.e. retentivity) differs widely between individuals and that this attribute is not closely correlated with either receptivity or adaptability (Reason and Brand, 1975).

The factors, receptivity, adaptability and retentivity all influence susceptibility but are not of equal importance when one attempts to assess if air-sickness is likely to be a problem to a particular aviator, or potential member of aircrew. Evidence of high receptivity implies that sickness will occur on initial exposure to unfamiliar motion, but if the individual is a fast adaptor and has good retention of adaptation, it is unlikely that air-sickness will be a persistent problem. On the other hand, a person with low adaptability and poor retention is likely to continue to be afflicted by sickness when exposed to provocative motion. Knowledge of these constitutional factors can thus be an aid in the prediction of motion-sickness susceptibility as well as the likely benefit to a particular individual of desensitization therapy (*see below*).

Laboratory techniques have been developed (Hemingway, 1946; Lansberg, 1960; Powell *et al.*, 1962; Kennedy and Graybiel, 1962; Guedry and Ambler, 1972) which assess a subject's susceptibility to provocative motion and which give some indication of receptivity, adaptability and retentivity. It should be noted, however, that none of the clinical vestibular functional tests differentiate the susceptible from the non-susceptible in a normal population (i.e. where there is no vestibular pathology). Early claims (de Wit, 1953) that high slopes ($^{\pi}/\Delta$ values) and low thresholds in the cupolometric test where indicative of high susceptibility have not been confirmed in longitudinal studies of large populations of student aircrew (Dobie, 1974).

Prevention and treatment

Behavioural measures

The simplest means of preventing air- or space-sickness, or indeed any type of motion-sickness, is to avoid exposure to the provocative motion. If he so wishes, man need not travel in an aircraft, or in any other vehicle, though in the modern world few can accept such a restriction of their mobility.

The role of head movement in the causation of motion-sickness is well established so any procedure which minimizes unnecessary motion of the head within the vehicle is likely to be beneficial. In the weightless environment sickness is prevented, but in conventional aircraft restriction of head movement will only reduce the incidence of sickness. The provision of a head support and good body restraint are of assistance and are further aided by the assumption of a reclined or supine position. Laboratory trials have shown that the incidence of sickness in subjects seated in a normal upright position was four times higher than when they were supine (Manning and Stewart, 1949).

Sickness is likely to be less when the aviator, or passenger, has a good view forward from the aircraft and hence reliable visual cues of motion. For those deprived of an external visual reference, closing the eyes reduces visual/vestibular conflict and allays the development of symptoms.

It is a common observation that mental activity and involvement in a task decreases susceptibility. Pilots rarely suffer from air-sickness except when travelling as passengers. In the laboratory it has been found that subjects exposed to provocative motion developed malaise more rapidly when their task was to introspect and report bodily sensations than when they had to carry out a mental task and were not asked about their symptoms (Guedry, 1970).

The measures described so far can be of immediate value to those who find themselves exposed to provocative motion, but in the long term adaptation is the most powerful prophylactic. It is 'Nature's own cure' and is the preferred method of preventing, or at least reducing susceptibility to, motion-sickness. It is of special importance to aircrew who, in general, should not fly when under the influence of anti-motion-sickness drugs. The basic principle governing the acquisition and maintenance of protective adaptation is that aircrew should be gradually introduced to the provocative motions of the aircraft, and that adaptation, once achieved, should be maintained by regular and repeated exposures. Inter-subject differences in receptivity, adaptability and retentivity do, however, imply that adaptation schedules must be tailored to the individual and preclude definition of the interval between exposures. Some aircrew are troubled by air-sickness if 2–3 days elapse between flights; others with better retentivity can spend several weeks on the ground without any increase in susceptibility.

There are, unfortunately, a small percentage of aircrew or student aircrew who do not develop sufficient adaptation during the course of their normal flying duties and have intractable air-sickness. Studies by Dowd (1972), Dobie (1974) and Cramer, Graybiel and Oosterveld (1976) have shown that the majority of those who fall into this category can be helped by a period of ground-based training involving graded incremental exposure to cross-coupled stimulation. This desensitization therapy, as it has come to be called, requires the subject to move (or be moved) in pitch and roll while rotating on a turntable. Initially the speed of rotation is low (30 degrees/s, 0.5 rad/s) and the number of movements made before symptoms of motion-sickness develop is quite often limited. But on successive days the patient is able to make more head movements or is able to tolerate a higher speed of rotation without loss of well-being, so that after 20, even 30, treatment sessions he can be rotated at 60 degrees/s (1.1 rad/s) and make many head movements without symptoms. Such an incremental adaptation schedule certainly reduces the patient's sensitivity to the specific canal/otolith mismatch produced by the cross-coupled stimulus but, and perhaps of no less importance, it also demonstrates to him that his tolerance has been increased; when he takes to the air again he will have greater confidence in his ability to cope with provocative motion. While the relative importance of vestibular and psychological factors in desensitization therapy is undetermined, it is known that the procedure is effective. A recent review of 57 aircrew treated over a ten-year period showed that 75 per cent had returned to operational flying duties without disability from air-sickness (Rance, 1978).

Drugs

Many studies, both in the laboratory and in the field, have clearly demonstrated that certain drugs can reduce the incidence of motion-sickness in a given population at risk. The number of drugs which have been assayed is large (*see* Brand and Perry, 1966; Wood, 1970; Lukomskaya and Nikol'skay, 1971), but relatively few are effective and none can completely prevent the development of the motion-sickness syndrome in every individual. Symptoms may be prevented or their onset delayed in some subjects, but in situations where the provocative motion is intense and a substantial proportion of subjects (say 80 per cent) vomit when no drug is administered, the exhibition of an anti-motion-sickness drug is likely to reduce incidence by only 10–20 per cent. It should be noted that none of the drugs of proven prophylactic value in motion-sickness are entirely specific; all have side-effects which substantially limit their utility in the aerospace environment. Both the antihistaminics (like promethazine and dimenhydrinate), and the parasympatholytics (like hyoscine) are central depressants and hence should not, in general, be taken by aircrew. There is a place, however, for the administration of anti-motion-sickness drugs to student aircrew, particularly in the early stages of flying training if air-sickness is a problem. But under no circumstances should drugs be taken by a pilot when he flies solo. Such restrictions do not apply to the use of drugs by passengers to alleviate air- (or space-) sickness, though where personnel are required to work at peak efficiency the possible decrement in performance due to sickness must be balanced against that which may be produced by medication.

The choice of prophylactic drug is, in part, dependent upon the duration of exposure to provocative motion and, in part, upon individual differences in tolerance (i.e. incidence of side-effects) and effectiveness (Graybiel *et al.*, 1975).

The response-time curves of effective drugs differ considerably. A single oral dose of 0.3–0.6 mg L-hyoscine hydrobromide acts in $\frac{1}{2}$–1 h and provides protection for about 4 h, whereas promethazine hydrochloride (25 mg) and meclozine hydrochloride (50 mg) take 1–2 h to act and are effective for 12 h or longer. The other useful antihistaminics, dimenhydrinate (50 mg) and cyclizine hydrochloride (50 mg), are absorbed at about the same rate as promethazine but their duration of action is shorter (*c.* 6 h). Thus for short exposure, as in training flights, L-hyoscine is the drug of choice; for longer journeys one of the slower acting drugs should be employed, with repeated dosage if indicated. Repeated administration of hyoscine at 4-hourly intervals is not recommended as certain side-effects of this drug, like dry mouth and impairment of accommodation, are cumulative and more disturbing effects such as hallucinations may develop.

The demonstration that D-amphetamine and ephedrine increased subjects' tolerance to cross-coupled stimulation (Wood, Graybiel and McDonough, 1966; Wood and Graybiel, 1969) led to the use of these drugs in combination with hyoscine and the antihistamines. It was found that there was a useful synergism of prophylactic potency with some reduction of side-effects, in particular drowsiness, except for the combination of these sympathomimetics with dimenhydrinate. A recent report (Graybiel *et al.*, 1975) claims maximal effectiveness for promethazine hydrochloride (25 mg) with ephedrine sulphate (25 mg), though in certain situations the shorter acting combination of L-hyoscine hydrobromide (0.3 mg) with ephedrine sulphate (25 mg) may be preferred.

Acknowledgements

Thanks are due to Professor J. Holmquist of Göteburg for permission to use his illustration from Chapter 17 of *Scientific Foundations of Otolaryngology*, edited by D. F. M. Harrison and R. Hinchcliffe (Heinemann Medical Books), and to Pergamon Press, for permission to use illustrations from *A Textbook of Aviation Physiology*, edited by J. A. Gillies.

References

Alt, F., Heller, R., Mager, W. and Von Schrötter, M. (1897). 'Pathologie der Luftdruckerkrankungen des Gehörorgans', *Mschr. Ohrenheilk*, **31**, 229

Anderson, H. G. (1919). 'Selection of candidates for aviation'. In *The Medical & Surgical Aspects of Aviation*, p. 33. London; Oxford Med. Publ.

Armstrong, H. G. and Heim, J. W. (1937). 'The effect of flight on the middle ear', *Journal of the American Medical Association*, **109**, 417

Aschan, G. (1954). 'Eustachian tube; histological findings under normal conditions and in otosalpingitis', *Acta Otolaryngologica*, **44**, 295

Aschan, G. (1955). 'The anatomy of the eustachian tube with regard to its function', *Acta Soc. Med. Upsal.*, **60**, 131

Ashley, K. F. (1977). 'Aerodontalgia — pain felt in the teeth during flight'. *Medical and Dental Newsletter*, London; Ministry of Defence (RAF), **26**, 15

Baker, C. H. (1966). 'Motion and human performance: review of literature', *Technical Report 770–1*, Goleta, Calif.; Human Factors Research Inc.

Barret, G. V. and Thornton, G. L. (1968). 'Relationships between perceptual style and simulator sickness', *Journal of Applied Physiology*, **52**, 305

Benson, A. J. (1977). 'Possible mechanisms of motion and space sickness'. In *Life-sciences Research in Space*, Report SP-130, 101–108, Paris; European Space Agency

Berry, C. A. (1973). 'Findings on American astronauts bearing on the issue of artificial gravity for future manned space vehicles'. In *Fifth Symposium on the Role of the Vestibular Organs in Space Exploration*, Report SP-314 Washington, D.C.; NASA; 15

Brand, J. J. and Perry, W. L. M. (1966). 'Drugs used in motion sickness', *Pharmacological Reviews*, **18**, 895

Brown, F. M. (1971). 'Vertigo due to increased middle ear pressure: six-year experience of the aeromedical consultation service', *Aerospace Medicine*, **42**, 999

Brown, H. H. S. (1965). 'The pressure cabin'. In *A Textbook of Aviation Physiology*, p. 152 (Ed. by Gillies, J. A.). Oxford; Pergamon Press

Campbell, P. A. (1944). 'Aerosinusitis — its cause, course and treatment', *Annals of Otology, Rhinology and Laryngology*, **53**, 291

Chinn, H. T. (1951). 'Motion sickness in the military service', *Military Surgeon*, **108**, 20

Chunn, S. P. (1960). 'A comparison of the efficiency of the valsalva manoeuvre and the pharyngeal pressure test and the feasibility of teaching both methods', ACAM Thesis, Texas; USAF School of Aerospace Medicine, Brooks AFB

Comroe, J. H. Jr., Dripps, R. D., Dumke, R. R. and Deming, M. (1945). 'Oxygen toxicity; effect of inhalation of high concentrations of oxygen for 24 hours on normal men at sea level and at simulated altitude of 18,000 feet', *Journal of the American Medical Association*, **128**, 710

Cramer, D. B., Graybiel, A. and Oosterveld, W. J. (1976). 'Successful transfer of adaptation acquired in a slow rotation room to motion environments in Navy flight training'. In *Recent Advances in Space Medicine*, Conf. Proc. 203, Neuilley sur Seine; AGARD, NATO

Dichgans, J. and Brandt, Th. (1972). 'Visual vestibular interactions and motor perception'. In *Cerebral Control of Eye Movements and Motion Perception, Bibl. Ophthal.*, **82**, 327

Dickson, E. D. D., McGibbon, J. E. G. and Campbell, A. C. P. (1947). 'Acute otitic barotrauma — clinical findings, mechanism and relationship to the pathological changes produced experimentally in the middle ears of cats by variations of pressure'. In *Contributions to Aviation Otolaryngology* p. 60 (Ed. by Dickson, E. D. D.). London; Headley Bros

Dickson, E. D. D., McGibbon, J. E. G., Harvey, W. and Turner, W. (1947). 'An investigation into the incidence of acute otitic barotrauma as a disability amongst 1000 aircrew cadets during a decompression test'. In *Contributions to Aviation Otolaryngology*, p. 104 (Ed. by Dickson, E. D. D.). London; Headley Bros

Dickson, E. D. D. and King, P. F. (1954). 'The incidence of barotrauma in present day service flying'. Flying Personnel Research Committee Report No 881, London; Air Ministry

Dobie, T. G. (1974). 'Air-sickness in aircrew', *Report – AG 177*. Neuilly-sur-Seine; AGARD, NATO

Dowd, P. J. (1972). 'The USAFSAM selection, test and rehabilitation program of motion-sick pilots'. In *Predictability of Motion Sickness in the Selection of Pilots*, Conf. Proc. 109. Neuilly sur Seine; AGARD, NATO

Duensing, P. and Schaefer, K. P. (1959). 'Uber die convergenz vershiedener labyrinthärer Afferenzen auf einzelne Neurone des Vestibulariskerngebietes', *Archiv für Psychiatrie, und Zeitschrift f.d. ges. Neurologie*, **199**, 345

Duvoisin, R. C., Kruse, F. and Saunders, D. (1962). 'Convulsive syncope induced by valsalva manoeuvre in subjects exhibiting low G tolerance', *Aerospace Medicine*, **33**, 92

Elner, A., Ingelstedt, S. and Ivarsson, A. (1971). 'The normal function of the eustachian tube. A study of 102 cases', *Acta Otolaryngologica*, **72**, 320

Enders, L. J. and Rodrigez-Lopez, E. (1970). 'Aeromedical consultation service case report: alternobaric vertigo', *Aerospace Medicine*, **41**, 200

Fraser, A. M. and Manning, G. W. (1950). 'Effect of variation of swing radius and arc on incidence of swing sickness', *Journal of Applied Physiology*, **2**, 580

Frenzel, H. (1938). 'Nasen-Rachendruckversuch zur Sprengung des Tubenverschlusses', *Luftfahrtmed.* Abh., **2**, 203

Frenzel, H. (1950). 'Otorhinolaryngology in German Aviation Medicine World War II'. *Washington: Government Printing Office*, **2**, 977

Goodhill, V. (1971). 'Sudden deafness and round window rupture', *Laryngoscope*, **81**, 1462

Graybiel, A. (1969). 'Structural elements in the concept of motion sickness', *Aerospace Medicine*, **40**, 351

Graybiel, A. and Knepton, J. (1976). 'Sopite syndrome; a sometimes sole manifestation of motion sickness', *Aviation, Space and*

Environmental Medicine, **47,** 873

Graybiel, A., Kennedy, R. S., Knoblock, E. C. *et al.* (1965). 'The effects of exposure to a rotating environment (10 rpm) on four aviators for a period of twelve days', Report No. 923. Pensacola, Fla.; U.S. Naval School of Aviation Medicine and National Areonautics and Space Administration

Graybiel, A., Miller, E. F. and Homick, J. L. (1974). 'Experiment M-131. Human vestibular function. 1. Susceptibility to motion sickness'. *Proceedings of Skylab Life Sciences Symposium*, Report TMX-58154, Houston. Texas; NASA; **1,** 169

Graybiel, A., Miller, E. F. and Homick, J. L. (1975). 'Individual, differences in susceptibility to motion sickness among six Skylab astronauts', *Acta Astronautica*, **2,** 155

Graybiel, A., Wood, C. D., Knepton, J., Hoche, J. P. and Perkins, G. F. (1975). 'Human assay of antimotion sickness drugs', *Aviation Space and Environmental Medicine*, **46,** 1107

Groen, J. J. (1960). 'Problems of the semicircular canal from a mechanico-physiological point of view', *Acta Otolaryngologica*, Supp. 163, 59

Guedry, F. E. (1970). 'Conflicting sensory orientation cues as a factor in motion sickness'. In *Fourth Symposium on the Role of the Vestibular Organs in Space Exploration*. Report SP-187, p.45, Washington, D.C.; NASA

Guedry, F. E. and Ambler, R. K. (1972). 'Assessment of reactions to vestibular disorientation stress for the purposes of aircrew selection'. In *Predictability of Motion Sickness in the Selection of Pilots*, Conf. Proc. 109, Neuilly sur Seine, AGARD, NATO; B5, 1

Guedry, F. E. and Benson, A. J. (1976). 'Coriolis cross-coupling effects: disorienting and nauseogenic or not?' *Aviation Space and Environmental Medicine*, **49,** 29

Hartmann, A. (1879). *Experimentelle Studien uber die Funtion der Eustachishen Rohre*, Leipzig

Harvey, W. (1944). 'Some aspects of dentistry in relation to aviation', *Proceedings of the Royal Society of Medicine*, **37,** 465

Head, H. (1920). 'The sense of stability and balance in the air', *Medical Research Council Special Report No 53*, 215, London; HMSO

Hemingway, A. (1946). 'Selection of men for aeronautical training based on susceptibility to motion sickness', *Journal of Aviation Medicine*, **17,** 153

Henn, V. S., Young, L. R. and Finley, C. (1974). 'Vestibular nucleus units in alert monkeys are also influenced by moving visual fields', *Brain Research*, **71,** 144

Hinchcliffe, R. (1972). 'Disorders of vestibular function'. In *Modern Trends in Diseases of the Ear, Nose and Throat*, Vol. 2, p. 47 (Ed. by Ellis, M.). London; Butterworths

Holmquist, J. (1976). 'Auditory tubal function'. In *Scientific Foundations of Otolaryngology*, p.254 (Ed. by Hinchcliffe, R. and Harrison, D. F. N.) London; Heinemann

Hughson, W. and Crowe, S. J. (1933). 'Experimental investigations of physiology of the ear', *Acta Otolaryngologica*, **18,** 291

Ingelstedt, S., Ivarsson, A. and Jonson, B. (1967). 'Mechanics of the human middle ear. Pressure regulation in aviation and diving. A non-traumatic method', *Acta Otolaryngologica*, Suppl., **228,** 1

Ingelstedt, S., Ivarsson, A. and Tjernström, O. (1974). 'Vertigo due to relative overpressure in the middle ear', *Acta Otolaryngologica*, **78,** 1

James, W. (1882). 'The sense of dizziness in deaf-mutes', *American Journal of Otology*, **4,** 239

Jones, G. M. (1958). 'Pressure changes in the middle ear after flight', Flying Personnel Research Committee Report No. 1059, London; Air Ministry

Jones, G. M. (1959). 'Pressure changes in the middle ear after simulated flights in a decompression chamber', *Journal of Physiology*, **147,** 43P

Kennedy, S. (1975). 'Motion sickness questionnaire and field independence scores as predictors of success in naval aviation training', *Aviation, Space and Environmental Medicine*, **46,** 1349–1352

Kennedy, R. S. and Graybiel, A. (1962). 'Validity of tests of canal sickness in predicting susceptibility to air-sickness and sea-sickness', *Aerospace Medicine*, **33,** 935

Kennedy, R. S., Moroney, W. F., Bale, R. M., Gregoire, H. G. and Smith, D. G. (1972). 'Motion sickness symptomatology and preference decrements occasioned by hurricane penetrations in C-121, C-130 and P-3 Navy aircraft', *Aerospace Medicine*, **43,** 1235

King, P. F. (1965). 'Sinus barotrauma'. In *A Textbook of Aviation Physiology*, p. 112 (Ed. by Gillies, J. A.). Oxford; Pergamon Press

King, P. F. (1966). 'Otitic barotrauma', *Proceedings of the Royal Society of Medicine*, **59,** 543

King, P. F. (1976). 'Aural problems in the armed services: otitic barotrauma and related conditions', *Proceedings of the Royal Society of Medicine*, **68,** 817

Lansberg, M. P. (1960). *A Primer of Space Medicine*. Amsterdam; Elsevier

Lederer, L. G. and Kidera, G. G. (1954). 'Passenger comfort in commercial air travel with reference to motion sickness', *International Medicine*, **167,** 661

Lukomskaya, N. Ya and Nikol'skay, M. I. (1971). In *Search for Drugs against Motion Sickness* (Ed. by Mikhel'son, M. Ya), Leningrad: Sechenov Inst. Evolutionary Physiol. & Biochem. (English Translation, published by Defence & Civil Institute of Environmental Medicine; Downsview, Ont. Canada. 1974)

Lundgren, C. E. G. (1965). 'Alternobaric vertigo — a diving hazard', *British Medical Journal*, **ii,** 511

Lundgren. C. E. G. and Malm, L. U. (1966).

'Alternobaric vertigo among pilots', *Aerospace Medicine*, **66,** 178

Macbeth, R. (1960). 'Some thoughts on the Eustachian tube', *Proceedings of the Royal Society of Medicine*, **53,** 151

McCauley, M. E., Royal, J. W., Wylie, C. D., O'Hanlon, J. F. and Mackie, R. R. (1976). 'Motion sickness incidence: exploratory studies of habituation, pitch and roll, and the refinement of a mathematical model', *Technical Report 1733–2*, Goleta, Calif.; Human Factors Research Inc.

McGibbon, J. E. G. (1942). 'Aviation pressure deafness', *Journal of Laryngology*, **57,** 14

McGibbon, J. E. G. (1947). 'Nasal sinus pain caused by flying'. In *Contributions to Aviation Otolaryngology*, p. 134 (Ed. by Dickson, E. D. D.). London; Headley Bros

McMyn, J. R. (1940). 'Anatomy of salpingo-pharyngeus muscle', *Journal of Laryngology*, **55,** 1

Manning, G. W. and Stewart, W. G. (1949). 'Effect of body position on incidence of motion sickness', *Journal of Applied Physiology*, **1,** 619

Melvill Jones, G. (1957). 'A study of current problems associated with disorientation in man-controlled flight', *Flying Personnel Research Committee Report No 1006*. London; Air Ministry

Miller, G. F. Jr. (1965). 'Eustachian tubal function in normal and diseased ears', *Archives of Otolaryngology, Chicago*, **81,** 41

Miller, J. W. and Goodson, J. E. (1960). 'Motion sickness in a helicopter simulator'. *Aerospace Medicine*, **31,** 204

Money, K. E. (1970). 'Motion sickness', *Physiological Reviews*, **50,** 1

Money, K. E. and Wood, J. D. (1970). 'Neural mechanisms underlying the symptomatology of motion sickness'. In *Fourth Symposium on the Role of the Vestibular Organs in Space Exploration*, Report SP-187. Washington, D.C.; NASA, 35

Money, K. E. (1972). 'Measurement of susceptibility to motion sickness'. In *Predictability of Motion Sickness in the Selection of Pilots*, Conference Proc. No. 109, Neuilly sur Seine; AGARD, NATO, B2, 1

Morrison, R. (1972). 'Radiotherapy of the larynx and laryngo-pharynx'. In *Modern Trends in Diseases of the Ear, Nose and Throat*, Vol. 2, p. 324 (Ed. by Ellis, M.). London; Butterworths

Noyek, A. M. and Zizmor, J. (1974). 'Pneumocele of the maxillary sinus', *Archives of Otolaryngology, Chicago*. **100,** 155

O'Hanlon, J. F. and McCauley, M. E. (1974). 'Motion sickness incidence as a function of the frequency of vertical sinusoidal motion', *Aerospace Medicine*, **45,** 366

Orban, B. and Ritchey, B. T. (1945). 'Toothache under conditions simulating high altitude flight', *Journal of the American Dental Association*, **32,** 145

Perlman, H. B. (1951). 'Observations on Eustachian tube', *Archives of Otolaryngology, Chicago*, **53,** 370

Perlman, H. B. (1967). 'Normal tubal function', *Archives of Otolaryngology, Chicago*, **86,** 632

Pestov, I. D. (1967). 'Cumulation of stimuli in motion sickness'. In *Problems of Space Biology* (Ed. by Sisakyan, N. M.). Moscow; Nauka Press, **6,** 191 (Translation. TT.F-528 Washington, D.C.; NASA, 1969)

Powell, T. J., Beach, A. M., Smiley, J. R. and Russell, N. C. (1962). 'Successful prediction of air-sickness in aircrew trainees', *Aerospace Medicine*, **33,** 1069–1076

Proctor, B. (1973). 'Anatomy of the eustachian tube', *Archives of Otolaryngology, Chicago*, **97,** 2

Rance, B. H. (1978). 'The assessment and treatment of air-sickness in the Royal Air Force', *Proceedings of the Royal Society of Medicine* (to be published)

Rayman, R. B. (1972). 'Stapedectomy: a threat to flying safety?' *Aerospace Medicine*, **43,** 545

Reason, J. T. (1967). 'An investigation of some factors contributing to individual variation in motion sickness susceptibility', *Flying Personnel Research Committee Report No 1277*. London; Ministry of Defence (Air)

Reason, J. T. (1968). 'Relations between motion sickness susceptibility, the spiral after-effect and loudness estimation', *British Journal of Psychology*, **59,** 385

Reason, J. T. (1970). 'Motion sickness: a special case of sensory rearrangement', *Advances in Science*, **26,** 386

Reason, J. T. and Graybiel, A. (1972). 'Factors contributing to motion sickness susceptibility: adaptability and receptivity'. In *Predictability of Motion Sickness in the Selection of Pilots*. Conf. Proc. 109, Neuilly sur Seine; AGARD, NATO, B4, 1

Reason, J. T. and Brand, J. J. (1975). *Motion Sickness*. London; Academic Press

Rich, A. R. (1920). 'A physiological study of the eustachian tube and its related muscles', *Bulletin of the Johns Hopkins Hospital*, **31,** 206

Rundcrantz, H. (1969). 'Posture and eustachian tube function', *Acta. Otolaryngologica*, **68,** 279

Schaefer, K-P., Schott, D. and Meyer, D. L. (1975). 'On the organisation of neuronal circuits involved in the generation of the orientation response (Visual Graspreflex)', *Fortschritte Zool.*, **23,** 199

Schöne, H. (1964). 'On the role of gravity in human spatial orientation', *Aerospace Medicine*, **35,** 764

Schwab, R. S. (1954). 'The non labyrinthine causes of motion sickness', *International Record of Medicine*, **167,** 631

Scott, S. (1919). 'The ear in relation to certain disabilities in flying'. In *Reports of the Air Medical Investigation Committee No 8 & 9*, p. 29, Special Report Series No. 37. London; Medical Research Council

Stevenson, R. Scott and Guthrie, D. (1949). *A History of Otolaryngology*. Edinburgh; E and S Livingstone

Thomson, K. A. (1958). 'Investigation on Toynbee's experiment in normal individuals', *Acta Otolaryngologica, Stockholm*, **140,** 263

Tingley, D. R. and MacDougal, J. A. (1977). 'Round window tear in aviators', *Aviation Space and Environmental Medicine*, **48,** 971

Tjernström, Ö. (1974). 'Middle ear mechanics and alternobaric vertigo', *Acta Otolaryngologica*, **78,** 376

Tjernström, Ö. (1977). 'Effects of middle ear pressure on the middle ear', *Acta Otolaryngologica*, **83,** 11

Tucker, G. J., Hand, D. J., Godbey, A. L. and Reinhardt, R. F. (1965). 'Air-sickness in student aviators', *Report NSAM*-939, Pensacola, Fla. ; US Naval School of Aviation Medicine

Van Wulfften Palthe, P. M. (1922). 'Function of the deeper sensibility and of the vestibular organs in flying', *Acta Otolaryngologica*, **4,** 415

Wang, S. C. and Chinn, H. I. (1954). 'Experimental motion sickness in dogs. Functional importance of chemoceptive trigger zone', *American Journal of Physiology*, **178,** 111

De Wit, G. (1953). 'Sea-sickness (motion sickness). A labyrinthological study', *Acta Otolaryngologica*, Suppl. 108

Wood, C. D. (1970) 'Anti-motion sickness therapy. In *5th Symposium on the Role of the Vestibular Organs in Space Exploration*, Report SP-314; Washington, D.C.; NASA, 109

Wood, C. D., Graybiel, A. and McDonough, R. C. (1966). 'Human centrifuge studies on the relative effectiveness of some antimotion sickness drugs', *Aerospace Medicine*, **37,** 187

Wood, C. D. and Graybiel, A. (1969). 'Evaluation of sixteen antimotion sickness drugs under controlled laboratory conditions', *Aerospace Medicine*, **39,** 1341

Wood, C. D. and Graybiel, A. (1972). 'Theory of antimotion sickness drug mechanisms', *Aerospace Medicine*, **43,** 249

Yemel'yanov, M. D. (1968). 'Some real problems of investigating the analyser function of astronauts in flight'. In *Physiology of the Vestibular Analyser* (Ed. Parin, V. V. and Yemel'yanov, M. D.). Moscow; Nauka Press. (Translation TTF-616. Washington, D.C.; NASA, 1970)

Zizmor, J., Bryce, M., Schaffer, S. L. and Noyek, A. M. (1975). 'Pneumocoele of the maxillary sinus', *Archives of Otolaryngology, Chicago*, **101,** 387

7 Physiological considerations of pressure effects on the ear and sinuses in deep water diving

P W Head

Introduction and general considerations

During the past two decades there has been an increasing awareness amongst medical authorities of the potentially damaging effects of diving on both the cochlea and vestibular apparatus. The simpler problems of sinus and otitic barotrauma have been long appreciated, but it is only in recent times that the full scope of the medical conditions that may be caused by exposure to a hyperbaric environment have become apparent (*Figure 7.1*). These conditions are not dissimilar from those encountered by aviators, but are more frequent due to the rapid changes in environmental pressure, the length of time under pressure, the respiratory gas

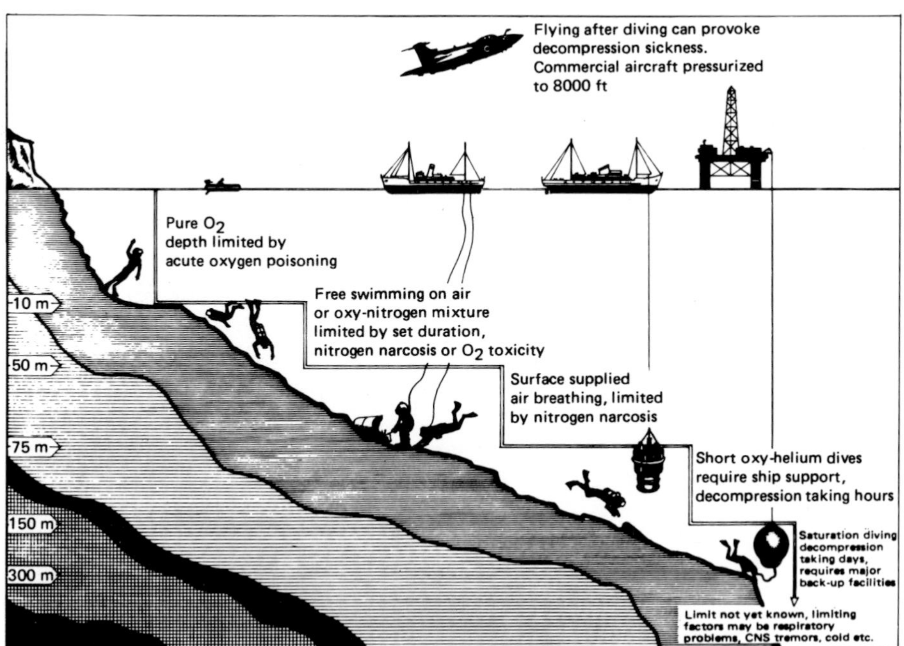

Figure 7.1 Some limiting factors in diving

mixture employed and the need for lengthy decompression. It has been difficult to evaluate the physiopathological problems (*Figure 7.2*) involving the ear and sinuses owing to the scattered nature of diving activities and their remoteness from skilled otological observers. Many of the symptoms and signs are transient and full subjective recovery may have taken place by the time a diver reaches the surface. It will be appreciated that from a deep saturation dive to 300 m it may be 9½ days before the diver is fully decompressed and in a situation where a complete otoneurological workout is feasible.

A limited knowledge of the physics involved in diving is essential to the clear understanding of how the middle ear, inner ear and sinuses may be involved in a

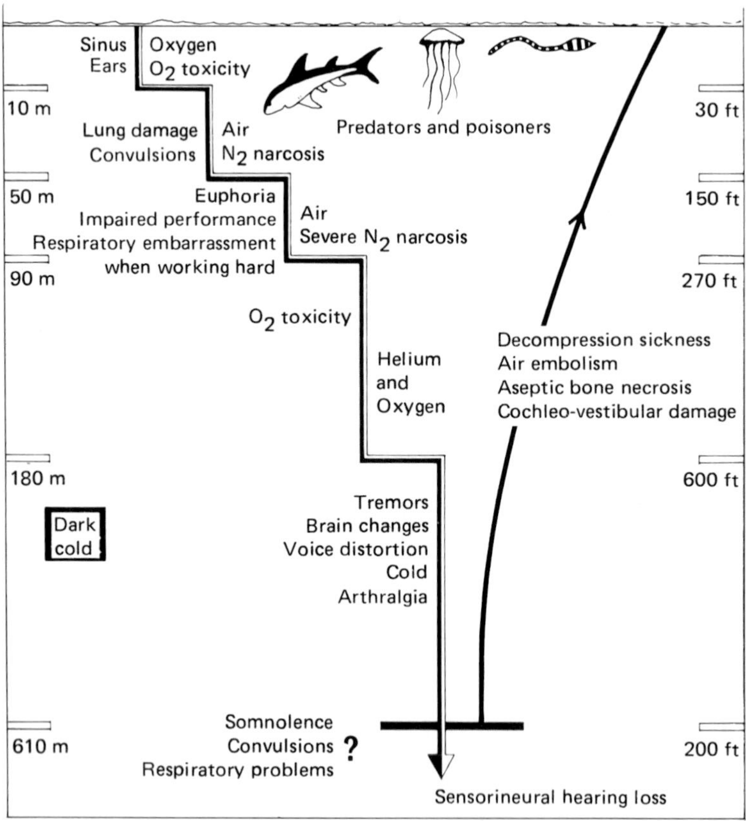

Figure 7.2 General physio-pathological effects which may result from diving

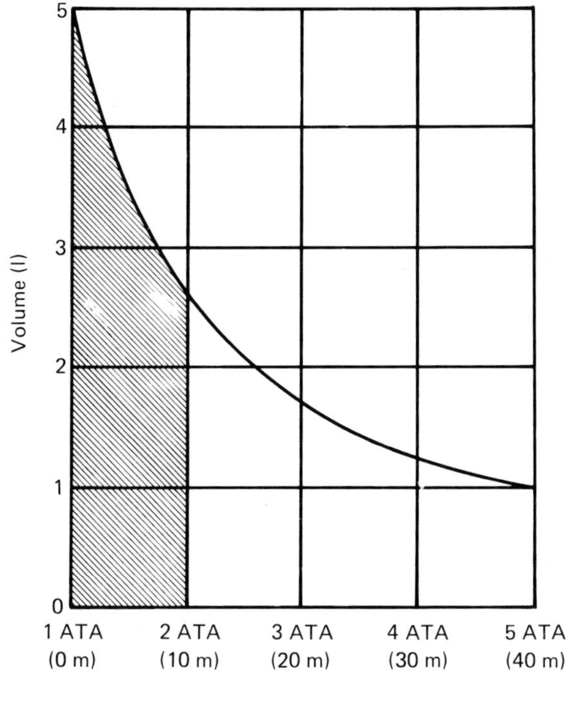

Figure 7.3 Pressure–volume graph showing that the maximum change occurs during the first 10 m of a dive

pathological process which itself may be temporary or permanent. At water surface the ambient atmospheric pressure is 14.7 pounds per square inch (psi); this is termed a pressure of 1 atmosphere. As one descends from the water surface this pressure increases in a rapid linear fashion due to the density of water. At 33 ft (10 m) the pressure is double that at the surface, i.e. 2 atmospheres. Contrast this with the aviator who has to ascend to 18 000 ft to experience a similar change in pressure, that is to 0.5 atmosphere. Every 33 ft (10 m) of descent underwater adds 1 atmosphere of pressure. According to Boyle's Law, assuming the temperature remains constant, the greater the pressure the smaller the volume of gas. A container of air which is open at the bottom will contain half as much at 33 ft (10 m) as it does at the surface (1 atmosphere pressure increased to 2 atmospheres). At 66 ft there is an increase to 3 atmospheres of pressure and therefore the volume of air in the container is reduced to one third of that at the surface (*Figure 7.3*).

The application of Boyle's Law to diving relates to all the air-containing spaces in the body. Through the open airway of the nose and mouth pressure changes are transmitted to the lung alveoli as well as to the paranasal sinuses and middle-ear cleft. Under normal circumstances equivalent pressure changes will occur in the external auditory meatus. The air-containing external auditory meatus, middle ear and paranasal sinuses require special consideration as they are inflexible bony cavities with openings which may not be patent and permit the easy equalization of pressure changes. The ambient pressure of the surrounding water is applied to the whole body, including the blood vessels.

Dalton's Law relating to partial pressures states that in a mixture of gases each gas exerts its own pressure independently of all other contained gases, and that the total pressure of the gas mixture is the sum of the partial pressures of all the constituent gases. The solubility of the various gases is proportional to their partial pressures. Oxygen constitutes approximately 21 per cent of air, but is the only part of the inspired air which is of use to the body. Nitrogen comprises some 70 per cent and is inert; however, at depth nitrogen dissolves in body tissues, especially fat. During decompression it may be released from these tissues faster than it can be carried by the blood to the lungs and dispersed. Bubbles of nitrogen may form in blood vessels and/or tissues leading to the condition known as 'bends'. Such bubbles may well occur in the inner ear resulting in cochlear or vestibular lesions. To reduce the likelihood of bends as well as nitrogen narcosis an oxyhelium gas mixture is commonly employed for deep and 'saturation' dives.

With the foregoing in mind it is convenient to describe the possible ENT pathology which may be associated with diving. Although it is more likely that such conditions will occur after prolonged, or deep dives, they have been found after a relatively shallow dive and short periods of exposure to the hyperbaric environment. In an initial evaluation of the aural problems caused by inadequate pressure equalization (barotrauma) it must be decided:

(1) Whether permanent or progressive hearing losses are present with greater frequency in divers than the general population.
(2) Whether these losses, conductive or sensorineural, are attributable to earlier obvious barotrauma.
(3) Whether other aetiopathological mechanisms related to underwater activity should be involved.

It may be that cochleo-vestibular problems could be initiated by:

(a) an increased endolymphatic fluid volume caused by osmotic pressure gradients related to dissolved inert gases; or dependent on insufficient decompression-time with bubble formation in the endolymphatic system;
(b) intravascular bubble formation or gas embolization in the inner-ear vessels;
(c) extravascular bubble formation in the inner-ear tissues.

A suitable classification for the study of ORL Diving Pathology is as follows:

(1) Barotrauma of descent (compression phase)	(a) Paranasal sinuses (b) Dental (c) External ear (d) Middle ear (e) Inner ear
(2) Lesions occurring at depth (steady hyperbaric state)	(f) Inner ear
(3) Barotrauma of ascent (decompression phase)	(g) Middle ear (h) Inner ear (cochlea and/or vestibule)
(4) Vascular	(i) Alteration in vessel walls and blood chemistry

(5) Acoustic hazard
(6) Miscellaneous

(j) Noise-induced hearing loss
(k) Apparently ORL symptoms not necessarily associated with abnormal vestibular or cochlear pathology

Paranasal sinuses

In diving or flying the paranasal sinuses may be subject to barotrauma similar to (but less commonly than) that experienced in the middle-ear cleft. Under normal circumstances the sinuses (and middle-ear cleft) contain air at the same pressure as that in the nose and nasopharynx. The sinus and nasal mucosae are contiguous through small ostia. These ostia vary in size and the smaller they are the more likelihood there is of obstruction by adjacent pathological changes in the mucosa. Adequate ventilation and pressure equalization within the sinuses is dependent to a large degree on nasal function. The situation is comparable with the middle-ear ventilation problem although there is no voluntary control over the diameter of the sinus ostia and therefore equalization of pressure may be difficult or impossible under certain circumstances. However, the Valsalva manoeuvre performed to inflate the middle-ear cleft will usually equalize the intra sinus and nasal pressures. Only the frontal and maxillary sinuses are involved in barotrauma. In the case of the frontal sinus there is the fronto-nasal duct, which could be compared with the eustachian tube, and in 80 per cent of subjects this duct opens into the anterior ethmoid cells presenting a rather long tortuous course subject to obstruction by mucosal oedema, polypi, new growth or infected secretions.

Figure 7.4 shows how on descent underwater (compression phase) antral barotrauma can be caused. With increasing environmental pressures congested mucous membrane, polypi, or new growths may be forced into the sinus ostium and at the same time the volume of air in the sinus decreases. With unrelieved obstruction and continuing descent this decrease in the volume of air in the sinus will exert a suction effect on the mucosa and enhance the blockage at the ostium. Similarly in the decompression phase (ascent to the surface) the reverse may occur and the sinus ostium may be blocked by polyploid sinus membrane or infected secretion. Unlike middle-ear barotrauma sinus barotrauma may equally occur during compression or decompression. Although some of the causes of sinus barotrauma have been mentioned, for the sake of completeness it should be pointed out that mechanical obstruction due to (1) old nasal injuries and (2) deviated nasal septum, is not infrequently a precipitating factor. In the trained diver, by far the commonest cause is exposure to pressure change during a coryzal state with or without sinus infection.

Mucosal swelling caused by vasomotor rhinitis or seasonal allergy may also lead to ostial obstruction and sequential barotrauma. Much depends on the size of the ostium or the tortuosity of the fronto-nasal duct – factors which may vary from person to person.

The pathological changes caused by sinus barotrauma can be described progressively. Assuming a blockage of the sinus ostium without variation in ambient pressure, there is some absorption of oxygen from the air within the sinus by the mucous membrane leading to the formation of a relative vacuum. The sinus lining

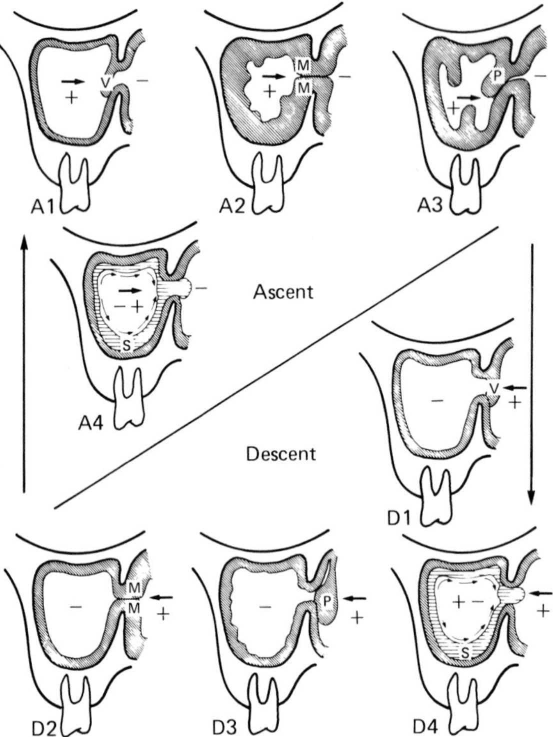

Figure 7.4 Some causes of antral barotrauma

membrane becomes oedematous and some degree of facial pain or discomfort may occur. In the diving situation the ambient pressure of the surrounding water is applied to all the body including blood vessels. As the diver descends the pressure

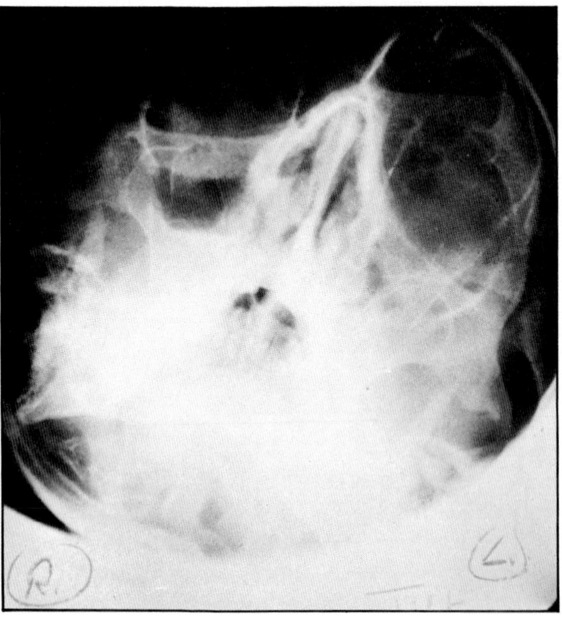

Figure 7.5 Tilt-x-ray – fluid level left frontal sinus and right antrum. Oedematous mucosal lining and fluid level left antrum

increases on all the tissues except the sealed off contents of the rigid middle-ear and paranasal sinuses. Therefore inside the sinus cavity there is a relatively reduced air pressure and blood will be forced into the vessels of the lining membrane. The vessels may swell with the overload of blood with the eventual formation of an oedematous membrane and serosanguinous transudate in the sinus cavity. Frank haemorrhage into the sinus may occur. The amount of pathological change is proportional to the degree of pressure differential and the length of time that the unequalized pressure exists. The fact that normal body tissue pressures are about 1/20 atmosphere greater than their environment increases the tendency towards transudate formation in the hyperbaric environment. During the period of reopening of the ostium or fronto-nasal duct it is common for the sufferer to experience a serosanguinous nasal discharge or frank epistaxis as the sinus contents are evacuated.

Figure 7.5 demonstrates the x-ray appearances of a severe case of sinus barotrauma in a diver. A fluid level in the antra and frontal sinuses is apparent. Although the clinical aspects of sinus barotrauma are dealt with elsewhere it should be pointed out that the presenting feature is of facial pain. It is not uncommon for pain caused by antral barotrauma to be referred to the frontal region via the nasociliary nerve.

Dental barotrauma of diving

In a number of normal subjects the roots of the upper premolar and first two molar teeth may impinge submucosally in the floor of the maxillary sinuses. Dental pain in these teeth can be caused by sinus barotrauma (similar to that which may be experienced in acute sinusitis). Gas spaces may exist near the roots of infected teeth or adjacent fillings which are no longer effective. Implosion of a tooth can occur in the presence of a cavity and thin cementum. This has been described by Carl Edmonds and colleagues.

Otitis barotrauma

It should be appreciated that in the underwater environment a diver wearing a Scuba suit has no connection with the surface and his appreciation of sound is achieved in a manner totally different from that of a person surrounded by air. Harris (1973) points out that the dominant route of normal reception must be via compression waves through the skull and contents to the cochlea. Acoustic energy in water is transmitted as waves of condensation and rarefaction to the skull. The surface area of the scala vestibuli is greater than that of the scala tympani and the round window is larger and more compliant than the oval window. As acoustic energy via the skull acts on both scalae equally, the basilar membrane is depressed into the scala tympani and sound is appreciated by the diver. This method of sound perception is complemented by the inertial route via the ossicles; the latter being suspended by ligaments and drum attachment can only move in a rocking motion around a fore-and-aft axis. When underwater energy strikes the skull vibration ensues but with some inertial lag of the ossicles due to their mass. However when they do move they do so in the only way anatomically possible, that is in the same fashion as when stimulated by normal air conduction. If the external auditory meatus contains water the compliance of the tympanic membrane is reduced and it has been shown that there is up to 20 dB reduction in bone conduction thresholds at low frequencies when the meatus is completely filled with water. With such situations there is liable to be loss of directional appreciation of incoming sound waves.

Whilst the sinus problems associated with barotrauma are well understood and the effects temporary, the physiology and pathology of the vestibular apparatus and cochlea in the hyperbaric environment are less clear. The clinical conditions encountered are more severe; and on occasion permanent loss of cochlear or vestibular function ensues. Much of the recent knowledge on the subject stems from the detailed investigations carried out by Edmonds and Freeman in Australia and Farmer, McCormick and colleagues in the United States.

Goodhill (1971) has also drawn attention to the possibility of round window fistula as the result of excess pressure in the CSF, or eustachian tube. Otitic barotrauma is arguably the commonest occupational disease of divers. Fortunately the more severe and permanent damage caused by otitic barotrauma is rare. Barotrauma will not occur providing the pressure within the middle-ear cleft and external auditory meatus remains the same as that surrounding a diver. With the ambient pressure changes experienced by a diver the presence of a pressure-sensitive middle ear is a potential hazard. Otitic barotrauma may result in either cochlear or vestibular lesions, comprising hearing loss, tinnitus and/or vertigo – less commonly a combination of all three.

External auditory meatus barotrauma: 'reversed ear'

This will occur if any obstruction prevents the increase in external canal water or air pressure whilst a diver descends, assuming that the middle-ear pressure does rise via the eustachian tube. Such obstruction may be caused by cerumen, ear plugs or even

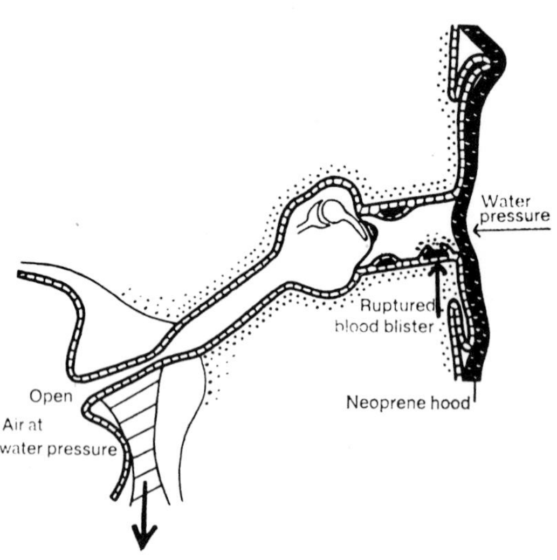

Figure 7.6 The development of 'Reversed Ear' (from Roydhouse, N. *Scuba Diving and the Ear, Nose and Throat.* Auckland, New Zealand; Roydhouse. Reproduced by permission of the publisher)

debris from an external otitis. Another cause is the compression of the soft hood of a Scuba suit against the pinna by the increasing surrounding water pressure (Jarrett, 1961). In such a situation the tympanic membrane will bulge laterally and eventually be lifted from the annulus posteriorly with the formation of a haemorrhagic bulla. After further generalized vascular congestion, mainly in the attic and along the handle of malleus, rupture occurs.

Middle-ear barotrauma

The middle-ear and mastoid air-cells normally contain air at atmospheric pressure air exchange occurring via the eustachian tube, i.e. the pressure on either side of the tympanic membrane, is atmospheric. A difference of only 0.25 atmosphere may cause otalgia. The eustachian tube is 3.7 cm long, the lateral 1/3 and middle ear are bony and incompressible. The medial 2/3 is cartilaginous and compressible. The isthmus or junction of the two parts is the narrowest point. The medial opening of the tube consists of cartilage, triangular in shape with the base folded over and projecting into the nasopharynx. The tubal orifice is slit-like and normally closed, but is opened by positive action of the tensor palati (*Figure 7.7*) and salpingo-pharyngeus muscles, e.g. yawning or swallowing. Increase in the ambient, and therefore nasopharyngeal pressure, when diving underwater tends to compress the eustachian tube orifice and this effect is enhanced by the corresponding increase in the surrounding tissue fluid pressures.

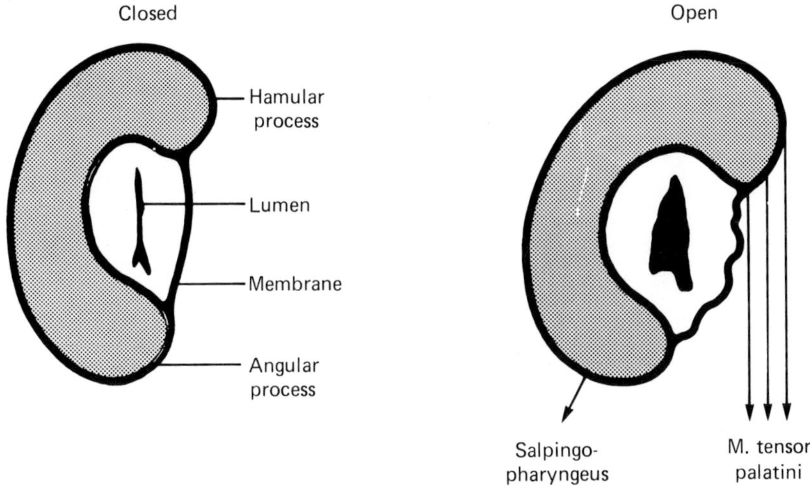

Figure 7.7 The mechanism of tubal opening (McGibbon, 1947)

Closure of the tubal orifice, 'locking', occurs in the frightened or inexperienced diver who allows tissue pressure to build up to an extent which renders clearance impossible without reduction in the ambient pressure. *Figures 7.8* and *7.9* illustrate the flutter valve mechanism of the medial end of the eustachian tube, and explain why barotrauma is more common in the compression phase rather than on ascent to the

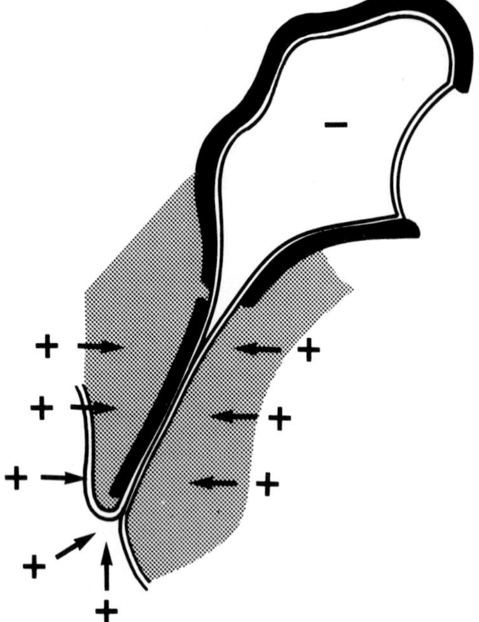

Figure 7.8 Diagrammatic representation of the middle ear and eustachian tube during descent. With increasing environmental pressure the TM is forced inwards and unless there is pressure equalization through the eustachian tube barotrauma will occur. (After McGibbon, 1947)

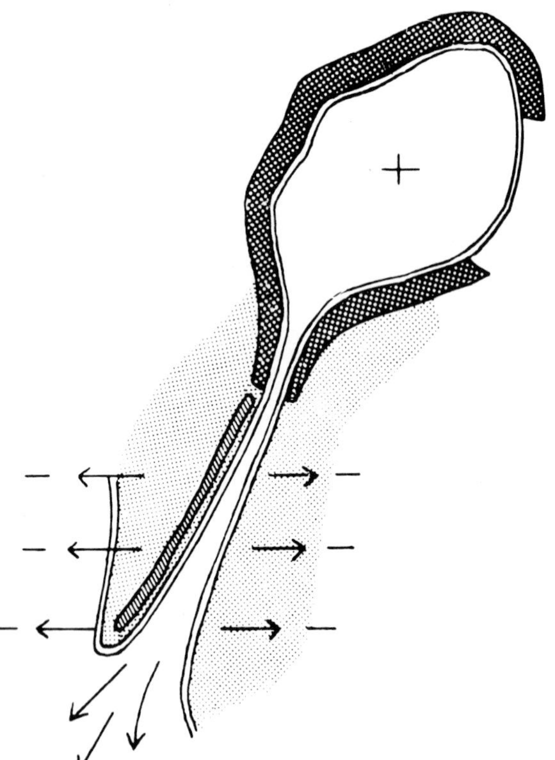

Figure 7.9 Passive escape of air from middle-ear cleft with reduction of environmental pressure (flutter valve effect)

surface. Venting of the middle-ear cleft is a passive affair, whereas to increase middle-ear pressure active movements such as yawning or swallowing are necessary. Normally the middle ear vents into the nasopharynx whenever the pressure in the former is 10–12 mmHg above the ambient. Underwater venting occurs every 0.5 m during the diver's rise to the surface. In 1 per cent of individuals the elastic resistance of the cartilaginous eustachian tube is high (> 60 mmHg) and these unfortunates may be subject to middle-ear barotrauma even on ascent.

Middle-ear barotrauma of descent is the most common aural disorder experienced by divers and is due to failure to equalize middle-ear pressure with that of the nasopharynx. The pathophysiological sequence of events within the middle-ear cleft is similar to that occurring in the paranasal sinuses, i.e. mucosal congestion and vascular engorgement which may be followed by a middle-ear transudate or frank haemotympanum. The tympanic membrane becomes progressively more indrawn with vascular engorgement first noted in the attic and along the handle of the malleus later spreading to involve the whole drum (*Figure 7.10*). At some stage perforation

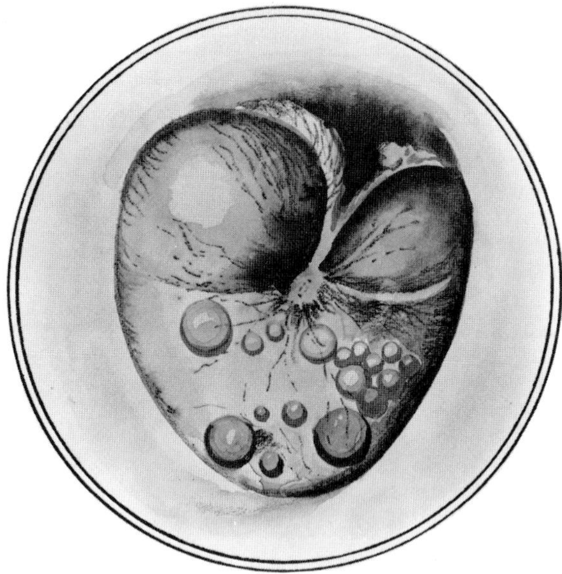

Figure 7.10 Appearance of otitic barotrauma with transudate and fluid level in the middle ear

(usually posterior) of the tympanic membrane occurs. This depends on the state of the membrane; in a healthy tympanic membrane rupture will occur with a differential pressure of 200 mmHg, or at a depth of 16 ft (4.8 m). The presence of a middle-ear transudate and change in the tympanic membrane will give rise to a variable degree of conductive hearing loss and there is evidence to prove that repeated middle-ear barotrauma with undue stretching of the tympanic membrane may lead to tympanosclerosis and loss of compliance of the structures involved. Occasionally underwater an early middle-ear barotrauma is relieved by a forceful Valsalva manoeuvre. Such sudden lateral movement of the tympanic membrane may be associated with ossicular disruption at the incudo-stapedial joint.

Inner-ear barotrauma of descent

Due to either sudden middle-ear barotrauma or forceful Valsalva manoeuvre to overcome this situation either the cochlea or the vestibular labyrinth may be damaged. Sudden uncontrolled medial movement of the stapes footplate may be associated with an equally sudden turbulence of the perilymph in the otic capsule. Such reaction can result in damage to the basilar membrane in the basal turn of the cochlea and permanent sensorineural high frequency hearing loss/tinnitus of variable

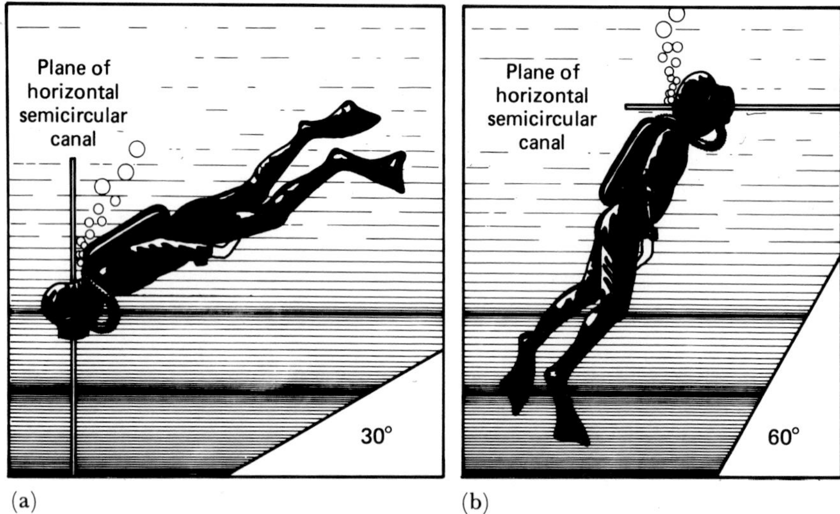

Figure 7.11 Potential caloric stimulation of the lateral semicircular canal whilst scuba diving (after Edmonds *et al.*, *Otological Aspects of Diving*)

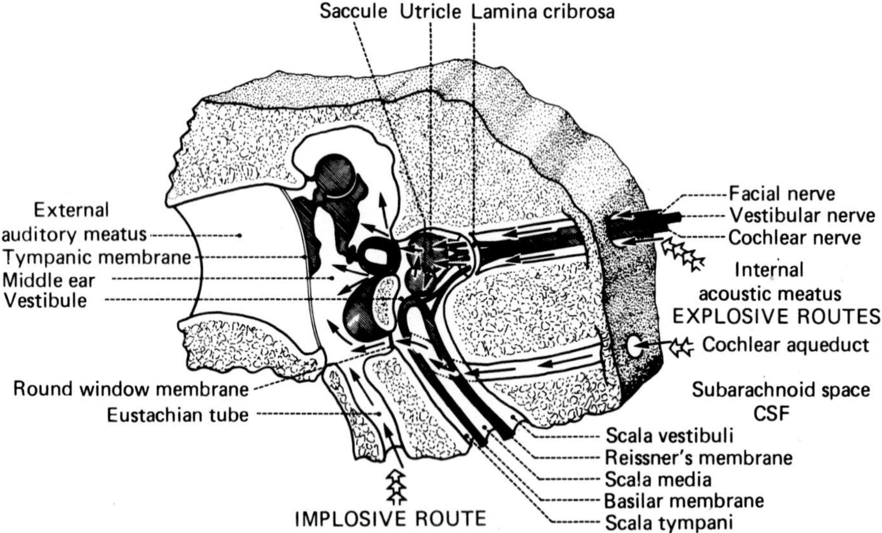

Figure 7.12 Possible pathways of implosive and explosive forces which may lead to inner-ear damage (After Goodhill (1971). *Laryngoscope*, **81,** 1462. Reproduced by permission of the publishers)

degree. Unilateral stapedial movement may also result in stimulation of the ipsilateral vestibule and sequential vertigo. Equally rapid lateral movement of the stapes (attached via incus and malleus to the TM) by forceful Valsalva manoeuvre may 'uncork' the stapes footplate from the oval window with perilymph leak leading to instant or progressive sensorineural hearing loss/tinnitus and/or vertigo. This 'uncorking' action is augmented by the increased middle-ear pressure on the thin round window membrane which then bulges medially and may rupture.

Under normal conditions an individual's spatial orientation is dependent on visual,

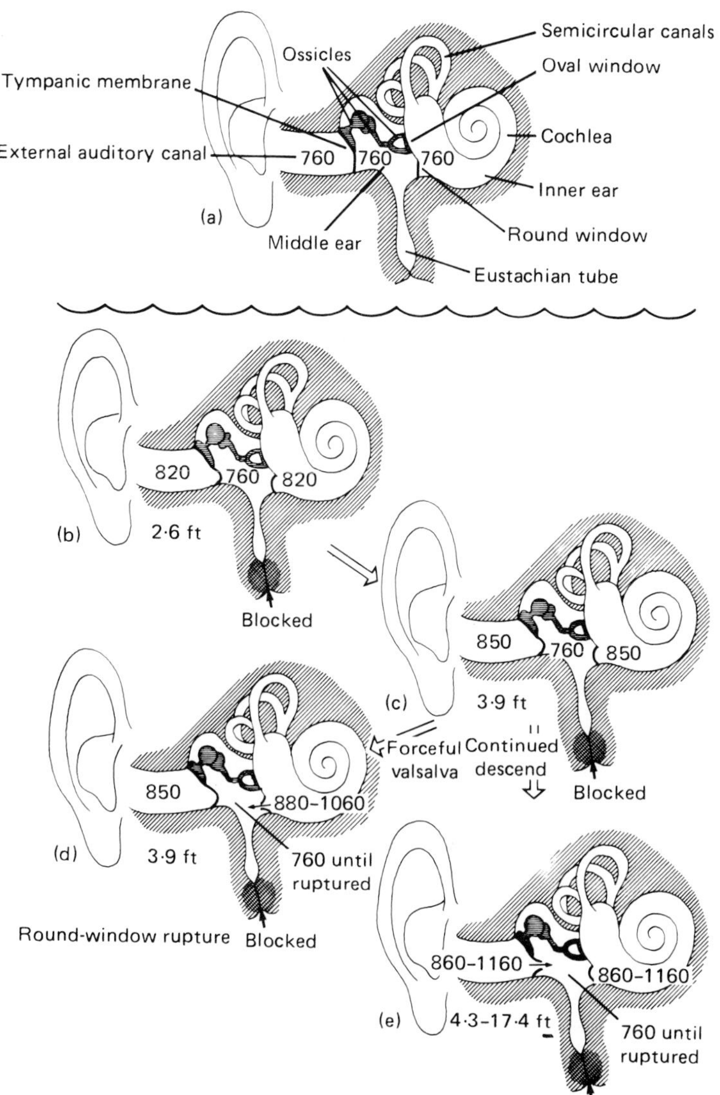

Figure 7.13 Round window fistula and TM rupture resulting from eustachian tube blockage (From Farmer, J. C. (1976). In *Diving Medicine*. Ed. by Strauss, R. New York; Grune and Stratton. Reproduced by permission of the author and publisher)

proprioceptive and vestibular information. Underwater, in the dark and with near zero gravity there is sensory deprivation of visual and proprioceptive input and the diver becomes more dependent on vestibular responses. Consider the diver descending underwater (*Figure 7.11a*); in this situation the lateral semicircular canal is orientated in the plane for maximum caloric stimulation. Therefore any unilateral stimulation by the ingress of water under a Scuba suit hood or via a perforated tympanic membrane might lead to subjective vertigo and disorientation with disastrous results. *Figure 7.11b* shows the reverse, i.e. on rising to the surface the lateral semicircular canal is in the position of minimal sensitivity.

The concept of round window fistula described by Goodhill (1971) is of particular relevance to the hyperbaric environment of the diver. The delicately balanced perilymph–endolymph system is intimately related to the hydrodynamic forces in the intracranial venous sinuses and the pressure variations in the cerebrospinal fluid. Goodhill suggested that the communicating channel between CSF and perilymph – the cochlear aqueduct, might vary in calibre and structure between individuals. The normal adult aqueduct is some 6 mm in length and 150 μm in diameter at its narrowest point and in 10 per cent of cases there is a barrier membrane at the junction with the scala tympani. The infantile aqueduct is only 3.5 mm long and of relatively wide bore. It was felt that in some adults the infantile type of aqueduct might persist. If so, the protective effect of the long narrow adult aqueduct on smoothing out and reducing the violent fluctuations in pressure differentials between the CSF and perilymph would be lost.

Any action therefore which increased CSF pressure could cause a sudden rise in perilymph pressure within the scala tympani leading to rupture of the round window membrane. This is possible when it is realized that the round window membrane although of three layers is only 4 or 5 cells thick with a middle layer of connective tissue. The thickness is not uniform, varying from 70 μm at the periphery to 10 μm at the centre (*Figures 7.12* and *7.13*).

Alternatively the pressure wave might rupture through the basilar and Reissner's membrane involving the utricle and saccule. In the former instance the perilymph leak into the middle ear via the round window perforation will lead to a sudden sensorineural hearing loss or a gradual loss over a few days. The loss of hearing may become total if treatment is not instituted, or may recover with spontaneous healing of the round window membrane. In the former case cochlear and vestibular damage is permanent. Physical exertion plus the hyperbaric diving environment will increase CSF pressure. In a susceptible diver an unexpectedly rapid uncontrolled increase in depth may be associated with middle-ear barotrauma of descent (low middle-ear pressure compared with ambient) and quick build up of perilymph pressure leading to either of the pathological conditions described above. Such cases have occurred and the diagnosis has been confirmed surgically.

Barotraumatic cochlear and vestibular lesions occurring at depth

These occur when the diver is in a hyperbaric environment which is not changing. They are more frequently associated with so-called saturation diving techniques where an oxyhelium mixture is breathed. Because of their fortunate infrequency and the difficulties in specialist medical examination in such circumstances knowledge is limited. Active research is being carried out in Australia by Edmonds, Freeman *et al.* (1973), the Royal Navy, US Navy and by Farmer, McCormick and colleagues in the United States. Most cases occur during deep dives where helium replaces nitrogen as the inert gas and it is apparent that either cochlear or vestibular lesions occur rather than both. The disorders are, or seem to be, precipitated by a change-over from an oxyhelium gas mix to compressed air at the beginning of decompression. Several possible physiological causes have been advanced to account for the occurrence of such lesions. Current opinion is that counter diffusion of two inert gases across a microscopically thin round window membrane may result in bubble formation at the interface between the middle and inner ear. This is logical when it is remembered that at the change-over of breathing mixtures the peri-endolymph is saturated with helium and that in a matter of seconds the middle-ear cleft is full of another breathing mixture, e.g. compressed air. Even without a pressure differential bubbling could be expected at or around the interface.

Otitic barotrauma of ascent (decompression phase)

Although the majority of the problems affecting either the cochlea or vestibular labyrinth during ascent are due to decompression sickness ('bends'), alternobaric vertigo described by Lundgren (1973) may occur. In addition otic pathology may be caused by changes in blood chemistry and structure of the blood vessels; these will be described under a separate heading. It has been noted earlier that the normal passive release of middle-ear air pressure by the flutter-valve mechanism of the medial end of the eustachian tube may be obstructed by an abnormally high elastic resistance of the cartilage. Lundgren has pointed out that this could account for a relative over-pressurization in one middle-ear cleft whilst a diver ascends (or by a forced Valsalva in an attempt to clear a 'sticky' eustachian tube). In such a unilateral circumstance the tympanic membrane bulges laterally together with an outward pull on the stapedial footplate and inward movement of the round window membrane with turbulence in the inner-ear fluids, unilateral vestibular stimulation and vertigo.

Decompression sickness affecting the ear

Decompression sickness in its various manifestations remains the major limiting factor for deep or prolonged saturation dives. As a diver increases his depth the respired gases are absorbed into the circulation and distributed through the body tissues. The amount of gas so absorbed depends on:

(1) Solubility.
(2) Partial pressure.
(3) Vascularity of tissue.
(4) Rate of tissue diffusion.

During decompression this dissolved gas must be returned to the gas state in the lungs by reversal of this process, or by the formation of gas bubbles in the tissues or fluids (e.g. blood, endolymph, perilymph). In the latter case bubbles obey Boyle's Law and increase in size as decompression proceeds. Divers are subject to a strict rate of

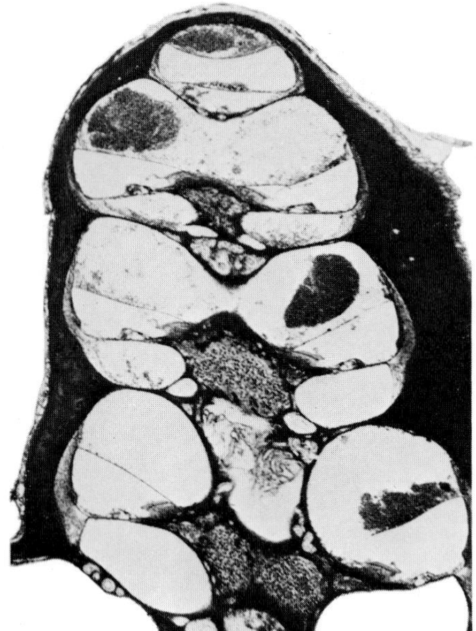

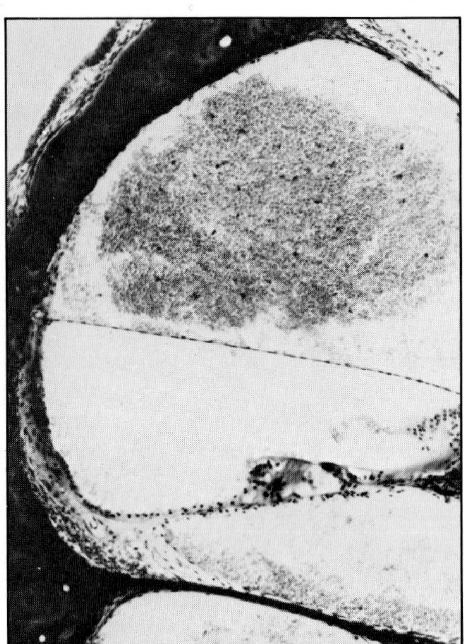

Figures 7.14 and *7.15* Haemorrhage into the cochlea of guinea-pig following simulated oxyhelium dive in a pressure chamber (From McCormick *et al.* (1973). *Laryngoscope*, **83**, 1483. Reproduced by permission of authors and publisher)

decompression by adherence to internationally recognized diving tables which equate the rate of ascent with original depth and length of the dive. Gas bubbles (of moist gas) may form in the part involved. Obesity, cold, dehydration and age are also predisposing factors. The production of a bubble is attended by alterations in the blood chemistry at the blood–bubble interface.

The blood supply to the cochlea and vestibule has been described elsewhere. The arteries are end-arteries with few anastomotic connections. Should obstruction to blood flow occur, severe and often permanent damage to the tissues supplied will result. In decompression sickness bubbles of nitrogen may present in any part of the tissues of the membranous labyrinth, or within the blood vessels themselves (bubble emboli). They may also form and involve the 8th nerve pathways and central connections in the brain stem. Bubble formation in the cerebellar pathways may produce a clinical picture superficially resembling a vestibular lesion. Animal experiments by McCormick reveal loss of hair-cells in the cochlea but with intact supporting cells. Haemorrhage into the perilymph of the cochlea and vestibule was noted (*Figures 7.14* and *7.15*).

Vascular and blood chemistry changes associated with hyperbaric states

It has been observed that as the result of exposure to a high ambient pressure certain changes occur in the blood vessel walls of the microcirculation, and also in the blood chemistry. Reduced capillary blood flow and random stasis in the microcirculation occurs (Lamberton *et al.*, 1976) and is not necessarily associated with bubble formation. There is general agreement that blood viscosity increases with haemoconcentration and the development of a hypercoaguable state. With stasis in the microcirculation oedema of the vessel walls is observed with possible changes in osmotic function. The serum lipid level is elevated, as is that of serum cholesterol. Philip and Martin at the Institute of Royal Naval Medicine have investigated the platelet concentration and find that after decompression there is a significant depression in circulating platelet level. This is due to platelet aggregation around the surface of developing nitrogen bubbles and the formation of platelet emboli. Bubbles in the blood have been shown to initiate clotting by their effect on Factor 12.

Although the foregoing changes are widespread it is clear that there is a potentially serious hazard to the micro-vasculature of the inner ear. There appears to be no particular part of the cochlea or vestibule which is more at risk. Degeneration of the neurosensory epithelium will occur as the result of lipid, bubble or platelet microemboli. It is of interest that whales and porpoises are probably protected from these hazards by possessing a potent heparin-like substance and a lack of Factor 12 in their clotting mechanism (McCormick, 1973).

Acoustic hazard in divers

Although many cases of sensorineural high-frequency hearing loss in divers can be explained by prior exposure to high-intensity noise (especially divers in the armed forces), there are others which are probably due to noise experienced during diving activities. Such losses may be permanent or temporary threshold shifts and in no way differ clinically from any other noise-induced hearing loss. A diver is unable to wear any form of ear muff or plugs whilst diving.

Within compression chambers and in some forms of diving helmets the noise level of the high-pressure inflow or exhausting mechanism has been recorded as high as

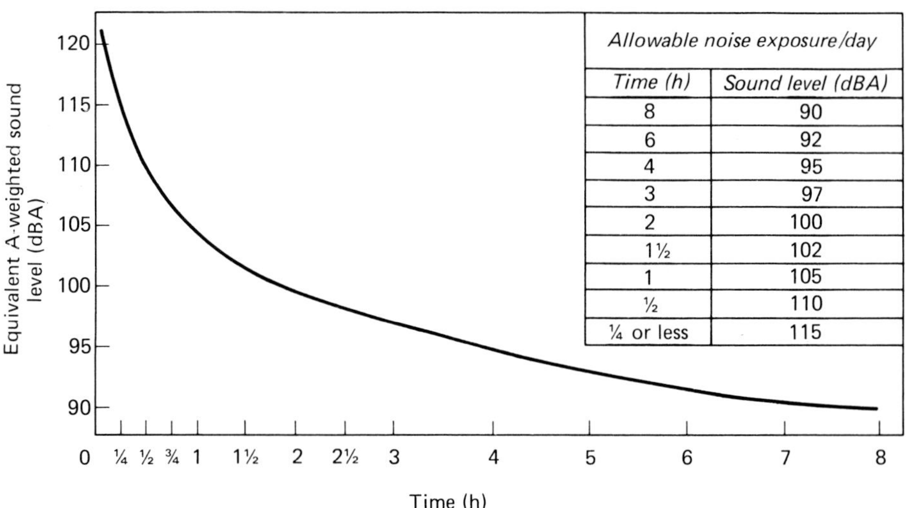

Allowable noise exposure/day	
Time (h)	Sound level (dBA)
8	90
6	92
4	95
3	97
2	100
1½	102
1	105
½	110
¼ or less	115

Figure 7.16 Acoustic trauma – damage risk level

120 dB at 1 khz. Divers may be exposed to such levels for fairly long periods during a working lifetime, certainly in excess of the level generally accepted for Damage Risk Criteria (*Figure 7.16*).

In addition divers' aural acuity may be at risk due to the proximity of underwater explosives involving both noise and blast (shock wave).

Miscellaneous

Under this heading are included a number of dissociated problems which might appear to be due to diving-induced damage to the cochlea or vestibule but in fact stem from other sources. Generalized hypoxia or anoxia may produce a subjective feeling of instability which must not be confused with labyrinthine dysfunction. Nitrogen narcosis and the high-pressure nervous syndrome present similarly.

The use of oxyhelium mixtures may provide communication problems. The pitch of the voice is determined by the vibration rate of the cords. Exhaled air rapidly passes through the glottic chink producing decreased pressure by the Bernoulli principle. Cord vibration produces sound. The three resonating frequencies for each pure tone produced by the vocal cord (formants) are altered by a helium environment. The lower density of the gas increases the speed of sound with resulting increase in the formant frequency and a 'Donald Duck' quality is imparted to speech.

References

Boot, G. W. I. and Shilling, C. (1913). *Annals of Otolaryngology*, **22,** 1121

Everly, I. A. (1942). *US Navy Medical Bulletin*, **40,** 664

Edmonds, C. (1976). *Diving Medicine* (Ed. by Straus, R.), p. 49. New York; Grune & Stratton

Edmonds, C., Freeman, P. *et al.* (1973). *Otological Aspects of Diving 1973*, Australian Medical Publishing Co.

Edmonds, C. and Freeman, P. (1972). *Archives of Otolaryngology*, **95,**

Farmer, J. (1977). *Annals of Otolaryngology*, **86,** Sup., 36

Goodhill, V. (1971). *Laryngoscope*, **81,** 1462

Harris, J. D. (1973). US Navy Medical Research Report 746

Head, P. W. (1973). *The Practitioner*, **211,** 738

Jarrett, P. (1961). *Journal of RN Medical Service*, **47,** 13

Lambertsen, Wells, *et al.* (1976). 5th Symposium on U W Physiology, Public Press Baltimore USA, 233

Lundgren, G. E. G. (1973). *Proceedings of the European Underseas Bio-Medical Society*, 406

Martin, K and Nichols, G. (1972). *Aerospace Medicine*, **43**(8), 827

McCormick, J. (1970). *Journal of the Acoustical Society of America*, **43**(6), 1418

McCormick, J. (1973). *Laryngoscope*, **33**(9), 1483

Morrison, L. (1969). *The eye & ENT Monthly*, **48,** 38

Murray, T. (1973). US Navy Submarine Centre Report 643

Philip, R., Schacham, P. and Gowdey, C. (1971). *Aerospace Medicine*, **42**(5), 494

Rawlins, J. S. P. (1961). MRC Report RN P61, 1011

Sivian, L. (1947). *Journal of the Acoustical Society of America*, **19,** 461

Summitt and Reimers, S. (1971). *Aerospace Medicine*, Nov., 1173

8 Anatomy of the mouth, pharynx and oesophagus

R F McNab Jones

Development

Towards the end of the first month, at the 10–14 somite stages, 23–25 days (Corner, 1929; Heuser, 1930), the foregut comes to lie dorsal to the developing heart tube (*Figure 8.1*), and to the developing septum transversum (developing diaphragm). Its anterior end is at this stage shut off by the buccopharyngeal membrane. At about the 20 somite stage, 26–27 days, the buccopharyngeal membrane ruptures and the ectodermally-lined stomatodaeum becomes continuous with the foregut. The

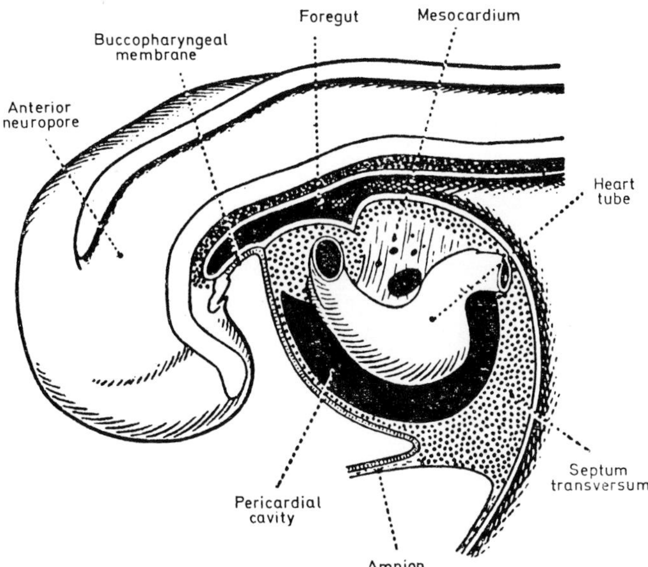

Figure 8.1 A schematic drawing of a longitudinal midline section through the cranial half of a 14-somite human embryo to show the rotation of the heart tube resulting from the formation of the head fold. The foregut is situated dorsal to the heart and pericardial cavity and the septum transversum lies caudal to the pericardial cavity; the mesocardium now shows fenestrations

endodermal lining of the foregut, once it is established, differentiates into a number of different structures (*Figure 8.2*). It gives origin to: (1) part of the nasal cavities; (2) the endodermally lined part of the buccal cavity; (3) the pharynx, and the glands and other structures derived from it, namely, the anterior lobe of the pituitary gland, the thyroid, thymus and parathyroid glands, the ultimobranchial body, the pharyngo-tympanic (eustachian) tube, the middle ear and the tonsils; (4) possibly the submandibular and sublingual salivary glands; (5) the larynx, trachea, bronchi and lungs; (6) the oesophagus; (7) the stomach; (8) the duodenum as far as the liver diverticulum. In the cranial portion of the foregut, in man, the branchial mesoderm does not split into splanchnopleuric and somatopleuric layers to form a coelom. The mesoderm adjacent to the caudal portion of the foregut splits on each side to form the pericardioperitoneal canals which later are to become the primitive pleural cavities. From a number of mesodermal condensations in the unsplit branchial mesoderm of the lateral wall and floor of the pharynx the branchial arches take origin (*Figure 8.3*). Between the arches successive grooves or clefts on the pharyngeal aspect are matched by corresponding grooves or clefts in the overlying ectodermal surface. Only a small amount of mesoderm separates the ectodermal and endodermal layers of the clefts. In normal development the clefts between the arches do not break down to form gill slits as occurs in fishes, but each groove becomes much modified and gives rise to a variety of structures. Occasionally the tissues of the cleft in the more cephalic of the pouches break down to form an open gill slit. Frequently this gill slit exists for a short period

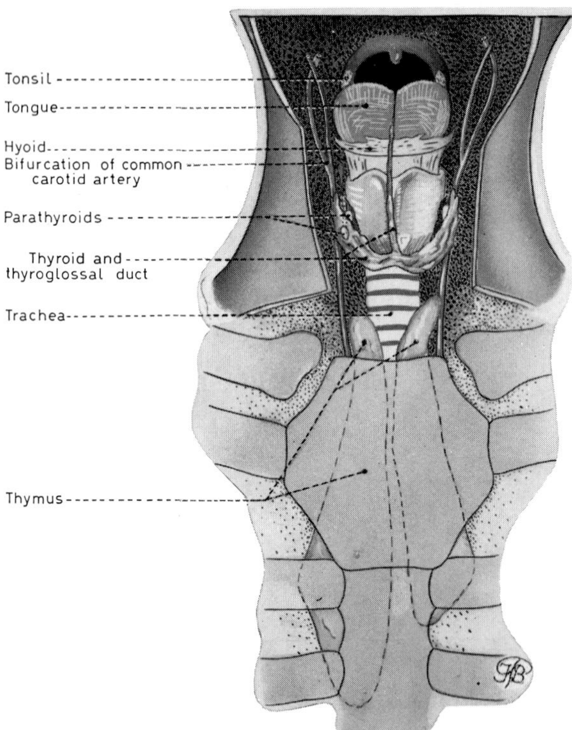

Figure 8.2 A diagram to show some of the derivatives of the endoderm of the primitive pharynx

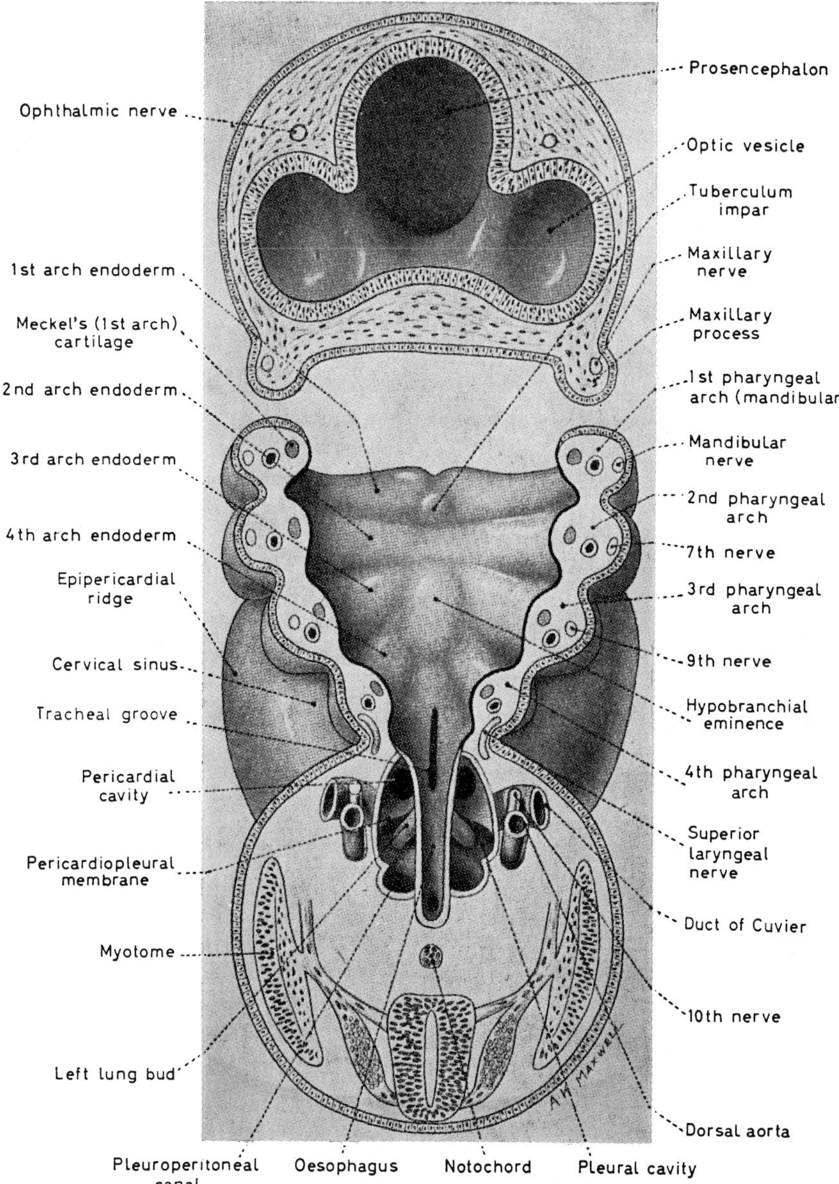

Figure 8.3 A section through the primitive pharynx of a 5-mm human embryo to show the pharyngeal arches and structures in the floor. (Reproduced by courtesy of Professors Hamilton, Boyd and Mossman)

during fetal life, and may remain in the adult as a branchial fistula or a persistent gill cleft.

A cartilaginous bar and branchial musculature, together with a branchial arch artery, differentiate in each mesodermal condensation. Each arch receives an afferent and an efferent nerve to supply the skin, the musculature and endodermal lining respectively of the arch concerned. In addition, each arch receives a branch from the nerve of the succeeding arch. This arrangement of the nerve supply to each arch is a relic of the pattern found in vertebrates when the nerve to the gill region was distributed cranial and caudal to the corresponding gill cleft. As a result, in man and the mammals, each arch receives a branch, called the post-trematic, from the nerve of its own arch and a second branch, called the pre-trematic, from the succeeding arch.

In an embryo at about the 5 mm stage (approximately 30–32 days) the floor of the foregut shows a number of elevations, produced by the mesodermal condensations, separated by depressions or grooves (*Figure 8.3*). The first arch of each side forms an elevation in the side wall of the foregut; the elevations meet in the midline. A small median elevation, the tuberculum impar, is seen immediately behind the middle part of the mandibular swelling. Behind the tuberculum impar a small median depression, the foramen caecum, marks the site of the invagination which gives rise to the median primordium of the thyroid gland. The second arch of each side is continuous across the midline of the foregut floor. Immediately caudal to the second arch a second and larger median swelling develops; this is the hypobranchial eminence. The third and fourth arches fail to reach the midline owing to the presence of the hypobranchial eminence; a fifth arch makes a transitory appearance. Caudal to the hypobranchial eminence a tracheobronchial groove develops, the lateral boundary of which is the rudimentary sixth arch. It is from this groove that subsequently there develop the lining epithelia and associated glands of the larynx, trachea, bronchi and possibly the respiratory epithelium of the alveoli themselves.

The development of the palate is described in Chapter 4. By definition the mandibular division of the trigeminal nerve is the post-trematic nerve of the first arch. The pre-trematic nerve going to the first arch is possibly represented by the chorda tympani branch of the facial nerve. The facial nerve itself is the post-trematic branch of the second arch, the pre-trematic nerve to this arch being derived from the tympanic branch (Jacobson's nerve) of the glossopharyngeal nerve. The glossopharyngeal is the post-trematic nerve of the third arch. The nerves of the remaining arches (fourth and sixth) are derived from the vagus and accessory nerves by their superior and inferior (recurrent) laryngeal branches, and from the pharyngeal branches. The pre-trematic nerves of these more caudal arches are not well defined in the human subject.

The tongue is initially represented by: (1) an anterior portion which arises from the tuberculum impar and the adjacent regions of both mandibular arches; (2) a posterior, paired, portion which arises from the ventromedial ends of the second (hyoid) arches; later, these paired portions fuse, in front of the hypobranchial eminence, to form a single swelling, sometimes known as the *copula*, to which the third arch mesoderm later contributes. The anterior two-thirds is derived from the first arch, the posterior one-third is derived mainly from the subepithelial overgrowth of second arch tissue by the third arch, the third arch coming into contact with first arch tissue and so obliterating the midline ventral portions of the first and second pharyngeal endodermal grooves. The development of the tongue thus explains its nerve supply in the adult. It should be noted that the extreme posterior part of the tongue, which forms the anterior wall of the valleculae, receives a nerve supply from the superior laryngeal branch of the vagus; this branch may represent the pre-trematic nerve of the third arch.

The growth forward and medially of the third arch mesoderm to the tongue at the 12 mm stage, 40–42 days, separates the hypobranchial eminence from the second

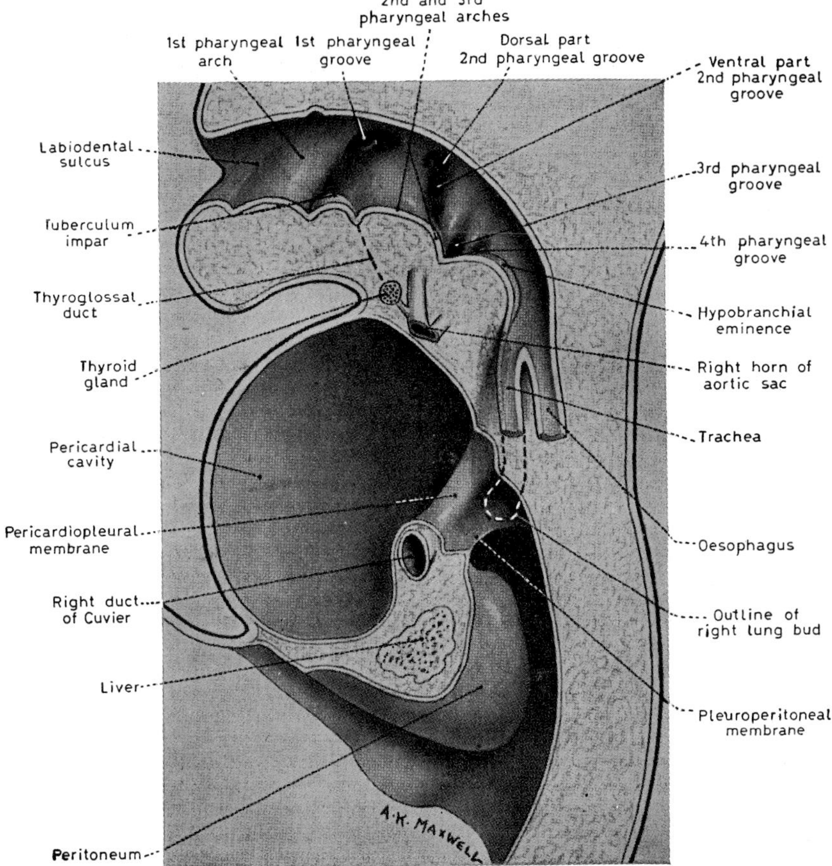

Figure 8.4 The lateral wall of the pharynx and pericardial region of a 7-mm human embryo, showing the pharyngeal grooves. (Reproduced by courtesy of Professors Hamilton, Boyd and Mossman)

arch. Simultaneously there is a caudal migration of the hypobranchial eminence and a relative reduction in its size. At the same time the hypobranchial eminence comes to be more transversely placed behind the tongue and still remains attached to the side wall of the pharynx by part of the third arch tissue; this, in fact, becomes the pharyngo-epiglottic fold of the adult. The groove between the dorsum of the tongue and the epiglottis, the glosso-epiglottic groove, is divided into the valleculae by the appearance of a median glosso-epiglottic fold. The poorly developed swellings which indicate the tracheal groove laterally become the arytenoid swellings.

In higher forms, including man, the pharyngeal grooves give rise to a series of structures which have functions very different from those of the primitive gill slits (*Figure 8.4*). Each groove differentiates into a ventral and dorsal pouch. A brief summary will be given of the derivatives of these pouches. The dorsal part of the first pouch, with the adjacent pharyngeal wall, together with part of the dorsal portion of the second pouch, gives origin to a diverticulum which becomes the pharyngo-tympanic (eustachian) tube (*Figure 8.5*), the middle ear and the mastoid antrum. The tubal (pharyngeal) tonsil arises as aggregations of mesenchymal cells, which later

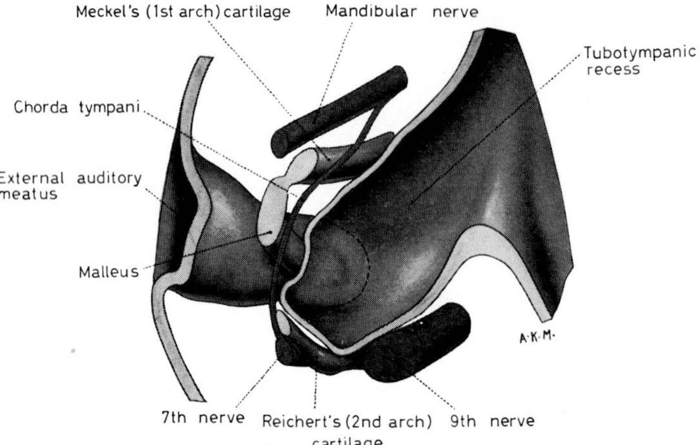

Figure 8.5 The middle-ear region of a 27 mm embryo to show the relationship of the chorda tympani. (Reproduced by courtesy of Professors Hamilton, Boyd and Mossman)

become invaded by lymphocytes, these having arisen *in situ* or having been derived from the blood stream. Similar aggregations of cells migrate into the endoderm of the dorsal pharyngeal wall to form the naso-palatine tonsil (adenoid). Further aggregations of lymphocytes occur in the dorsum of the tongue (second and third arch) to form the lingual tonsil.

The ventral part of the first groove is completely obliterated by the development of the tongue. A portion only of the dorsal part of the second pouch, as already stated, gives rise to the pharyngotympanic tube; the remainder of this pouch is absorbed into the dorsal pharyngeal wall. The ventral pouch of the second arch is almost completely obliterated by the proliferation of its endodermal lining; this is later invaded by mesodermal tissue to form the primordium of the palatine (faucial) tonsil. The unobliterated part of the pouch persists as the intratonsillar cleft or fossa (*Figure 8.13*).

The dorsal pouch of the third arch gives origin to parathyroid III (lower) whilst the ventral part gives rise to the thymus gland (*Figure 8.6*). The dorsal pouch of the fourth arch gives origin to parathyroid IV (upper). The fate of the ventral part of this pouch has been much debated. It is considered by Weller (1933) and Norris (1937) to fuse with the median thyroid diverticulum and to give rise to part of the lobe of the thyroid gland. Gilmour (1937), on the other hand, believes that it contributes to the thymus gland. Kingsbury (1939) and Godwin (1940), while believing that it fuses with the thyroid diverticulum, contend that it retrogresses and does not give rise to thyroid tissue. Occasionally it may persist and give rise to ultimobranchial cysts.

The thyroid gland first appears as a midline thickening of the endoderm in the floor of the pharynx caudal to the tuberculum impar. The anterior lobe of the pituitary gland develops from the roof of the pharynx just in front of the anterior end of the notochord. After separation of these various diverticula the remainder of the primitive pharynx may now be called the definitive pharynx.

The first arch cartilage gives origin to a number of different structures. The mandibular cartilage and its perichondrial capsule (Meckel) become the adult incus,

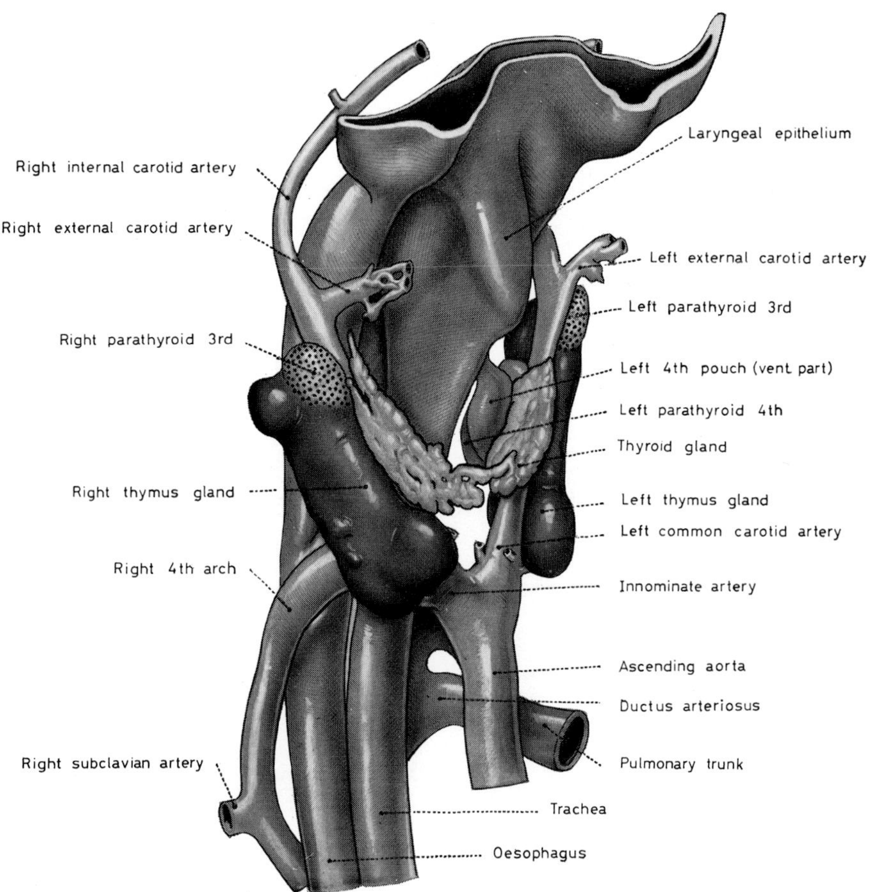

Figure 8.6 A drawing of a reconstruction of the pharyngeal region with associated pharyngeal derivatives and arteries. (Reproduction by courtesy of Professors Hamilton, Boyd and Mossman)

malleus and its anterior ligament, the sphenomandibular ligament. The remainder of the cartilage is absorbed into the mandible. The second cartilage (Reichert) gives rise to the stapes, the styloid process of the temporal bone, the stylohyoid ligament, the lesser cornu and upper part of the body of the hyoid bone. The caudal part of the third arch cartilage disappears, the anterior portion becomes the greater cornu and the lower part of the body of the hyoid bone. The fourth, fifth and sixth arch cartilages also only persist in their anterior part. They give rise to the thyroid cartilage and possibly to the other laryngeal cartilages and tracheal rings.

The caudal part of the foregut extends from the tracheobronchial groove to the dorsal margin of the septum transversum and gives rise to the oesophagus, stomach and part of the duodenum. It is only the development of the more cephalic portion of this part of the foregut, which gives rise to the oesophagus, that will be described here.

The oesophagus comes to lie dorsal to both the developing heart and the septum transversum as a result of the folding under of the anterior part of the early embryo. It is embedded in visceral mesoderm, without any true mesentery. The pericardio-peritoneal canals (into which are invaginated the primitive lung buds – themselves, of course, foregut derivatives) lie one on either side of the self-defining and self-definitive oesophagus. It is at first a short tube extending from the tracheal groove to the fusiform dilatation of the foregut which becomes the stomach.

The oesophagus lengthens rapidly at the time of the caudal migration of the developing heart and respiratory system, and at the same time there may be a temporary obliteration of the lumen. The obliteration has been denied by some recent investigators. It is of interest to note, as Streeter (1945) has pointed out, that there is a marked proliferation and differentiation in the respiratory diverticulum at this time, whereas that of the oesophagus appears to lag behind. The oesophageal endodermal lining is at first of the columnar type, but gradually becomes of the stratified squamous variety. There is some doubt as to the origin of this epithelium; it may become stratified squamous by metaplasia of the existing cells, or there may be migration of cells from the buccal cavity. The smooth muscle fibres develop from the visceral mesoderm, but the origin of the striated muscle, which is found in the upper and middle portions of the tube, is still in doubt.

The mouth

The cavity of the mouth is divided into a vestibule, or labial cavity, between the lips, cheeks, gums and teeth, and a posterior buccal cavity, bounded by the dental arches consisting of the teeth, gums and alveolar processes. The *lips* enclose the anterior part of the vestibule and contain a voluntary sphincter, the *orbicularis oris* muscle. The external surfaces of the lips are covered with skin; the free margins and inner aspects are covered with mucous membrane. As the latter is more transparent than skin, the underlying capillaries give these parts their reddish-pink colour (sometimes referred to as the vermilion of the lip). The submucosa contains small mucus-secreting labial glands. The tortuous labial arteries are embedded in each lip with anastomoses across the midline. The sensory nerve supply of the lips is derived from the labial branches of the maxillary and mandibular branches of the trigeminal nerves. The lymphatic vessels pass into the anterior auricular, submandibular and submental nodes and thence into the deep cervical nodes.

Vestibule

This is a narrow cleft (*Figure 8.7*) unless the cheeks are distended by food, or air, or through paralysis of the musculature in their walls. The main boundary walls of the vestibule are partly muscular and partly osseous. The lateral walls are formed by the *cheeks*, which have the same general structure as the lips, the *buccinator* muscle forming the main muscular component. This muscle is strengthened externally by a strong fascial layer, the *buccopharyngeal* fascia (*Figure 8.7*). Racemose buccal mucous glands lie between the buccinator and the mucous membrane. In young infants a considerable amount of fat, the '*suctorial pad*', is usually present over the posterior part of the muscle, giving the cheeks a rounded appearance. It has been suggested that the fat provides a mechanical support for the cheek in the action of sucking. When this fat

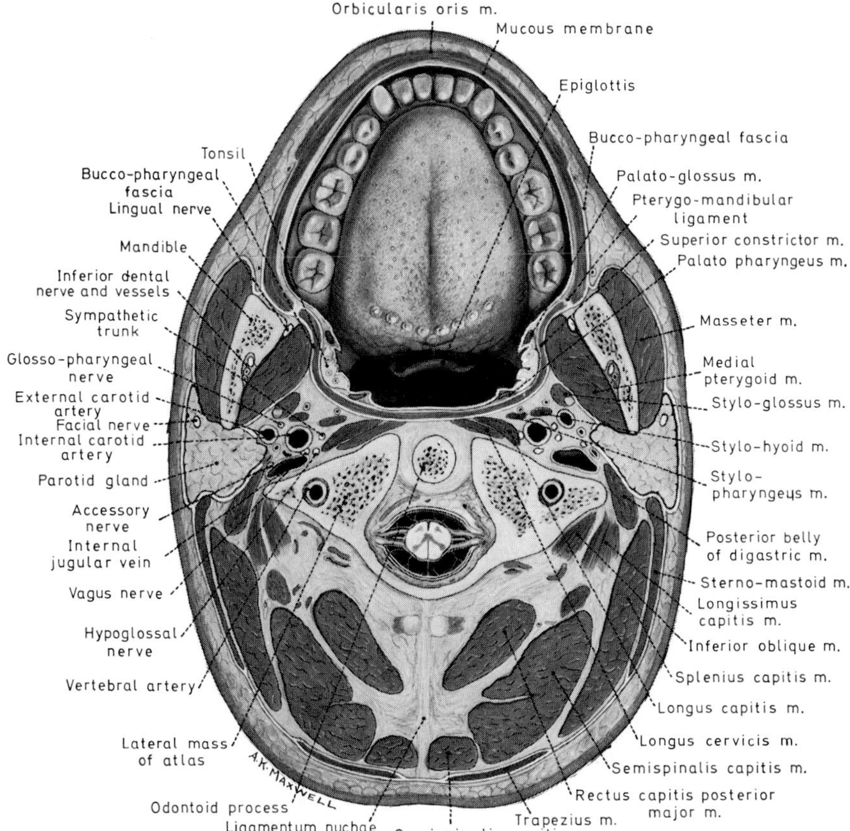

Figure 8.7 Transverse section through the head at the level of the atlas to show the relations of the mouth and pharynx

becomes deficient in the adult, there is a characteristic depression of the facial contour. At its upper and lower limits the mucous membrane is reflected from the lips and cheeks to the gums. In the midline, both superiorly and inferiorly, there is a small vertical fold (frenulum) of mucous membrane from each lip to the anterior incisor region. When the mouth is closed and the teeth are in apposition, the vestibule at each side communicates with the buccal cavity behind the last molar tooth. The duct of the parotid gland opens into the vestibule opposite the crown of the second upper molar tooth.

Buccal cavity

This cavity lies within the dental arches and communicates posteriorly with the oral pharynx (*Figures 8.7* and *8.8*) through the oropharyngeal isthmus at the level of the palatoglossal arches. The roof of the buccal cavity is formed by the hard palate and the anterior part of the soft palate. The floor is formed by the dorsal surface of the anterior two-thirds of the tongue and by the reflection of the mucous membrane from the under-surface and sides of the tongue to the inner side of the gums. A prominent

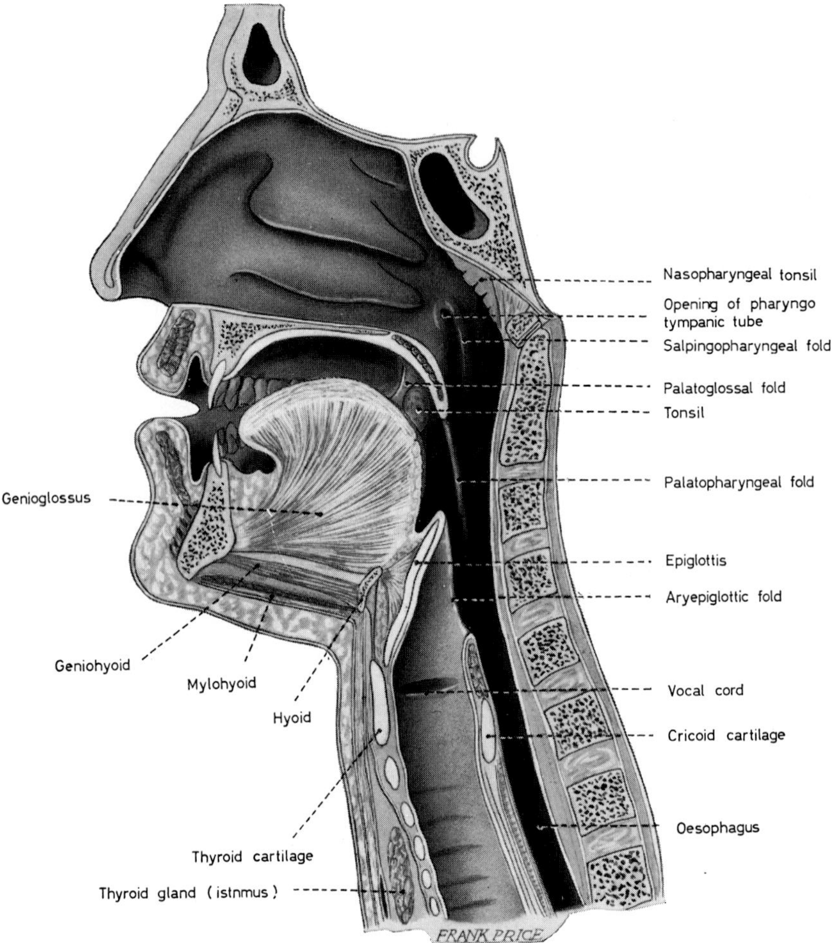

Figure 8.8 A drawing of a sagittal section through the nasal cavity, pharynx and larynx in the adult

median fold of the mucous membrane, the *frenulum linguae*, passes downwards and forwards from the under-surface of the tongue to the floor of the anterior part of the buccal cavity. A second fold, the fimbriated fold, is found on the under-surface of the tongue on each side of the frenulum. Between the frenulum and the fimbriated fold the profunda artery of the tongue can be seen through the mucous membrane (*Figure 8.9*).

In the floor of the buccal cavity on either side of the frenulum of the tongue an elevation, the *sublingual fold*, is produced by the underlying *sublingual salivary* gland. The orifice of the submandibular duct opens at the *sublingual* papilla at the side of the frenulum. The sublingual gland and its duct are supported by the mylohyoid, geniohyoid and genioglossus muscles, and the anterior belly of the digastric muscle (*Figure 8.10*). (For details of the histology of the mouth, see Sicher, 1966.)

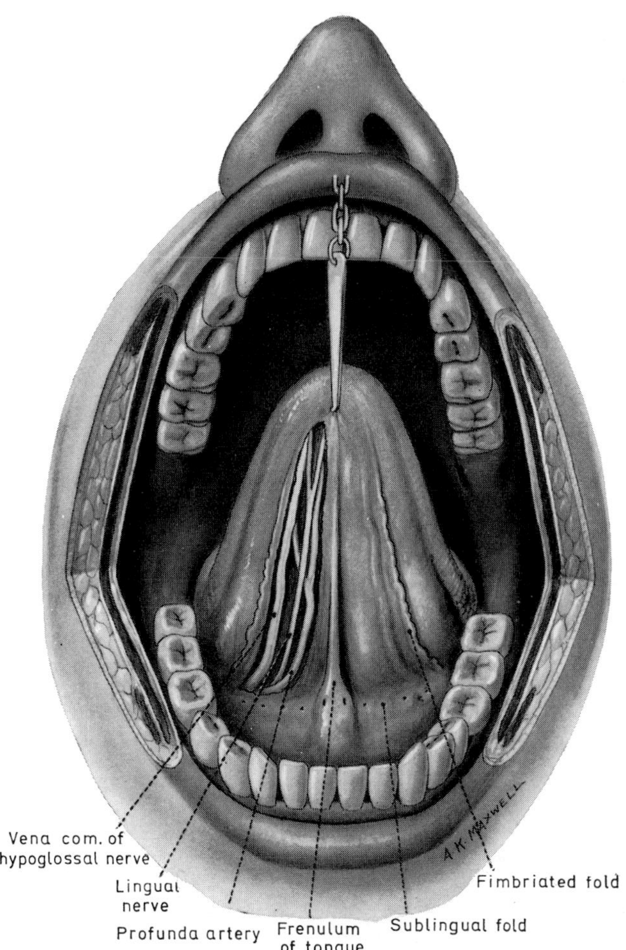

Figure 8.9 The inferior surface of the tongue. Part of the mucous membrane has been removed to expose the vessels and nerve

Blood supply, innervation and lymphatic drainage of the mouth

The mouth is supplied mainly by the superior and inferior labial arteries, the lingual branch of the inferior alveolar artery, and branches of the greater palatine, infra-orbital and posterior superior alveolar arteries.

The *inferior labial artery*, a branch of the facial artery, supplies the glands, mucous membranes and muscles of the lower lip and anastomoses with the artery of the opposite side and with the mental branch of the inferior alveolar artery. The *lingual branch* of the inferior alveolar artery supplies the mucous membrane of the mouth. The *superior labial artery*, another branch of the facial artery, supplies the upper lip.

Branches of the *greater artery*, itself a branch of the maxillary artery, supply the palate, mucous membrane of the roof of the mouth, and gums. The branches of the *infra-orbital* and of the *posterior superior alveolar arteries* supply the upper lip and gums respectively.

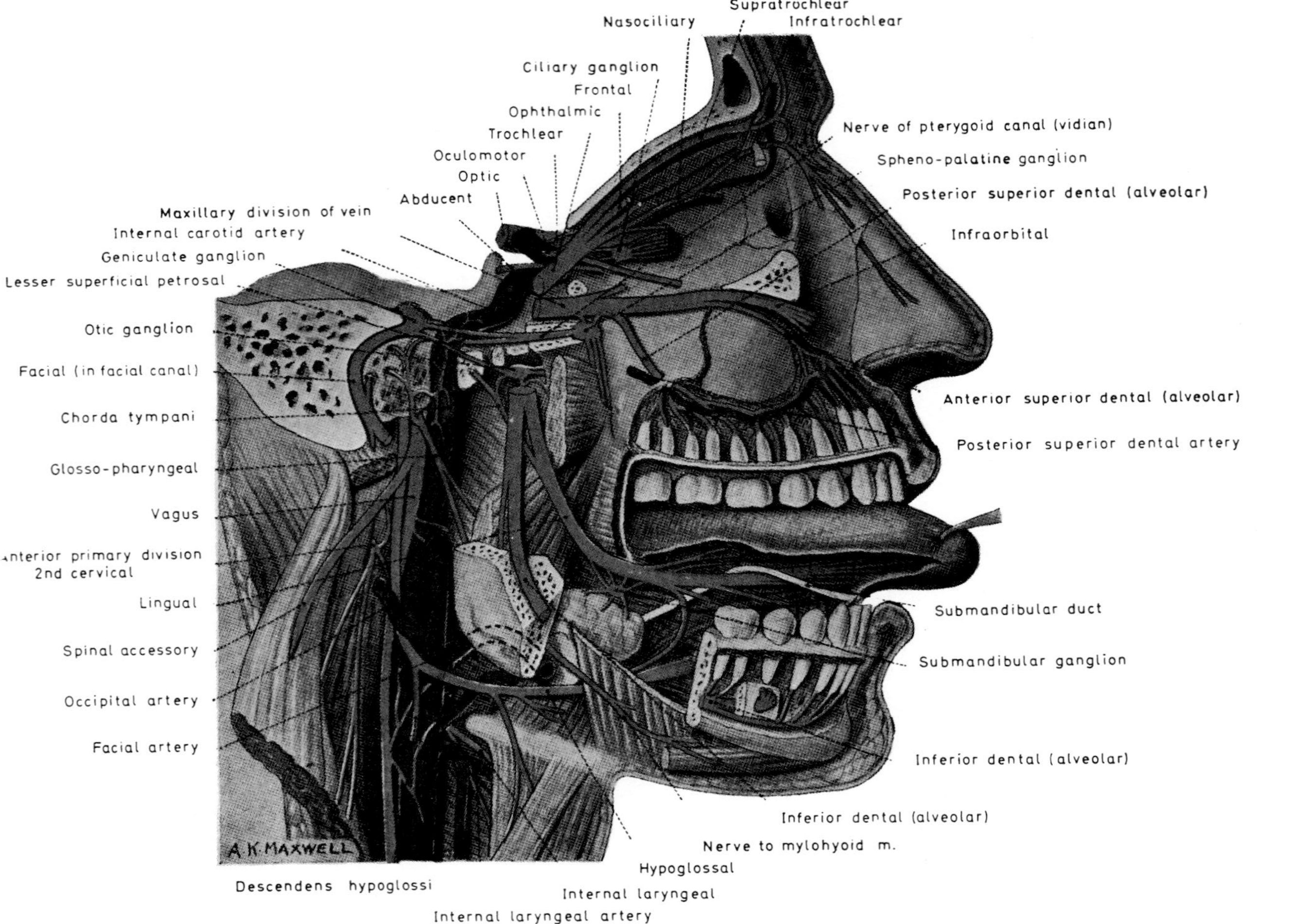

Figure 8.10 A deep dissection to show the distribution of the trigeminal and hypoglossal nerves. The mouth has been opened and

The nerves supplying the upper gum are derived from the maxillary nerve through its anterior palatine, naso-palatine and anterior, middle and posterior superior alveolar branches. The mandibular nerve innervates the lower gum by its inferior alveolar, lingual and buccal branches, the last two supplying the corresponding surfaces of the gum (*Figure 8.10*).

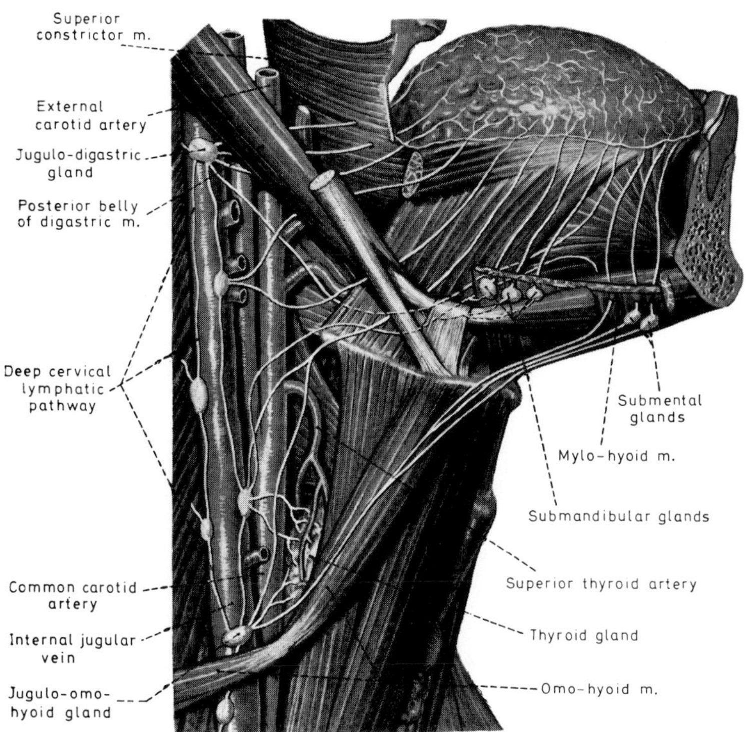

Figure 8.11 Lymph pathways of the tongue

The lymph vessels of the outer (buccal) aspect of both the upper and lower gums drain, with the deeper tissues of the cheek, into the submandibular nodes. The inner (lingual) aspect of the lower gum also drains into the submandibular group, but the inner aspect of the gum of the upper jaw drains, with the vessels of the hard and soft palates, directly into the upper deep cervical nodes; sometimes vessels may pass into the retro-pharyngeal nodes. The gum round the lower incisor teeth sometimes drains into the submental nodes (*Figure 8.11*).

Dental arches

Each dental arch is made up of the alveolar process, the gum and the teeth.

The alveolar processes are formed by the alveolar portions of the maxilla and mandible. In each process there is a series of sockets (alveoli) for the roots of the teeth. The alveolar processes are covered by the gums which consist of vascular mucous membrane supported by dense fibrous tissue firmly adherent to the underlying periosteum. At the neck of each tooth the gum forms a collar which is attached to the enamel of the tooth.

The number of teeth present in the different mammalian groups shows considerable variation; even amongst the primates the number is not constant. The generalized type of dentition which probably gave rise to that of the mammals had on each side of the jaw: three incisors, one canine, four pre-molars and three molars. Such a dentition is indicated by the dental formula

$$\text{I. } \frac{123}{123}, \quad \text{C. } \frac{1}{1}, \quad \text{P. } \frac{1234}{1234}, \quad \text{M. } \frac{123}{123}.$$

In Man and other primates some teeth have been suppressed. There is a tendency in 'modern man' to a further reduction in the number and size of the teeth.

In the *human temporary dentition*, completed during the first two years of life, there are ten teeth in each jaw. In each half of each jaw the dentition consists of two incisor teeth (medial and lateral), one canine and two molar teeth. The temporary teeth are gradually replaced by the *permanent teeth*, which number sixteen in each jaw (*Figures 8.7* and *8.9*). In each half of each jaw there are two incisors (medial and lateral), one canine, two pre-molars and three molars (first, second and third or wisdom tooth). The first tooth of this set (first molar) is erupted at about the sixth year, and the others at varying intervals until the age of 17 to 25 years.

Development and eruption of the teeth

The teeth begin to develop early in fetal life. (For a full description of the human dentition before birth *see* Kraus and Jordan, 1965.) The tooth is first represented by a crown; the root grows rapidly before the tooth is erupted and then slowly over a period of years. At birth the crowns of the temporary teeth, and of the incisors, canines and first molars of the permanent set, are well developed but none have erupted. The germs of the pre-molars and the second permanent molar teeth are only present in a rudimentary state, but those of the third molars do not appear until after birth. The crowns of all the temporary teeth have commenced to calcify before birth, but the process is not completed until later. In the permanent dentition, calcification begins in the crown of the first lower molar tooth before birth and shortly after birth in the first upper molar. About six months after birth the incisors become calcified, followed soon by the canines. Calcification does not commence in the pre-molars and second molar teeth until the second to fourth year. The third molar does not show calcification until about the tenth year. About six months after calcification has commenced in a tooth the crown will cast a shadow on a radiograph.

During the period that the teeth are developing and growing (i.e. during fetal life and childhood), an adequate supply of calcium and phosphates is required; in addition, vitamins A and D are essential for proper formation of the teeth. The diet of the mother during pregnancy may have a profound influence on the subsequent condition of the teeth of the child. The salts of calcium and phosphorus are essential for the formation of both enamel and dentine, while vitamin D is required for the utilization of these substances. When vitamin D is deficient, the surface of the teeth is rough instead of smooth and shiny, and the teeth erupt irregularly. If there is a deficiency of vitamin A, the ameloblasts fail to differentiate properly, and as a consequence their organizing influence upon adjacent dentine is disturbed, and so dentine is formed in an atypical manner. A tooth which is badly formed is more susceptible to caries than a normal tooth. (For details of the structure of enamel *see* Stack and Fernhead, 1965; Miles, 1967.)

The *eruption* of the teeth may be considered as part of the general process of body growth, and the times at which different teeth erupt therefore gives an indication of the physical state of a growing individual. The times of eruption of different teeth are subject to individual variations. It appears that the normal sequence of eruption is of greater importance than the precise time. Both the deciduous and permanent teeth erupt in moderately consistent sequence, but certain general conditions may cause considerable variation. Some of the deciduous teeth erupt earlier in boys than in girls, but many permanent teeth erupt earlier in girls. In taller children eruption tends to be accelerated.

A disturbance in the eruption sequence commonly results in malocclusions. (For descriptions of irregularity and malocclusion of teeth *see* Brash, 1956.)

Disturbances of the endocrine system, such as hypothyroidism, or nutritional deficiencies, such as vitamin D deficiency, may cause a marked delay in the eruption times of deciduous or permanent teeth (Miles, 1967).

Of the temporary dentition the first teeth to appear are the central incisors. The range of ages for eruption are as follows:

Lower central incisors	6–9 months
Upper incisors	8–10 months
Lower lateral incisors and first molars	15–20 months
Canines	16–20 months
Second molars	20–24 months

Of the permanent dentition the first molars erupt at about the sixth year, and the second at the twelfth year. The molars at the sixth year provide for mastication of food while deciduous teeth are being shed. The eruption of the other permanent teeth follows in a fairly regular sequence. The times at which the various teeth appear are:

First molar	end of 6th year
Median incisors	end of 7th year
Lateral incisors	end of 8th year
First pre-molars	between 10th and 11th years
Canines	between 11th and 12th years
Second pre-molars	between 11th and 12th years
Second molars	between 12th and 13th years
Third molars	between 17th and 25th years

During the eruption of the teeth important growth changes occur in both jaws, and more especially in the alveolar processes which must increase in size to accommodate the developing roots. The relations of the teeth to the jaws are also altered, and the alveolar process of the maxilla grows downwards, forwards and laterally, and the teeth show a concomitant movement. The relationship of the roots of the teeth to the floor of the enlarging maxillary sinus are altered as the roots increase in size; some roots eventually project into the sinus when it is fully developed. The growth of the jaws is a continuous process, but is accelerated at definite periods. In the first five years of life when the deciduous teeth are erupting there is an antero-posterior growth of the face. From the age of five to fifteen, during which period the deciduous teeth are shed and all the permanent teeth except the third molars are erupted, there is an extensive lateral and vertical growth of the face. This is associated with spurts of growth in all the air sinuses (Scott, 1967). The changes which occur in the proportions of the jaw bones are the result of the deposition of new bone in certain regions, and the absorption of bone in other areas. For example, the first lower permanent molar tooth lies during its development in the ramus of the mandible at the base of the coronoid process; in order to make room for this tooth, the mandible is remodelled by the absorption of the anterior part of the ramus, and the deposition of new bone on its posterior border. Space for the second and third molar teeth is obtained by a further remodelling of the bone as these teeth are erupted.

Arrangement of the teeth

The teeth are normally arranged in each jaw to form an arched curve without projections inwards or outwards of individual teeth. The arch formed by the teeth in the upper jaw is elliptical, while that in the lower jaw is parabolic.

In certain individuals the teeth may show irregularities in their arrangement, a condition termed *malocclusion*. This may be caused by irregularities in the arrangement of individual teeth or discord in the growth of the jaws. If the dental arches are narrowed with poorly developed alveolar processes, there is not sufficient space for the teeth, and so they become crowded and irregularly spaced. It is generally believed that these conditions are brought about by genetic factors rather than factors of post-natal origin. Local conditions, however, may also cause malocclusion, such as may result from injudicious extraction of teeth. Malocclusion is said to be more common in modern highly civilized people than in the more primitive races. This has been attributed to the less vigorous use of the jaws required with modern diet, though the evidence given to support such a view is in no way conclusive (Brash, 1956; Scott, 1967).

The nerve supply of the teeth of the upper jaw is by the alveolar branches of the maxillary nerve and those of the lower jaw by the inferior alveolar branch of the mandibular division of the trigeminal nerve.

Irritation of a decayed tooth usually causes pain which is felt in the tooth itself, but the sensation of pain may be referred to definite regions of the face and neck, associated chiefly with the distribution of the trigeminal nerve (*Figure 8.10*).

Palate

The palate, as already stated, forms the roof of the mouth and the floor of the nasal fossae (*Figures 8.8* and *8.12*). The anterior two-thirds is rigid and is distinguished as the *hard palate*. It is formed, for the greater part, by the palatine processes of the maxillae

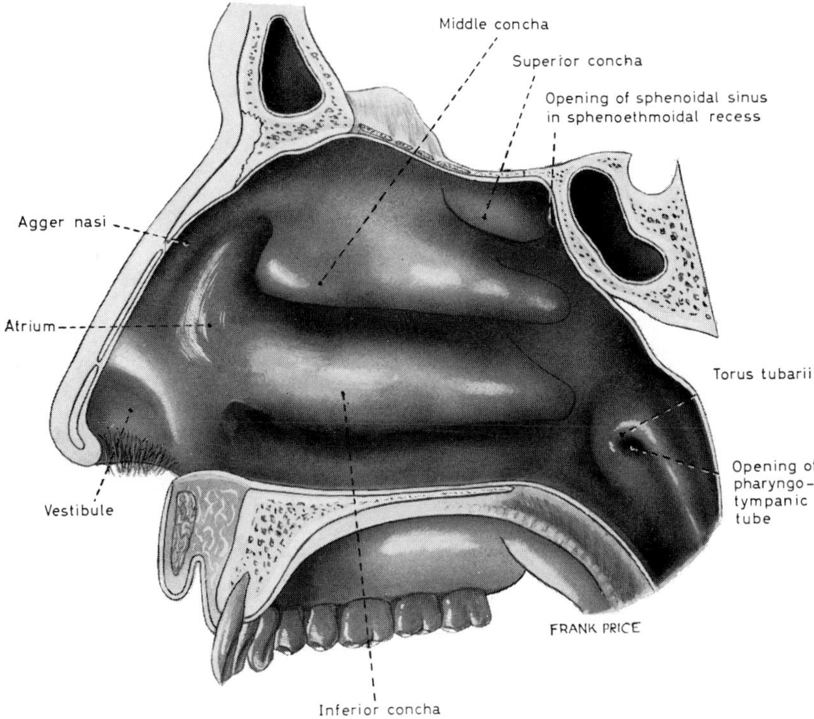

Figure 8.12 The lateral wall of the nasal cavity in the recent state

and the horizontal plates of the palatine bones (*Figure 8.12*). The posterior one-third constitutes the *soft palate*, a movable fibro-muscular partition which is attached to the posterior margin of the hard palate and to the side wall of the pharynx (*Figure 8.13*).

The shape of the normal palate varies in different individuals. In primitive man it was low and relatively flat, similar to that found in many living native races. During the last 500 years the form of the palate in Europeans has gradually changed and has tended to become highly vaulted and narrow; this has caused a crowding and misplacement of the teeth, and has altered the shape of the lower jaw so that the 'bite' is horseshoe-shaped with the teeth arranged in arches. This change in the form of the palate has been attributed to enlargement of the nasopharyngeal tonsils and consequent mouth breathing. Statistical analysis, however, reveals that a high palate is equally frequent in normal children.

Hard palate

The hard palate shows a faint median ridge (*Figure 8.14*) at the site of fusion of the original palatal processes of maxillary mesoderm. It ends anteriorly at the incisive fossa in a small elevation, the incisive papilla. Failure of fusion or incomplete fusion of the process gives rise to varying degrees of cleft palate. There is a number of transverse ridges on the anterior part of the palate. A midline hard swelling, the *torus palatinus*, is

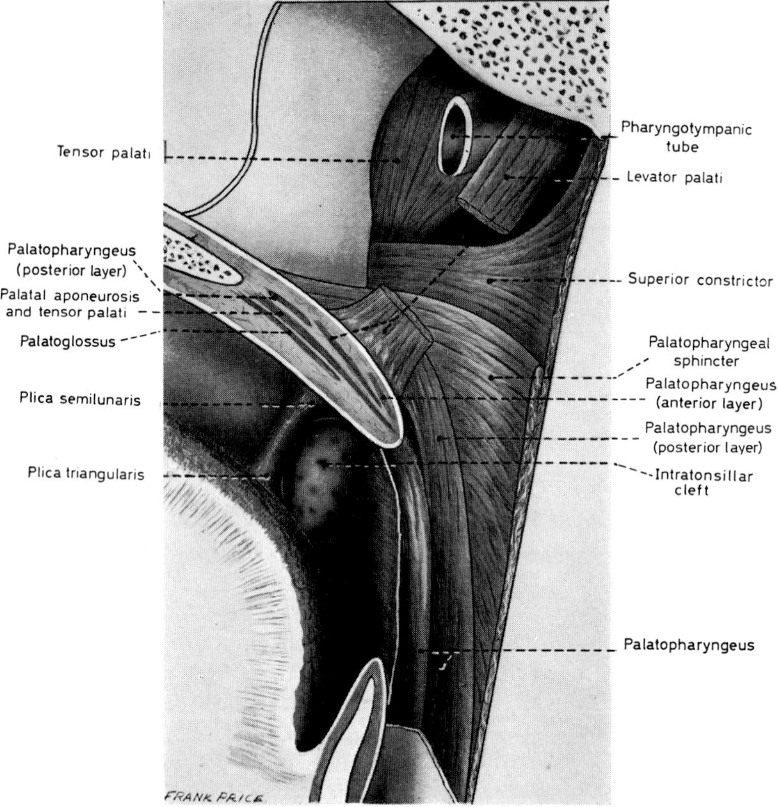

Figure 8.13 A drawing of the tonsil and the muscles of the palate (based on Browne, 1928, and Whillis, 1930)

occasionally mistaken when present for an exostosis or tumour. The mucous membrane of the hard palate is firmly united to the periosteum to form a mucoperiosteum, which posteriorly contains a large number of mucous glands.

Soft palate

The soft palate consists of a dense fibrous framework called the palatine aponeurosis, formed by the expanded tendons of the tensor palati muscles. To this aponeurosis the other palatine muscles are attached. The inferior surface, posterior margin, and to a variable extent the superior surface, are covered with stratified squamous epithelium. Columnar pseudo-stratified ciliated epithelium (respiratory epithelium) covers the rest of the superior surface. Much of the substance of the soft palate consists of mucous glands, and diffused amongst them is lymphoid tissue. Laterally the soft palate blends with the pharyngeal wall. Passing downwards from the palate are two folds – an anterior one to the side of the tongue, the *palatoglossal fold* formed by the palatoglossus muscle, and a posterior one to the pharyngeal wall, the *palatopharyngeal fold*, formed by the palatopharyngeus muscle (*Figures 8.8* and *8.13*). The soft palate is attached to the base of the skull on each side by two muscles, the tensor palati and the levator palati.

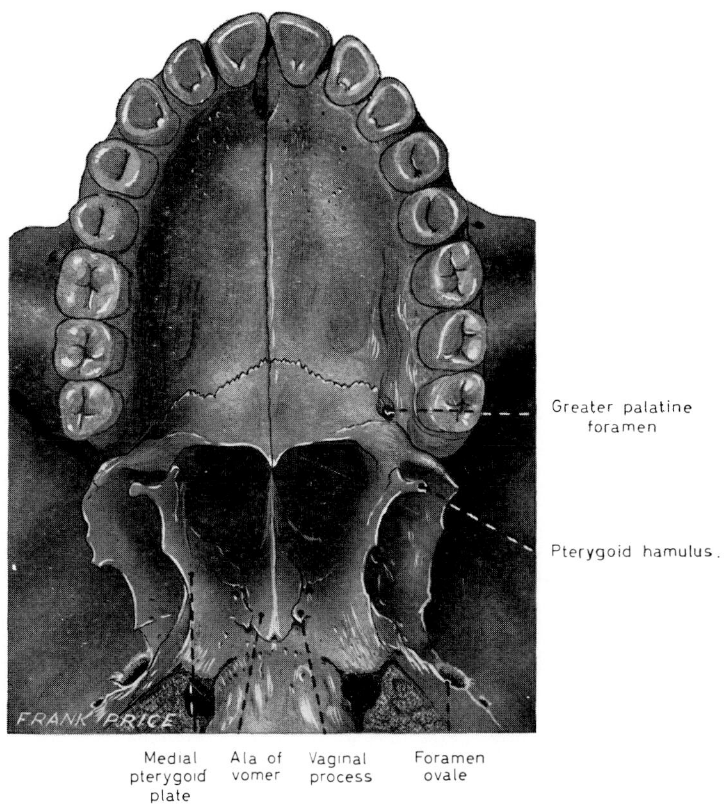

Figure 8.14 The palate and posterior nasal apertures seen from below

These muscles come into action in swallowing, breathing and phonation. Posteriorly the soft palate has a free margin which is prolonged downwards and backwards in the midline as a rounded projection of varying size, the *uvula*. Changes in the position of the soft palate, together with contraction of the superior constrictor muscle of the pharynx, regulate the size of the communication between the nasopharynx and the oropharynx. The nasal part of the pharynx can be completely shut off from the oral part. The movements of the soft palate can be appreciated better after the attachments of the muscles have been described.

Muscles of the soft palate

Tensor veli palatini (tensor palati)

Each muscle is fan-shaped and arises from the spine of the sphenoid bone, from the scaphoid fossa and from the lateral surface of the cartilaginous part of the pharyngotympanic tube. The muscle passes down on the lateral surface of the medial pterygoid plate to end in a tendon which passes round the pterygoid hamulus. The tendon spreads out and it forms the palatine aponeurosis, the anterior part of which is attached to the posterior edge of the hard palate (*Figure 8.13*).

Levator veli palatini (levator palati)

This muscle arises from the medial surface of the cartilaginous part of the pharyngotympanic tube and from the adjacent area of the petrous part of the temporal bone in front of the carotid canal. As the muscle passes downwards to the palate it lies on the medial side of the upper part of the superior constrictor muscle (*Plate 5, facing page 302* and *Figure 8.13*). The muscle of each side is inserted into the palatine aponeurosis and blends with its fellow of the opposite side in the middle line of the palate.

Palatoglossus

This muscle has attachments to the side of the tongue and the soft palate. The fibres pass from the tongue in the palatoglossal fold and end in the anterior part of the palatine aponeurosis. The fibres of each muscle are inserted into the other in the middle line.

Palatopharyngeus

This muscle arises from the pharyngeal aponeurosis and from the posterior border of the thyroid cartilage. (The origin is commonly described as the insertion of the muscle.) The muscle fibres pass almost vertically upwards to the palate in the palatopharyngeal fold (*Plate 5*). As the muscle passes forwards to the palate it divides into two strands (*Figure 8.13*). One strand passes anteriorly and laterally to the levator palati and is inserted into the anterior part of the superior surface of the palatal aponeurosis and the posterior edge of the hard palate. This strand lies above the musculus uvulae. The other more inferior strand passes medial to the levator and blends with its fellow of the opposite side in the middle line. In the palate this strand lies below the musculus uvulae.

Musculus uvulae

The muscle of each side arises from the posterior nasal spine and passes backwards between the two layers of the palatopharyngeus and above the levator veli palatini muscle. The muscles of each side unite as they are inserted into the mucous membrane of the uvula.

Nerve and blood supply

The muscles of the soft palate, except the tensor palati, are all supplied by the pharyngeal plexus. The motor fibres in the pharyngeal plexus are mainly derived from the cranial root of the accessory nerve. They are carried by the vagus and are distributed to the pharyngeal plexus by the pharyngeal branch of the vagus. The tensor veli palatini is supplied by fibres from the mandibular division of the trigeminal nerve which pass through the otic ganglion. Phylogenetically the tensor veli palatini was originally a muscle of mastication.

The sensory nerves of the soft palate are derived from the lesser palatine branches of the spheno-palatine ganglion and from branches of the glossopharyngeal nerve.

The blood supply of the soft palate is from branches of the ascending palatine branch of the facial artery, the lesser palatine branches of the greater palatine branch of the maxillary artery and the palatine branch of the ascending pharyngeal artery.

The ascending palatine branch of the facial artery runs on the side wall of the pharynx and sends a branch over the upper free edge of the superior constrictor muscle to pass down on the inner aspect of the pharynx to supply the soft palate. The palatine branch of the ascending pharyngeal artery follows a similar course, and running parallel to the levator palati enters the inner aspect of the pharynx. The greater palatine branch from the maxillary artery runs through the greater palatine canal and gives off several lesser palatine arteries which pass through small canals to reach the soft palate.

The venous drainage runs mainly into the tonsillar and pterygoid plexuses, and from there to the anterior facial vein through the deep facial vein. The pterygoid plexus is also connected with the cavernous sinus by emissary veins passing through the foramina in the base of the skull. The lymphatic drainage of the soft palate is partly to the retropharyngeal nodes and partly direct to the upper deep cervical nodes.

Tongue

The tongue is a muscular organ situated in the floor of the mouth and the anterior wall of the pharynx (*Figures 8.7* and *8.8*). It is concerned with mastication, deglutination, phonation, touch and taste. There is a free portion or tip, and a main mass or body with a free rounded border as far back as the last molar tooth. It is attached by muscles to the hyoid bone below, the mandible in front, the styloid process behind, and the palate above, and by mucous membrane to the floor of the mouth, the lateral walls of the pharynx and the epiglottis (*Figures 8.7* and *8.15*). When the mouth is closed the anterior two-thirds of the upper surface or dorsum is convex

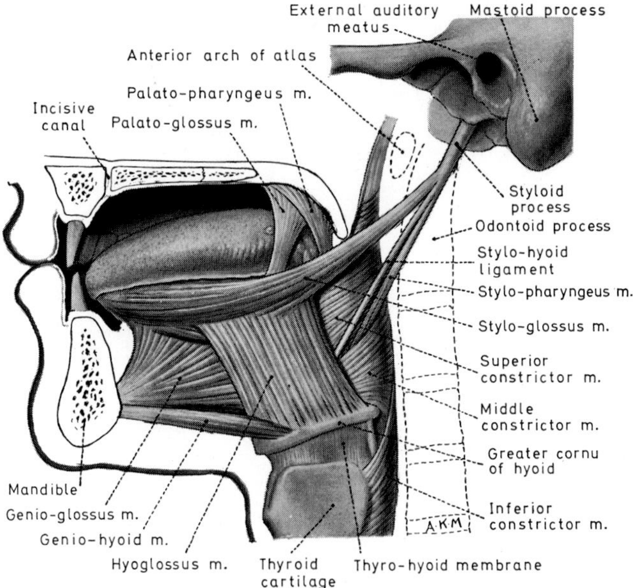

Figure 8.15 Lateral view of the muscles of the tongue and upper part of the pharynx

from before backwards and from side to side, and it is moulded into the vault formed by the superior dental arch and palate.

The dorsum of the tongue is subdivided by a 'V-shaped' groove, the *sulcus terminalis*, into an anterior palatine part and a posterior pharyngeal part. Anterior to the groove are the vallate papillae (*Figure 8.7*). At the apex of the sulcus terminalis which is directed backwards, there is a depression, the *foramen caecum*. This foramen indicates the site of origin of the thyroid downgrowth from the floor of the mouth. The anterior portion of the tongue is developed from the first pharyngeal arch and is supplied by the nerves associated with that arch, namely, the lingual branch of the trigeminal nerve, the post-trematic nerve of the first arch and the chorda tympani, a branch of the nerve of the second arch. The pharyngeal portion arises from the second and third pharyngeal arches. The third, however, grows over the second arch, separating the tissues of the second arch from the surface epithelium. The nerves to this part are from the third arch nerve, the glossopharyngeal, and the internal laryngeal branch of the vagus nerve from the fourth arch.

Structure

The tongue consists of: (a) a mucous membrane which is shaped like an inverted shoe covering the organ except at the root where the muscles, vessels and nerves enter; (b) mucous glands; (c) lymphoid tissue and fat; (d) interlacing bundles of striated muscle fibres, which constitute the greater part of the tongue; (e) fibrous tissue. A median connective tissue septum divides the tongue into right and left halves. The septum is of surgical importance, since an abscess on one side of the tongue is thus confined to that side.

Mucous membrane

The mucosa of the tongue is firmly adherent to the underlying muscle tissue and is covered by stratified squamous epithelium. The superficial cells are continuously being cast off and replaced by cells of the deeper layer. In living subjects the appearance of the tongue varies in different regions. In healthy individuals the oral part of the mucous membrane is pink and studded with numerous small projections, the papillae, which give it a velvety appearance; the pharyngeal part is smoother and shows nodular elevations due to the underlying lymphoid nodules and mucous glands. The mucous membrane, however, of the posterior part of the oral surface of the tongue may be covered by a thin whitish fur. A median fold, the *glosso-epiglottic fold*, passes backwards from the root of the tongue to the epiglottis, and laterally, the *pharyngo-epiglottic folds* pass from the sides of the tongue and pharyngeal wall to the *epiglottis*. Between the glosso-epiglottic fold and the pharyngo-epiglottic fold of each side there is a depression, the *vallecula*. On the inferior surface of the tongue the mucous membrane is thin and smooth and more loosely connected to the underlying muscle. In the median line below the tip of the tongue the mucous membrane is raised into a sagittal fold, the frenulum linguae (*Figure 8.9*), on each side of which there is a second fold, the fimbriated fold.

Papillae

These are projections consisting of a connective tissue core covered with stratified squamous epithelium. Three varieties can be recognized – *vallate* (circumvallate), *fungiform and filiform.*

Vallate papillae
These are the largest and most distinct. They vary from 7 to 12 in number and are arranged in a row parallel to and in front of the sulcus terminalis (*Figure 8.7*). These vallate papillae are so called because they are surrounded by a circular groove round

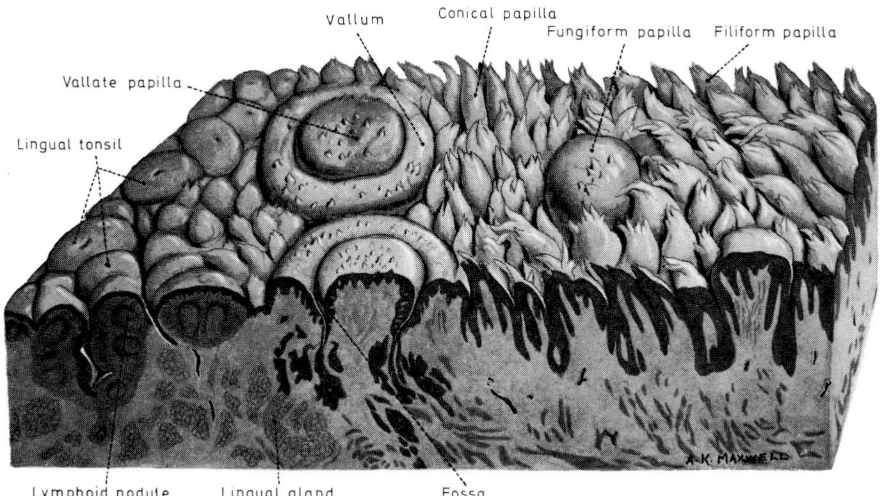

Figure 8.16 Surface view of the tongue at the junction between the anterior two-thirds and the posterior one-third to show the papillae (based on Braus)

which is an annular fold, the vallum, of the mucous membrane (*Figure 8.16*). Ducts of one or more serous glands open into the groove. Each papilla projects slightly above the general surface level.

Fungiform papillae
These are smaller and more numerous than the vallate papillae. They are somewhat globular in form with a slightly constricted stalk (*Figure 8.16*), and are especially numerous near the tip and margins of the tongue. They can be distinguished in the living individual by their bright red colour, due to their rich blood supply and comparatively thin epithelial covering.

Filiform papillae
These are the most numerous of the papillae, and are found on the dorsum of the tongue arranged in rows parallel to the sulcus terminalis. At the tip, however, they are arranged transversely. Each consists of a central connective tissue core, the summit of which shows several secondary papillae with pointed tips (*Figure 8.16*). The epithelial covering follows the outlines of the central core. The superficial cells are

transformed into hard scales. In the general disturbances which accompany disease processes, but also even in quite healthy individuals, the scales may accumulate on the tongue and, together with disintegrating lymphocytes and other debris, give it a 'coated' appearance.

Taste buds

Associated with the papillae are the microscopic taste buds, each of which is somewhat flask-shaped, with a wide base and a short narrow neck opening at the taste pore. Each bud has two kinds of cells – supporting and neuro-epithelial taste cells (*Figure 8.17*). The supporting cells are elongated and spindle-shaped, but vary

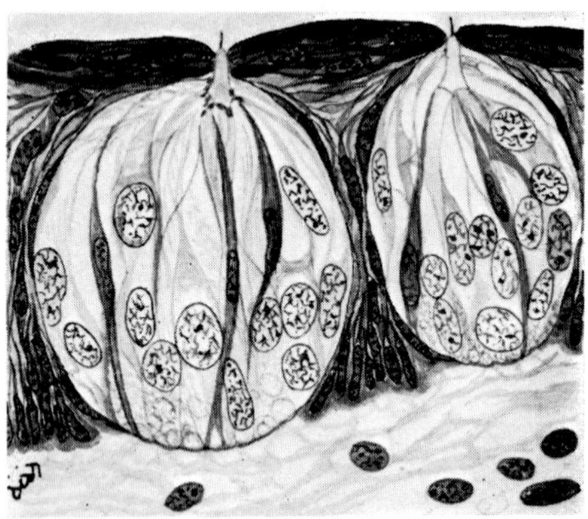

Figure 8.17 A semi-schematic drawing of two taste buds. The peripheral processes of the taste cells pass through the taste pores

somewhat in shape according to their position. The taste cells are in the centre of the bud amongst the supporting cells. Each of the taste cells is spindle-shaped, and from the peripheral extremity of the cell, a fine hairlike process projects on to the surface through the taste pore. Centrally, each cell ends in a fine filament. The terminal branches of the taste nerve fibres terminate in relation to the taste cells.

Glands

Many serous and mucous glands are situated behind the sulcus terminalis. Others are embedded in the muscle on the under-surface of the apex of the tongue, where they constitute the anterior lingual glands.

Lymphoid tissue

Numerous lymphoid masses, the *lingual tonsils*, are found in the posterior third of the tongue, to which they impart an irregular nodular appearance (*Figures 8.7* and *8.16*). Between the nodules are irregular spaces or *crypts*.

Muscles

The muscles of the tongue are paired and are grouped into an *extrinsic* and an *intrinsic* set, and by their action they move the tongue and alter its shape. They comprise, on each side, the genioglossus, the hyoglossus and the styloglossus.

Genioglossus

This is a fan-shaped muscle which arises from the corresponding upper genial tubercle of the mandible and is inserted into the tongue from its tip to its root (*Figure 8.15*). Acting in conjunction the two genioglossi protrude the tongue, but each genioglossus acting by itself draws the tongue forwards, and over to the opposite side. Hence if one muscle is paralysed, the protruded organ deviates to the paralysed side.

Hyoglossus

This is a flat quadrilateral muscle arising from the greater cornu of the hyoid bone and passing upwards to be inserted into the side of the tongue (*Figure 8.15*). By its contraction the side of the tongue is depressed.

Styloglossus

This is a slender muscle arising from the styloid process near the tip, and passing forwards and downwards, is inserted into the side of the tongue (*Figure 8.15*). By its contraction the tongue is drawn upwards and backwards.

The palatoglossus muscle is described with the muscles of the palate.

The intrinsic muscle fibres are arranged in four groups, superior and inferior longitudinal, transverse and vertical. By their actions they alter the shape of the tongue.

Vessels and nerves

Arteries and veins

The tongue has a rich blood supply. Hence when it is injured there may be profuse bleeding, but wounds heal rapidly on account of the vascularity. There is practically no communication between the arteries of the right and left halves of the tongue except at its tip. The lingual artery is the main blood supply of the tongue. The artery runs forward immediately above the hyoid bone, passing deep to the hyoglossus, and continues to the tip of the tongue as the profunda artery. At its termination the artery is quite superficial, covered by the mucous membrane on the inferior surface of the tongue. In this situation the pulsation of the artery may be seen, and can usually be felt on holding the tongue between the thumb and the index finger. Bleeding from the tongue may easily be controlled by pulling the tongue forwards and downwards over the lower jaw. The veins from the tongue drain eventually into the internal jugular vein.

Lymphatics

The lymph vessels of the tongue all drain finally into the deep cervical nodes (*Figure 8.11*). Those from the tip of the tongue usually pass first to the submental nodes, whereas those from the remainder of the anterior two-thirds usually traverse the submandibular lymph nodes, having pierced the mylohyoid muscle. From the posterior one-third of the tongue lymph passes to the upper nodes of the deep cervical chain, and that from the anterior two-thirds passes to nodes at a level below this. There is a varying degree of communication between lymphatics from the right and left halves of the tongue.

Nerves

The muscles, intrinsic and extrinsic, with the exception of the palatoglossus, are supplied by the hypoglossal nerve (*Figure 8.10*).

The sensory nerves are those of taste and common sensation. The sensation of taste from the anterior two-thirds of the tongue is conveyed by the chorda tympani branch of the facial nerve, and from the posterior one-third, by the glossopharyngeal nerve, and by the internal laryngeal nerve, a branch of the vagus. The nerves of common sensibility are the lingual branch of the mandibular division of the trigeminal nerve from the anterior two-thirds of the tongue, and the glossopharyngeal nerve from the posterior one-third.

Salivary glands

The salivary glands consist of:

(1) A number of small glands, situated in the mucosa and submucosa of the buccal cavity, which are given special names according to their situation, e.g. labial glands in the lips, lingual glands beneath the mucous membrane of the tongue, and palatine glands on the under-surface of the palate. These glands probably secrete more or less continuously and their secretion moistens and lubricates the oral mucous membrane.

(2) Three pairs of large glands – the *parotid*, *submandibular* and *sublingual* glands. These glands open by ducts into the mouth cavity. They do not secrete continuously but only when the sensory nerve-endings in the oral mucous membrane are activated by mechanical, chemical or thermal stimuli. They also secrete as the result of 'psychic' or olfactory stimulation. The glands may be classified according to the type of their secretory epithelium. The parotid gland is composed of serous cells and secretes a watery saliva; the submandibular and sublingual glands are described as mixed glands since they have both mucous and serous cells.

Parotid gland

This is the largest of the salivary glands. It has a lobulated appearance, and an irregular wedge shape (*Figure 8.7*) in conformity with the retromandibular space which it occupies. The gland is covered by a capsule, the parotid sheath, a prolongation upwards of the investing fascia of the neck (*Figure 8.7*). The strong sheath covering the superficial surface offers considerable resistance to swelling of the gland.

The parotid gland is divided into two lobes, a superficial lobe and a deep lobe, by the main branches of the facial nerve which pass through it in a fascial plane. The facial nerve enters the upper part of the posteromedial surface and divides within the gland into the terminal branches which appear at the anterior border (*Figure 8.20*). Immediately deep to the branches of the facial nerve lie the posterior facial vein and its tributaries. The vein passes downwards roughly parallel to the posterior border of the vertical ramus of the mandible. On a slightly deeper plane still lies the external carotid artery which divides in the substance of the gland into its terminal branches, the superficial temporal and internal maxillary arteries. The former continues upwards through the gland to become superficial in the temporal region just anterior to the tragus, and the internal maxillary passes inwards towards the pterygo-maxillary fissure. A detailed description of the surgical anatomy of the parotid gland will be found in Volume 4.

Three main surfaces can be recognized – a superficial, an anteromedial and a posteromedial. The superficial surface of the gland is somewhat triangular in outline. It extends upwards to the zygomatic arch, backwards to the external auditory meatus and the anterior border of the sternomastoid muscle, and forwards over the surface of the masseter muscle. The anteromedial surface is in contact with the posterior surface of the ramus of the mandible, and with the masseter and medial pterygoid muscles. The posteromedial surface lies against the mastoid process, the sternomastoid and the posterior belly of the digastric muscle (*Figure 8.7*). The deepest part of the gland is related to the styloid process with its attached muscles, the internal carotid artery and the internal jugular vein. The lower part of the gland extends downwards into the neck, between the angle of the mandible and the sternomastoid muscle. In addition to

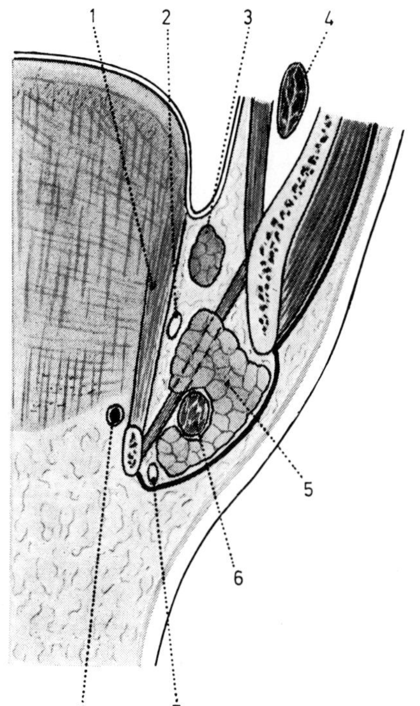

Figure 8.18 Submandibular gland. (1) Hyoglossus muscle; (2) lingual nerve; (3) sublingual gland; (4) internal pterygoid muscle; (5) submandibular gland; (6) digastric muscle; (7) hypoglossal nerve; (8) lingual artery

the three main surfaces there is a limited superior surface in contact with the cartilaginous and bony floor of the external auditory meatus. The *parotid duct* arises from the most prominent part of the anterior border of the gland, passes forwards on the masseter muscle, and then turns round its anterior border to pierce the buccinator muscle (*Figure 8.20*). It enters the vestibule of the mouth at the level of the crown of the second upper molar tooth. Associated with the duct is an accessory parotid gland.

The external carotid artery divides within the gland into the maxillary artery, which passes from the anteromedial surface of the gland and the superficial temporal artery which emerges from the upper border. The posterior facial vein is formed within the gland.

Submandibular gland

This gland has a lobulated appearance; it consists of an oval-shaped main part, situated superficially in the digastric triangle partly under cover of the body of the mandible, and a small deep part lying in the floor of the mouth, above the mylohyoid muscle (*Figure 8.20*). The two portions are continuous around the free posterior border of this muscle. The superficial portion of the gland extends as far backwards as the lower part of the parotid, from which it is separated by a layer of fascia. The superficial portion has a superficial and a deep surface. The upper part of the superficial surface is related to the submandibular fossa of the mandible and the medial pterygoid muscle. The lower part is relatively superficial, being covered by the deep fascia, platysma, subcutaneous tissue and skin. Some submandibular lymph nodes lie superficial to the gland, or may be actually embedded in it, and near its posterior part the anterior facial vein passes backwards and downwards. Below, the medial surface overlaps the posterior belly of the digastric and the stylohyoid muscles.

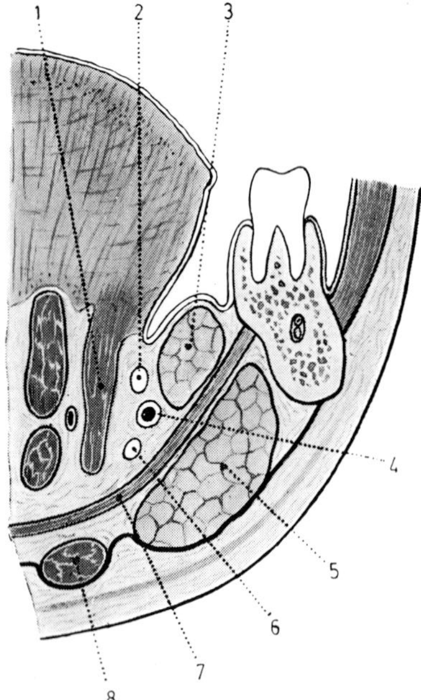

Figure 8.19 Submandibular gland. (1) Hyoglossus muscle; (2) lingual nerve; (3) sublingual gland; (4) submandibular duct; (5) submandibular gland; (6) hypoglossal nerve; (7) mylohyoid muscle; (8) anterior belly of digastric muscle

Above, the gland rests on the mylohyoid muscle in front, and the hyoglossus muscle behind (*Figure 8.19*). The facial artery grooves the posterior part of the gland and emerges between it and the mandible. The deep portion of the gland extends forwards on the upper surface of the mylohyoid muscle as far as the posterior border of the sublingual gland. Above, it is covered by the mucous membrane of the mouth. Medially, it is related to the hypoglossal and lingual nerves as they lie on the hyoglossus muscle. The *submandibular duct* is formed in the superficial part of the gland; it passes into the deep portion from which it extends forwards to open in the mouth at the anterior edge of the sublingual fold at the side of the frenulum of the tongue. As the duct passes forward it lies above the lingual nerve. Both the hypoglossal nerve and the submandibular duct may be accompanied by venae comitans.

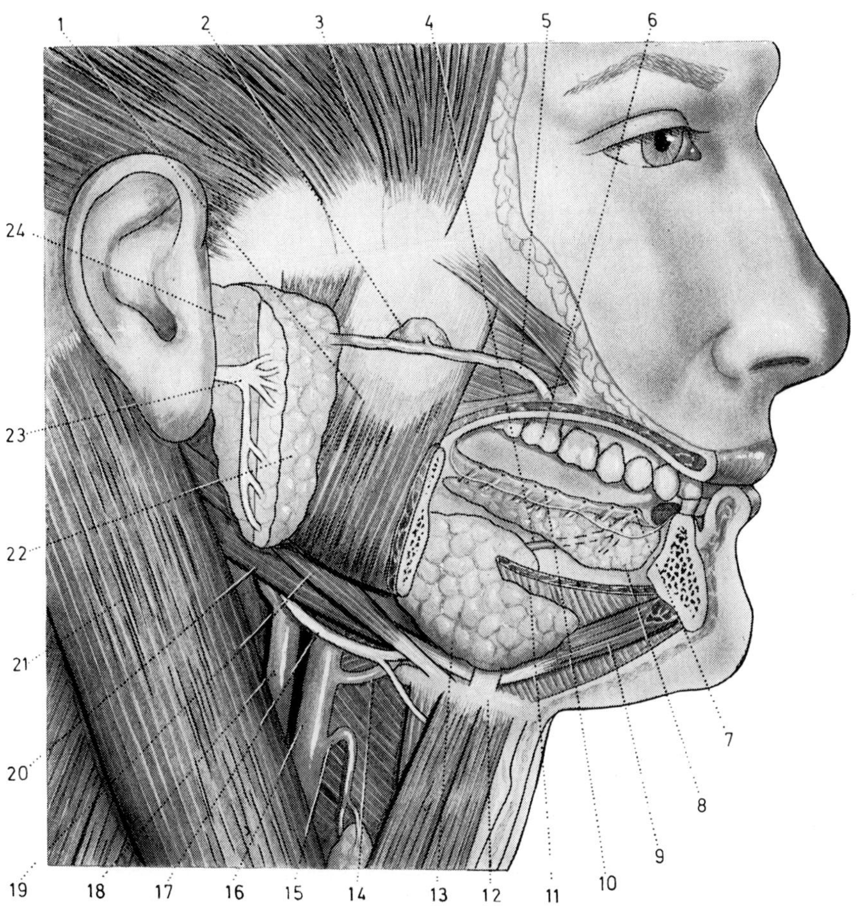

Figure 8.20 A lateral view of the face to show the relationships of the salivary glands. Portions of the mandible and the parotid gland have been removed. (1) masseter muscle; (2) accessory lobe of parotid gland; (3) temporalis muscle; (4) submandibular duct; (5) parotid duct; (6) second molar tooth; (7) smaller sublingual duct; (8) sublingual gland; (9) anterior belly of digastric muscle; (10) sublingual fold; (11) mylohyoid muscle; (12) hyoid bone; (13) submandibular gland; (14) lingual artery; (15) superior thyroid artery; (16) external carotid artery; (17) hypoglossal nerve; (18) internal carotid artery; (19) stylohyoid muscle; (20) posterior belly of digastric muscle; (21) sternomastoid muscle; (22) parotid gland; (23) facial nerve; (24) parotid gland (cut surface)

Sublingual gland

This, the smallest of the main salivary glands, is almond-shaped. It is situated in the floor of the mouth, where it produces an elevation, the sublingual fold, between the tongue and the mandible (*Figures 8.19* and *8.20*). The gland extends backwards and outwards from the frenulum of the tongue, and comes into contact posteriorly with the deep part of the submandibular gland. Below, the gland rests on the mylohyoid muscle. Above, it is separated from the buccal cavity by mucous membrane. Medially, it is related to the genioglossus muscle, and laterally to the sublingual fossa of the mandible. The lobules of the gland are loosely held together by connective tissue. The anterior part of the gland is compact and has a duct called the greater sublingual, which opens into the submandibular duct. The posterior lobules are loosely arranged and have several ducts, the lesser sublingual, opening separately into the mouth on the side of the sublingual fold.

Structure of salivary glands

The parotid, submandibular and sublingual glands are compound tubulo-alveolar glands. They consist of glandular tissue or parenchyma, supported by an interstitial connective-tissue framework through which blood vessels and nerves are distributed. The parenchyma is composed of branching duct systems and the secretory epithelium of the alveoli (acini). As already stated, the cells lining the alveoli may be all of the serous type, all mucous, or mixed. In sections stained with haemotoxylin and eosin, the mucous cells are light in colour, whereas the serous cells are dark. The mucous cells appear empty, but special staining methods (e.g. mucicarmine) show that they contain mucinogen granules, the precursors of mucus.

The parotid gland has serous alveoli only, the submandibular gland is formed mainly of serous alveoli, while in the sublingual gland mucous and mixed alveoli predominate. The cells of the serous alveoli are tall and pyramidal, with a spherical nucleus, and surround a narrow lumen. Fine intercellular secretory canaliculi penetrate between the cells and may even extend into the cells as intracellular

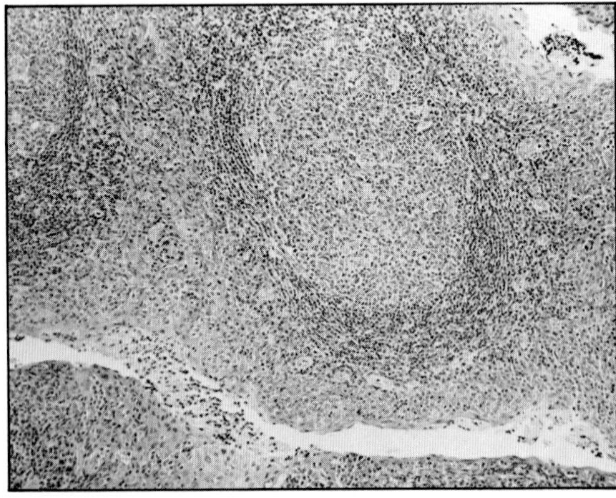

Figure 8.21 Section of submandibular gland showing serous and mucous acini and a minor duct

canaliculi. In the mixed alveoli of the sublingual gland especially, and also in the submandibular, the serous cells form *demilunes* (Heidenhain) or *crescents* (Gianuzzi) on one side of the wall of the alveolus. The demilunes are frequently separated from the lumen by the mucous cells, and communicate with it by intercellular canaliculi. The mucous alveoli have a distinct lumen; the nuclei of the cells stain deeply and are flattened and compressed against the basement membrane (*see Figure 8.21*).

The alveoli in the parotid and submandibular glands are joined to the salivary ducts by the so-called intercalated ducts, which are lined with a low epithelium. The intercalated ducts are well developed and branched in the parotid gland, short in the submandibular, but absent in the sublingual.

The salivary ducts are easily recognized by their intense staining with eosin, and by the acidophilic striation in the deeper part of the cells between the nuclei and the basement membrane. There is evidence that the cells lining the salivary tubules can contribute water and certain salts from the surrounding tissue fluids to the secretion of the alveoli.

Blood supply of salivary glands

The parotid gland derives its arterial supply from branches of the maxillary and superficial temporal arteries. The submandibular gland is supplied by branches from the facial artery and the sublingual gland by branches from the sublingual and submental arteries.

Nerves

Each of these glands receive parasympathetic (secretomotor), sympathetic and sensory fibres. The parotid gland derives its secretomotor fibres from the tympanic branch of the glossopharyngeal nerve through the otic ganglion from which fibres are distributed through the auriculo-temporal nerve to the gland. The sympathetic fibres are derived from the plexus surrounding the external carotid artery and the sensory fibres from the auriculo-temporal nerve. The submandibular and sublingual glands receive their parasympathetic secretomotor fibres via the chorda tympani nerve and their sympathetic innervation from the sympathetic plexus on the facial artery. The sensory fibres are carried by the lingual nerve.

Lymphatic drainage

The lymph vessels of the parotid pass to the pre-auricular and upper deep cervical nodes. The submandibular and sublingual glands drain into the submandibular and upper deep cervical nodes (*Figure 8.11*).

The pharynx

Descriptive anatomy

The pharynx is a cone-shaped space, bounded by fibromuscular walls. It extends from the base of the skull, to which its walls are firmly attached, as far as the lower border of the cricoid cartilage, where it becomes continuous with the oesophagus at the level of the sixth cervical vertebra. The walls of the pharynx are formed from within outwards by the mucous membrane, the pharyngobasilar fascia, a muscular coat and the pharyngeal part of the buccopharyngeal fascia. Anteriorly the pharyngeal wall is deficient so that the cavity is in free communication, from above downwards, with the nasal cavity through the posterior nasal apertures, with the buccal cavity by the oropharyngeal isthmus, and with the larynx by the laryngeal aditus.

Interior of the pharynx

The cavity of the pharynx is incompletely divided by the soft palate, except during swallowing, into an upper part, the nasopharynx, and a lower part, which is further subdivided into an oral part, behind the oropharyngeal isthmus, and a laryngeal part behind the larynx (*Figure 8.8*). The pharynx in the adult measures 12–14 cm in its greatest length. The width of the pharynx is greatest in the nasal part, where it measures about 3.5 cm; in the oral part it is about 1 cm. At the junction of the pharynx with the oesophagus the width is reduced to less than 1.5 cm. This junction of the pharynx with the oesophagus is the least dilatable part of the alimentary canal, with the exception of the appendix.

Nasal part of the pharynx

The nasopharynx lies behind the nasal cavities and above the soft palate. Anteriorly, as already stated, it is in free communication with the nasal cavities on each side of the free edge of the nasal septum. The roof of the nasopharynx abuts against the under-surface of the basi-sphenoid and the basi-occipital as far back as the pharyngeal tubercle. The upper part of the posterior wall of the pharynx lies in front of the anterior arch of the atlas.

A collection of lymphoid tissue, the nasopharyngeal tonsil, is found embedded in the mucous membrane at the junction of the roof with the upper and posterior part of the nasopharynx. In a young child the nasopharyngeal tonsil is almost triangular in shape, with the apex extending forwards towards the back of the nasal septum. The pharyngeal bursa, appearing as a blind recess, lies close to the base of the nasopharyngeal tonsil. The lymphatic tissue of the nasopharyngeal tonsil grows rapidly until about the age of six years, after which it usually shows retrogressive changes. On each lateral wall there is the narrow pharyngeal orifice of the pharyngotympanic tube. This orifice is situated 1.25 cm behind the inferior concha (tubinate), and is partially surrounded postero-superiorly by the torus. The latter is formed by the medial cartilaginous part of the pharyngotympanic tube. Immediately behind the torus there is a narrow vertical depression, the pharyngeal recess (Rosenmüller). This recess passes laterally above the upper edge of the superior constrictor muscle of the pharynx and corresponds to the position of the sinus of Morgagni. A ridge in the mucous membrane, produced by the underlying salpingopharyngeus muscle, passes down from the lower edge of the torus of the tube and gradually fades out on the pharyngeal wall. A less well defined ridge passes from the anterior opening of the tube to the upper surface of the soft palate. The levator palatai muscle produces this elevation. Both ridges are more prominent when their respective underlying muscles contract.

Oral part of the pharynx

The oropharynx extends from the soft palate to the inlet of the larynx (*Figure 8.8*). It communicates with the buccal cavity at the oropharyngeal isthmus. The lateral boundary between the buccal cavity and the oropharynx is marked by the palatoglossal fold, which passes from the under-surface of the palate to the side of the mucous membrane of the tongue a little posterior to its middle. The palatoglossus muscle lies in this fold. A second fold, the palatopharyngeal, passes downwards and backwards from the posterior edge of the soft palate to the side wall of the pharynx. This fold is produced by the underlying palatopharyngeus muscle. The faucial tonsil lies in a somewhat triangular tonsillar fossa, bounded by the antero-superior and palatopharyngeal folds, and the posterior part of the side of the tongue. A thin triangular fold of mucous membrane, the plica triangularis, passes backwards from the palatoglossal fold and frequently partially covers the tonsil; the antero-superior part of the edge of this fold is free, while the lower border is attached to the tongue. A further thin triangular fold of mucous membrane, the plica semilunaris, is frequently found connecting the palatoglossal and palatopharyngeal folds above the tonsil. The tonsil itself may thus project into the cavity of the pharynx.

The tonsil

The tonsil is usually described as an oval mass of lymphoid tissue, but as it occupies a triangular space, which it completely fills (Browne, 1928), it follows that its deep part is almost triangular in shape in its normal state (*Figure 8.13*). The free surface varies so enormously in its appearance that it is almost impossible to give an adequate description; furthermore, it presents varying appearances in different subjects and in the same subject at successive ages. It may, and frequently does, bulge into the pharynx, or it may be sessile and limited to the tonsillar fossa. Usually, in the upper part of the tonsil, an intratonsillar cleft is found. In the past this has often been inaccurately called the supratonsillar fossa. The intratonsillar cleft represents the remains of the ventral part of the second pharyngeal pouch. In addition to the intratonsillar cleft, the surface shows a large number of narrow crypts, the tonsillar crypts. The upper part of the tonsil, which passes deep to the plica semilunaris, reaches to, and frequently extends into, the soft palate. The inferior part of the tonsil comes into contact with the tongue and is often attached to its base. The deep or lateral surface of the tonsil is covered by a fibrous tissue capsule from the inner surface of which fibrous septa pass into the tonsil. The fibres of the palatoglossus and palatopharyngeus muscles are attached to the capsule.

Structure As already indicated, the tonsil is broken up into a series of lobules by fibrous tissue septa that arise from the capsule. From the septa a network of reticular connective tissue permeates the entire organ. The reticulocytes are probably part of the reticulo-endothelial system. Amongst this network are lymphoid follicles composed of aggregations of lymphocytes. In each follicle there is a germinal centre which is the site of active proliferation of the lymphocytes. Taillens (1944) has given an extensive review on the activity of the germinal centres. He agrees with the theory of Hellman (1930) that these are centres of reaction rather than areas of lymphocytic proliferation. In the atrophic tonsil the centres are reduced in size or may be absent.

The free surface of the tonsil is covered with stratified squamous epithelium which also lines the tonsillar crypts. Frequently these crypts contain lymphocytes, leucocytes and desquamated epithelial cells. In some crypts the epithelial wall is deficient so that organisms can readily invade the underlying lymphatic tissue (*see Figure 8.22*).

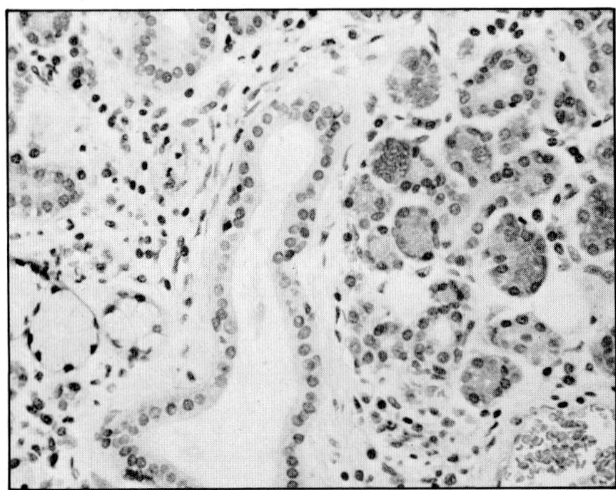

Figure 8.22 Section of tonsil showing crypt and adjacent lymphoid follicle

The size of the tonsil varies at different periods of life. After birth and for the first five or six years of life the tonsil increases rapidly in size. Its involution begins at puberty when the lymphoid tissue undergoes atrophic changes; in old age little lymphoid tissue remains.

The main artery to the tonsil is derived from the tonsillar branch of the facial artery. This artery ascends on the outer surface of the pharyngeal wall and pierces the superior constrictor muscle opposite the tonsillar fossa to enter the lateral surface of the tonsil. Additional small branches are derived from the ascending pharyngeal and dorsalis linguae arteries, from the greater palatine branch of the internal maxillary artery and from the ascending palatine branch of the facial artery.

The veins from the tonsil emerge from its lateral surface as two branches, the paratonsillar veins, which pierce the superior constrictor muscle to end in the common facial vein and pharyngeal plexus. Lymphatic vessels from the tonsil commence in a closed plexus around each follicle. The main vessels pass to the lateral surface of the tonsil and then pierce the pharyngeal wall to end in the upper deep cervical nodes and especially in the jugulodigastric nodes. This node is related to the internal jugular vein where it is crossed by the posterior belly of the digastric muscle.

Laryngeal part of the pharynx

This part of the pharynx is in free communication with the oropharynx above and is continuous with the oesophagus below the lower border of the cricoid cartilage (*Figure 8.8*). The laryngopharynx lies behind and partially surrounds the larynx. The inlet of the larynx is obliquely placed on the upper part of this region of the pharynx. It is bounded anteriorly by the upper part of the epiglottis and posteriorly by the elevations produced by the arytenoid cartilages surmounted by the corniculate and cuneiform cartilages.

The aryepiglottic fold unites the arytenoid cartilage to the upper part of the side of the epiglottis and forms the lateral boundary of the inlet of the larynx. The lower portion of the laryngeal part of the pharynx has in its anterior wall the posterior surfaces of the arytenoid and cricoid cartilages.

On the lateral side of the aryepiglottic fold and the lateral surface of the arytenoid cartilage there is a recess, the piriform fossa. The lateral boundary of this fossa is formed by the mucous membrane covering the inner surface of the posterior part of the medial surface of the lamina of the thyroid cartilage and thyrohyoid membrane.

Structure of pharynx

The pharyngeal aponeurosis

This aponeurosis forms an incomplete coat of varying thickness in the lateral and posterior walls of the pharynx. It is thick in its upper part, especially where the muscular wall is absent, and it is thin below. The aponeurosis blends with the periosteum of the under-surface of the basilar part of the occipital bone in front of the pharyngeal tubercle. It is attached to the spine of the sphenoid bone and laterally to the inferior surface of the petrous temporal bone medial to the carotid canal. Above the level of the upper border of the superior constrictor muscle of the pharynx, the pharyngeal aponeurosis is firmly united to the buccopharyngeal fascia, thus here forming a single layer. The tensor palati and levator palati muscles together with the cartilaginous part of the pharyngotympanic tube pass through this part of the pharynx to reach the palate and lateral wall of the pharynx respectively. Anteriorly the fascia is attached from above downwards to the posterior edge of the medial pterygoid plate, the pterygomandibular raphe and the posterior part of the mylohyoid ridge of the mandible. Below this level it becomes thinned and disappears as a distinct layer as it gains attachment to the posterior part of the tongue.

The muscles of the pharynx

The muscles of the pharynx are arranged into longitudinal and circular layers (*Plate 5, facing page 302*). The circular layer comprises the superior, middle and inferior constrictor muscles of the pharynx. Each of these muscles is a fan-shaped sheet, and together they form an almost complete coat for the side and posterior walls of the pharynx. In their posterior parts the muscles are so arranged that they overlap each other from below upwards. At their attachments in the front of the pharynx an interval separates the edges of the muscles from each other. There is also an interval between the upper border of the superior constrictor and the base of the skull (sinus of Morgagni). Through these various intervals structures can pass from the exterior of the pharynx into its cavity or to the mucous membrane. The longitudinal muscle layer includes the stylopharyngeus and the palatopharyngeus muscles. The longitudinal muscles are essentially elevators of the pharynx during swallowing.

The superior constrictor muscle

This muscle arises successively from above downwards from the posterior border of the lower part of the medial pterygoid plate, the hamular process, the pterygomandibular raphe, the posterior one-fifth of the mylohyoid ridge of the mandible and from the musculature of the tongue and the adjacent mucous membrane. The fibres pass backwards to be inserted into the pharyngeal tubercle and into the median pharyngeal raphe. The upper border of the muscle is free and, as stated above, forms the lower boundary of the sinus of Morgagni. A band of muscle fibres, the palatopharyngeal sphincter (Whillis, 1930) passes forwards from the superior constrictor muscle parallel with its upper fibres to be inserted into the palatal aponeurosis (*Figure 8.13*). This muscle corresponds to the position of the ridge of Passavant in the living subject. Contraction of the palatopharyngeal sphincter assists in closing off the nasopharynx.

The middle constrictor muscle

This muscle arises from the posterior edge of the lower part of the stylohyoid ligament and from the greater and lesser cornua of the hyoid bone. The fibres spread out as they pass backwards to be inserted into the whole length of the pharyngeal raphe. The upper fibres overlap superficially the lower part of the superior constrictor muscle, while the lower fibres are overlapped by the upper edge of the inferior constrictor muscle. The stylopharyngeus muscle and the glossopharyngeal nerve pass into the pharyngeal wall anteriorly between the lower border of the superior constrictor and the upper border of the middle constrictor.

The inferior constrictor muscle

This muscle arises from the oblique line of the thyroid cartilage, from the side of the cricoid cartilage and the fascia covering the posterior part of the cricothyroid muscle. The upper fibres ascend obliquely upwards to be inserted into the pharyngeal raphe (thyropharyngeus). The transverse fibres are continuous with the circular fibres of the oesophagus (cricopharyngeus). This part of the inferior constrictor plays an important role in the pharyngo-oesophageal sphincter mechanism and is normally in tonic contraction. In the triangular interval between the middle and inferior constrictors and the thyrohyoid muscle anteriorly, the internal laryngeal nerve and artery pierce the thyrohyoid membrane. The recurrent laryngeal nerve passes upwards beneath the lower edge of the inferior constrictor behind the articulation of the inferior horn of the thyroid cartilage with the cricoid cartilage.

Stylopharyngeus muscle

This muscle arises from the medial side of the base of the styloid process of the temporal bone. It passes downwards between the superior and middle constrictors of the pharynx to enter the wall of the pharynx. The muscle spreads out on the medial side of the inferior constrictor and is also inserted into the superior and posterior border of the thyroid cartilage. Some of the fibres are inserted with the palato-pharyngeus on the wall of the pharynx.

Palatopharyngeus muscle

This muscle is described on p. 282.

The buccopharyngeal fascia

This fascia forms a thin fibrous layer on the external surface of the muscular coat. Posteriorly the fascia is loosely attached to the pre-vertebral fascia covering the pre-vertebral muscles. At the sides it is loosely connected to the styloid process and its muscles, and to the carotid sheath.

Blood vessels, lymphatic drainage and nerve supply

The blood supply of the pharynx is derived from the ascending pharyngeal artery, the ascending palatine branch of the facial and the greater palatine branch of the maxillary artery. In addition small twigs are derived from the dorsalis linguae, the tonsillar artery and the artery of the pterygoid canal.

The ascending pharyngeal artery arises from the medial side of the external carotid artery just above its origin. It passes upwards behind the carotid sheath and immediately against the pharyngeal wall. Branches are distributed to the wall of the pharynx and the tonsil; the palatine branch passes over the upper free edge of the superior constrictor muscle to supply the inner aspect of the pharynx and the soft palate. A small branch supplies the pharyngotympanic tube.

The details of the distribution of the veins of the pharynx have been described by Batson (1942). The veins are arranged in two well-defined plexuses, an internal submucous and an external pharyngeal, with numerous communicating branches. The submucous plexus drains definite areas of the mucous membrane; in addition the plexus forms, in several places, an extensive network, found on the posterior wall of the pharynx and around the entrance to the larynx. These networks communicate with the veins of the dorsum of the tongue, the superior laryngeal veins, the oesophageal veins, and with the external pharyngeal plexus. The latter drains to the internal jugular and the anterior facial veins. The pharyngeal plexus is also closely connected to the cavernous sinus through emissary veins.

The lymphatic vessels of the pharyngeal wall can be divided into three groups: superior, middle and inferior. The superior vessels drain by main trunks which pass to the retropharyngeal and upper deep cervical nodes. The vessels of the middle group pass to the jugulodigastric nodes of the upper deep cervical group. The inferior group of vessels pass to the inferior deep cervical nodes.

The motor and sensory nerve supply of the pharynx is derived from the pharyngeal plexus. This is formed by the pharyngeal branches of the vagus nerve, branches of the glossopharyngeal nerve and sympathetic fibres. The pharyngeal branch of the vagus carries the main motor supply. These fibres (branchiomotor) arise from the cranial root of the accessory nerve and join the vagus at the level of its superior ganglion. They form an extensive plexus on the lateral surface of the middle constrictor and also supply the muscles of the soft palate, except the tensor palati. The pharyngeal branches of the glossopharyngeal nerve arise as three or four filaments which join the pharyngeal branches of the vagus. The sympathetic component of the pharyngeal plexus is derived from the superior cervical ganglion by a series of laryngopharyngeal branches. From this extensive plexus branches are distributed to the muscles of the pharynx, except the stylopharyngeus, which is supplied directly by the glossopharyngeal nerve. In addition a twig is given off from the recurrent laryngeal nerve to the inferior constrictor of the pharynx.

Movements of palate, tongue and pharynx

Palate

Many of the movements of the soft palate can be seen by inspection through the open mouth. In quiet respiration the soft palate hangs down above the posterior part of the tongue, leaving an interval between its posterior edge and the pharyngeal wall. Normal deglutition and speech depend upon the efficient closure of this interval by movements of the palate and the related part of the pharyngeal wall.

During swallowing the anterior part of the soft palate is lowered and made tense by the contraction of the tensor palati muscles, while the posterior part is elevated against the posterolateral part of the pharyngeal wall by the upward and backward pull of the levator palati muscles. Simultaneously the upper fibres of the superior constrictor and the palatopharyngeus muscles contract to form a ridge on the posterior pharyngeal wall, with which the posterior edge of the elevated palate comes into contact so closing the nasopharynx. After the bolus of food has passed into the pharynx the oropharyngeal isthmus is narrowed by the contraction of the palatoglossus muscles. In phonation the size of the nasopharyngeal isthmus changes according to the sound produced. In producing the sound ‘Ah’, and during the production of the palatal consonants, such as ‘K’, the palate is elevated so that the nasopharyngeal isthmus is closed. During blowing, or in retching and vomiting, the nasopharyngeal isthmus is also closed.

If the motor nerve supply is interrupted on one side the affected side of the palate cannot move. If both nerves are interrupted the nasopharyngeal isthmus cannot be closed, the individual has a nasal intonation, and, while eating, food may regurgitate through the nose.

Tongue

The tongue is used extensively in phonation, mastication and deglutition.

The voice is mainly produced by vibrations of the vocal cords, but the sounds employed in speech are modified by changes in the shape of the passage through which the expired air carrying the sound passes. The tongue plays an important role in the modification of the sounds, as it is capable of adopting an indefinite number of positions due to the arrangement of the muscle fibres arising within it and inserted into it. The entire organ may be moved within the cavity, thereby altering the capacity of the cavity, and at the same time the tongue can be bent upwards or downwards, made broad or convex, or its tip may be carried to any point of the teeth, gums or palate.

By virtue of these many movements the tongue is capable of checking the flow of expired air at different positions, and this checking is responsible for the formation of many of the consonants.

Mastication

During mastication food in the buccal cavity is pressed outwards between the teeth by the elevation of the tongue. The masticated food is finally formed into a bolus by the tongue and cheeks preparatory to swallowing.

Deglutition

The act of swallowing, although described in three stages, is a continuous process. The first stage is voluntary and the other two stages involuntary. In the first stage the food is carried into the pharynx, in the second through the pharynx and, during the third, through the oesophagus into the stomach. The movements of the tongue are concerned only with the first stage. At the beginning of this stage the flooor of the mouth, the hyoid bone and the larynx are raised by the contraction of the mylohyoid muscles. The tip of the tongue first comes into contact with the hard palate, and then successive parts of the dorsum rise to the hard palate. The effect is to force the bolus of food through the oropharyngeal isthmus into the pharynx. The upward and backward movements of the tongue are assisted by the simultaneous contraction of the styloglossus muscles and the palatoglossus muscles. The contraction of the latter muscles also narrows the oropharyngeal isthmus and prevents the return of food into the mouth (Whillis, 1946).

Pharynx

As the bolus of food passes down from the buccal cavity into the oropharynx, the oropharyngeal isthmus is reduced in size by the contraction of the palatoglossus muscle. As already stated the larynx has been elevated and at the same time the inlet to the larynx has been reduced in size so that the aditus to the larynx becomes triradiate. This opening is closed by the elevation of the larynx against the epiglottis, which is thrust backwards and downwards, through a right angle, by the movements of the base of the tongue (Johnstone, 1942). The backward thrust of the tongue, due to the contraction of the mylohyoid and styloglossus muscles, causes the bolus to be passed into the pharynx. The subsequent progress of the bolus depends on its nature;

if fluid, or semi-fluid, the momentum given by the thrust of the tongue is sufficient to project it into the oesophagus. If the bolus is solid there are successive contractions of the pharyngeal muscles and the bolus is carried into the oesophagus. Barclay (1930, 1936) has demonstrated that the pharyngeal space is obliterated just before the bolus passes into the pharynx; subsequently the space re-appears. Barclay states that 'the bolus as it travels gives the impression of being sucked rather than pushed down'.

The movements of the palate in speech are referred to in the section on the larynx.

The oesophagus

Descriptive anatomy

The oesophagus extends from the lower border of the cricoid cartilage, at the level of the sixth cervical vertebra, to the cardiac orifice of the stomach at the side of the body of the tenth or eleventh thoracic vertebra (the level of the cardiac orifice is subject to variation in the living subject on account of the movements of the diaphragm). In the newborn infant the upper limit of the oesophagus is found at the level of the fourth or fifth cervical vertebra, whereas inferiorly it terminates higher at the level of the ninth thoracic vertebra.

The oesophagus is approximately 23–28 cm long (the average length is 25 cm or 10 in) in the adult. At birth the oesophagus varies in length from 8 to 10 cm and by the end of the first year it has increased to 12 cm. Between the first and fifth years it reaches a length of 16 cm; the increase from the fifth year until puberty is slow as the oesophagus measures only 19 cm by the fifteenth year.

The greatest diameter of the empty oesophagus is about 20 mm; however, when distended it may be as much as 30 mm. At birth the diameter is about 5 mm, but this dimension almost doubles in the first year (9 mm) and by the age of 5 years it has attained a diameter of 15 mm. In the cadaver the oesophagus is usually flattened from before backwards, and the lumen in sections appears as a transverse slit, except immediately above the diaphragm, where it may be stellate in shape. The diameter of the oesophagus is not uniform throughout its length; it has three constrictions, upper, middle and lower, with slightly elongated dilatations between them. The upper constriction is immediately below the cricoid cartilage, the middle one is found where the oesophagus is crossed by the aorta and left bronchus, and the lower one where it pierces the diaphragm.

The course pursued by the oesophagus is not straight from its origin to its termination, but shows three curves. One lies in the sagittal plane, the other two are in the coronal plane. The sagittal curve is the most prominent and runs parallel with the contour of the anterior aspect of the vertebral column as far as the seventh thoracic vertebra. Beyond this point the oesophagus comes forward to lie in front of the descending thoracic aorta. The first of the coronal curves, which has a slight amplitude to the left, begins a little below the commencement of the oesophagus and ends where the oesophagus reaches the midline at the level of the fifth thoracic

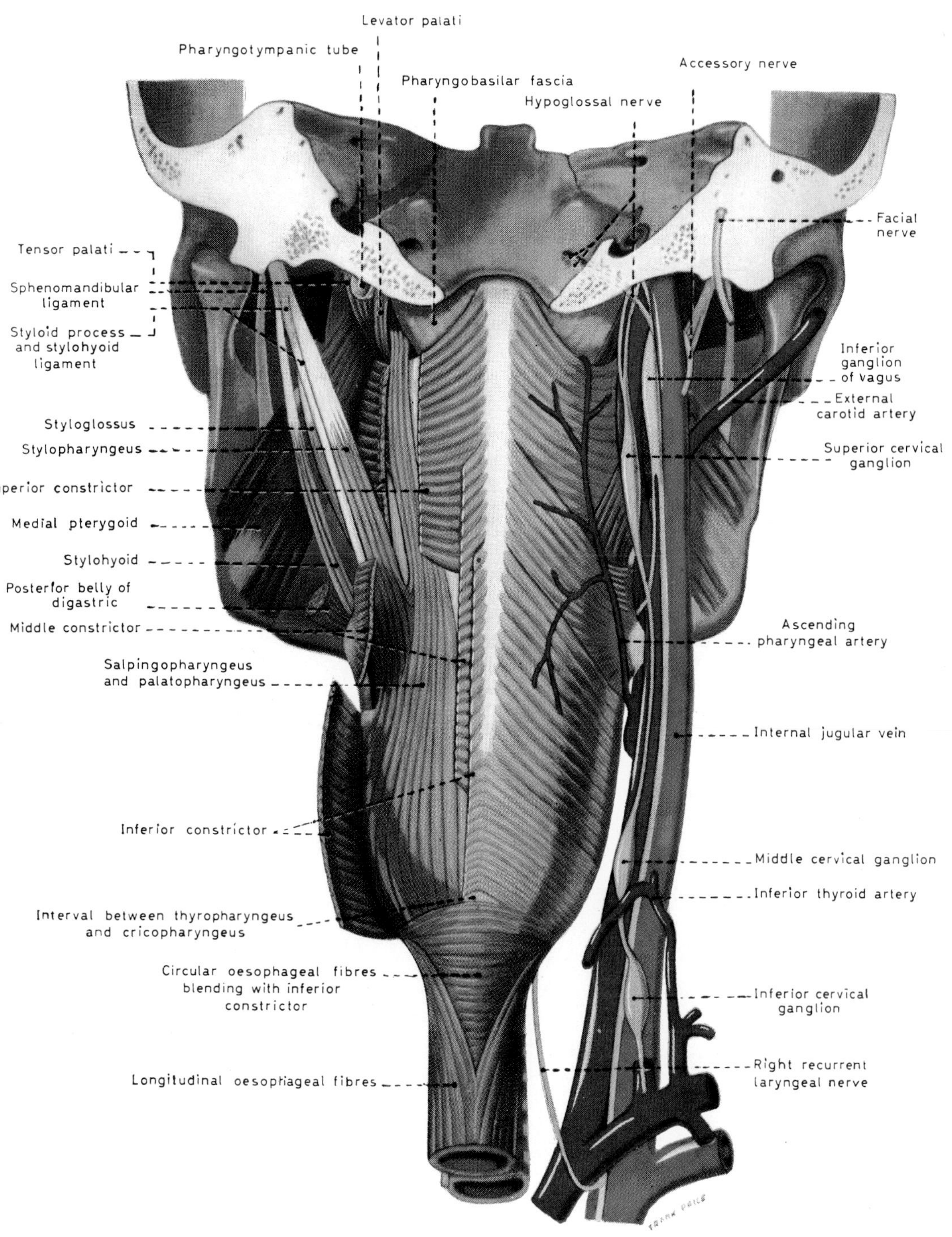

Plate 5 A drawing of the pharynx and associated structures as seen from the back

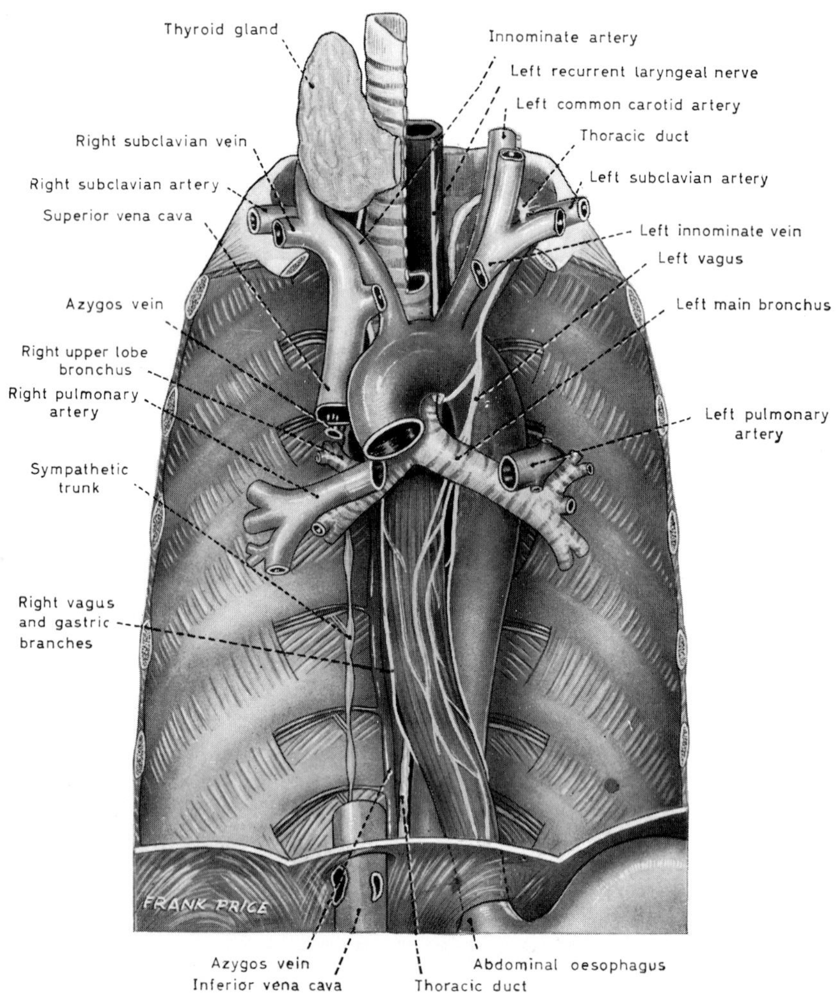

Plate 6 A drawing of a dissection to show the main relations of the oesphagus

vertebra. This curve is therefore found in the lower part of the neck and upper part of the thorax. At the point of maximum deflection of the curve the oesophagus projects 4–6 mm beyond the left margin of the trachea. The second coronal curve is formed by a bend to the left as the abdominal part of the oesophagus passes to the left to enter the stomach (*see Figure 8.23*).

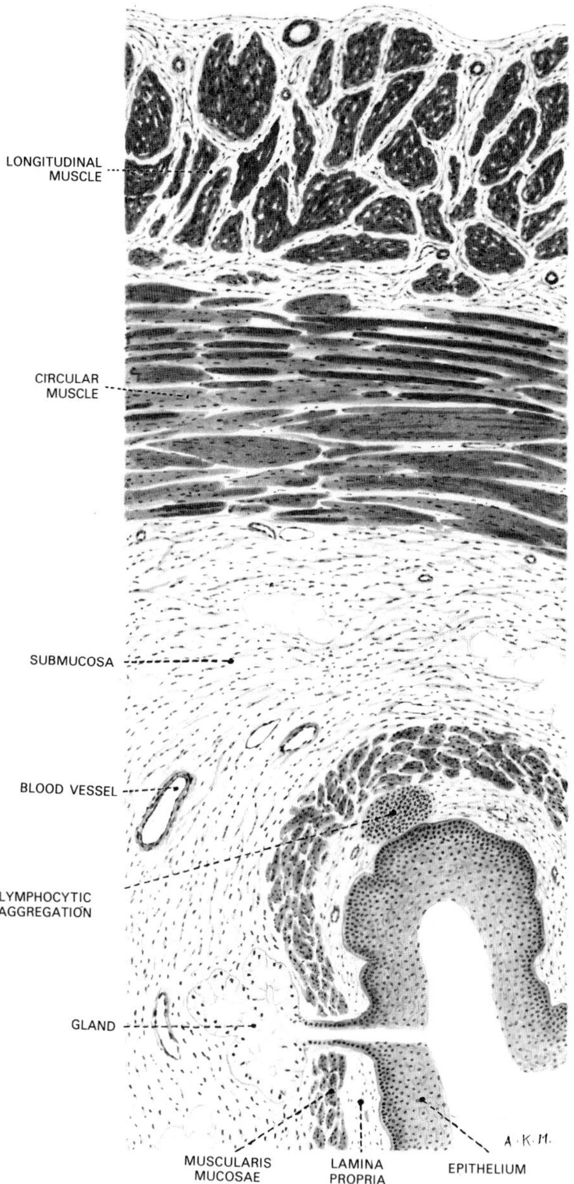

Figure 8.23 High-power view of transverse section of the oesophagus. (From *Textbook of Human Anatomy*, 1976. Edited by W. J. Hamilton, London, Macmillan. Reproduced by kind permission of the publishers)

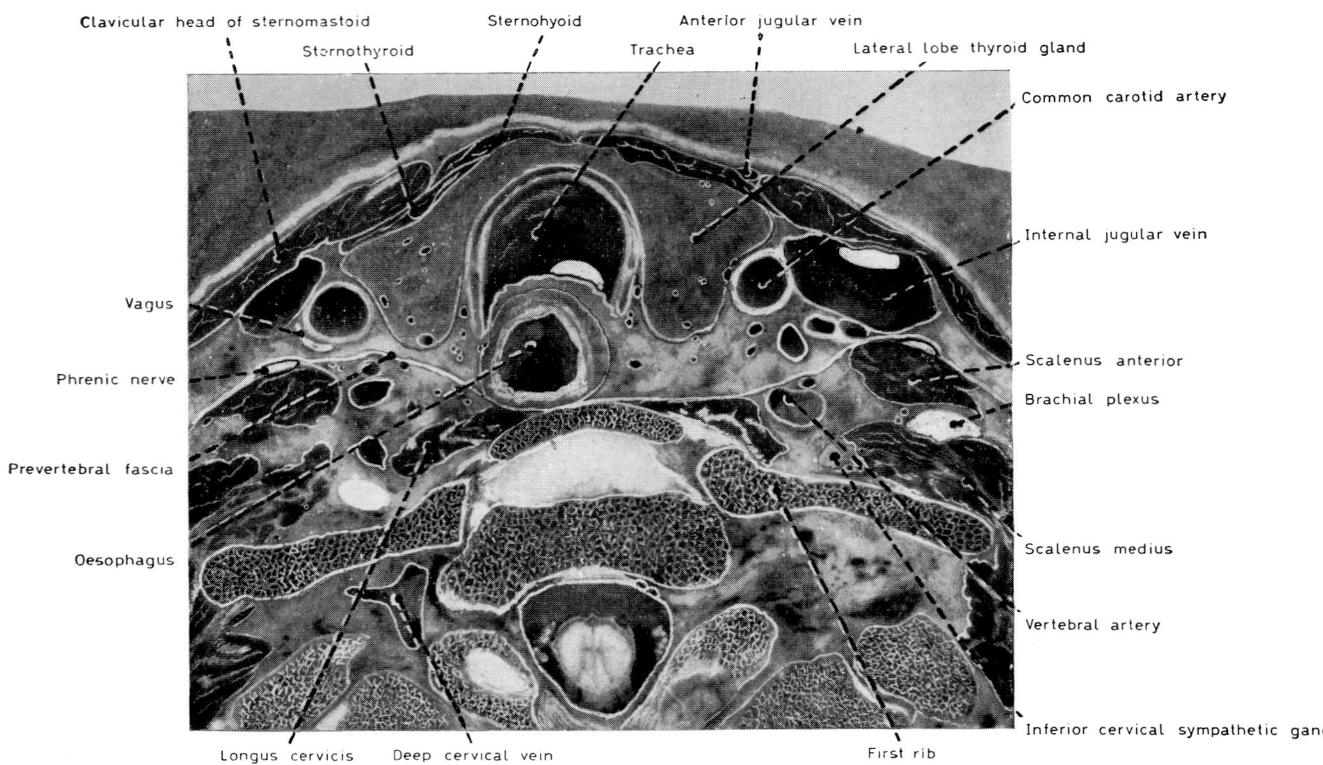

Figure 8.24 Retouched photograph of a transverse section through the level of the first thoracic vertebra

Anatomical relationships

The oesophagus has relations in the root of the neck, the superior and posterior mediastina and in the abdomen. The relations are shown in *Plate 6 (facing page 302)* and can also be seen in the cross-sections of the neck and thorax shown in *Figures 8.24–8.28*.

The oesophagus is separated from the vertebral bodies and intervening intervertebral discs by the anterior longitudinal ligaments from the seventh cervical to the seventh thoracic vertebrae. The longus cervicis muscle, covered by the pre-vertebral fascia (*Figures 8.24* and *8.25*), intervenes betwen the oesophagus and the vertebral bodies, the ligaments and muscles in the neck and the superior mediastinum. Below the level of the seventh thoracic vertebra the aorta passes behind the oesophagus and forms a right relation to it in the lower thorax and abdomen. The thoracic duct (*Plate 6, facing page 302*) lies immediately to the right of the lower part of the oesophagus up to the level of the fifth thoracic vertebra; it then passes behind the oesophagus and ascends as a left relation of the oesophagus lying between it and the left pleura. The vena azygos (*Plate 6, facing page 302*) lies to the right of the thoracic duct and accompanies it until the latter crosses the midline. The upper five right intercostal arteries and the transverse parts of the hemi-azygos veins pass behind the oesophagus (*Figure 8.26*). As the oesophagus passes through the diaphragm it lies first on the decussating muscular fibres of the right crus and then on the left crus of the diaphragm.

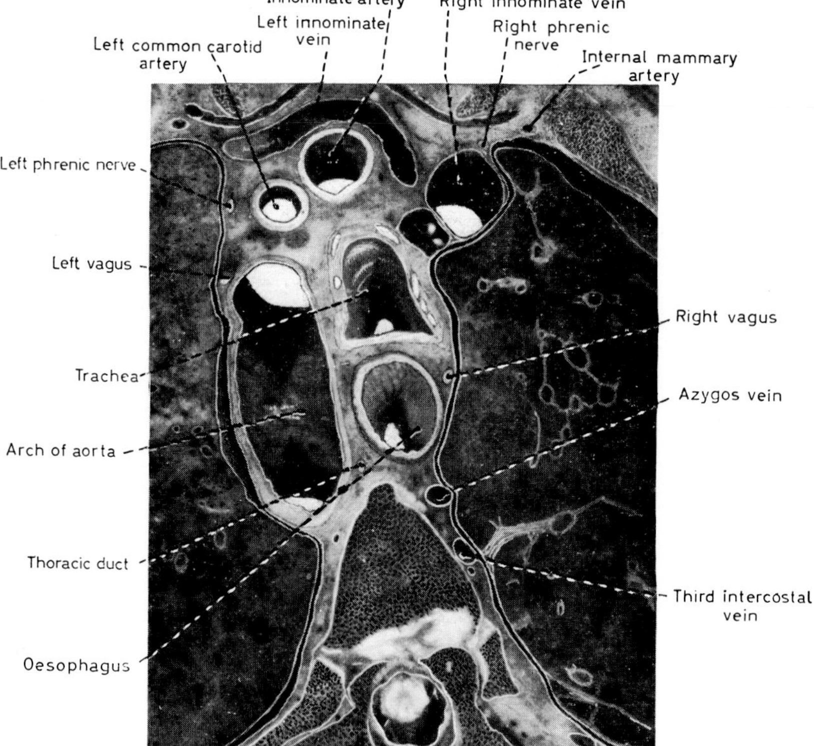

Figure 8.25 Retouched photograph of a transverse section through the level of the fourth thoracic vertebra

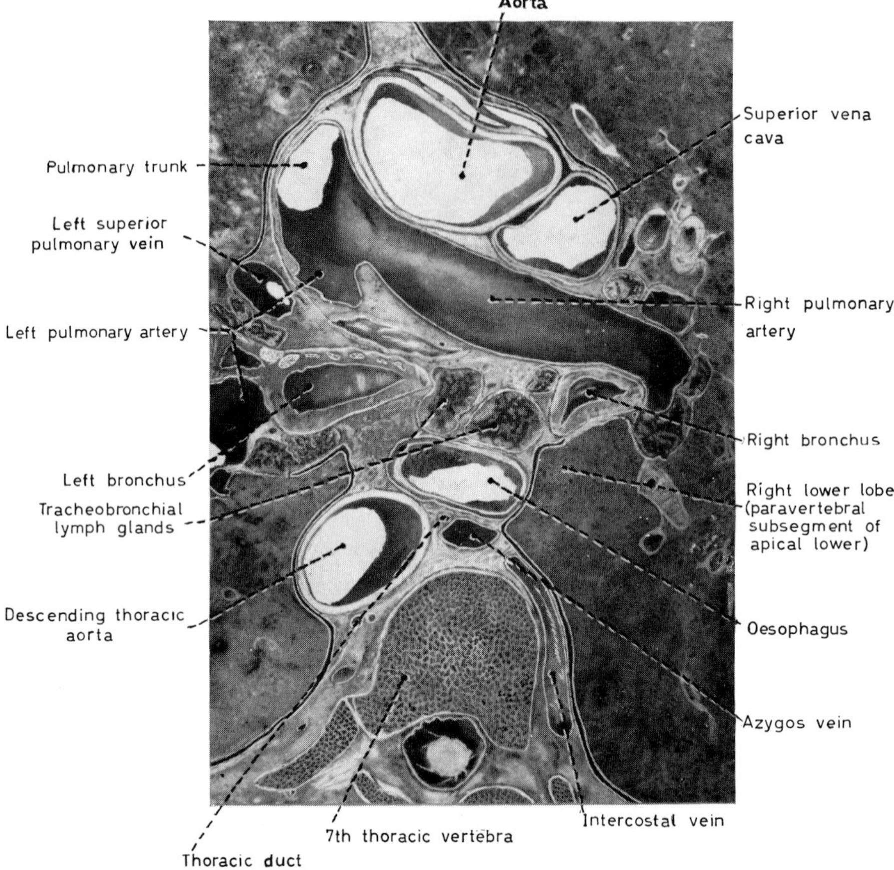

Figure 8.26 Retouched photograph of a transverse section through the level of the seventh thoracic vertebra

The trachea lies in front of the oesophagus as far as the fifth thoracic vertebra, at which level it is loosely connected to the oesophagus by the pre-tracheal fascia. As the oesophagus descends it gradually inclines to the left so that it projects at the side of the trachea at the lowest level of the latter. The left recurrent laryngeal nerve thus lies on the anterior aspect of the oesophagus as the nerve starts to ascend. Immediately below this level the oesophagus is crossed by the left bronchus and the right pulmonary artery (*Figure 8.26*). The inferior tracheobronchial lymph nodes are interposed between the bifurcation of the trachea and the oesophagus (*Figure 8.26*). Below this level, the convexity of the left atrium, covered by the pericardium, lies in direct relationship with the front of the oesophagus (*Figure 8.27*). At this point the descending aorta lies to the left and somewhat posteriorly, separating the oesophagus from the left lung and pleura. At the level of the seventh thoracic vertebra the oesophagus lies behind and to the left of the inferior vena cava and the coronary sinus (*Figure 8.28*). Just before the oesophagus pierces the diaphragm it lies immediately behind the decussating fibres of the crura as they enter the central tendon. In the abdominal cavity the oesophagus grooves the upper part of the left lobe of the liver.

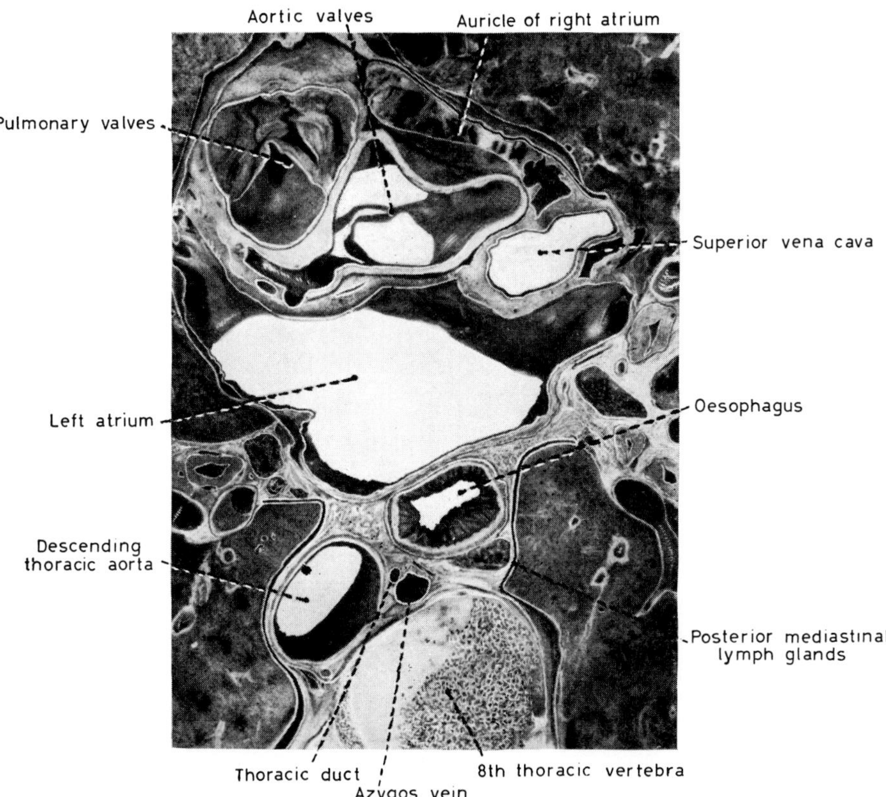

Figure 8.27 Retouched photograph of a transverse section through the level of the eighth thoracic vertebra. The thoracic duct and vena azygos are somewhat to the left of this section

In the cervical part of its course the lateral lobe of the thyroid gland, the carotid sheath and its contents, and the oesophageal branch of the inferior thyroid artery lie lateral to the oesophagus. The recurrent laryngeal nerve of each side ascends between the trachea and the oesophagus to enter the larynx. Owing to the deviation of the oesophagus to the left in the upper part of its course, the thyroid gland with the related inferior thyroid artery lies anterior and lateral to it in this situation. On the left side also lie the left subclavian artery, the thoracic duct and the left pleura.

In the thoracic part of its course the oesophagus is related on its right side to the mediastinal pleura, which separates it from the mediastinal aspect of the right lower lobe behind the hilum of the lung and the pulmonary ligament, and also to the arch of the azygos vein (*Figures 8.26* and *8.27*). The latter curves against the side of the oesophagus and then passes above the root of the lung to join the superior vena cava. Just before the oesophagus pierces the diaphragm the pleural cavity on the right-hand side frequently forms a small diverticulum which passes to the right side of the oesophagus, and into which a portion of the cardiac segment* projects. On the left

* This segment was formerly referred to as the azygos lobe (lobus impar or infracardiac lobe [Narath]) as it apparently corresponded to a similar lobe found in other mammals. The term azygos in its modern sense is used to refer to that part of the upper lobe which may be separated from the rest of that lobe by the vena azygos.

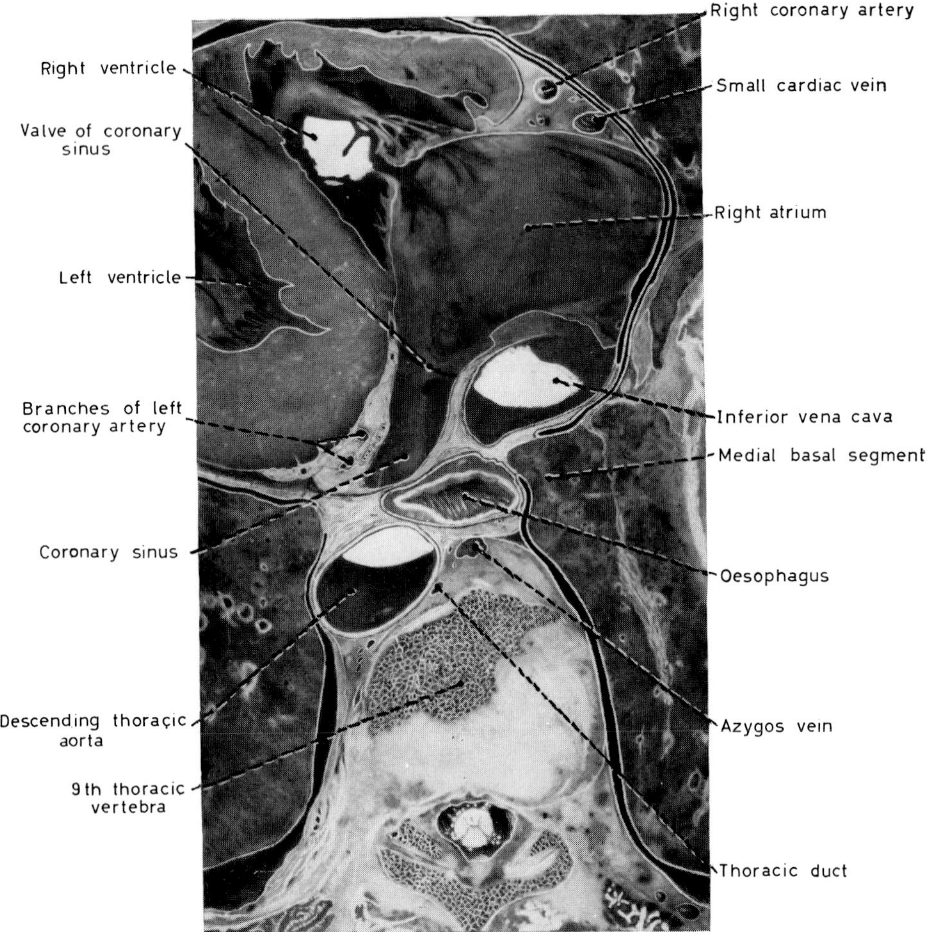

Figure 8.28 Retouched photograph of a section through the level of the ninth thoracic vertebra. The thoracic duct has crossed low down to the left-hand side

side, in the upper part of its course, the pleura, subclavian artery and thoracic duct separate the oesophagus from the left lung. The arch of the aorta passes backwards above the level of the root of the lung to become continuous with the descending aorta. Above the diaphragm the oesophagus grooves the medial side of the lower lobe of the left lung just below the pulmonary ligament.

The vagi nerves are intimately related to the oesophagus in the posterior mediastinum. Posterior to the root of the lung each nerve breaks up to form the posterior pulmonary plexus, from the lower part of which two nerves arise and pass to the oesophagus. The nerves of each side divide and communicate with each other to form an oesophageal plexus. At the oesophageal opening of the diaphragm each vagus nerve becomes reconstituted, the left nerve passing in front of the oesophagus, and the right nerve behind it, to become the anterior and posterior gastric nerves.

Structure

The wall of the oesophagus has four layers; from without inwards these are the fibrous, muscular, submucous and mucous layers.

Fibrous layer

The fibrous layer forms a loose covering which allows the oesophagus to move freely on the adjacent structures.

Muscular layer

The muscular layer is composed of an outer longitudinal and an inner circular coat. In the upper part of the oesophagus the two coats are well developed but are not clearly defined. The longitudinal coat is as thick as the circular coat except posteriorly at the beginning of the oesophagus. In this situation the longitudinal coat is deficient since the upper fibres of the longitudinal coat diverge as they pass upwards and forwards to gain attachment to the posterior surface of the cricoid cartilage. The area between the diverging fibres is a potentially weak region in the wall of the oesophagus and pre-disposes in certain conditions to the formation of oesophageal diverticula. On the corresponding area on the anterior surface of the upper part of the oesophagus there may also be a deficiency of longitudinal fibres.

The circular coat forms a complete investment, continuous above with the inferior constrictor of the pharynx and below with the circular and oblique muscle coats of the stomach. The circular fibres at the lower end of the oesophagus and adjacent part of the stomach act as a functional sphincter. According to Shattock (1916) there is a widespread thickening of the circular muscle into a sphincter; on the other hand, Whillis (1931) could not find any histological evidence of the cardiac sphincter in man.

The muscle fibres of both coats in approximately the upper third of the oesophagus are striated; in the middle third the striated fibres are progressively replaced by unstriated muscle fibres, whereas in the lower third only unstriated muscle fibres are present.

Submucous layer

The submucous layer consists of connective tissue made up of collagenous and elastic fibres. The deep part of the oesophageal glands proper are situated in this layer. Together with the muscularis mucosae, the submucous layer produces longitudinal folds in the lumen of the oesophagus which form the irregularities of the lumen seen in transverse section; these folds disappear upon distension of the oesophagus.

Mucous layer

The mucous membrane is covered with non-cornified stratified squamous epithelium with a deep germinal layer. The epithelium is continuous above with that of the mucous membrane of the pharynx, but is paler in colour; at the cardio-oesophageal junction it is abruptly succeeded by the columnar epithelium of the stomach. The lamina propria contains many ridges projecting into the epithelium as papillae, which do not produce elevations on the free surface of the mucous membrane. The lamina propria consists of loose connective tissue and a very fine network of elastic fibres. In early embryonic life the epithelium of the oesophagus is composed of columnar epithelium, many of the cells of which are ciliated. At the time of birth the ciliated cells are isolated in small groups and eventually disappear, and the oesophagus is now lined with stratified squamous epithelium of 5–6 cell layers in thickness. Soon after birth the epithelium thickens rapidly to assume its adult appearance.

Oesophageal glands

Two kinds of gland, the oesophageal glands proper and the cardiac glands, are found in the oesophagus. The oesophageal glands are compound glands; the tubulo-alveolar secretory portion contains only mucous cells. The bases of these glands are situated in the submucosa and are irregularly distributed. The glands communicate with the lumen of the oesophagus by means of ducts, the distal parts of which are lined with three or four layers of stratified squamous epithelium. At the junction of the duct and the gland there is a gradual transition from the stratified epithelium to low cuboidal epithelium. The oesophageal cardiac glands resemble the cardiac glands of the stomach; they are found in the upper part of the oesophagus and in the lower part near the cardia. Unlike the oesophageal glands, they do not penetrate the muscularis mucosae. Some of the glands may contain typical zymogenic and parietal cells, and some investigators consider them to be areas of heterotopic gastric mucosa.

Blood vessels

The arteries of the oesophagus are derived from the inferior thyroid artery in the neck, the descending thoracic aorta in the thorax and the left gastric artery in the abdomen; additional twigs are also derived from the left phrenic artery. An extensive venous plexus is formed on the exterior of the oesophagus and drains into the inferior thyroid veins in the cervical region, and the azygos system of veins in the thorax. At the cardia, many small thin-walled subepithelial veins connect the oesophageal veins with the gastric veins. The oesophageal veins form an extensive and free communication between the systemic and portal circulations and frequently become varicose in portal obstruction. Cranially the longitudinal submucous oesophageal veins enter the pharyngolaryngeal plexus situated in the dorsal and ventral walls of that part of the pharynx opposite the cricoid cartilage. The larger dorsal plexus forms a triangular rete mirabile or even a cavernous sinus which projects ventrally towards the cricoid cartilage when distended. It is larger in the newborn than in the adult (Butler, 1949; *see also* Kegaries, 1934).

Nerve supply

The upper third is supplied by the recurrent laryngeal nerve and the lower two-thirds by branches from the vagus and the inferior cervical sympathetic ganglion. In the lower two-thirds there are two nerve plexuses in the oesophageal wall. Auerbach's plexus lies between the longitudinal and circular muscle coats and Meissner's in the submucosa.

Lymphatic drainage

Two networks of lymphatic capillaries are found in the oesophagus (Rouvière, 1932). A plexus of fairly large capillaries is found in the mucous layer, and is continuous above with those of the pharynx and below with those of the gastric mucosa. A second plexus of finer capillaries is present in the muscular coat, and although this may be independent of the mucous plexus it drains by the same collecting vessels. The latter leave the oesophagus in two ways. They may pierce the muscular coat immediately and drain into neighbouring nodes (posterior mediastinal nodes), or ascend or descend beneath the mucosa. The superior vessels drain into the paratracheal, lower deep cervical glands or the tracheobronchial nodes. The lower vessels pass to the posterior mediastina nodes and to the left gastric nodes.

References

Barclay, A. E. (1930). *British Journal of Radiology*, **3**, 534

Barclay, A. E. (1936). *The Digestive Tract*. 2nd edn. London; Cambridge University Press

Batson, O. V. (1942). *Archives of Otolaryngology*, **36**, 212

Brash, J. C. (1956). *The Aetiology of Irregularity and Malocclusion of the Teeth*. London; Dental Board of the United Kingdom

Browne, D. (1928). *Journal of Anatomy, London*, **63**, 82

Butler, H. (1949). Personal communication

Corner, G. W. (1929). *Contributive Embryology, Carnegie Institute*, **20**, 81

Gilmour, J. R. (1937). *Journal of Pathology and Bacteriology*, **45**, 507

Godwin, M. C. (1940). *American Journal of Anatomy*, **66**, 51

Hellman, T. (1930). *Handbuch der mikroskopischen Anatomie* (Ed. by von Möllendorf, Vol. 6, p. 233). Berlin; Springer

Heuser, C. H. (1930). *Contributive Embryology, Carnegie Institute*, **21**, 135

Johnstone, A. S. (1942). *Journal of Anatomy, London*, **77**, 97

Kegaries, D. L. (1934). *Surgery of Gynecology and Obstetrics*, **58**, 46

Kingsbury, B. F. (1939). *American Journal of Anatomy*, **65**, 333

Kraus, B. S. and Jordan, R. E. (1965). *The Human Dentition Before Birth*. London; Kimpton

Miles, A. E. W. (1967). *Structural and Chemical Organization of Teeth* (Vols. 1 and 2). New York; Academic Press

Norris, E. H. (1937). *Contributive Embryology, Carnegie Institute*, **26**, 247

Rouvière, H. (1932). *Anatomie des lymphatiques de l'homme*. Paris; Masson

Scott, J. H. (1967). *Dento-facial Development and Growth*. Oxford and London; Pergamon Press

Shattock, S. G. (1916). *Proceedings of the Royal Society of Medicine*, **10**, 16

Sicher, H. (1966). *Orban's Oral Histology and Embryology*. Saint Louis; Mosby

Stack, M. V. and Fernhead, R. W. (1965). *Tooth Enamel*. Bristol; Wright

Streeter, G. L. (1945). *Contributive Embryology, Carnegie Institute*, **31**, 27

Taillens, J. P. (1944). *Acta otolaryngologica*, Suppl. 56

Weller, G. L. (1933). *Contributive Embryology, Carnegie Institute*, **24**, 93

Whillis, J. (1930). *Journal of Anatomy, London*, **56**, 92

Whillis, J. (1931). *Journal of Anatomy, London*, **66**, 132

Whillis, J. (1946). *Journal of Anatomy, London*, **80**, 115

9 Physiology of the mouth, pharynx and oesophagus

R F McNab Jones

Mouth

Physiology of the salivary glands

The glandular parenchyma consists of acini with a tubular system and excretory ducts leading to the main duct. Acinus → intercalated duct → intralobular duct → interlobular (excretory) duct.

Acinar structure

Each acinus is a spherical or elongated ovoid with a central lumen. The acinar walls are composed of pyramidal-shaped cells surrounding a minute central lumen which leads into the duct system. The acinar cells rest on a homogeneous basement membrane.

The secreting epithelium of the acini may be one of two types of cell – mucous or serous. The mucous cells contain large translucent refractile mucinogen globules which can be seen in fresh preparations. The serous cells have a large number of smaller more opaque acidophilic-staining secretion granules. These are zymogen granules, i.e. the precursors of the salivary amylase.

The mucinogen granules discharge mucin into the saliva, thus contributing largely to its viscosity, while the fine zymogen granules of the serous cells discharge the enzymes of the salivary secretion.

In the resting gland these granules accumulate and fill the cell so that the nucleus is not readily seen. With secretion, the serous granules decrease in number and size and are left only at the apical end of the cell. Histochemical studies have suggested that possibly three types of cell can be identified, depending on the relative proportions of neutral and acidic polysaccharides. Serous cells contain mainly neutral polysaccharides, while mucous cells have a high proportion of acidic polysaccharides and seromucinous cells have both neutral and acidic polysaccharides.

The myoepithelial 'basket' cells

These are flattened stellate cells with a central nucleated body and elongated branching radiating processes. The cytoplasm has poorly-defined longitudinal striations. This fibrillar cytoplasm resembles that of smooth muscle. These cells lie between the bases of the acinar cells and the basement membrane. They are found also in a similar location on the intralobular salivary ducts. They are regarded by most investigators as contractile in function and functionally analogous to the myoepithelium of the mammary gland.

These myoepithelial cells are contracted by sympathetic stimulation or adrenaline. This accounts for the sudden spurt of a small volume of saliva produced when the sympathetic salivary nerve supply is stimulated – probably indicating expression of saliva from the ducts by myoepithelial contraction.

Duct system

The duct system leading from the secreting segments or acini can be differentiated into three structural regions on the basis of histological and electron microscopical appearances. These are: (1) intercalated ducts with epithelium of cubical cells; (2) striated intralobular ducts with larger lumen and cells characterized by basal striations due to mitochondria enclosed in folds of the basal cell walls; and (3) excretory ducts lined by clear cubical cells resting on flattened cells. The terminal part of the main excretory duct has a stratified squamous epithelium.

The intercalated ducts are shorter in the submandibular gland than in the parotid.

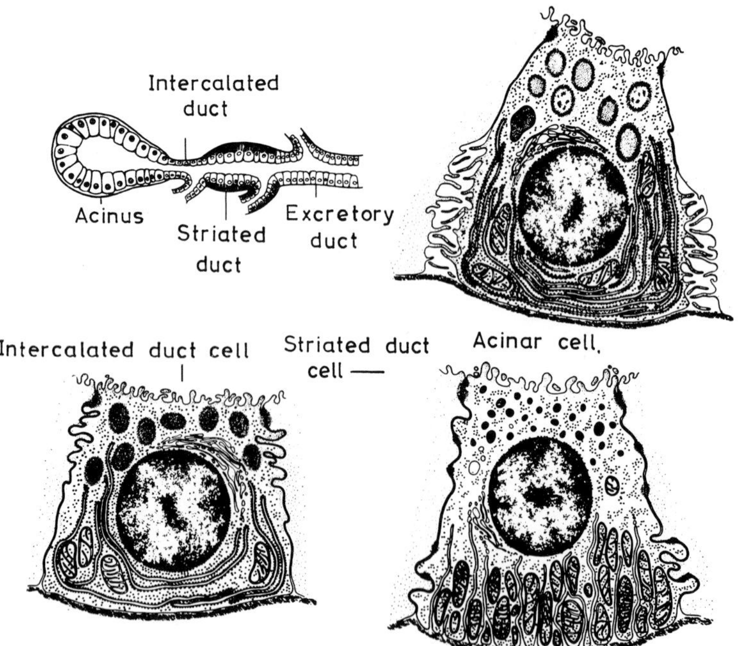

Figure 9.1 Diagrammatic representation of the fine structural characteristics of the various cell types in the mouse submandibular gland. (After Rutberg)

The sublingual gland has no intercalated ducts and the striated ducts also are practically absent, being represented by only a few groups of rodded cells scattered in the walls of the excretory ducts.

The general arrangement of the complex duct system is shown in *Figure 9.1*.

Secretory acini are continuous with narrow necks or intercalated ducts. These join to form intralobular ducts. Each intralobular duct with its tributary intercalated ducts and their acini form a secretory lobule. The 'striated' intralobular ducts lead into interlobular excretory ducts. These successive generations of ducts finally drain into the main excretory duct of the gland.

The epithelial lining of the duct system exhibits a progressive change from columnar to pseudostratified columnar to stratified columnar to stratified squamous type.

The acinar and the duct epithelium rests on a basal basement membrane. Scattered basal 'basket' or myoepithelial cells are interposed between the epithelial cells and this basement membrane.

Special features of individual glands

Parotid In man as in most mammals the secretory acini of the parotid gland consist entirely of serous cells. The parotid secretion is accordingly a watery serous secretion low in mucin and high in enzymes. The intercalated ducts are long and there are numerous striated ducts.

Submandibular This is a mixed gland with predominantly serous secretory units. Some of the mucous acini have serous cells at their terminal ends, some have serous demilunes. The ratio of serous to mucous cells is 4:1. The intercalated ducts are short and narrow. The intralobular ducts are branched, longer and more numerous than in the parotid duct system and are lined by two types of cell.

Sublingual gland This is a complex of small glands although described as a single gland. The acini are mainly pure mucous though some have large serous crescents. There are a very few pure serous acini. The ratio of serous to mucous cellular elements is 1:4. The intercalated ducts are very short and some acini open directly into striated intralobular ducts. These intralobular ducts have only one type of 'striated' cell. The glands open by some extralobular ducts into the floor of the mouth.

Accesory salivary glands

Many small glands are present in the mucosa and submucosa of the oral cavity. These include:

(1) In the oral vestibule: labial glands in the upper and lower lips and buccal glands in the cheeks. These have mixed serous and mucous cells.
(2) In the floor of the mouth cavity: small sublingual and glossopalatine glands.
(3) On the tongue: anterior lingual (Blandin or Nuhn) glands, and posterior lingual glands. The former have tubules or mucous cells with small demilunes. The latter group includes serous glands (von Ebner) opening in the floor of the groove around the circumvallate papillae and some mucous glands at the root of the tongue. The secretion of the serous glands in the circumvallate furrow serves to wash out the region of the taste buds.

(4) On the palate; glands of mixed type are present.

In general these accessory glands seem to be the source of the basal or resting secretion.

Histochemistry

Histochemical techniques have been used for the identification of chemical substances and their location within the acinar and duct cells of the salivary glands.

The periodic acid-Schiff reaction is a histochemical group reaction for the presence of carbohydrates. This stain gives a positive reaction with glycogen, mucins, neutral polysaccharides and glycoproteins. If a positive staining reaction is prevented in a parallel slide by previous digestion by amylase then glycogen is present.

Carbohydrates

An amylase-resistant, PAS-positive, polysaccharide material can be demonstrated in acinar cells. This material is more evident in mucous than in serous cells. The salivary glands of some species form sulphated mucins; others do not but form sialomucin; and yet others produce both kinds of mucin.

Duct cells have a high glycogen content.

Enzymes

Acid phosphatase has been shown to be present in both duct and acinar cells of the salivary glands of some species of animals. Alkaline phosphatase has also been demonstrated in myoepithelial cells.

Cholinesterase is present in low concentration in the basal cytoplasm and nuclei of acinar cells. Other enzymes which have been demonstrated by histochemistry are succinic dehydrogenases and aminopeptides in duct cells.

Physiology of circulation

Blood supply

The blood supply to the salivary glands is described in Chapter 8. The main arteries of supply of the submandibular and sublingual glands enter at the hila of the glands; some smaller vessels enter through the capsule. The parotid gland has no hilum and the vessels pierce the gland surface without any constant pattern.

The vascular distribution and arrangement within the gland and the regulation of blood flow in these glands has special physiological significance in relation to the mechanism of formation of saliva.

The general vascular pattern is that the arterial branches accompany the extralobular and interlobular ducts into the gland lobules. In the lobules these arteries feed into arterioles and thence into a dense capillary network around the intralobular ducts. The rich vascularity of the ducts is related to the active transport functions which take place in the ducts. From the capillary plexus on the ducts, vessels pass to a second capillary bed around the acinar cells. From the capillary beds the venous drainage passes alongside the ducts out of the lobules. Spanner (1937) described arteriovenous anastomoses within the glands and large sacculated veins in the hilar region. He proposed that these veins had a reservoir function and served as a 'throttle' mechanism to raise the pressure in the capillary bed during secretion.

There may be a portal circulatory arrangement in this circulation akin to that in the kidney. Burgen and Seeman (1957) claimed that the greater part of the blood flow was distributed to the duct system and that the flow in the duct capillaries was countercurrent to, i.e. opposite to, the flow of saliva in the duct.

Control of salivary blood flow

Extensive investigations of the neural regulation of the vasculature of the salivary glands have been carried out.

The circulatory responses to sympathetic and parasympathetic stimulation vary with the gland and with the species, as do the secretory responses. The submandibular glands of both the dog and the cat respond to parasympathetic stimulation with vasodilatation and secretion. On the other hand sympathetic stimulation in the dog induces vasoconstriction and a scanty salivary flow while in the cat it produces an abundant flow of dilute saliva accompanied by alternating vasoconstriction and vasodilatation.

Changes in blood flow produced by the two autonomic routes of stimulation are not primarily the cause of the particular changes in composition and rate of secretion which occur. However, variations in blood flow can to some extent secondarily influence the secretory rate and the specific composition of saliva.

Composition of saliva

Saliva is a colourless opalescent viscous liquid. It consists of water, inorganic constituents of the extracellular fluid, and organic compounds, notably the protein enzymes and mucin.

Its composition shows a great variability in the concentration of the chief individual constituents. This variability is a consequence of the following: (1) The composition of the secretion of the different salivary glands varies. This is determined by the proportion of serous and mucus-secreting cells. Mucous acini elaborate a viscid secretion of high mucin content. (2) The final secretion is adjusted in composition and volume flow to the different types of stimuli used to elicit the secretion. (3) The concentration of many of the constituents bears a specific relationship to the rate of secretory flow. (4) The salivary concentration of some constituents varies with the plasma concentration.

The 'normal' composition of saliva therefore covers a wide range depending on the relative contributions of the different glands, the proportions of mucous and serous cells activated, the nature of the stimulus, the flow rate, the composition of the plasma and the method of collection.

The 'mixed' saliva collected from the mouth is a mixture of the secretions of main and accessory glands and thus is not very constant in composition. Also it must be realized that the addition of bacterial products of fermentation and putrefaction, food debris, desquamated epithelial cells, and evolution of carbon dioxide into the atmosphere will further modify the composition of the saliva in the mouth.

Inorganic constituents

The main cations of saliva are sodium, potassium, calcium and magnesium and the principal anions are chloride, bicarbonate with smaller concentrations of phosphate and sulphate and traces of thiocyanate, iodide, fluoride and nitrite. The levels of these ions may be influenced by gland of origin, age, sex, rate of secretion, nature of stimulus, plasma concentration, diet and disease.

In general, distinctive characteristics of human saliva are its hypotonicity, and the lower sodium and higher potassium levels relative to the extracellular fluid concentrations. In this latter respect saliva approximates the composition of intracellular rather than extracellular fluid in its cationic components. Another special feature of saliva is that the sodium and chloride concentrations are flow-dependent; with increased secretory rate the sodium level rises and the chloride concentration increases. These changes in ionic concentrations are linearly related to the rate of salivary flow (*Figure 9.2*). Potassium concentration is only very slightly changed with increase of flow.

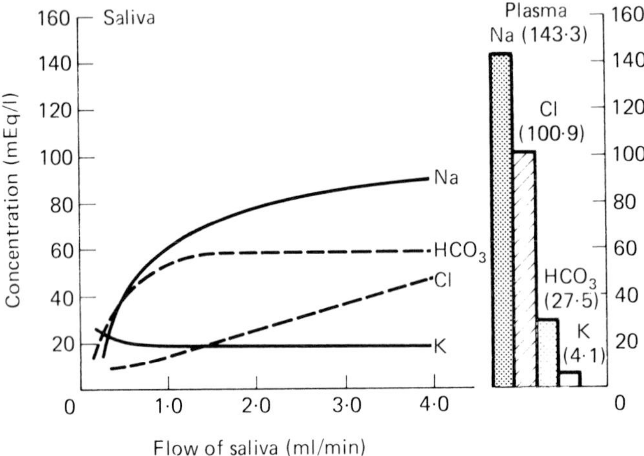

Figure 9.2 Changes in electrolyte concentration in human parotid saliva, with rate of salivary flow. (From Thaysen, Thorn and Schwartz, 1954, reproduced by courtesy of the Editor of *American Journal of Physiology*)

The salivary calcium is usually below that of the plasma but the resting concentration varies with the plasma calcium. It is not affected by the dietary intake of calcium. Some of the salivary calcium is protein-bound, some is colloidal calcium phosphate and some is complexed with carbon dioxide. As with sodium, the calcium concentration rises with the flow rate. Saliva is supersaturated with respect to calcium and phosphate. This is a factor in the formation of tartar on teeth and salivary calculi. The greater incidence of calculus formation in the submandibular gland is probably related to the difference in calcium concentration in parotid and submandibular saliva. There is some evidence of a raised calcium percentage in the saliva in caries-resistant subjects, but no convincing evidence that salivary calcium is of importance in relation to the development of caries.

Saliva collected from different glands shows a wide range of variation in chloride content. The percentage chloride is higher in sublingual and palatal gland secretions than in parotid or submandibular saliva. The chloride content of both parotid and submandibular saliva increases linearly with flow rate.

Both inorganic and organic phosphates are present in saliva. Approximately 20 per cent is organic and 80 per cent inorganic phosphate. The organic phosphate includes hexose phosphate, phospholipids, phosphoproteins and nucleic acids. The concentration of phosphate in mixed saliva is twice that present in the blood plasma.

In parotid and submandibular saliva the bicarbonate concentration at low flow rates is less than in the plasma. As the flow increases the bicarbonate rises and exceeds the plasma level. On the other hand the bicarbonate of the sublingual saliva is very low. The fact that the salivary bicarbonate may be higher than in the plasma implies that some bicarbonate may be formed in the gland cells. Thus the bicarbonate present in saliva is derived both from the blood plasma and interstitial fluid and also from metabolic processes in the gland cells.

The salivary glands have the capacity of 'trapping' iodides from the circulating blood plasma and excreting this ion in the saliva. The iodide concentration in resting saliva is much higher than in plasma. This concentration falls with increasing rates of flow. Thus the effect of changes of flow rate on iodide concentration is different from that observed for other ions.

Secretion of bromide in saliva resembles that of chloride, with a slightly higher saliva-to-plasma ratio.

The concentration of fluoride in the saliva varies with the fluoride content of the drinking water. Knowledge of the factors influencing salivary fluoride is very incomplete. This aspect of the subject is specially significant because fluoridation of water supplies has been advocated for reducing the incidence and the severity of dental caries.

Thiocyanate is present in saliva, particularly in heavy smokers.

Organic constituents

The organic constituents of saliva include proteins, polypeptides, amino acids, urea, uric acid, creatinine, cholesterol, citrate, thiocyanate, vitamins C and B complex. The proteins present are mainly mucin and amylase. In addition many other enzymes, group-specific agglutinogens, albumin, globulin, including blood clotting factors, have been demonstrated in saliva.

Proteins Human saliva contains approximately 0.3 g per cent protein. The salivary proteins determine its physical properties of viscosity and adhesiveness.

These proteins comprise a complex group of several classes of proteins. Electrophoretic patterns of saliva show differences in the saliva from different glands. The main peak in parotid saliva is due to amylase, while in submandibular saliva the principal component is a low-mobility mucoprotein.

In animal experiments the protein percentage was found to increase linearly with secretory rate. Thus the total protein per minute rises sharply with increase of flow. However the protein content of human parotid saliva is less clearly altered by changes in flow rate. In the submandibular gland saliva in response to sympathetic stimulation the protein concentration is high. Increasing the strength of parasympathetic stimulation increases the number of different proteins as well as increasing initially the amount of those which were present in the saliva before stimulation. The total protein and the proportions of protein present are both different in saliva elicited by sympathetic stimulation from that evoked by para-sympathetic stimulation. Further, although the protein concentration rises at first with increasing flow, it later decreases. With prolonged stimulation the total protein output per minute becomes steadily reduced.

Mucins These mucins are mucoproteins, mainly sialomucins. The mucin content is greatest in the sublingual saliva and the palatal and other accessory salivary glands. Mucins are present in lower concentration in the secretion of the submandibular gland and least in the parotid saliva. Thus the mucin content shows a correspondence with the percentage population of mucous acinar cells, in the different glands.

Mucins determine the viscosity of saliva. This accounts for the more viscous property of submandibular saliva in contrast with the low-viscosity, more watery, character of parotid saliva.

The mucins provide the physical and chemical basis of many of the functions of the saliva which are referred to in the section on functions of saliva (p. 324).

Amylase This enzyme belongs to the globulin class of proteins. It is present in highest concentration in parotid saliva; lower levels are found in the submandibular and sublingual saliva.

Its concentration is independent of the rate of secretion. It is highest in subjects who have been for prolonged periods on a high carbohydrate diet.

Other proteins In addition to mucin and amylase other proteins identified in saliva include albumin and globulin.

Other enzymes Besides amylase many other enzymes have been demonstrated in saliva. These may be constituents of the secretion of the gland cells, or derived from desquamated cells from the oral mucosa, or from bacteria or digested food. These enzymes include acid and alkaline phosphatases, cholinesterase, lipase, carbonic anhydrase, peroxidase, glycuronidase, dehydrogenase, sulphatase, kallikrien and lysozyme.

Isohaemagglutinogens The mucopolysaccharide agglutinogens A and B which determine the blood group of the ABO system are found not only on the red cell membrane but also in other tissue and body fluids of some individuals. The so-called 'secretors', 80 per cent of the population, have in their saliva the haemagglutinogen corresponding to their individual ABO grouping. In the 'non-secretor' 20 per cent of the population, the saliva and other body fluids do not contain the AB agglutinogens.

In the saliva of 'secretors' the concentration of agglutinogen is more than 100 times that of the erythrocytes. The distribution of these agglutinogens in human salivary glands has been explored using fluorescent antibody techniques. The A, B and H antigens are present in high concentration in the mucous acinar cells and not in duct cells of salivary glands of 'secretors'. They are absent in non-secretors. The concentration of these antigens is highest in the sublingual glands, less in the submandibular gland and very low in the parotid. This secretor status is genetically determined. The H and Le (Lewis) antigens may also be secreted in the saliva. Other blood group antigens of the Rhesus (C, D, E) system or M and N systems are never normally found in saliva.

Gases in solution

Oxygen, carbon dioxide and nitrogen are present in solution in saliva, as in all the body water compartments and secretions.

The enzyme carbonic anhydrase is also present in saliva, and it accelerates the combination of water with carbon dioxide to form carbonic acid.

Cellular constituents

Saliva collected from the mouth contains desquamated epithelial squames, lymphocytes from lingual and faucial tonsils, polymorphs and the bacterial flora of the mouth.

Physical properties

The physical properties of saliva vary greatly with changes in chemical composition and are affected by the nature of the stimulus, method of collection, gland of origin, and action of bacteria.

Reaction of saliva

The reaction of saliva has been extensively studied both in health and disease. Salivary hydrogen ion concentration has been implicated in various ways as a vital factor in the pathogenesis of dental caries. The reaction of saliva is markedly affected by flow rate, by the source of the saliva, and by the method of collection of saliva.

The human unstimulated mixed saliva as secreted is just on the acid side of neutrality. The mean pH is 6.7, with a range from 5.6 to 7.6. Submandibular resting saliva has a slightly less acid reaction than parotid saliva.

The pH of saliva is extremely sensitive to changes of flow rate. With increased flow in stimulated glands the pH rises and the salivary reaction approximates to the slightly alkaline reaction of plasma.

Viscosity of saliva

The viscosity of saliva is largely a function of its mucin content. The viscosity varies therefore in the secretion of the different glands in relation to the relative proportions of mucous and serous elements in their cell population.

The relative viscosities are: parotid 1.5; submaxillary 3.4; sublingual 13.4.

Processes of secretion

The mechanism of production of the secretion of salivary glands involves three main processes.

(1) Transport of water and some crystalloids from the plasma via the tissue fluid into the saliva. This involves processes of (a) active secretion, (b) active reabsorption, and (c) passive reabsorption.
(2) Synthesis, storage and secretion of colloidal organic molecules such as mucins and salivary enzymes.
(3) Diffusion and excretion of some organic electrolytes.

Saliva is formed by (1) acinar secretion and (2) tubular duct activity. The acinar secretion is an active transport of electrolytes with a secondary transport of water. In the acini also, protein enzymes, mucin and other organic substances are synthesized and excreted.

The cells of the duct system modify the acinar fluid to form the ultimate hypotonic saliva. This ductal activity includes in the main active reabsorption, active secretion and passive transport.

The mechanism of formation of acinar fluid is essentially an active secretory process and not merely a physical process of ultrafiltration. The acini are the main source of the water content of all saliva. Saliva contains substances, e.g. amylase and mucins, which are not present in plasma and are therefore synthesized in the gland cells.

The saliva is the end result of the functional activity of several types of cell, particularly (a) serous and mucous acinar cells; (b) striated intralobular duct epithelium; (c) cells of the main ducts. It is produced by acinar secretion, followed by active ductal reabsorption and secretory activity.

Factors influencing salivary secretion

Resting or basal secretion

The maintenance of the normal lubrication and moist surface of the mucosal epithelium of the tongue, mouth and pharynx is dependent on the continuous secretion of a small volume of saliva. This secretion also serves for cleansing and antibacterial activity and is one component in the thirst mechanism. This function is especially important during waking hours between meals and in sleep. The salivary output in these periods of minimal stimulation is referred to as the resting or basal secretion. This small continuous secretion can be demonstrated in any normal individual in health.

The contributions of the different salivary glands to the total resting secretion is shown in *Figure 9.3*. The resting secretory rate of the submandibular gland is three times that of the parotid. Sublingual secretion is less than 5 per cent of the total submandibular and sublingual resting secretion.

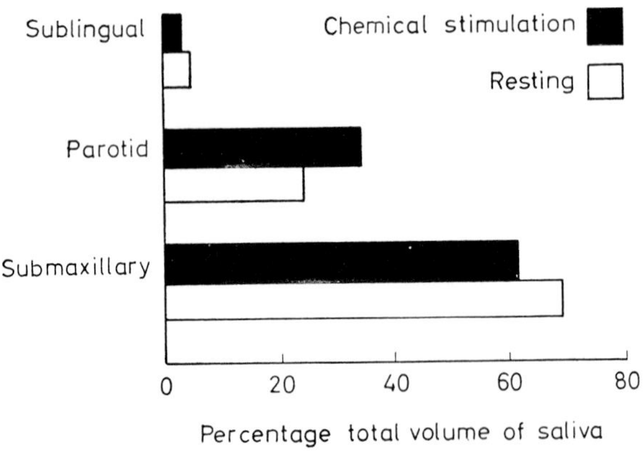

Figure 9.3 Relative percentage contribution from the main salivary glands to the volume of basal salivary secretion and to the total volume of saliva excited by acid stimulation. (From data of Schneyer and Levin)

The resting secretion is almost completely absent in sleep, and it is decreased by dehydration. Violent muscular exercise, mental effort and fear will also decrease the basal secretion. Movements of the mouth and jaws, as in jaw opening and closing, yawning and swallowing will cause small transient increases in secretion followed by a compensatory decrease. This effect may be due to a mechanical expression of saliva by compression of the gland or by reflex stimulation of a contractile mechanism within the gland. It is not due to any increase in secretory rate.

Mechanism of basal secretion The resting secretion may be attributed to any of the following mechanisms.

(1) Reflex stimulation from drying of the oral and pharyngeal mucous membranes.
(2) Reflex stimulation by other unknown stimuli.
(3) Some secretory cells may secrete continuously as an inherent spontaneous activity, independently of any extrinsic nervous or hormonal excitation.

The so-called basal or resting secretion could thus include both 'spontaneous' secretory activity and secretion due to tonic discharge from salivary nerve centres or to reflexes elicited by mucosal drying or some other not yet recognized stimuli.

The *accessory salivary glands* of the mouth have this capacity of spontaneous secretion.

Stimulated secretion

Against the background of spontaneous and 'resting' secretion there is superimposed the increased salivary secretion elicited reflexly by the ingestion of food and mastication, thermoregulation and other bodily activities.

Salivary secretion in response to taking of food The main peaks of salivary secretion occurring against the background of the basal or resting secretion are associated with the taking of food. These peaks of secretion are the result of a series of reflexes occurring in sequence. These are: (1) a conditioned reflex secretion in response to the thought, sight or smell of food; (2) inborn reflex secretion evoked by chewing; (3) reflex responses to stimulation of taste receptors and oral tactile receptors; (4) a further secretion during the passage of the bolus down the oesophagus and into the stomach – the oesophagosalivary and gastrosalivary reflexes.

Masticatory salivary reflex The chewing of insoluble tasteless substances, e.g. paraffin wax, will cause salivary secretion. Individuals with a low resting secretion respond usually with a smaller salivation response to chewing than those with a high resting secretory rate. Lashley (1916) showed in man that when chewing is restricted to one side, the salivary output from the glands on that side was much larger than from the glands of the other side. Thus the glands on the chewing side secrete actively while the glands of the opposite side produce only a small secretion. Pressure on the teeth did not elicit secretion. Pressure on the teeth together with mechanical stimulation of oral mucosa resulted in less secretion than with an object held between the teeth. The closure of the teeth of upper and lower jaws on an object appears to be the adequate stimulus for this reflex.

This masticatory–salivary secretion reflex is influenced by the size and consistency of the bolus. With constant size and physical characteristics of the bolus a constant volume of saliva was produced, with any given material increasing the size of the bolus chewed increased the secretion of saliva. There was a linear relation between the weight of the bolus and the salivary output. This may be due to the greater mass of the bolus increasing the area of receptor field stimulated, thus more receptors are fired and at a greater frequency of discharge. The greater afferent impulse stream to the salivary centres results in a greater reflex secretory response.

These experimental findings demonstrated that the important factors in initial stimulation of the reflex receptors are the rate of change of pressure and the duration of the cycle of pressure on the teeth during mastication.

The receptors for the masticatory–salivary reflex are probably mechanoreceptors in the periodontal membrane, and receptors of the oral mucous membrane and tongue.

Gustatory salivary reflex Saliva secretion occurs in response to stimulation of the taste receptors in the oral cavity. The morphology and physiology of these gustatory cells is discussed on p. 337.

Oesophagosalivary reflex Stimulation of the mucosa of the oesophagus or distention of this structure results in a well-marked reflex salivary flow. The swallowing of this saliva sets up oesophageal peristaltic stripping waves which assist in ensuring the effective passage of swallowed material along the oesophagus. Excessive salivation is often a symptom of chronic oesophagitis or cancer of the oesophagus.

Total volume

The total volume of saliva secreted per day is 0.5–1 litre.

This is calculated on the basis of 15 h at 20 ml/h of resting flow, together with 2 h for meals producing 300 ml of saliva and 7 h of sleep accounting for 20 ml of secretion. Measurements from patients with oesophageal fistula gave an average volume secreted of 500 ml per day.

Functions of saliva

Saliva fulfils a number of functions. These include moistening of the mouth, cleansing action, lubrication in swallowing and speech, buffering, diluent and solvent action, digestive action, thirst mechanism and antibacterial activity.

Moistening

The saliva keeps the mucous membrane of the mouth and pharynx moist. This is important in oral hygiene. When saliva is inadequate or absent the oral mucosa becomes dry and cracked leading to invasion by bacteria. This is an important aspect of the routine management of oral hygiene especially in the early post-operative period. In mouth-breathers the saliva becomes dehydrated, thick and viscous; and ropy sticky strands may form on the teeth and oral mucous membrane.

Lubrication for mastication and swallowing

The saliva moistens the food and facilitates the action of mastication and the movements of the tongue in manipulating and forming the soft mass of the bolus. The presence and taste of food in the mouth together with the masticatory movements causes increased secretion of saliva for this lubrication of the bolus – an action which is essential for normal swallowing. The water and mucin are the constituents of saliva which are especially concerned in this function.

Lubrication for speech

The moistening and lubrication of the mouth are essential for speech. The complex movements of the tongue and lips in the production of speech sounds necessitates normal oral lubrication. When the mouth is dry, clear speech is difficult. Xerostomia thus results in difficulty in swallowing and speech. Prolonged talking requires repeated sipping of water, because of the excessive evaporation of the saliva.

Role of mucins

In the above functions the mucins play a significant role. These substances assist in oral cleansing and lubrication, prevention of lodgement of food particles, formation of the soft bolus and facilitation of the movements of the lips, cheeks and tongue. In addition mucins slow down the rate of water evaporation and thus delay drying of the oral cavity. They suppress the action of some proteolytic enzymes and make a minor contribution to the buffering capacity of the saliva.

Buffer action

Saliva is a buffered fluid. Buffer solutions will prevent or minimize any change in reaction when acids or alkalis are added to the solution. This serves as a defence against any significant change in hydrogen ion concentration, and ensures the maintenance of the reaction of the fluids in the mouth within the range optimal for the activity of the salivary enzymes.

The maintenance of the constancy of the pH of the oral fluids is also important in relation to the bacterial flora of the mouth and to the development of dental caries.

The bicarbonate is the major buffer in saliva. This is convincingly demonstrated by the striking reduction of buffering power which follows removal of the bicarbonate from saliva.

The salivary proteins (mainly mucins) do not apparently contribute significantly to the buffering capacity of the saliva.

Solvent action

Soluble substances ingested and retained in the mouth will dissolve in the saliva, and can be swallowed in liquid form. This function of saliva is also important in relation to stimulation of taste receptors.

Digestion of starch

Salivary amylase (ptyalin) acts on the polysaccharides starch, dextrin and glycogen. Starch must be cooked so that the insoluble layer on the outer surface of the starch granule is first disrupted.

Antibacterial activity

Saliva exerts an effective action in suppressing the growth of micro-organisms in several ways.

(1) Saliva has a purely mechanical function of washing bacteria off the teeth and oral mucosa and holding these in suspension. This bacteria-laden saliva is swallowed

and the organisms are destroyed by the acid pepsin of the gastric juice.

(2) Leucocytes in the saliva can ingest bacteria by phagocytosis and destroy them by intracellular enzymes.

(3) The bacteriostatic properties of saliva include the following:

(a) Salivary leucotaxin exerts a chemotactic attraction for leucocytes into the saliva. This is especially evident in the presence of damaged oral mucosa.

(b) Opsonins are present in saliva and they increase the susceptibility of organisms to phagocytosis.

(c) Lysozyme and other antibacterial substances are present in saliva.

(d) Antibodies have been demonstrated in saliva.

The list of organisms normally resident in the mouth is very great. The warm moist environment of the mouth provides favourable conditions for the growth of organisms. The saliva contains amino acids and many nutrients essential for bacterial culture. Further the ingestion of food and the inspiration of air through the mouth (especially in mouth-breathers) means that many different organisms repeatedly gain access to the oral cavity.

The bacterial flora of the mouth in health and disease and their biochemistry are of importance in relation to the aetiology of dental decay, periodontal disease, and as a source of focal sepsis. The effects that follow the administration of oral antibiotics also have special interest. Several varieties of bacteria isolated from the mouth have been suggested as implicated in the aetiology of dental caries.

Salivary component in thirst mechanism

In thirst the mouth and pharynx feel dry and there is decreased salivary secretion. Normally drying of the oral mucosa is an effective stimulus promoting salivary secretion. However, in speaking for prolonged periods excessive evaporation of saliva from the mouth may exceed salivary secretion.

Dehydration due to water deprivation or excessive water losses, as in prolonged vomiting, diarrhoea, fistulae or excessive sweating, results in decreased salivary secretion.

Excretory function

Several substances are excreted in the saliva. However this is only a temporary means of removing these substances from the extracellular fluid. The saliva is normally swallowed and these excreted substances are then reabsorbed from the intestine. Thus only substances which are destroyed or digested in the alimentary tract after swallowing can be regarded as effectively cleared from the body by excretion into the saliva.

Saliva and taste

Substances can only excite taste cells in the oral cavity when they are in solution. Saliva by providing an aqueous solvent for solid foods plays a role in the sensory appreciation of eating and also serves to stimulate reflex secretions of saliva and gastric and pancreatic juices.

Dilution and cooling
Saliva poured out in response particularly to acid solutions will serve to dilute these solutions. Hot foods are cooled and cold foods are warmed by saliva before swallowing.

Cleansing action
The saliva serves to wash food particles and other solid material from the surface of the teeth and the gums, cheeks and tongue. This prevents stagnant food residues forming and acting as media for the growth of micro-organisms.

Anticaries activity
The possible importance of saliva in relation to the causation of dental caries has been extensively investigated. In rats excision of the salivary glands results in marked increase in dental caries. The gums especially around the incisor teeth show marked recession with exposure of cementum and caries.

Middle-ear pressure adjustment
The repeated swallowing of the basal secretion of saliva opens with each swallow the pharyngeal ostium of the pharyngotympanic tube and thus maintains the pressure equilibrium on the two surfaces of the tympanic membrane.

Neural control of salivary secretion

Salivary glands are under nervous control. This is a consequence of the need for the salivary secretory response to be rapid, since food is normally in the mouth for a brief period of time. Denervation of a salivary gland results in cessation of secretion and disuse atrophy.

The peripheral neural pathways are described in outline below.

Innervation of salivary glands
The major salivary glands have a double autonomic supply from the parasympathetic and sympathetic divisions of the autonomic nervous system.

Parasympathetic supply The three main salivary glands and the small glands of the oral and pharyngeal mucosa receive a nerve supply from the cranial division of the parasympathetic nervous system, distributed along the branches of the fifth, seventh, ninth and tenth cranial nerves.

This parasympathetic supply is the chief secretory supply of the salivary glands, and constitutes the final common path of efferent neurones of all the reflex arcs of the salivary response to the taking of food and many other stimuli.

The pre-ganglionic nerve cells of the parasympathetic salivary innervation are in the superior and inferior salivary nuclei in the medulla. The superior salivary nucleus activates secretion of the submandibular and sublingual glands while the inferior salivary nucleus regulates secretion of the parotid gland.

The pre-ganglionic fibres from the superior salivary nucleus pass out in the pars intermedia of the facial nerve and through the geniculate ganglion and leave the trunk of the facial nerve in the chorda tympani. The fibres then join the lingual branch of the trigeminal nerve and leave this to enter the submandibular ganglion. They synapse here. Axons of some post-ganglionic neurones of the submandibular ganglion pass directly to the submandibular gland, others pass back into the lingual nerve and are distributed to the sublingual gland complex. A few pre-ganglionic fibres pass through the submandibular ganglion and relay on ganglion cells in the hilum of the submandibular gland.

The pre-ganglionic axons of the cells of the inferior salivary nucleus emerge from the medulla in the glossopharyngeal nerve. They leave this nerve at its tympanic branch to pass to the tympanic plexus of the middle ear and then through the lesser superficial petrosal nerve to the otic ganglion. These fibres synapse here with post-ganglionic neurones. The fibres of these post-ganglionic neurones pass to the auriculo-temporal nerve and thus are distributed to the parotid gland.

Stimulation of the parasympathetic causes active secretion of a profuse watery fluid. This outflow of saliva is accompanied by vasodilatation and increased blood flow. The parasympathetic is the chief secretory supply of the salivary glands.

The parasympathetic nerve fibres supply acinar and duct cells and each secretory cell is innervated by terminal endings from several parasympathetic nerve fibres.

Parasympathetic transmitter The chemical transmitter at the post-ganglionic parasympathetic endings is acetyl choline.

Sympathetic supply Pre-ganglionic cells innervating the salivary glands are located in the lateral horn of grey matter of the first and second thoracic segments of the spinal cord. Pre-ganglionic axons arising from these cells emerge from the spinal cord in the ventral nerve roots of these segments and then pass along the corresponding mixed spinal nerves, anterior primary rami and white rami communicants to the first and second thoracic ganglia of the sympathetic trunk. These pre-ganglionic fibres ascend in the cervical sympathetic chain to synapse with cells of the superior cervical ganglion.

From these superior cervical ganglion cells, post-ganglionic fibres pass to the plexus around the external carotid artery and its branches and thus reach the salivary glands along their vascular supply.

In man sympathetic nerve impulses have been described as producing a small volume of viscid saliva in striking contrast with the profuse watery secretion of parasympathetic stimulation. Further it is claimed that stimulation of the cervical sympathetic chain will cause secretion by the submandibular gland but not by the parotid gland.

The secretion due to sympathetic stimulation may be attributed to the mechanical expression of secretion as a result of contraction of the myoepithelial cells.

The adrenergic transmitter The transmitter of the post-ganglionic sympathetic impulses is noradrenaline.

Dual innervation of individual secretory cells

The sympathetic and parasympathetic may both have the effect of stimulating salivary secretion. The existence of this double excitatory nerve supply raises the question whether each secretory cell has a double innervation or whether each cell is supplied by only one division of the autonomic nervous system, either parasympathetic or sympathetic.

Investigation of the electrical changes and pharmacological and histological studies support the first of these views, i.e. that each acinar gland cell is supplied by both sympathetic and parasympathetic nerve fibres. There is abundant other experimental evidence that each individual secretory cell is influenced by both sympathetic and parasympathetic nerve fibres.

While these experiments and histological studies show that acinar cells have a dual nervous control, the duct cells are apparently innervated only by the parasympathetic.

Medullary salivary reflex centres

Salivary secretion can be reflexly evoked by afferent stimulation, e.g. of taste receptors in the decerebrate animal. The gustatory–salivary reflex acts therefore through brain stem reflex centres.

The general salivatory reflex area is constituted by a pool of neurones in the reticular formation of the brain stem extending from the facial nucleus to the nucleus ambiguus.

The rostral portion of this area consists of the cell bodies of the pre-ganglionic neurones of the parasympathetic nervous system which regulate the submaxillary and sublingual glands. This is the superior salivatory nucleus. The caudal portion or the inferior salivatory nucleus is the pre-ganglionic neurone pool of the parasympathetic innervation of the parotid gland. The localization of the salivatory centres for the different glands is shown in *Figure 9.4*.

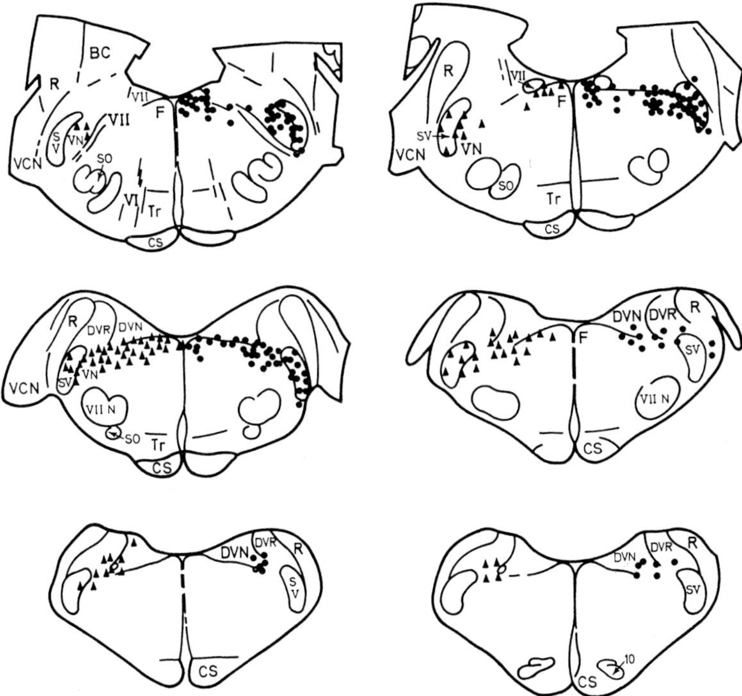

Figure 9.4 Diagrammatic representation of areas in medulla controlling salivation. Circles indicate responses from the ipsilateral submandibular gland and triangles responses from the ipsilateral parotid gland. (From Wang, 1943, reproduced by courtesy of the Editor of *Journal of Neurophysiology*)

The axons from these salivatory nuclei in the lateral portion of the reticular formation pass first rostrally and then dorsolaterally to emerge from the brain stem in the pars intermedia of the facial nerve and in the glossopharyngeal nerve.

These medullary secretory centres regulate mainly but not exclusively the salivary glands of the same side.

Afferent impulses from the mouth receptors will reflexly stimulate superior and inferior salivatory nuclei of both sides but mainly on the same side. In the same way stimulation of the central end of the sectioned lingual nerve may cause secretion of both sides.

Impulses from taste receptors in the anterior part of the tongue mediated along fibres of the lingual nerve excite the superior more than the inferior salivatory nucleus and thus cause salivary flow mainly from the submandibular gland.

Stimulation, on the other hand, of taste cells in the posterior part of the tongue initiates impulses transmitted along glossopharyngeal fibres to excite the inferior salivatory nucleus and produce parotid gland secretion.

Supramedullary control

The medullary salivary centres are under constant regulation from the hypothalamus and cerebral cortex.

This diencephalic and cortical control may in some instances be excitatory, in others inhibitory.

Inhibition from these 'higher' levels is seen in sleep, fear and in hypnosis. The salivary secretion produced reflexly in association with feeding, i.e. conditioned reflex responses to sight or smell of food, and inborn reflex secretion to taste, involves parasympathetic salivary secretory centres. This is a localized response to normal environmental stimuli. In contrast the emotional responses to fear, i.e. the 'fight and fright' reaction, is accompanied by massive widespread sympathetic discharge. This is a generalized response to the abnormal stress situation.

Increased salivation is a prominent symptom of the tremor–rigidity syndrome (parkinsonism) resulting from lesions in the basal ganglia. Cases of epilepsy also may show hypersalivation.

Hypothalamus Electrical stimulation through electrodes implanted in various areas of the hypothalamus can elicit salivary secretion.

Cortical control Salivation can be produced by stimulation of several areas of the grey cortex of the frontal lobe of the brain (*Figure 9.5*). Stimulation of the face area of the motor cortex at the lower part of the pre-central gyrus causes salivation. This forms one element in a complex reaction including licking movements of the tongue, movements of the lips and lower jaw and salivation.

Salivation may also be induced by excitation of the superior frontal gyrus and the region of the orbital gyri of the frontal lobe and from olfactory areas of the brain, especially the pyriform lobe and amygdaloid nucleus.

Cortical control is represented in the conditioned reflexes exciting salivary secretion.

In summary, the brain stem salivary centres are activated reflexly and are also controlled by cortical hypothalamic and amygdaloid centres in the execution of an integrated normal pattern of responses to the taking of food. The supramedullary

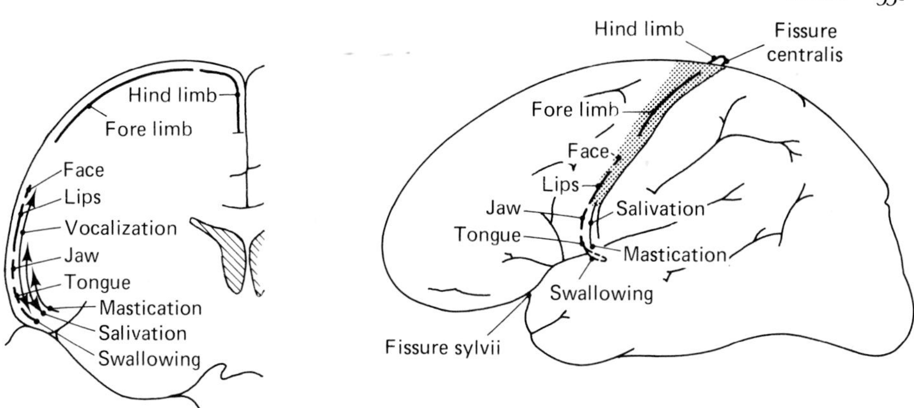

Figure 9.5 Diagram of the motor representation on the cerebral cortex in man indicating localization of cortical areas for salivation, mastication and swallowing (after Babkin and Van Buren, 1951)

centres also regulate the salivary responses to emotional stress, fear or rage and as part of the response of thermal regulation in maintaining the relative constancy of body temperature.

Drugs affecting salivary secretion

Drugs stimulating or inhibiting salivary secretion may act on (1) peripheral receptors of reflex arcs eliciting salivary secretion; (2) salivary secreting centres, either directly or from other areas in the central nervous system; (3) autonomic ganglia; (4) autonomic neuro-effector junctions in salivary glands; (5) salivary gland secretory cells; (6) myoepithelial cells; (7) vascular supply of the glands.

Stimulation of peripheral receptors

Taste receptor stimulation The salivary response to substances which excite taste receptors has been described in a previous section. Sucrose and acetic acid solutions cause an increase in secretion, and bitter tasting alkaloids also stimulate gustatory chemoreceptors and reflexly excite salivary secretion.

Irritation of oral mucosa Profuse salivation is a feature of mercury poisoning. This effect is due in part to irritation and stomatitis caused by the mercury excreted in the saliva. This irritation reflexly excites salivary secretion. Smoking also induces salivation by the irritant effect of tobacco fumes on the mucosal nerve endings. Some anaesthetics such as ether, chloroform and cyclopropane cause salivation. This effect decreases as deeper planes of anaesthesia are reached. This salivation is absent if the volatile anaesthetic is administered through a tracheal tube, or when the mucosa of the upper respiratory tract is anaesthetized by a local anaesthetic. Thus the receptors responsible for this secretion are located in the upper respiratory tract. Intranasal menthol or some alcohol vapours will cause ipsilateral parotid secretion. This reflex is still present in cases of complete anosmia. The receptors are therefore not olfactory but trigeminal nerve endings.

Drugs acting centrally

Central stimulants Nikethamide, picrotoxin, or cocaine will increase salivary flow. Reserpine also stimulates parasympathetic centres to produce increased secretion.

Drugs inducing nausea and vomiting Increased salivation is usually an accompaniment of nausea. Drugs causing vomiting also induce salivation. These may act (1) reflexly; (2) on the medullary vomiting centre; (3) on the chemoreceptor trigger zone for vomiting.

This group of emetic drugs includes apomorphine, morphine, digitalis and quinidine. Salivation accompanying nausea may be alleviated by antihistaminic and other anti-emetic drugs.

Drugs affecting temperature regulation Salivary secretion is especially notable with hyperthermia in dogs. Sweat glands are absent, and salivation and panting breathing form part of the physiological bodily response to rising body temperature. Drugs which have a calorigenic effect and tend to raise the basal metabolic rate will increase salivatory flow. The increase in secretory rate is proportional to the rise in body temperature.

Anaesthetic agents Salivary reflexes are readily suppressed by many anaesthetic agents.

Drugs with ganglionic action

Transmission of nerve impulses is cholinergic at parasympathetic and sympathetic ganglionic synapses as well as at parasympathetic peripheral post-ganglionic neuroglandular junctions. Thus acetylcholine and related choline-esters could stimulate secretion at any of these three sites. The threshold of response of the gland cells is however much lower than that of ganglionic synapses. The concentration of acetylcholine that will excite secretion by peripheral action is considerably less than that required to stimulate ganglionic nerve cells. Thus acetylcholine acts by its peripheral parasympathomimetic action; its effects are not significantly reduced by ganglionic blockade.

Drugs stimulating the autonomic ganglia can excite salivary glands through both parasympathetic and sympathetic post-ganglionic fibres. The parasympathetic effect always predominates.

Ganglion blocking drugs will prevent transmission at both parasympathetic and sympathetic pre-ganglionic–post-ganglionic synapses. As the physiological regulation of salivary secretion acts chiefly through the parasympathetic outflow as a final common path, the more important action of these drugs is in the parasympathetic synapses.

Salivary secretory activity is one of the autonomic responses which is most sensitive to the action of these blocking drugs. Parasympathetic salivary ganglia are the first of the autonomic ganglia at which transmission is suppressed by ganglion blocking drugs, e.g. hexamethonium.

Drugs acting at neuro-effector endings

Parasympathetic mimetic drugs These drugs can cause as large a volume of secretion from a salivary gland as that of maximal stimulation of the parasympathetic nerve supply of that gland.

In this group of parasympathomimetic drugs are included acetylcholine, mecholyl and pilocarpine.

Parasympatholytic drugs Atropine will completely block the secretory response to parasympathetic stimulation. In very large doses it can also inhibit sympathetic ganglionic synapses and can block peripheral sympathetic neuroglandular transmission. This group of drugs includes scopolamine and methylscopolamine. Some of these chemicals are more potent inhibitors of salivary secretion than atropine.

Some antihistaminic drugs have a peripheral parasympathomimetic action. This effect is additional to the inhibition of secretion by a central anti-emetic and sedative action. Barbiturates also have an antisialogogue effect.

Sympathomimetic drugs Sympathomimetic drugs elicit a much less marked response than the parasympathomimetic drugs.

Many sympathomimetic amines have been studied and they show differences in their stimulatory capacity. In order of potency, they are adrenaline, noradrenaline, ephedrine, isoprenaline, and amphetamine.

These drugs also induce vasoconstriction and this may secondarily effect a reduction of salivary secretion.

Sympatholytic drugs The normal response to sympathetic nerve stimulation can be abolished by ergotamine and dibenamine. Priscol blocks the vasoconstrictor response while chlorpromazine abolishes both secretion and vasomotor effects.

Other drugs

Histamine In large doses histamine increases salivary secretion.

Histamine has a stimulating action on salivary gland cells and on myoepithelial contractile elements. In addition histamine has a central action and also causes a release of adrenaline from the adrenal medulla.

Atropine blocks the action of histamine on salivary gland cells but does not prevent its action on myoepithelium.

Mercury Hypersalivation is a distinctive feature of mercury poisoning. Several factors produce this effect. Stomatitis causing reflex secretion, central action on salivatory nuclei and inhibition of cholinesterase at peripheral parasympathetic endings, may all play a part in this excessive salivation.

Potassium Potassium salts have a slight sialogogue effect. This is due to a local release of acetylcholine since the response to close arterial injection of potassium salts can be potentiated by eserine.

Nitrogen mustards These produce a two-phase response; an initial increase is followed by a period of cessation of flow. Then a second secretion occurs. This rises to a maximal rate which is then maintained for hours. Atropinization will prevent this effect of nitrogen mustard but only if the atropine is given before the nitrogen mustard.

Analysis of the mechanism of this secretory response to nitrogen mustards has demonstrated that it is due mainly to a peripheral parasympathetic stimulation. The two-phase response has not been explained nor is there any satisfactory explanation of the failure of atropine to block this action.

Salivary secretagogues A substance stimulating salivary secretion has been demonstrated in saliva. When saliva is injected into the blood supplying a salivary gland, secretion results. This substance could be an intermediary between the released neurochemical transmitter and the salivary gland cell.

Physiology of taste

Taste is a chemical sense. It is a sensory experience produced by appropriate stimulation of specific chemical receptors in the oral cavity.

Distribution of taste receptors

The receptors for taste are located in taste buds, present mainly on the tongue, but also sparsely distributed in the mucous membrane of the palate, fauces and epiglottis. Their distribution is described in Chapter 8.

The taste buds total about 9000 in the adult. They are embedded in the stratified epithelium mainly in relation to fungiform and vallate papillae. There are no taste buds in the central part of the dorsal surface of the tongue of the adult. Taste buds are more numerous in children and they are distributed more widely, being found in the whole of the dorsal surface of the tongue, the hard and soft palates and the mucosa of the cheeks. In old age the taste buds undergo regression; and they are markedly reduced in number. There is a corresponding decrease in the sensitivity of the taste mechanism in the elderly.

Taste bud structure

Each taste bud consists of supporting cells and taste cells. The peripheral supporting cells are arranged like the segments of an orange to form the walls of a small oval chamber. This central chamber opens through a circular opening, the inner taste pore, into a short canal which in turn opens superficially through an outer taste pore. The cavity of the taste bud is occupied by some 5–20 taste receptors or gustatory cells, together with a filling of central supporting cells. Each gustatory cell is spindle-shaped. Its outer apical end extends through the inner pore and has numerous microvillous processes. At this gustatory pore, substances in solution in the saliva come into contact with the receptor cell.

Electron microscopic studies by Murray, Murray and Fujimoto (1969) of the ultrastructure of the taste bud showed that the cells within each taste bud can be divided into three distinct types (*Figure 9.6*). Type I cells are slender and dark and are presumed to be supportive in function. Type II cells are pale and slender. The apical ends of these have minute villous processes. Type III cells resemble type II in shape and cytoplasmic density but they have characteristic aggregates of synaptic vesicles in the central part of the cell. One variety of these vesicles resembles those which have been postulated to contain acetylcholine. Another type of vesicle is larger, with a dense core, and has the features of vesicles which have been shown to store catecholamines. They also have no microvilli.

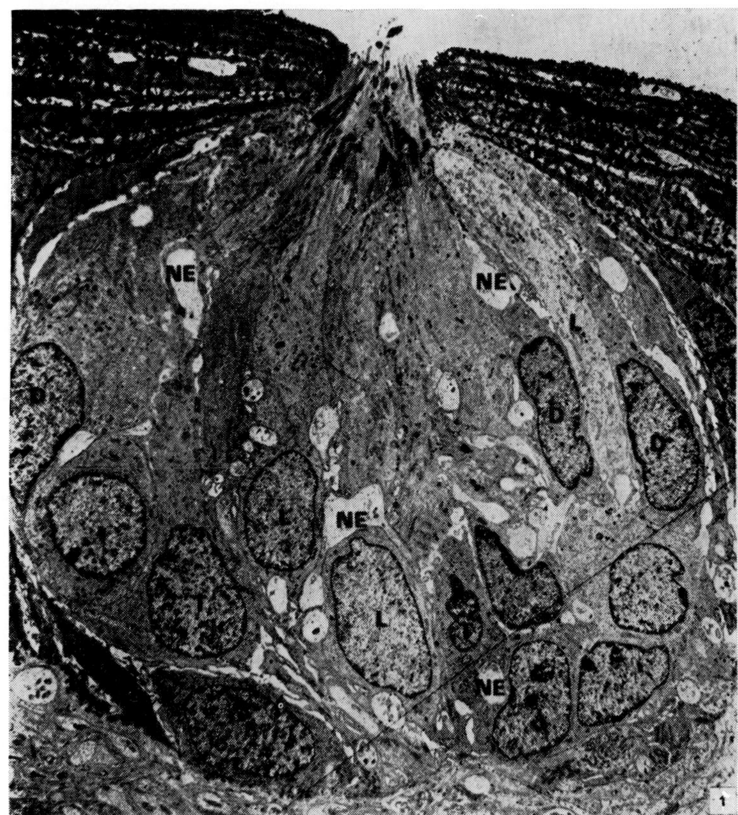

Figure 9.6 Survey view of entire taste bud. Rabbit foliate papilla (× 3000). (From Murray, Murray and Fujimoto, 1969, reproduced by courtesy of the Editor of *Journal of Ultrastructure Research*)

Each taste cell is innervated by nerve fibrils at its basal end. These fibrils are derived from a subepithelial nerve plexus and terminate in invaginations of the membrane of the receptor cell.

The receptor cells for taste are constantly degenerating and being replaced. This replacement is effected by mitotic division of epithelial cells adjacent to the taste cells. This rapid turnover of taste receptors has been investigated by determining the mitotic rate after arresting cell division by colchicine, and has been confirmed by radio-autographs after tagging these cells with radio-isotopic labelled thymidine.

Taste buds on the anterior two-thirds of the tongue are innervated by fibres from cells in the geniculate ganglion of the facial nerve. These fibres reach the taste cells through the facial nerve and thence mainly via the chorda tympani and the lingual nerve. The taste cells of the posterior third of the tongue are supplied by fibres with cell bodies in the petrous ganglion of the glossopharyngeal nerve. The taste receptors on the soft palate, pharyngeal surface of the tongue and the epiglottis are innervated by vagal fibres.

No taste afferent fibres are present in the trigeminal nerve which however mediates general somatic sensation from the tongue and mouth. Gasserian ganglionectomy does not cause loss of taste sensation. However, impulses subserving tactile, pressure, thermal and other common sensations from the oral cavity, do contribute with taste to the total sensory complex we imply by the expression 'flavour' of food, and are mediated along trigeminal sensory neurones. The nervous pathway for taste is described in a later paragraph. Taste buds gradually degenerate when their afferent nerve fibres are sectioned. When the sectioned nerve regenerates, the taste buds may also be regenerated.

Basic modalities of taste

Four primary submodalities of taste sensations are normally recognized – sweet, salt, sour (acid) and bitter. Two additional basic sensations are accepted by some – alkaline and metallic tastes.

The numerous identifiable tastes are due to combinations of stimulation, at varying intensities, of one or more of the primary taste sensations or to association of these primary taste combinations with sensations resulting from stimulation of the non-gustatory nerve endings of the lingual and oral mucosa, and of the olfactory receptors. Olfaction forms a large element in some of the flavours that are commonly regarded as tastes. The flavour of many foods is due to both their gustatory and olfactory components. Depression of the olfactory sense, for example during a cold, leads to impairment of the appreciation of the flavour of food. Taste and smell are functionally linked in the regulation of food intake and are associated in the reflex control of the glandular secretions of the alimentary tract. Tactile sensation, the smooth or rough quality, the degree of hardness or softness of the food together with its temperature also contribute to the flavour of the food. Stimulation of nerve endings by irritants like mustards and peppers partly accounts for their characteristic effects. These tactile and pressure receptors and free nerve endings in the oral mucous membranes discharge along fibres in the trigeminal nerve. Dentures, by preventing contact of food with the tactile and thermal sensory receptors in the palatal mucosa, cause a diminished appreciation of 'taste'.

Thus the great number of different tastes can be explained as varying permutations of different intensity and duration of stimulation of the primary peripheral taste receptors and supplemented by stimulation to varying extents of chemical, tactile, thermal, pressure and olfactory receptors, together with, in some instances, the inductive effect of simultaneous and successive contrast.

Distribution of primary taste sensations

The basic taste sensations are spatially distributed in different parts of the tongue. Sweet taste is located mainly at the tip of the tongue which, however, also responds to the other submodalities. The tongue margins are most sensitive to acid but also to salt. The posterior and basal part of the tongue and the epiglottis have taste receptors for bitter.

The intensity threshold, i.e. the lowest concentration that can be identified, consequently shows a regional distribution over the tongue.

There may be a functionally specific receptor for each primary taste. This is confirmed by recording action potentials in nerve fibres from individual taste buds. No histological features have been found to differentiate taste cells into types corresponding to the functional types.

Electrophysiology of taste receptors

Taste receptors are gustatory transducers. Action potential studies recording from single *taste fibres* show that stimulation by more than one taste can excite impulses in a single fibre. Impulses can be produced in some fibres more readily by one specific taste. In other fibres impulses can be recorded when any of several taste stimuli are applied to the tongue.

Intracellular micro-electrode recording from single *taste cells* indicated that from some of these cells, changes in membrane potential could be detected with several kinds of taste stimuli. These findings suggest that some taste cells have the ability to be excited by more than one type of taste stimulus. This concept would imply that different taste sensations would be signalled to the brain by differences in the pattern of nerve fibres conducting impulses, and thus would be recognized by the pattern of the arrival sites at which these impulses end in the cortical taste centre.

Investigations of individual *taste buds* reveal that in some taste buds, all the taste cells respond only to one of the primary stimuli. Some others contain cells serving more than one modality of taste but no one taste bud responds to all four primary tastes.

When *individual papillae* are tested it is found that taste buds on *fungiform* papillae respond to sweet and salt or acid and sweet or to bitter and acid. A few papillae have a complement of taste buds subserving each of the primary tastes. All the taste buds on *vallate* papilla are responsive only to bitter substances.

Taste receptors adapt fairly rapidly. The intensity of a taste decreases although the stimulus is maintained constant.

When a sweet substance is kept in contact with an area of the tongue the sweet taste gradually decreases. Moving the sweet to another unstimulated area of the tongue immediately restores the original taste intensity. An area adapted to acid will fail to respond to all acid stimuli; but adaptation to one bitter or sweet substance will not necessarily modify the taste of other bitter or sweet substances.

One physiological problem is whether there are four types of taste receptors, each single receptor responding to one of the four primary stimuli or alternatively whether each taste cell may respond to more than one or to all of the stimuli. On the first view taste 'analysis' takes place peripherally and is signalled to the brain by whichever receptors are stimulated, and therefore which part of the taste centre is the final arrival platform for these impulses. Strength of taste would be signalled by the frequency of the train of impulses. On the second view, each receptor would have to signal differently in some unknown way when stimulated by different tastes.

Although there appears to be some evidence from membrane potential and action potential studies and histology supporting the single receptor type hypothesis there is also considerable evidence for the multiple receptor theory. This latter view conforms with the mechanisms established for all other peripheral sensory receptors. Further evidence is provided by the localization of taste sensations on the tongue and in separate taste buds, the recording of action potentials in single fibre preparations and the selective suppressor effect of drugs on taste sensations.

Mechanism of stimulation

The mechanism of stimulation and initiation of impulses from taste receptors is unknown. One suggestion is that the sapid substances act by affecting the activity of enzymes in the taste receptor cells. Taste substances may theoretically act by enhancing or suppressing the velocity of action of the enzymes. Quinine for example will inhibit phosphatase and nucleotidase but potentiates other enzymes. Thus the spectrum of influence of taste substances in different directions on various enzymes would determine its capacity to stimulate different receptors. Phosphatases, esterases and other enzymes have been demonstrated histochemically in the lingual epithelium and taste buds.

Another theory is that sapid substances become bound to a surface film of electrolyte on the receptor cell. This produces a change in the surface charge on the cell. This causes a 'generator' potential which results in 'depolarization' of the nerve axon and a self-propagated nerve action potential along the nerve fibre.

Chemical constitution and taste

Correlation of taste and chemical constitution has been attempted.

Sweet Sweet tasting substances are organic compounds. These include the sugars, e.g. sucrose, glucose, some polysaccharides, glycerol, some alcohols and ketones, saccharine, cyclamates and chloroform. However, a few inorganic salts like lead acetate and dilute alkalis also are sweet. It has been postulated that sweetness depends on the presence in the molecular structure of two types of radical or atom. One of these is 'glucophore' and the other 'auxogluc'. The presence of both a glucophore and an auxogluc in the molecule is necessary to confer a sweet taste on a substance.

Salt Salty substances are mainly inorganic salts. Notable examples are the chlorides of sodium, potassium, magnesium and ammonium, and some sulphates and iodides, and the nitrates of sodium and potassium. The salty taste is due to the anion. The halogens in particular taste salty. The threshold dilution at which this taste of the halogens can just be detected is greatest for chloride, next for bromide and lowest for iodide. A few organic compounds have a saline taste.

Sour This taste is a property of acids and acid salts. The adequate stimulus for these acid receptors is the hydrogen ion. The intensity of the sour taste is normally directly related to the hydrogen ion concentration for any particular acid. Nevertheless some organic acids (acetic, citric, tartaric) are several times more acid in taste than solutions of mineral acids of the same hydrogen ion concentration. This difference is thought to be due to the greater penetrating power of the organic acid into the taste cells.

The ability to recognize differences in the taste of different organic acids, e.g. acetic and citric acids, may be due to the additional effect of the acid anion.

Bitter Most of the substances which have a bitter taste are organic compounds. These include the alkaloids, quinine and strychnine and morphine, nicotine, and caffeine, urea and bile salts. Some inorganic salts of magnesium, ammonium and calcium also taste bitter due to the cation.

Some substances may stimulate more than one primary receptor, for example sodium salicylate stimulates sweet and bitter receptors and magnesium sulphate excites both salt and bitter taste cells.

Neural pathways for taste

The fibres from the taste cells of the anterior two-thirds of the tongue pass into the lingual nerve. They leave this nerve and enter the chorda tympani and join the facial nerve in the facial canal.

An alternative pathway is from the chorda tympani by a communicating branch to the otic ganglion and from there in the greater petrosal nerve to the geniculate ganglion and the facial nerve trunk.

The cell bodies of all these fibres are in the geniculate ganglion of the facial nerve. The central processes of these ganglion cells run in the pars intermedia to enter the brain stem at the sulcus between the pons and medulla. They terminate by synapsing on the cells of the cephalic part of the nucleus solitarius.

From the posterior third of the tongue the taste fibres are in the glossopharyngeal nerve. The cell bodies are in the petrous ganglion. The central processes of these first order neurones enter the brain stem and terminate on the cells of the lower part of the nucleus solitarius.

Impulses from taste cells in the pharyngeal mucosa and on the epiglottis pass in fibres of the vagus nerve. Their cell bodies are located in the nodose ganglion.

All taste impulses are of low amplitude and slow velocity of conduction indicating small diameter fibres less than 4 μm.

Central connections

The taste fibres in the facial, glossopharyngeal and vagus nerves enter the medulla, descend in the solitary tract and terminate on the cells of the nucleus of the tractus solitarius.

The 'taste' fibres in these three cranial nerves relay at different levels in the nucleus solitarius; those in the facial and glossopharyngeal nerves end in the rostral part of this nucleus and those in the vagus end in the caudal region of this nucleus.

From the nucleus solitarius two main sets of connections are made:

(1) To the preganglionic parasympathetic cells in the superior and inferior salivatory nuclei and the dorsal vagal nuclei. These constitute interneurones in gustatory reflex pathways. Inborn reflex responses to taste include salivary secretion and secretion of gastric and pancreatic juice. The reflex gastric response to taste is an important component in the cephalic phase of gastric secretion.
(2) Second-order ascending neurones subserving the taste sensation. This bulbo-thalamic pathway crosses to join the medial lemniscus of the opposite side. These fibres ascend and relay in the thalamus.

In the thalamus these fibres relay on cells close to where fibres of somatic sensation from the face relay.

From the arcuate nucleus of the thalamus a final third-order neurone conducts 'taste' impulses to the cortical taste centre. Bornstein has produced evidence that the centre is in the inferior part of the cortex of the parietal lobe adjacent to the somatosensory area for the tongue and face. This area extends into the lateral fissure and on to the insula. Electrophysiological studies have shown potential changes in the inferior part of the post-central gyrus in the region of the cortical sensory area for the face and tongue, when the taste receptors are stimulated. The cortical centre for taste and that for somatic sensation of the face and tongue are intermingled and overlap.

In primates the taste threshold was raised when the cortex around the insula was damaged. Stimulation of the insular region in man caused hallucinations of taste. Bornstein showed a contralateral decrease of gustatory perception in patients with bullet wounds of the inferior post-central area of the cerebral cortex. This close association with the area for common sensation for the mouth is relevant to the contribution made to some flavours by stimulation of non-gustatory endings in the oral mucous membrane.

Taste sensitivity

The intensity taste threshold for any substance can be investigated by determining the minimum concentration at which its taste can be appreciated. Some examples of this minimum detectable concentration for each of the four primary taste groups are listed in *Table 9.1*.

Table 9.1

Substance		*Minimum detectable concentration*
Sweet:	Cane sugar	0.01 M
	Saccharin	0.000023 M
Salt:	Sodium chloride	0.02 M
Sour:	Hydrochloric acid	0.0001 M
Bitter:	Strychnine	0.0000016 M

Intensity discrimination

When the strength of a sensory stimulus is gradually increased the smallest change in stimulus intensity which can be perceived as a change in sensation intensity, is a constant fraction of the preceding intensity. This Weber–Fechner law applies to all senses including the special senses of vision, hearing, olfaction and taste. In general terms the smallest increment in stimulus intensity (ΔI) which will produce a just perceptible difference in sensation (S) bears a fixed ratio to the initial stimulus intensity; thus $\Delta I/I = K$ (a constant).

In the case of taste, the ability to discriminate differences in taste intensity is poorly developed. The stimulus must be increased by 30 per cent at any given intensity, before it is consciously recognized as an increase in taste.

Taste contrasts

The effect of different modalities of taste either successively or simultaneously excited from the tongue, induces changes in perception responses. Thus the taste sensation manifests the phenomena of successive and simultaneous contrast.

Successive contrast The taste of a sweet substance is intensified if preceded by tasting a substance of salty or bitter taste. The latter tastes are similarly enhanced if preceded by sweet. The same kind of successive contrast applies to sour and sweet stimuli, for example lemon juice preceded by sugar. This is a form of temporal induction.

Simultaneous contrast Salt applied to one border of the tongue increases the sweet sensation to a sweet-tasting substance simultaneously applied to the opposite border. This spatially-induced enhancement of response can also be demonstrated with salt and acid, but no simultaneous contrast can be shown for the bitter taste.

Selective suppression

Some drugs can specifically block particular taste sensations. Such a selective effect is one action of Gymnemic acid. Local application of this extract of the leaves of *Gymnema sylvestre* to the tongue abolishes sweet and decreases bitter while salt and acid tastes persist. Local anaesthetics will suppress all taste and common sensibility. These various sensations are abolished in the following order: pain – bitter – sweet – salt – acid and touch.

'Taste blindness'

'Taste blindness' is an inherited mendelian recessive trait characterized by an inability to taste phenylthiocarbamide. This chemical is a sulphur containing a derivative of the extremely sweet dulcin, which is 500 times more sweet than sucrose. Phenylthiocarbamide tastes very bitter to 70 per cent of individuals. It is tasteless for the other 30 per cent who are 'taste blind'.

Physiology of mastication

Mastication of solid food is usually an essential preliminary to deglutition.

By breaking up solid food and assisting the solution of its soluble constituents in the saliva, chewing has a subsidiary physiological role in relation to taste and reflex secretion of saliva, and gastric and pancreatic secretion.

The food is crushed and disintegrated in the mouth by the action of the teeth and jaws, moved by the muscles of mastication and assisted by tongue, lips and cheeks. These movements involve rhythmic separation and approximation of the jaws, together with some forward and backward and lateral movements. The tongue and cheeks serve to keep on placing the food between the occlusal surfaces of the teeth.

The main power of the movements in mastication is provided by the muscles of mastication bringing about movements of the mandible at the temporo-mandibular joint. Three main varieties of movement occur at this joint: (1) hinge-like movement; (2) protrusion and retrusion; (3) lateral movement.

The hinge movement is used in biting while the lateral movement provides the grinding motion for crushing the food.

The lateral movement is roughly symmetrical in its amplitude in most normal subjects. Normal mastication is achieved by a complex pattern of movements involving all three types of joint movement, to varying extents and in a varying force, sequence and duration of movement.

The movements of mastication vary with the nature of the food. In biting soft foods most individuals employ a slight protrusion together with a hinge movement for closing the jaws. When biting harder foods the jaws are closed and then a retrusive movement of the lower jaw follows. In chewing the chief crushing activity consists of a combination of lateral movements with forceful opening and closing actions.

Role of the lips and tongue in mastication

The tongue The tongue has several functions in relation to mastication. It assists in the process of thoroughly mixing the food with mucinous saliva during chewing and preparatory to swallowing. Very soft foods can be broken up by pressure between the hard palate and the tongue. The rugae of the anterior part of the hard palate serve to arrest any tendency for the food to slip during this lingual compression. During mastication the tongue consistently pushes food between the occlusal surfaces of the teeth and also moves the food from one masticating surface to another. In the later stages of chewing, the tongue explores the chewed masses in the mouth and assesses which portions are adequately disintegrated and ensalivated to be ready for swallowing. The tongue further separates and forms these portions into a bolus for swallowing. In these actions the afferent innervation of the tongue, both sensory and proprioceptive, must play an important part. The presence of muscle spindles in the lingual musculature in man has been confirmed. The high innervation density and fine tactile sensitivity of the mucosa of the hard palate suggests that this region also contributes to the assessment of the firmness and texture of the chewed food in the mouth, and thus the decision as to when it is ready for swallowing. The tongue provides part of the propulsive force in the oral phase of swallowing.

Tactile sensibility and appreciation of temperatures by the tongue also forms part of the complex sensation of 'taste'. This explains the decreased taste sensation when wearing dentures which cover the palate.

The lips and cheeks The lips are used in the transfer of fluid and solid food into the mouth and to retain the food in the oral cavity during mastication. The lips and cheeks assist the tongue in ensuring the replacement of food between the teeth during chewing. Their high neural sensitivity both thermal and tactile help in the entry of food into the mouth and preventing the cheeks coming between the teeth during the masticatory strokes. Occasionally some food may be held in the oral vestibule between the cheeks and the alveolar ridge and teeth called the 'parking bolus'. The lips also close and provide an anterior oral seal during the initial oral phase of deglutition.

Frequency of chewing movements

The number of chewing movements per minute tends to be a fixed characteristic of each individual. On the average the frequency is higher in the male than in the female. The masticatory stroke frequency is also affected by gross differences in the consistency of the food; greater toughness is compensated by a greater chewing frequency.

Occlusal contact

The masticatory surfaces of the teeth do not necessarily make contact with each chewing movement. Anderson and Picton (1957) studied tooth contact and correlated this with simultaneous electromyographic records. The percentage of masticatory strokes in which the tooth surfaces came into actual contact varied with the physical nature of the masticated food. In chewing meat or bread 50 per cent of chewing strokes were completed by tooth contact while in the chewing of biscuits contact took place very seldom.

Masticatory force

The masticatory stroke of the jaws comprises initially an isotonic contraction of the jaw-closing muscles as the lower jaw is elevated, accompanied by reciprocal relaxation of the antagonistic muscles. This is followed by an isometric contraction of the jaw elevators after the teeth are in contact.

The maximum biting force is about 45 kg for the molar teeth and is lower in the female than the male. On the incisor teeth the force is identical for male and female. In the normal chewing of food the masticatory force applied to the teeth is about one-third of the maximum. This force varies in different parts of the dental arch. It is greatest at the first molars, slightly less on the second and third molars and lower still at pre-molars and incisors. This differential distribution of force is probably a consequence of the occlusal areas of the teeth and the position of the teeth relative to the insertions of the jaw-elevating muscles.

Relation of mastication to digestibility

The need for thorough chewing to ensure the effective digestion of the food has been studied by the examination of the faeces of individuals with abnormal dentition or in individuals with normal dentition after swallowing food without preliminary chewing. These are controlled by comparison with normal individuals chewing normally. It might be expected that inadequate chewing would impair digestion but Farrell (1956) has shown that this is not so for many foods.

Mastication has an effect on gastric emptying time, and also serves reflexly to promote salivary and gastric secretion.

Relation of mastication to health of oral tissues

Chewing may be relatively unimportant as a preliminary for adequate enzyme degradation of modern soft foods, but it has a definite role in maintaining the integrity and health of oral tissues. Mastication of coarse food has an action in promoting the blood flow and keratinization of the epithelium of the gums. Masticatory pressure on the teeth results in increased thickness of the periodontal membranes. Mastication is a factor during the growth period, in determining growth of the jaws.

Neural mechanism of mastication

Rest position of the mandible

In the normal resting position of the mandible the teeth are not in contact. A 'free-way' space of 2–3 mm exists usually between the upper and lower pre-molars. This position is the equilibrium position maintained by the tone in the jaw-closing muscles balancing the gravitational pull of the weight of the lower jaw, tending to cause the mandible to fall. This tone is maintained by a monosynaptic reflex pathway from muscle spindles in the jaw-closing muscles.

Reflex control

Mastication may be voluntary or reflex. As long as food is present in the mouth the alternate opening and closing of the jaws will continue automatically.

The stimulus of food contact with the gums and palate evokes reflex opening of the mouth. This movement is mainly a result of inhibition of the resting tone in the jaw-closing muscles and an active contraction of the jaw-opening muscles. This reflex opening can be excited also by mechanical stimulation of jaws, pressure on teeth or stimulation of the anterior part of the palate. Following this reflex opening of the jaws, as the stimulus ceases there occurs a rapid rebound movement. Repetition of alternation of this cycle of a jaw-opening reflex followed by jaw-closing with a powerful rebound, continues until all the solid food is masticated and removed by swallowing.

Central control

This masticatory reflex is unilateral. After section of the symphysis, stimulation of the gingival or palatal mucosa on one side causes jaw movements on the stimulated side only.

Although the cerebrum is not essential for the chewing reflex, the jaw opening and closing movements can be produced on stimulation of the amygdaloid nucleus region. These movements are also represented in the pre-central and post-central areas of the cerebral cortex in man. Chewing movements are produced when specific areas in this part of the cortex are stimulated. There is thus a dual neural control, voluntary from the cerebral cortex and reflex through a medullary reflex 'centre'. The medullary centre is supervised by the cortical centre which controls the finer details of the masticatory movements. Destruction of the appropriate cortical areas results in reduction of the efficiency of reflex chewing.

Pharynx

Introduction

The pharynx is a chamber with bony and fibromuscular walls serving as a thoroughfare common to the respiratory and alimentary systems. It functions both as a conducting airway for the ventilation of the lungs, and as a channel for fluids and food and other swallowed materials down to the oesophagus. At the lower end of the pharynx the pathways of the respiratory and digestive tracts separate into the larynx and the oesophagus.

Thus the pharyngeal cavity communicates with the nasal chambers, the pharyngotympanic tubes, the oral cavity, the larynx and the oesophagus. These openings are guarded by functional muscular mechanisms including: (1) the palatal and salpingo-pharyngeal muscles at the pharyngeal ostium of the eustachian tube; (2) the soft palate and sphincter muscle of the nasopharyngeal isthmus; (3) the base of the tongue and the palatoglossal folds; (4) the aryepiglottic folds and muscles which form the first of the triple sphincters of the larynx; (5) the cricopharyngeal sphincter.

The pharyngeal wall is formed essentially from within outwards of a mucous membrane, a fibrous pharyngeal aponeurosis, a muscle coat and a lamina of fibrous tissue. The epithelial lining of the pharynx varies in its different regions in accordance with their varying physiological functions. The section normally traversed only by air, that is, the nasopharynx as far as the level of the lower border of the soft palate, is lined by a pseudostratified columnar ciliated epithelium. The regions subject to the abrasive wear of contact with food, or where surfaces rub together, have an epithelial covering of stratified squamous non-keratinizing type. In the border zone between these different epithelia there may be a narrow zone of the stratified columnar variety. A striking feature of the pharyngeal mucosa is the presence of masses of lymphoid tissue forming part of Waldeyer's ring of lymphoid tissue. The subepithelial connective tissue is dense. In some regions, particularly in the nasopharynx close to the pharyngotympanic tubal opening, racemose mucous glands are present in this layer. External to this is the muscle coat of the longitudinal muscles and the three constrictor muscles of the pharynx. These are lined externally by a stratum of fibrous tissue.

Functions of the pharynx

The pharynx is involved in a number of physiological activities. It is a part of the pathway for air and food. The pharyngeal muscles are concerned in the movements of the pharyngeal phase of swallowing. They are also concerned in other acts like sneezing, coughing and vomiting. The pharynx forms part of the chamber whose variations in shape is intimately concerned with speech sounds. The considerable aggregations of lymphoid tissue form part of the general lymphoid organ of the body and may have special functions. Sensory receptors are located in the pharyngeal mucosa. These include those of general somatic sensations like touch, pain and temperature and occasional special receptors of taste. Afferent receptors are also present concerned with the reflexes of swallowing and vomiting. Thirst sensation, in conditions of depletion of body water, is usually associated with or referred to the pharynx. The pharynx is related to the opening of the eustachian tube and the equalization of pressure on the two surfaces of the tympanic membrane. Some of these functions are considered in this chapter.

Lymphoid tissue

Pharyngeal lymphoid tissue

A considerable amount of lymphoid tissue is distributed within the pharyngeal mucous membrane, especially at the so-called Waldeyer's ring around the pharynx and across the base of the tongue. This includes the distinct masses of lymphoid tissue of the nasopharyngeal tonsil or adenoids, the faucial tonsils, the lingual tonsils, and a collection of scattered smaller nodes in the pharyngeal mucous membrane. The pharyngeal lymphoid tissue has no afferent lymph channels. Numerous efferent lymphatics drain from this tonsillar tissue to the superior cervical lymph nodes.

Faucial tonsils

The faucial tonsils are bilateral ovoid masses of lymphoid tissue deep to the epithelium extending between the anterior and posterior faucial pillars. This stratified squamous epithelium is folded into the lymphoid tissue as 10–30 primary crypts in each tonsil. These recesses extend through almost the whole depth of the lymphoid tissue and, from them, epithelium-lined extensions project out into the adjacent lymphoid tissue as secondary crypts.

These crypts, which provide a great expansion of the tonsillar surface, have narrow necks and broader bodies. The secondary crypts are also club-shaped. Normally the crypts are collapsed forming fissure-like spaces. The cellular tissue of the tonsils abuts directly against the epithelium. The effect of this anatomical arrangement is to increase the area of contact between these subepithelial lymphoid aggregations and the environment of the oral and pharyngeal cavities. The crypts often contain desquamated cells, food debris, concretions and organisms.

Microscopically, the lymphoid tissue is arranged in nodules which may have germ centres. Between these nodules is loose internodular lymphatic tissue. The surface epithelium is infiltrated with lymphocytes. This invasion may be so dense as to obscure the deeper parts of the epithelium. From this infiltrate, lymphocytes escape into the oral cavity and form the so-called salivary corpuscles found in saliva collected from the mouth. Mucous glands are present but their ducts do not open at the base of the crypts as in the lingual tonsil. The flushing action attributed to these glands in the lingual tonsil of washing debris out of the crypts is thus absent, and this may contribute to the greater predisposition to stagnation of materials in the crypt with resulting tendency to infection.

Nasopharyngeal tonsils
The nasopharyngeal lymphoid tissue is made up of structurally similar masses of subepithelial tissue forming a series of parallel ridges. This again provides an enlarged surface of contact with the air traversing the nasopharynx.

Lingual tonsil
Collections of lymphatic nodules in the subepithelial tissue of the root of the tongue comprise the so-called 'lingual tonsil'. Here again, the epithelium dips into the lymphatic tissue as crypts, the walls of which are infiltrated by lymphocytes.

Lymphoid tissue organ

Structure of lymphoid tissue
Lymphoid tissue consists essentially of: (1) a supporting framework of reticular fibres with reticulum cells and some collagenous and elastic fibres and a few muscle cells; (2) a cellular mass of free lymphocytes, large and small, and their precursor cells.

Lymphatic tissue aggregations are sometimes described as comprising cortical and medullary portions but these two portions are continuous and the boundary is not clear. The predominant cell of the lymphoid tissue cell population is the small lymphocyte. The other cell types present include primitive reticular cells, macrophages and occasional plasma cells. The phagocytic macrophages are both fixed and free types and include reticulum cells, the lining endothelial cells of the lymph sinuses and free macrophages.

The lymphocytic cells are often arranged in groups with a central region of clear, actively multiplying cells, and a peripheral zone of lymphocytes produced from the central precursors or lymphoblasts. This is the 'germinal centre' of Flemming. Hellman believes that these centres are reaction zones representing the reaction of this tissue to toxic substances.

Lymphoid tissue may be broadly classified into three groups.

(1) Lymph nodes. These are the familiar 'lymph glands' dispersed along the lymphatic system with afferent and efferent lymph vessels. These lymph vessels begin as a network of minute lymph capillaries in relation to the extracellular tissue space. They form peripheral plexuses and drain along lymph vessels into lymph nodes. The efferent vessels from lymph nodes may drain to other nodes and ultimately into the main lymph ducts, thoracic duct and right lymph duct and thence into the venous system at the root of the neck.
(2) Epithelial lymphoid tissue. This group embraces all the lymphoid tissue lying in

contact with the epithelial lining of the mucous membranes of the alimentary and upper respiratory tracts. It includes the pharyngeal lymphoid tissue (faucial, lingual and nasopharyngeal tonsillar tissue) solitary and aggregated lymphoid nodules in the small intestine (Peyer's patches) and the lymphoid tissue of the appendix and small solitary nodules in the colon. These tissues are characterized by their subepithelial location and the absence of afferent lymphatic vessels.

(3) Lymphoid tissue in haemopoietic organs. The lymphoid tissue scattered in spleen and bone marrow form this group. Here there are neither afferent nor efferent lymphatic vessels. The tissue is related intimately to blood vascular sinusoids.

Total mass of lymphoid organ

Approximate determinations have been made based on the dissection and measurement of all the major discrete masses of lymphoid tissue, and the calculation of the volume of smaller scattered nodules from histological preparations. The total lymphoid tissue of the body may form about 1 per cent of the body weight.

Lymphoid tissue shows a characteristic growth curve. It increases in size in early years until puberty, then decreases to adult level and finally undergoes physiological involution in old age (*Figure 9.7*).

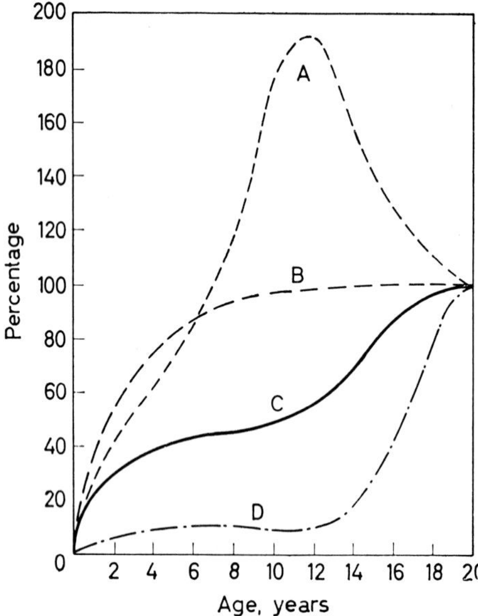

Figure 9.7 Curves of the comparative rate of growth of different types of tissue (A = lymphoid; B = neural; C = general; D = reproductive)

Starvation leads to atrophy of lymphoid tissue and disappearance of germ centres, while a high calorie diet and especially a high fat diet leads to hyperplasia of the pharyngeal and intestinal lymphoid tissue.

Functions of lymphoid tissue

Methods of study

The investigation of the functions of lymphoid tissue in health and disease presents special difficulty because of its scattered widespread distribution in the organs and tissues of the body. Removal of the entire 'lymphoid organ' to disclose the effects consequent upon such an extirpation is not possible. Further, partial excision or destruction is compensated by hyperplasia of the remaining lymphoid tissue.

A great variety of experimental methods have been applied to the exploration of this problem. These include: (1) Experimental destruction or involution produced by external sources of radiation, by administration of radioactive isotopes causing selective damage to the more sensitive lymphocytic series of cells, or by cytotoxic chemicals with a specific toxic effect on lymphoid tissue. (2) Tissue culture and histological studies including electron microscopy and histochemical examination of the enzyme content of cells of lymphoid tissue. (3) Collection and analysis of lymph from different parts of the body and the comparison of the composition of lymph leaving lymph nodes with the afferent lymph. (4) Lymphatic fistulae, and diversion or obstruction of lymph drainage into the vascular system. (5) Quantitative studies of clearance of inert particles. (6) Blockage of cells of reticulo-endothelial system. (7) Studies of antibody synthesis by electrophoresis and fluorescence techniques.

General functions of lymphoid tissue

Numerous functions have been attributed to lymphoid tissue, but despite extensive experimental and clinical research, considerable gaps still exist in our knowledge of the precise physiological role of this tissue. Some of these functions proposed for lymphoid tissue in general are considered and the specific role of the pharyngeal part of this tissue indicated in the following paragraphs.

Formation of lymphocytes

Lymphoid tissue is the site of formation of lymphocytes. They are derived from the primitive reticular cells in the germinal centres. The first cell in the series of transitional stages of development from the reticulum cell to the small lymphocyte is the lymphoblast. This is a large rounded cell (20–25 μm) with round or slightly indented vesicular nucleus and basophilic cytoplasm. This cell, by successive mitoses, gives rise to the large lymphocyte about 15 μm diameter, having a nucleus with deeper chromatin and considerable cytoplasm. The large lymphocyte undergoes a process of maturation involving progressive decrease in size, decrease in cytoplasm and in its degree of basophilia, and increased condensation and clumping of nuclear chromatin, to become the mature small lymphocyte.

The small lymphocyte is about 10 μm in diameter with a rounded deeply staining nucleus and a thin rim of cytoplasm. The lymphocyte is not phagocytic. It is motile with a characteristic slow amoeboid movement with the nucleus preceding the cytoplasm. This cell forms 30 per cent of the leucocytes of the blood as well as being the distinctive cell of lymphoid tissue. Electron-microscopic studies reveal the special characteristic of these cells, as clear cytoplasm and conspicuous mitochondria. Cytochemical investigations have demonstrated the localization within lymphocytes of several enzyme systems, including oxidases and dehydrogenases.

Lymph collected from the efferent lymphatics of a lymph node always contains more lymphocytes than the lymph entering that node. Lymphocytes produced in lymph nodes, and doubtless also those from subepithelial lymphoid tissue, pass via lymph channels to the blood. On the other hand, some lymphocytes from bone marrow and spleen pass directly into the blood.

Daily lymphocyte turnover The relative constancy of the absolute lymphocyte count of the blood indicates that lymphocytes are leaving the blood as rapidly as they are being discharged into the blood. Further, some mechanism must maintain this balance of production and destruction of lymphocytes. The daily production of lymphocytes has been calculated from measurements of the volume and cell content of the thoracic duct lymph. This indicates a replacement rate of all the lymphocytes of the blood varying from every 2 h in the rabbit to every 12 h in the dog. These calculations may indicate an excessive turnover rate since lymphocytes may be continuously re-circulating.

Thus the daily replacement factor is difficult to assess with accuracy, and varies with all species. Further experiments, to measure the life span of the lymphocyte and its intravascular survival time, have been carried out using a transfusion with lymphocytes labelled with radioactive tracers or fluorescent dyes. Studies of the survival time of small lymphocytes labelled by incorporation of radioactive nucleic acid has shown that there may be two distinct populations of these cells. One group has a short mean circulating life span of 2–3 days, while the other group has a much longer intravascular life of about 200 days; 20 per cent of small lymphocytes belong to the first group; the remaining 80 per cent constitute the second group.

Fate of lymphocytes The high rate of entry of lymphocytes into the blood implies an equally rapid rate of elimination or destruction of these cells. The removal of lymphocytes from the blood has been attributed to five different mechanisms.

(1) Ageing and dissolution of lymphocytes in the circulation. This process is increased in states of stress as a result of increased secretion of adrenal cortical hormones. Injection of adrenal glucocorticoids such as cortisone will result in a lymphopenia.
(2) Migration of lymphocytes into the lumen of the alimentary tract from the pharyngeal and intestinal lymphoid nodules. Only a relatively small proportion are excreted by this method. Excision of the alimentary tract does not significantly reduce the loss of lymphocytes from the blood.
(3) Migration of lymphocytes into bone marrow. Lymphocytes have been proved to pass out of the sinusoids into the bone marrow. Thus small lymphocytes are found in the marrow extravascular cell population. Yoffey and others (1956, 1958) have shown that, when labelled lymphocytes are transfused into the blood stream, large numbers of these cells can be found in bone marrow. The ultimate fate of these migrated lymphocytes is not known. They may be phagocyted and used as raw material for the formation of other cells. The view that these lymphocytes may act as stem cells for the formation of red blood cells and other leucocytes has been disputed.
(4) Continuous re-circulation of lymphocytes. Lymphocytes in the circulating blood may wander out into the extravascular tissue spaces and, from here, pass back into the lymphatic system and re-enter the blood stream. Experiments using labelled lymphocytes (with ^{32}P or ^{54}Cr or ^{3}H) have demonstrated that these cells leave the blood in lymph nodes and are carried back to the blood in the efferent

lymph. This has been confirmed by electron microscopy. The lymphocytes penetrate the endothelium of the post-capillary venules in lymph nodes. Not all the cells in the lymph leaving a lymph node are newly formed cells; a proportion of these lymphocytes are re-circulating cells. Thus the apparent extremely high rate of discharge of small lymphocytes from lymph nodes is not necessarily indicative of an equally high rate of new formation of these cells. A considerable fraction of these small lymphocytes are re-circulating and a smaller proportion are new cells. In contrast large lymphocytes are relatively infrequent in lymph and they do not re-circulate from the blood.

(5) Destruction of lymphocytes in germinal centres. It has been suggested that the lymphocytes may be disintegrated in the germinal centres of lymphoid tissue. The numerous macrophages in these centres ingest and digest effete lymphocytes. The cytoplasmic constituents may be released into the general plasma protein pool and have been suggested as a source of circulating gamma globulin and antibodies.

Control of lymphocyte production The maintenance of the constancy of the lymphocytes in the blood implies some mechanism, presumably chemical or hormonal, regulating the balance of destruction and new formation of these cells. Since removal or destruction of part of the lymphoid tissue in the body results in compensatory enlargement of the remainder, some unknown factor must regulate the demand for a minimal total amount of functioning lymphoid tissue.

Lymph filtration: barrier function

This 'filtration' mechanism is one of the methods by which the lymphoid tissue serves as a major component in the body's defences against invasion by micro-organisms. Lymph nodes can clear the lymph percolating through the gland of particulate matter such as micro-organisms and also of colloidal molecules such as bacterial toxins or other proteins and dyes.

The lymph node is structurally adapted for this filtering activity. Several afferent lymphatics open through its capsule on the convex border into a cortical marginal sinus. This sinus is traversed by fibrous trabeculae and a delicate reticular meshwork. These are covered by very numerous actively phagocytic cells.

From the marginal sinus the lymph permeates through narrow channels within the lymphoid tissue to leave by the usually single efferent lymph vessel. The effect of this structural arrangement is that: (1) the rate of lymph flow is sharply reduced within the node, thus providing more time for filtration processes; (2) the lymph is exposed in the node to a relatively enormous surface covered with highly active phagocytic cells of the reticulo-endothelial system. These nodes have been described as 'settling chambers' and filters acting to clear the lymph of extravascular proteins, micro-organisms, bacterial toxins and inert foreign particles. The remarkable efficiency of lymph nodes in arresting the passage of bacteria or macromolecules has been repeatedly proved experimentally, and is clinically obvious in the characteristic lymphangitis and lymphadenitis seen in the spread of some infections. Although in animal experiments this clearance is normally quite adequate to prevent spread of infection beyond the area of lymphatic drainage, acceleration of lymph flow, for example by movement of an inflamed area, will increase the danger of bacteria penetrating the lymph node–phagocyte barrier and escaping beyond that node.

Inflammatory reaction in a lymph node appears to enhance the efficiency of clearance of bacteria from the lymph by that lymph node.

Cancer cell emboli in the lymph stream become arrested in lymph nodes with the development of metastatic growths.

The pharyngeal lymphoid ring, in common with other subepithelial lymphoid tissue, has no afferent lymph channels and is therefore unlikely to exercise this barrier function of clearing the lymph stream. There is no evidence that they exert any protective action based on filtration.

Reaction centres: toxin clearance from blood

Hellman and his associates postulated that lymph nodes had a twofold clearance or filtration function. In addition to the filtration of lymph, discussed above, by the reticulo-endothelial cells of the sinuses of the lymph nodes, there was also the clearance of toxins from the blood by the cells in the so-called germ centres which they regard as 'reaction centres'. This view obtains some support from the facts that, in bacteria-free animals bred and maintained in a pathogen-free environment, the total lymphoid tissue developed is only 25 per cent of that in the control animals kept in a normal laboratory environment, and that no 'germ centres' are present. However, the bulk of the experimental evidence is against this view that these clear zones in lymphoid tissue indicate a reaction to circulating toxins.

Body's cellular defence to infection

Lymphocytes, together with their derivative plasma cells, form part of the cellular response characteristic of chronic inflammations and chronic granulomata, and are also found as a small round cell infiltration around tumours. Their precise significance in the chronic inflammatory exudate is not clear. It has been suggested that: (1) they play a minor but definite phagocytic role and provide proteolytic enzymes which assist in removal of fibrin and other cellular debris; (2) they are a source of other cells becoming transformed into plasma cells, fibroblasts and macrophages; (3) they are a source of antibodies.

Humoral response to infection: antibody synthesis

In addition to the purely mechanical aspects of physical clearance of micro-organisms and toxins from the lymph and blood, and in addition to the function of increasing production of lymphocytes in some infections, lymphoid tissue has a third most important role in response to infections. This is the synthesis of antibodies and their transport and release into the circulation.

There is unequivocal experimental evidence that lymph nodes can produce antibodies. After the injection of an antigen the lymph leaving a lymph node has a higher titre of antibody than the lymph entering that node. Sedimentation of the cellular elements in this efferent lymph by centrifuging shows that the antibody is chiefly in the lymphocyte layer and not in the supernatant fluid. Extracts of washed cells from lymph nodes have a high antibody content. Administration of adrenal cortical steroids to immunized animals, causes an increased destruction of lymphocytes and a rise in the antibody concentration of the plasma. Destruction of lymphoid cells by irradiation decreases the amount of antibody produced in response to an antigenic stimulus. All these experiments support the view that the important cell in the formation and transport of antibody is the lymphocyte. Recent experiments, and in particular those using the fluorescent antigen–antibody techniques, demonstrate that the cell type concerned in antibody synthesis is the plasma cell. Other experiments show that lymphocytes can become differentiated into plasma cells and that this metamorphosis occurs during antibody synthesis.

The part played by lymphoid tissue in the humoral mechanism of defence can be summarized as follows. The bacterium or its toxin is ingested by the macrophage cells of the lymph node. The bacterial protein or mucopolysaccharide complex acts as an antigen and starts the process. The antigen becomes 'modified' and, in one view, is transferred to adjacent mesenchymal cells where active synthesis of gamma globulins takes place and these cells become plasma cells. Another view is that the gamma globulin antibody is made to a great extent by lymphocytes which then become transformed into plasma cells.

Other reticulo-endothelial functions

Lymphoid tissue contains reticular cells of the reticulo-endothelial system which share with the rest of that system the common physiological property of active phagocytosis. Other cells of this system are scattered in various tissues. They include fixed phagocytic endothelial cells lining blood sinusoids of liver, spleen, bone marrow and lymphatic channels of lymph nodes, reticular cells of bone marrow and lymphoid tissue, connective tissue histiocytes and macrophages in the stroma of many tissues and organs and also the microglia of the nervous system and the wandering macrophages and monocytes of the blood. Most of these reticulo-endothelial functions have already been mentioned. Others are:

(1) Destruction of red blood cells and iron storage. The cells of the reticulo-endothelial system are involved in the ingestion of effete red blood cells and of their products after haemolysis. Arising from this physiological activity, these cells: (a) store iron bound to the globulin apoferritin, as the storage form of iron called ferritin; (b) form the pre-hepatic bile pigment. Lymphoid tissue can only be concerned in these functions to a minor extent, mainly in the so-called haemolymph glands.

(2) Relation to lipids and vitamins. Fat and other lipids can be taken up by reticulum cells of lymphoid tissue. Disturbance of this function is seen in a group of conditions where various types of lipids accumulate in the reticular cells called the lipid storage diseases. Vitamin A deficiency leads to reduction of lymphoid tissue while vitamin D deficiency is associated with lymphoid hyperplasia.

Control of lymphoid tissue

Lymphoid tissue is under the control of several endocrine glands, notably the cortex of the adrenal gland. There is a reciprocal relationship between the amount of adrenal cortical tissue and the mass of lymphoid tissue. Injections of cortisone or of ACTH result in degenerative changes in small lymphocytes. Mitosis ceases, and the nuclei become pyknotic and break up. The fragments of the lymphocytes are taken up by macrophages. Consequent upon this decreased formation of lymphocytes there is a lymphopenia. Stress reaction, such as occurs in trauma, operations and exposure, also results in involution of lymphoid tissue and lymphopenia. This response does not occur in adrenalectomized animals and is due to secretion of adrenal corticosteroids as a result of release of ACTH from the pituitary gland by the stress stimulus.

Sex hormones, both male and female, also bring about slight involution of lymphoid tissue. Thyrotrophic hormone or thyroxin produces an increase in lymphoid tissue, and clinically lymphoid hyperplasia accompanies hyperthyroidism.

Special role of pharyngeal lymphoid tissue

Knowledge of any specific role for the pharyngeal lymphoid tissue is very fragmentary and not based on any unequivocal experimental evidence. It might be assumed that all or most of the functions assigned to lymphoid tissue in general are also fulfilled to a lesser or greater extent by this subepithelial lymphoid tissue. However, this tonsillar tissue, while basically resembling the structure of lymph nodes, is differentiated by its subepithelial location and the consequent absence of any afferent lymph vessels. Because of these features its functions may well differ in some respects from those of lymph nodes. The absence of any filtering function, because there are no incoming lymphatics, is referred to on p. 351. It has been suggested that, because the pharyngeal lymphoid tissue is so frequently involved in recurrent and chronic infections, it cannot be regarded as exerting any protective function. However, there is no general agreement on this point. Certainly virus particles and some organisms have been shown experimentally to be capable of penetrating the mucous membrane of the nasopharynx.

The fact that this lymphoid tissue is strategically stationed at the gateway to the respiratory and alimentary tracts, has led to the proposal that it protects the delicate respiratory ciliated epithelium, and the mucosa of the stomach and intestines which, in differentiating for the specialized function of absorption, has become more vulnerable. Undoubtedly these regions at the commencement of the respiratory and alimentary tracts are areas of high bacterial content. The nasopharyngeal adenoids come into contact with the inspired air streams. The raised parallel ridges on these bodies may help to increase the surface area for 'sampling' the bacteria in this air. Further ciliary clearance in the nasopharynx sweeps nasal mucus, with its contained random sample of the bacterial content of the air and nose, over the adenoids. Similarly the faucial tonsillar recesses, it is suggested, provided an extension of the surface concerned in an identical 'sampling' activity in relation to the bacterial flora of the food and oral cavity. Not only are they ideally situated for this activity, but the contraction of the superior constrictor muscles with each swallowing movement pushes the tonsils from their beds into the pharynx and their surfaces become bathed with the fluid in the mouth and pharynx. It is postulated that in this way the lymphoid tissue monitors continuously the different varieties of bacteria in air and food, and a steady stream of samples trickles through the lymphoid tissue. This results in the automatic elaboration in the body of antibodies to these organisms from the nose and mouth. Antibody formation by the tonsil has been established in several investigations, including the use of fluorescent microscopy and the measurements of the antibody content of extracts of tonsillar tissue. It is perhaps also significant that the tonsils are minute at birth and increase at 1–3 years at the time when active immunity is being established. It is thus suggested that the tonsils probably collect micro-organisms from the mouth and, in addition to forming their own small complement of antibodies, may modify these micro-organisms and release them or their toxins to the reticulo-endothelial system of the body as an antigenic stimulus for exciting active immunization. The tonsillar tissue is thus intimately involved in the mechanism of production of natural immunity.

Motor activity of the pharynx

Mechanism of deglutition

The act of swallowing is a complex co-ordinated reflex action which is usually initiated voluntarily but is for the most part completed as an orderly sequence of reflexes. The primary function of deglutition is the transfer of solid and liquid food from the buccal cavity to the stomach. Two subsidiary functions are of importance. First, swallowing completes the disposal of the dust- and bacteria-laden mucus which is conveyed by ciliary action to the pharynx from the nasal passages and sinuses, tympanic cavities, larynx and tracheobronchial tree. Secondly, the opening of the pharyngeal ostia of the pharyngotympanic tubes, which accompanies deglutition, serves periodically to establish equalization of pressure on the outer and inner surfaces of the tympanic membranes.

Following the classical account of deglutition by Magendie, it is convenient for descriptive purposes to divide the act into three stages: (1) oral; (2) pharyngeal; (3) oesophageal. These three stages correspond to the three anatomical regions through which the swallowed material passes. It must be emphasized, however, that swallowing is a continuous and integrated act; the initiation of the first phase inevitably leads to the automatic completion of the whole process.

Oral stage

This is a voluntary stage and involves the propulsion of the bolus of food from the mouth through the isthmus of the fauces into the oral pharynx.

Solids Solid food is first disintegrated by chewing. This mastication may be voluntary or reflex. As long as food is present in the mouth the alternate opening and closing of the jaws continues automatically. The physiology of mastication is discussed on p. 342. This sequence of alternation of opening and closing of the jaws continues reflexly until all the food is swallowed. The reflex nature of chewing is shown by the fact that in the decerebrate animal food in the mouth still excites chewing movements. The reflex is unilateral. After separation of the mandible into two halves, unilateral oral stimulation causes chewing movements only on the stimulated side. During mastication lubrication of the bolus by admixture with viscid saliva is achieved. The importance of lubrication is shown by the great difficulty in attempts at swallowing dry solids from a dry mouth.

The lubricated fragments are moulded into a bolus by the tongue, cheeks and hard palate, and collected on the dorsum of the tongue preparatory to swallowing. A small inspiratory movement of the diaphragm occurs known as the respiration of swallowing. The lips are closed and the buccinator muscles contract compressing the cheeks against the teeth. The bolus is forced backwards by a piston-like movement of the tongue resulting from elevation of the floor of the mouth combined with a backward movement of the base of the tongue. The anterior part of the tongue is elevated and pressed against the hard palate. The elevation of the floor of the mouth is mainly due to contraction of the mylohyoid muscles; the hyoid bone is drawn forwards and upwards and fixed by contraction of geniohyoid, stylohyoid, mylohyoid and digastric muscles. This elevation of the floor of the mouth compresses the tongue against the palate and forces the posterior part to bulge into the pharynx. In addition, the posterior part of the tongue is drawn backwards by the hyoglossus and styloglossus muscles. The retraction of the tongue temporarily obliterates the lumen of the oropharynx. This backward displacement of the tongue propels the bolus into the oropharynx. At the same time the faucial opening is narrowed by contraction of the palatoglossus muscles approximating the anterior pillars of the fauces. Total removal of the tongue does not prevent swallowing; the muscles of the cheeks and floor of the mouth can compensate.

Fluids Fluid is drawn into the mouth by creating a subatmospheric pressure in the mouth by retraction of the tongue in contact with the palate. After fluid has been sucked in, the succeeding swallowing movements have been described by Whillis (1946) as consisting of two components. This analysis of the movements of the tongue in swallowing is based on a careful study of a case in which a part of the left cheek had been removed.

In the first phase with the mouth closed the contraction of the extrinsic muscles of the tongue brings the tip of the tongue against the palate just behind the incisive papilla. The upper surface of the tongue is moulded to form a longitudinal groove completing, with the hard palate, a tubular space containing the fluid. The margins of the tongue are pressed against the lingual surface of the gums and teeth. This moulding of the tongue is due to the contraction of the superior longitudinal and genioglossus muscles (*Figure 9.8a*). The dorsum of the tongue is next forced upwards. This commences at the anterior end and extends backwards. This movement is brought about by contraction of the inferior part of the transverse lingual muscles and results in a progressive obliteration of the tubular space between the tongue and palate. The effect of this is that the fluid is 'squirted' backwards into the oral pharynx.

In the second phase the teeth are brought into occlusion and the mylohyoid muscles contract, raising the floor of the mouth. Consequently the posterior part of the tongue is forced backwards into the pharynx, pushing the fluid into the laryngeal part of the pharynx (*Figure 9.8*). In the swallowing of solids this second phase alone is responsible for thrusting the bolus from the mouth into the pharynx.

Muscular forces of the oral phase The muscular forces developed in this oral phase may be significant factors in determining the occlusion of the teeth. Abnormal swallowing has been suggested as playing a role in the pathogenesis of dental malocclusion. The total force to which the teeth and alveolar arches are subjected is the product of (a) the force on the lingual and on the labial aspects of the jaws per swallow, and (b) the daily frequency of swallowing.

Frequency of swallowing Lear and Mooress recorded the frequency of swallowing over a complete 24 h period, in healthy subjects with normal dental occlusion. They found a mean frequency of 600 swallows per day, with a range of variation from 200 to 1000 per day. The frequency was highest during meals and least during sleep.

Pressures of swallowing (a) Lingual pressure. The pressures exerted on the palate by the tongue have been measured with pressure transducers. These pressures are greater on the anterior and lateral palatal areas, than on the central part of the palate. In spontaneous swallowing the mean pressures were approximately 40 g/cm^2

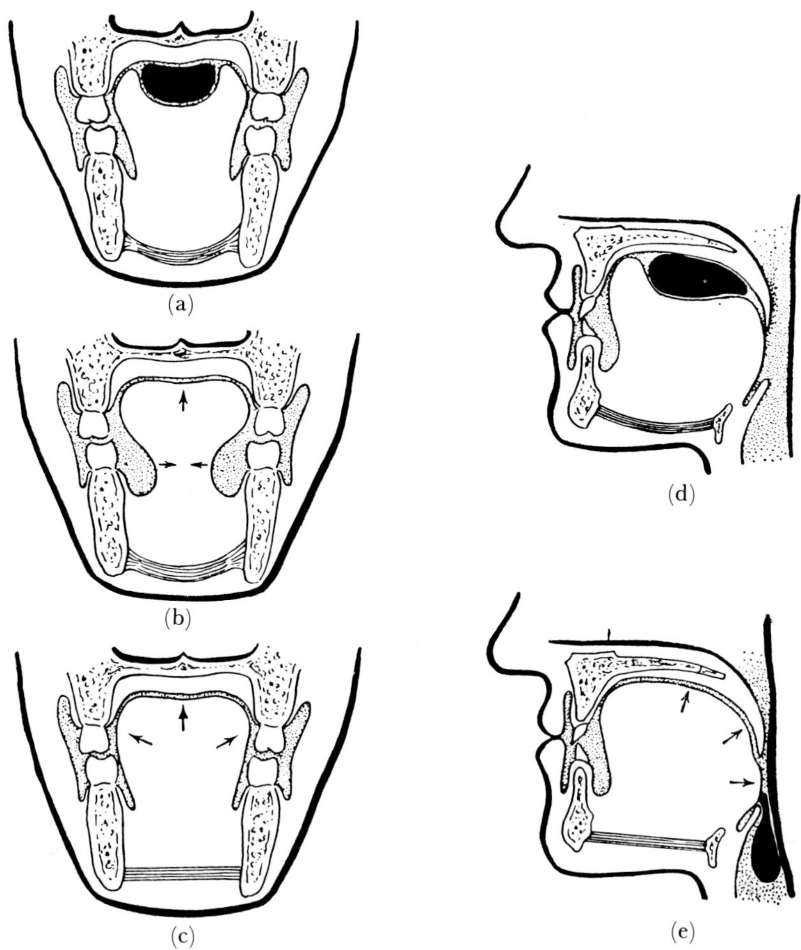

Figure 9.8 Diagram of the oral phase of swallowing (after Whillis, 1946)

as compared with 50 g/cm² for drinking water, and 95 g/cm² for 'dry' swallowing of saliva. Individuals with narrow high palates exert greater pressure on lateral palatal areas than those with rounded or flat palates. It has been calculated by Lear and Mooress that the average lingual pressure on the dental arch per day due to swallowing is equivalent to 0.1 g acting continuously. The resting pressure between swallows is 2–4 g. Normal swallowing therefore makes no significant supplement to the total lingual pressure on the alveolar arch. (b) Pressure by the lips and cheeks. The peri-oral muscles of the cheeks and lips exert pressure on the teeth. This pressure was measured by Winders (1958), who found mean resting pressures on the molars of 4 g/cm², on the upper incisors of 6 g/cm² and on the lower incisors of 8 g/cm².

Pharyngeal stage

In this stage the food passes through the pharynx to the upper end of the oesophagus. As the pharynx is common to both the respiratory and alimentary passages, the transference of the bolus is accompanied by closure of the nasal, oral and laryngeal openings into the pharynx. The nasal, oral, laryngeal and oesophageal openings of the pharynx are provided with sphincteric mechanisms. The nasopharyngeal hiatus is controlled by the combined action of the palatopharyngeal sphincter muscles and the elevators of the mobile soft palate. The palatoglossus muscles of the anterior pillars of the fauces exert in some measure a sphincteric action at the oropharyngeal isthmus. The laryngeal inlet is equipped with three successive sphincteric defences: (1) the aryepiglottic muscles at the inlet; (2) the thyro-arytenoid muscles and the false vocal folds; (3) the adductors of the vocal cords. The oesophageal end of the pharynx is controlled by the cricopharyngeus muscle.

This phase of swallowing is a reflex mechanism elicited from receptors in the mucosa of the posterior part of the buccal cavity and the posterior pharyngeal wall. These receptors are stimulated by contact of the bolus of food.

The complex contractions which comprise the reflex response in this stage may be summarized as follows.

Closure of nasopharyngeal hiatus During deglutition the nasopharyngeal aperture is closed by the co-ordinated action of several muscles. The levator palati muscles pull the soft palate upwards and backwards towards the posterior wall. The tensors of the palate tighten the soft palate and depress its transverse arch, at the same time opening the pharyngeal ostium of the pharyngotympanic tube. Coincident with this elevation of the soft palate the palatopharyngeus muscle contracts and acts as a sphincteric mechanism of the nasopharyngeal hiatus. The contraction of this sphincter approximates the walls of the opening and raises a rounded ridge (Passavant's bar) on the posterior pharyngeal wall. The upper surface of the elevated soft palate makes contact with this ridge. Thus the passage of food into the nasopharynx is prevented. Paralysis of the palatal muscles interferes with effective closure of the entrance to the nasopharynx, and regurgitation of food into the nose results.

Closure of oropharyngeal isthmus Maintained contraction of the lingual muscles keeping the tongue against the palate and the sphincteric action of the palatoglossus muscles prevent the bolus returning into the oral cavity.

Closure of laryngeal inlet The bolus of food is prevented from passing into the larynx by the following factors:

(1) During the second stage of swallowing respiration is inhibited.
(2) The larynx is suddenly and forcibly elevated into apposition with the base of the tongue. The entrance to the larynx is thus drawn upwards under the shelter of the backward projecting base of the tongue. This powerful elevation is effected mainly by the stylohyoid, stylopharyngeus, digastric and mylohyoid muscles. The thyrohyoid muscle also contracts, pulling the thyroid cartilage upwards. The upper border of the thyroid cartilage may be drawn upwards well behind the hyoid bone. Fixation of the thyroid cartilage, preventing elevation of the larynx, renders deglutition impossible.
(3) Closure of the laryngeal sphincters. The laryngeal closure mechanism consists of a triple tier of sphincters. In swallowing all three sphincters close. The aryepiglottic folds are approximated by the sphincteric action of the aryepiglottic and oblique arytenoid muscles. This closure is completed anteriorly by the tubercle of the epiglottis. At a lower level the thyro-arytenoid muscles

approximate the false vocal cords or ventricular folds and provide a second line of defence. The thyro-arytenoid and interarytenoid muscles also cause sliding of the arytenoid cartilages forwards and towards one another. The apices of the cartilages are tilted towards the epiglottic cushion. The laryngeal aperture thus becomes a T-shaped opening well protected under the projecting base of the tongue. The rima glottidis is closed by the adduction of the vocal cords produced by the lateral crico-arytenoid muscles, and by the approximation of the arytenoid cartilages.

(4) The action of the epiglottis. The classical view was that the epiglottis turned over during swallowing and thus served to guard the laryngeal vestibule. The radiological studies of Barclay (1936) led to the conclusion that the epiglottis did not close like a lid over the laryngeal aperture (*Figure 9.9*). It remained upright and was cushioned between the base of the tongue and the upper boundary of the larynx. The erect epiglottis and aryepiglottic folds diverted swallowed fluids through the piriform fossae on each side of the laryngeal aperture. Johnstone (1942), on the other hand, produced evidence from a radiological study that the epiglottis may turn over during swallowing (*Figure 9.10*). High speed cine-radiography, coupled with X-ray image intensification has made possible the precise analysis of the details of the action of the epiglottis during swallowing. Ardran and Kemp (1951) and other investigators have demonstrated unequivocally that retroversion of the epiglottis occurs during swallowing closing over the approach to the laryngeal inlet. This inversion is attributed to the operation of the following mechanical factors: (a) the upper free part of the epiglottis is forced downwards and backwards by the thrust of the base of the tongue against its anterior surface; (b) the lower attached end of the epiglottis is carried upwards and forwards by the marked elevation of the thyroid cartilage; (c) the epiglottis is forced backwards by the bulging of the pad of fat at its base as the thyroid cartilage is elevated and simultaneously the arytenoid cartilages move forwards. The arytenoid cartilages meet the epiglottic tubercle and serve as the fulcrum about which the epiglottis is rolled over, thus covering the laryngeal ostium. The anterior surface of the epiglottis directs the stream of fluid into two lateral channels leading to the piriform fossae. If several successive swallows are made the epiglottis remains turned over.

Pharyngeal peristalsis and elevation of the pharynx The bolus is passed very rapidly through the pharynx, the openings to the nose and larynx having been closed off as described above. The pharyngeal musculature involved in this action may be considered in two functional groups: (1) the longitudinal and vertically disposed elevator group of muscles; and (2) the more or less circular and horizontally disposed pharyngeal constrictors. Contraction of the elevator group of pharyngeal muscles, that is, stylopharyngeus and palatopharyngeus, together with the elevators of the hyoid bone and larynx, decreases the vertical length of the pharynx. This facilitates the passage of the bolus because the pharyngeal wall is, as it were, pulled up over the descending bolus, and the pharyngo-oesophageal opening is pulled upwards to meet the descending bolus.

This contraction of the elevator muscles is followed by a progressive wave of contraction over the middle and inferior constrictor muscles.

Electromyographic recording from the individual muscles has revealed the

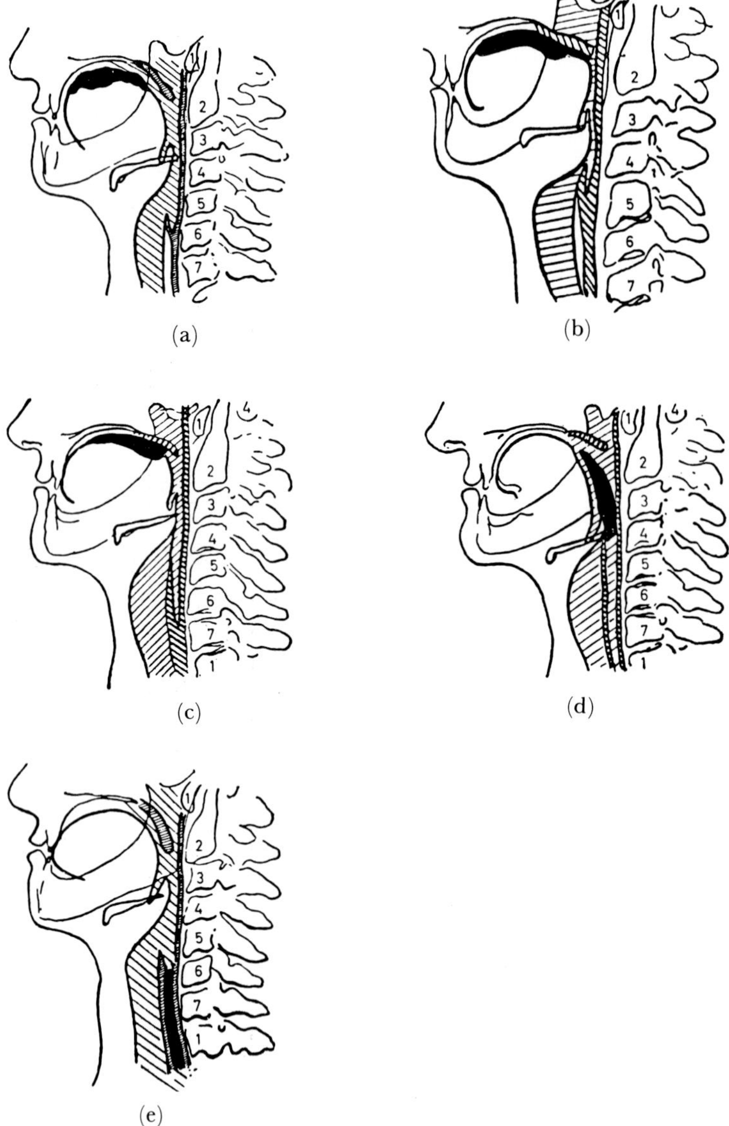

Figure 9.9 Diagram of radiographic study of pharyngeal phase of swallowing (after Barclay, 1936): (a) commencement of swallowing – bolus between tongue and palate, soft palate elevating, larynx rising; (b) nasopharynx closed off – pharynx and larynx closed; (c) pharynx opening in upper part – laryngeal pharynx drawn up; (d) bolus passing through the pharynx – sliding past epiglottis; (e) larynx and pharynx return to normal position – bolus enters pharyngeal end of oesophagus

sequence of contraction of the various muscles as well as their duration of contraction. The pattern of motor activity is summarized in *Figure 9.11*. It is seen that the muscles contracting initially include the mylohyoid, geniohyoid, posterior lingual muscles and palatopharyngeus. The superior constrictor contracts with the palatopharyngeus. This is followed in sequence by the thyrohyoid and middle constrictor. Next,

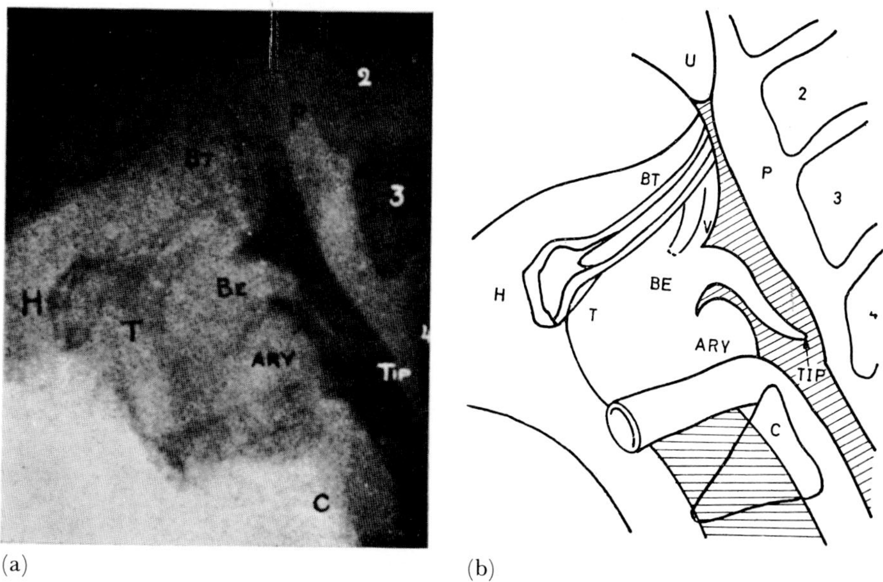

Figure 9.10 Movement of epiglottis in swallowing (after Johnstone, 1942): (a) radiograph taken during pharyngeal stage; (b) outline drawing to show position of epiglottis and related structures. C = cricoid cartilage; H = hyoid bone; U = uvula; V = vallecula; ARY = arytenoid cartilage; BT = base of tongue; P = posterior pharyngeal wall; BE = base of epiglottis; TIP = tip of epiglottis

the cricothyroid contracts and relaxes abruptly and then the inferior constrictor contracts. These electrical studies correlate well with the sequence of events described above.

Bilateral paralysis of the pharyngeal muscles causes inability to swallow; unilateral paralysis is associated with considerable difficulty in swallowing.

The pressure changes, recorded by transducer technique, in the pharynx and at the pharyngo-oesophageal sphincter during deglutition are shown in *Figure 9.12*.

The oesophageal phase of swallowing is considered in the next section.

The oesophagus

Structure

The anatomy and structure of the oesophagus have been described in the previous chapter. Only a few points of physiological significance need be mentioned. The oesophagus, like the mouth and pharynx, is lined except at its termination by a stratified squamous epithelium. This is correlated with the fact that the oesophagus is the only part of the alimentary tract from which no absorption normally occurs. Numerous mucous glands are present to lubricate the surface for free passage of swallowed material, and for protection. Squamous epithelium is very susceptible to damage by acid regurgitated from the stomach. No enzyme-secreting glands

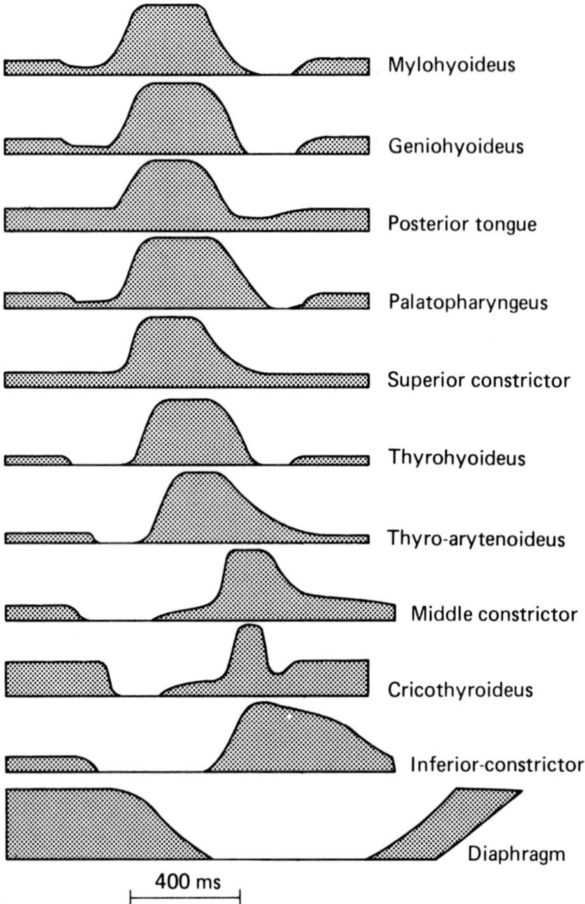

Figure 9.11 Summary of the temporal sequence of outflow from the deglutition centre, based on electromyographic recordings from the muscles involved in swallowing. (From Doty and Bosma, 1956, reproduced by courtesy of the Editor of *Journal of Neurophysiology*)

discharge into the lumen of the oesophagus. The mucosal epithelium rests on loose areolar tissue separating it from the muscle layer. The mucosa of the empty oesophagus is thrown into long folds which flatten out when the oesophagus distends. The muscle of the oesophageal wall is striated in the upper one-third. This is followed by a transitional portion and then the lower half of the oesophagus which has only plain muscle in its wall. The muscle is composed of an inner coat of 'circular' muscle arranged as short horizontal spirals, and an external coat of 'longitudinal' or vertical spiral fibres. The motor nerve supply is derived from the vagus and recurrent laryngeal nerves which form with post-ganglionic sympathetic fibres of the oesophageal plexus. Two intramural plexuses are present in the oesophagus – the myenteric plexus (Auerbach) between the two muscle coats and Meissner's plexus in the submucous layer.

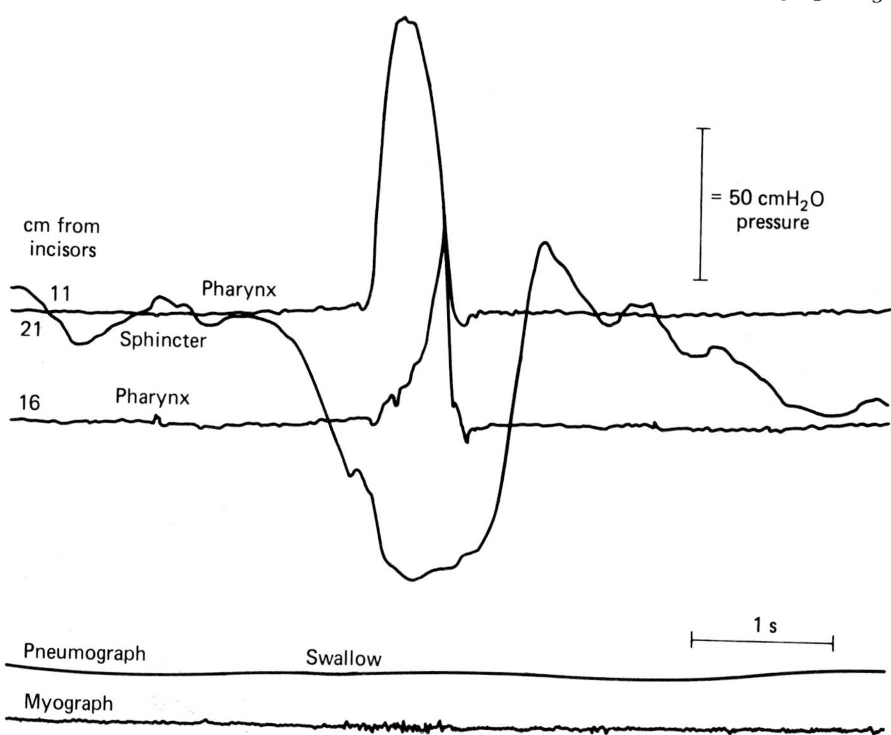

Figure 9.12 Pressure changes in pharynx and pharyngo–oesophageal sphincter during swallowing. Figures indicate distance from incisors. (From *Surgical Physiology of Gastro-intestinal Tract*, reproduced by courtesy of The Royal College of Surgeons of Edinburgh)

The oesophagus functions essentially as a conducting tube for conveying substances to, and occasionally from, the stomach.

Motor activity of the oesophagus

Methods

Knowledge of the physiological mechanisms of the oesophagus especially at the oesophagogastric junction, is essential as a basis for understanding their derangement in disease, and for rational medical or surgical treatment of disorders of the oesophagus. Investigation of the oesophagus by oesophagoscopy, radiology, and by recording of intraluminal pressures, has assumed special importance not only in physiological research but also in clinical diagnosis.

The methods used in the study of the oesophagus include anatomical methods such as dissections of the normal and abnormal human oesophagus, histology, embryology and comparative anatomy. Radiology has proved specially valuable in the investigation of oesophageal activity. Examination of the rapid sequence of events in the oesophagus has been facilitated by cine-radiography. Radio-opaque markers have been inserted in the oesophagus to make possible localization of various structures during x-ray studies. Pharmacological studies have been made *in vitro*, using strips of oesophageal muscle to record the effects of autonomic drugs. The study of oesophageal motility has been greatly advanced by the introduction of modern electronic techniques for recording pressure changes. The use of these pressure transducers has revolutionized our knowledge of the movements of the oesophagus. These transducers transform pressure changes into electrical signals which can be recorded, and permit continuous and accurate measurement of intraluminal pressures.

Normal oesophageal pressures

The intra-oesophageal pressure is fairly uniform throughout the oesophagus, except for about 3 cm at each of its proximal and distal ends.

Pharyngo-oesophageal junction

The resting intrapharyngeal pressure is equal to the atmospheric pressure. During swallowing there is a transitory rise of about 40 mmHg.

At the pharyngo-oesophageal junction there is a region of raised pressure about 3 cm in length. The pressure profile in this region as recorded by pressure transducer shows in the first centimetre of this zone a rising pressure, followed by 1 cm of peak pressure reaching about 35 mmHg. This region of peak pressure corresponds to the position of the cricopharyngeus muscle. Beyond this is a distal centimetre in which the pressure decreased to atmospheric pressure. These recordings demonstrate the existence of a tonic sphincter of considerable competence. During swallowing pressure in this zone falls abruptly just before the pharyngeal peristaltic wave reaches this zone. This indicates relaxation of the sphincter so that the entrance to the oesophagus opens before the arrival of the bolus and the pharyngeal contraction wave (*Figure 9.12*). Immediately after the bolus has passed, the sphincter contracts strongly with a rise of pressure to 50–100 mmHg. This abrupt contraction has the function of preventing reflux while peristalsis is occurring in the upper oesophagus. When the bolus passes further down the oesophagus, the pressure in the pharyngo-oesophageal zone returns to normal, that is, the sphincter returns to its normal state of tonic contraction.

Oesophagus

Resting pressures In the intrathoracic oesophagus the muscle coat is relaxed and the intraluminal pressure corresponds to the intrapleural pressure. With normal breathing at rest this pressure is subatmospheric.

At the end of expiration this intra-oesophageal pressure is −5 mmHg, and with inspiration it falls to −10 mmHg. During a powerful inspiration with the glottis closed the pressure may decrease to 30 mmHg below atmospheric pressure. Expiration against resistance or with the glottis closed, as in coughing or straining during defaecation, parturition or physical effort such as weight-lifting, raises the intrathoracic and therefore the intra-oesophageal pressure. During maximal expiratory effort with the glottis closed, pressures of 40 mmHg above atmospheric may be reached.

Oesophageal peristalsis during deglutition During swallowing peristaltic waves pass down the oesophagus and are recorded as waves of positive pressure. The rise of pressure with each peristalsis may reach 50–100 mmHg. This peristalsis begins immediately beyond the pharyngo-oesophageal junction.

Primary peristaltic wave The peristaltic pressure wave varies somewhat with the nature of the swallowed substance. With a dry swallow there is a simple wave with a smooth rise and fall of pressure. With liquid or semi-solid swallowing the pressure wave is more complex. This pressure recording has four components. First there is an initial negative wave which is most evident in upper oesophageal records; it is probably due to elevation of the larynx drawing on the cervical oesophagus. This is followed by an abrupt positive wave; this coincides with the entry of the bolus into the oesophagus. Next comes a slow rise of pressure or a maintained plateau of raised pressure, succeeded by a final large positive pressure wave which rises and falls rapidly. This is the peristaltic stripping wave. Its amplitude and duration are least in the proximal oesophagus and increase progressively to the lower end. In addition the extent of the contracted portion is longer in the distal than in the proximal oesophagus.

Secondary and tertiary contractions Secondary peristaltic waves arise locally in the oesophagus in response to distension and they serve to complete the transportation of bolus portions which have been left after the passage of the primary peristaltic wave. Tertiary oesophageal contractions are recorded occasionally. These are irregular non-propulsive contractions involving long segments of the oesophagus. They are more frequent in situations of emotional stress. A characteristic x-ray appearance called 'curling' may be due to these contractions.

Velocity of oesophageal transport The transit of the primary oesophageal peristalsis has been timed by Hightower and Salem. It traverses the oesophagus in 8–12 s. This peristalsis is more rapid in the upper part of the oesophagus than in the distal half. This is correlated with the differences in muscle type and in the neural mechanism of the propagation of the peristalsis.

Oesophagogastric junction

The resting pressure in the stomach beyond the oesophagogastric junction is positive and about 5–10 mmHg above atmospheric pressure. This intragastric pressure rises with inspiration and falls with expiration. This respiratory variation is opposite in its direction to the rhythmic respiratory variation in intra-oesophageal pressure which falls with inspiration and rises with expiration. Intragastric pressure is lower in the erect than in the supine position. It increases sharply with coughing and other forced expiratory acts, e.g. sneezing, blowing and also whenever the anterior abdominal wall muscles contract, as in micturition, defaecation, parturition and vomiting, or during abdominal compression.

At the oesophagogastric junction there is a zone of raised pressure about 3 cm in length and extending above and below the diaphragm. The mean pressure here is approximately 8 mmHg higher than the intragastric pressure. Although this pressure is only slightly in excess of that in the stomach, regurgitation of gastric contents does not occur normally. This region of the oesophagus with an intraluminal pressure higher than that in the rest of the oesophagus or in the stomach, must be regarded as the location of the 'physiological sphincter' of the oesophagogastric zone.

Above this high pressure zone the intra-oesophageal pressure approximates to the negative subatmospheric intrapleural pressure fluctuating with the inspiratory and expiratory phases of respiration.

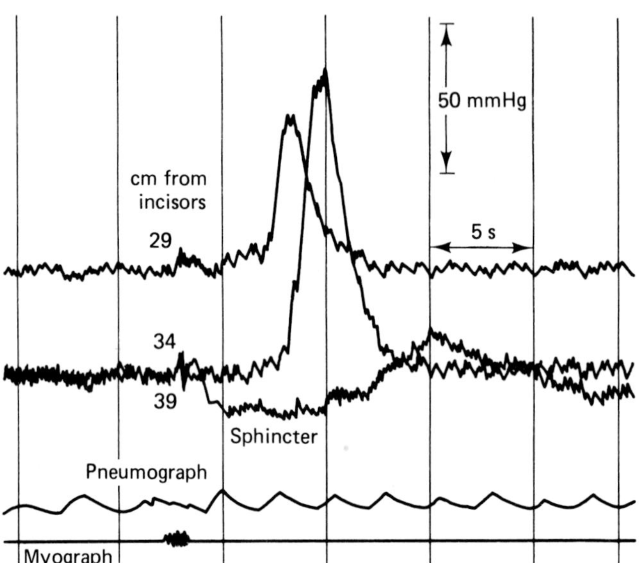

Figure 9.13 Pressure changes in the lower oesophagus during swallowing. (From Davenport's *Physiology of the Digestive Tract*, reproduced by courtesy of Year Book Medical Publishers)

The muscle of this 'sphincteric' region is thus normally in slight tonic contraction. Before the oesophageal peristalsis commences in the cervical oesophagus the oesophagogastric zone pressure falls indicating relaxation of its muscular wall. This relaxation persists for several seconds and then when the peristaltic wave reaches this physiological sphincter the pressure rises above the normal resting pressure. This contraction persists for 5–10 s, after which the pressure returns to the normal resting level. Thus, as with the pharyngo-oesophageal sphincter, at the upper end of the oesophagus, the oesophagogastric sphincter normally in tonic contraction undergoes relaxation before the peristalsis reaches it and similarly a reflux-preventing contraction occurs immediately the bolus has passed into the stomach (*Figure 9.13*).

Oesophageal stage of swallowing

During this stage the food passes along the oesophagus and through the cardiac sphincter to enter the stomach. The physical consistency of the swallowed material determines to some extent the mechanism involved in its passage through the oesophagus.

When fluid is swallowed the force of the initial contractions in the buccal stage may be sufficient to project the fluid through the pharynx and oesophagus to its lower end.

The fluid reaches the oesophagogastric junction in 1 s if the subject is standing. Even in the supine position the fluid arrives at the stomach ahead of the oesophageal peristalsis. When studied under radiological visualization the rapid passage of swallowed fluid down the oesophagus may be followed by temporary arrest at the cardiac orifice of the stomach. The fluid then enters the stomach in a narrow stream. In consequence of this rapid passage, the swallowing of corrosive fluids causes burns localized mainly to the regions in which the fluid tends to be held up by reason of narrowing of the oesophageal lumen. These sites are: (1) where the left bronchus crosses in front of the oesophagus; (2) at the pharyngeal end, that is, the cricopharyngeal sphincter; (3) at the oesophageal hiatus in the diaphragm.

When the bolus is solid or semi-solid it is passed down the oesophagus by a peristaltic contraction of the oesophageal musculature.

Entry of bolus into pharyngeal end of oesophagus: relaxation of pharyngo-oesophageal sphincter

The pharyngeal end of the oesophagus is guarded by a cricopharyngeal sphincter. This is formed by the lowest fibres of the inferior constrictor of the pharynx arising from the cricoid cartilage. This sphincter is normally in a state of tonic contraction while the rest of the inferior constrictor (thyropharyngeus) is relaxed. Thus it prevents the inspiratory increase in capacity of the thoracic cage drawing air into the oesophagus. Such oesophageal ventilation would result in some of the increase in the capacity of the thorax in inspiration being taken up by air drawn into the oesophagus, in effect increasing the dead space and thus diminishing the effective ventilation of the pulmonary alveoli.

This sphincter may be detected as a slight resistance during the passage of an oesophagoscope.

The cricopharyngeal sphincter has a double autonomic innervation. Post-ganglionic sympathetic fibres are derived from the superior cervical ganglion. Parasympathetic vagal fibres reach the muscle in the recurrent laryngeal nerve. Stimulation of the vagus causes relaxation, and sympathetic excitation causes contraction of the sphincter. The main propulsive part of the inferior constrictor – thyropharyngeus muscle – and the cricopharyngeal sphincteric portion are reciprocally innervated. The cricopharyngeal sphincter is inhibited when the main part of the inferior constrictor contracts in the reflex response constituting the pharyngeal stage of deglutition. Thus the arrival of the bolus at the oesophageal opening is preceded by relaxation of the tonically contracted cricopharyngeal sphincter. Relaxation of this sphincter occurs very early at the commencement of swallowing when the bolus is propelled from the mouth. Thus the pharyngo-oesophageal junction is open well in advance of the arrival of the bolus. This relaxation further permits a forward movement of the larynx, increasing the capacity of the laryngeal end of the pharynx and facilitating the passage of the bolus. Reflex inhibition of the tonus of the oesophagus is described as accompanying the relaxation of the sphincter. Thus the 'mouth' of the oesophagus opens to receive the bolus.

Recordings of intra-oesophageal pressures have shown that after the bolus has passed beyond the relaxed sphincter, the latter contracts powerfully. This has the effect of preventing reflux during peristalsis in the upper oesophagus. As the bolus passes beyond the proximal oesophagus the contraction decreases and the sphincter returns to its normal resting tone.

This sequence of automatic sphincter relaxation at the commencement of deglutition well in advance of the arrival of the bolus, and the prolonged strong contraction after its passage may be the general pattern of the mode of action of other sphincters in the alimentary tract. A similar mechanism has been demonstrated at the oesophagogastric junctional zone.

Failure of relaxation of the sphincteric mechanism may be an important aetiological factor in the production of pharyngeal diverticula. Herniation occurs at the relatively weak part of the wall between the inferior border of the thyropharyngeal and the superior border of the cricopharyngeal portions of the inferior constrictor. Loss of normal tonic contraction of the sphincter may lead to air swallowing and dilatation of the oesophagus.

Passage through the oesophagus: oesophageal peristalsis

The bolus is passed down the oesophagus by coordinated waves of peristalsis. Gravity normally plays little part in the process as the rate of movement of the bolus along the oesophagus is not significantly affected by changing from the erect to the supine position. In marked dilatation of the oesophagus, peristalsis may be ineffective as a propulsive mechanism and the descent of the bolus is dependent to some extent on gravity.

The muscular coat of the upper one-third of the oesophagus is composed of striated muscle. The lower half has unstriated muscle while the intervening zone is mixed. Correlated with the differences in type of musculature there are differences in motor activity. In the upper part of the oesophagus the peristaltic wave progresses rapidly, solid food passing through the upper third in 1 s. In the lower one-third the contraction wave is more sluggish, the bolus passing through in 3 s. Reverse peristalsis in the oesophagus does not normally occur in man although it has been reported during heartburn with acid regurgitation.

Oesophagogastric sphincter

The mechanism preventing reflux at the oesophagogastric junction and regulating the entry of food into the stomach has been the subject of considerable research. The numerous theories which have been proposed include: (1) an anatomical sphincter; (2) pinch-cock action of the diaphragm; (3) gastric muscular loop of Willis; (4) oblique angle of entry of oesophagus into stomach; (5) mechanical valve mechanism by mucosal folds or rosette; (6) difference in external pressure on supradiaphragmatic and infradiaphragmatic parts of the oesophagus with a flutter valve effect; (7) physiological intrinsic muscle sphincter. Some of these theories are discussed briefly below.

Anatomical sphincter Early descriptions of a thickening of the circular muscle forming an anatomical sphincter were based on autopsy or cadaver dissections. Most recent investigators have failed to confirm the existence of this muscle.

Sling fibres of Willis The portion of the stomach adjacent to the oesophageal opening has a definite collar of muscle (Willis' loop). This is part of the internal muscle layer of the stomach, the fibres sweeping up from the lesser curvature to encircle the terminal oesophagus. These muscular fibres form the only structure that could be regarded as an anatomical sphincter in this region. However, this 'sling' does not correspond in position with the 'sphincter mechanism', as determined by x-rays or by manometric pressure studies, for the pressure barrier at the oesophagogastric junction extends above as well as below the diaphragm, and in man the sling fibres surround only part of the intra-abdominal oesophagus. Further, the anti-reflux mechanism has been shown to be competent after section of these sling fibres.

Oesophagogastric junctional angle The oesophagus opens obliquely into the lesser curvature of the stomach so that a sharp angle is formed between the oesophagus and the greater curvature of the fundus of the stomach. It has been suggested that the fold thus formed could act as a mechanical flap valve. With a rise of intragastric pressure the fundus compresses the adjacent part of the terminal oesophagus and prevents reflux. The higher the pressure in the stomach the more securely will this flap valve be closed. But this angle of entry is very variable in man and some patients suffer from reflux despite a normal oesophagogastric angle.

Change in direction of the oesophagus The oesophagus, after passing through the diaphragm and under the liver, turns to the left across the left crus to reach the stomach. Mosher claimed that this change in direction acts as a mechanical closure of the lower oesophagus, unfolding as the stomach descends with inspiration.

Role of the diaphragm Since the oesophagus passes through the hiatus in the muscular part of the diaphragm, a significant role in the closure mechanism at the gastric end of the oesophagus has often been attributed to this muscle. Jackson described this as the pinch-cock effect of the diaphragm. This view is supported by a puckering of the inner wall of the oesophagus at this level seen during oesophagoscopy. Further supporting evidence is the brief arrest of swallowed food and liquids at this diaphragmatic level and the prolongation of this arrest by a maintained deep inspiration. But this hold-up could equally be a result of the increased intra-abdominal pressure. Furthermore, the zone of raised intra-oesophageal pressure extends beyond the hiatus for an equal distance above and below the diaphragm, and paralysis of the diaphragm by muscle relaxants or phrenic nerve section does not lower this pressure, nor does it cause reflux or impair the sphincteric mechanism. Although the diaphragm undoubtedly does not constitute the main sphincter, it may play an auxiliary role.

Pressure gradient: flutter valve The supradiaphragmatic part of the oesophagus is subject externally to the negative subatmospheric intrathoracic pressure tending to separate its walls, while the walls of the infradiaphragmatic abdominal portion of the oesophagus are pressed together by the positive intra-abdominal pressure. Creamer, Donoghue and Code (1958) pointed out that the oesophagus is a flaccid tube passing through the narrow diaphragmatic opening from a region of lower to a region of higher pressure, and that this pressure gradient would lead to collapse of the intra-abdominal segment and act as a pneumatic anti-reflux mechanism. Edwards (1961) modified this theory, following a study by radiology and by pressure measurements of patients with hiatus hernia and others with gastric reflux. He suggests that the mechanism works on the principle of the mechanical flutter valve, as used in physiological respiratory apparatus. The essential part of the flutter valve is a soft rubber tube flattened at the end so that air passing down the tube separates the walls, while air tending to pass back will draw the walls together and close the tube. The soft compressible oesophagus, with its walls flattened by intra-abdominal pressure and by the intrinsic muscle sphincter, could behave like a flutter valve and ensure unidirectional flow.

Mucosal folds or rosette The concept that folds of the oesophageal mucosa may act as anti-reflux valves, akin to valves in the vascular system, has been supported by several observers, since it was first proposed by Magendie. Prominent mucosal folds are present in some species and absent in others. Dornhorst and others (1954) have demonstrated mucosal folds in man. They are present in most subjects, though varying greatly in their arrangement. Smooth muscle has been described in these folds, and by tonic contraction this muscle may help to close the folds and prevent retrograde flow (*Figure 9.14*). It is suggested that, even in the presence of a

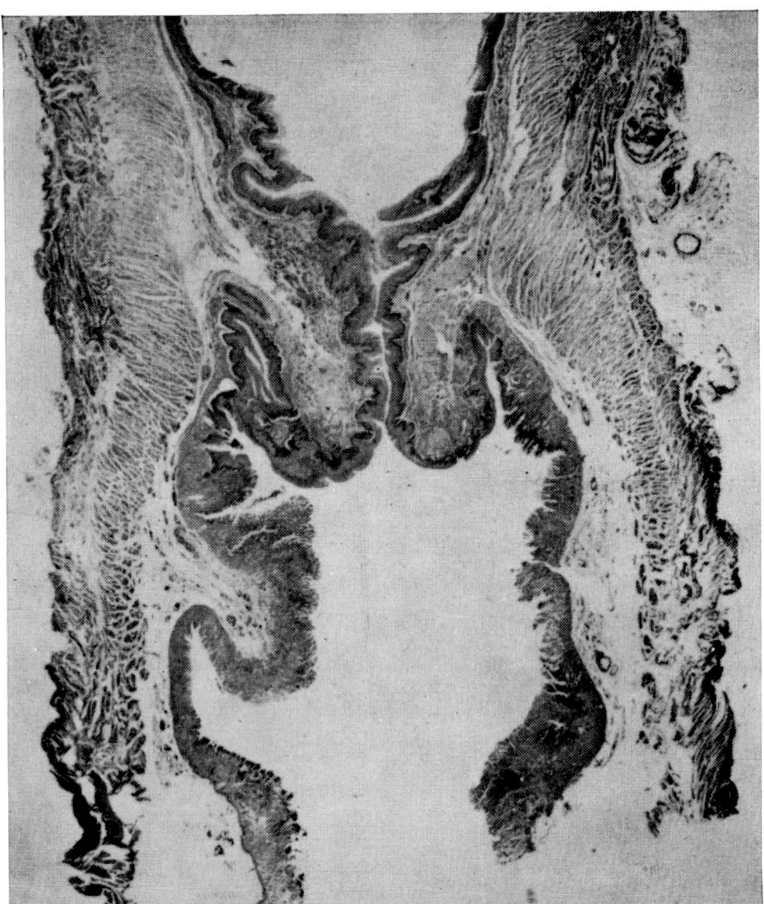

Figure 9.14 Section of oesophagogastric junction showing mucosal folds forming a valve. (From Creamer, 1955, reproduced by courtesy of the Editor of *Lancet*)

physiological muscular sphincter, epithelial folds forming a sort of 'rosette' could act as a plug completing the sealing of the opening at its centre. This would seal the opening even against the passage of air.

Intrinsic physiological sphincter The absence of a structural sphincter, that is, a thickening of the circular muscle, does not preclude the possibility of a functional sphincter. If the intrinsic muscle of the terminal part of the oesophagus is normally in a state of resting tonic contraction while the rest of the muscle above this is relaxed and if reciprocal innervation of these two portions exists, then an effective physiological sphincter is present. Manometric studies in man have demonstrated that, at the oesophagogastric junctional zone, there is a region of raised intraluminal pressure extending above and below the diaphragm. As described in a previous paragraph on oesophageal pressures this zone of raised pressure is clearly demonstrated when a catheter for pressure transducer recording is gradually withdrawn from the stomach into the lower oesophagus. Such manometric studies by Fyke and Code (1953), Atkinson, Edwards and Rowlands (1957) have established clearly the presence of this 'sphincter' region of raised pressure and its functional importance in providing a competent antireflux mechanism. Relaxation or denervation of the muscle of the lower part of the oesophagus produces a reduction of this high pressure; stimulation of this muscle causes an increase in this barrier pressure. The pressure here falls, as we have seen, with swallowing, indicating reduction or inhibition of the tonic contraction of the sphincter. The existence of this functional sphincter in the intrinsic muscle of the oesophagus is supported by pharmacological evidence. Parasympathomimetic drugs cause an increase in tone while adrenergic drugs relax the circular muscle of the 'sphincter' zone.

The sequence of pressure changes in the pharynx and oesophagus during swallowing, is shown diagrammatically in *Figure 9.15*.

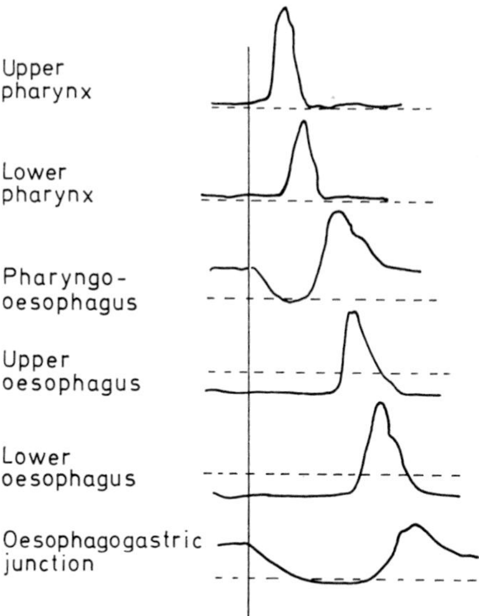

Figure 9.15 Diagram to illustrate pressure factors during swallowing

Summary of above theories It is generally accepted that an anatomical sphincter cannot be demonstrated in man. A physiological 'sphincter' or antireflux mechanism is present and this is believed to be due to several factors, some mechanical, some physiological, some acting on the oesophagus externally and others intrinsic in the muscle or mucosal lining. The extent to which each factor contributes is not agreed. The diaphragm is not the main component of this reflux-preventing mechanism although it can influence oesophageal emptying by changes of the intrapleural and intra-abdominal pressures. A mucosal rosette or larger mucosal folds may help to complete the plugging of the lumen, but can only subserve this function, provided the muscle of the wall is in tonic contraction. The pressure difference in the environment of the portions of the oesophagus above and below the diaphragm may have a flutter valve action. The main bulk of the evidence supports the view that the chief component of the 'sphincter' is a segment of intrinsic muscle of the oesophagus close to the oesophagogastric junction which is normally in tone and which contracts and relaxes as a single functional unit.

Some of the suggestions as to the nature of the oesophagogastric mechanism are shown diagrammatically in *Figure 9.16*.

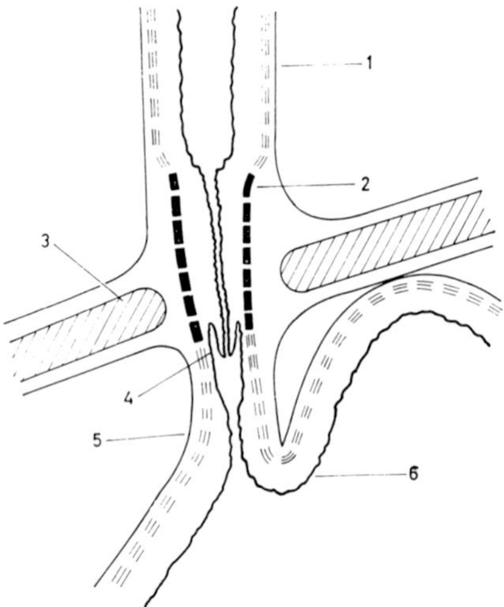

Figure 9.16 Diagram to illustrate factors involved in the oesophagogastric antireflux mechanism. (1) Negative intrathoracic pressure; (2) intrinsic physiological muscular sphincter; (3) pinch-cock effect of diaphragm; (4) mucosal folds; (5) positive intra-abdominal pressure; (6) oesophagogastric angle

Sounds during deglutition

Two sounds can be heard on auscultation over the oesophagus during swallowing. They can be recorded electrically. The first sound occurs immediately after the commencement of the act and is probably due to the fluid impinging on the posterior pharyngeal wall. The second sound resembles a bubbling or trickling noise, occurs at a variable interval of 4–10 s after the first sound and persists for 2–3 s. It is heard most clearly over the epigastrium. In the recumbent subject the second sound is replaced by a few discrete squirting sounds each of 1 s duration. When a solid bolus is swallowed, the second sound may be absent.

Nervous regulation of deglutition

From the neural aspect deglutition involves two components: (1) a buccopharyngeal component; (2) an oesophageal and oesophagogastric stage.

Swallowing can first be elicited about the twelfth week of fetal life. This early appearance suggests that swallowing is a brain stem reflex. This is confirmed by the persistence of a swallowing reflex in the decerebrate animal. From the twenty-fourth week the fetus swallows amniotic fluid.

The orderly sequence of muscular responses which constitute the act of swallowing is reflex in origin. The stimulus eliciting the reflex is usually the contact of a bolus of food or saliva with the posterior pharyngeal wall.

The *sensory receptors* from which the reflex can be most readily evoked are concentrated mainly in sensitive areas of the mucosa of the posterior pharyngeal wall, anterior and posterior pillars of the fauces, and the base of the tongue (*Figure 9.17*). The normal swallowing reflex is disrupted by local anaesthesia of these trigger zones in the pharynx and mouth.

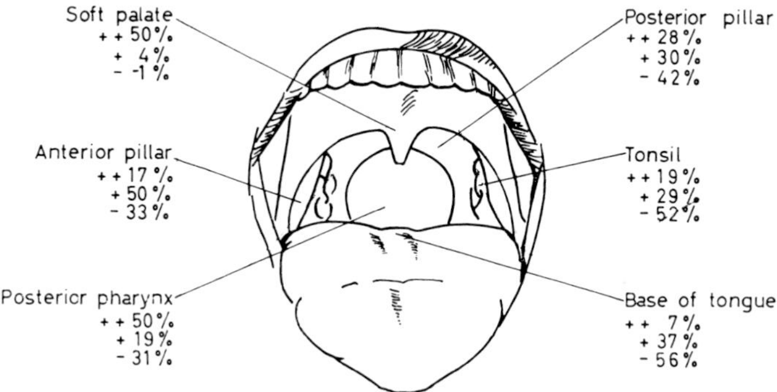

Figure 9.17 Diagram of sensory receptor area for the deglutition reflex (after Pommerenke, 1928)

Swallowing can also be excited by dipping the face or nose in cold water.

The *afferent pathways* of this reflex arc are fibres of the nerves innervating the mucosa of these receptive areas of the back of the mouth and pharynx. These are the glossopharyngeal nerve, the pharyngeal and internal laryngeal branches of the vagus, and the trigeminal nerve. Electrical stimulation of the central end of the internal laryngeal nerve and, less constantly, the glossopharyngeal nerve in animals will excite reflex swallowing movements.

The *afferent impulses* have been traced along thick rapidly-conducting fibres to the solitary fasciculus of the brain stem. This is supported by the following evidence. Stimulation of the laryngeal branch of the vagus produces electrical activity in the fasciculus solitarius. Electrical stimulation of the region of this fasciculus causes swallowing. Destruction of the rostral end of this fasciculus abolishes the swallowing response to stimulation of laryngeal nerves. Action potential and electromyographic studies, and experimental lesions produced in the brain stem have also confirmed that the afferent impulses of swallowing pass to the lateral part of the solitary fasciculus and from there are relayed into a specific section of the neurone population of the reticular formation in the medulla. This area constitutes a 'swallowing centre'.

The *efferent limb of the reflex arc:* (1) The motor neurones supplying the *striated* muscles of swallowing, i.e. the buccal, oral, pharyngeal muscles and the striated muscle coat of the upper oesophagus, are located in the motor cranial nuclei of the trigeminal, facial, glossopharyngeal and hypoglossal nerves, together with the nucleus ambiguus of the vagus. The rostral part of the nucleus ambiguus innervates the palatal, pharyngeal and oesophageal muscles, while the caudal part controls the laryngeal muscles. Thus in bulbar poliomyelitis, if the cephalic portion of this nucleus is affected severe dysphagia results – but when the disease involves the caudal part, dysarthria is produced. (2) The neurones supplying the plain muscle of the distal oesophagus are in the dorsal nucleus of the vagus.

A *swallowing centre* in the functional sense is located in the medulla. This 'centre' is in close relation to but distinct from the 'respiration centre' in the reticular formation. Lesions in the medulla may abolish the swallowing reflex without inhibiting respiration. Central depression of breathing as a result of trauma, the administration of drugs or reflex inhibition does not necessarily disturb swallowing. However these centres are interconnected and respiration is always inhibited during swallowing.

Serial sections of the brain stem in animals provide evidence that the deglutition centre lies close to the midline, dorsal to and between the facial nucleus and the inferior olive.

The centre is bilateral and consists of two half centres. Destruction of the half centre on one side eliminates the response of the muscles of that side in swallowing. The two half centres are linked by interneurones thus ensuring the normal integrated bilateral response of the muscles of the mouth, pharynx and larynx in swallowing. Experimentally a short midline incision in the appropriate region of the medulla results in only a unilateral response of the swallowing muscles with the exception of the inferior constrictor muscles. Stimulation of the 'centre' on one side in this experimental preparation causes a contraction of the muscles of that side except for the inferior pharyngeal constrictors which contract on both sides.

This deglutition centre may be regarded as a coordinating and distributing centre. The afferent impulse stream is relayed from the deglutition centre in orderly timed sequence along association fibres to the appropriate motor neurones supplying the muscles involved in the reflex stages of deglutition (*Figure 9.18*).

The efferent motor fibres concerned in the swallowing reflex are mainly in the hypoglossal, spinal accessory, vagus (pharyngeal and laryngeal branches), glossopharyngeal and trigeminal nerves. The efferent impulses are mediated through these nerves to the muscles of the tongue, fauces, palate, pharynx, larynx and oesophagus concerned in the reflex stages of deglutition.

The reflex stimulation of the deglutition centre results in a coordinated motor discharge producing contraction of the elevators and tensors of the palate, palatoglossus, the palatopharyngeus muscles, the elevators of the larynx and pharynx, the sphincteric muscles of the larynx, adductors of the vocal cords, and the elevators of the pharynx. It also produces a coordinated peristaltic wave of contraction of the pharyngeal constrictors and the oesophageal musculature. The propagated 'peristaltic' contraction of the pharyngeal constrictors is accompanied by inhibition of the cricopharyngeal sphincter. This sphincter is innervated by the recurrent branch of the vagus and by post-ganglionic sympathetic fibres from the superior cervical ganglion. Vagal stimulation causes relaxation and sympathetic stimulation causes contraction.

The orderly progress of the peristaltic wave in the upper oesophagus is part of the reflex response excited by the initial stimulation of the sensory receptors in the pharynx. Thus, upper oesophageal peristalsis is mediated through the extrinsic nerves and is dependent on the integrity of the vagal oesophageal plexus. Evidence for

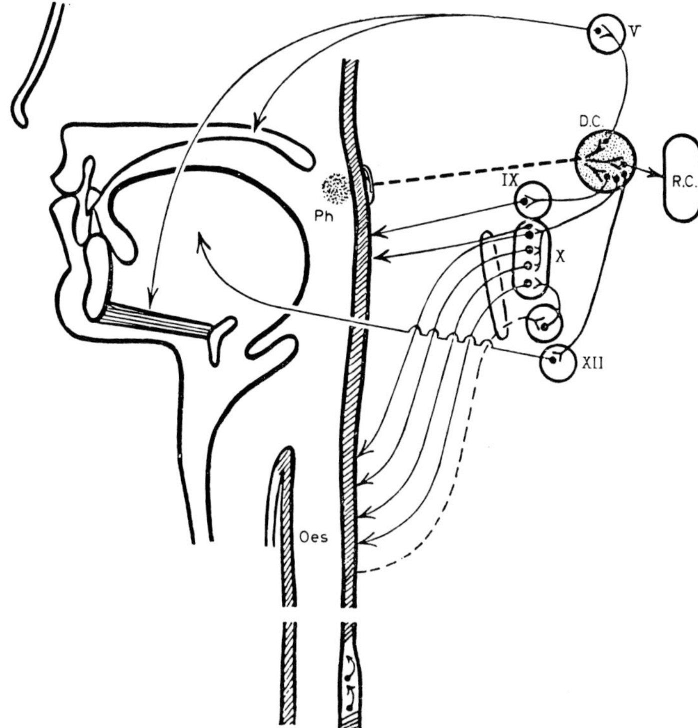

Figure 9.18 Diagram of the neural mechanism of the deglutition reflex

this is provided by the following experiments. Transection of the oesophageal wall or removal of an entire segment of the oesophagus does not prevent the peristaltic wave passing across the break in continuity of the oesophageal wall, provided the extrinsic vagal plexus is intact. Section of the oesophageal plexus without division of the oesophageal wall results in arrest of peristalsis at the site of the nerve section. This mechanism is illustrated by the classical case cited by von Mikulicz. A part of the oesophagus was resected and a fistulous opening into the oesophagus was established in the lower cervical region. Food introduced into the fistulous opening did not move until the patient swallowed.

This main reflex mechanism excited from the pharynx at the beginning of the act is supplemented by secondary reflex responses. These are initiated by the stimulation of sensory endings in the oesophageal mucosa by the bolus of food. Afferent impulses from these receptors evoke reflexly, via the vagi and the medullary deglutition centre, a strong contraction of the pharyngo-oesophageal sphincter and a peristaltic contraction of the oesophageal muscle above the bolus. This peristalsis pushes the bolus onward. Thus the bolus of food itself causes a series of reflex contractions, by local stimulation of sensory endings in the oesophagus. In this way each contraction provides the stimulus for the reflex contraction of the succeeding segment of the oesophagus. If the propulsion of the bolus to the stomach is not effected by the initial peristaltic wave of the deglutition reflex, then this accessory reflex mechanism will complete the transportation through the upper oesophagus.

In the lower oesophagus, in which the muscle coat is composed of smooth muscle, the propagation of the wave of peristalsis is independent of the extrinsic nerve supply. The coordination of peristaltic contraction is dependent here on the intramural myenteric plexus.

Pharyngeal dysphagia The cranial nuclei containing the cell bodies of the neurones supplying the muscles involved in swallowing lie close together in the medulla. Lesions in this region such as those of bulbar poliomyelitis, motor neurone disease or thrombosis of the posterior cerebellar artery may cause dysphagia. The palatal and pharyngeal muscles may be paralysed, but the cricopharyngeus is usually not affected. The palatal paralysis results in nasal regurgitation, and the absence of adequate closure of the laryngeal inlet causes coughing on swallowing.

Peripheral lesions of the glossopharyngeal or vagus nerves, if unilateral, do not produce any serious disorder of swallowing.

Dysphagia is a common symptom in myasthenia gravis. Here transmission of motor nerve impulses at the motor end-plates of the neuromuscular junction is defective. In this disorder the cricopharyngeus muscle is also affected as well as the other muscles of the pharyngeal phase of swallowing. Difficulty in swallowing may also be a feature of the increased motor neurone excitability in tetanus.

'Globus hystericus' describes a sensation of a lump in the throat without apparent cause. Malcomson carried out a clinical and radiological investigation of 300 globus patients. In 80 per cent organic lesions in the foregut were found. These patients did not display any manifestations of hysterical personality. True dysphagia was absent; the symptom was more prominent between meals than during eating. Malcomson (1968) explains this symptom as an example of referred sensation or hypertonus of the pharyngeal musculature reflexly induced by distal lesions, e.g. hiatus hernia, duodenal ulceration or gastric lesions. He suggests that since in the majority of cases hysteria is not present the diagnosis 'globus hystericus' could be replaced by the term 'globus pharyngis' which correctly describes the symptom without implying diagnosis of its cause.

Pharyngeal and oesophageal sensation

The pharynx is innervated by glossopharyngeal, vagal and sympathetic fibres from the pharyngeal plexus. The glossopharyngeal nerve is distributed mainly to the upper one-third while the middle and lower thirds are supplied by pharyngeal branches of the vagus. The sympathetic supply is from the superior cervical ganglion. The oesophagus is supplied by vagus and sympathetic. The parasympathetic supply to the cervical oesophagus is from the recurrent laryngeal nerves. The intrathoracic part is supplied by both vagal trunks; the left vagus is distributed mainly anteriorly and the right vagus posteriorly. Sympathetic supply to the oesophagus is mainly from the inferior cervical ganglion.

Touch

Touch sensation is present in the pharynx as far as the level of the cricoid.

Thermal sensation

Thermal sensation is present in the pharynx and throughout the whole length of the oesophagus.

Thirst

This sensation is made up of two components. The first is a pharyngeal sensory element. This is due to dehydration causing decreased salivary secretion and drying of the pharyngeal mucosa with consequent stimulation of special sensory receptors. Impulses from these receptors are conducted along fibres in the glossopharyngeal and vagus nerves. This pharyngeal component can be abolished by stimulating salivary secretion or by local anaesthesia of the pharyngeal mucous membrane.

There is considerable evidence for an additional extrapharyngeal component or 'thirst drive'. Although thirst is generally associated with a dry mouth, the latter can be present without thirst. Inhibition of salivary secretion by atropine or the xerostomia due to disease produces a dry mouth but not the full thirst sensation with the urge to drink. Furthermore, neither sensory denervation of the pharynx nor removal of salivary glands influences significantly the volume of water taken in. The intensity of this extrapharyngeal drive to increase water intake is closely related to the magnitude of the water depletion of the body. The mechanism of this central component is not agreed, although it seems clearly related to the intracellular osmolarity. Intravenous hypertonic saline or a high intake of salt with low water intake, causing intracellular dehydration and a rise in intracellular crystalloid osmotic pressure, produces thirst. Water depletion accompanied by an equivalent loss of salt does not cause thirst. This osmotic effect is believed to act on osmoreceptor neurones in the hypothalamus because stimulation through implanted electrodes or by micro-injections of hypertonic saline in the hypothalamus causes excessive water drinking.

Pain

Pain receptors in the form of free naked nerve terminals are present in the pharynx and oesophagus.

Pharyngeal pain is produced by the usual noxious traumatic stimuli, cutting, crushing, burning and inflammation, which also cause cutaneous pain. Inflammation of the pharynx lowers the pain threshold locally and light contact or swallowing movements will cause pain from the inflamed mucosa.

Oesophageal pain is not readily elicited experimentally by the usual cutting or crushing stimuli. The adequate stimuli which excite oesophageal pain are distension and muscular spasm. In this respect the oesophagus resembles the stomach and the rest of the hollow muscular viscera. Chemical stimulation by acid gastric reflux may under certain conditions cause pain.

Oesophageal pain also resembles visceral pain in being often poorly localized and referred. Pain produced by experimental oesophageal distension, is localized anteriorly in the midline of the body over the sternum. The area of reference to which the pain is projected corresponds roughly with the level of the part of the oesophagus being distended (*Figure 9.19*).

Various types of pain originating in the oesophagus have been described. In diffuse spasm of the oesophagus a prominent symptom is acute substernal pain. In this condition prolonged and strong contractions of the whole lower half of the oesophagus occur. These contractions produce a rise of intraluminal pressure of up to 300 mmHg. Spasm limited to the oesophagogastric region will also cause some pain or discomfort. This type of pain produced by marked spasm may be referred to the epigastric region and simulate the pain of peptic ulceration or of disease of the gall bladder. Occasionally the pain is severe and retrosternal and resembles cardiac pain. This reference seems to suggest that the pain impulses may be mediated along nerve fibres entering the spinal cord through the posterior nerve roots of the upper thoracic segments of the cord.

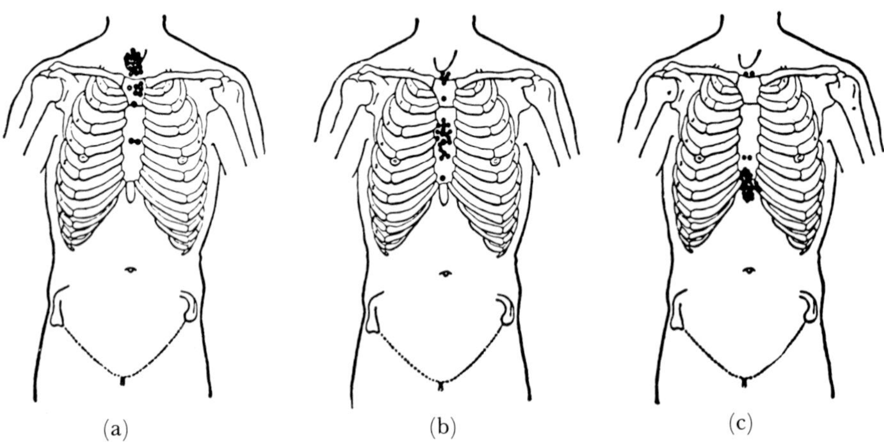

Figure 9.19 Areas of reference of pain produced by distension of the oesophagus at different levels: (a) upper oesophagus; (b) mid-oesophagus; (c) lower oesophagus and cardia. (From Jones *Digestive Tract Pain*, reproduced by courtesy of The Macmillan Co.)

Another variety of oesophageal pain, commonly called heartburn, is a burning, hot sensation felt under the lower part of the sternum and radiating sometimes up into the neck and jaws. This sensation may be accompanied by regurgitation of acid fluid, and is not relieved by taking food. Heartburn has been attributed to regurgitation of acid gastric contents into the lower oesophagus. However, heartburn has been reported in patients with achlorhydria, and N/10 acid introduced into a normal oesophagus probably does not cause this sensation. On the other hand, a burning sensation similar to heartburn has been produced by inflation of a balloon introduced into the lower oesophagus in normal subjects. Furthermore, x-ray studies have shown that, during an attack of heartburn, the lower oesophagus is often in spasm. This suggests that the cause of heartburn is not acid reflux primarily, but a prolonged spastic contraction of muscle comparable to that causing the pain of intestinal colic. In patients with some inflammation of the oesophageal mucosa with its attendant lowering of the pain threshold, gastric reflux may well cause heartburn. In cases with heartburn and gastric reflux, oesophagoscopy often reveals an oesophagitis. The acid irritant in these cases may nevertheless be producing this burning sensation by exciting a local muscle spasm. The distribution of pain produced in patients by acid perfusion of the oesophagus is shown in *Figure 9.20*.

Sensory receptors in the pharynx and oesophagus also subserve reflexes. The afferent limbs of these reflex arcs are mediated along fibres passing in the ninth and tenth cranial nerves. These reflexes include swallowing, gagging, retching, vomiting and salivation.

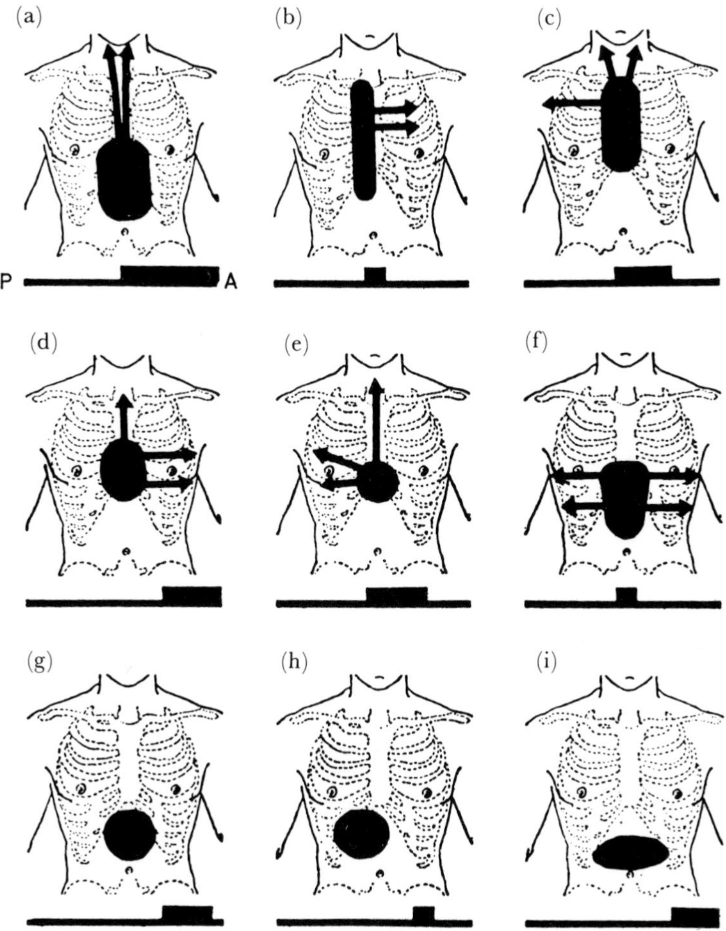

Figure 9.20 Areas of distribution of pain produced by acid perfusion of the oesophagus. Black areas = main area of pain; arrows = direction of pain radiation. The black rectangle on the line P–A indicates the approximate antero-posterior localization of the pain

Manometry in oesophageal disorders

Recording of oesophageal motility by manometry has now been developed into a useful method in the full clinical investigation of disorders of oesophageal musculature. This has proved particularly useful in the diagnosis of achalasia, diffuse spasm, scleroderma and oesophagitis. In these conditions characteristic patterns of pressure-change profiles have been described (*Figure 9.21*) (Creamer, Harrison and Pierce, 1959; Olsen and Schlegel, 1965).

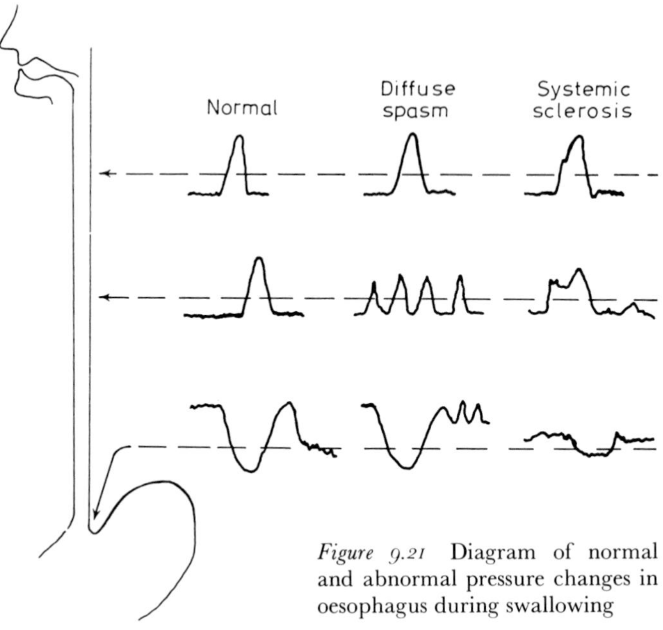

Figure 9.21 Diagram of normal and abnormal pressure changes in oesophagus during swallowing

Achalasia of the oesophagogastric junction

This condition is usually due to degeneration of the ganglion cells of Auerbach's plexus at this region. The oesophagus is dilated and its muscle hypotonic. Radiological studies show that in swallowing, the oesophageal peristalsis is weak or absent. Feeble non-propagated contractions occur simultaneously in different parts of the oesophagus. Manometric investigations reveal that with very few exceptions the resting tone is not raised. However, the complete usual relaxation of tone in the high-pressure zone of the oesophagogastric junction during swallowing does not occur. Instead the upper and lower segments of the oesophagogastric sphincter respond differently. The lower half relaxes normally during deglutition, but the upper half fails to relax and manifests instead premature and repeated series of contractions.

Thus the disorder is a true achalasia or failure of relaxation and not a cardio-spasm or hypertonus of the musculature of the lower oesophagus. In addition to the absence of the normal initial relaxation there is a premature onset of contraction which would normally follow the arrival at the cardia of the oesophageal peristaltic wave.

Pressure records from transducers show that peristaltic waves are not present in the oesophagus. The high pressure oesophagogastric zone is only forced open when the pressure of the oesophageal contents exceeds the resistance of the normal tone of the 'sphincter'. Manometry is especially useful in the identification of early cases before oesophageal dilatation is present.

Diffuse spasm This disorder is associated with distinctive radiological appearances. With a barium swallow the lower oesophagus presents a segmented or serrated outline. When fully developed this has been termed the 'cork-screw oesophagus'.

A characteristic abnormal motility pattern is revealed by manometry: (1) the resting pressure at the oesophagogastric region is raised in the lower half; (2) in a high proportion of these cases the zone of higher pressure is supradiaphragmatic as there is an associated hiatus hernia; (3) the lower oesophageal peristalsis is abnormal. The normal peristaltic wave is replaced by repeated premature sustained high-pressure contractions.

Hiatus hernia In hiatus hernia the high pressure zone of the oesophagogastric junction is some distance from the point of respiratory reversal. The point of respiratory reversal is where the fluctuations of intra-oesophageal pressure with the inspiratory and expiratory phases of respiration change from those reflecting the changes in intrathoracic pressure to those characteristic of the variations of intra-abdominal pressure during the respiratory cycle. This point indicates the position where the oesophagus passes through the diaphragm.

Scleroderma In systemic sclerosis affecting the oesophagus, the muscle coat of this organ is progressively replaced by fibrous tissue. In the initial stages of this progressive fibrosis, oesophageal peristalsis is diminished in duration and power of contraction but the oesophagogastric sphincter is normal. In the late stages the sphincter is affected and fails to relax during swallowing. One characteristic feature of diffuse scleroderma is that the peristaltic waves of the upper third of the oesophagus are not affected.

References

Alvarez, W. C. (1940). *An Introduction to Gastroenterology*. New York; Hoeber

Anderson, D. J. (1953). *Journal of dental Research*, **32,** 785

Anderson, D. J. (1956). *Journal of dental Research*, **35,** 664, 671

Anderson, D. J. and Picton, D. C. G. (1957). *Journal of dental Research*, **36,** 21

Adran, G. M. and Kemp, F. H. (1951). *Proceedings of the Royal Society of Medicine*, **44,** 1038

Ardran, G. M. and Kemp, F. H. (1952). *British Journal of Radiology*, **25,** 406

Atkinson, M., Edwards, D. A. W., Honour, A. J. and Rowlands, E. N. (1957). *Lancet*, **2,** 918

Barclay, A. E. (1936). *The Digestive Tract*. London; Cambridge University Press

Blomquist, A. J., Benjamin, R. M. and Emmers, R. E. (1962). *Journal of comparative Neurology*, **118,** 83

Bosma, J. F. (1957). *Physiology Review*, **37,** 25

Botha, G. S. M. (1958). *British Journal of Surgery*, **45,** 569

Bruce, J. and Smith, A. N. (1962). *Surgical Physiology of Gastro-intestinal Tract* (Symposium)

Burgen, A. S. V. (1956). *Journal of Physiology*, **132,** 20

Burgen, A. S. V. and Seeman, P. (1957). *Canadian Journal of Biochemical Physiology*, **35,** 481

Burgen, A. S. V. and Emmelin, N. G. (1961). *Physiology of the Salivary Glands*. London; Edward Arnold

Burgen, A. S. V., Terroux, K. G. and Gonder, E. (1959). *Canadian Journal of Biochemical Physiology*, **37,** 359

Code, C. F. and Schegel, J. F. (1968). *Handbook of Physiology*. Vol. IV, p. 1828. Baltimore; Williams and Wilkins

Code, C. F., Creamer, B., Schegel, J. F., Olsen, A. M., Donaghue, F. E. and Anderson, H. A. (1958). *Atlas of Oesophageal Motility*. Springfield, Ill.; Thomas

Coons, A. H., Leduc, E. H. and Connolly, J. M. (1955). *Journal of experimental Medicine*, **102,** 61

Cooper, S. (1953). *Journal of Physiology*, **122,** 193

Creamer, B., Olsen, A. M. and Code, C. F. (1957). *Gastroenterology*, **33,** 293

Creamer, B., Donoghue, F. E. and Code, C. F. (1958). *Gastroenterology*, **34,** 782

Creamer, B., Harrison, G. K. and Pierce, J. W. (1959). *Thorax*, **14,** 132

Davenport, H. W. (1961). *Physiology of the Digestive Tract*. Chicago; Year Book Medical Publishers

Dornhorst, A. C., Harrison, K. and Pierce, J. W. (1954). *Lancet*, **1,** 695

Doty, R. W. and Bosma, J. F. (1956). *Journal of Neurophysiology*, **19,** 44

Dougherty, T. F., Chase, J. H. and White, A. (1944). *Proceedings of the Society of experimental and biological Medicine,* **67,** 295

Edwards, D. A. W. (1961). *British Journal of Radiology,* **34,** 474

Edwards, D. A. W. (1967). *American Journal of digestive Diseases,* **12,** 267

Ellis, F. G. (1962). *Annals of the Royal College of Surgeons of England,* **30,** 155

Elsberg, C. A. (1955). In *Medical Physics.* Ed. by O. Glasser. New York; Lloyd-Luke

Elsberg, C. A., Spotnitz, H. and Strongin, E. I. (1942). *Archives of Neurology and Psychiatry,* **47,** 707

Emmelin, N. G. (1953). *Acta physiologica scandinavica,* **30** (Suppl. 3) 34

Emmelin, N. G. (1967). *Handbook of Physiology.* Vol. 11, p. 595. Baltimore; Williams and Wilkins

Erickson, R. P. (1963). In *Olfaction and Taste.* Ed. by Y. Zotterman. New York; Macmillan

Ericsson, Y. (1959). *Acta odontologica scandinavica,* **17,** 131

Faaborg-Anderson, K. (1957). *Acta physiologica scandinavica,* **41** (Suppl.) 140

Fagreus, A. (1958). *Acta haematologica,* **20,** 1

Farrell, J. H. (1956). *British dental Journal,* **100,** 149

Fritz, M. E. and Botelho, S. Y. (1969). *American Journal of Physiology,* **216,** 1392

Fyke, F. E. Jnr. and Code, C. F. (1955). *Gastroenterology,* **29,** 24

Gowans, J. L. (1959). *Journal of Physiology,* **146,** 54

Greenfield, B. E. and Wyke, B. D. (1956). *British dental Journal,* **100,** 129

Hilton, S. M. and Lewis, G. P. (1955a). *Journal of Physiology,* **128,** 235

Hilton, S. M. and Lewis, G. P. (1955b). *Journal of Physiology,* **129,** 253

Hurst, A. F. (1934). *Journal of the American medical Association,* **102,** 582

Hurst, A. F. (1942). *Proceedings of the Royal Society of Medicine,* **36,** 93

Ingelfinger, F. J. (1958). *Physiology Review,* **38,** 533

Johnstone, A. S. (1942). *Journal of Anatomy, London,* **77,** 97

Jones, C. M. (1938). *Digestive Tract Pain.* London; Macmillan

Kawamura, Y. (1961). *Journal of the American dental Association,* **62,** 545

Kawamura, Y. (1964). *Advances in oral Biology,* **1,** 77

Kerr, A. C. (1961). *Salivary Secretion in Man.* London; Pergamon

Kimura, K. and Beidler, L. M. (1961). *Journal of comparative Physiology,* **58,** 131

Kydd, W. L. and Toda, J. M. (1962). *Journal of the American dental Association,* **65,** 319

Kydd, W. L. and Neff, C. W. (1964). *Journal of dental Research,* **43,** 363

Lashley, K. S. (1916). *Journal of experimental Psychology,* **1,** 461

Lundberg, A. (1957). *Acta physiologica scandinavica,* **40,** 21

Lundberg, A. (1958). *Physiology Reviews,* **38,** 21

Malcomson, K. G. (1968). *Journal of Laryngology and Otology,* **82,** 219

Marchand, P. (1955). *British Journal of Surgery,* **42,** 405

Martinez, J. R., Holzgreve, H. and Frick, A. (1966). *Archiv gesamte Physiologie,* **290,** 124

Meltzer, S. J. (1899). *American Journal of Physiology,* **2,** 266

Mosher, H. P. (1927). *Laryngoscope,* **37,** 235

Mosher, H. P. (1930). *Journal of Laryngology,* **45,** 161

Murray, R. G., Murray, A. and Fujimoto, S. (1969). *Journal of Ultrastructural Research,* **27,** 444

Negus, V. E. (1929). *The Mechanisms of the Larynx.* London; Heinemann

Negus, V. E. (1942). *Proceedings of the Royal Society of Medicine,* **36,** 85

Oakley, C. L., Warrack, G. H. and Batty, J. (1954). *Journal of Pathology and Bacteriology,* **67,** 485

Ottesen, J. (1954). *Acta physiologica scandinavica,* **32,** 75

Patton, H. D. and Amassian, V. E. (1952). *Journal of Neurophysiology,* **15,** 245

Patton, H. D., Ruch, T. C. and Walker, A. E. (1944). *Journal of comparative Physiology,* **7,** 171

Pfaffman, C. (1963). In *Olfaction and Taste.* Ed. by Y. Zotterman. New York; Macmillan

Pommerenke, W. J. (1928). *American Journal of Physiology,* **84,** 36

Schlegel, J. F. and Code, C. F. (1958). *American Journal of Physiology,* **193,** 9

Schneyer, L. H. (1955). *Journal of dental Research,* **34,** 257

Schneyer, L. H. and Levin, L. K. (1955). *Applied Physiology,* **7,** 609

Schneyer L. H. and Schneyer, C. A. (Eds.) (1967). *Secretory Mechanisms of Salivary Glands.* New York; Academic Press

Scott, B. L. and Pease, D. C. (1959). *American Journal of Anatomy,* **104,** 115

Scott, B. L. and Pease, D. C. (1964). In *Salivary Glands and their Secretions.* Ed. by L. M. Screebny and J. Meyer. London; Pergamon.

Screebny, L. M. and Meyer, J. (Eds.) (1964). *Salivary Glands and their Secretions.* London; Pergamon

Sherrington, C. S. (1916). *Quarterly Journal of experimental Physiology,* **9,** 147

Sherrington, C. S. (1917). *Journal of Physiology,* **51,** 420

Spanner, R. (1937). *Zeitschrift fur Anatomie und Entwicklungsgechichte,* **107,** 124

Tateda, H. and Beidler, L. M. (1964). *Journal of general Physiology,* **47,** 479

Thaysen, J. H., Thorn, N. A. and Schwartz, I. L. (1954). *American Journal of Physiology,* **178,** 155

Wang, S. C. (1943). *Journal of Neurophysiology*, **6**, 195

Whillis, J. (1946). *Journal of Anatomy, London*, **80**, 115

Winders, R. V. (1958). *Angle Orthodontist*, **28,** 226

Wright, A. J. (1950). *Journal of Laryngology and Otology*, **64,** 1

Yoffey, J. M. and Courtice, F. C. (1956). *Lymphatics, Lymph and Lymphoid Tissue.* London; Edward Arnold

Yoffey, J. M. and Hanks, G. A. (1958). *Annals of the New York Academy of Sciences*, **73,** 47

Young, J. A., Fromter, E., Schogel, E. and Hamann, K. F. (1967). In *Secretory Mechanisms of Salivary glands.* Ed. by L. H. Schneyer and C. A. Schneyer. New York; Academic Press

Zotterman, Y. (Ed.) (1963). *Olfaction and Taste.* New York; Macmillan

10 Anatomy of the larynx and tracheobronchial tree

P M Stell and B J Bickford

The larynx

Development

The larynx, trachea, bronchi and lungs arise from a midline ventral respiratory diverticulum of the foregut known as the laryngotracheal groove (a full description of the foregut is given in Chapter 8). The groove first appears, posterior to the hypobranchial eminence, in the 3-millimetre stage at 25–28 days. The portion of the foregut posterior to the diverticulum later becomes elongated and gives rise to the oesophagus. Two ridges, running longitudinally, appear on the inner and ventral surface of the oesophagus, their upper ends lying just below the diverticulum. The edges of the two ridges approach each other and eventually close, thus leaving a separated canal anterior to the oesophagus. The ridges gradually extend cranially, their edges fusing, until the opening to the diverticulum is closed off except for a small orifice just behind the hypobranchial eminence. This opening represents the primitive aditus to the larynx. The diverticulum is now in the form of a tube, which elongates rapidly and branches dichotomously at the caudal end to become bilobed. Each lobe later becomes a primary bronchus and gives rise to the rest of the bronchial tree and alveoli. Streeter (1942) has commented on the greater epithelial proliferation of the primitive respiratory system as compared with that which occurs in the oesophagus at this time, although the two are not only in proximity but also in communication. The greater activity of the respiratory system is not, in his opinion, related to an environmental stimulus.

The lower portion of the diverticulum above its bifurcation becomes the trachea and the upper part gives rise to the larynx. At first the opening to the laryngeal cavity is bounded above by the hypobranchial eminence and posteriorly by the fused upper extremities of the two longitudinal ridges in the ventral wall of the oesophagus. In the upper edge of the fused ridges two swellings appear, the arytenoid swellings, and a small cleft is present between them (*Figure 10.1*). The cleft usually remains occluded until the third month of intra-uterine life.

The epiglottis develops from the posterior part of the hypobranchial eminence and is connected to the arytenoid swelling by the aryepiglottic fold.

The laryngeal cartilages develop during the second month of fetal life. They appear in the branchial mesoderm where it surrounds the upper part of the respiratory diverticulum. The thyroid cartilage develops from the fourth arch cartilage and the fifth and sixth arch cartilages possibly form the other cartilages of the larynx and the rings of the trachea. The branchial nerves of the fourth and sixth arches, that is the superior laryngeal and the recurrent laryngeal nerves, supply the larynx. The nerve to the fifth arch does not persist in the adult. It must be noted, however, that on the left side the recurrent laryngeal nerve passes posterior to the ductus arteriosus, which is the sixth arch artery.

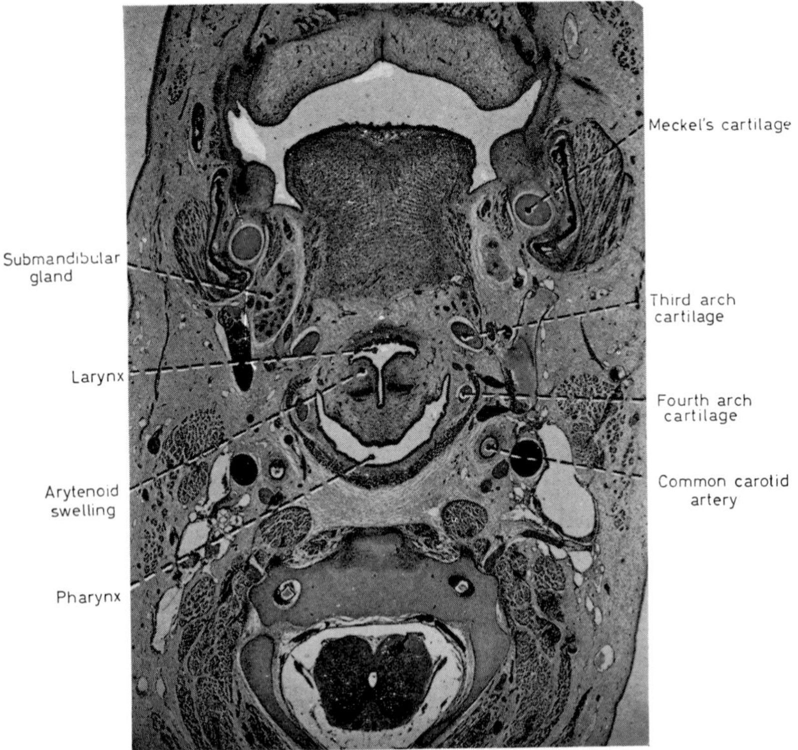

Figure 10.1 A photograph of a section through the laryngeal region of a 50 mm human embryo

In this connection it will be remembered that each branchial arch receives a branch from the nerve to that arch, this branch being the post-trematic nerve of the arch since it lies posterior to the gill-slit (*trema* = a slit). Further, each arch receives a branch from the nerve of the succeeding arch; this branch is pre-trematic since it passes above and in front of the gill-slit. The artery of each arch lies caudal to, or behind, the main post-trematic nerve of the arch. Therefore, since the recurrent laryngeal nerve is caudal to the sixth arch artery, the ductus arteriosus, it follows that the recurrent laryngeal nerve is probably not a nerve of an arch, but may be a post-branchial nerve.

Descriptive anatomy

The larynx is situated at the upper end of the trachea and, in adult men, lies opposite the third to sixth cervical vertebrae. It is somewhat higher in children and in women. It is composed of a number of articulated pieces of cartilage, inter-connected by ligaments, and moved by muscles. The larynx may be moved in relation to surrounding structures and also individual cartilages move one upon another; thus there are intrinsic and extrinsic muscles attached to the cartilages. In adult men the larynx is about 4.4 cm long, 4.3 cm across and 3.5 cm in its antero-posterior extent. In adult women it is altogether smaller, but more so in its length, 3.5 cm, and antero-posterior diameter, 2.5 cm, than in its breadth which is nearer that of men, 4.1 cm. These dimensions are average ones and may well be exceeded. There is little difference in the size of the larynx in boys and girls until after puberty when the increase in the antero-posterior diameter becomes apparent within a few years.

The cartilages

Thyroid cartilage

The largest cartilage is the thyroid, which consists of two main flattened quadrilateral pieces, the laminae, fused for most of their extent anteriorly in the midline, but diverging as they extend backwards (*Figure 10.2*). The subtended angle made by the two laminae is about 90 degrees in men and up to 120 degrees in women. In the male the fused anterior borders form a projection, which can be seen subcutaneously on the front of the neck as the laryngeal eminence or Adam's apple. The eminence is generally absent in women, due to the wider angle made by the laminae. A small narrow strip of cartilage, the intrathyroid cartilage, separates the two laminae anteriorly in childhood. The laminae are attached to it by strong connective tissue. The superior part of the cartilage is most prominent, and the two laminae separate above the eminence to form the thyroid notch, readily felt by the examining finger. The upper and lower posterior angles of the lamina continue respectively upwards and downwards as the superior and inferior horns. The superior horn passes upwards and backwards and ends in a rounded knob to which is attached the lateral thyrohyoid ligament. The short inferior horn is turned slightly medially and articulates on its inner aspect with the lateral surface. It is concave posteriorly, and to it is attached the lower border of each half of the thyrohyoid membrane. The lower border is slightly concave, but has the inferior thyroid tubercle projecting downwards in the middle. The conus elasticus is attached to the anterior part of each lower border. The posterior border of the lamina has a rounded edge and is directed slightly backwards.

The outer lateral surface of the thyroid lamina is marked by an oblique line, extending from the superior thyroid tubercle, which lies anterior to the superior horn on the lateral surface, to the inferior tubercle. This line marks the attachments of the thyrohyoid, sternothyroid and inferior constrictor muscles. The inner aspects of the laminae are mainly covered by loosely attached mucous membrane. At the junction of the laminae anteriorly and in the angle thus formed the thyro-epiglottic ligaments are attached. The vestibular and vocal ligaments, and the thyro-arytenoideus, thyro-epiglotticus and vocalis muscles are attached to the back of the laminae close to the

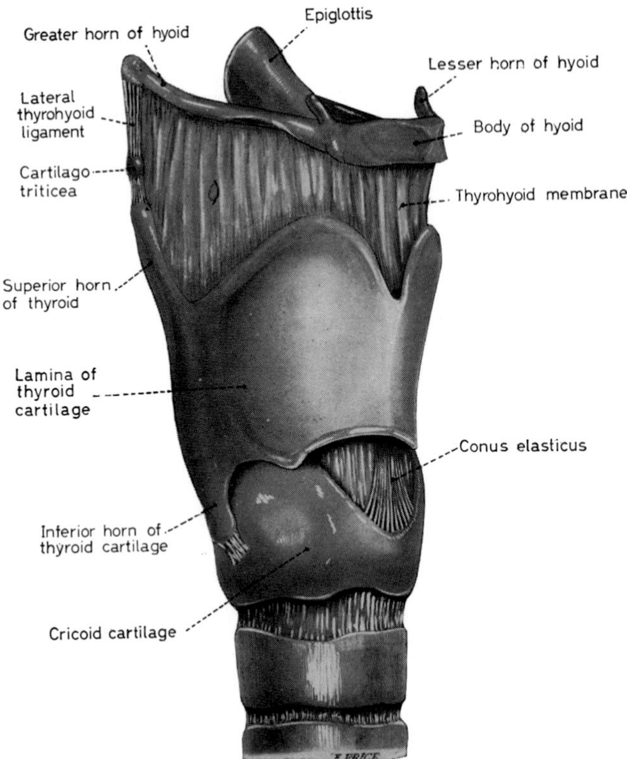

Figure 10.2 A drawing of the cartilages and ligaments of the larynx

origin of the thyro-epiglottic ligament (*Figure 10.4*). One of these is particularly important: the anterior commissure tendon which is formed by the fusion of the anterior ends of the two vocal ligaments (Broyles, 1943). This tendon is an important route of spread of carcinoma.

Cricoid cartilage

Immediately inferior to the thyroid cartilage, and articulating with it, is the smaller cricoid cartilage (*Figures 10.2* and *10.3*). The cartilage possesses a narrow anterior arch and a broad, almost quadrilateral posterior lamina. The cartilage forms the lower part of the larynx and its broad lamina contributes to the major part of the posterior wall of the larynx.

The arch is narrow, being about 6 mm in its vertical extent, but is wider at the sides where it is continuous with the lamina. The cricothyroid muscles are attached to the anterior and lateral aspects of each side of the arch, and the inferior constrictor of the pharynx arises slightly behind the attachment of the former muscles. At the site of the junction of the arch with the lamina, on each side and slightly nearer the inferior margin than the superior, is the circular facet for articulation with the inferior horn of the thyroid cartilage. At the upper extent of the junction of the arch with the lamina is a second facet, oval and convex, for articulation with the arytenoid cartilage.

The inferior margin of the cartilage is placed almost horizontally in the erect position of the body. The upper ring of the trachea is connected to it by the cricotracheal ligament. The superior margin of the cartilage is directed anterosuperiorly in the erect posture owing to the greater vertical extent of the lamina (25 mm) over that of the arch. Anteriorly, the conus elasticus is attached to the superior border of the arch. On each side are attached the cricothyroid ligament (cricovocal membrane) and the lateral crico-arytenoid muscle.

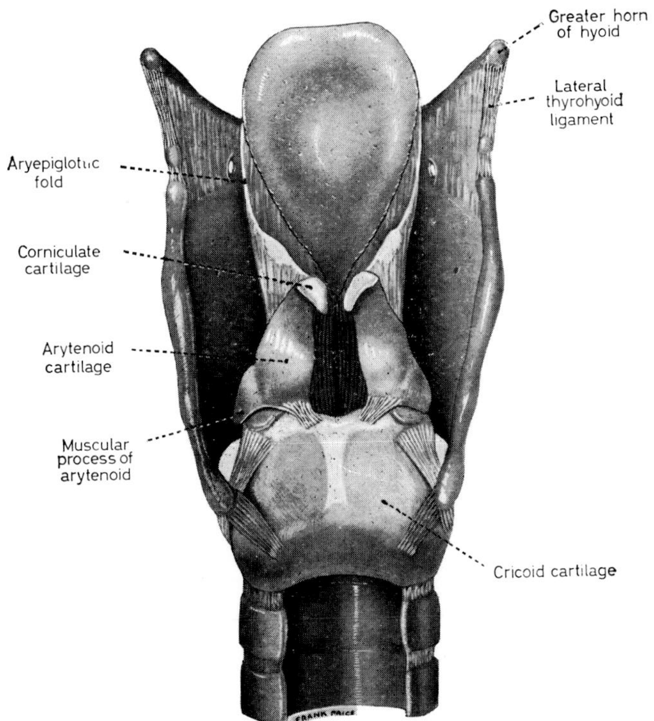

Figure 10.3 A drawing of the cartilages and ligaments of the larynx seen from behind

The lamina is broader at its base and its sides curve gently medially to the narrower, slightly concave superior border. There is a median vertical ridge passing down the back of the lamina to the upper half of which are attached some longitudinal fibres of the oesophagus, the so-called tendon of the oesophagus. On each side of the ridge the posterior crico-arytenoid muscle arises. The entire interior surface of the cricoid cartilage is lined with mucous membrane.

The joints between the thyroid cartilage and the cricoid cartilage are synovial with a capsular ligament strengthened by some fibrous bands. A rotation of the cricoid cartilage on the thyroid cartilage can occur about an axis passing transversely through the joints. A small degree of gliding movement can occur in various directions.

Arytenoid and smaller cartilages

The two arytenoid cartilages are placed close together on the upper and lateral borders of the cricoid cartilage (*Figure 10.3*). Each is an irregular three-sided pyramid in shape, the base articulating with the cricoid cartilage. The apex is curved backwards and medially and is flattened for articulation with the corniculate cartilage. The medial surfaces are smooth, are covered with mucous membrane and the fold passing between the two cartilages forms the posterior boundary of the rima glottidis. The smooth posterior surface is entirely covered by the transverse arytenoid muscle. The anterolateral surface is irregular and is divided below into two fossae by a crest which runs downwards from the apex with a curve to the vocal process (*Figure 10.4*). The upper triangular fossa marks the attachment of the vestibular ligament, and into the lower oblong fossa are attached the vocalis and lateral crico-arytenoid muscles.

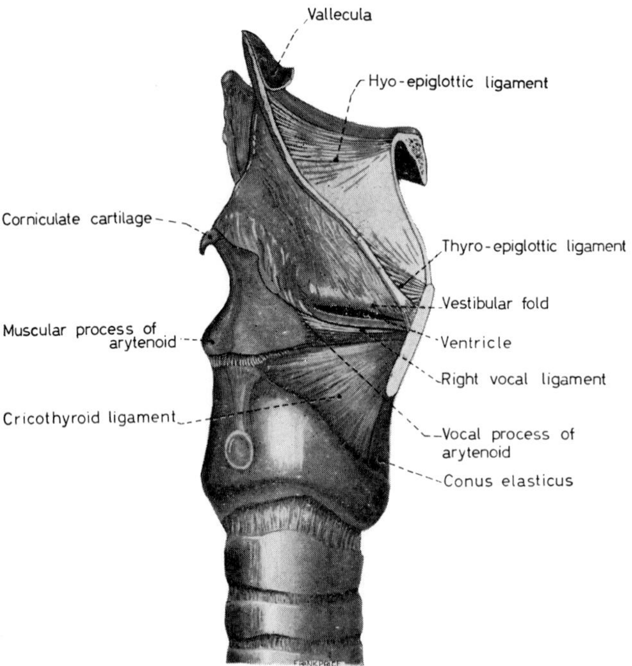

Figure 10.4 A drawing of the lateral aspect of the larynx; the right-hand side has been dissected to show the right arytenoid cartilage and the right vocal ligament

The lateral angle is prolonged posteriorly and laterally to form the muscular process which gives attachment to the posterior crico-arytenoid muscle behind, and in front to the lateral crico-arytenoid muscle. The anterior angle is prolonged forwards to form the vocal process, to which the vocal ligaments are attached.

Each arytenoid cartilage articulates with the cricoid cartilage by means of a synovial joint, which is strengthened by capsular ligaments and by the firm posterior crico-arytenoid ligament; the latter prevents forward movement of the arytenoid cartilage. This cartilage can rotate on the cricoid cartilage round an axis passing not quite vertically through the arytenoid (Frable, 1961). It may also glide laterally and downwards following the slope of the cricoid facet, or medially towards the other arytenoid cartilage. The two movements usually occur together, thus medial rotation about the vertical axis occurs together with a gliding movement in a medial direction (von Leden and Moore, 1961).

A small nodular corniculate cartilage, composed of elastic cartilage, articulates with each flattened medially directed apex of the arytenoid cartilages. A synovial joint may be present, or the two cartilages may be fused. A small elongated cuneiform cartilage is placed slightly in front of each corniculate cartilage. Both corniculate and cuneiform cartilages are enclosed within the mucous membrane of the aryepiglottic folds to form two swellings on each side of the posterior part of the rima glottidis. A Y-shaped ligament extends from the apices of the two corniculate cartilages down to the cricoid cartilage and reinforces the restraining action of the posterior crico-arytenoid ligaments. The capsules of the laryngeal joints contain abundant free nerve endings and lamellated corpuscles: these sensory endings are probably involved in the essential muscle co-ordination required during phonation (Kirchner and Wyke, 1965).

Epiglottis

The epiglottis is a flattened leaf-like sheet of elastic fibrocartilage projecting upwards behind the tongue and hyoid bone (*Figure 10.3*). The narrow lower part is attached by the thyro-epiglottic ligament to the angle between the thyroid laminae, below the thyroid notch. The upper broad part is directed upwards and backwards; its superior margin is free. The posterior surface of the epiglottis is concave and smooth but a small central projection, the epiglottic tubercle, is present in its lower part. Mucous membrane passes from the tongue on to the anterior surface of the epiglottis. The mucous membrane in the midline is raised to form the median glosso-epiglottic fold, and on each side two further folds, the lateral glosso-epiglottic folds, pass to the pharyngeal wall. The depression thus formed on each side of the median glosso-epiglottic fold is the vallecula. An elastic ligament, the hyo-epiglottic ligament, connects the epiglottis to the hyoid bone in front. From each side of the epiglottis the mucous membrane is continued as a fold passing down towards the arytenoid cartilages. This is the aryepiglottic fold, which together with its fellow and the free edge of the epiglottis forms the anterior boundary to the inlet of the larynx. A number of mucous glands are present in the mucous membrane of the posterior surface. The epiglottis is not functionally developed in man in that respiration, deglutition and phonation can take place almost normally even if it has been destroyed.

Calcification of the laryngeal cartilages

Calcification of the thyroid cartilage begins in the region of the inferior cornu in the late 'teens'. It then proceeds anteriorly and superiorly until the entire rim is calcified. A central radiolucent 'window', sometimes divided by a vertical bar, persists into old age (*Figure 10.5*).

Calcification of the cricoid cartilage begins in the superior border of the lamina, in the late teens and proceeds anteriorly. Calcification of the posterior part of the lamina may be confused at radiography with a foreign body (*Figures 10.6* and *10.7*).

Calcification of the apex, body and muscular process of the arytenoid begins later, but the vocal process does not ossify (Hately, Evison and Samuel, 1965).

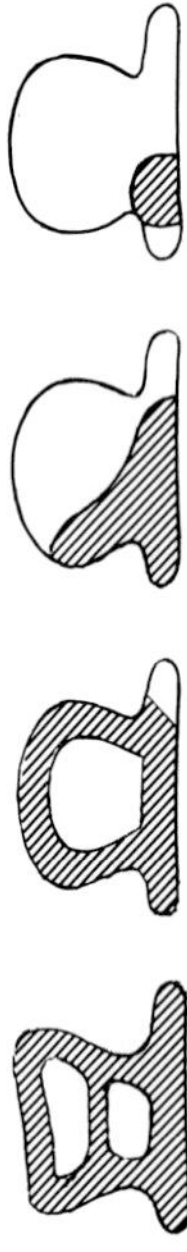

Figure 10.5 Stages in ossification of the thyroid cartilage

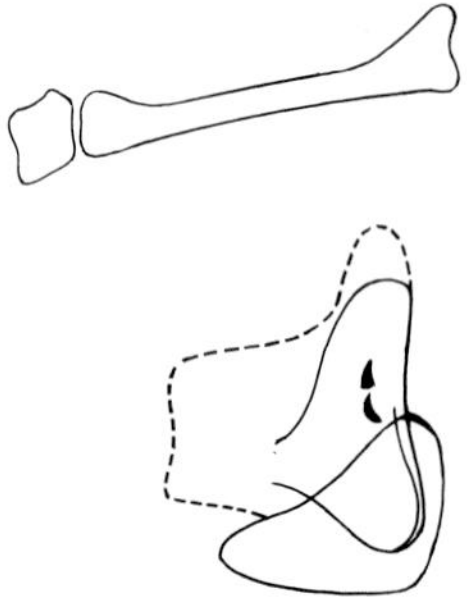

Figure 10.6 Ossification in tip of cricoid which may mimic a foreign body

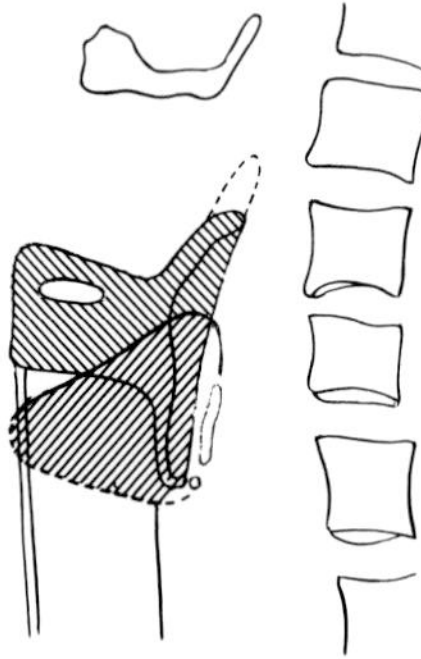

Figure 10.7 Ossification in posterior lamina of cricoid which may mimic a foreign body

The ligaments

Extrinsic ligaments connect the cartilages to the hyoid and trachea, and intrinsic ligaments connect the cartilages themselves. The lateral thyrohyoid ligaments connect the tips of the superior horns of the thyroid cartilage to the posterior ends of the greater horns of the hyoid and each often contains a small nodule, the cartilago triticea. The cricotracheal ligament has already been described. The thyrohyoid membrane stretches from the upper border of the body of the thyroid cartilage and the anterior borders of the superior horns to the 'upper' border of the posterior surface of the body and greater horns of the hyoid bone. The membrane is composed of fibro-elastic tissue and is in the form of a broad curved sheet. A bursa is often found on the posterior surface of the body of the hyoid bone, between it and the upper part of the thyrohyoid membrane. The central part of the membrane is condensed to form the median thyrohyoid ligament and is pierced on each side by the internal laryngeal nerve and the superior laryngeal artery. Anterior to the membrane lie the thyrohyoid and the omohyoid and sternohyoid muscles; posteriorly, loose connective tissue separates the membrane from the epiglottis.

The intrinsic ligaments and membranes of the larynx consist of those ligaments that strengthen the capsules of the intercartilaginous joints and the parts of the fibro-elastic membrane of the larynx (*Figure 10.4*). The latter is a broad sheet of fibro-elastic tissue lying beneath the mucous membrane, divided into an upper and lower part by the laryngeal ventricle. The upper quadrangular membrane extends between the border of the epiglottis and the arytenoid cartilage. It is poorly developed and extends downwards to the vestibular fold, in which a thickening of fibrous tissue forms the vestibular ligament. The lower part of the membrane is well developed and forms the cricothyroid ligament (cricovocal membrane). The anterior middle part is thick and forms the strong conus elasticus, which stretches from the lower border of the thyroid cartilage to the upper border of the cricoid cartilage. The lateral parts of the membrane extend upwards on each side from the upper border of the cricoid cartilage to be attached in front to the inner surface of the thyroid angle and behind to the tip of the vocal process of the arytenoid cartilage. The superior edge of this lateral part of the cricothyroid ligament is free and thickened to form the vocal ligament.

The muscles

The muscles of the larynx may be divided into extrinsic, which attach the larynx to neighbouring structures, and intrinsic, which move the various cartilages of the larynx.

Extrinsic muscles

The extrinsic muscles are the sternothyroid, thyrohyoid, the stylopharyngeus, palatopharyngeus (pharyngopalatinus) and the inferior constrictor. The sternothyroid muscle arises from the posterior surface of the manubrium of the sternum and the edge of the first and occasionally the second costal cartilage. It is inserted into the oblique line on the anterior lateral surface of the thyroid lamina. It is supplied by the ansa cervicalis (C.2), and its action is to draw the larynx downwards. The thyrohyoid muscle arises from the oblique line of the thyroid lamina and is inserted into the lower border of the greater horn of the hyoid bone. It is supplied by the hypoglossal nerve, although the fibres innervating it are derived from the first cervical nerve. The muscle raises the larynx, if the hyoid is fixed, or depresses the hyoid if the larynx is fixed. The stylopharyngeus muscle arises from the inner surface of the base of the styloid process of the temporal bone. It passes between the superior and middle constrictors of the pharynx and spreads out beneath the mucous membrane. Many of its fibres blend with the inferior constrictor and the palatopharyngeus or are lost in the pharyngo-epiglottic fold. Some fibres are, however, inserted into the posterior border of the thyroid cartilage. The stylopharyngeus muscle is supplied by the glossopharyngeal nerve, and although the main action is to raise the lateral wall of the pharynx, it also raises the larynx. The detailed origins of the palatopharyngeus are described in the section on the pharynx; this muscle is inserted close to the stylopharyngeus into the posterior border of the thyroid cartilage. It is supplied by the accessory nerve through the pharyngeal plexus. The main action of the muscle is to raise and then shorten the wall of the pharynx. At the same time, however, it probably helps in tilting the larynx forward, thus enabling food to pass straight into the oesophagus during the act of swallowing. The inferior constrictor muscle can be divided into two parts. The cricopharyngeus arises from the cricoid cartilage on the lateral surface of the arch between the origin of the cricothyroid in front and the articular facet for the inferior horn of the thyroid cartilage behind. The thyropharyngeus arises from the oblique line on the thyroid lamina, from a tendinous band crossing over the cricothyroid muscle and stretching to the cricoid cartilage, and from the inferior horn of the thyroid cartilage. The fibres pass backwards and are inserted into the median fibrous raphe at the back of the pharynx. The cricopharyngeus acts as a sphincter during swallowing movements (Fuller, Fozzard and Wright, 1959) of the pharynx and the thyropharyngeus provides a propulsive thrust. The inferior constrictor muscle does not move the larynx. It is supplied by the pharyngeal plexus from fibres of the cranial root of the accessory nerve, which enter the vagus nerve and are distributed to the plexus by the pharyngeal branch of the vagus nerve. The inferior constrictor is also supplied by fibres from the external branch of the superior laryngeal nerve and from the recurrent laryngeal nerve.

Other movements of the larynx are brought about by virtue of the ligamentous and muscular connections of the larynx to the hyoid bone. Thus muscles which raise the hyoid, such as the mylohyoid, geniohyoid and stylohyoid, will raise the larynx, and the sternohyoid and omohyoid will depress it. For an account of the effects of the extrinsic laryngeal muscles on voice production the reader is referred to an article by Sokolowsky (1943).

Intrinsic muscles

The intrinsic muscles of the larynx may be divided into those that open and close the glottis, namely the lateral and posterior crico-arytenoids and the transverse and oblique arytenoids; those that control the tension of the vocal ligaments, the thyro-arytenoids, the vocales and the cricothyroids; and those that alter the shape of the inlet of the larynx, the aryepiglotticus and the thyro-epiglotticus. All these muscles are paired, with the exception of the transverse arytenoid. Neuromuscular spindles and other types of nerve ending are found in all human laryngeal muscles (Keene, 1961).

The lateral crico-arytenoid muscle arises from the upper border of the lateral part of the arch of the cricoid cartilage and is inserted into the anterior surface of the muscular surface of the arytenoid cartilage (*Figure 10.8*). The posterior crico-arytenoid muscle arises from the lower and medial surface of the back of the cricoid

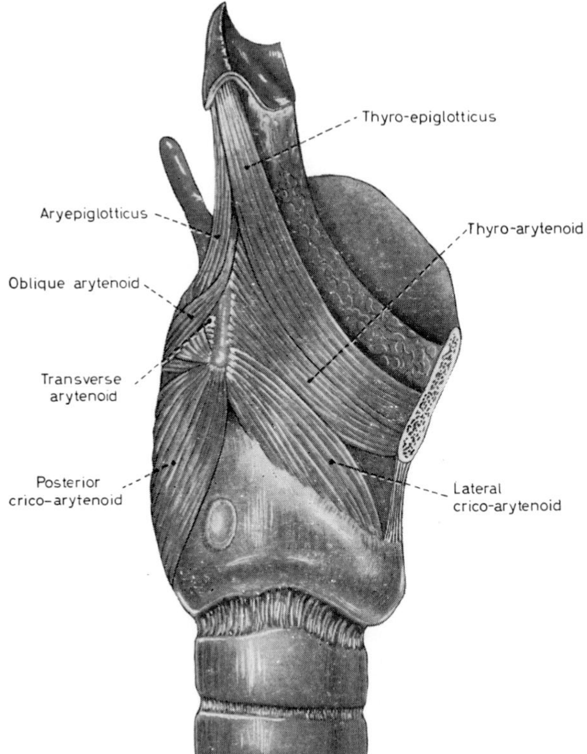

Figure 10.8 A drawing of a dissection of the larynx to show the muscles on the right-hand side

lamina and is inserted into the back of the muscular process of the arytenoid cartilage of the same side (*Figure 10.9*). The muscle is broad at its origin and thus the upper, middle and lower fibres converge as they pass to the insertion, the lower fibres passing almost vertically. The lateral and posterior crico-arytenoid muscles act in opposition to each other: the lateral crico-arytenoid muscles approximate (adduct) the vocal ligaments by rotating the arytenoid cartilages medially; the posterior crico-arytenoid muscles rotate the cartilages laterally and thus abduct the vocal processes. Negus (1947, 1950) further investigated the action of the posterior crico-arytenoid muscle. He found that the lateral fibres of the muscle are attached to the body of the arytenoid cartilage and that on contraction they slide the arytenoid cartilages laterally and thus separate the two cartilages. They also brace the arytenoid cartilages during phonation. The weight of the abductor muscles of the larynx is less than 25 per cent of that of the adductors (Withington, 1960), which may explain the greater vulnerability of the abductors in partial injury to the recurrent laryngeal nerve (Semon's law).

Each oblique arytenoid muscle passes from the posterior aspect of the muscular process of one arytenoid cartilage to the apex of the other. The two muscles thus cross each other. The transverse arytenoid muscle, the only unpaired intrinsic muscle, lies deep to the oblique pair, arises from the posterior surface of the muscular process and outer edge of one arytenoid cartilage and passes to similar attachments on the other cartilage. The action of both muscles is to approximate the arytenoid cartilages and thus close the intercartilaginous part of the rima glottidis.

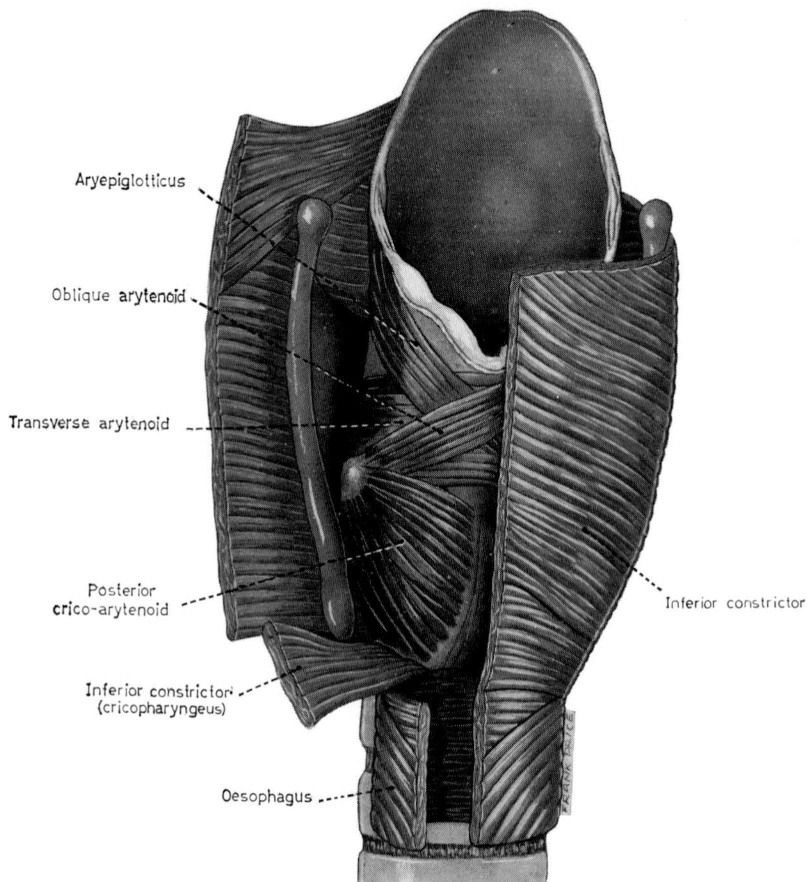

Figure 10.9 A drawing of a dissection of the larynx to show the muscles from the back

The thyro-arytenoids arise from the back of the inferior part of the angle made by the thyroid laminae and from the cricothyroid ligament below this. The muscles are inserted into the anterolateral surface of each arytenoid cartilage. Each muscle passes lateral to the vocal ligaments and cricovocal membrane, and is in the form of a broad sheet. The lower part of the muscle is thicker and forms a distinct bundle called the vocalis muscle. Each vocalis muscle is attached posteriorly to the vocal process of the arytenoid cartilage and to the lateral surface of the body of the cartilage. Many of the fibres arise from the vocal ligament and thus the muscle is more pronounced posteriorly. Occasionally a small slip of muscle, the superior thyro-arytenoid, extends from the superior and upper aspects of the back of the thyroid lamina and passes down to the arytenoid cartilage. The muscle fibres of the thyro-arytenoid muscle vary greatly in size and structure; some resemble Purkinje fibres (Konig and von Leden, 1961). Numerous sensory endings are present in the muscle. Sonesson (1960) states that no fibres of the vocalis muscle are inserted into the vocal ligament. He has also studied vibratory patterns of the vocal folds by photo-electric methods. The parts of the vocalis muscle that directly adjoin the vocal cord have a better capillary circulation than the rest of the muscle and may have a special function (Ganz, 1962).

The cricothyroid is a fan-shaped sheet of muscle that arises from the lateral surface of the anterior arch of the cricoid cartilage. The fibres spread out and pass backwards in two main groups. The straight part ascends to the posterior part of the lower border of the thyroid lamina, whereas the oblique part passes backwards and laterally to the anterior surface of the inferior horn of the thyroid cartilage. The cricothyroid acts in opposition to the thyro-arytenoid and the vocales muscles. The cricothyroid muscle rotates the cricoid cartilage about the horizontal axis passing through the joints between the inferior horns of the thyroid and the cricoid cartilages. Negus (1947), however, believed that during phonation the cricoid cartilage is held immovably against the front of the vertebral column by the cricopharyngeal sphincter, and that the thyroid cartilage moves on the stationary cricoid cartilage. In swallowing, the cricoid does move on the thyroid cartilage. Thus contraction of the muscle results in elevation of the anterior arch and backward rotation of the superior border of the lamina. In this way the arytenoid cartilage is also carried backwards and the vocal ligaments are tightened and elongated; at the same time the cricovocal membrane becomes slack in its anterior part. The thyro-arytenoid muscles cause the approximation of the arytenoid cartilages to the thyroid angle and thus slacken the vocal ligaments; the cricovocal membrane, however, becomes taut during this movement. The vocalis muscle, by virtue of its origin from the vocal ligament, can tighten the anterior part of the ligament, and at the same time can release the posterior part when it contracts. Both the thyro-arytenoid muscles and the vocales muscles rotate the vocal process of the arytenoid cartilages medially about their vertical axes, adducting the vocal ligaments and thus opposing the action of the posterior crico-arytenoid muscles. The classification of the positions of the vocal cords has been the subject of much disagreement. Six positions are described (Clerf and Suehs, 1941; Negus, 1947) and *Figure 10.10* illustrates nomenclature and briefly indicates the function. The sixth

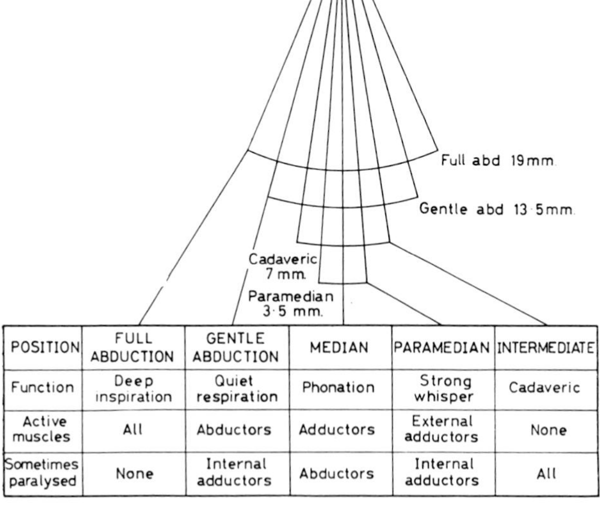

POSITION	FULL ABDUCTION	GENTLE ABDUCTION	MEDIAN	PARAMEDIAN	INTERMEDIATE
Function	Deep inspiration	Quiet respiration	Phonation	Strong whisper	Cadaveric
Active muscles	All	Abductors	Adductors	External adductors	None
Sometimes paralysed	None	Internal adductors	Abductors	Internal adductors	All

Figure 10.10 Diagram to illustrate positions assumed by the vocal cords in health and disease. In addition to the five illustrated, a sixth, the 'glottic chink', is assumed in some cases of double abductor paralysis. (Reproduced by courtesy of Sir Victor Negus)

position, the abductor or glottic chink, not shown in the diagram, is assumed in double abductor paralysis. Movements of the vocal folds during phonation have been investigated by high-speed cinematography.

The aryepiglotticus muscle is a continuation of the fibres of the oblique arytenoid muscle and passes round the apex of the arytenoid cartilage into the aryepiglottic fold. In the same way the fibres of the thyro-arytenoid muscles are continued above the vocal process and lateral border of the arytenoid cartilage into the aryepiglottic fold to form the thyro-epiglottic muscle. Many fibres reach as far as the lateral border of the epiglottis. The aryepiglottic and the oblique arytenoid muscles tend to narrow the inlet of the larynx by acting as a sphincter. Besides acting on the aryepiglottic fold they approximate the arytenoid cartilages and the tubercle of the epiglottis. The thyro-epiglottic muscles tend to widen the inlet of the larynx by pulling the aryepiglottic folds slightly apart.

All the intrinsic muscles of the larynx, except the cricothyroid, are supplied by the recurrent laryngeal nerves from the two vagi. The fibres arise from neurones localized in the lower part of the nucleus ambiguus (Negus, 1947). These nerves pass into the larynx from below, having passed posteriorly round the ligamentum arteriosum on the left and the first part of the subclavian artery on the right. They ascend to each side of the trachea and then lie in the groove between the trachea and the oesophagus, closely related to the medial surface of the thyroid gland. The nerve at this point may be enclosed within the pretracheal fascia and it may lie behind or in front of the inferior thyroid artery (Reed, 1943). In rare instances the recurrent laryngeal nerve comes off the vagus near the level of the cricoid cartilage and crosses almost at once to the larynx. It enters the larynx under the lower border of the inferior constrictor muscle immediately behind the articulation of the inferior horn of the thyroid cartilage with the cricoid cartilage. The cricothyroid muscle is supplied by the external branch of the superior laryngeal nerve from the vagus. The internal laryngeal branch is said to carry some motor fibres to the transverse arytenoid muscle, but this is denied by Negus (1947). All the muscles of the larynx contain neuromuscular spindles.

The interior of the larynx

The cavity of the larynx

When examined in the recent state with the mucous membrane *in situ*, the cavity of the larynx is seen to extend from the pharynx at the laryngeal inlet to the commencement of the lumen of the trachea at the lower border of the cricoid cartilage. The cavity of the larynx can be divided into a superior vestibule above the vestibular folds, a middle part, the ventricle or sinus of the larynx, between the vestibular and vocal folds, and a lower part extending from the vocal folds to the lower border of the cricoid cartilage (*Figure 10.11*). The fissure between the vestibular folds is called the rima vestibuli, that between the vocal folds is the rima glottidis.

The pharynx opens into the laryngeal cavity by the inlet of the larynx. The plane of the inlet is directed backwards and slightly upwards. The inlet is bounded superiorly by the free edge of the epiglottis and on each side by a fold of mucous membrane, the aryepiglottic fold, extending from the lateral edges of the epiglottis to the arytenoid cartilage. Posteriorly the inlet is completed by the mucous membrane that passes between the two arytenoid cartilages. In the posterior part of each aryepiglottic fold two swellings, separated by a narrow sulcus, are formed by the corniculate and cuneiform cartilages. The aryepiglottic folds contain within them the upper parts of the elastic lamina of the larynx and some muscular fibres. Mucous glands are present in considerable number in the margins of the aryepiglottic folds.

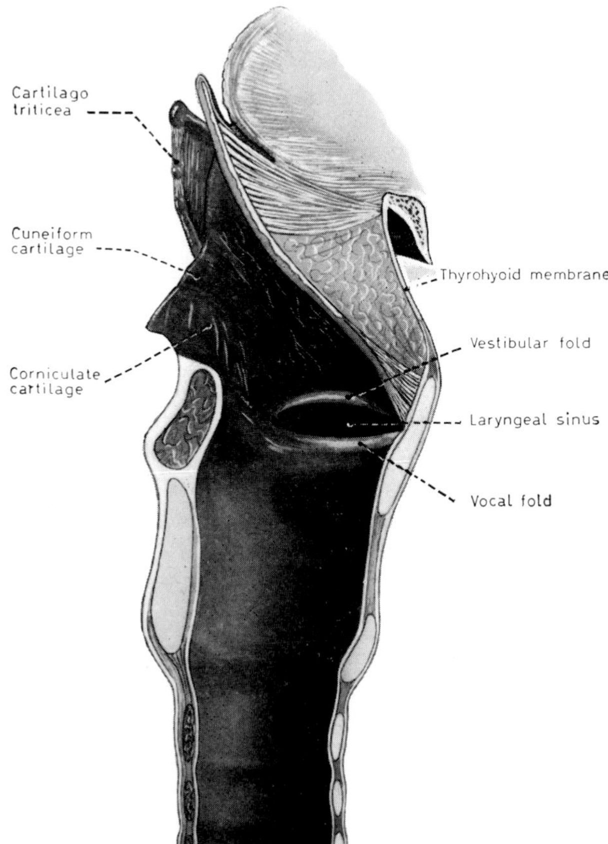

Figure 10.11 A drawing of a midline sagittal section of the larynx in the recent stage

The superior vestibule The vestibular part of the laryngeal cavity lies between the inlet of the larynx and the level of the vestibular folds. It narrows as it extends downwards and its anterior wall is much longer than the posterior wall since the former consists of the posterior surface of the epiglottis. The lower part of the epiglottis, the tubercle, projects backwards into the vestibule. The lateral wall of the vestibule is formed by the inner aspect of the aryepiglottic fold, and the posterior wall is formed by the mucous membrane covering the anterior surface of the arytenoid cartilages.

The middle part of the cavity (and the ventricle) The middle part of the cavity lies between the vestibular and vocal folds, which cover over the ligaments of those names. Between the two folds a narrow horizontal slit opens into the ventricle (sinus) of the larynx. The ventricle is an elongated recess which extends for a short distance above and lateral to the vestibular fold. From the anterior part of the ventricle a pouch, the saccule of the larynx, ascends between the vestibular folds and the inner surface of the thyroid cartilage. It may extend as far as the upper border of the cartilage, and in some monkeys and apes extends even further into the neck and as far as the axilla. The mucous membrane lining the saccule contains numerous mucous glands, lodged in the submucous tissue. Fibrous tissue surrounds the saccule and a limited number of muscle fibres pass from the apex of the arytenoid cartilage across the medial aspect of the saccule to the aryepiglottic fold. Presumably the function of the glandular mucous membrane of the saccule is to provide lubrication for the vocal folds; the muscular tissue may well aid in the expression of mucus from the saccule.

The lower part of the cavity The lower part of the laryngeal cavity extends from the level of the vocal folds to the lower border of the cricoid cartilage and is sometimes known as the infraglottic larynx. The vocal folds are formed by the sharp reflexion of the mucous membrane over the vocal ligaments. These latter are the free upper edges (internal part) of the cricovocal membrane and they extend from the angle of the thyroid cartilage anteriorly to the vocal process of the arytenoid cartilage posteriorly. The mucous membrane over the vocal ligaments is closely attached and the epithelium is of the stratified squamous type with no submucous layer. There is therefore a poor blood supply to the vocal folds, and their appearance in the living subject is of two shining white cords. The vocal ligament contains numbers of elastic fibres and is therefore capable of slight stretching, which causes the folds to be intimately concerned in the production of the voice sounds. Distinct changes are seen in the distribution of the elastic fibres in the vocal cords in elderly subjects (Mayet, 1962).

The rima glottidis

The elongated fissure between the vocal cords anteriorly and the vocal processes and bases of the arytenoid cartilages posteriorly is known as the rima glottidis. About three-fifths of its length is called the intermembranous part since it lies between the vocal cords, and the remainder is termed the intercartilaginous part. Posteriorly the rima glottidis is limited by the mucous membrane that stretches between the two arytenoid cartilages. The average length of the rima glottidis varies from 23 mm in men to 16 mm in women. In the resting state the anterior intermembranous part is triangular in shape, the base being posterior and extending from the tip of one vocal process of the arytenoid cartilage to the tip of the other. The posterior portion is, however, rectangular, due to the medial surfaces of the arytenoid cartilages being parallel. They are usually about 8 mm apart in the resting state. In adduction, the apposition of the vocal processes of the arytenoid cartilages, which are medially rotated, results in the intermembranous part being reduced to a narrow slit, whilst the intercartilaginous part becomes triangular since the arytenoid cartilages remain separated posteriorly. In abduction, the intermembranous part is triangular, but the intercartilaginous part becomes triangular with the apex directed backwards, due to the apposition of the posterior edges of the arytenoid cartilages. Thus in abduction the outline of the rima glottidis is lozenge-shaped.

Mucous membrane

The mucous membrane lining the larynx is continuous above with that of the pharynx and below with that of the trachea. It is loosely attached to the walls, except over the posterior surface of the epiglottis, over the corniculate and cuneiform cartilages, and over the vocal ligaments, where it is firmly adherent to the underlying structures.

The *epithelium* of the larynx is of three types:

(a) squamous;
(b) ciliated columnar;
(c) transitional (stratified ciliated epithelium).

The posterior surface of the epiglottis has a rim of squamous epithelium which occupies about one-third of the entire surface of the epiglottis. In the healthy adult the remaining part of the epiglottis is columnar ciliated in type, with small islands of squamous epithelium especially over the tubercle of the epiglottis. The false vocal cords are covered by columnar ciliated epithelium but patches of squamous epithelium are common even in the healthy non-smoking adult and occur in as many as half of the specimens examined.

The true vocal cords are covered by squamous epithelium which has a fusiform outline. Towards the anterior end of the vocal cords the inferior border of the cord slopes upwards (*Figure 10.12*) so that the vertical height of the vocal cord is least at this

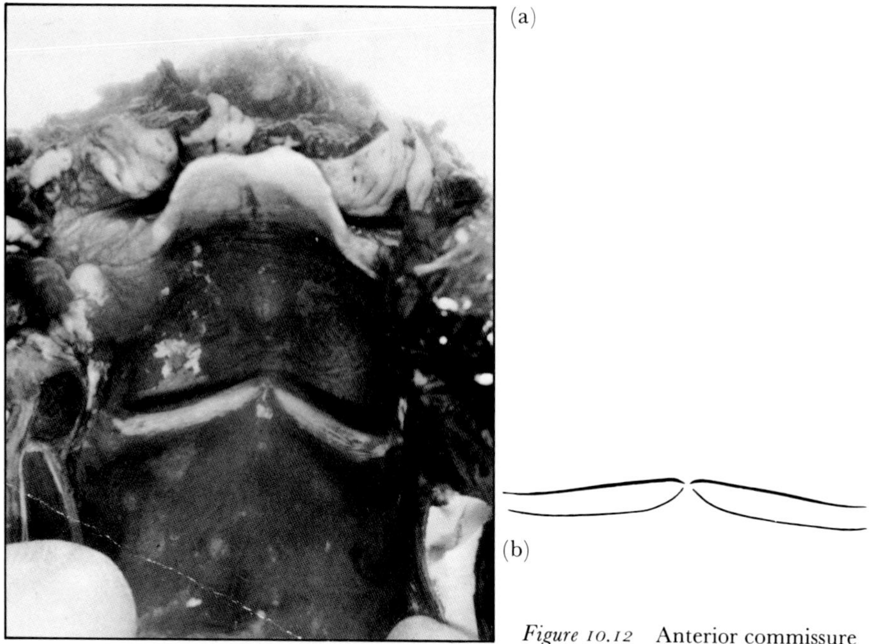

Figure 10.12 Anterior commissure

point. Indeed, in approximately 20 per cent of specimens the anterior ends of the vocal cords are separated by a narrow strip of non-squamous epithelium; this strip of epithelium may consist of transitional epithelium (Tucker *et al.*, 1976). Posteriorly, the band of epithelium widens out to its greatest vertical height at the centre of the vocal cords and then narrows again over the vocal processes; the individual heights in men and women are given in *Table 10.1*. The collar of squamous epithelium is then

Table 10.1 Mean heights of the vocal cord (mm)

	Anterior commissure	*Quarter way along the cord*	*Half way along the cord*	*Three quarters along the cord*	*Posterior end*
Men	4.8	5.0	5.5	5.3	5.0
Women	2.8	3.4	4.2	4.3	4.2

continued posteriorly over the posterior commissure where it forms a large saddle-shaped area of squamous epithelium which has a distinct inferior border in the normal larynx (*Figure 10.13*).

The subglottic space is normally lined entirely by columnar ciliated epithelium but islands of transitional or squamous epithelium are found in at least half of healthy non-smoking adults and their size and extent increases in those who smoke (Stell and Watt, 1977).

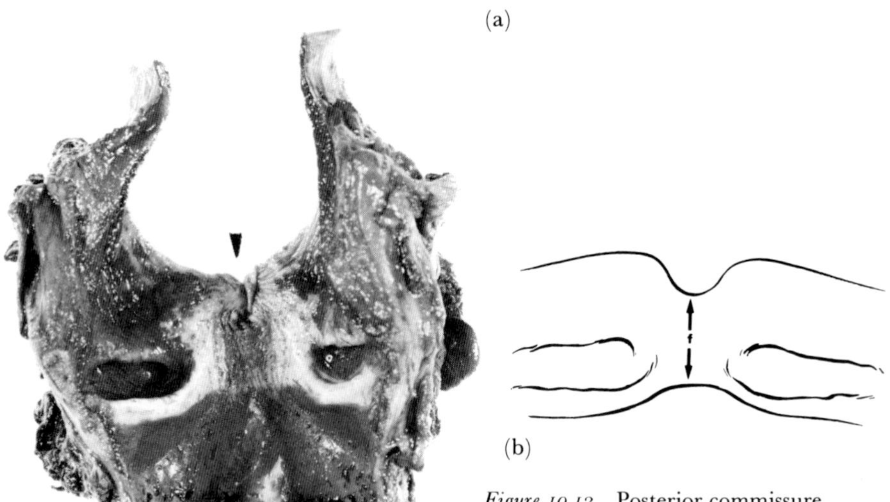

Figure 10.13 Posterior commissure

Mucous glands are freely distributed throughout the mucous membrane and are particularly numerous on the posterior surface of the epiglottis, where they form indentations into the cartilage, and in the margins of the lower part of the aryepiglottic fold, and in the saccules. The vocal folds do not possess any glands, and the mucous membrane is lubricated by those in the saccule. Some taste buds have been found in the region of the epiglottis.

Spaces of the larynx

There are two potential spaces within the larynx, which are important in the spread of tumours: the paraglottic space, and the pre-epiglottic space.

The paraglottic space is bounded by the thyroid cartilage laterally, the conus elasticus and the quadrangular membrane medially and the anterior reflection of the pyriform mucosa posteriorly; it embraces the ventricles and saccules.

The pre-epiglottic space is bounded by the hyo-epiglottic ligament, the epiglottis and the quadrangular membrane and the thyrohyoid ligament. It is continuous laterally with the paraglottic space (*Figure 10.14*).

Reinke's space is defined elsewhere.

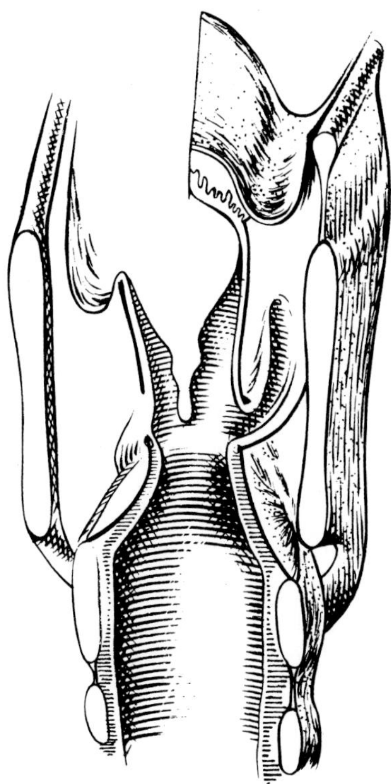

Figure 10.14 Paraglottic space

Blood supply

The blood supply is derived from the laryngeal branches of the superior and inferior thyroid arteries and the cricothyroid branch of the superior thyroid artery. The superior thyroid artery arises from the external carotid artery below the level of the greater horn of the hyoid bone, and the inferior thyroid artery arises from the thyrocervical trunk of the subclavian artery. The superior laryngeal artery passes deep to the thyrohyoid muscle together with the internal laryngeal nerve. It pierces the thyrohyoid membrane below and in front of the internal laryngeal nerve. The artery supplies the muscles and mucous membrane of the larynx and anastomoses freely with the branches of the artery of the opposite side and with those of the inferior laryngeal artery. The inferior thyroid artery ascends in front of the scalenus anterior muscle, passes medially, and in front of the vertebral vessels, behind the carotid sheath. The thoracic duct is an important relation of the commencement of the inferior thyroid artery on the left-hand side of the body. The duct usually lies in front of the artery, or of the thyrocervical trunk, crossing them from the medial to the lateral side. The inferior laryngeal artery is given off about the level of the lower border of the thyroid gland, or at the point where the middle cervical ganglion lies on the inferior thyroid artery. The inferior laryngeal artery ascends on the trachea together with the recurrent laryngeal nerve. It enters the larynx beneath the lower border of the inferior constrictor muscle, supplies the muscles and mucous membrane and anastomoses freely with the branches from the superior laryngeal artery. The cricothyroid artery passes from the superior thyroid artery across the upper part of the cricothyroid ligament and anastomoses with the branch of the other side. The veins leaving the larynx accompany the arteries; the superior vessels enter the internal jugular vein *via* the superior thyroid or facial vein; the inferior vessels pass *via* the inferior thyroid veins into the brachiocephalic veins. Some veins from the larynx also pass by the middle thyroid vein which drains into the internal jugular vein.

Lymphatic drainage

The lymphatic drainage of the larynx passes *via* two main systems of vessels to end in the deep cervical nodes. That part of the larynx above the vocal cords is drained by vessels which pierce the thyrohyoid membrane, accompany the superior laryngeal vessels and end in the upper deep cervical nodes near the bifurcation of the common carotid artery. The part of the larynx below the vocal cord is drained by vessels which may pierce the cricovocal membrane and, after passing to the pre-tracheal and pre-laryngeal nodes, enter the lower deep cervical nodes. Further vessels pass below the cricoid cartilage and above the first tracheal ring to enter the deep cervical nodes directly.

Nerve supply

The nerve supply to the mucous membrane is from the superior and recurrent laryngeal nerves. The superior laryngeal nerve arises from the inferior ganglion of the vagus and it also receives a branch from the superior cervical sympathetic ganglion. The nerve descends lateral to the pharynx, behind the internal carotid, and, at the level of the greater horn of the hyoid, divides into an internal and external branch. The internal laryngeal branch descends to the thyrohyoid membrane, pierces it above the entrance of the superior laryngeal artery, and divides into two main branches. The upper branch supplies the mucous membrane of the lower part of the pharynx, epiglottis, vallecula and vestibule of the larynx. The lower branch passes medial to the pyriform fossa beneath the mucous membrane and supplies the aryepiglottic fold and the mucous membrane of the posterior part of the rima glottidis. Terminal branches from the nerve end in the inferior constrictor muscle of the pharynx. The mucous membrane below the level of the vocal folds is supplied by branches of the recurrent laryngeal nerves.

Trachea, bronchi and lungs

Development

The respiratory system develops from a midline diverticulum in the foregut called the laryngotracheal groove, which first appears in embryos of about 3 mm crown-rump length (about 25 days), and is found immediately caudal to the hypobranchial eminence. The formation and eventual fusion of the two longitudinal ridges on each side of the groove separate the respiratory tract from the foregut proper. The fusion gradually extends cranially, and by the fifth week the respiratory diverticulum that has by now been formed communicates with the foregut by the narrow opening of the primitive laryngeal aditus. The caudal end of the diverticulum divides into two lobes, each of which will form the endodermal lining of the main bronchus, bronchial tree and alveoli of a lung. The cranial portion of the diverticulum does not divide, and becomes the larynx and trachea.

The trachea increases rapidly in length from the fifth week, and at about 48 days, when the embryo is about 20 mm in length, its cartilaginous rings make their appearance in the surrounding mesoderm. At first the bilobed caudal extremities of the respiratory diverticulum are symmetrically disposed, but at the 5 mm stage (32 days) the left lobe lies more transversely. At the 8 mm stage (38 days) the lobes divide again, each giving origin to a ventral diverticulum. On the right side a separate craniodorsal diverticulum is the rudiment of the upper lobe of the lung. At this stage, therefore, the primary pattern of the bronchial tree has already appeared, with three divisions on the right and two on the left. The basic pattern of further septation is present in the 18-week-old fetus (Reid and Rubino, 1959), but it is uncertain whether lung-budding determines the septal pattern or whether the development of the connective tissue septa controls the final form of the lung (Emery, 1969). Each primary bronchus continues to divide dichotomously until by birth some 18–23 generations of divisions have appeared. These are not necessarily equal in the several lobes. Several important events in the development of the lung occur almost simultaneously at about the sixth month of intra-uterine life. Three periods have been recognized (Emery, 1969); a 'glandular' period when the primitive bronchi ramify through the mesenchyme (up to 4 months); a 'canicular' period when the primitive respiratory bronchioles, recognized by the presence of cuboidal cells, are generated from the terminal bronchi (4–6 months); and an 'alveolar' period from 6 months onwards when further respiratory bronchioles and the terminal alveoli, which will be the functional airspaces with their blood–air barriers, are formed.

The number of generations, or divisions, in the bronchial tree has been the subject of a good deal of discussion. Some observers (Broman, 1923; Engel, 1947) considered that growth and continued branching of the bronchi took place after birth. However, later work has caused this view to be modified and in similar fashion the work of Short (1952) who thought that the post-natal increase in the size of the lung was mainly due to distension of already formed alveoli, has not been substantiated by later observations.

Reid and her co-workers (Bucher and Reid, 1961a and b; Davies and Reid, 1970), have produced convincing evidence that all post-natal growth of the lung occurs in the distal portions of the respiratory tract, that is in the acinar parts of the air-passages beyond the terminal bronchioles, which are the last air-passages with an intact epithelium and which have muscle but no cartilage in their walls. She later expressed the essence of her investigations into lung growth in the form of three 'laws' of lung development (Reid, 1967). These are:

(1) The bronchial tree is developed by the 16th week of intra-uterine life.
(2) Alveoli, as commonly understood, develop after birth, increasing in number until

the age of 8 years and in size until growth of the chest wall is finished;

(3) Blood vessels are remodelled and increase, certainly while new alveoli are forming, and probably until growth of the chest is complete.

Bucher and Reid (1961a and b) showed that all the bronchial generations were complete by the 16th week of intra-uterine life, and that they may even be slightly more numerous at this age than in the adult. Cudmore, Emery and Mithal (1962) confirmed that the number of generations in the bronchial tree of the human right upper lobe did not differ to a significant degree from a mean of 18 in specimens taken from subjects at the 37th week of intra-uterine life up to the 6th decade of adult life. Hayward and Reid (1952) found that the number of generations of the bronchial tree was different in the various parts of the lung; for example there were as many as 25 generations in the posterior basal segments of the lower lobes, with lowest counts of 8–10 elsewhere.

There is now general agreement that almost all of the increase in size of the post-natal lung is due to an increase in the number of alveoli in the first years of life, and that thereafter there is a great increase in the size of the alveoli. Dunnill (1962) estimated that the number of alveoli in the two lungs increased from about 24 million at birth to the adult figure of about 300 million at the age of 8 years. Davies and Reid (1970), repeating this work, came to the conclusion that these figures were an under-estimate by about 10 per cent. Studies by Loosli and Potter (1959), Emery and Mithal (1960), Weibel (1961), Hieronymi (1960) and Weibel and Gomez (1962) all lead to similar conclusions.

The trachea

The trachea extends downwards from the lower part of the larynx, at the level of the sixth cervical vertebral body, into the mediastinum, where it bifurcates into the right and left main bronchi. The bifurcation is described as being at the level of the upper border of the fifth thoracic vertebra, but a more practical, because easily determinable, level is that of the 2nd costal cartilage, or the manubrio-sternal angle. There is, in fact, a certain amount of movement on the part of the trachea during respiration and deglutition. The bifurcation moves appreciably upwards on swallowing, and downwards and forwards during inspiration. The diameter of the air-passages increases appreciably during inspiration, and decreases during expiration. This change in diameter makes it easier to engage a foreign body with forceps during bronchoscopic manipulations. The membranous posterior wall of the trachea and main bronchi is a good deal more mobile than the cartilaginous portion and this contributes largely to the alterations in diameter. This movement can be readily appreciated during bronchoscopy, especially under a local anaesthetic.

The trachea of the child is relatively smaller than that of the adult, and the bifurcation is at a higher level until the age of 10–12 years. The length of the trachea is about 11 cm, with a range of 9–15 cm. The carina is a convenient practical point at which the bifurcation can be localized, and is usually 25–27 cm from the upper incisor teeth or alveolar margin. Being D-shaped in cross section rather than cylindrical, the transverse diameter is greater than the antero-posterior (about 20 mm in the adult male compared with 15 mm). The exact dimensions of the major air-passages have, rather surprisingly, been the subject of few detailed investigations, and the figures available vary considerably in different series. Thus Engel (1962) (*Table 10.2*) gave the internal diameters of the trachea as measured in histological preparations as averaging 16.5 mm in the sagittal (transverse) plane and 14.4 in the coronal (antero-posterior) whereas Jesseph and Merendino (1957), taking the dimensions of fresh post-mortem specimens, found the average diameter in the adult male to be 22 mm and in the female 17 mm.

Table 10.2 The internal dimensions of the trachea (after Engel, 1962)

Age	*Average length*	*Average diameter*	
		Sagittal	*Coronal*
	(cm)	(mm)	(mm)
0–1 months	4.0	5.7	6.0
1–3 months	3.8	6.5	6.8
3–6 months	4.2	7.6	7.2
6–12 months	4.3	7.0	7.8
1–2 years	4.5	9.4	8.8
2–3 years	5.0	10.8	9.4
3–4 years	5.3	9.1	11.2
6–8 years	5.7	10.4	11.0
10–12 years	6.3	9.3	12.4
14–16 years	7.2	13.7	13.5
Adult	9.15	16.5	14.4

The cartilaginous 'rings' of the trachea and main bronchi are incomplete segments of a circle, so that the trachea in cross-section is shaped like the letter D, the straight limb being posteriorly situated and formed by the membranous wall. The lumen of the trachea is indented on the left and anteriorly in its lower portion by the arch of the aorta, this deformity being exaggerated if the aorta is dilated. The rings of the trachea can easily be seen in outline beneath the mucosa during endoscopy; they cause a distinct, if slight, elevation and pallor of the mucosa.

Relations (*Figure 10.15*)

The cervical portion of the trachea is covered anteriorly by the skin, superficial and deep fascia, and the sternohyoid and sternothyroid muscles. The isthmus of the thyroid gland covers a variable number of the uppermost rings, usually 2 or 3 in number. Although in the thin subject the trachea can be readily palpated in the neck and seems to be a very superficial structure, the surgeon will find that in order to expose the trachea he has to incise a surprisingly large number of fascial condensations. A communicating branch between the anterior jugular veins crosses in front of the trachea. The right and left lobes of the thyroid gland lie on either side of the trachea, as does the carotid sheath enclosing the common carotid artery, the internal jugular vein and the vagus nerve. The inferior thyroid vessels are anterolateral relations, and the recurrent laryngeal nerve, which lies in the groove between the trachea and the oesophagus, is a close relation to these vessels. The only important posterior relation of the trachea is the oesophagus.

In the mediastinum the trachea lies behind the manubrium sterni and is crossed anteriorly by the arch of the aorta. The brachio-cephalic (innominate) artery is closely related to the trachea which it crosses anteriorly from its aortic origin to become a right-sided relation. The left brachio-cephalic (innominate) vein crosses in front of the trachea at a more superficial level. The thymus gland, which is usually small and insignificant in the adult, but relatively large and fleshy in infancy and childhood, is an anterior relation. Other anterior relations from above down are the arch of the aorta and the origin of the left common carotid artery, the deep part of the cardiac plexus and a variable number of pre-tracheal and para-tracheal lymph nodes.

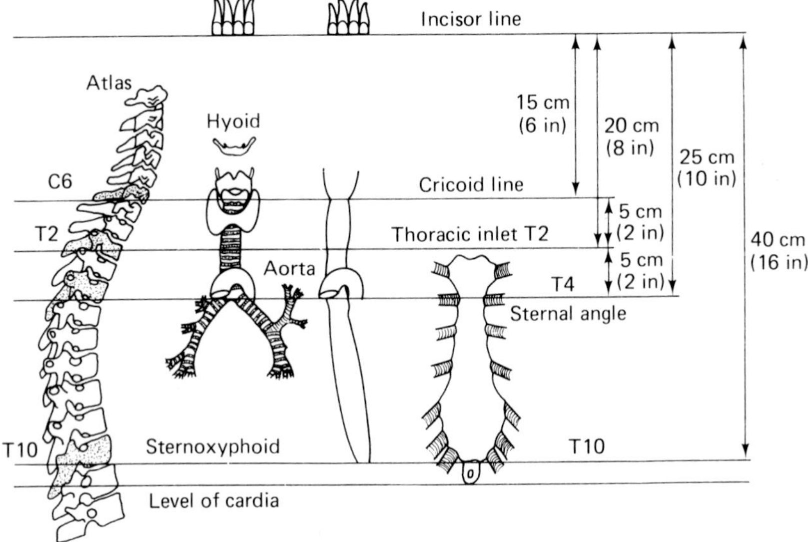

Figure 10.15 Diagram to indicate some important anatomical levels

On the left side of the mediastinal part of the trachea are the left common carotid and left subclavian arteries, the left vagus nerve and the descending part of the arch of the aorta. The left recurrent laryngeal nerve passes upwards deep to the arch of the aorta and then between the trachea and the oesophagus. On the right side the trachea is related to the pleura and the upper lobe of the right lung as well as to the right vagus nerve and the arch of the azygos vein. It should be noted that the right recurrent laryngeal nerve has only a very small course in the mediastinum proper as it hooks under the right subclavian artery before passing upwards in the neck.

Structure

The trachea is a membranous tube about 11 cm in length and containing about 16–20 incomplete rings of cartilage which serve to stiffen its wall anteriorly and laterally. The wall consists of a mucosal layer, a submucosal layer and an outer layer composed of fibrous tissue, smooth muscle and the cartilages (*Figure 10.16*).

The mucosa consists of a pseudostratified ciliated columnar epithelium with numerous goblet cells resting on a broad basement membrane. Beneath the membrane is a layer of reticular tissue containing lymphocytes and, outside this, in a position comparable to the muscularis mucosae of the gut, lies a dense layer of interlacing longitudinal elastic fibres. These are continuous lower down with the elastic tissue about the alveoli.

The submucosa consists of a layer of loose fatty connective tissue which extends to the perichondrium of the tracheal rings. The bodies of the compound tracheal glands are in this layer, and the glands contain both mucous and serous elements. It is probable that the serous secretion forms a film of fluid in which the cilia can move freely as they sweep the mucus upwards to the larynx and pharynx. The secretions of

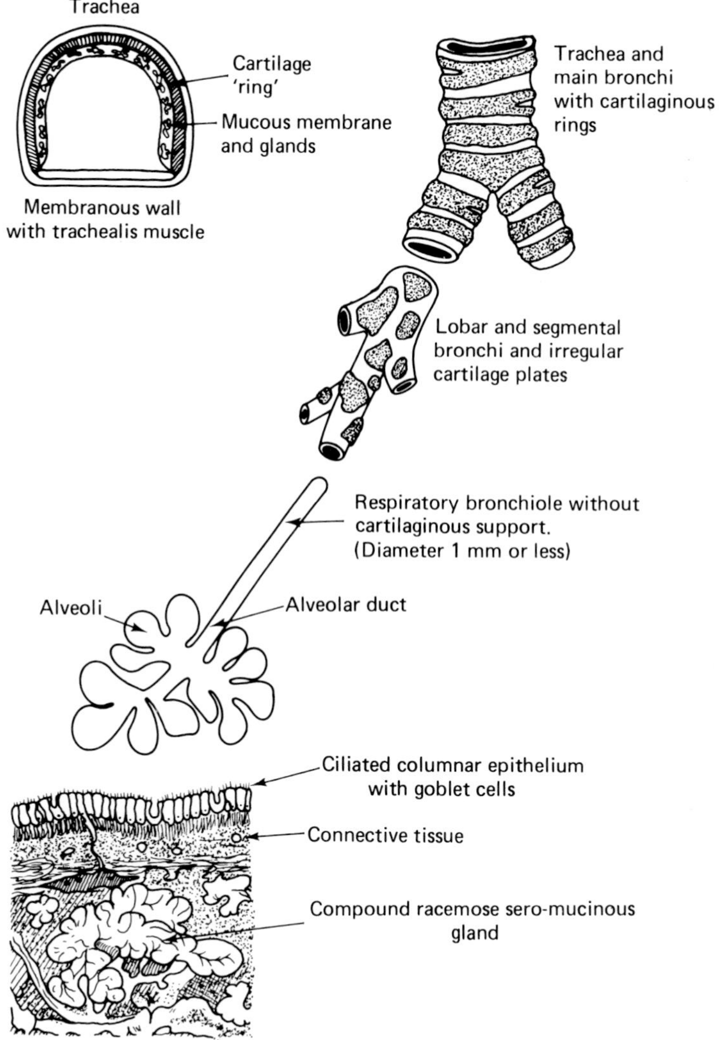

Figure 10.16 Diagram to show the histological characteristics of the respiratory tract and histological structure of mucous membrane of trachea and bronchi

the tracheal glands and the addition of transudate raises the relative humidity of the air reaching the alveoli to 100 per cent (Negus, 1958).

The outer fibrous and muscular layer is continuous with the loose areolar tissue of the mediastinum and contains blood and lymphatic vessels as well as nerves. It is continuous with the perichondrium of the cartilages. The latter are incomplete rings occupying the anterior two-thirds of the circumference of the trachea. The ends of the rings project towards each other posteriorly and the gap is closed by fibrous tissue with smooth muscle, the transverse fibres of which constitute the trachealis muscle. The whole is enclosed in a tough membrane. The cartilages are about 3–4 mm wide and 1 mm thick. They exhibit frequent branching and interconnection in a manner which is very inconstant; it is hardly an exaggeration to say that the perfectly formed ring is the exception rather than the rule.

It needs hardly to be said that the function of the cartilaginous skeleton of the tracheobronchial tree is to prevent collapse of the walls of the air-passages during respiration.

Jelihovsky (1972) has drawn attention to the fact that the elastic tissue tends to be concentrated into longitudinal bands which are most numerous in the membranous posterior wall of the trachea. These bands are continued down into the major bronchi, more entering the right than the left main bronchus. The elastic bundles become prominent in chronic bronchiectatic lungs, and are readily apparent to the bronchoscopist.

Blood and nerve supply

The blood supply of the trachea is derived from branches of the inferior thyroid arteries; at the lower end branches from bronchial arteries also contribute. The tracheal veins drain into the thyroid venous plexus. The lymphatic drainage is to the pre-tracheal and para-tracheal groups of nodes. The muscle fibres of the trachea, including the trachealis muscle, are innervated by the recurrent laryngeal nerves, which also carry sensory fibres from the mucous membrane. Sympathetic nerve fibres come mainly from the middle cervical ganglion and they also have connections with the recurrent laryngeal nerves.

Fisher (1964) describes the intrinsic innervation of the trachea.

The bronchi and the bronchial tree

In the adult the trachea bifurcates into the right and left main bronchi at the level of the second costal cartilage. The main bronchi are separated at their origin by the narrow ridge called the carina from its fancied resemblance to the keel of an upturned boat. The carina always contains cartilage, though the actual dividing ridge is frequently membranous. The anatomy of the tracheal bifurcation has been studied in detail by Vanpeperstraete (1973), who has shown that it is difficult to state with accuracy precisely where the boundary lies between trachea and main bronchus. The usual landmark is given as the angle between trachea and bronchus. This is always obtuse and may be non-existent. Von Luschka (1863) gave the first satisfactory description of the anatomy of the tracheal bifurcation and introduced the term 'carina' for the dividing ridge. Both workers conclude that it is most logical to consider that the carina belongs always to the main bronchi and never to the trachea proper. Obviously this is to a great extent a problem of nomenclature only as the main bronchi are a direct continuation of the trachea.

Nomenclature of the bronchial tree

The question of devising a satisfactory and universally acceptable system of names for the various portions of the bronchial tree is a difficult one and it cannot be said that it has yet been settled. It was a somewhat academic matter until modern thoracic surgery had developed to the point of needing more precise knowledge about bronchopulmonary anatomy. The earliest reasonably accurate description of the tracheobronchial tree was given by Diemerbroeck of Utrecht in the 17th century (Diemerbroeck, 1685). Aeby (1880) made a basic study of the comparative anatomy of the lungs, noting the asymmetry of the two lungs. Hasse (1892) modified Aeby's views and Felix adapted them in the first important textbook on modern thoracic surgery by Sauerbruch (1920, 1928).

In Britain, Ewart (1882, 1889) laid down a basic system of subdivisions of the bronchial tree and the lungs, which is little different in essence from that currently in use. His diagrams were, however, too complicated to be of easy practical value and were not easy to understand. Later, with Huntington (1920), Ewart maintained that early descriptions of the anatomy had been made with other mammals too much in mind and Huntington noted that the variations to be found in different animals were largely adaptations to differing life-styles.

In pre-antibiotic days, the exact localization of lung abscesses was of great importance to surgeons who had the difficult task of draining them externally. Kramer and Glass (1932) conducted fundamental studies on methods of localization and advanced the concept that there were smaller and relatively constant units of lung structure than the lobes. They introduced the term 'broncho-pulmonary segment' as an anatomical and pathological entity, and this concept has remained in use to the present day.

Nelson (1932, 1934), who was concerned with developing a precise and practical method for postural drainage for the treatment of bronchiectasis published clear and simple diagrams of the pulmonary lobes and segments. This work was elaborated by Lucien and Weber (1936) and Neil and his co-workers (1937). Churchill and Belsey (1939) established the concept that the main broncho-pulmonary segments could be identified by the surgeon at thoracotomy and could be selectively removed in bronchiectasis; this principle was later extensively utilized in the treatment of partially healed tuberculous lesions in the lungs.

Foster-Carter (1942), on the basis of the preparation of celloidin casts of the bronchial tree, inflation of segments of the lungs with air, dye injection and bronchography gave what is basically the current account of the anatomy of the lungs and bronchi, recognizing ten major segments in the right lung and eight in the left. As a result of these studies it became possible to correlate bronchograms and bi-plane radiographs with pathological lesions in the lungs and to localize them with considerable accuracy. Jackson and Huber (1943) were able to correlate the bronchoscopic appearances of the lobar and segmental bronchial orifices with the corresponding areas of the lungs, and described accurately the more usual dispositions of these structures in the clinical situation. They also proposed a simplified nomenclature.

Further basic work on the anatomy of the bronchial tree was done by Brock (1946) in this country and by Boyden (1955) in the USA. Boyden's book, 'Segmental Anatomy of the Lungs', is a standard reference work which describes the anatomy of the lung in great detail.

The nomenclature of the portions of the bronchopulmonary anatomy have, unfortunately, been the subject of much discussion and constant change over the years. As it had become urgently necessary for a common terminology to be established, recommendations were made by an International Committee which met in London in 1949 (reported in *Thorax*, 1950). With certain small exceptions related to usage in the USA this terminology has been generally adopted by clinicians and remains in common use at the present day. In anatomical circles this terminology has since been altered in small respects, notably by the use of the words 'principal' for 'main', and 'superior and inferior' for 'upper and lower'. The actual anatomical description has not been affected by this, however, and in this chapter it has seemed best to conform to the standard terms in everyday use by clinicians working in the field of thoracic disease. The bronchopulmonary segments were also given numbers, which are not much used, but which will be indicated in the text and figures.

The right main bronchus

The right main bronchus is wider and more nearly vertical than the left, being much more nearly a continuation of the line of the trachea. The exact definition of the main bronchus has been a matter of some confusion. Some workers refer to the main bronchus as being that portion of the bronchus between the tracheal bifurcation and the orifice of the right upper lobe bronchus, while others consider that the term should include the more distal part of the airway as far as the orifices of the right middle lobe bronchus and the apical segment of the right lower lobe.

It is proposed to adopt the latter course in this chapter, and to refer to an upper portion of the right main bronchus between the tracheal bifurcation and the upper lobe orifice, and a lower portion between the upper and the middle lobe openings. If the main bronchus is taken as extending only to the upper lobe orifice, the term 'bronchus intermedius' is used for the distal part of the bronchus. This is quite commonly used by clinicians and has a certain merit in terms of easy description. It will not, however, be used in the present text (*Figures 10.17* and *10.18*).

The right main bronchus, then, ends at the orifice of the middle lobe bronchus and is about 5 cm in length. It has a posterior membranous wall, and a series of cartilage rings very similar in structure though smaller in size than those of the trachea. The right upper lobe bronchus opens almost directly laterally about 1.25–2.0 cm from the carina. The average angle made by the right main bronchus with the trachea is given by Turner (1962) as about 30 degrees, with a range of 13–44 degrees.

The precise diameters of the bronchi have been studied by different workers with surprisingly different results, as has already been noted in the case of the trachea. There is little doubt that the figures given depend very much on the method of investigation and they must therefore be interpreted with some caution. Engel (1962)

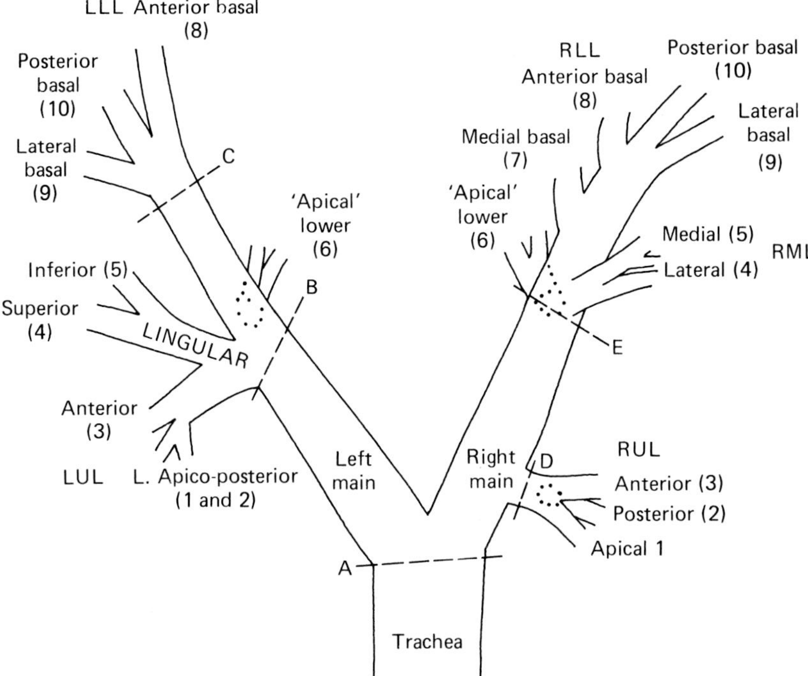

Figure 10.17 Diagram of the bronchial tree (after Stradling, P., (1976). *Diagnostic Bronchoscopy*, 3rd edn. London; Churchill Livingstone)

Table 10.3 Diameter of main bronchi taken from casts of Wood's metal (after Engel, 1962)

Age	*Right Main Bronchus*		*Left Main Bronchus*	
	Sagittal	*Coronal*	*Sagittal*	*Coronal*
(Months)	(mm)	(mm)	(mm)	(mm)
1	4.4	4.1	4.0	3.8
3	5.6	4.7	4.0	4.1
5	6.1	5.9	4.9	4.3
12	6.5	6.8	4.5	5.6
Years				
2	7.5	7.3	4.9	5.2
3	7.4	7.3	7.0	5.5
4	8.4	9.1	6.0	6.8
5	8.7	8.1	6.4	7.0
7	9.0	9.3	6.9	8.2
10	8.6	9.2	7.3	8.4
13	9.6	10.9	8.5	8.5
Adult	14.0	14.4	11.5	11.1

made casts of the trachea and main bronchi by pouring Wood's metal into the trachea of cadavers with the chest unopened. Figures which he obtained for both main bronchi in subjects of various ages are given in *Table 10.3*. No indication of sex is given by Engel, and the size of the main bronchi given by his method is distinctly

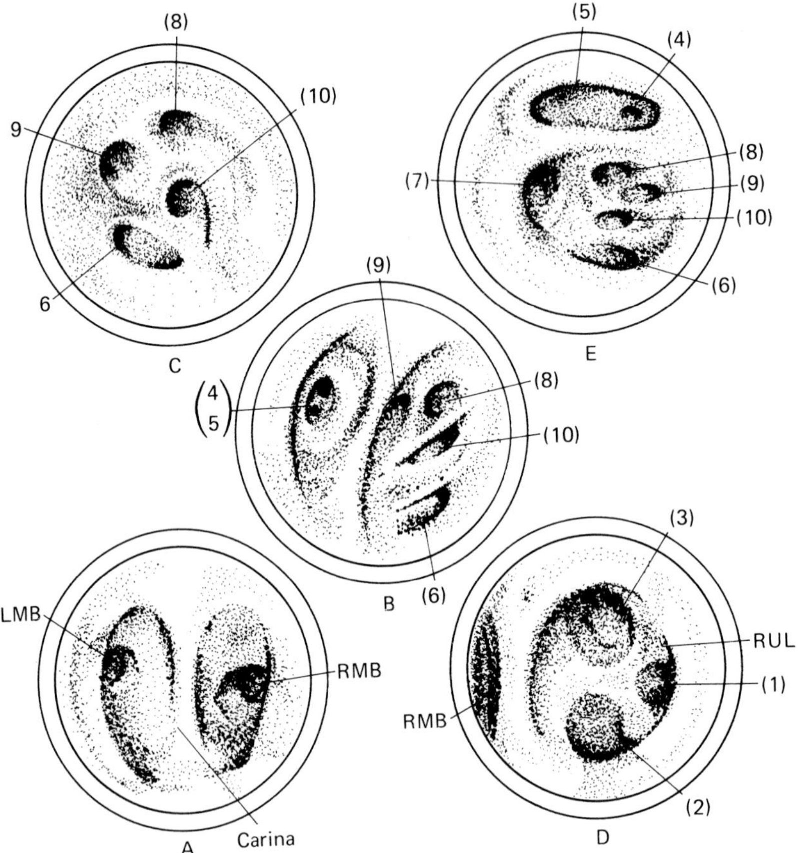

Figure 10.18 Subdivisions of bronchial tree as seen at bronchoscopy. (A) Carina and main branch (from lower end of trachea); (B) left upper and lower lobe bronchi (from left main bronchus); (C) left lower lobe segmental bronchi; (D) right upper lobe segmental bronchi (through 90 degree telescope); (E) right middle and lower lobe bronchi (from right main bronchus)

smaller than that given by Jesseph and Merendino (1957) who measured the coronal diameter of the main bronchi in 21 male and 36 female subjects soon after death. The figures given by these workers indicated an average coronal diameter of the right main bronchus of 1.7 cm (range 1.2–2.1 cm) in the male; in the female the average diameter was 1.5 cm, with a range of 1.1–2.0 cm. For the left main bronchus the figures for the male were: average 1.5 cm with a range of 1.0–1.8 cm; in the female the average was 1.2 cm and the range 0.9–1.5 cm.

In view of the conflicting information, which is presumably due to experimental error from the method used, it seems reasonable to say that the coronal diameter of the right main bronchus is about 17 ± 4 mm in the male and about 15 ± 4 mm in the female; the corresponding diameter on the left side is 2–3 mm less.

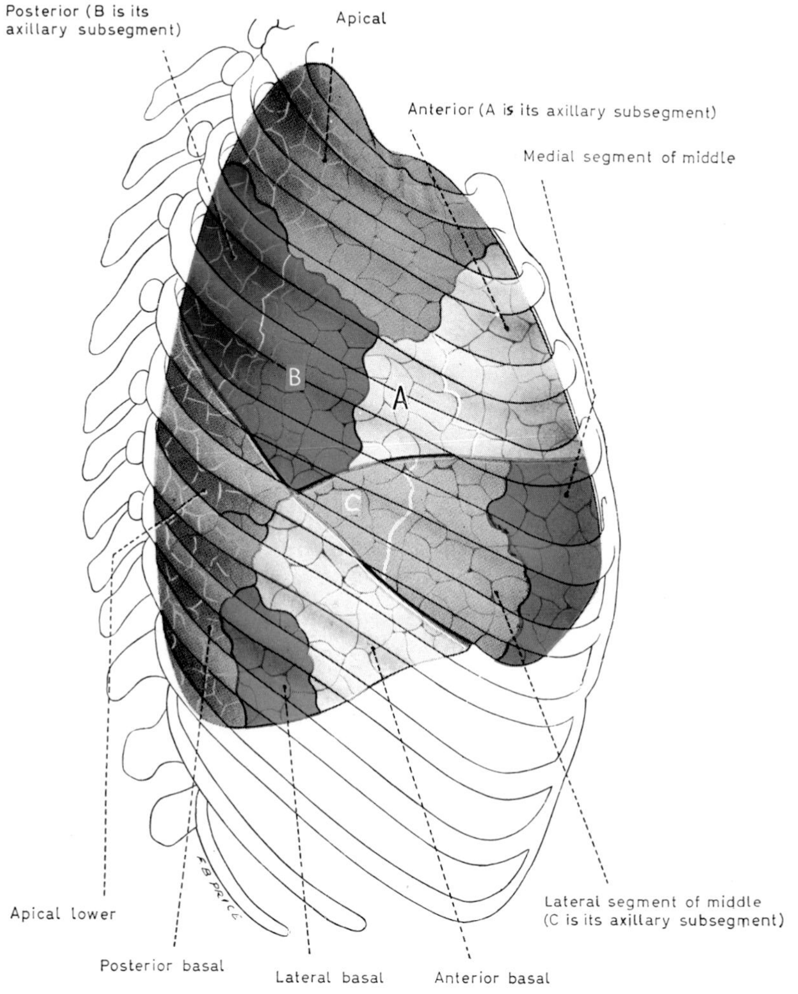

Plate 7 A drawing of the bronchopulmonary segments as seen on the lateral aspect of the right lung

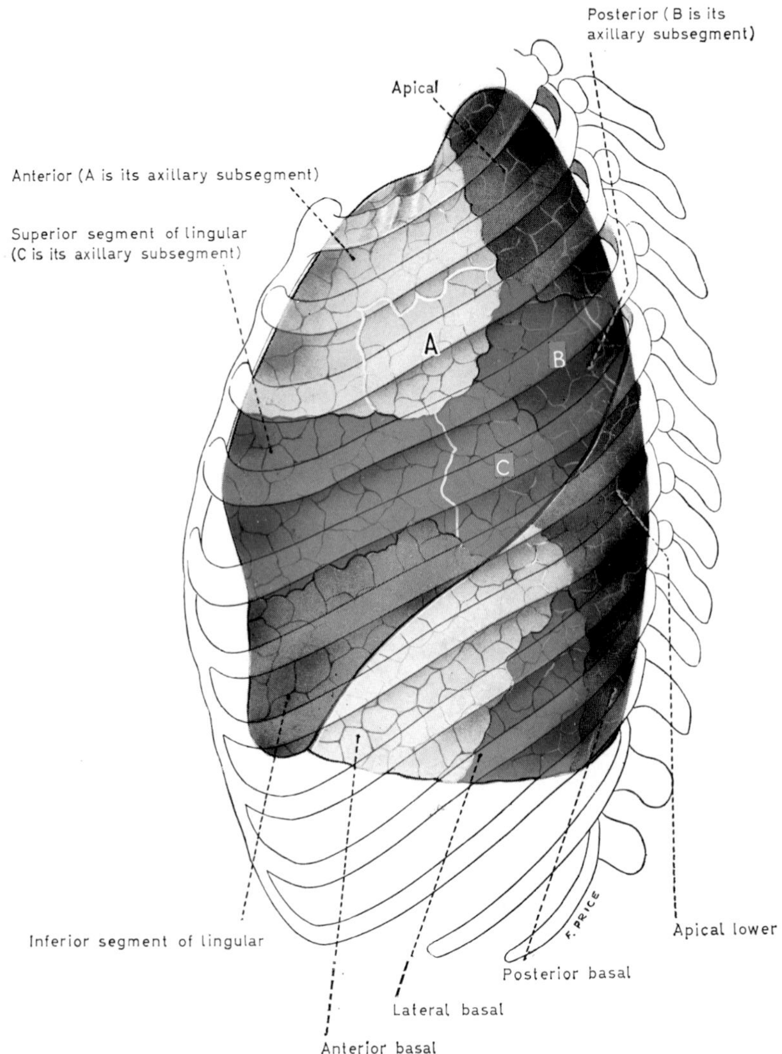

Plate 8 A drawing of the bronchopulmonary segments as seen on the lateral aspect of the left lung

The right upper lobe bronchus

The right upper lobe bronchus (commonly abbreviated to RUL) arises from the right lateral aspect of the right main bronchus about 12–20 mm from the carina. It passes for a very short distance almost at right angles to the line of the main bronchus, that is in a lateral and slightly upward direction. It is seldom more than 10 mm in length and very constantly divides into three component segmental divisions, each of approximately equal size. These divisions supply the anterior, apical and posterior segments of the upper lobe. This trifurcate division cannot be appreciated with the rigid straight-viewing bronchoscope unless for some reason the bronchus should be much displaced-downwards. It is, however, readily seen with a right-angled telescope, and with the fibre-optic instrument.

The *apical segmental bronchus* (1) passes upwards and after about 1 cm divides into apical and anterior subsegmental branches.

The *posterior segmental bronchus* (2) runs backwards and somewhat upwards parallel to the line of the oblique fissure of the lung. It divides into lateral (or axillary) and posterior subsegmental bronchi.

The *anterior segmental bronchus* (3) passes forwards, downwards and somewhat laterally, dividing after a short distance into lateral (or axillary) and anterior subsegmental branches.

This trifurcation of the right upper lobe bronchus is a typical and remarkably constant pattern; variations do occur, however, and most often take the form of an early bifurcation of the bronchus before the subsegmental divisions have arisen. An interesting but unusual variant is when an apical segment or a subsegment of the apical segment is supplied by a 'tracheal' bronchus which arises from the lateral (right) aspect of the lowest part of the trachea just above the carina. Such a displaced bronchus has naturally only a small orifice and it is not difficult to fail to observe its presence on bronchoscopy. Its chief clinical importance is the confusion that it may cause during a resection of the lung, e.g. for carcinoma.

It has already been noted that the right main bronchus is more nearly in line with the trachea than is the left. For this reason it is easier for inhaled foreign bodies or fluids such as gastric contents to enter the right rather than the left bronchial tree. If the patient should be lying on his side it is natural for fluids, including infected mucus from the upper respiratory tract, to enter the upper lobe bronchi. It is also easier for such material to enter the lateral or 'axillary' subsegments of the anterior and posterior segments of the lobe. They thus have considerable clinical importance as being frequent sites for the development of a lung abscess or inhalational pneumonitis (*see Figure 10.19*).

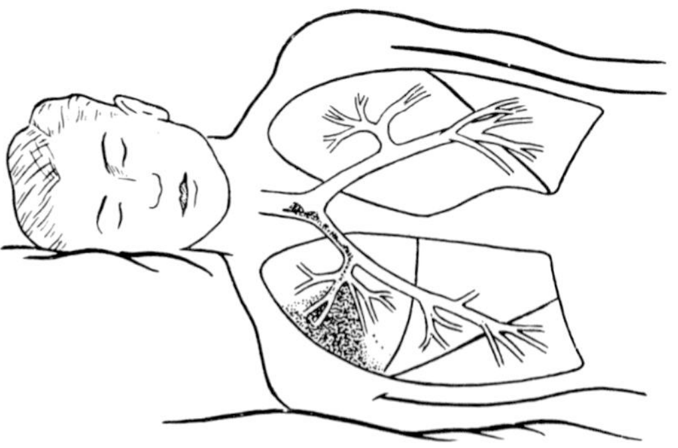

Figure 10.19 Diagram to show inhalation of infected material into the posterior bronchus of the right upper lobe by an unconscious patient lying on his right side (after Brock)

The right middle lobe bronchus (4 and 5)

The origin of the right middle lobe (RML) bronchus is about 2.5–3 cm beyond that of the upper lobe and it marks the definitive end of the right main bronchus, or, in the alternative terminology, of the bronchus intermedius. The orifice is on the anterior aspect of the bronchus and has a characteristic and unmistakable appearance at bronchoscopy, with its secondary carina lying horizontally across the field of vision. The middle lobe bronchus is directed forwards, downwards and somewhat laterally almost parallel to the lower part of the oblique fissure of the lung. In fact, in the right lateral bronchogram the bronchi of the anterior segment of the upper lobe, the right middle lobe and the anterior basal segment of the lower lobe are seen to lie almost parallel to one another somewhat resembling the tiers of a wedding cake.

After a short course of 1–1.5 cm the middle lobe bronchus divides into lateral (4) and medial (5) subsegments. On occasion these segments have more of a superior and inferior disposition.

The right lower lobe bronchus (6, 7, 8, 9 and 10)

The right lower lobe (RLL) bronchus supplies five segments of the lung; on the left side there are only four, as will be seen. The apical segment of the lower lobe on each side has a special status on account of the origin and disposition of its bronchus. In fact it is not uncommon for this segment to have a more or less well developed fissure which at any rate partially demarcates it from the remainder of the lobe. Its importance having been described by Nelson (1932) it is sometimes referred to in Continental European literature as Nelson's lobe, and it has the added distinction of being sometimes referred to as the 6th segment.

The *apical segmental bronchus* (6) arises rather confusingly from the posterior aspect of the termination of the right main bronchus, its orifice being opposite to and only a very short distance lower than that of the right middle lobe. There is also some disagreement as to its nomenclature, the term 'apical' being in common use in Great Britain, while 'superior' is favoured in the USA. The bronchus and its segment are commonly referred to as the 'apical lower' in this country, a concise and accurate but somewhat ungrammatical term. The apical segmental bronchus divides into medial and lateral subsegments, but a subapical or subsuperior bronchus is not uncommon and may arise from the posterior basal segment. The apical lower segment of either lung is another part of the lung in which aspirated material may readily collect and cause a pneumonitis, segmental collapse or an abscess. It was formerly also a not uncommon site for a tuberculous cavity (*Figure 10.20*).

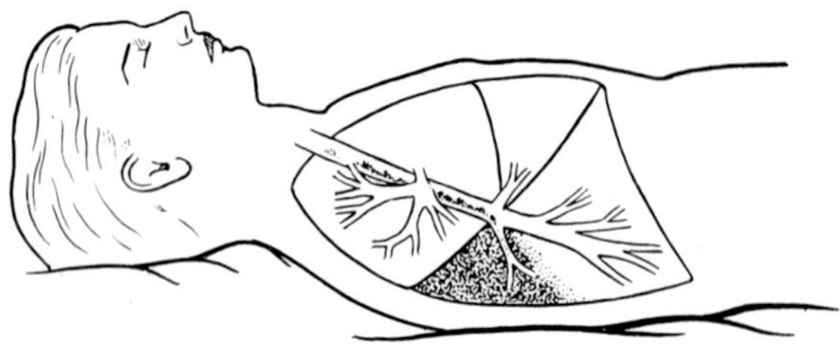

Figure 10.20 Diagram to show inhalation of infected material into the apical bronchus of the right lower lobe by an unconscious patient in the supine position (after Brock)

There are four *basal segmental bronchi* in the right lower lobe. They supply corresponding segments which occupy the lower portion of the lobe and are related to the dome of the diaphragm. The *medial basal* bronchus (7) has a higher point of origin than the other basal bronchi; it also has a characteristic appearance in the bronchogram as it curves downwards parallel to the right border of the heart. For this reason it is often referred to as the 'cardiac' segment. The other basal segmental bronchi are the anterior (8), lateral (9) and the posterior (10). They occupy corresponding positions in relation to the diaphragmatic surface of the lobe. These three bronchi may arise together as a trifurcation, or the anterior segmental branch may have a separate origin 1–2 cm above the other two.

The left main bronchus

The left main bronchus is longer and narrower than the right and it curves markedly away from the line of the trachea as it passes downwards and somewhat laterally beneath the arch of the aorta. Turner (1962) gives its angle with the trachea as being on average 43.8 degrees, with a range of 25–58 degrees (*Figure 10.17*). There is thus a very marked degree of variation in alignment. Estimates of the diameter of the left main bronchus have already been given in connection with those of the right side, and again it is to be noted that there is a very considerable amount of variation.

The left main bronchus has a posterior membranous wall, and is supported anteriorly and laterally by a series of incomplete cartilaginous rings very much as on the right side. It is about 5.5 cm in length and ends by division into upper and lower lobar divisions. It enters the lung at about the level of the 6th thoracic vertebra, and lies beneath the left pulmonary artery, behind the superior pulmonary vein and above the inferior pulmonary vein of the corresponding side.

Being at more of an angle to the line of the trachea than the right main bronchus, foreign bodies enter it less readily; probably because it is longer, narrower and more curved it seems that it is more difficult for infected secretions to be expectorated, and this may well account for the greater liability of the left lung to become bronchiectatic compared with the right.

The left upper lobe bronchus

The left upper lobe (LUL) bronchus arises as the lateral element of the bifurcation of the left main bronchus about 5.5 cm from the carina. The bronchus passes antero-laterally to the left, downwards and forwards, giving rise to four distinct segmental elements, apical (1), posterior (2), anterior (3) and lingular (4 and 5). There is a good deal of variation in the manner in which the segmental bronchi arise. It is usual for the apical and posterior segmental bronchi to come from a common stem – the apico-posterior segmental bronchus. The manner in which the anterior segmental and the lingular bronchi arise is less uniform, as is the size of the subdivisions of these segments. There may be a common anterior and lingular branch; Boyden (1955) noted that in about a quarter of the specimens he examined there was a trifurcate pattern to the upper lobe bronchi on the left involving the apico-posterior and the anterior segmental bronchi.

While the other three segments of the left upper lobe are very similar to the corresponding segments of the right upper lobe, the lingular bronchus is a separate entity which has no precise parallel on the right side. It is a long, rather thin segment which occupies the portion of the upper lobe adjacent to the lower part of the interlobar fissure. It received its name from its fancied likeness to the tongue, and first attracted attention of clinicians when Churchill and Belsey (1939) showed that it was frequently involved in bronchiectatic change; they also observed that failure to remove it with the involved lower lobe at operation led to subsequent deterioration of the segment and recurrence of symptoms.

The bronchoscopist easily recognizes the left upper lobe orifice as it opens anteriorly and to the left at the bifurcation of the left main bronchus. With the rigid instrument it is seldom possible to obtain a good view of the segmental branches with the exception of the lingular and perhaps the anterior. A better view can be obtained with an oblique-viewing telescope, and an excellent view is gained of all the segmental divisions with the fibre-optic instrument.

The lingula is sometimes regarded as the analogue of the middle lobe on the right. There is, however, no real need to draw such analogies. The left lung is smaller than the right because of the space occupied by the heart in the left hemithorax. Also the left upper lobe bronchus must have a lower point of origin than the right because of the fact that the arch of the aorta overlies the left main bronchus. There does not, in fact, appear to be any entirely typical model of the two lungs in all mammals. Much appears to depend on the particular circumstances of life-habits, body-shape and function of the animals concerned. Most of the differences between the two lungs in man seem to be related to the constant asymmetry of the viscera with a left-sided heart and descending aorta. The left upper lobe is larger than the right, but the right lung is larger than the left, with about 55 per cent of the total lung volume.

The segments of the left upper lobe are subdivided in much the same manner as on the right, and there are well-marked lateral or axillary subsegments in both the anterior and posterior segments. The lingula is also divided into superior (4) and inferior (5) segments.

The left lower lobe bronchus

The left lower lobe bronchi follow very much the same pattern as on the right side, but in mirror-image disposition. The left lower lobe (LLL) is, however, smaller than the right in that it has no medial basal segment.

The *apical segmental bronchus* (6) takes its origin posteriorly from the left lower lobe bronchus about 1 cm or a little more below the upper lobe orifice. In contrast to the situation on the right side it is very definitely a branch of the lower lobe bronchus, but, as on the right side, it opens posteriorly and has in most instances a medial and a superolateral trunk (Boyden, 1955). It has a length of 0.5–1 cm before it divides.

There are three *basal segmental bronchi* in the left lower lobe, the anterior (8), lateral (9) and posterior (10). It is usually stated that the left lower lobe bronchus divides by trifurcation about 1.5–2 cm below the origin of the apical segmental bronchus. However, Boyden (1955) who has conducted the most meticulous studies into the anatomy of the bronchial tree, points out that 77 per cent of his specimens showed that there was a pattern of bifurcation of the basal segmental trunk into antero-medial and posterolateral subdivisions. He further considers that there is a definite and identifiable medial basal segmental bronchus in most specimens on the left side as well as on the right. He also notes that there is frequently a recognizable subapical – or, in his terminology, subsuperior – bronchus both on the left and the right side, supplying a posterolateral portion of the upper part of the lower lobe. At the same time, it must be said that these fine distinctions are of more importance to the anatomist than to the practising clinician. It is certainly possible to resect individual segments of the lung in certain places, especially in the upper lobes, but it is seldom either feasible or needful to attempt resection of individual basal segments of the lower lobes.

The pulmonary fissures and the bronchopulmonary segments

It has been pointed out above that the divisions of the bronchi and the lobes and segments of the lungs cannot be considered in isolation from each other.

Some idea of the arrangement of the lobes and segments may be obtained from *Figures 10.21* and *10.22* and *Plates 7 and 8 facing page 414.*

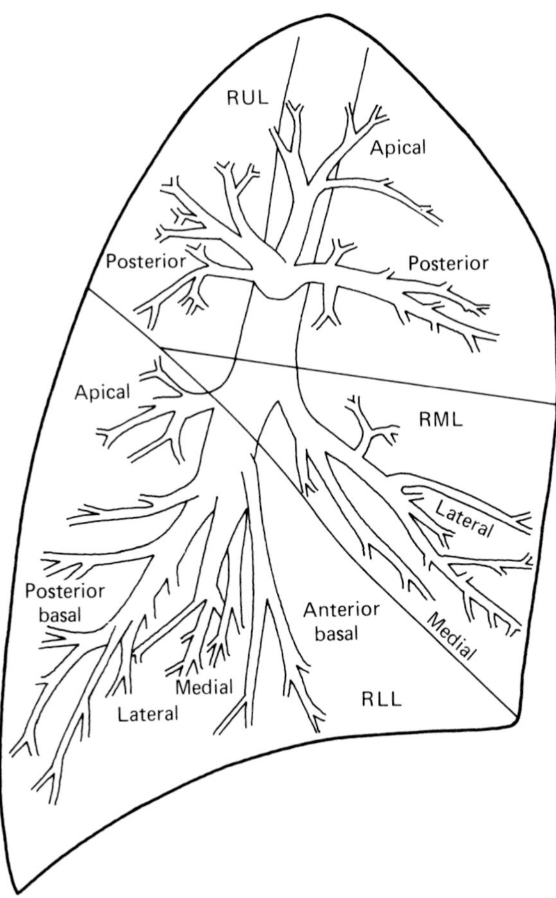

Figure 10.21 Bronchi and segments of right lung – lateral aspect (diagrammatic)

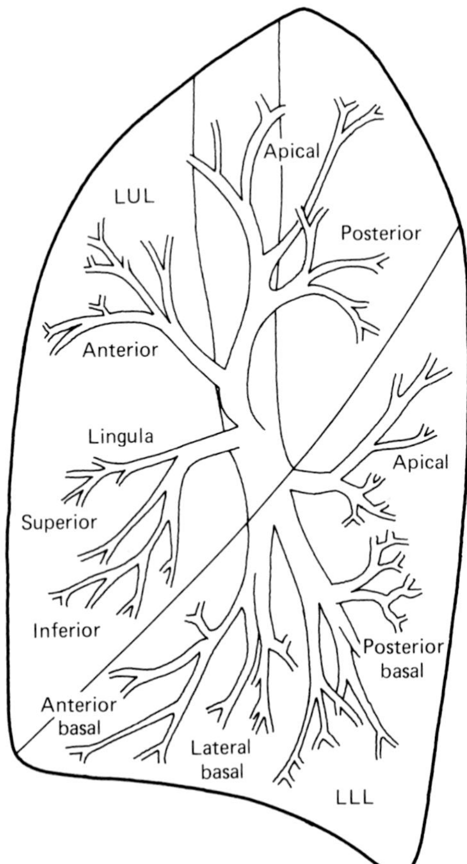

Figure 10.22 Bronchi and segments of left lung – lateral aspect (diagrammatic)

It may be helpful to tabulate (*Table 10.4*) the divisions of the lungs once more together with the numbers allocated to the individual segments by the International Committee (1950).

Table 10.4

Right lung		*Left lung*	
Right Upper Lobe (RUL)		Left Upper Lobe (LUL)	
Apical segment	(1)	Apico-posterior segment	(1 + 2)
Posterior segment	(2)		
Anterior segment	(3)	Anterior segment	(3)
Right Middle Lobe (RML)		Lingula	
Lateral segment	(4)	Superior segment	(4)
Medial segment	(5)	Inferior segment	(5)
Right Lower Lobe (RLL)		Left Lower Lobe (LLL)	
Apical segment	(6)	Apical segment	(6)
Medial basal segment	(7)		
Anterior basal segment	(8)	Anterior basal segment	(8)
Lateral basal segment	(9)	Lateral basal segment	(9)
Posterior basal segment	(10)	Posterior basal segment	(10)

The numbers attached to the individual segments have found little use practically with the exception, as mentioned, of the 'apical lower' segment, which is not infrequently referred to as the 6th segment in European literature.

The lungs are divided into two more or less equal portions on each side by the oblique fissure. This, however, is not always completely developed; on rare occasions it is completely absent, and frequently there is failure of the fissure to develop fully, especially towards its upper end. The oblique fissure on the right side separates the upper and middle lobes above from the lower lobe below. On the left side the fissure separates the upper from the lower lobe, and on the right there is the short horizontal fissure which is often incompletely developed. It separates the middle from the right upper lobe. It is not uncommon for there to be at least a partially developed fissure between the apical and basal segments of the lower lobe, and between the lingula and the remainder of the left upper lobe.

The usual description of the oblique fissure (Brock, 1954) is that it follows the line of the sixth rib on the right side and approximately the fifth rib on the left. The upper end of the fissure is one or two ribs or spaces higher than this, and tends to be somewhat higher on the left than on the right side.

The most important feature of the interlobar fissures is that when they are well developed they greatly facilitate segmental resection or pulmonary lobectomy. If absent they may make these operations difficult, especially on the right side. Loculated effusions or collections of pus occasionally form in the fissures.

Readers who are interested in obtaining more detailed information about the anatomy of the lung and bronchial tree are recommended to consult the classical and authoritative work of Boyden (1955) on the subject.

The pulmonary vascular system

The foregoing description of the bronchial tree and the lungs perhaps suffers from considering the latter as being in some sense mere appendages of the former. In reality nothing could be further from the truth, and it is best to think of the lungs as organs of gas exchange in which the inspired air is brought into intimate contact with the blood circulating in the pulmonary capillaries. In addition to the bronchial tree with its subdivisions ending ultimately in the alveoli, each lobe and each bronchopulmonary segment has its pulmonary arterial tree which subdivides in the same manner as the bronchial tree, and ends in the capillaries in the alveolar walls. In the subsegments of the pulmonary lobes the anatomy of the arterial tree closely parallels that of the bronchial tree. At lobar and segmental level, however, there is no such parallelism, although the arterial supply to these larger portions of the lungs has a reasonably standard anatomical pattern. The pulmonary veins which return the blood from the alveolar capillaries eventually into the left atrium tend to run between the bronchopulmonary segments rather than in their substance. This peculiarity is made use of in performing a segmental resection of the lung, when it is only necessary to secure the corresponding artery and bronchus and to exert traction on this. Separation of the segment from the remainder of the lung will take place in a plane in which there is little air-leak and only a few small venous radicals will have to be secured.

The pulmonary arteries

The main pulmonary artery, often referred to as the pulmonary artery trunk, arises from the right ventricle and passes upwards and a little to the left, close to and on the left side of the aorta. It is as large as the aorta in diameter, and the output from the right ventricle is, of course, the same as that from the left. The blood is desaturated and as the pulmonary vascular resistance is much lower than that in the systemic circulation the pressure in the pulmonary artery (about 25 mmHg) is much lower than in the aorta.

The pulmonary artery trunk divides into the *right* and *left pulmonary arteries* beneath the arch of the aorta. The right pulmonary artery makes an angle of rather less than 90 degrees with the pulmonary artery trunk; the left pulmonary artery makes a definitely obtuse angle at its take-off. Each artery conveys blood to the corresponding lung, forming a major component of the pulmonary hilum. The *right pulmonary artery* is longer than the left. It turns sharply to the right beneath the arch of the aorta and enters the right lung hilum after passing posterior to the ascending aorta and the superior vena cava. As it enters the lung it lies above the superior pulmonary vein and anterior to the right main bronchus. It divides into a smaller superior and a larger inferior division before it enters the substance of the lung. The superior division or trunk usually divides to supply the apical and anterior segments of the right upper lobe. The inferior trunk passes downwards and crosses in front of the lower portion of the right main bronchus below the upper lobe bronchus and above the middle lobe bronchus. It gives one or two branches to the middle lobe and one or two to the posterior segment of the upper lobe. It is now in the depths of the oblique fissure and shortly enters the substance of the lower lobe where it gives a major branch to the apical segment and individual branches to each of the four basal segments. There is a good deal of possible variation in this distribution of branches, but the main pattern is remarkably constant.

The *left pulmonary artery* runs to the left through the hollow of the arch of the aorta and enters the hilum of the left lung after passing in front of the descending aorta. It lies above the left main bronchus and curves round to descend in the depths of the interlobar fissure. Typically, its first branch is a large one to the apical and anterior segments of the upper lobe. It then supplies a very variable number of branches to the remaining segments of the upper lobe, often to the anterior segment also. There is a constant large branch to the apical segment of the lower lobe; the artery then enters the substance of the lower lobe to distribute branches to the individual basal segments. There may be two or three large branches to the upper lobe or as many as seven or eight smaller ones.

The pulmonary veins

The oxygenated venous blood returns from the alveoli in venules and veins which lie for the most part in the peripheral parts of the lobules and segments. The terminal arrangement of the veins is remarkably constant. On the right side the veins from the upper lobe join a single trunk to which the middle lobe vein is added just outside the pericardium. This superior pulmonary vein lies anterior to the right main bronchus and to the inferior division of the right pulmonary artery. After a short course it enters the pericardium and drains into the left atrium. The middle lobe vein sometimes does not join the upper lobe veins and enters the left atrium independently. There is a well-marked vein from the apical segment of the lower lobe; this joins a vein draining the basal segments of the lobe and forms the inferior pulmonary vein. This is the lowest major structure in the right pulmonary hilum and lies below the lower part of the right main bronchus. It has a short course outside the pericardial cavity and after an equally short intrapericardial course it enters the left atrium below the superior vein.

On the left side there is a superior vein which drains the upper lobe, and an inferior vein which drains the lower lobe. The latter again has a well-marked apical segmental branch. The superior vein lies anterior to the left main bronchus at the point where the upper lobe bronchus takes off; the inferior vein is again the lowest major structure in the pulmonary hilum and lies below the left main bronchus and its lower lobe branches.

There are thus normally four pulmonary venous orifices into the left atrium, which occupies the posterior portion of the heart. On occasion the two pulmonary veins from one lung fuse into a common venous trunk which enters the left atrium by a single orifice; this appears to be more common on the left side.

Structure of the bronchi and lungs

The successive divisions of the bronchial tree are the main bronchi, lobar and segmental bronchi, bronchioles, terminal bronchioles, respiratory bronchioles, alveolar ducts and alveoli (*Figure 10.16*). It has been shown by Lambert (1955) that there are accessory communicating canals between bronchioles and alveoli; it is also well known that there is 'collateral ventilation' between adjacent groups of alveoli within the same lobule of the lung (Van Allen, Lindskog and Richter, 1929–30) through the pores of Kohn. This may reach considerable proportions on occasion and varies a good deal in different species of mammal (Baarsma, Dirken and Huizinga, 1948). It does mean that obstruction of a segmental bronchus does not necessarily lead to de-aeration of the segment it supplies.

It is a common impression that the whole bronchial tree is supported by cartilage rings as in the trachea and the main bronchi. This is, however, not the case, as a detailed investigation of the exact anatomy of the cartilaginous skeleton of the bronchial tree has shown (Vanpeperstraete, 1973). Most earlier work had been done with the aid of bronchial casts, but Vanpeperstraete showed that, with appropriate staining of the cartilages of the air-passages, the anatomy was considerably different from that which had been generally supposed. Hayward and Reid (1952) made an important contribution to knowledge about the bronchial cartilages when they investigated the distribution of the cartilages in bronchi in connection with changes in the lung in bronchiectasis and massive collapse. Vanpeperstraete found that the C-ring pattern was present in both main bronchi, and that it persisted down to the origin of the apical segmental bronchus of the lower lobe on each side. There were about 10 rings on each side (average 9.9 on the right and 10.2 on the left). In this way a fundamental symmetry of the major airways on each side is demonstrated.

The C-ring structure persisted into the left upper lobe bronchus in almost all instances, but into the right upper lobe in only 73 per cent of specimens. There was only rarely any ring-shaped cartilage in the right middle lobe bronchus, and never any in the lower lobe bronchi; instead, the wall of these bronchi is supported by numerous cartilaginous plates of very varied shape and size. Whereas there was always a membranous wall in the bronchi with C-rings there was none in the bronchi with plates in their walls. Vanpeperstraete came to the conclusion that the C-ring structure with a well-marked membranous wall is only present in the extrapulmonary portion of the bronchial tree where the walls need to be relatively rigid. This does not apply to those parts of the bronchial tree which are within the substance of the lung, where the walls need to be relatively mobile and have less tendency to collapse.

The trachea is lined, as already stated, with pseudostratified ciliated columnar epithelium with numerous goblet cells. The same type of epithelium is present in the bronchi, but as the passages become smaller with repeated branching the epithelium becomes thinner and is eventually single-layered. There are fewer goblet cells, and a narrower basal membrane in the smaller air-passages.

The cartilage plates also gradually become smaller and fewer in number and are not found in bronchioles, where the diameter is less than 1 mm. Some elastic fibres are found in the cartilages of smaller bronchi. Circular muscle fibres almost completely surround the tube inside the cartilages, replacing the elastic layer found in the trachea. Numerous elastic fibres are present amongst these muscle fibres. The latter are arranged in an interlacing network, partly circular and partly diagonal, so that their contraction constricts and shortens the tube. Muscle fibres are found as far distally as the alveolar ducts, where they condense to form slight sphincters.

The branched tubulo-racemose glands are less numerous in the smaller bronchi and are not present in the bronchioles. Lymphoid tissue is found diffused throughout the mucosa of the bronchi, often in solitary nodules; it is particularly abundant at points of bifurcation.

The respiratory bronchioles are about 0.5 mm in diameter and are short tubes. Their first part is lined with ciliated columnar epithelium as in the bronchioles but without goblet cells. The epithelium more distally changes to a low cuboidal type without cilia (*Figure 10.16*). The walls are composed of collagenous connective tissue containing numerous bundles of interlacing muscle and elastic fibres. A few alveoli arise from the side of a respiratory bronchiole opposite to that along which the branches of the pulmonary artery run.

Each respiratory bronchiole branches into two or three alveolar ducts which radiate out for short distances. The ducts are thin-walled tubes which pursue a tortuous course and have several branches. Numerous thin-walled alveolar sacs open off the ducts; elastic, collagenous and muscle fibres surround their mouths, and 2–4 alveoli open from them. The walls of the alveoli contain a dense capillary network with very free and close anastomoses; there are also branching reticular fibres and fine elastic fibres. These fibres occupy the central part of the septa which intervene between the alveoli; the capillaries pass among and between the fibres so that part of their wall lies close to the alveolar lining. The considerable quantity of elastic tissue in the lung is arranged in four interconnected complexes (Emery, 1969). There is a plexus of elastic fibres within the pleura with projections into the septa. A second plexus surrounds the airways and connects distally with that of the alveoli. A third plexus is that of the tunica adventitia of blood vessels which extends into the septa and connects distally with other complexes. The fourth complex is an extensive network of fine isolated fibres in the alveolar walls and a denser arrangement of fibres around the alveolar mouths. This complex becomes more marked as the lung grows.

The number of alveoli in the lungs is approximately 300 million (Hayek, 1960; Weibel, 1961). Estimates of the actual surface area of the alveolar walls – the alveolar respiratory surface – may be put at about 90 m^2, or 50 times the total surface area of the body. Hayek (1960) estimated that the respiratory surface area varied from 30 m^2 in expiration to as much as 100 m^2 in full inspiration. Weibel (1961) gives slightly smaller figures with a maximum of 80 m^2.

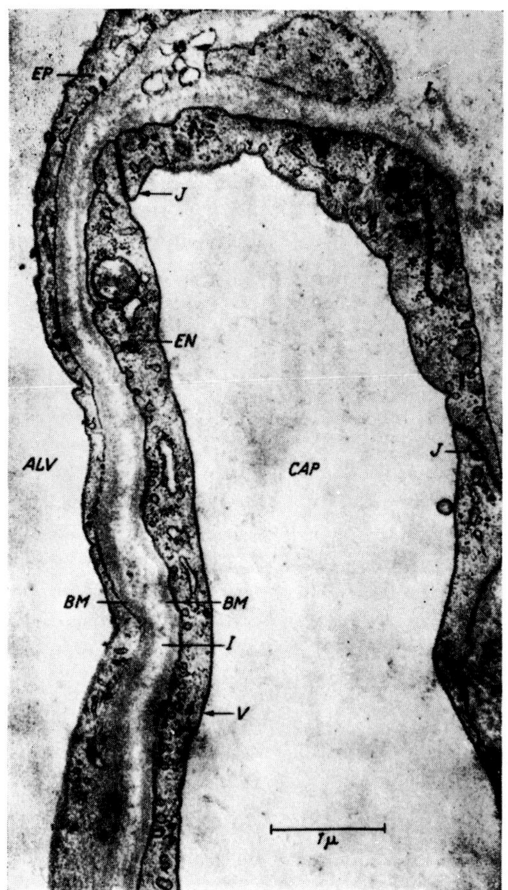

Figure 10.23 Electron micrograph of an alveolar capillary (CAP) from the human lung showing the components of the air-blood barrier. ALV = alveolus, EP = epithelial and EN = endothelial cells. BM = basement membranes, I = interstitial space. V = pinocytotic vesicles. J = junction between endothelial cells (×23000). (From Weibel, E.R., *Morphometry of the Human Lung*, 1963, reproduced by courtesy of Springer-Verlag)

There has been much discussion about the exact nature of the lining of the alveoli and in particular as to whether there is a continuous membrane lining the interior of each alveolus. Important papers which may be referred to are those of Low (1953), Bertalanffy and Leblond (1955), Karrer (1956), Schulz (1959), Low (1961) and Weibel (1963). It is certain from electron-microscopy studies that the membrane which forms the actual blood–air barrier in the walls of the alveoli is composed of three distinct layers – epithelial and capillary endothelial layers separated by a basement membrane which derives from both the other layers and which may itself be separated into two thin layers by interstitial substance. In the normal lung the thickness of the alveolar wall varies from 0.36 to 2.5 μm and approximately two-thirds of the lining surface of the alveolus acts as the gas-exchanging respiratory surface. The electron-microscopic appearances of the alveolar wall are illustrated in *Figure 10.23*.

The continuity of the alveolar walls is interrupted here and there by the pores of Kohn; there has been considerable controversy about these in the past. They have been thought to be artefacts, or the result of disease processes, but are now known to be normal features in the alveolar walls. It is through these pores that collateral ventilation of lung tissue can occur even if the bronchial passage to the portion of lung concerned should become obstructed. It is also known that phagocytes can pass through the pores.

The cells lining the alveoli are designated Type I and Type II pneumocytes. The Type I cells are exceedingly thin, and have deep cytoplasmic processes which enable one cell to pass between the alveolar capillaries and form part of both sides of the alveolar wall. The Type II cells are rounded and are attached to the basement membrane of the alveolar epithelium. The Type I pneumocytes are unable to regenerate if damaged and appear to be unable to proliferate. The Type II pneumocytes can proliferate to take the place of Type I cells and probably can become transformed to Type I cells (Spencer, 1977). They also appear to be to some extent phagocytic. It is possible that the Type II pneumocytes are the source of alveolar surfactant (Scarpelli, 1968), though others think that the Clara cells perform this function (Niden and Yamaha, 1966; Azzopardi and Thurlbeck, 1968; Smith, Heath and Moosavi, 1974).

Other cellular systems

It has already been mentioned that the large air-passages are lined by ciliated columnar epithelium. There are mucus-secreting goblet cells between the ciliated cells, and there are also glands of the mixed salivary type down as far as bronchi of the order of 1.0 mm in diameter. There are other cells in the lining of the air-passages, and since the advent of electron microscopy these have been studied in some detail.

At all levels of the bronchial tree 'brush' cells are found, and with the electron microscope it can be seen that their domed surfaces project above the level of the rest of the epithelium. They have microvilli on their free surface and they may be the source of the watery element of the bronchial mucus (Spencer, 1977), but little is known for certain about their function. They are much less numerous than the other cells.

The basal layers of the epithelium consist of cells which are presumed to develop into the other types of cell. There are also pale-staining cells described by Fröhlich (1949). They may be argentaffin or argyrophilic and are possibly sensory nerve endings of some kind. They are sometimes known as Feyrter cells and are found also in the gastro-intestinal tract (Feyrter, 1953). Carcinoid tumours are derived from these cells.

As in other structures derived from the fetal endodermal canal, and as in the adrenal medulla and structures deriving from the neural crest, Kulschitzky cells ('K-cells') are to be found in the epithelium of the bronchial tree. These cells contain numerous neuro-secretory granules and appear to be related to the mucus-secreting elements of the mucosa. They are probably related to the APUD cellular system (Pearse, 1966), and were first described by Bensch *et al.* (1968).

Other cells, which are found in the terminal bronchioles, are the Clara cells, named after the worker who first described them in detail (Clara, 1937). Electron microscopy leads to the supposition that they are actively secretory and it is possible that they are an important – perhaps the only – source of surfactant in the alveoli. It is, however, uncertain how much the Type II pneumocytes contribute to this process.

The bronchial arteries and veins

The only means by which oxygenated blood is carried to the tissues of the air-passages and the lungs is by the bronchial arteries; if the blood-flow through the pulmonary arteries is interrupted, the lung does not suffer in its nutrition. The existence of the bronchial arteries appears to have been known to Galen in antiquity; the bronchial circulation has been studied in recent years with sometimes conflicting results. Important contributions to our knowledge have been made by Berry and Daly (1931), Berry (1935), Daly (1935–6), Miller (1947) and Cauldwell *et al.* (1948). It is generally agreed that the main bronchial arteries come from the aorta, either from the under-side of the arch, or from the descending aorta distal to the origin of the left subclavian artery. On occasion they may be branches of an intercostal artery or an internal thoracic artery (Miller, 1947; Marchand, Gilroy and Wilson, 1950). There are from one to three arteries on each side. Cudkowicz and Armstrong (1951) observed that branches of the bronchial arteries went to the oesophagus, the mediastinum, the hilar lymph nodes and the vagus nerves. They also supply branches to the visceral pleura and act as vasa vasorum to the larger pulmonary arteries. There has been some difference of opinion as to whether there are pre-capillary anastomoses between the bronchial and the pulmonary arteries. Such anastomoses, if they exist, cannot be of any great importance but they are certainly present and responsible for the maintenance of life in certain forms of congenital heart disease in which the pulmonary artery or the pulmonary valve is atretic, and may well be of importance in some adult lungs with chronic respiratory disorders (Liebow, 1962).

The bronchial arteries follow the ramifications of the bronchial tree, finally entering the interlobar septa and ending in the supporting tissue of the walls of the alveoli (Cudkowicz and Armstrong, 1951).

There is some uncertainty whether true bronchial veins exist. Marchand, Gilroy and Wilson (1950) appear to have demonstrated definite venous channels which either entered the left atrium directly or joined major pulmonary veins near their entry into the left atrium. However, other workers such as Cudkowicz and Armstrong could not demonstrate any bronchial veins and were of the opinion that the blood from the bronchial arteries eventually entered pulmonary venous channels in the lungs and returned through them to the left atrium. Thoracic surgical experience would favour real doubt that bronchial veins exist as a definite entity.

Nerve supply

The nerves to the lungs are derived from the parasympathetic and sympathetic divisions of the autonomic nervous system. The posterior pulmonary plexus is formed in the posterior portion of each pulmonary hilum by a number of fibres from the vagus nerve and also from the second to fifth thoracic ganglia of the sympathetic chain. Fibres sometimes come from the first (stellate) ganglion also. Fibres also come from the deep cardiac plexus and from the left recurrent laryngeal nerve. There are a few anterior pulmonary branches from the vagus nerves which combine to form the anterior pulmonary plexus which also has connections with the deep cardiac plexus and, on the left side, with the superficial cardiac plexus. From these plexuses nerves pass into the lungs along the bronchi and the branches of the pulmonary arteries. Small collections of nerve cells are present near the root of the lung: the efferent vagal fibres from the dorsal nucleus synapse on them. These fibres supply the bronchiolar muscle; they are secretomotor to the bronchial glands and vasodilator. Afferent fibres are involved in the cough reflex and perhaps in the Hering–Breuer reflex. There is considerable evidence (Campbell and Howell, 1962; Widdicombe, 1961) that the Hering–Breuer reflex is either very weak or non-existent in man, however. The cells of the afferent vagal fibres are in the inferior vagal ganglion. The efferent sympathetic fibres dilate the bronchioles and constrict blood vessels. Some afferent sensory sympathetic fibres innervate the visceral pleura and the air-passages.

The lymphatic drainage

The lymphatics of the lungs are abundant and have been described by Miller (1947) as two almost completely isolated systems; a superficial or pleural system lying beneath the visceral pleura (Simer, 1952) and a deep or alveolar system arising from capillaries in the interalveolar septa and in the intersegmental connective tissue of the lungs. Trapnell (1963) describes the peripheral lymphatics. The two lymphatic systems have some intercommunication about 3 mm beneath the visceral pleura and also at the hilum (Tobin, 1954, 1957). The lymphatic flow in the lung appears to be relatively greater in infancy than at any other age (Emery, 1969).

The superficial or pleural lymphatic system forms a plexus of lymphatics beneath the pleura and is provided with numerous valves. These lymphatics unite and form a variable number of trunks which enter the hilar lymph nodes.

The lymphatics of the deep or alveolar system form trunks which accompany the pulmonary and the bronchial arteries, and convey lymph from the interior of the lung to the hilar nodes. They have few valves except where they anastomose with the pleural lymphatics and at the hilum. The bronchial lymph vessels originate in plexuses beneath the mucous membrane. The lymphatics penetrate the muscle coat and form a second plexus in the outer fibrous coat, often incorporating nodules of lymphoid tissue.

The distribution of the tracheal and bronchial lymph nodes is shown in *Figure 10.24*. There are pulmonary groups of nodes around the smaller bronchi, bronchopulmonary nodes mainly beneath the points of division of the intrapulmonary air-passages, inferior tracheobronchial nodes beneath the divisions of the larger bronchi and a subcarinal group of nodes beneath the bifurcation of the trachea. From this group of nodes lymphatics pass either to the right or the left para-tracheal nodes. There are more lymphatic channels on the right than on the left side, and as always in the lymphatic system a proportion of the vessels by-passes every group of nodes (*see also* Dickey, 1911; Nelson, 1932).

The right superior tracheobronchial nodes lie in relation to the right upper lobe bronchus and the right side of the lowest portion of the trachea. Lymphatics from all parts of the right lung drain into these nodes, and there are communications with the left upper lobe also. Lymphatics pass from these nodes to the right para-tracheal group of nodes, and into the right lymph duct. Some enter directly into the region of the junction of the internal jugular and right subclavian veins.

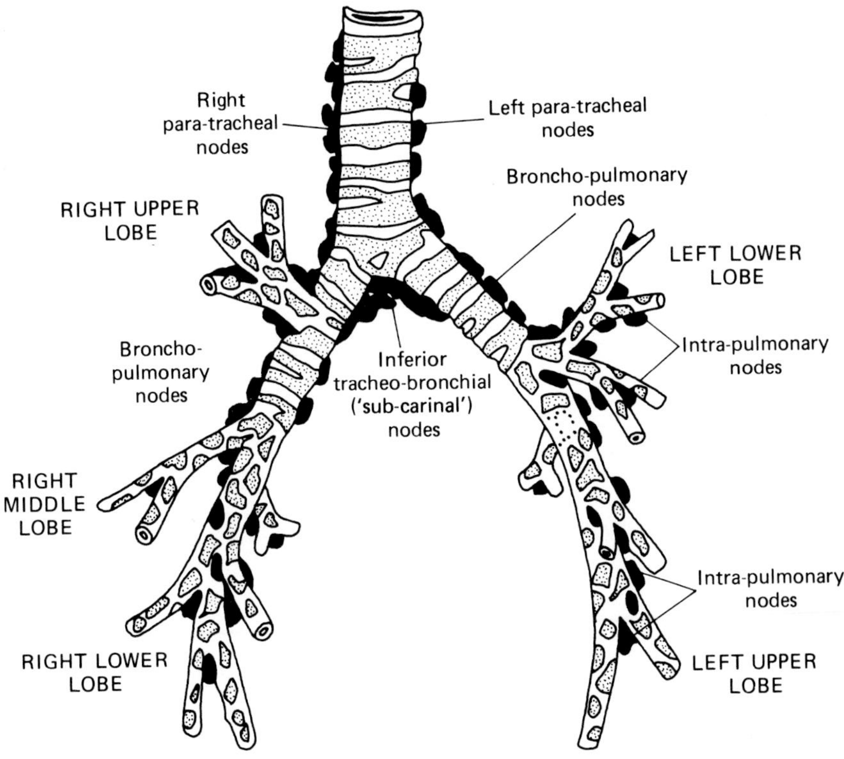

Figure 10.24 Diagram to show the distribution of pulmonary and tracheobronchial lymph nodes

The left superior tracheobronchial nodes lie in close relation to the left main bronchus, the left pulmonary artery and the arch of the aorta. They drain lymph from the greater part of the left lung, and lymphatics from these nodes pass mainly into the left paratracheal nodes.

The important inferior tracheobronchial group of nodes lies between the two main bronchi, and is often referred to as the subcarinal group. There are usually 3–5 nodes in this group; one, which lies immediately beneath the carina and in close relation to the right main bronchus is usually larger than the others, which are related to both main bronchi. The importance of these nodes is that they drain lymph from both lungs, and also that lymphatics from them pass to the paratracheal nodes on both sides. From the clinical aspect, if these nodes become greatly enlarged they will cause widening of the carina and an increase in the interbronchial angle which will be evident to the bronchoscopist. This can be of crucial importance in considering whether a patient with a lung cancer can be offered surgical treatment; if these nodes should be occupied by tumour metastases a curative operation becomes unfeasible.

The right paratracheal group of nodes lies to the right of the trachea in the upper mediastinum and is closely related to the azygos vein and the superior vena cava. They are larger and much more numerous than the left para-tracheal nodes which lie to the left of the trachea and are related to the lower surface and posterior aspect of the arch of the aorta. Both groups drain for the most part into the broncho-mediastinal trunk.

From the above description it will be obvious that it is impossible to determine with any accuracy the area of drainage of any particular group of nodes. The clinical importance of this is that metastases from bronchial carcinoma may cross the midline and appear in lymph nodes on the opposite side of the mediastinum from the primary tumour. It is much more common for a carcinoma of the left lung, and especially the left lower lobe, to cross to the right para-tracheal nodes than for the opposite to occur.

References

Aeby, C. (1880). *Der Bronchialbaum der Saügethiere und der Menschen, nebst Bemerkungen über den Bronchialbaum der Vögel und Reptilien.* Leipzig; Engelman

Azzopardi, A. and Thurlbeck, W. M. (1968). *American Review of Respiratory Disease*, **97**, 1038

Baarsma, P. R., Dirken, M. N. J. and Huizinga, E. (1948). *Journal of Thoracic Surgery*, **17**, 252

Bensch, K., Corrin, B., Pariente, R. and Spencer, H. (1968). *Cancer (Philadelphia)*, **22**, 1163

Berry, J. L. (1935). *Quarterly Journal of Experimental Physiology*, **24**, 305

Berry, J. L. and Daly, I. de B. (1931). *Proceedings of the Royal Society*, B, London, **109**, 319

Bertalanffy, F. D. and Leblond, C. P. (1955). *Lancet*, **2**, 1365

Boyden, E. A. (1955). *Segmental Anatomy of the Lungs.* New York; McGraw-Hill

Braus, H. (1934). *Anatomie des Menschen*, 2nd edn, Vol. 2, Berlin. Quoted by Marchand *et al.* (1950)

Brock, R. C. (1946). *The Anatomy of the Bronchial Tree.* London; Oxford University Press

Broman, I. (1923). *Verhandlung der Anatomische Gesellschaft* (Jena), **23**, 83

Broyles, E. N. (1943). 'The anterior commissure tendon', *Annals of Otology, Rhinology and Laryngology*, **52**, 342

Bucher, U. and Reid, L. (1961a). *Thorax*, **16**, 207

Bucher, U. and Reid, L. (1961b). *Thorax*, **16**, 219

Campbell, E. J. M. and Howell, J. B. L. (1962). *Pulmonary Structure and Function* (Ciba Foundation Symposium). London; Churchill

Cauldwell, E. W., Siekert, R. G., Lininger, R. E. and Anson, B. J. (1948). *Surgery, Gynecology and Obstetrics*, **86**, 395

Churchill, E. D. and Belsey, R. (1939). *Annals of Surgery*, **109**, 481

Clara, M. (1937). *Zeitschrift für mikroskopisch-anatomische Forschung* **41**, 321

Cudkowicz, L. and Armstrong, J. B. (1951). *Thorax*, **6**, 343

Cudmore, R. E., Emery, J. L. and Mithal, A. (1962). *Archives of Disease in Childhood*, **37**, 481

Daly, I. de B. (1935–6). *Harvey Lecture*, **31**, 235

Davies, G. and Reid, L. (1970). *Thorax*, **25**, 669

Dickey, J. S. (1911). *Applied Anatomy of the Lungs and Pleural Membranes.* Belfast; Mayne and Boyd

Diemerbroeck, I. van (1685). *Opera omnia, anatomica et medica*, Utrecht

Dunnill, M. S. (1962). *Thorax*, **17**, 329

Emery, J. (1969). *The Anatomy of the Developing Lung.* London; Heinemann

Emery, J. L. and Mithal, A. (1960). *Archives of Disease in Childhood*, **35**, 544

Engel, S. (1947). *The Child's Lung.* London; Arnold

Engel, S. (1962). *Lung Structure.* Springfield, Ill.: Thomas

Ewart, W. (1882). *British Medical Journal*, **i**, 453

Ewart, W. (1889). *The Bronchi and Pulmonary Blood Vessels; their Anatomy and Nomenclature.* London; Baillière, Tindall and Cox

Felix, W. (1920). In *Die Chirurgie der Brustorgane*, 2nd Edn (Ed. by Sauerbrach, F.). Berlin; Springer

Felix, W. (1928). In *Die Chirurgie der Brustorgane*, 3rd Edn (Ed. by Sauerbrach, F.). Berlin; Springer

Feyrter, F. (1953). *Über die peripheren endokrinen (parakrinen) Drüsen des Menschen.* Wien, Düsseldorf; Maudrich

Fisher, A. W. F. (1964). *Journal of Anatomy, London*, **98**, 117

Foster-Carter, A. F. (1942). *British Journal of Tuberculosis*, **36**, 19

Fröhlich, F. (1949). *Frankfurter Zeitschrift für Pathologie*, **60**, 517

Hasse, C. (1892). *Archiv für Anatomie und Entwicklungsgeschichte.* 324

Hately, W., Evison, B. and Samuel, E. (1965). 'The

pattern of ossification in the laryngeal cartilages', *British Journal of Radiology*, **38**, 585
Hayek, H. von (1960). *The Human Lung*. New York; Hafner
Hayward, J. and Reid, L. M. (1952). *Thorax*, **7**, 89
Hieronymi, G. (1960). *Verhandlung der deutschen Gesellschaft für Pathologie*, **44**, 129
Huntington, G. S. (1920). *American Journal of Anatomy*, **27**, 99
International Committee (1950). *Thorax*, **5**, 222
Jackson, C. L. and Huber, J. E. (1943). *Diseases of the Chest*, **9**, 319
Jelihovsky, T. (1972). *Pathology*, **4**, 65
Jesseph, J. E. and Merendino, K. A. (1957). *Surgery, Gynecology and Obstetrics*, **105**, 210
Karrer, H. E. (1956). *Journal of Biophysical and Biochemical Cytology*, **2**, 241
Kramer, K. and Glass, A. (1932). *Annals of Otology, Rhinology and Laryngology, St. Louis*, **41**, 1210
Lambert, M. (1955). *Journal of Pathology and Bacteriology*, **70**, 311
Liebow, A. A., Hales, M. R. and Lindskog, G. E. (1949). *American Journal of Pathology*, **25**, 211
Liebow, A. A. (1962). *Medicina Thoracalis*, **19**, 609
Loosli, C. G. and Potter, E. L. (1959). *American Review of Respiratory Diseases*, **80**, 5
Low, F. N. (1953). *Anatomical Record*, **117**, 241
Low, F. N. (1961). *Anatomical Record*, **139**, 105
Lucien, M. and Weber, P. (1936). *Archives d'Anatomie d'Histologie et-d'Embryologie*, **21**, 109
Luschka, H. von (1863). *Die Anatomie der Brust des Menschen*, Tübingen: Laupp and Siebeck
Marchand, P., Gilroy, J. C. and Wilson, V. H. (1950). *Thorax*, **5**, 207
Miller, W. S. (1947). *The Lung*, 2nd Edn. Springfield, Ill.; Thomas
Negus, V. E. (1958). *The Comparative Anatomy of the Nose and the Paranasal Sinuses*. Edinburgh; Livingstone
Neil, J. H., Gilmour, W., Gwynne, F. J., Main, W. and Fairclough, W. A. (1937). *Annals of Otology, Rhinology and Laryngology, St. Louis*, **46**, 338
Nelson, H. P. (1932). *Journal of Anatomy, London*, **66**, 228
Nelson, H. P. (1934). *British Medical Journal*, **ii**, 251
Niden, A. H. and Yamaha, E. (1966). *Proceedings of the VIth International Congress for Electron Microscopy*. Tokyo; Maruzen
Pearse, A. G. E. (1966). *Nature, London*, **211**, 598
Reid, L. (1967). In *Development of the Lung* (Ciba Foundation Symposium), p. 109. London; Churchill
Reid, L. and Rubino, M. (1959). *Thorax*, **14**, 3
Reuck, A. V. S. de and Porter, R. (1967). *Development of the Lung*. London; Churchill
Richards, D. (1962). In *Pulmonary Structure and Function* (Ciba Foundation Symposium), p. 26. London; Churchill
Scarpelli, E. M. (1968). *The Surfactant Systems of the Lung*. Philadelphia; Lea and Fibinger
Schulz, H. (1959). *Submicroscopy of the Lung*. Berlin; Springer
Short, R. H. D. (1952). *Proceedings of the Royal Society*, B, **140**, 432
Simer, P. H. (1952). *Anatomical Record*, **113**, 269
Smith, P., Heath, D. and Moosavi, H. (1974). *Thorax*, **29**, 147
Spencer, H. (1977). *Pathology of the Lung*, 3rd Edn. Oxford; Pergamon Press
Stell, P. M. and Watt, J. (1977). 'Morphology of the laryngeal epithelium', *Clinical Otolaryngology* (in press)
Tobin, C. E. (1954). *Anatomical Record*, **120**, 625
Tobin, C. E. (1957). *Anatomical Record*, **127**, 611
Trapnell, D. H. (1963). *British Journal of Radiology*, **36**, 660
Tucker, J. A., Vidic, B., Tucker, G. F. and Stead, J. (1976). 'Survey of the development of laryngeal epithelium', *Annals of Otology, Rhinology and Laryngology*, Supplement 30
Turner, R. S. (1962). *Anatomical Record*, **143**, 189
Vanpeperstraete, F. (1973). 'The cartilaginous skeleton of the bronchial tree', *Advances in Anatomy, Embryology and Cell Biology*, **48**, 3
Van Allen, C. M., Lindskog, G. E. and Richter, H. G. (1929–30). *Yale Journal of Biology and Medicine*, **2**, 297
Weibel, E. R. (1961). *Federation Proceedings: Federation of American Societies for Experimental Biology*, **20**, 425
Weibel, E. R. (1963). *Morphometry of the Human Lung*. Berlin; Springer
Weibel, E. R. and Gomez, D. M. (1962). *Science, New York*, **21**, 163
Widdicombe, J. G. (1961). *Clinical Science*, **21**, 163

11 Physiology of the larynx and tracheobronchial tree

P M Stell and C C Evans

The larynx

Introduction

The comparative anatomy of the larynx exhaustively studied by Negus (1929) is described in his classic monograph. With the first development in evolution of primitive lung buds arising from the floor of the pharynx in lung fish, a protective sphincter of circular muscle appears to protect the lungs from the entry of water. This protective mechanism is represented at first by the contraction and relaxation of a circular muscle band encircling the mouth of this pulmonary outgrowth. When the fish is on land the sphincter relaxes to allow air to be taken in. Later, in higher forms, the mechanism becomes more complex and separate dilator muscles are evolved. These increase the efficiency of opening of the narrow aperture in the pharynx leading to the air-passages. Cartilaginous structures are later evolved as points of origin for these muscles. Further, the larynx acquires function as a check valve to retain air that has been taken in. In certain species, but not in man, the larynx is concerned in olfaction. In these animals the upper larynx and epiglottis extend into the nasopharynx. A backward extension of the soft palate is developed. This makes contact with the upward projecting epiglottis, thus separating the nasal and laryngeal airway from the oral and pharyngeal food channel. This makes it possible for respiration and olfaction to continue during feeding. To these respiratory, protective, valvular, and olfactory functions, the highly complex physiological activity of sound production or phonation is added much later in evolution. This attains its highest development in human speech.

Functions of the larynx

The physiology of the larynx has been comprehensively reviewed by Pressman and Kelemen (1955) who have made notable contributions to knowledge in this field.

The functions of the larynx may be broadly classified:

(1) Respiratory air channel and air flow regulation.
(2) Circulatory function in promoting venous return.
(3) Sphincteric functions:
  (a) fixation of thorax;
  (b) tussive and expectorative;
  (c) protective closure in swallowing and vomiting.
(4) Receptive field for reflexes, for example cough reflex.
(5) Phonation and speech.

Respiratory function

The larynx is part of the tubular system of airways for the passage of air to and from the lungs in breathing. Within the larynx, at the glottis, the cross-sectional area of the respiratory airway is smaller than at any other level. It thus plays a role in determining the resistance to air flow which is related inversely to diameter. During normal respiration the cords are relaxed and halfway between adduction and full abduction. The vocal folds in some individuals abduct slightly in inspiration and adduct slightly during expiration. Thus the lumen of the larynx at this point narrows in expiration and widens in inspiration. This movement of the vocal cords is usually very slight in the resting subject but increases in amplitude with increasing depth of breathing. With very deep breathing, as in violent exercise, the cords may be abducted almost flush with the lateral wall so that the resistance to air flow is reduced to a minimum. It has also been suggested that the larynx has a more intimate relation to the chemical regulation of breathing than the function of serving as a conduit for air. It is claimed that the glottis is under constant reflex adjustment in response to changes in the chemical composition of the blood. In particular, the factors suggested as controlling the position of the cords are the pH and the pCO_2 of the blood. In this way the larynx could serve, to a minor extent, as a supplementary control of the ventilation of the alveolar surface of the lungs, to maintain the constancy of the acid–base equilibrium of the body fluids.

In addition to these intralaryngeal movements of the vocal cords, a slight motion of the larynx as a whole during breathing has been described. During inspiration the larynx descends due to contraction of the infrahyoid muscles and to the descent of the diaphragm and the increased negative pressure in the thorax. At the same time the hilum of the lung moves downwards and forwards to facilitate ventilation of the apical and paravertebral parts of the lung. The larynx also sometimes is displaced slightly backwards in inspiration. There may also be present in some subjects a lateral deviation, invariably to the left.

Sphincteric functions

Laryngeal sphincters

The sphincter mechanisms of the larynx have been divided, from the functional viewpoint, into three successive physiological sphincters superimposed at different anatomical levels. These sphincters in cephalocaudal order are:

(1) The aryepiglottic folds.
(2) The ventricular folds or false vocal cords.
(3) The vocal folds or true vocal cords.

These sphincters are structurally adapted for each to serve a distinctive specialized function, while functioning collectively to prevent ingress of foreign material.

Aryepiglottic inlet sphincter The first tier of the triple laryngeal sphincter mechanisms lies at the level of the superior inlet of the larynx. This sphincter separates the pharynx from the vestibule of the larynx. The aditus to the larynx which it guards faces posteriorly and is almost vertically placed. This is the aryepiglottic sphincter consisting of a pair of thick fibromuscular, vertical aryepiglottic folds extending from the arytenoid cartilages posteriorly to the lateral border of the epiglottis. The muscle component within these folds is derived from the thyro-arytenoid, and the interarytenoid muscles. When this muscle of the epiglottic folds contracts the folds are approximated into contact to close the laryngeal inlet (*Figure 11.1*). The closure of these folds is stabilized by the presence within each fold posteriorly of a vertical rod of yellow elastic cartilage (cuneiform cartilage), acting as props. This sphincteric closure is completed anteriorly by the tubercle of the epiglottis and posteriorly by the bodies of the arytenoid cartilages. Thus the contraction of the muscle brings the aryepiglottic folds together. This sphincter closes during deglutition and vomiting. It prevents the entry of food, fluid, other accidentally swallowed material, or vomitus, into the respiratory tract.

False vocal cord sphincter (ventricular folds) The false vocal cord, on the lateral wall of the laryngeal cavity on each side, is a horizontal fold between the supraglottic part or vestibule of the larynx and the ventricle of the larynx. Each fold has a free medial border which slopes lightly downwards. The folds extend from the angle of the thyroid cartilage above the attachment of the true vocal cords, to the anterolateral surface of the arytenoid cartilages. At rest the folds do not project as far medially into the laryngeal cavity as do the true vocal cords. The inferior surface of the folds is flat while the superior surface slopes obliquely upwards and outwards fiom the medial free margins. The main substance of the fold is fibrous and elastic tissue, covered with ciliated pseudostratified columnar epithelium with mucous glands. The fibrous tissue of the fold is thickened to form a ventricular ligament. When the muscle fibres external to the ventricular ligaments contract the medial borders of the folds are approximated into contact. At the same time the bodies of the arytenoid cartilages also approximate. This constitutes the false vocal cord sphincter.

The muscular closure of this sphincter is shown in *Figure 11.2* from the detailed cinematographic study by Pressman. The true vocal folds close first. These establish contact progressively from before backwards. This is followed by a similar adduction and closure of the false vocal folds. Short segments of the most posterior part of the false vocal cords first come together representing the initial approximation and inward rotation of the arytenoid cartilages by the interarytenoid muscle, together with the thyro-arytenoid and the lateral crico-arytenoid muscles. Then the false vocal cords approximate and their edges make contact, beginning at their anterior ends and progressing smoothly along the folds to the posterior end. The closure is finally completed by a forward tilt of the arytenoids plugging the small gap at the posterior end of the folds.

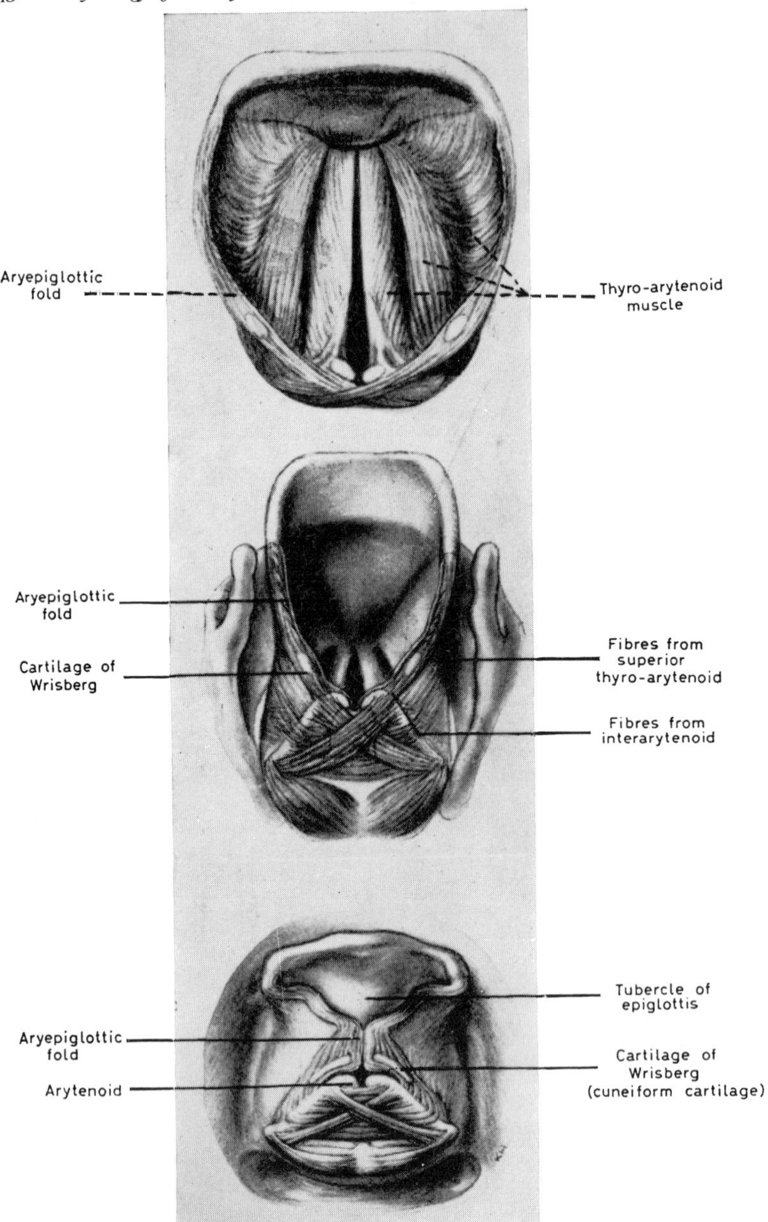

Figure 11.1 Closure of aryepiglottic sphincter. (From Pressman, 1954, reproduced by courtesy of the Editor of *Archives of Otolaryngology*)

The time relations of this laryngeal closure naturally vary with its cause. In the cough reflex the approximation of the false vocal folds is very rapid and the period of closure is very brief. In voluntary closure, as in thoracic fixation, the movements are slow and the closure persists as long as the act is maintained.

The design of the ventricular folds indicates that they could also function as purely mechanical exit valves preventing the outflow of air from the lungs. By virtue of their

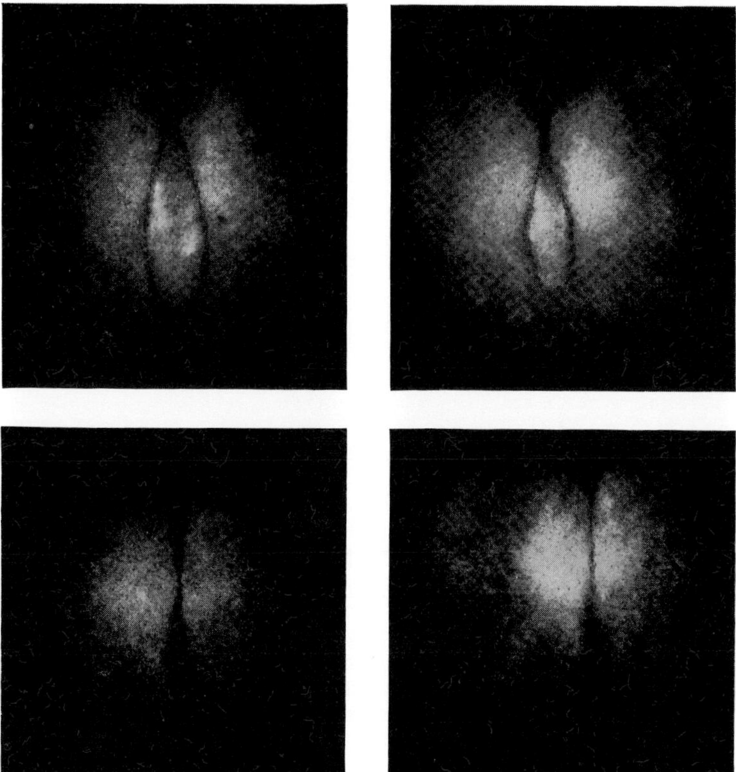

Figure 11.2 Closure of false vocal cord sphincter (modified from Pressman, 1954).

shape the folds, acting as flaps of the valve, would become more firmly wedged together the greater the rise of intratracheal pressure. The greater the pressure gradient between the inferior or glottic and the superior or vestibular surfaces of these folds, the more securely the valve is sealed. On the other hand the position and shape of the valves precludes any effective action as a mechanical valve preventing air entry in the opposite direction, i.e. when the pharyngeal pressure increases or the infraglottic pressure decreases. Closure of this sphincter is invariably accompanied by the preceding closure of the true vocal folds. This latter valve at the true vocal cords is mechanically ineffective if the intratracheal pressure is raised.

The physiological role of the false vocal cords can be considered under two headings.

(1) The main function is as part of the mechanism for increasing the intrathoracic pressure, by blocking the outflow of air while the air trapped in the lungs is compressed by contraction of the muscles of expiration. This serves to produce the pressurized air for the high velocity blast of air in coughing and sneezing. This mechanism is also an essential part of thoracic fixation when the intra-abdominal pressure is raised, as in physiological acts of micturition, defaecation, parturition and vomiting. This action is more dependent on the mechanical valve effect, based on the physical design of the folds, than on muscular contraction. But the

valvular mechanism requires for its effective operation that the margins of the valve are apposed by active muscular contraction.

(2) A supplementary function is as a second line of defence beyond the aryepiglottic inlet sphincter, in preventing by reflex closure, ingress of foreign material or food into the lower respiratory airway.

The efficiency of this sphincter is demonstrated by the fact that it forms an adequate sphincter mechanism even after excision of the true vocal folds.

The true vocal cord sphincter (*vocal folds*) These fibromuscular folds extend from the angle between the laminae of the thyroid cartilage just above its midpoint, to the vocal processes of the arytenoid cartilages. The fibrous element is condensed at the medial border of the vocal fold with the elastic tissue of the upper thickened border of the conus elasticus. The muscular element is the thyro-arytenoid muscle. The upper surface of the shelf-like vocal fold is flat, while the lower surface is curved with the concavity directed downwards. This shape provides a more efficient valve for preventing entry than a simple circular sphincter muscle alone. However, the dome-shaped under-surface of the folds concentrates the infraglottic air-pressure on to the sloping free margins of the folds. This has the effect of readily forcing the cords apart. Thus on a purely mechanical basis the true vocal cords cannot serve as an efficient valve preventing outflow of air, although extremely effective as a sphincter preventing inflow of air (*Figure 11.3*).

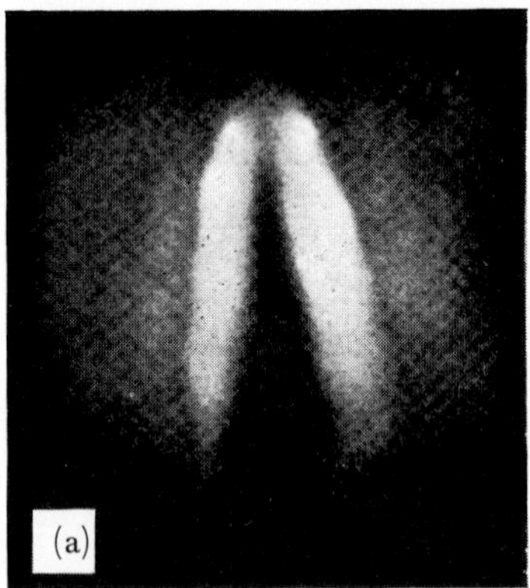

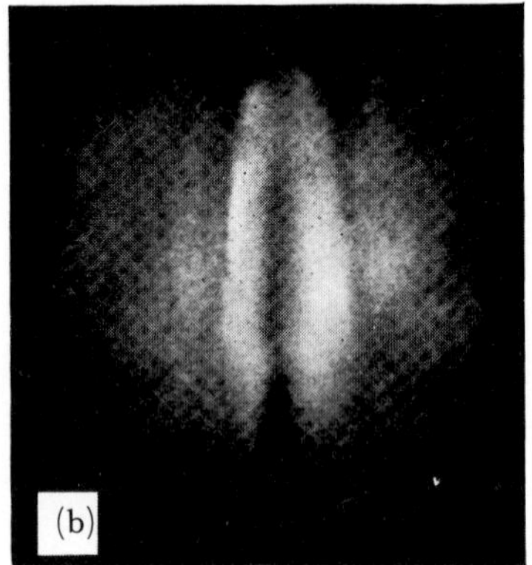

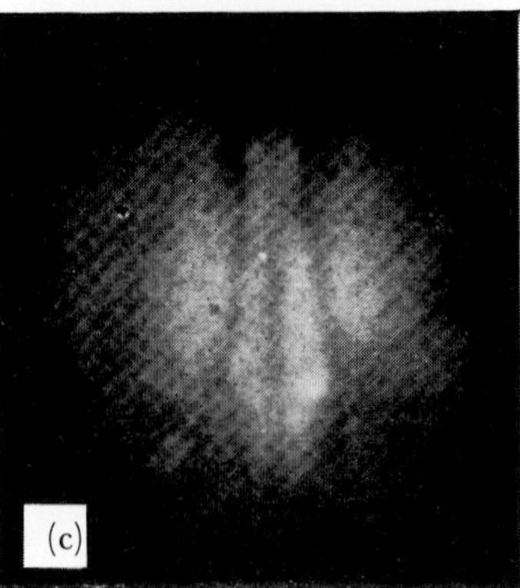

Figure 11.3 Closure of true vocal cord sphincter. (From Pressman, 1954, reproduced by courtesy of the Editor of *Archives of Otolaryngology*)

Summary of mechanisms of laryngeal closure

The laryngeal apparatus can be divided into three parts, situated at three anatomical levels: (a) the aryepiglottic sphincter at the laryngeal inlet; (b) the ventricular folds at the lower border of the vestibule of the larynx, and separated by the ventricle of the larynx from (c) the vocal folds which form the lower border of the ventricle separating it from the infraglottic larynx.

The operation of these 'sphincters' depends on either one or both of two mechanisms. These are (a) physiological, that is, a sphincter based on the functional activity of muscle; (b) mechanical, that is, a valve mechanism based on the physical shape, position and design of the valvular folds.

A muscular sphincter is present in each of the three tiers or levels in the larynx. These may contract together or independently. All three may act together, as for example, during deglutition. The false and true vocal folds may close together without closure of the aryepiglottic sphincter, as is observed during laryngoscopy. The false vocal cords cannot be closed independently of the true vocal cords. On the other hand the true vocal cords adduct without closure of the other two sphincters during phonation.

Mechanical valvular mechanisms are present at the false and true vocal folds but not at the aryepiglottic sphincter level. This mechanical action provides a more resistant and powerful valve than the contraction of the sphincter muscle alone. But muscle contraction is essential for effective operation of the folds as a mechanical valve.

In the false vocal cords the effect of the mechanical valve is to prevent outflow of air. The greater the outflow pressure applied to the valve the greater is its resistance. They have no useful mechanical action in impeding inflow.

In the true vocal folds the mechanical principle acts in the opposite direction, preventing inflow. They can resist inflow against pharyngeal pressures of 150 mmHg, but they offer no significant mechanical barrier to the outflow of air.

The unidirectional nature of these valves is a property of their shape. The false vocal cords have flat lower surfaces and pressure on this surface is uniformly distributed. Their upper surfaces slope obliquely. Pressure applied from above to this surface is maximally deflected onto the free margins which are therefore readily forced apart. The true vocal cords have flat upper surfaces while the lower surfaces are curved and sloping and thus not designed to resist pressures from below.

Functions of the sphincter mechanisms

Functions of the sphincter mechanisms include:

(1) Reflex protection against entry of foreign material into the tracheobronchial tree by closure of the sphincters.

(2) Inlet check valve to permit thoracic fixation during the contraction of the muscles of the pectoral girdle arising from the ribs. This ensures that the force of contraction of these muscles, during such voluntary acts as pulling on a rope or pulling the trunk upwards to the arms as in climbing, is applied effectively to achieving the desired movement and is not partially dissipated in expanding the chest. This function has however been disputed.

(3) Outlet check valve in the production of raised intrathoracic and intra-abdominal pressure: (a) this function is seen in the building up of intratracheal pressure for explosive release in reflex coughing and sneezing; (b) the outlet sphincter closes to prevent air being forced out during contraction of the muscles of the anterior abdominal wall with the attendant rise of intra-abdominal pressure in defaecation, micturition, parturition and straining, as in lifting very heavy weights. Here the laryngeal closure traps the air in the lungs and ensures that the force of contraction of the abdominal muscles is devoted to raising the intra-abdominal pressure and is not dissipated in causing a forcible ascent of the diaphragm and forcing air out of the lungs. X-ray studies have confirmed that an increased elevation of the domes of the diaphragm is produced during straining, if the laryngeal sphincters are prevented from effective closure by intubation or tracheotomy. With the larynx open, the capacity to raise the intra-abdominal pressure by active contraction of the abdominal muscles is reduced by 20 per cent.

Function in deglutition

The changes in the larynx which occur in deglutition may be briefly summarized here.

(1) Elevation of the larynx towards the base of the tongue is brought about by the contraction of the inferior constrictor, palatopharyngeus and stylopharyngeus muscles. This laryngeal elevation may help to grasp the bolus and to bring the pharyngo-oesophageal opening up towards the bolus.
(2) Cessation of laryngeal airflow by reflex inhibition of respiration.
(3) Contraction of the three-tiered muscular sphincter mechanisms in the larynx. This is part of the reflex response to the stimulation of the pharyngeal deglutition receptors. This reflex laryngeal closure may be further reinforced by reflex sphincter contraction from stimulation of mechanoreceptors in the mucosa in the region of the laryngeal inlet.
(4) The epiglottis tilts over to close the opening to the larynx, and the shape of its upper surface assists in deflecting and guiding the swallowed material onwards.

Phonation

The human larynx is a highly modified portion of the airway, extending between the pharynx and the trachea. Voice can be produced in this tubular organ by the vocal cords vibrating in an expiratory blast of air. This vibration of the cords effectively chops the air stream into a series of rhythmical segments or puffs. This produces a complex motion of the air column consisting of a fundamental tone and overtones. This complex of sound frequencies is modified by the resonators and vocal cavities to impart to it its characteristic quality or wave-form. Changes in the shape of the resonating vocal cavities can transform the laryngeal sound into the various vowel and consonant sounds which constitute the vocal components for speech. In this way man has utilized sound production in the larynx to provide an elaborate communication code for conveying thoughts and information to others. This power of speech has contributed greatly to man's ascendancy over other species, and to his commanding position in the animal kingdom.

Before considering the phonatory function of the larynx some elementary points about the physics of sound must be very briefly mentioned, since any acceptable explanation of the mechanism of phonation must accord with these known physical facts about sound.

Sounds are vibrations which excite the peripheral auditory apparatus and evoke an auditory sensation. They are alternate phases of compression and rarefaction of the particles of the air or other medium through which the sound is being conducted. These particles vibrate longitudinally, that is, their motion is forward and backward in the direction of propagation of the sound.

These phases of compression and rarefaction are conventionally represented as a 'wave', with the horizontal axis representing time, and the displacement of the curve above the mean line representing the period of compression and the portions of the curve below the line representing the phase of rarefaction. The amplitude of the displacement above or below the mean line denotes the intensity or energy level of the sound.

These sound 'waves' which produce a sensation we call hearing are divided into two classes: (1) sounds which are quite irregular in character called noise; and (2) sounds of smooth and regular rhythmic changes called musical sounds.

Vibratory movements and the sound waves they produce can vary in: (a) amplitude; (b) frequency; (c) wave-form; (d) duration; (e) phase.

These physical properties of sound are important in the production of sound by the larynx because they determine the loudness, pitch and quality (or timbre) of the laryngeal sound.

The *intensity* of a sound is the physical force or strength of the sound, and is a function of the total amount of energy or absolute pressure of the phases of compression and rarefaction constituting the sound. This intensity may be expressed quantitatively as the power measured in watts/unit area of 1 cm^2, or as a pressure determined in dynes/cm^2. This property of sound is conventionally denoted by the amplitude of the sound 'waves'. The intensity range of the sounds produced by the human larynx is from 0.001 mW/cm^2 in whispering, to 1000 mW/cm^2 in loud shouting. The width of this range can be appreciated from the fact that the standard threshold of hearing for the human ear is taken as corresponding to 0.0002 dynes/cm^2 at a frequency of 1000 Hz.

Loudness is a physiological attribute equivalent to the physical property of intensity of sound. This sensory experience called loudness is the basis of the sensory judgment involved in assessing the relative physical power of the sound, that is, in placing the sound in a scale from soft to very loud. When the intensity of a sound is very low the sound gives rise to no sensory percept and is inaudible. As the intensity of the sound is gradually increased, then a threshold value is reached when the sound is just perceived. As the physical intensity is further increased the progressive increments in intensity of the note are recognized as progressive increases in loudness.

The relation between intensity and loudness is not completely independent of other factors, for the pitch of a note modifies its loudness. When two sounds of different pitch are matched by the human ear as being of equivalent loudness, they will not be of the same intensity. The threshold intensity of sound as perceived by the human auditory apparatus varies with the frequency of the sound as shown in the chart of the intensity and frequency characteristics for the human ear. The loudness of a sound is usually expressed in clinical practice by the logarithm of the ratio of the energy of the sound to the energy of a reference sound which is taken as a tone of 1000 Hz at the audibility threshold for the human ear. The unit in this range for some more common sounds is shown in *Figure 11.4*. An increase of 1 dB implies a 26 per cent increase in power, while 10 dB means a tenfold increase in power and 20 dB is equivalent to a one hundred times increase in power. The minimum increase in power which can be perceived as an increase in loudness is approximately 1 dB at about 1000 Hz.

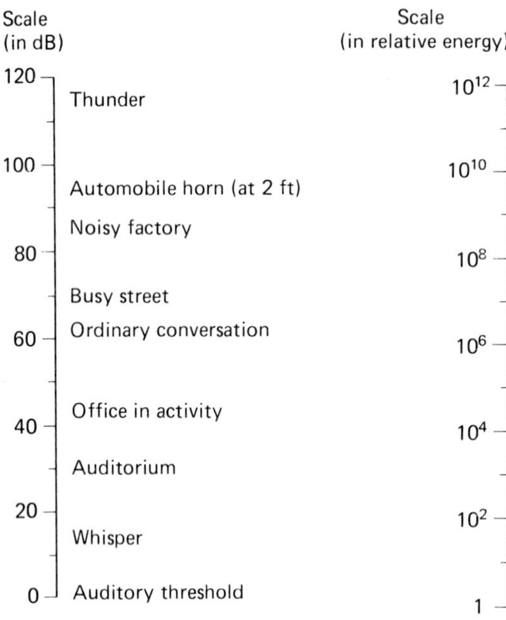

Figure 11.4 Intensity of human voice relative to some common sounds

Pitch is the physiological property which permits the placing of a note in the scale from low to high. It is related to the frequency of the vibrations expressed in cycles per second (Hz). This frequency is the rate of repetition of the vibrations. The time duration of one complete cycle is called the period of the vibration. This period is the reciprocal of the frequency since the greater the number of cycles per second, the shorter is the duration of each cycle. The relation between pitch and frequency is not absolute, for the intensity of a sound modifies the pitch. This is seen when a tuning fork vibrating at a steady frequency is moved gradually closer to the ear, the increase in intensity resulting from the inverse square law (intensity is inversely proportional to the square of the distance), is accompanied by a fall in the pitch of the sound.

Normal human voices cover a pitch range from 82 to 1175 Hz (about 4 octaves) (*Figure 11.5*). Musical instruments produce sounds ranging in pitch over 7 octaves from 25 to 8500 Hz. The auditory pitch spectrum for the human ear extends from 16 to 20 000 Hz; that is, 11 octaves.

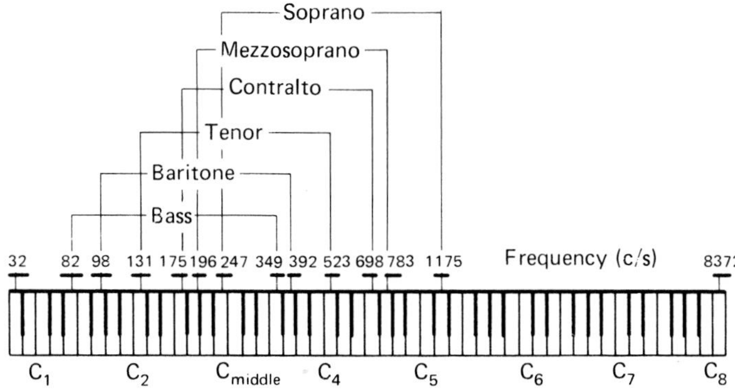

Figure 11.5 Range of pitch of human voice

Quality or timbre Musical notes of the same pitch and intensity when produced by different instruments can be distinguished. Timbre is that quality of a sound by which this distinctiveness is perceived. Sound produced by a vibrating body is seldom of a single frequency. It is invariably a complex of several tones. The tone of lowest frequency and greatest amplitude or intensity is the fundamental tone. In addition overtones or harmonics are present. They are of higher frequency (that is, low integral multiples of the fundamental frequency) and are of lesser intensity. The characteristic quality or timbre depends on the number, frequency and relative intensity of these overtones. The quality of a sound is represented diagrammatically by its wave-form.

Resonance
When sound waves of a particular pitch reach any structure or cavity, whose natural fundamental frequency of vibration is the same as that of the incident sound, then that structure will vibrate. In this way a sound vibration of low intensity may become amplified in volume, or reinforced, by causing a large cavity to vibrate by resonance. Some resonators are of limited sensitivity range, vibrating only to a narrow range of frequencies; others may respond to a wider range.

Voice production

The production of voice by the larynx requires three mechanisms.

(1) The respiratory bellows, which produce the expiratory blast of a high-pressure column of air.
(2) The vibrating mechanism in the larynx.
(3) The resonating chambers in the thorax and pharynx, mouth and nasal chambers.

The mechanism of voice production with particular reference to singing is described in Volume 4.

The respiratory bellows: high pressure subglottic column of air

The high-pressure column of air is essential to phonation. This is provided by the contraction of the muscles of expiration in the thorax and abdominal wall. Immediately before phonation the cords are adducted and tensed. The muscles of expiration contract and compress the thorax, with a rise in the thoracic and infraglottic pressures. These contractions of the abdominal and thoracic muscles have been studied by electromyography. When the pressure reaches an adequate level the cords are set vibrating with the production of a laryngeal sound.

The essential nature of this high-pressure subglottic column of air is confirmed by several facts. Sounds can be produced in the excised or cadaver larynx, if the cords are artificially tensed and adducted and then a blast of air of adequate pressure forced through. In patients with an open tracheostomy, where this pressure of air cannot be achieved, phonation is not possible unless the stoma is closed.

The force or magnitude of the air pressure generated in the subglottic space determines the intensity or volume of sound produced. The loudness of the sound is almost directly proportional to the force of the blast of air.

The vibrating mechanism: the vocal folds of the larynx

The larynx is the modified upper portion of the trachea extending to the pharynx. The vibrating structures essential for phonation are the true vocal folds. In some respects the larynx resembles a reed instrument in which a moving column of air forces an elastic tongue to vibrate. In this musical instrument the frequency of vibrations, and therefore the pitch of the note, is determined by the length of the reed and by the length of the tube of the instrument. In the larynx the pitch of the note produced depends on the period of vibration of the cords. This is varied by a number of factors.

(1) Regulation of the tension of the vocal cords.
(2) Variation in the length of the segment of the vocal folds that is actually vibrating.
(3) Adjustment of the shape of the free margins of the vocal cords. These may vary from broad and thick to thin and narrow. This alteration of the contour of the cord margins, which is a feature of the different registers of the voice, is accomplished by the action of the internal fibres of the thyro-arytenoid muscles.
(4) The pressure of the infraglottic column of air being forced through the vibrating cords. The pitch of the laryngeal tone rises with increasing force of the blast if the cord tension remains constant. Hence when a sustained note is increased in loudness, the increasing pressure for the crescendo must be precisely compensated by a reduced tension in the cords.

Resonating mechanism

The tone produced in the larynx is weak and non-resonant. Modification and enhancement of the overtones in the laryngeal tone is produced by the resonating mechanisms. This gives the voice its characteristic richness and fullness of quality. The resonators are the air-spaces of the lungs and trachea, and the supralaryngeal resonators of the pharynx, oral cavity, nasal chambers and sinuses. These resonators increase the volume of the feeble laryngeal sound, reinforce some of its overtones and thus give the voice its individual quality. This is represented by the complex waveform of the sound. Thus the voice of any individual has its characteristic timbre by which it is recognized by those who have heard it previously. In this way too the voice of two individuals singing the same note can be distinguished. Thus speech involves a complex integrated neuromuscular mechanism combining the muscles involved in phonation, articulation and resonance. The quality of the voice alters with disease or malformation of the resonators. Characteristic defects in the quality of voice and speech occur in hyperplasia of nasopharyngeal lymphoid tissue, cleft palate, hare lip and dental malocclusion.

The walls of these resonators are partly mobile, as in the soft palate, tongue, cheeks and lips. The resonators are consequently not static but dynamic. The shape and volume of the resonators can be changed by voluntary contractions of appropriate muscles. Modification of these resonators of the pharynx and mouth by the lips, tongue and palate is a mechanism in the articulation of vowels and consonant sounds that constitute speech. A characteristic shape of the resonating chamber for each vowel sound has been described. In formation of some consonants the laryngeal tone amplified in the resonators is modified by various stops, partial or complete, of the blast of expired air at some point in the airway as at the palate, teeth or lips. In others the vibrating column of air is forced through a narrow passage between tongue and palate. In each case the laryngeal tone may be present or absent. In nasal consonants the mouth is closed and the vibrating column of air is blown out through the nasal chambers. The complex adjustments of the position of the tongue, palate and lips involved in adjusting the shape and volume of the supralaryngeal resonants during articulation, are studied by combining x-rays of different regions outlined by radio-opaque materials, with cinematographic films and oscillographic sound recordings. Such studies have shown that there are, for example, considerable individual differences in the position of the tongue in pronouncing the same sound. Furthermore there appears to be greater variability in these movements in the same individual than had been previously believed.

Speech may be summarized as the production of sound by the larynx (phonation), and the modification of this sound by resonance of the supralaryngeal air spaces (articulation).

Methods of study

Knowledge of the mechanism of the larynx has been considerably advanced in the last 30 years by the application of modern techniques of observing and recording its movements. These methods include laryngoscopy, stroboscopy, cineradiography, cinematography, radiology, tape recordings, phonography, spirometry, glottography, oscillography and electromyography. A notable contribution was the slow motion film of *The Human Vocal Cords* by the laboratories of the Bell Telephone Company. In this slowing, by a factor of 1 to 250, the movements of the true vocal cords were clearly demonstrated.

Vocal cords during phonation

The production of a laryngeal tone is associated with vibration of the cords. The cords are first approximated and rendered tense by contraction of the intrinsic and extrinsic musculature of the larynx. This adduction of the cords is due to the approximation of the arytenoid cartilages by the transverse arytenoid muscles and by medial rotation of the arytenoid cartilages by the lateral crico-arytenoid and thyro-arytenoid muscles. The arytenoid cartilages are supported, and the thyroid and cricoid cartilages are maintained in their correct relative positions, by the tonic contraction of the posterior crico-arytenoid and cricothyroid muscles. Thus four basic movements are involved in the adduction of the vocal cords for phonation, as for closure of the sphincter at this level. (1) The external fibres of the thyro-arytenoid muscle and the lateral crico-arytenoid inserted on the muscular process of the arytenoid will rotate the cartilage and so adduct the vocal processes and their attached vocal ligaments. (2) the arytenoid cartilages are approximated by the interarytenoid muscles. (3) The tension of the vocal cords is increased by contraction of the cricothyroid muscle. Contraction of this muscle draws the anterior ring of the cricoid up under the lower margin of the anterior part of the thyroid cartilage, so that the cricoid lamina behind (with the arytenoid cartilages) is drawn backwards, so increasing the length and tension of the vocal cords. (4) During these movements the arytenoid cartilages are kept firmly on the articular facets on the thyroid laminae, against the pull of the thyro-arytenoids, by the posterior crico-arytenoid muscles; and the cricoid itself is braced by contraction of the inferior pharyngeal constrictor. The infraglottic pressure rises as a result of contraction of expiratory muscles.

The adducted tense vocal cords are set vibrating during phonation. Studies with high-speed cinematography at 4000 frames per second (Bell Telephone Company) have demonstrated that the vibrations of the vocal folds in phonation are not merely simple horizontal separations and approximations of the vocal folds (*Figure 11.6*). The vocal folds are seen in slow motion to execute a movement in which the cord margins are rolled outwards and upwards. The movement suggests that the surfaces of contact of their margins are being forced apart from below. The lower parts of their apposed margins are separated before the upper. This sequence is more distinctly observed when the medial margins of the cords are thick with a relatively large surface of contact, as occurs during the production of low tones. Thus the cord movement has a vertical as well as a horizontal component, the cord edges moving along an elliptical path with its long axis horizontal and its short axis vertical. This eversion of the lips of the vocal folds has been picturesquely described as 'creating the illusion of a pair of soft flexible hands rhythmically and gracefully supinating and pronating to show first the palms and then the backs in a continuous flowing movement'.

These vibrations may involve the entire lengths of the cords or segments of their anterior ends, varying with the pitch of the laryngeal tone. The time relations of the opening and closing phases of the cycle of vibration vary with the pitch of the sound. Thus the duration of closed contact of the margins of the cords as a proportion of the total time of the whole vibratory cycle varies with the pitch. The lower the pitch, the longer the period of closure. At the lower limit of the vocal range the period of cord contact is equal to, or more than, half of the total time. With increasing pitch the period of closure becomes progressively shorter than the duration of the opening phase.

The effect of this vibratory cycle, during which the cords make contact and then separate, is that the column of expired air is cut up into a series of rhythmical short

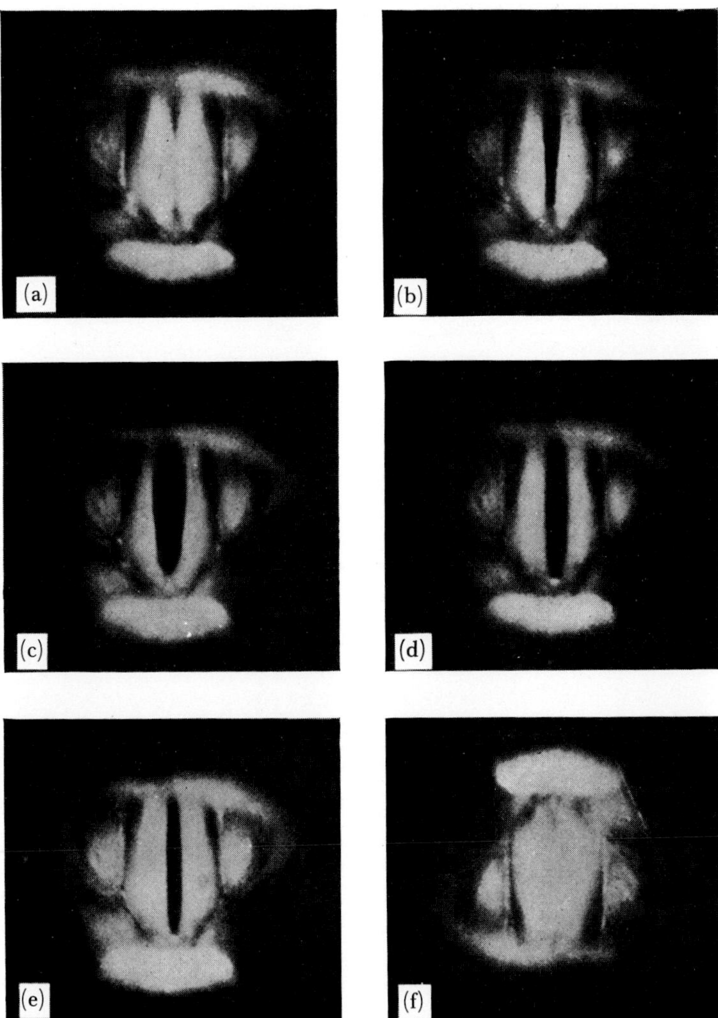

Figure 11.6 High-speed action photographs of vocal cords through one complete cycle of vibration at a frequency of about 125 Hz. (From Farnsworth, 1940, reproduced by courtesy of the Editor of *Bell Laboratories Record*)

columns of air. Thus a rapid series of phases of compression and rarefaction of air is produced which constitutes sound. The frequency of these phases, or alternations of pressure change, determines the pitch of the tone. The force or power of the air stream determines the volume or intensity.

Electromyography of the laryngeal muscles has confirmed the pattern of activity of these muscles in relation to phonation.

At rest a tonic discharge is recorded from the cricothyroid, arytenoid and thyro-arytenoid muscles. This tonic activity maintains the resting position of the vocal cord. It fluctuates in phase with the respiratory cycle, increasing with inspiration and decreasing with expiration. The resulting motion of the cords, of abduction in inspiration and adduction in expiration, produces rhythmic fluctuations in the laryngeal resistance to airflow.

The production of a laryngeal tone is preceded by about 0.5 s by a marked increase in activity of the adductor muscle group, together with an inhibition of the resting tone of the abducting posterior crico-arytenoid muscle. This interval represents the period during which the infraglottic air pressure, necessary to produce sound by forced vibration of the cords, is being developed. The frequency of the muscle action potentials, recorded from single motor units in these contracting muscles, is of the order of 15–50/s (Faaborg-Andersen, 1957). The concept that the frequency of contraction of the laryngeal muscles is the same as the frequency or pitch of the sound produced has not been confirmed.

With an increase in the intensity of sound, the pattern and amplitude of electrical activity in the laryngeal adductors does not change. This confirms the view that intensity of sound is dependent not on a laryngeal muscle change but on the pressure of the expiratory air current.

With a rise in pitch of the laryngeal tone, electrical activity recorded from the adductor muscles increases, as more motor units are recruited into active contraction to effect a greater tension, and a change of shape, of the true vocal folds.

Even the anticipatory process of thinking about producing a particular tone, without actual sound production, is accompanied in the larynx by the pattern of motor activity normally characteristic of the utterance of that particular sound. Thus the shape and tension of the vocal folds is adjusted to the pitch of sound before the sound is actually produced.

Mechanisms of pitch variation

Alteration in pitch of the laryngeal tone by the individual is achieved by regulation of several processes in the larynx. These are the length and tension of the vibrating segments of the cord, the shape and size of the contact areas of the cord edges, and the air pressure.

Length and tension of vocal cords The fundamental frequency of vibration of a string depends on its length and tension. The shorter the vibrating segment and the greater the tension, the higher is the frequency.

Length and tension changes in the vocal cords are controlled by the thyro-arytenoid muscles, and indirectly by active contraction of the external laryngeal muscles, especially the cricothyroids. These latter muscles appear to be involved only in the production of high-pitched notes (above 650 Hz).

Shape of vocal cords The vocal cords are altered in shape from thin and sharp edges, to thick, rounded or flattened margins. In the production of low tones (chest register) the vocal folds are broad and vibrate as a whole along their entire length, and their tension is relatively low (*Figure 11.7*). As the vocal scale is ascended, the rising pitch is achieved not only by increased tension (by contraction of more motor units of the thyro-arytenoid muscle) but also by a change in shape of the cord margins. In the upper range of the vocal scale (head register) the edges of the cords are thin and the areas in contact are reduced. This is brought about by the lower parts of the original rounded edges being pulled apart. During normal conversational speech, the usual range of pitch utilizes only two mechanisms, i.e. changes in the tension and shape of

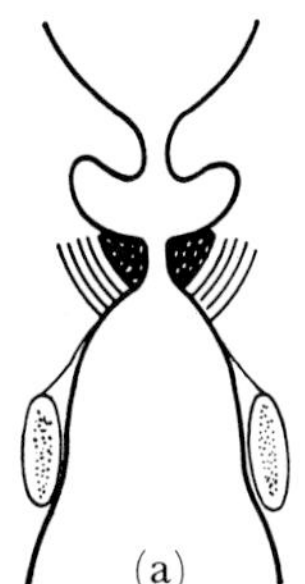

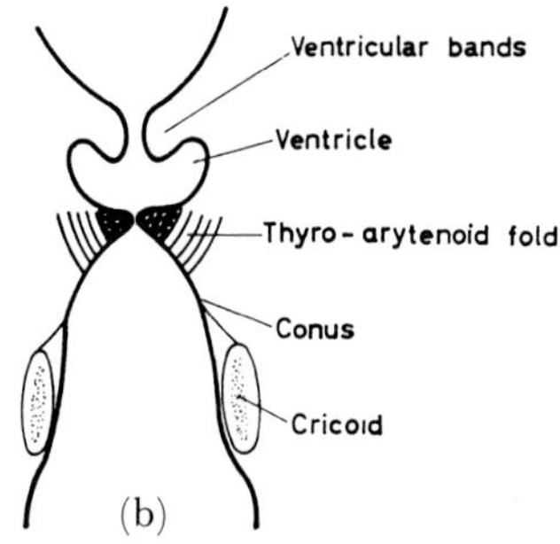

Figure 11.7 Contour of margins of vocal folds in phonation of low- and high-pitched tones: (a) low tone; (b) high tone. (From Houssay's *Human Physiology*, reproduced by courtesy of McGraw-Hill Book Co.)

the cords. In singing, however, as demonstrated by slow-motion cinematography, the cords also lengthen as the pitch rises. This lengthening is a consequence of the tilting of the cricoid cartilage in relation to the thyroid cartilage. This increase in length is compensated by a further increase in tension.

Subglottic air pressure The force of the expiratory blast of air, as well as determining directly the volume of sound, also influences slightly the pitch. With an increase in the pressure of the air stream, the resulting increment in intensity is accompanied by a slight rise in pitch. Thus there is a tendency for a sustained note to rise in pitch when it is increased in volume ('swelling on a note'). Experienced singers learn to compensate for this tendency for the pitch of the note to become sharp, by continuous reduction of the tension of the cords.

Conversely when the pitch of a note is raised by increasing tension in the cords, the greater resistance to the infraglottic air stream tends to reduce the loudness of the sound. This is automatically adjusted by increasing the air pressure to maintain a constant volume of sound.

It has been suggested that in the production of very high notes the false vocal cords come into contact with the upper surface of the vocal cords and thus raise the frequency of their vibrations.

Whispering In whispering (*Figure 11.8*) the interarytenoid muscles do not contract and so the arytenoid cartilages are not approximated, although their vocal processes are rotated medially as in normal speech.

In a weak whisper the cords only meet in their central portions so that there is an aperture anteriorly and also posteriorly between the arytenoids. As the whisper is increased in volume the anterior aperture is closed but the posterior opening persists

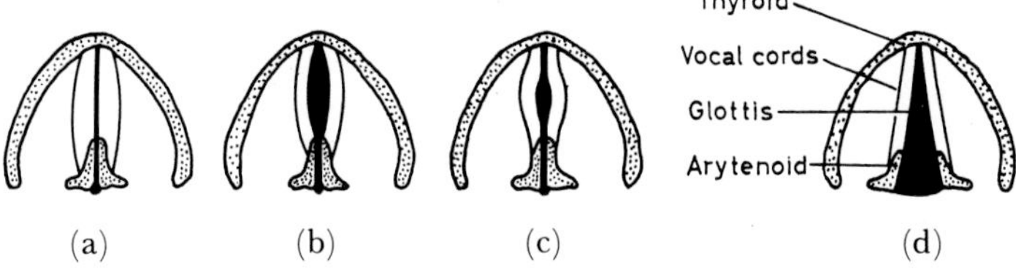

Figure 11.8 Diagram of shape of glottis during phonation: (a) closed phase of phonation; (b) low voice; (c) falsetto voice; (d) whispering. (From Houssay's *Human Physiology*, reproduced by courtesy of McGraw-Hill Book Co.)

thus allowing the escape of air and preventing the build-up of pressure. This imparts to the sound its characteristic aspirate quality.

Actions of the laryngeal muscles

The intrinsic muscles of the larynx are described in detail in Chapter 10, 'Anatomy of the Larynx and Tracheobronchial Tree'.

The actions of these muscles determine the position, the shape and the tension of the vocal cords which are significant factors in influencing the pitch of the laryngeal sounds. Those actions of physiological importance are considered below.

(1) Abduction of the vocal cords with widening of the glottis is produced by contraction of the paired posterior crico-arytenoid muscles (*Figure 11.9*). Contraction draws the muscular process backwards and rotates it medially, so that the vocal process with the attached posterior end of the vocal ligament is rotated laterally and slightly upwards. This muscle contracts in phase with inspiration producing the abduction of the vocal cords which accompanies this part of the respiratory cycle. Its function is thus primarily concerned with respiration. In phonation this muscle braces the arytenoid by its backward pull, so that contraction of the thyro-arytenoid will tense the cords and not be dissipated in pulling the arytenoid forward.

(2) Adduction of the vocal cords and closure of the glottis is produced by contraction of the lateral crico-arytenoid, the interarytenoid and the lateral thyro-arytenoid muscles. Contraction of the lateral crico-arytenoid muscle rotates the arytenoid cartilages around a vertical axis, sweeping the vocal processes medially and adducting the vocal cords. This rotation is thus in a direction opposite to the rotation produced by the posterior crico-arytenoid muscles. In addition to its action in phonation this muscle contracts in deglutition as part of the laryngeal sphincteric mechanism described earlier.

The unpaired interarytenoid muscle consists mainly of transverse fibres, with some more superficial oblique decussating fibres. This muscle extends directly between the posterior surfaces of the arytenoid cartilages. Contraction of the muscle draws these cartilages together, thus approximating the vocal cords. This muscle also assists in closure of the glottis, in deglutition and thoracic fixation.

The lateral fibres of the thyro-arytenoid muscles draw the arytenoids forwards and rotate these cartilages medially, thus adducting the cords. An indirect action on the cricothyroid joint has also been attributed to this muscle; it tends to tilt the cricoid cartilage forwards.

(3) The tension of the vocal folds is increased by the contraction of the cricothyroid muscles and the medial fibres of the thyro-arytenoid muscles (*Figure 11.10*).

Contraction of the cricothyroid muscle raises the anterior arch of the cricoid upwards, reducing the cricothyroid gap. The posterior lamina of the cricoid is tilted backwards. The arytenoids superimposed on the cricoid lamina are carried backwards, thus elongating and stretching the cords and increasing their tension. Apart from this role in phonation, this muscle is also described as contracting during glottic closure for thoracic fixation, and relaxing during deglutition.

The medial fibres of the thyro-arytenoid muscle lie within the vocal folds and are called the vocalis muscle. In view of the very special role of the thyro-arytenoid

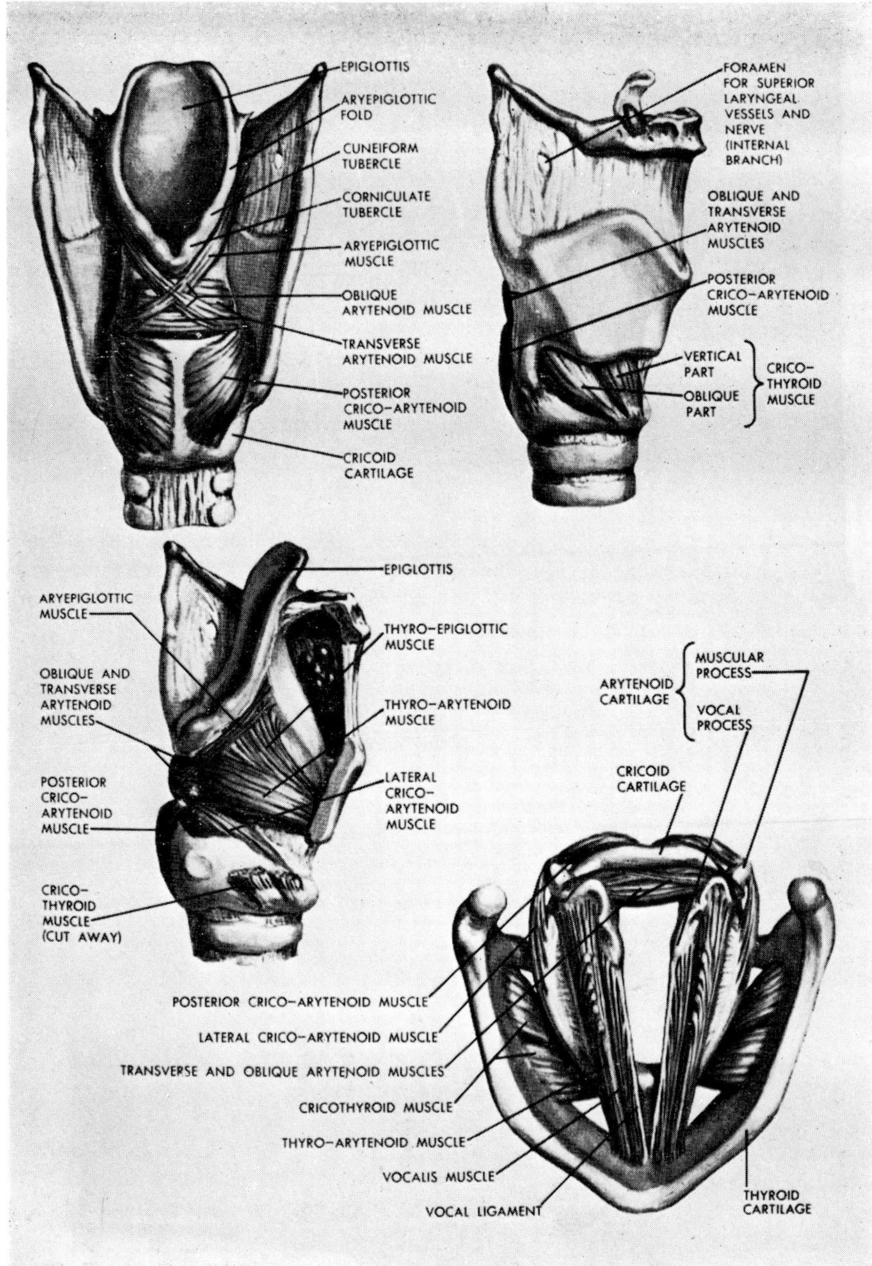

Figure 11.9 Intrinsic muscles of larynx. (Reproduced by courtesy of the Ciba Foundation)

muscle in relation to the mechanism of phonation, the architectural arrangement of the bundles of muscle fibres in this muscle has been the subject of detailed study. Two main groups of fibres are described, forming a criss-cross pattern in relation to one another. One group takes origin from the vocal process of the arytenoid cartilage and runs anteriorly. The bundles of fibres of this part pass successively inwards to attach to the vocal ligament. A second group of muscle bundles are disposed in a similar manner but pass posteriorly from their anterior origin on the lower half of the inner aspect of the angle of the thyroid cartilage. These bundles pass successively medially (the more medial groups first, followed by the more lateral fibres) to be attached to the vocal ligament. A third group of intrinsic muscle fibres in the fold are described. These are shorter and form successive overlapping curves both arising from and being

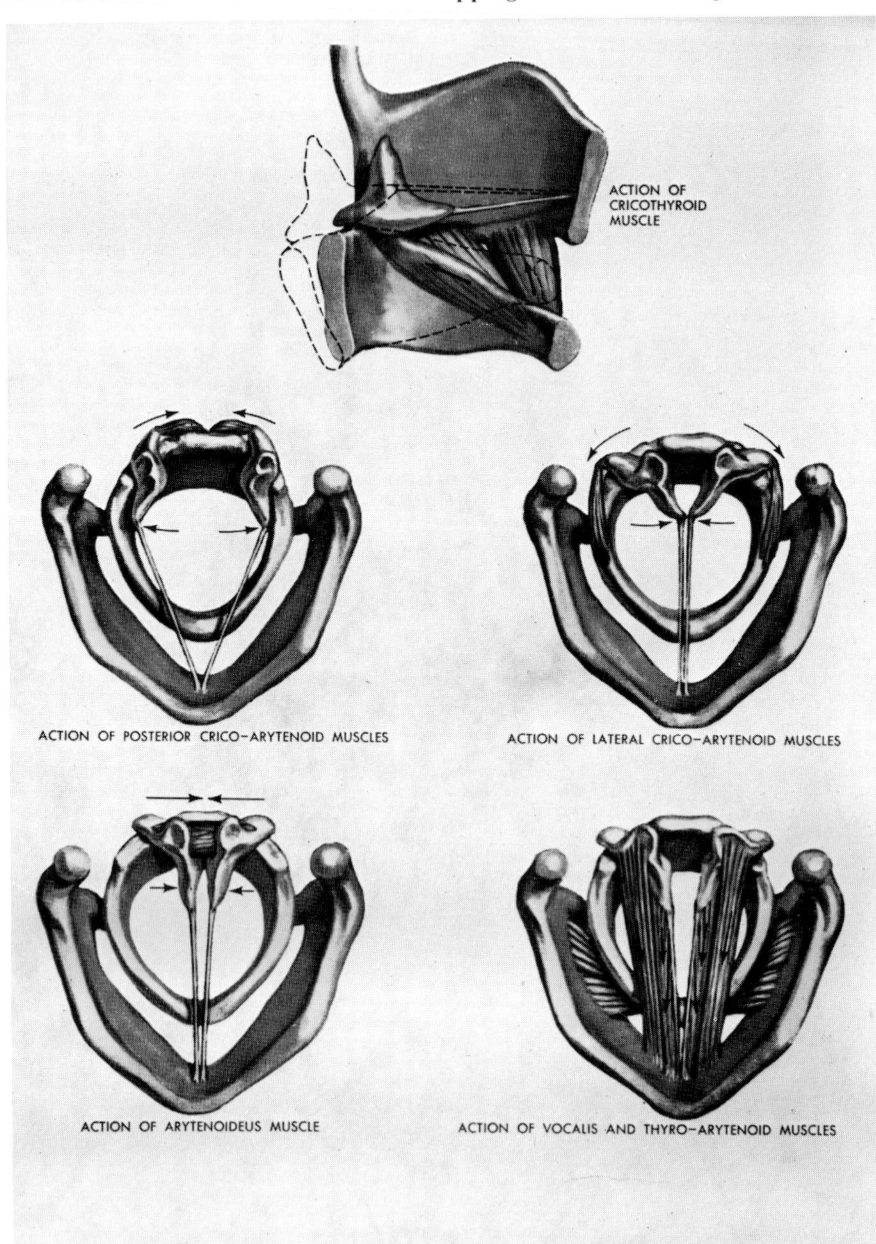

Figure 11.10 Actions of intrinsic muscles of the larynx. (Reproduced by courtesy of the Ciba Foundation)

inserted into the vocal ligament. This has not been confirmed. This systematic arrangement of muscle fibres provides an important part of the complex peripheral neuromuscular apparatus essential for the execution of the numerous, fine, precise changes in the contour, shape, tension and length of the vocal cords which are effected in the larynx in the performance of the skilled voluntary act of producing laryngeal tones over the human vocal range.

Control systems in speech

The following is adapted from a review by Wyke (1974).

A speaker may be regarded as proceeding through a sequence of precisely controlled neuromuscular events which begins with his decision on the sounds he wishes to make. This is followed by voluntary pre-phonatory posturing of the vocal fold musculature to achieve that objective, and then by voluntary setting in motion of the expiratory air flow – at which point, sound emission commences. These voluntary operations are then followed and accompanied during each utterance by the subconscious operations of a triad of reflex systems that control the state of the intrinsic laryngeal musculature, whose activity may be further modified in response to the singer's acoustic automonitoring of his own vocal output.

Translating these proposals into the wider and more realistic context of the practical experience of the singer in performance, it would appear that the accurate production of each phonemic utterance in speech depends upon the efficient and precisely timed sequential operations of the following three sets of neuromuscular control systems.

Pre-phonatory tuning This is effected *voluntarily* through the projections from the inferior paracentral regions of the cerebral cortex in the corticobulbar tracts to the motoneurone pools controlling the laryngeal muscles. It should be emphasized in the present context that this pre-phonatory tuning process involves not only the intrinsic laryngeal muscles but also the intercostal and abdominal muscles and the external laryngeal muscles as well as the middle-ear (stapedius and tensor tympani) muscles, and the oropharyngeal musculature, and is set in train immediately after each voluntary interphrase inspiration.

Electromyographic studies of the intrinsic laryngeal muscles of normal human subjects during phonation have shown that motor unit activity increases briefly but substantially in all the vocal fold adductor muscles just before each phonemic utterance (accompanied by an equally brief decrease in the activity of the abductor posterior crico-arytenoid muscles) with an interval that varies (in different individuals and circumstances of utterance) from 50 to 500 ms. Other aerodynamic studies of subjects speaking and singing have shown that the expiratory air flow commences, and the subglottic air pressure begins to rise, also just before each audible utterance – but some 50–100 ms after the pre-phonatory changes in laryngeal muscular activity described above have begun.

It is suggested that the transient burst of motor unit potentials that occurs in the vocal fold adductors just prior to each phonemic utterance (and also prior to the increase in subglottic pressure), and which is accompanied by an equally brief reduction in vocal fold abductor (posterior crico-arytenoid) activity, indicates that the tension, length, mass, and mutual posture of the vocal folds are repeatedly pre-set during running speech and song to the required values just before the production of each audible sound. It is further suggested that this *pre-phonatory tuning* of the laryngeal musculature is the principal voluntary contribution to the control of the larynx during speech and singing, operating in concert with voluntary control of the respiratory musculature; and that it is effected through the bilateral corticobulbar tract projections from the inferior paracentral regions of the cerebral cortex to the laryngeal motoneurones in the nucleus ambiguus. In other words, it seems that a subject, having decided upon the sequence of sounds that he wishes to make, *voluntarily pre-sets* the tension pattern of his laryngeal musculature into a state that his past experience (acquired during the period of infantile speech maturation and refined by subsequent training in elocution or singing) leads him to believe will produce the desired sounds, just prior to each phonemic utterance.

Because this process is voluntary, its precision can be improved markedly by specific training in elocution and singing, both in respect of the efficiency of control of the intrinsic and extrinsic laryngeal muscles and of that of the respiratory, tongue and oropharyngeal musculature.

Laryngeal reflex control systems But once the expiratory column of air is set into motion through the larynx – in consequence of the rise in subglottic air pressure resulting from the elastic recoil of the previously inflated lungs aided by the voluntarily controlled contraction of the internal intercostal and abdominal musculature in the presence of a now relaxed diaphragm, it is apparent that the vocal folds would be deflected upwards and outwards from their pre-set posture, in the absence of some rapidly acting and continuously operating stabilizing mechanism. Consideration of the time relations involved in such a correcting process, and of the fact that speakers and singers have no conscious awareness of the state of their laryngeal musculature, makes it clear that it cannot be effected voluntarily and must therefore be dependent on the operation of some rapidly acting reflex system or systems. As the laryngeal tissues themselves (muscles, mucosa and intercartilaginous joints) are each provided with low-threshold mechanoreceptor reflexogenic systems, it is therefore proposed that their integrated facilitatory and inhibitory reflex effects on the laryngeal motorneurones provide the basis for the unconscious modulation of laryngeal muscular activity that occurs throughout each phonemic utterance in speech and song.

Of this triad of laryngeal reflex systems, the most important appears to be that operated from the low-threshold, stretch-sensitive *myotatic mechanoreceptors* located in each of the intrinsic laryngeal muscles. During phonation, these slowly-adapting receptors are continuously stimulated by the varying stretching forces applied to the vocal folds from below by the elevated (but fluctuating) subglottic air pressure, and their afferent discharges thus evoked reflexly modulate the activity of the vocal fold adductors and abductors throughout each utterance, thereby contributing to the unconscious maintenance of the desired (and consciously pre-set) tension and mutual posture of the vocal folds during the period of phonatory air flow.

During each phonemic utterance, the subglottic pressure is maintained between 3 and 10 cm H_2O in normal conversational and declamatory speech, at about 10–20 cm H_2O when singing with moderate loudness at *mezzo forte* (about 60–70 dB, A), and reaches peak values of between 50 and 70 cm H_2O when singing *fortissimo* (about 100–110 dB, A). At the same time, i.e. again throughout each utterance, the vocal fold adductors show irregularly augmented motor unit activity (which is, however, less than that seen in the pre-phonatory phase), as do the previously inhibited posterior crico-arytenoid muscles, to degrees determined by the pitch and phonetic nature of the sounds being uttered. The maintenance of the subglottic phonatory pressure head (whose magnitude is the principal determinant of the loudness of the voice) depends largely upon the coordinated activity of the abdominal and internal intercostal muscles operating against the glottic resistance provided by the already adducted and tensed vocal folds.

Next in importance to this myotatic reflex stabilization of vocal fold muscle activity, is the coincident, supplementary reflex influence on the laryngeal motorneurones exerted from the low-threshold *mucosal mechanoreceptors* in the subglottic mucosa. Their threshold is such that they are readily stimulated by the range of subglottic pressures that obtain during singing, so that their afferent discharges are continuously delivered at varying frequency throughout phonation to the laryngeal motorneurones. Clear evidence of the relevance of these rapidly- and slowly-adapting mucosal receptors to control of the laryngeal muscles during phonation is provided by the vocal effects of topical anaesthesia of the infraglottic mucosa.

Finally added to the foregoing influences are the arthrokinetic reflex effects on the laryngeal motorneurones of the *articular mechanoreceptors* located in the fibrous capsules of the intercartilaginous joints of the larynx, whose (mainly) rapidly-adapting afferent discharges are repeatedly provoked by the rapid movements of the laryngeal (especially the cricothyroid and crico-arytenoid) joints that occur throughout phonation.

The irregularly maintained motor unit activity that is seen in the intrinsic laryngeal musculature (both adductor and abductor) throughout each audible utterance results in large measure from the tonic reflex operations of the laryngeal myotatic mechanoreceptor system, supported by tonic and phasic reflex contributions from the subglottic mucosal mechanoreceptors and by phasic reflex contributions from the laryngeal articular mechanoreceptors, in response to the variations in subglottic air pressure that occur during speech and song. In this way, the triad of intrinsic laryngeal reflex systems that control the laryngeal musculature exercises a rapidly operating, subconsious, stabilizing or smoothing influence on the activity of all the muscles controlling the status of the vocal folds throughout phonation, in the presence of the less smooth voluntary control of the abdominal and intercostal muscules that modulates the expiratory air flow.

The laryngeal muscular activity that has been described above results from, and is continuously controlled by, the interaction of a triad of intrinsic laryngeal *reflex* systems with the *voluntary* cortical projection systems at the level of the laryngeal motorneurone pools located in the nucleus ambiguus in the medulla oblongata.

Acoustic automonitoring Once a sound begins to be uttered, the subject's acoustic monitoring of his own on-going vocal output – either directly, or indirectly from the reverberations in a room, concert hall or opera house – may lead to further fine readjustments of the motor unit activity obtaining in the laryngeal (as well as in the respiratory and oropharyngeal) musculature. Empirical evidence of the operation of this acoustic automonitoring process is provided by the disturbing effects of delayed or distorted auditory feedback upon the phonatory processes of normal speakers and singers, and by the experience of singers and their teachers that additional voluntary control of the phonatory process (often of a high order of precision) in response to acoustic monitoring of the vocal output may be acquired in the course of the specific musical and acoustic training that professional singers undergo.

Theories of the mechanism of vocal cord vibration

Two theories of the nature of the mechanisms producing the vibrations of the vocal cords must be briefly discussed. These are: (a) neuromuscular or clonic or neurochronaxic theory; and (b) aerodynamic or tonic theory.

Neuromuscular or clonic theory

This theory postulates that the vibrations of the vocal cords are a direct result of active muscle contractions. The vibrations are brought about by a rapid series of separate active contractions of the thyro-arytenoid muscles. These muscular contractions occur at the frequency of the laryngeal tone produced. The vibrations of the cords are not dependent on the air stream through the larynx. It is claimed that the thyro-arytenoid muscle contains special transverse fibres. The contraction of these transverse fibres separates the approximated cords, while their relaxation allows the cords to recoil by virtue of their inherent elasticity, and to close the glottis. The opening phase of the cycle of cord movement is thus effected by muscle action; the closing phase is due to elastic recoil.

The essential postulate of this theory is therefore that the cord vibrations are maintained by rhythmical cycles of active contraction and relaxation of the thyro-arytenoid muscles. These rhythmic contractions are the result of excitation by a rhythmic discharge of impulses, from the motor neurons whose axons pass in the vagus nerves and their recurrent laryngeal branches, to innervate the motor units of the transverse fibres of the thyro-arytenoid muscles. These lower motor neurones, in their turn, are stimulated during phonation by rhythmic bursts of impulses, which like the muscle contractions they excite, are at the frequency of the laryngeal tone produced.

The pressure of the blast of air expelled in phonation is held – by supporters of this theory – to play no role in setting the cords into vibration. They claim further, that the laryngeal air pressure has no modifying effect on the frequency of the movements of the vocal cords produced by the clonic muscular contractions, although it may have a supplementary action in varying the amplitude of these cord movements. This summary states, in outline, what may be termed the neuromuscular or clonic theory of cord vibration. Husson, who re-introduced this theory in 1950, refers to it as the neurochronaxic theory, because he claims that the refractory period of the thyro-arytenoid muscle is approximately equal to that of the motor nerve fibres innervating that muscle.

On this theory, for the production of a laryngeal tone of any specific frequency or pitch within the vocal range, the train of impulses generated in the cerebral cortex, relayed in the vagal nucleus and conducted along the fibres of the recurrent laryngeal nerve to the thyro-arytenoid muscle, must be at that same specific frequency. This stream of impulses stimulates the transverse fibres of the thyro-arytenoid muscle which then contracts rhythmically at that same frequency. This clonic contraction produces vibrations of the cords at this particular frequency. The end-result of this is that the series of puffs of air emerging from the larynx are also at this self-same frequency, resulting therefore in the production of a tone of the intended specific frequency or pitch.

On a first analysis, this theory assumes:

(1) That the motor fibres of the recurrent laryngeal nerve to the thyro-arytenoid muscles can conduct impulses at a frequency up to 2048/s, which corresponds to the pitch of the highest note recorded for the human voice.
(2) That the transverse fibres of the thyro-arytenoid muscles can contract repetitively at up to 2048 separate contractions per second without the genesis of tetany, that is, without the contractions becoming fused into a constant steady and unvarying state of sustained contraction, which is called tetany.

Supporting evidence

Husson based his support of this theory on stroboscopic observations on himself, and on other experimental evidence, some of which is listed below. Many of these supporting experiments or the conclusions drawn from them have been challenged.

(1) Goettler (1951) described the presence in the thyro-arytenoid muscle of transverse fibres capable of abducting the vocal cords. This has subsequently been denied by several investigators.
(2) Electrical excitation of the recurrent laryngeal nerve in the dog at frequencies up to 400 Hz produced cord movements, observed by stroboscopy, at frequencies identical with the rate of electrical stimulation. These cord vibrations, synchronous with the applied stimulation, were still present when the laryngeal air stream was diverted or abolished by tracheostomy. With stimulation rates above 400/s, cord vibrations could be elicited only by very intense stimulation, and the resulting vibrations were small in amplitude (Laget, 1953).
(3) During the operation of laryngectomy under local anaesthesia, if the infraglottic space was closed with an inflated rubber cuff and the patient was asked to attempt to sing, then the cords vibrated although no air stream was passing between the vocal folds. This was verified by slow-motion cinematography and these cord vibrations also occurred when the larynx had been separated from both the trachea and the pharynx as long as the nerve supply was still intact.
(4) Electromyographic tracings from the thyro-arytenoid muscles demonstrated motor unit action potentials at the frequency of the sound during phonation. It was assumed, therefore, that the muscle was necessarily contracting at the same frequency as that of the motor unit electrical potentials which were recorded. This is not a valid assumption as will be discussed below.
(5) Moulonguet (1954) claimed that records of the nerve action potentials in the recurrent laryngeal nerve made during operation on the human larynx, revealed that the nerve impulse frequency corresponded with the vibration frequency of the vocal cords.

The upper limit of the frequency of impulses which can be conducted along a single nerve fibre depends on the absolute refractory period of the fibre which is in turn correlated with the fibre diameter. Neurophysiological research has established unequivocally that individual nerve axons cannot transmit impulses at a frequency equal to that of the vibratory movements of the vocal cords at the upper limit of the vocal scale. Husson endeavoured to overcome this fundamental objection by postulating a polyphasic organization of the laryngeal motor impulses, similar to that proposed in the volley theory of conduction of sensory impulses in the fibres of the auditory nerve.

Incorporating this volley modification the neuromuscular theory proposes that in the production of sounds involving vibrations of the cords at frequencies below 400–500 Hz, each active motor unit of the muscle responds by a single contraction to each individual nerve impulse reaching it. With vibration frequencies in the range 500–1000 Hz, the impulses are conducted in two separate groups of nerve fibres out of phase with one another. Two distinct groups of motor units in the muscle therefore contract alternately. Similarly, in the vibration frequency ranges 1000–1500 Hz and 1500–2000 Hz, the nerve fibres conduct out of phase in three and four groups respectively volleying in succession. Vibrations of the vocal cords at frequencies above the maximal conduction frequency for nerve is thus explained by the suggestion that the different groups of motor units contract asynchronously. Each group contracts in phase with the impulses transmitted down its motor nerve fibres. The muscle as a whole therefore contracts at some mutliple of the frequency of impulses volleying down the motor nerve fibres.

Evidence refuting neuromuscular theory

The evidence against this view of a neuromuscular mechanism based on active voluntary clonic contractions of the thyro-arytenoid muscles is impressive.

Anatomical and histological studies of the thyro-arytenoid muscle fails to confirm the existence of transverse fibres in the thyro-arytenoid muscle. The presence of these fibres is essential to this theory in which they constitute the active contractile elements causing the vibrations of the cords. The arrangement of the collagenous and elastic fibres in the vocal folds is not consistent with that required for this theory. Further, it seems very improbable that active contraction of such short muscle fibres, as these supposed transverse fibres must inevitably be, could achieve the observed amplitude of vibration of the vocal cords. Neurohistological investigations show no unusual features of the motor innervation of this muscle, as might be anticipated if it possessed the unique response characteristics required by this theory.

The vocal range of the normal human larynx is usually regarded as covering 82 Hz to 1175 Hz; the extreme limits recorded are 44 Hz and 2058 Hz. The neuromuscular theory requires therefore that the thyro-arytenoid muscle must be capable of making discrete contractions separated by intervals of relaxation at up to 2000 contractions/s. Repetitive stimulation of other striated mammalian muscle at any frequency of over 100 stimuli/s results in a fusion of the mechanical contractions. The muscle remains, during the period of stimulation, in a state of sustained contractile tension called tetany. The experiments of Floyd and others (1957) demonstrate that this physiological principle applies also to the laryngeal muscles. The movements of the vocal cords of the cat are recorded by piezo-electric transducer and the muscle action potentials of the thyro-arytenoid muscle by electromyography from concentric needle electrodes in that muscle. The recurrent laryngeal nerve is stimulated with varying stimulus parameters. With stimulation rates of up to 100/s, the records show separate clonic contractions of the muscle. With stimulation at 110/s or higher, fusion of contractions occurs and the muscle passes into a steady tetanic contraction maintained for the duration of stimulation. Other investigators report that the critical frequency of stimulation for the genesis of full tetany in the thyro-arytenoid muscle of the dog is about 60 stimuli/s. These experimental findings are in accord with the physiological response of skeletal muscle in general to repetitive stimulation. They are incompatible with the requirements of the neuromuscular theory for a very rapid series of separate active contractions of the muscle of the vocal cord.

The reports of the demonstration of nerve action potentials in the recurrent laryngeal nerve at the frequency of the laryngeal sound may be susceptible of alternative explanations. The first is that these impulses may not all be motor impulses, but a proportion may be afferent proprioceptive impulses from laryngeal joint capsules, ligaments and muscle spindles. The presence of sensory receptors in and around the laryngeal joints has been demonstrated by several investigators, and nerve impulse discharges have been recorded in fibres of the articular nerves. The second explanation is that the electrical activity recorded is in the nature of a microphone effect due to the vibrations of the cords and the oscillations of other parts, close to the recording electrodes.

Electromyographic investigations apparently supporting the neuromuscular theory are not confirmed by others. The claim – that in patients phonating during laryngeal operations under local anaesthesia, the muscle action potentials observed by electromyograph from the laryngeal muscles are at a frequency equal to that of the tone produced – does not necessarily prove that the muscle is contracting rhythmically at this frequency. If a skeletal muscle is stimulated experimentally at a frequency of over 100/s, a steady tetanic contraction results; nevertheless electromyographic recordings from this muscle in tetany will show the separate electrical muscle potentials at a frequency corresponding to the rate of stimulation. The experiments of Floyd, Negus and Neil (1957) show that when the recurrent laryngeal nerve in the cat is stimulated at a rate in excess of 250 stimuli/s, there is no correlation between the frequency of the muscle potentials and the nerve stimulation frequency. Faaborg-Andersen (1957) finds that the highest frequency of motor unit electrical activity, observed in electromyographic records from the human larynx during phonation, is 30/s.

The vocal cord movements can be recorded by high-speed cinematography in patients with a normal larynx and a tracheostomy. Rubin (1960) finds that with the tracheostomy closed, the vocal cords approximate and vibrate normally during phonation. When the stoma is open, the cords remain immobile even when the subject is attempting phonation. Closure of the tracheal opening during this attempted phonation is followed immediately by resumption of vibration of the cords. As long as the stoma is open, however, the cords, during attempts at phonation, are tightly approximated but do not vibrate. If the neuromuscular theory were correct the cords should vibrate whenever a subject endeavours to produce a laryngeal tone, whether the air stream is passing through the larynx, or is diverted to the exterior from the infraglottic tracheal stoma.

The aerodynamic or tonic theory

This is the classic, and at present still the most acceptable, theory of the mechanism of phonation. The effective force setting the cords into vibration is the pressure of the infraglottic air column. This pressure acts on the vocal cords which are first approximated and tensed by a steady tonic contraction of laryngeal muscles. In this theory the opening and closing of the glottis are a passive result of the raised pressure of the air stream, while a tonically contracted muscle maintains apposition of the cords. This contrasts with the neuromuscular theory which supposes that the cord vibrations are actively produced by clonic muscle contractions and are independent of the air pressure.

Production of a laryngeal tone involves, first, contraction of the thyro-arytenoid muscles and other laryngeal muscles, approximating the vocal cords and adjusting their length, shape and tension, to the particular sound it is intended to produce. The muscles of the abdominal wall and thorax contract to force a column of air out of the respiratory passages against the resistance of the closed cords. This raised subglottic air pressure forces the vocal cords apart, allowing some of the column of air to escape through the glottic chink. The subglottic pressure falls with this escape of air, and so the cords are forced into apposition again by elastic recoil and by the tone in the still contracted thyro-arytenoid muscles. It is probable that when the cords are forced apart, the elastic tissue of the cords, and the thyro-arytenoid muscle fibres are stretched and this may increase their recoil force. The vocal cords, now again in contact, prevent the escape of air. The subglottic pressure rises again until the vocal cords are again forced apart, and this cycle repeats itself.

The vibrations of the vocal cords are thus a direct result of the infraglottic air pressure. They are a consequence of the competition between the infraglottic air pressure, tending to force the cord margins to separate, and the contracted thyro-arytenoid muscles tending to prevent this displacement of the cords. Thus there results a rapid sequence of opening and closing of the glottis. The frequency of vibration of the cords thus induced determines the number of successive phases of air compression released per second, which in turn, determines the pitch of the sound produced.

In phonation the expired stream of air is precisely adjusted in its force to the intensity of the sound it is desired to produce. This is achieved by regulation of the strength of contraction of the expiratory muscles of the abdominal wall and the thorax. The air pressure provides the mechanism causing the vibration of the cords and determining the loudness of the sound. The frequency of the vibrations produced by the air pressure is determined by variations of the shape, the length and the tension of the vibrating portions of the vocal cords, and is influenced to a lesser extent by the air pressure. The moving column of expired air is separated by the vibrating vocal cords into a series of rhythmical puffs. These alternating sections of condensed and rarefied air constitute the laryngeal note consisting of a fundamental tone and a series of overtones.

Evidence for aerodynamic theory

This aerodynamic theory is supported by the experimental findings discussed before as evidence refuting the neuromuscular theory. A few other points may be mentioned.

(1) Models can be constructed demonstrating the production of vibrations by air pressure as in a clarinet.
(2) An artificial larynx can be constructed of two adjacent strips of muscle over the end of a tube. When air is pumped down the tube the muscle strips are forced

apart and recoil rhythmically. These vibrations of the muscle strips result in the production of a sound. Stimulation of the muscle strips to increase their tension and speed of recoil causes a rise in the pitch of the sound produced.

(3) When the cords of an excised or cadaver larynx are artificially approximated and tensed, then air forced through the larynx produces a sound. Experiments with these models demonstrate that the pitch of the sound produced varies with the tension of the cords. Further, a rise of air pressure causes an increase in loudness and also a slight rise in pitch. Because of this rise in pitch with increase of air pressure in this excised human larynx model, maintenance of a constant pitch with increasing intensity of sound requires that the tension of the cords is adjusted by a corresponding decrease in tension. This is described as the 'law of compensation of forces in the larynx'. The direction of this pitch change applies only in the upper part of the vocal frequency range, that is, the head register. In the lower frequencies, that is, the chest register, an increase in infraglottic pressure lowers the pitch of the tone produced.

(4) Sudden pressure on the abdomen, causing a rise of the pressure of the expired air stream, during phonation of a constant note, not only increases its loudness but also changes its pitch.

(5) Slow-motion cinematography has revealed the complex pattern of changes in the vibratory motion of the vocal cords. This vibration is not a simple horizontal movement as would be anticipated on the neuromuscular theory. The vocal folds are rolled upwards as well as outwards, giving the definite impression that they are being forced apart from below. The lower portions of their surfaces of contact are separated before the upper parts. This is even more apparent when the apposed surfaces of the cords are relatively thick, as during the phonation of low tones.

(6) The effects of neurological lesions involving the motor innervation of the laryngeal muscles, support the aerodynamic theory. These effects of unilateral and bilateral cord paralysis on phonation can be adequately explained by this theory.

(7) The aerodynamic concept of the mechanism of phonation is also supported by the fact that voice can be produced after laryngectomy, as in oesophageal speech. The essential requirements are a blast of air from the oesophagus and a tonically contracted muscle to close the upper opening to the oesophagus. Air is drawn into the oesophagus to provide a form of 'bellows', and the vibration is produced at the edges of the oesophagus. The cricopharyngeal sphincter plays an important role in this form of extralaryngeal speech. The sphincter is first relaxed. The oesophagus then fills with air due to the negative intrathoracic pressure. This pressure gradient drawing air in, is increased by a strong voluntary inspiratory effort. The sphincter is then closed. Strong contraction of the muscles of expiration follows. This causes a rise of the intrathoracic pressure and therefore of the intra-oesophageal pressure. This intra-oesophageal head of pressure forces air through the sphincter. The edges of the oesophagus at the level of the sphincter vibrate in a manner similar to that envisaged at the vocal cords by the aerodynamic theory. The sound produced by this oesophageal vibrating mechanism is modulated by the tongue, palate and lips to produce speech sounds as with a normal laryngeal vibrating mechanism.

Neural regulation of the larynx

The anatomy of the motor and sensory nerve supply of the larynx is described in Chapter 10.

Afferent innervation

From the physiological point of view the more important sensory receptors of the larynx are: (a) mucosal receptors subserving pain; (b) mechanoreceptors concerned with the cough reflex and the control of the laryngeal sphincter; (c) receptors in relation to the muscles, ligaments and joints related to proprioceptive control of laryngeal motor activity. Considerable importance is attached to this last group of articular nerve endings in the precise regulation of the fine skilled movements of the laryngeal muscles.

The structure and functional activity of receptors at the thyro-epiglottic joint are described by Andrew. These receptors are of the slow-adapting type, similar in response characteristics to those found at the joints of the limbs. These receptors presumably signal the position and movement of the epiglottis.

Experimental displacement of laryngeal cartilages produces reflex responses mediated by afferent impulses in fibres of the laryngeal nerves. The pattern of these proprioceptive impulses in the internal laryngeal nerve is the subject of researches of Martenson and other investigators. Artificially produced joint movements cause discharges of afferent impulses followed by a post-excitatory inhibition. Comparison of the discharge of impulses induced by contraction of the laryngeal muscles, with that produced by passive movement at the laryngeal joints, shows that the receptors stimulated are not in the muscles, but mainly in the ligaments, capsules and peri-articular tissues of the joints, especially in the lateral epiglottic folds and close to the arytenoid cartilages. The proprioceptive reflexes are initiated from receptors around the joints and mediated along afferent fibres in the internal laryngeal nerve. Martenson uses records of action potentials from single nerve fibre preparations of the internal laryngeal nerve to analyse these proprioceptive responses to the particular movement produced when each individual laryngeal muscle is stimulated to contract. All these receptors are of the slow-adapting type. The impulses transmitted in the internal laryngeal nerve are from the upper half of the larynx. Some receptors respond reciprocally in the movements produced by contraction of the posterior crico-arytenoid and of the thyro-arytenoid muscles. Since these muscles oppose one another in their actions on the crico-arytenoid joint, these particular receptors are doubtless located around this joint. Histological and action potential studies have demonstrated a rich sensory innervation of the capsule of the crico-arytenoid joint. Also, a dense sensory innervation and numerous muscle spindles are described in the thyro-arytenoid muscle.

Other receptors fire when either abduction or adduction of the cords is produced. These receptors are probably located at sites where either abduction or adduction causes a similar pressure effect. Mechanoreceptors from the region of the cricothyroid joint do not discharge along the internal laryngeal nerve. Presumably they discharge along afferent fibres in the recurrent laryngeal nerve.

The extensive proprioceptive innervation of the laryngeal joints and muscles provides the neural basis for a sensory feedback mechanism for the sensory guidance of the motor cortex in the execution of the precisely co-ordinated, minute contractions of the laryngeal muscles which are accurately graded for force, sequence and duration of contraction, in phonation.

Motor supply

The laryngeal muscles, with the exception of the cricothyroid muscles, are innervated by the recurrent laryngeal branch of the vagus nerves. The cricothyroid muscle is supplied by the external branch of the superior laryngeal branch of the vagus. These motor fibres have their cell bodies in the nucleus ambiguus in the medulla. Nuclear and peripheral infranuclear lesions of the recurrent laryngeal nerve causes unilateral paralysis of the vocal cords with hoarse voice and difficult ineffective cough. Bilateral lesions result in paralysis of both cords and shortness of breath. Cerebellar lesions result in explosive slurring scanning speech with a staccato character. This is a result of the loss of sensory guidance of the motor centres in carrying out this voluntary muscle activity, that is, the sensory 'feedback' from the muscles and joints of the larynx is no longer operating effectively.

Laryngeal lubrication

The mucous membrane of the larynx is covered by a ciliated columnar epithelium except over the true vocal folds. It varies in thickness in different areas. The thickest regions are on the aryepiglottic folds, and the epithelium is thinnest over the laryngeal surface of the epiglottis and the false vocal folds. The alveolar tissue of the aryepiglottic folds is loose, permitting free movement of the arytenoid cartilages and these folds. The mucosa of the margin of the true vocal folds, because it is involved in firm vibratory contact at high frequency with the opposite cord, is covered by stratified squamous epithelium.

Mucus-secreting glands are found scattered generally in the laryngeal mucous membrane except in that covering the true vocal cords. These glands are most densely concentrated in the walls of the ventricle of the larynx and its anterior extension as the saccule of the ventricle. They are also relatively plentiful around the false vocal cords and the laryngeal inlet, that is, the lower part of the epiglottis and aryepiglottic folds. These glands provide the mucous film for the action of the intralaryngeal ciliated epithelium. The saccule is described as the 'oil-can of the vocal cords'. The mucus, secreted by the glands in its walls, accumulates in the cavity of the saccule, retained by the valvular action of two crescentic folds of mucous membrane at its opening into the ventricle. This reservoir of mucus is expressed by the contraction of some fibres of the thyro-arytenoid and interarytenoid muscles acting as the compressor muscle of the laryngeal saccule. The expressed mucus flows over the vocal cords and serves to lubricate these constantly and rapidly moving surfaces.

Tracheobronchial tree

Introduction

The main function of the tracheobronchial tree is to provide a channel for the passage of air from the exterior to the terminal gas exchanging units of the lung. It is essential that this upper air channel provides structural rigidity necessary for the bidirectional passage of air during the respiratory cycle and at the same time permits free movement of the head and neck.

Relationship between structure and function

The 16–20 horseshoe-shaped tracheal cartilages and the smooth muscle and alveolar tissue of the posterior tracheal wall prevent collapse of the intrathoracic portion of the air channel during expiration when the intrathoracic pressure is greater than atmospheric. The connective tissue and elastic fibres between adjacent tracheal rings allow free movement of the head and neck and limit tracheal movements during coughing, swallowing, and vomiting without obstruction of the airway.

Like the trachea, all the bronchi contain some cartilage offering rigidity to the air channel. The bronchioli are those air channels distal to the last plate of cartilage and there are approximately 10 generations of these ending in a terminal bronchiolus which is immediately proximal to a respiratory bronchiolus into which alveolar ducts and alveoli open. The small bronchi and more peripheral subdivisions of the bronchial tree do not stay patent in massive lung collapse and apposition of the walls of the terminal bronchioli is responsible for air-trapping during expiration in subjects with airways obstruction such as emphysema.

The airway is lined with ciliated epithelium continuous from the larynx to the respiratory bronchioli and many cell types are interspersed in this mucous membrane presenting a pseudostratified appearance. These histological elements and their secretions may alter the calibre of the airway but the main control of this is bronchial muscle occurring along the whole tracheobronchial tree. The physiology of this bronchial muscle is considered on p. 468.

Lung volumes and dead space

The respiratory tract may be divided functionally into the conducting passages and the gas-exchanging surface. The former consists of the nose, mouth, pharynx, larynx and tracheobronchial tree as far as the terminal bronchiole and the latter includes respiratory bronchioles, alveolar ducts and alveoli of which there are some 300 million in the adult with a total gas-exchanging area of approximately 70–80 m^2.

At the end of a normal breath, the volume of air in the chest and the upper air passages is known as the functional residual capacity (FRC). At the limit of maximum inspiration the volume of air in the chest is known as the total lung capacity (TLC) whilst the residual volume (RV) is the volume of air in the chest at the end of a maximum forced expiration (*see Figure 11.11*). The vital capacity (VC) is the maximum amount of air which can be exhaled after a maximum inspiration. The other subdivisions of lung volume are shown in the spirogram and it should be noted that the values given are very approximate since they alter according to the subject's age, sex and height. It will be obvious that the RV and hence the FRC and TLC cannot be measured if only a spirometer is available and these absolute gas volumes of the lung can be obtained using inert gas dilution, whole body plethysmography or radiological techniques (Cotes, 1975).

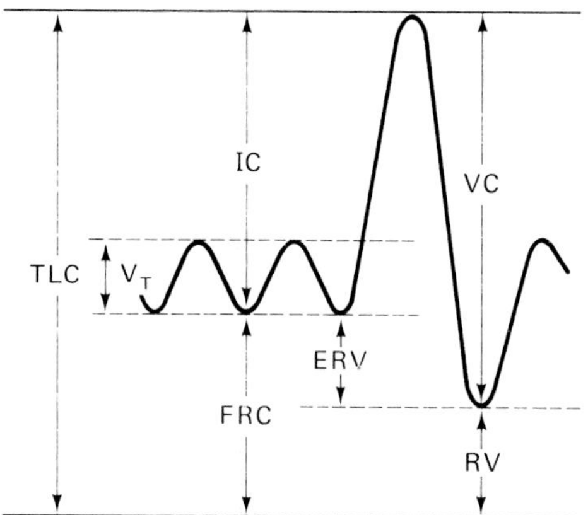

Figure 11.11 The subdivisions of lung volume and approximate normal values

Subdivisions of lung volume

TLC	=	Total lung capacity	4–7l
FRC	=	Functional residual capacity	2.5–4l
VC	=	Vital capacity	3–5l
ERV	=	Expiratory reserve volume	1–2l
RV	=	Residual volume	1–2l
IC	=	Inspiratory capacity	2–3l
TV	=	Tidal volume	0.4–0.6l

The tidal colume (V_T) usually amounts to 500 ml and, since the respiratory frequency (f) is normally 12–15/min, the overall minute ventilation (V_E) is 6–8 litres. However, about 150 ml of each breath remains within the upper airway and the tracheobronchial tree and does not reach the gas-exchanging surfaces in the alveoli and does not contribute to exchange of oxygen and carbon dioxide. This part of the airway is known as the anatomical dead space (V_D). Thus alveolar ventilation (V_A) is assessed by the expression: $V_A = V_E - fV_{D\,anat}$ and is between 4 and 6 litre/min in adults.

During shallow respiration, as the tidal volume decreases, the wasted dead space assumes a greater fraction of the inspired air, whereas when the depth of breathing is increased a greater proportion of the inspired volume contributes to alveolar ventilation. Thus an increase in minute ventilation by increase in depth of respiration is more effective in gas exchange than by an increase in frequency of respiration. For this reason during induction of anaesthesia deep breathing produces a more rapid rise in anaesthetic concentration than an increase in the rate of breathing and similarly deep breathing is more effective in accelerating the elimination of volatile anaesthetics from the body.

It is also important to reduce the dead space of any anaesthetic or respiratory apparatus to a minimum. Some of the value of tracheostomy in subjects with respiratory failure may be attributed to a reduction in their anatomical dead space.

The physiological dead space may be calculated from measurements of the output of carbon dioxide and the carbon dioxide content of the alveoli. The physiological dead space is of similar volume to the anatomical dead space in normal subjects but is greater in lung disease due to the non-uniformity of mixing of alveolar ventilation with alveolar perfusion.

Tracheobronchial tree and air flow

Weibel (1963) and Horsfield and Cumming (1968) have shown that although the bronchi branch repeatedly there is only a small change in total cross-sectional area until the eighth and ninth generation when individual bronchi have a diameter of about 2 mm. Macklem and Mead (1967) showed that approximately 75 per cent of the pressure drop between the trachea and the alveoli occurred in these larger airways whereas only 25 per cent occurred in the numerous smaller peripheral branches with a greater cross-sectional area and therefore lower linear velocity of airflow. The velocity of air flow is therefore greatest in the upper tracheobronchial tree and narrowing in the calibre of this portion of the airway will have considerable effects on airway resistance (see below).

Measurement of air flow

It was originally proposed that the maximum volume of air that a subject can breathe per minute was a reliable index of pulmonary performance. This maximum breathing capacity and maximum voluntary ventilation may be measured with a spirometer or with a mouthpiece, valve and collecting bag and the subject breathes maximally for 15 or 30 s. Although dependent on lung flow resistance this measurement is influenced by non-pulmonary factors such as endurance and motivation so that single breath determinations, less dependent on the subjects' co-operation, are now commonplace.

The forced expiratory volume in 1 s (FEV_1) is the volume of gas expelled from the lungs over 1 s when the subject makes a maximal expiratory effort from a position of full inspiration and is best obtained using a bellows spirometer. The forced expiratory volume may be expressed as a percentage of the vital capacity ($FEV_1/VC) \times 100$) and in normal subjects 70–80 per cent of the vital capacity can be expired in the first second, a smaller proportion implying airways obstruction.

Another commonly used index of airways obstruction is the peak expiratory flow rate (PEFR) delivered from a position of full inspiration into a Wright's Peak Flow Meter which records the maximum rate of expiratory air flow sustained for 10 ms (Wright and McKerrow 1959).

Miller and Hyatt (1969) have popularized the flow-volume loop as a means of assessing intrathoracic and extrathoracic airflow. During inspiration air flows into the lungs because the pressure within the thoracic cavity is lowered below atmospheric. During expiration intrathoracic pressure exceeds atmospheric and gas flows out of the lungs. The large airways within the thorax are subject to these pleural pressure changes and they will thus dilate in inspiration and narrow in expiration providing the airway wall maintains some mobility. The extrathoracic airway however is surrounded by atmospheric pressure throughout the respiratory cycle and during inspiration when the pressure within the airway is below atmospheric the lumen will narrow and will tend to dilate during expiration when the airway pressure is greater than atmospheric. Thus if the airway wall is mobile obstructing lesions of the extrathoracic airway limit inspiratory flow more than expiratory, whereas obstructing lesions of the intrathoracic main airway reduce expiratory flow more than inspiratory.

The flow–volume loop is constructed by recording the lung volume and air flow at the mouth during a maximum forced expiratory vital capacity followed by a maximum forced inspiratory vital capacity.

Examples of a normal flow–volume loop and in intrathoracic and extrathoracic tracheal obstruction are shown in *Figure 11.12*.

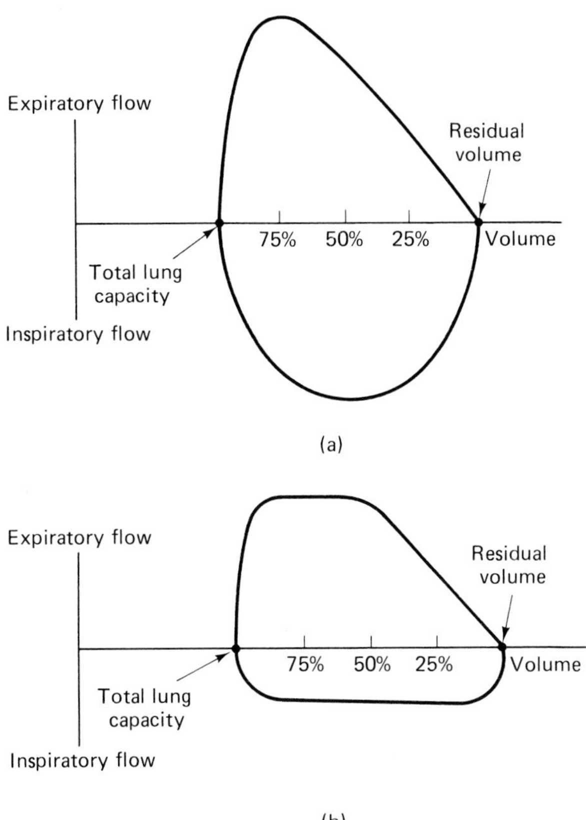

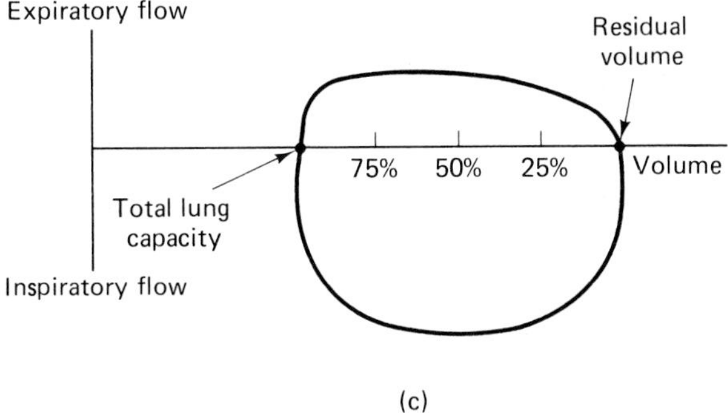

Figure 11.12 (a) A normal flow–volume loop. (b) Flow–volume loop in extrathoracic upper airway obstruction. (c) Flow-volume loop in intrathoracic upper airway obstruction

Tracheobronchial muscle

Smooth muscle fibres disposed in an oblique plane are found in a continuous network from the trachea to the bronchioles and when they contract the airways narrow. In the trachea the posterior ends of the cartilages are approximated whilst more peripherally muscle contraction not only narrows the lumen but shortens the bronchi. Simultaneously the mucous membrane becomes folded and puckered, further narrowing the airway. Elastic tissue is also present in the bronchial walls and provides the recoil force when muscle contraction is relaxed. The elastic tissue is also a major factor in determining distensibility of the airway.

Resting bronchomotor tone and nerve supply

The tracheobronchial tree is innervated by the vagus and sympathetic fibres derived from the cardiac and pulmonary plexuses. The two groups of nerves are inter-related and the precise anatomy is obscure. The smooth muscle is in a state of partial tonic contraction mediated through the vagus which may be blocked by atropine and abolished by vagotomy which produces bilateral bronchial dilation after unilateral section. Stimulation of the sympathetic nerves relaxes bronchial smooth muscle. Bronchomotor tone is controlled by many factors and much of the experimental work is inconclusive. Some of the reflexes involved are given below but for a more detailed account, the reviews of Widdicombe (1954, 1966) should be consulted.

Central and reflex nervous control of bronchial muscle

The tracheobronchial muscle is influenced by the cerebral cortex; stimulation of the cortical area of the frontal lobe controlling the facial muscles causes bronchoconstriction. Reflexes mediated through centres in the brain stem influence the width of the respiratory airway.

Nasobronchial reflex
Stimulation of nasal mucosa results in reflex bronchoconstriction. This reflex can be elicited by cold air, irritant gases, smoke fumes and by mechanical and electrical stimulation.

Laryngobronchial and cough reflex
Irritation of the laryngeal mucosa causes contraction of bronchial muscle. During the expiratory phase of the cough reflex the capacity of the tracheobronchial airway is greatly decreased. This is a pressure effect and not due to increased bronchial muscle tone.

Pulmonary inflation bronchial reflex
Inflation of the lung causes reflex bronchodilation which is prevented by vagotomy. The receptors for this reflex may be those concerned with the reflex apnoea following pulmonary inflation, that is the Hering–Breuer reflex. Inert dust particles, introduced into the lower respiratory tract of man, tend to cause bronchial constriction. Irritant gases and inhalation anaesthetics also stimulate bronchoconstriction.

Hypoxia and hypercapnia

Reflex bronchoconstriction with reduction of volume and increased resistance of the airway, is produced by hypoxia. This action is reflex from the arterial chemoreceptors of the carotid and aortic bodies. A rise of CO_2 tension also produces bronchial constriction but this effect is probably mainly direct on the medullary centres.

Baroreceptor reflexes

The reflex effect of stimulation of the carotid and aortic arterial baroreceptors on bronchomotor tone is not agreed. Some observers have found that increased blood pressure in the carotid sinus causes powerful reflex bronchoconstriction. Others have failed to confirm this effect; some claim that the reflex changes are confined to the smooth muscle of the pulmonary vascular bed.

Nociceptive reflex

Bronchial constriction or dilation accompanies somatic or visceral pain. Stimulation of cutaneous afferent fibres or of the central end of the splanchnic nerve causes contraction of bronchial muscle, and this effect is probably due to stimulation of pain fibres.

Other reflexes

Pulmonary embolism is associated with bronchoconstriction. This effect may be reflex but it can also be partly due to the release of 5-hydroxy-tryptamine, histamine and other kinins from the intravascular thrombus formation.

Local chemical regulation of bronchial muscle

The effect of hypoxia is entirely reflex; a decrease in oxygen tension has no notable direct effect on bronchial muscle. Carbon dioxide, on the other hand, does exert a direct local effect on bronchial muscle.

Tracheobronchial secretions

Our knowledge of the secretions of the respiratory tract is incomplete. Numerous branched tubular-acinar submucosal glands are present in the trachea and bronchi but not in those terminal air-passages lacking cartilage. The secretions of goblet cells are discharged along ciliated ducts opening on to the surface epithelium which are found as far down as the bronchiole. They also produce mucus. In the submucosal glands there are three types of cell – mucus cells with basophilic cytoplasm and granular cells some of which are smaller and eosinophilic, and others basophilic.

In the terminal bronchiole the surface epithelium becomes cuboidal but scattered peg-shaped cells with domed non-ciliated laminal surfaces project above the epithelial cells. These are known as Clara cells and electron microscopy has confirmed their apocrine nature. It is believed that they are responsible for the bronchiolar secretion of surfactant whilst the alveolar source of this phospholid is thought to be the type II granular pneumocyte.

Nerve supply

The glands and their ducts are surrounded by a network of myoepithelial cells and electron microscopy suggests that these cells are under neural control. Vagal stimulation and parasympathomimetic drugs excite secretion of the glands which can be blocked by atropine.

There is no known nerve supply to goblet cells, Clara cells or type II granular pneumocytes.

Argyrophyl cells are found sparsely throughout the large bronchi and they contain neurosecretory intracytoplasmic granules. No neural connections with these cells have yet been demonstrated but it is suspected that they fulfil a chemoreceptor function.

Volume of secretion

The volume of mucus secretion in man is approximately 100–200 ml per day of which a substantial majority comes from the mucous glands rather than the goblet cells. Diffusion of water through the mucosal epithelium contributes to the overall volume.

Composition of secretion

The normal bronchial secretion is 95 per cent water. The mucus secretion consists mainly of sialic acid or sulphate and neutral polysaccharides. Albumen and immunoglobulins, especially secretory immunoglobulin IgA, are also present. The pH is neutral and the concentration of potassium and sodium mid-way between serum and cellular level. Specific antibodies have been shown to be present in nasal secretions and reaginic antibody IgE in tracheobronchial secretions of allergic subjects. Other substances such as lysozyme and transferrin may have an anti-infective function.

Pulmonary surfactant

Pulmonary surfactant is a phospholipid synthesized from glycerol in Clara cells and type II granular pneumocytes. It is responsible for stabilizing the surface tension of the alveolar surface such that the pressure within and between alveoli is equalized as they expand and contract. Without surfactant many alveoli are collapsed and the work of breathing greatly increased, which is the case in premature infants with the neonatal respiratory distress syndrome or hyaline membrane disease.

Functions of bronchial mucus

Tracheobronchial mucus does not humidify the inspired air, for in its passage through the nose this air becomes 90–95 per cent saturated with water vapour. External humidification is necessary when endotracheal intubation or tracheostomy has been performed. Mucus merely diminishes water loss from the respiratory tract and this effect is known as 'water proofing'. Tracheobronchial mucus provides a surface protection or physical barrier to inhaled organisms, chemicals and mechanical irritants. The secretions provide the necessary mucous blanket for the protective trapping of particles including micro-organisms, which are conveyed upwards and out of the respiratory tract by the ciliary mechanism and cough. In local infection bronchial mucous secretion is increased and an anti-infective action exerted by antibodies and non-specific substances such as lysozyme.

Hypersecretion and chronic bronchitis

Prolonged mild irritation results in an increase in the mucus-secreting cell population. Ciliated epithelial cells become replaced by goblet cells. In patients with a long history of chronic bronchitis this transformation is marked; the mucosal epithelium may become almost entirely composed of mucus-secreting cells. The deep mucous glands also become strikingly increased in size. The increase in thickness of this glandular layer may be up to threefold, which represents an increase in the volume of secreting tissue of over 25 times normal.

Reid (1960) has proposed that hypertrophy of what may be called the 'mucus secretory cell mass' represented by the sum total of all mucin secreting cells in the tracheobronchial tree, is the essential feature of 'chronic bronchitis', characterized by bronchial hypersecretion. This hypertrophy may result from chronic irritation by any of several irritants including infection, irritant and noxious gases, for example, smoke fumes or sulphur dioxide laden air in industrial zones. The increased secretion from the hypertrophic secreting cell mass results in failure of clearance of mucus from the bronchi, because the production of mucus exceeds the clearance capacity of the ciliary escalator. This mechanism may be further embarassed by the increased viscosity of the secretions and by the destruction of cilia by the inflammatory processes. The stagnant secretion becomes infected, and this has the effect of: (1) acting as an additional chronic irritant, causing further glandular hypertrophy; (2) decreasing the potential clearance capacity of the cilia, by further destruction of cilia and by depressing the efficiency of the surviving cilia. The stagnant secretion will tend to accumulate in and plug smaller bronchioles and even to enter the alveolar area, thus reducing the effective surface for gaseous exchanges. This hypersecretion leads to the sputum which is the clinical feature of this respiratory disorder.

Absorption from tracheobronchial mucosa

Absorption through the mucous membrane of the trachea and bronchial tree is slight. This is in striking contrast with the extensive absorption from the mucosa of the nose and nasopharynx, although the bronchial tree has, like the nasopharynx, a very rich network of capillary vessels. Water and crystalloids readily diffuse through the nasal mucosa.

When dyes which are readily absorbed from the nasopharyngeal mucosa (such as Evans blue) are introduced into the trachea only very small amounts are absorbed. Inhaled soot if it reaches the bronchial tree is mainly filtered out by adhering to the mucous blanket and then eliminated by ciliary action or expelled by the cough reflex.

A very minor amount is taken up by phagocytes and penetrates the bronchial mucous membrane.

Mucociliary mechanism

The inspired air which comes into contact with the lining mucosa of the tracheobronchial tree often has suspended particles, both inert and living and of varying size. Several defences exist to prevent these particles reaching the depths of the lung. The first line of defence provided by the mucociliary mechanism in the nose and nasopharynx has been discussed in Chapter 5. A similar protective mechanism for the arrest and disposal of bacteria and particulate matter is found in the trachea and bronchial tree. In the larynx and trachea the mucosa is lined by ciliated epithelium except over the vocal cords. The columnar ciliated epithelium is covered by a thin mucous film, which is maintained by ciliary action in constant motion, and which floats on an underlying fluid layer. The mucous blanket is steadily renewed by the secretion of the mucous glands.

Ultrastructure of cilia

Viewed with the light microscope cilia appear structurally homogeneous, with a small granule or basal body at the attached end of each cilium. Electron microscopy has revealed that each cilium has an external plasma membrane enclosing its central cytoplasm. Further, within the cytoplasm, are nine longitudinal electron-dense filaments or fibres, arranged around the periphery of the cilium, and two centrally placed longitudinal filaments. These structures are shown in cross-section in *Figure 11.13*. Each of the peripheral fibres is double. One of the two parts appears to be

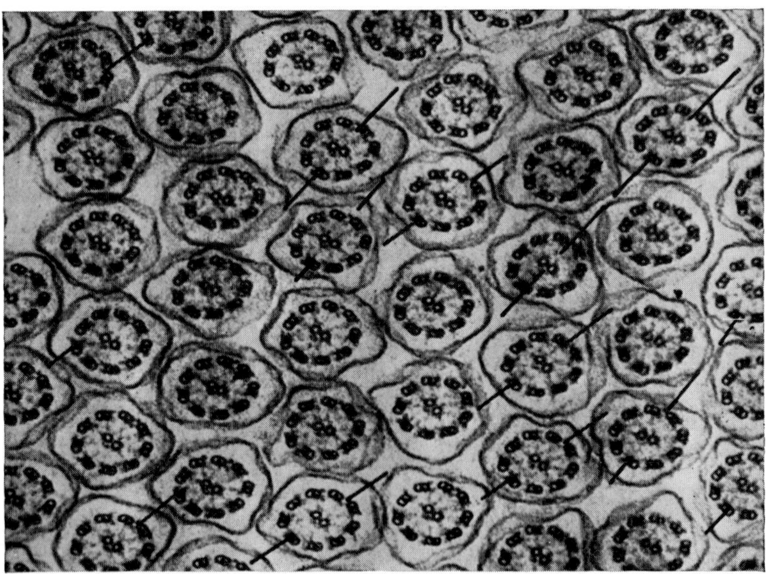

Figure 11.13 Cross-section of cilia. (From Satir, 1963, reproduced by courtesy of the Editor of *Journal of Cell Biology*)

tubular and the other more solid, and this solid subfibre has short projections or 'arms'. One pair of the nine peripheral fibres are joined by a bridge. The two central fibres are enclosed in a sheath. Radial sheets pass from this central sheath to the outer fibres and on each of these there is a secondary longitudinal fibre. This complex intraciliary arrangement is shown diagrammatically in *Figure 11.14*. The basal body

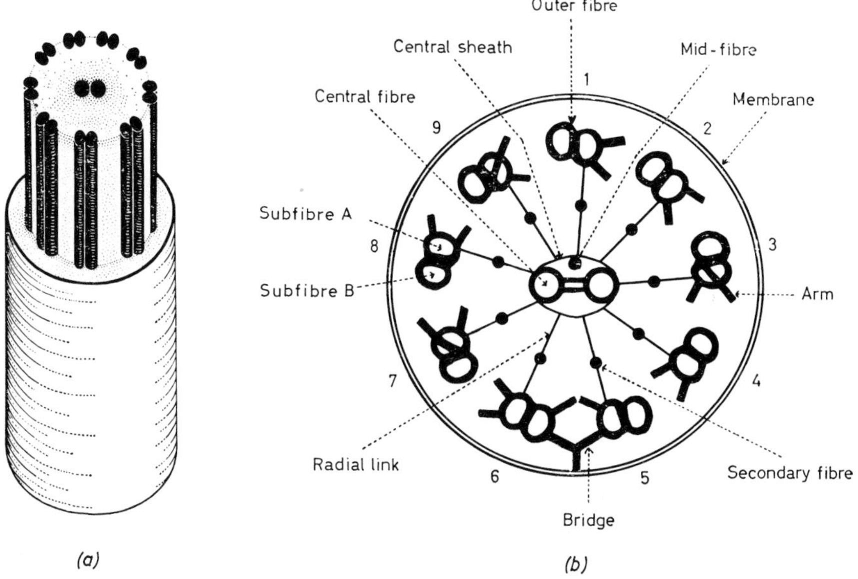

Figure 11.14 (a) Simplified diagrammatic representation of structure of a cilium. (From Fawcett, 1954, reproduced by courtesy of the Editor of *The Laryngoscope*. (b) Diagrammatic representation of transverse section of cilium showing detail of internal fibre organization. (From Gibbons, 1961, reproduced by courtesy of the Editor of *Journal of Biophysical and Biochemical Cytology*)

at the base of each cilium also has a complex internal organization consisting of a cylinder of nine fibres each, composed of three subfibres. It also has a dense cone-shaped foot-like projection with a system of fine tubules. This basic pattern of ultrastructure as displayed by the electron microscope is found to be universal in the cilia and flagella of all animal species. Between the cilia are scattered slender projections up to 1 μm in length called microvilli. Each ciliated cell is furnished with approximately 250 cilia and 150 microvillous processes.

Mechanism of ciliary motion

The movements of these ciliary processes are described in Chapter 5. The internal structure exposed by electron microscopy has made it possible to offer some suggestion as to the mechanism of ciliary movement. The ciliary beat could result from shortening, by internal molecular changes, of longitudinally disposed contractile elements. The rapid propulsive stroke may be explained as due to initial shortening of intraciliary contractile elements on one side only, and the recovery stroke as resulting from a later contraction of contractile structures on the opposite side. The dense peripheral fibres seen under the electron microscope may represent these contractile elements.

Cilia move in a constant direction and are found to beat uniformly along a plane perpendicular to the plane of the two central fibres. The effective stroke is towards the two peripheral fibres joined by a bridge. This is also the direction in which the basal foot is pointing. It has been suggested that the basal foot is the site of initiation of the excitation which produces the contraction of the bridged fibres. The excitation may then spread round the cilium to the other fibres. The basal foot is thus the 'pacemaker' of the ciliary cycle.

Ciliary streams

The mucus streams, produced by ciliary movement in the trachea and bronchi, flow in spirals towards the larynx and the pharynx. The speed of the movement of the mucus layer may reach 1–3 cm/min. The ciliary mechanism is highly efficient in the removal of organisms, dust and other particulate matter from the inspiratory air stream. This is of considerable significance in the polluted air of modern industrialized towns and in the dusty atmospheres of mining and allied occupations and in dusty climates. The efficiency of the nasal and tracheobronchial mucociliary mechanisms in removing bacteria from the inspired air is shown by the fact that in health air in the bronchi is free of micro-organisms.

Effective ciliary motion is dependent on normal composition and viscosity of the mucus; changes in viscosity readily affect ciliary propulsion. Drying causes degeneration and destruction of cilia. Ciliary beating is also inhibited by thermal changes, by changes of pH from the normal, and by hypertonic and hypotonic solutions. Ether and chloroform vapour in anaesthetic concentrations do not affect ciliary action.

References

Buchtal, F. (1960). *Experimental Physics*, **44**, 137

Campbell, E. J. M., Dickenson, C. J. and Salter, J. D. H. (1963). *Clinical Physiology*. Oxford; Blackwell

Comroe, J. H. J. (1962). *The Lung*. Chicago; Year Book Publishers

Cotes, J. E. (1975). *Lung Function*. Oxford; Blackwell

Engström, H. (1951). *Acta otolaryngologica, Stockholm*, **39**, 364

Faaborg-Andersen, K. (1957). *Acta physica Scandinavica*, **41**, (Suppl.) 140

Farnsworth, D. (1940). *Bell Laboratory Record*, **18**, 203

Fawcett, D. W. (1954). *Laryngoscope*, **64**, 557

Fletcher, H. (1953). *Speech and Hearing* (2nd edn.). New York; van Nostrand

Floyd, W. F., Negus, V. E. and Neil, E. (1957). *Acta otolaryngologica, Stockholm*, **48**, 16

Gibbons, I. R. (1961). *Journal of Biophysical and Biochemical Cytology*, **11**, 179

Goettler, K. (1951). *Forsching Anatomie*, **115**, 352

Horsefield, K. and Cumming, G. (1968). 'Functional consequences of airway morphology', *Journal of Applied Physiology*, **24**, 384

Husson, R. (1950). *Revue of Laryngology*, **78**, (Suppl.) 515

Laget, P. (1953). *Revue of Laryngology*, **74**, (Suppl.) 132

Macklem, P. T. and Mead, J. (1967). 'Resistance of central and peripheral airways measured by a retrograde catheter', *Journal of Applied Physiology*, **22**, 395

Miller, R. D. and Hyatt, R. E. (1969). 'Obstructing lesions of the larynx and trachea: Clinical and physiological considerations', *Mayo Clinic Proceedings*, **44**, 145

Moulonget, A. (1954). *Revue of Laryngology*, **75**, (Suppl.) 110

Negus, V. E. (1929). *The Mechanism of the Larynx*. London; Heinemann

Negus, V. E. (1956). *Lectures on the Scientific Basis of Medicine*, **4**, 332

Portmann, G. (1957). *Journal of Laryngology and Otology*, **71**, 1

Pressman, J. J. (1941). *Archives of Otolaryngology*, **33**, 351

Pressman, J. J. (1944) *Archives of Otolaryngology*, **39**, 14

Pressman, J. J. (1954). *Archives of Otolaryngology*, **59**, 221

Pressman, J. J. and Kelemen, G. (1955). *Physiology Review*, **35**, 506

Reid, Lynne (1960). *The Scientific Basis of Medicine*, **8**, 235

Rubin, H. J. (1960). *Archives of Otolaryngology*, **71**, 913

Satir, P. (1963). *Journal of Cell Biology*, **16**, 345

Weibel, E. R. (1963). *Morphometry of the Human Lung*. Berlin; Springer-Verlag

Weiss, D. A. (1959). *Archives of Otolaryngology*, **70**, 609

Widdicombe, J. G. (1954). *Journal of Physiology*, **123**, 71

Widdicombe, J. G. (1966). 'The regulation of bronchial calibre'. In *Advances in Respiratory Physiology* (Ed. by Caro, C. G.). London; Arnold

Wright, B. M. and McKerrow, C. B. (1959). 'Maximum forced expiratory flow rate as a measure of ventilatory capacity', *British Medical Journal*, **2**, 1041

Wyke, B. D. (1974). 'Laryngeal neuromuscular control systems in singing', *Folia Phoniatrica*, **26**, 295–306

12 The generation and reception of speech

A Fourcin and D B Fry

Introduction

Speech is beyond question the most complex and highly organized voluntary activity in which man indulges; and in the course of it he makes use of a number of mechanisms which also serve more vital physiological purposes – those of breathing, swallowing and hearing. The anatomy and physiology of many parts of the speech mechanism are dealt with in detail in other chapters of this book. There are, however, some parts of the mechanism, particularly those in the cerebral cortex, of which we are not as yet able to give an adequate description; they perform functions which we can describe only in psychological terms by referring to memory stores, language units, information, and so on; the most we can say at present is that operations of a given kind are carried out during speech communication, and there must be neural circuits in the brain which perform them. The purpose of this chapter is to give a brief functional account of the whole speech mechanism, including those elements of which we can make working drawings and circuit diagrams and those of which we cannot.

Both the sending of speech and its reception are necessary parts of the process of communication by speech, and the fact that the rôles of speaker and listener are combined in each individual has an important bearing on the consideration of the speech mechanism. In ordinary conditions, a speaker is certainly listening to his own speech while he is talking and it is not really possible to separate entirely the mechanism used for generating speech from that used for receiving it, since much of the machinery is used in both processes. In the following description of the speech mechanism, however, it will be convenient to deal separately with the two aspects of the process – generation and reception.

The generation of speech

The function of the brain

Communication by speech begins with some activity in the brain of the speaker, activity which is concerned with having something to say and with finding a way to say it. The 'something to say' may come from different sources, which we may characterize (to borrow Hughlings Jackson's terms) as propositional or affective (emotional) sources; the 'finding a way to say it' consists in organizing an appropriate language-form for the message, and it is with this part of the brain's activity that we shall be most concerned here.

In order that people may communicate with each other by speech they must have a common language. This means that the brain of each individual must be furnished with a memory store of certain linguistic material relevant to the language being used – whether it be English, or French, or any other language. Every language is a system of units which has certain properties, and it is a knowledge of what these properties are that constitutes the linguistic information which must be stored in the brain of speaker and listener alike.

Linguistic systems

All natural languages have the common property that their systems have a hierarchical structure, that is to say the system includes small units which are combined together to form units of the next higher level, and so on. In spoken English, for example, the smallest unit is the phoneme, in much the same way as the letter is the smallest constituent of the written language. Just as the written word *bat* consists of three letters, so when this word is spoken it is made up of three sounds. It is possible to draw up a complete inventory of the phonemic classes in a language by going systematically through the possible substitutions in phoneme sequences. For instance, in addition to the sequence /bat/*, the sequences /bad/, /bag/, and so on, also occur in which a substitution has been made in the third position in the sequence. Further possibilities are found by making a change in the first place, as in /pat/, /sat/, and so

Table 12.1 (a) English vowel phonemes

Symbol	Key word	Symbol	Key word	Symbol	Key word	Symbol	Key word
i:	heed	o	hod	ə:	herd	au	how
i	hid	o:	hoard	ə	hard<u>er</u>	oi	toy
e	head	u	hood	ei	hay	iə	here
a	had	u:	whom	ou	hoe	eə	hair
a:	hard	ʌ	hum	ai	high	uə	tour

(b) English consonant phonemes

Symbol	Key word	Symbol	Key word	Symbol	Key word	Symbol	Key word
p	pip	tʃ	church	s	sip	n	neat
b	bib	dʒ	judge	z	zip	ŋ	si<u>ng</u>
t	tit	f	first	ʃ	ship	l	<u>l</u>ip
d	did	v	verse	ʒ	measure	r	rip
k	kick	θ	thick	h	hip	j	yet
g	gig	ð	then	m	meat	w	wet

* Letters printed between oblique strokes represent sequences of phonemes.

on, or in the second place, as in /bit/, /bet/. The number of phonemes in the English system, arrived at in this way is just over 40, of which about 20 are the vowel phonemes and the rest the consonant phonemes. A list of the phonemes, with key words illustrating their occurrence, is given in *Table 12.1*.

Sequences of phonemes make up the morphemes, which are the next order of units and which have a grammatical function. It is important to realize that each type of linguistic unit is distinguished by its function rather than its form. The word *bat* was used as an example in talking about the phoneme system. This is one of the words which consists of only one morpheme; in fact there are two English morphemes /bat/, one which functions as a noun and one which functions as a verb. The latter may have another morpheme added to it, for example the morpheme /iŋ/, in the sentence 'He's been batting for an hour'; or the morpheme /id/, in the sentence. 'He batted for an hour'. In this way morphemes are put together to make words, which are the next order of units; but there are a great many cases in which one morpheme also forms a word in English, and there will be in addition a small number of morphemes which do not constitute words. The total number of English words in use at one period is very large; Daniel Jones' *English Pronouncing Dictionary*, for example, gives about 55 000 words.

It is one of the features of the economy of natural languages that a small basic repertory of phonemic units is used to give a very large store of words. This is an important fact in the learning of a language; a child, by the time he is five or seven years old, has learned the whole of the phonemic system and for the rest of his life has no need to add to his inventory of phonemes (as far as his native language is concerned), yet he will continually add to his stock of words.

The stringing together of words to make sentences needs little comment, except that in the spoken language any complete remark constitutes a sentence and hence it is very common for a single word to function as a sentence.

Knowledge of a language, then, means first of all a knowledge of what units are available at the various levels; but it also means a knowledge of the rules which govern the combination of units on one level into units on the next level. At the phonemic level, the language-user knows the complete inventory of phonemes and knows what sequences of phonemes are likely to occur in the composition of morphemes and words; the English speaker knows, for example, that a word may well begin with the sequence /pr/ but that it will certainly not begin with the sequence /pf/. He also knows what morphemes may or may not follow each other in his own language. The village child who was heard to say ''Er bain't a-calling we, us don't belong to she' was applying rules of morpheme combination just as surely as another child brought up in a different language environment who might say 'She's not calling us, we don't belong to her'. That is to say, the word 'rules' in this connection is related not to any notion of 'correctness', but only to usage.

In a similar way, most of the information concerning the sentence-level is stored in the form of rules for combining words into sequences that are possible in the language.

On the morpheme and word levels, the language-user will have a fairly large vocabulary of units which he can recognize (his passive vocabulary) and a much more restricted list of units which he himself will utter (his active vocabulary).

No communication by speech is possible without recourse to the kind of information which has just been briefly sketched. The first operation on the part of the speaker is to formulate what he has to say in language form. He chooses certain key words (content words) which embody the substance of what he wants to say, and intersperses them with words that settle the grammatical form of the sentence (form words). The choice of words in itself implies the choice of the proper morphemes, and this in its turn dictates the string of phonemes to be selected. Phoneme selection is a vital part of the process of speech-generation because upon it depend the operating instructions fed forward to the muscles used in speech.

Rhythm, intonation and voice quality

A great deal of the information contained in a message is carried by the phoneme-string, but there are other factors which play a part in speech communication. These are rhythm, intonation and voice quality. In language systems generally all these may have a function; in the English system, rhythm and intonation have an important rôle. An example of a rhythmic difference which has a linguistic function in English is to be found in pairs of words such as con*trast* and *con*trast; the first has iambic rhythm and is a verb; the second is trochaic and is a noun; and the distinction of rhythmic pattern regularly accompanies the difference in grammatical function. A difference in intonation pattern may similarly be linked with a difference of function.

In addition to their possible function in the language system, however, rhythm, intonation and voice quality all serve to convey information about the speaker as an individual. Indeed, part of the function of the speech centres in the brain is to control the muscular mechanisms in such a way that the personal voice quality of the speaker, his mannerisms of intonation and pronunciation, his habitual rhythm and tempo of speech, and also his more ephemeral changes of mood appear whenever he speaks.

Motor control of speech

It is clear from what has been said already that even the shortest utterance demands intense internal activity on the part of the speaker. The effects of this activity are passed on to the outside world by means of muscular actions which in turn give rise to sound waves. Respiration, phonation and articulation are the three main aspects of this muscular activity and, in each of these, many different muscles are employed. Since the movements in speech are so complex, so highly co-ordinated and so precisely timed, the brain must contain a motor control mechanism; and we may regard this as a very complicated 'phase control' which determines the exact moments at which different muscles begin their action, how long the action shall continue, and the moments at which it shall cease or be modified.

The instructions issued by this cerebral mechanism include the command to take in breath rapidly at appropriate moments in the stream of speech, and the paying out of breath as the utterance proceeds. As the phonemic units succeed each other in the message, they will call for the switching on of the laryngeal mechanism for all voiced sounds, and the switching off for all voiceless sounds and for silences.

The articulation of the sounds requires complex actions by the muscles of the pharynx, the various parts of the tongue, the soft palate and the facial muscles. Changes in the syllabic rate and in rhythm are implemented in part by the chest muscles; changes in the volume of the speech and in intonation are brought about very largely by the laryngeal muscles, which are also mainly responsible for changes in the quality of the voice.

The schematic diagrams shown in *Figures 12.1* and *12.2* indicate, in two stages, the control circuits which the speech centres of the brain must contain. *Figure 12.1* covers the formulation of a message in linguistic form and the feeding of information to the motor control mechanism; *Figure 12.2* shows the various muscular actions governed by this mechanism.

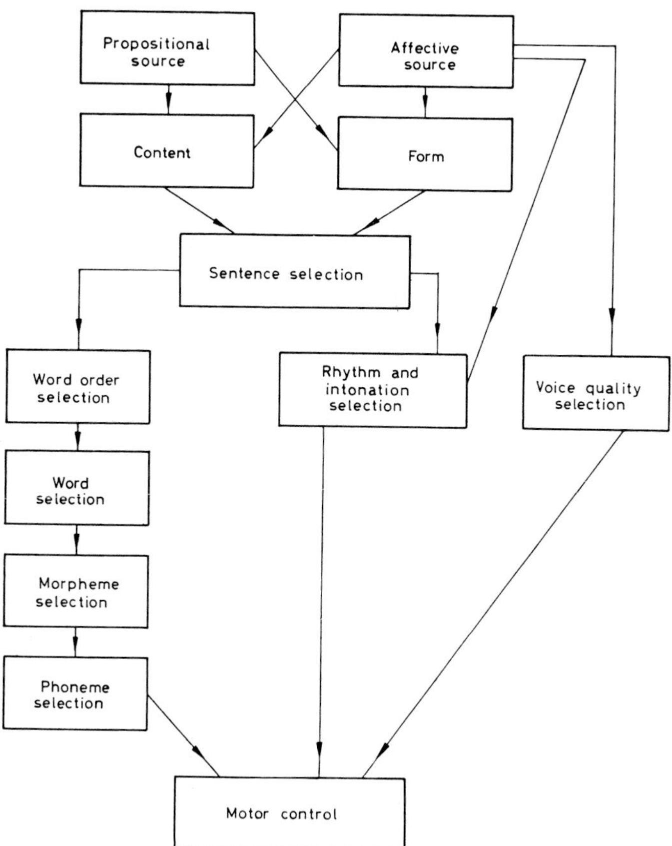

Figure 12.1 Schematic diagram showing the flow of information in the linguistic organization of the utterance

Feedback control of speech movements

It is clear that the motor control mechanism is a vital unit in the speech mechanism as a whole and that it is responsible for very highly co-ordinated and accurately timed movements. This degree of control is in fact never found, either in nature or in man-made machines, associated with systems in which instructions are simply fed forward to effector mechanisms. To achieve it, it is necessary to have recourse to feedback

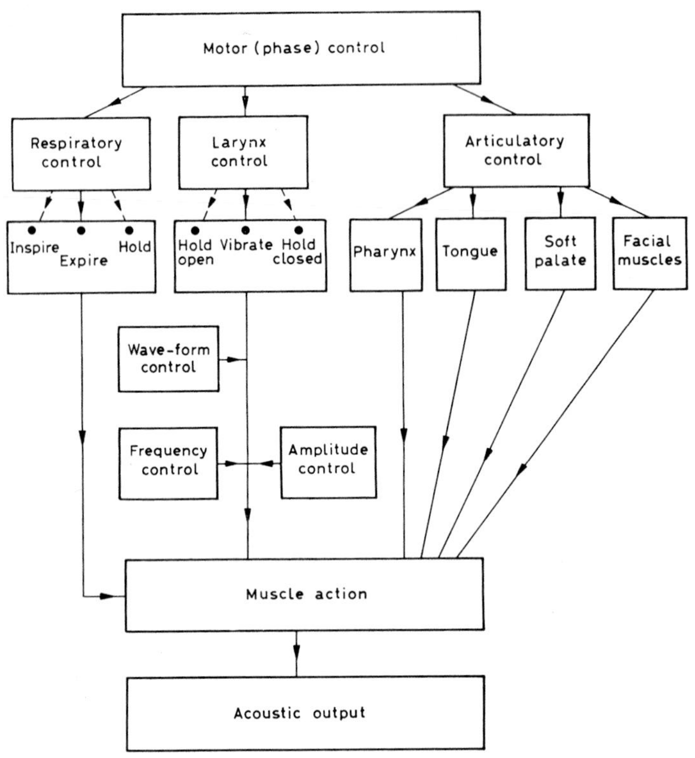

Figure 12.2 Schematic diagram of the motor control system used in speech

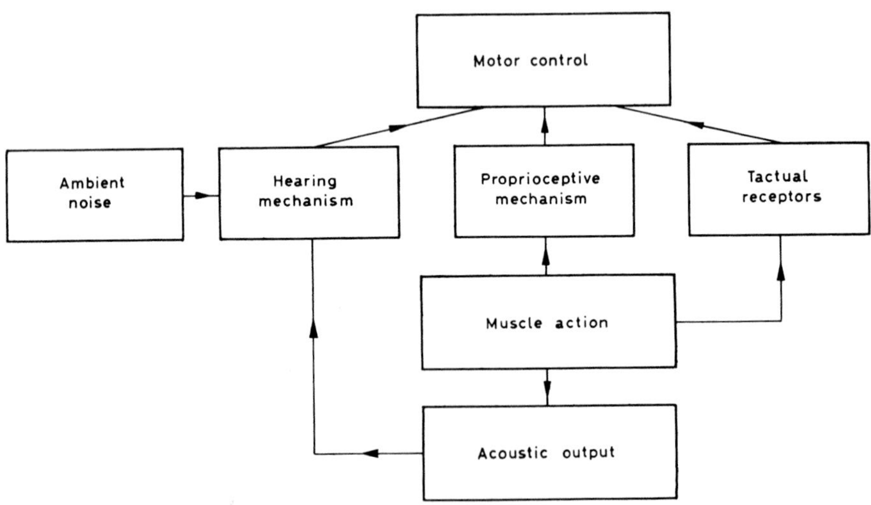

Figure 12.3 Feedback circuits used in the control of speech movements

loops, that is, to devices by means of which the output of the system is used in part to control the activity of the system itself.

In the control of speech movements, three feedback loops normally operate. These are shown schematically in *Figure 12.3*.

The first is the auditory feedback loop. The sounds which a speaker generates are transmitted to his own hearing mechanism as well as to the outside air. In the course of the learning process in childhood and during subsequent years, a firm association is established between variations in the sound heard and the articulatory movements which produce the sound, so that the information fed back to the speaker's brain by his hearing mechanism provides a continuous report on the progress of the movements. This information is important for the timing of an utterance, in order to 'programme' subsequent sections. This fact is very well demonstrated by the effects of delayed auditory feedback, that is, delaying the arrival of the sound of the speaker's voice to his own ear. For many speakers, a delay of about 0.1 s produces a marked disruption of the flow of speech movements, an artificial stammer.

It seems that the false information fed to the motor control mechanism in the case of delayed auditory feedback is more upsetting to the programming than a total lack of auditory information. If a very loud masking noise is fed into the ears of a speaker, many changes will take place in his speech, but he will continue to time the movements very much as he did when there was no masking noise. One change that takes place immediately when noise is fed into a speaker's ears is that the intensity of his speech rises. This indicates a very important function of the auditory feedback, which is to maintain as far as possible a satisfactory ratio between any noise that reaches the speaker's ears and the loudness of his own speech.

Much of the acoustic information that a speaker receives from his own voice reaches his hearing mechanism through the bones and other tissues of his head. This transmission path has very different characteristics from the air transmission path through which listeners hear the speaker's voice; consequently, a speaker's impression of his own voice quality is very different from his hearer's impression. For this reason it is difficult for a speaker to recognize his own voice the first time he hears it recorded, because the idea of his own voice that each individual builds up over the years is coloured above all by the bone-conducted sound.

It is evident, however, that the auditory feedback loop is not the only means of exercising control over the speech movements. If it were, we should expect to find a serious deterioration of speech when the speaker is in the presence of a loud noise, but such is not the case. It is true, of course, that in some patients who become very deaf in adult life, the prolonged absence of auditory feedback may eventually produce some deterioration of speech. A great measure of control is assured, however, through the medium of the kinaesthetic feedback loop, the circuit by means of which the brain receives information about the course of muscular actions, through the proprioceptive mechanism. In the period of learning in infancy and childhood, the use of the auditory feedback loop is of the utmost importance (Whetnall and Fry, 1964); and the control of speech movements without the aid of auditory feedback is possible only after the habits of movement have been thoroughly established. All habitual movements, including those of speech, are based on stored kinaesthetic patterns, and in normal conditions the control of speech is shared between the auditory and the kinaesthetic feedback loops, and the information from the two sources is complementary. The reason why delayed auditory feedback is disrupting to speech is that it causes the information fed back from the hearing mechanism to contradict that from proprioception.

A third circuit which contributes to the control of speech is the tactual feedback loop. Marked sensations of touch are obtained from various points in the speech mechanism – the tongue tip, the gums, the inside of the lips, and so on; and information which reaches the brain in this way plays some part in the control of speech.

In normal speech, these three feedback loops work together to produce the fine control of movement which speech demands.

The muscular speech mechanism

From the motor control mechanism of speech, there is a flow of instructions to the various muscles which carry out the movements of speech. Three main muscular systems are involved in this activity – respiration, phonation and articulation.

Respiration in speech

The transmission of speech from speaker to listener depends upon the generation of sound waves by the speaker. The source of energy for this acoustic output is provided by the flow of air from the lungs and therefore speech occurs only during the expiratory phase of breathing.

During quiet breathing, it is usual for the inspiratory and expiratory phases to occupy approximately equal amounts of time. If this regular rhythm of intake and output were preserved during speech, this would mean that half the speech time was used for breathing in; speech, however, makes much more economical use of the expired air and the typical rhythm of breathing for speech is a very rapid inspiration followed by a much longer period of expiration during which the breath is paid out more or less slowly.

The control of breathing for speech is affected by a number of factors which influence both the frequency of inspiration and also the amount of speech given out on each breath. The amount of time that intervenes in speech between one inspiration and the next is determined approximately by the individual habits of the speaker and by the demands of the situation. However, the exact moment at which breath is taken is dictated by the language system, because a breath-pause is made to coincide with the end of a syntactic group; without being at all aware of it, speakers carry in their brains a complete knowledge of the syntactical structure of their language and use this knowledge in the control of the speech mechanism.

In spontaneous speech, as distinct from reading aloud or reciting a prepared text, there are 'hesitation-pauses' in addition to 'breath-pauses'. These occur when the speaker needs additional time in which to find the word that appropriately conveys his meaning; consequently, they tend to happen just before content words, particularly the more uncommon ones. The incidence of hesitation-pauses in spontaneous speech is very much greater than any individual speaker or listener realizes, and a survey of a large body of material in English has shown that the mean number of words uttered consecutively without a pause is no more than four. From the point of view of the breathing mechanism, the pause forms a part of the speech output.

The action of the breathing muscles

The first task of the breathing muscles in speech is to take in air rapidly; their second task is to regulate the outflow of air from the lungs in such a way as to maintain the subglottic pressure at a level requisite for the production of voice by the larynx and of sounds articulated (in various ways) above the larynx. In quiet breathing the act of expiration is largely passive and is brought about in part by the tendency of the elastic material of the lungs to return to its unexpanded state – that is, by the relaxation pressure. The relaxation pressure depends in turn upon the amount of air taken in, that is, on whether the subject has breathed deeply or not so deeply. For a considerable proportion of the time, the relaxation pressure itself is enough to provide the necessary subglottic pressure for speech, but activity of the respiratory muscles may be necessary for two specific purposes. First, at the beginning of an utterance it may be necessary to counteract the effect of the relaxation pressure if it is too high. This is done by activity of the muscles used in inspiration – mainly the external intercostals, or the diaphragm, or both. The function of these muscles is to enlarge the thoracic cavity, thereby reducing the intrathoracic pressure; in speech they simply check the reduction in volume of the cavity. Second, towards the end of a long utterance on a single breath, when the relaxation pressure is no longer enough to produce the required subglottic pressure, muscular activity may be necessary to increase this pressure. Here the muscles of expiration, mainly the internal intercostals and the abdominal muscles, come into play and reduce still further the size of the thoracic cavity, thus increasing the pressure.

Amongst individuals, there is a well-known variation in the proportion of thoracic to abdominal muscular activity. It is generally said that women tend more to thoracic breathing and men to abdominal, but many examples of both kinds of breathing are to be found in both sexes. The statement refers, of course, to quiet breathing. The balance of evidence seems to be that speakers of either sex who show any degree of diaphragmatic activity during speech are in a very small minority. In the majority of speakers and the majority of utterances, the subglottic pressure is regulated entirely by the internal intercostal muscles, but at the end of a long utterance the abdominal muscles may be used to supplement the effort of the intercostals.

In addition to providing the reservoir of air and regulating its outflow, the breathing muscles also play some part in the articulation of the stream of speech sounds and, in particular, in the division of the stream into syllabic sequences.

The mechanism of phonation

The respiratory system affords the power supply for the acoustic speech output. In order that the sounds themselves should be generated, the flow of air in one direction from the lungs has to be used to produce alternating pressure changes. The larynx is the principal source of these pressure changes which are set up by the act of phonation, that is to say, by the vibration of the vocal cords.

In the production of voice, the pressure in the trachea is applied to the closed vocal cords, which are brought together by the action of the intrinsic laryngeal muscles.

The mechanics of the muscular actions are described in Chapter 10.

The breathing mechanism continues to build up the subglottic pressure, which is withstood for a certain time by the vocal cords but eventually overcomes the resistance offered by the obstruction, thus forcing the cords apart. There is an immediate outflow of air through the glottis and this gives rise to a fall in pressure on the underside of the cords (the Bernoulli effect). The return of the vocal cords to their closed position is due, therefore, to the combined effects of the restoring force of their own elasticity and the rarefaction due to the Bernoulli effect. This cycle of opening and closing continues as long as muscular action is maintained to adduct the cords, and the subglottic pressure is high enough to force them apart.

An important aspect of laryngeal activity during phonation is the changing of the period of vibration of the vocal cords which regulates the fundamental frequency of the sound produced. In speech, the frequency of the laryngeal tone changes continuously, whilst in singing it is held constant for some appreciable time, although even here the frequency is generally subject to the rhythmic fluctuations introduced by vibrato.

The frequency of the cord vibrations at any given moment is determined by the mass, length and tension of the cords and these physical characteristics are regulated by various muscular actions in the larynx. Increase in mass and length, and decrease in tension, will all lower the frequency of vibration. The control mechanism adjusts the activity of all the various muscles concerned, so as to produce the desired frequency when the prevailing subglottic pressure is applied to the cords.

Functions of the laryngeal mechanism

The primary function of the sound of voice in speech is to make speech audible. It acts as a carrier-wave on which intelligence may be imposed and conveyed to the listener, and it is not surprising, therefore, that phonation should be maintained during a good proportion of the time occupied by an utterance. The importance of phonation can be judged from the fact that the replacement of ordinary voice by whisper reduces the audibility of speech very drastically.

Laryngeal action is the vehicle for many of the differences between speakers, particularly in voice quality, and also for many of the temporal changes required by a given language system. The size and shape of the larynx, the properties of the vocal cords and the way in which the laryngeal muscles are employed all contribute to the quality of voice which we take to be characteristic of an individual speaker.

As far as the linguistic system is concerned, laryngeal activity plays an important rôle in conveying differences in intonation, in rhythm and syllabification, and in phonemic sequence. In normally-voiced speech, intonation patterns are associated mainly with patterns of variation in the frequency of the laryngeal tone.

We have already noted that the breathing muscles play some part in syllabification. Laryngeal action also contributes something to the syllabic character of speech, although the work of the articulatory mechanism is the main factor here. From this point of view, the switching on and off of phonation is important; for example, the word ‘potato’ has three syllables and the larynx is switched on and off three times during its utterance; but in the expression ‘good morning’, the larynx is simply switched on at the beginning and off at the end of the three syllables. The rhythmic pattern, in English particularly, is often established by the amount of time for which the larynx is switched on; the difference between the two words ‘*per*fect’ (adjective) and 'per*fect*' (verb) depends to a great extent on whether the larynx is switched on for a longer time in the first or in the second syllable.

We shall be dealing in the following section with the phonemic differences that depend on articulation. Presence or absence of phonation, however, is also a factor that distinguishes between sounds belonging to different phonemic classes. For example, in the pair of voiced and voiceless consonants /d, t/, the first is marked by some slight laryngeal activity, the second by the absence of laryngeal vibration; and the length of time for which the larynx is switched on may be significant. For instance, in the word 'bead' phonation will continue longer than in 'beat', even though it may cease before the articulation of /d/ is completed.

The articulatory speech mechanism

Respiration provides the power supply for speech; phonation is the process by which the power is used to generate a train of pulses which constitute the carrier-wave; it is the action of articulation that imposes on this carrier the intelligence which is conveyed to the listener. The pharynx, the soft palate, the tongue and the lips (that is to say, the whole of the vocal tract above the larynx) play a part in the articulation of the various sounds that make up speech.

The first major effect of articulation is to modulate the amplitude of the carrier-wave and thus to impart to speech its syllabic structure. Switching off the laryngeal mechanism, as we have already seen, is one way of marking a syllabic boundary; this reduces the amplitude of the carrier to zero. In other cases, the amplitude is simply decreased by using the articulatory mechanism to constrict or to close down completely the air-passage at some point above the larynx. A syllable consists of that section of an utterance during which the carrier-amplitude is high, with a section of low amplitude on either side. The high-amplitude sections correspond to the occurrence of vowels in the phoneme sequence, the low-amplitude sections to the occurrence of consonants.

The sounds of speech are classified in accordance with the articulatory movements that give rise to them. The two basic classes are those of the vowel (in which the vocal tract is relatively open above the glottis) and the consonant (in which it is constricted or completely obstructed for some time). Within these classes, much of the differentiation is based on the action of the tongue (*Tables 12.2* and *12.3*).

In uttering vowels, the movement of the tongue may carry it towards the front of the oral cavity, giving rise to front vowels, towards the back of the cavity, back vowels, or to the middle part of the cavity, central vowels. In addition, the tongue may rise to a relatively high point in the mouth, in which case the vowel is a close vowel; or it may be kept low in the mouth, in which case it is an open vowel. The terms half-close and half-open are used for movements of intermediate extent.

Classification of the articulatory movements that give rise to consonant sounds requires a somewhat more complex system. We have already noted that some consonants are voiceless and some are voiced. In *Table 12.3*, which gives a complete list of English consonants, the voiced consonants are shown in bold type. The other dimensions used with regard to consonants are first, the place in the vocal tract at which the constriction or closure is made; and second, the way in which the

Table 12.2 Classification of English vowels

	Front	Central	Back
Close	i:		u:
Half-close	i		u
Half-open	e	ə:, ə, ʌ	o:
Open	a		a:, o

Table 12.3 Classification of English consonants

Manner of articulation	Place of articulation						
	Bilabial	Labiodental	Dental	Alveolar	Palatal	Velar	Glottal
Plosive	p **b**			t **d**		k **g**	
Affricate				tʃ **dʒ** tr **dr**			
Fricative		f **v**	θ **ð**	s **z** ʃ **ʒ**			h
Nasal	**m**			**n**		**ŋ**	
Lateral				**l**			
Semi-vowel				**r**	**j**	**w**	

articulation is carried out – that is, the combination of movements or the time sequence of movements.

In the columns of *Table 12.3* are shown the sounds which are made at approximately the same place in the vocal tract. Bilabial sounds require a movement bringing together the two lips; labiodental sounds are made by approximating the upper teeth and the lower lip; in alveolar sounds the tongue movement brings the edge of the tongue into contact with the upper alveolar ridge, in front and at the sides; the articulation of palatal sounds carries the front of the tongue up under the hard palate, and of the velar sounds, the back of the tongue under the soft palate; in glottal sounds, the point of articulation is actually at the glottis.

The mode of articulation provides the horizontal dimension in *Table 12.3*. Plosive consonants are those in which the vocal tract is completely obstructed for a short time; during this time, since air is still issuing from the lungs, pressure builds up behind the obstruction. There is then a rapid separation of the parts which are causing the obstruction – the two lips in bilabial articulation, the edge of the tongue and the alveolar ridge in alveolar sounds, and so on. If instead of a complete closure, the articulatory movement narrows the vocal tract at some point, the resulting sound is a fricative. In making these sounds, especially the voiceless ones, the volume of air flowing past the point of constriction has to be higher than would be provided by the normal outflow of air for other sounds; and the respiratory muscles therefore come into play to increase the flow. Affricates require a combination of plosive and fricative movements; first there is a complete closure of the vocal tract, with a building-up of pressure, but the movement of release is slower than in the plosive consonant; hence, as the pent-up air escapes, it gives rise to a fricative sound produced at the same point of articulation as the stop.

The lower three rows of *Table 12.3* refer to modes of consonant articulation which are of rather different character. In nasal consonants, the oral branch of the vocal tract is completely obstructed but the airway through the nasopharynx is open and there is therefore no building-up of pressure above the glottis. This is the only class of articulation in which the soft palate is not raised to shut off the nasal branch from the oral branch of the vocal tract. Lateral articulations are those in which an open air-passage is maintained along the side or sides of the tongue; the tip of the tongue makes contact with the upper alveolar ridge in the front, but the sides of the tongue are withdrawn from contact through the contraction of the transverse fibres of the tongue. Semi-vowels, as the name suggests, consist in the brief articulation of a vowel.

The production of running speech requires the stringing together of all these types of articulatory movement, in a great variety of sequences, each movement running smoothly into the next. The system of classification gives an oversimplified impression of the articulatory movements, since it suggests a progression from one articulatory position to another. In fact, there are no positions, only continuous movement. In addition to the features of articulation that form the basis of classification, there are others (such as the action of the lips and facial muscles) which accompany all articulations but do not happen to play a part in the English system of distinctive differences. The variety and complexity of these concomitant movements is demonstrated by the fact that people are able to lip-read speech.

The acoustic output

We will turn now from the consideration of the physiological aspect of the muscular speech mechanism to a discussion of this mechanism as a physical system for producing sound waves. As such, it consists of two elements; a sound-producing source – the larynx for the greater part of the time; and placed on top of the source, an irregularly-shaped tube whose acoustic properties modify the character of the waves coming from the source, and so give rise to the sound waves which issue from the mouth of the speaker. It will be clear that all the changes that take place in the larynx will introduce modifications in the source; on the other hand, most of the articulatory movements affect mainly the size and shape of the tube. An exception to this division of functions has to be noted in the case of certain consonants, in which the articulatory mechanism itself provides a source of sound.

The source function

The vibrations of the vocal folds set up cycles of pressure change at the lower end of the vocal tract. Whilst the folds are apart, the subglottal airways are in communication with the vocal tract and the egressive pulmonic air flow which maintains normal vocal fold vibration occurs. For normal phonation, vocal fold closure occurs much more rapidly than fold separation. This is a result of the Bernoulli effect which requires that, in the absence of any external force, the total energy in the air particles flowing through the glottis should be constant. Since adduction of the vocal folds reduces glottal area the consequent increase in air particle velocity is associated with a complementary reduction in air pressure. This is a positive feedback process which gives a shock excitation to the vocal tract. The resulting acoustic response of the vocal tract for a typical vowel sound is illustrated in *Figure 12.4 (a)*. Each complex oscillatory cycle corresponds to one complete vocal fold vibration. A convenient way

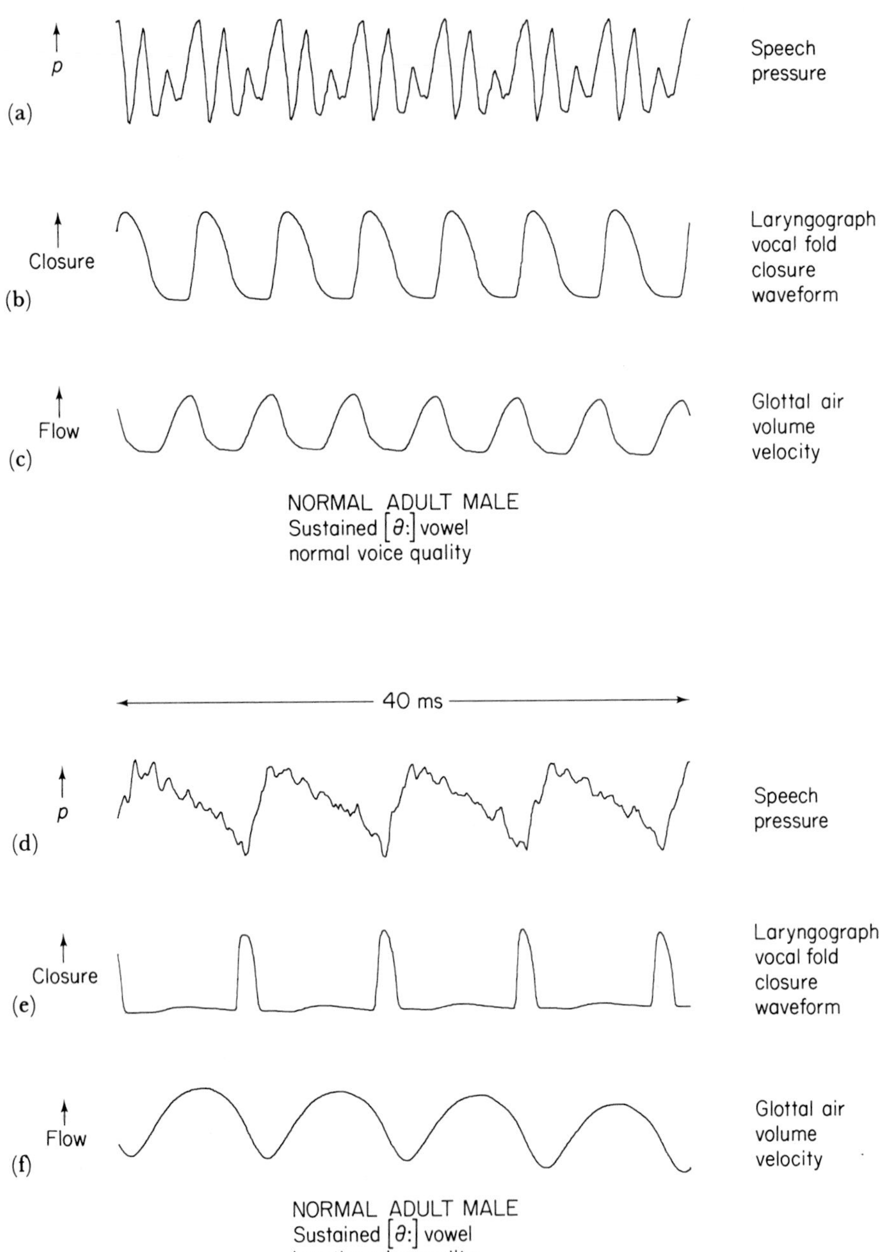

Figure 12.4 Sustained [ð:] vowel, in the normal adult male. (a)–(c) normal voice quality; (d)–(f) breathy voice quality

of examining vocal fold activity is provided by the laryngograph (Fourcin, 1974), and its output, *Lx,* is shown in *Figure 12.4 (b)*. The peak of speech pressure activity clearly follows the sharply defined closure of the vocal folds and acoustic response continues during the closure phase. During the open phase, however, the coupling of the subglottal cavities to the vocal tract reduces its acoustic response. Good voice production depends on three factors, which are clearly shown in *Figure 12.4 (a)* and *(b)*. First, there must be a sharply defined closure of the vocal folds. Second, closure must be maintained for an appreciable proportion of the vibratory cycle. Third, the closure of the vocal folds must occur regularly. *Figure 12.4 (c)* shows how the glottal air flow is related to these acoustic pressure and vocal fold contact wave-forms. *Figure 12.4 (d), (e)* and *(f)* shows the same wave-form conditions when the speaker uses a breathy voice quality. Here the increased length of the open phase introduces a marked increase in vocal tract damping and the resonances of the vocal tract are far less well defined. These examples have important implications in an understanding of voice pathology.

Regular vocal fold closure not only gives a coherent excitation to the resonances of the vocal tract, but also defines the pitch of the speaking – and singing – voice. *Figure 12.5* illustrates the way in which the controlled adjustment of the laryngeal musculature by a normal adult male speaker can result in changes in vocal fold frequency which are significant in speech. On the left a citation question form is shown, corresponding to rising voice pitch whilst on the right a falling statement form is shown. These apparently smooth curves are obtained by the direct, unsmoothed measurement of successive vocal fold periods from the closures detected in the

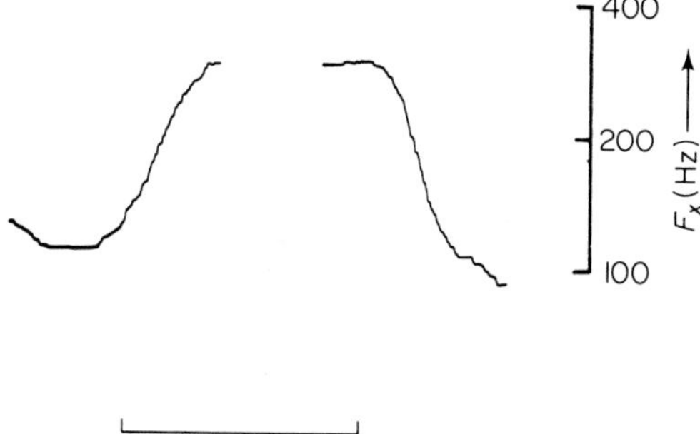

Figure 12.5 Adult male rise–fall intonation contrast, measured directly from *Lx* wave-forms

speaker's laryngograph wave-forms. This provides a very accurate basis for the measurement of the frequency, *Fx,* with which the vibrating vocal folds excite the resonances of the vocal tract. This combination of precision and simplicity makes the laryngograph a useful tool for both clinical work and research. A particular example of *Lx* and *Fx* is shown in the contribution by E. E. Douek* (Fourcin and Abberton, 1971). This apparatus is routinely employed for therapy in cases of voice production disorder in several centres. It is also possible to provide a basis for the quantitative assessment of treatment by the use of this approach. Speech and *Lx* recordings can be made on a standard stereo recorder and the *Lx* information analysed to provide a graphical representation of the patient's voice condition which may be included in the case notes.

* Volume 2

A particularly useful, and simple, representation of this type is shown in *Figure 12.6*. *Figure 12.6 (a)* shows the distribution of voice frequencies in the speech of a normal woman whilst *Figure 12.6 (b)* gives the result of similar analysis for a normal adult male speaker. These distributions are typical of normal phonation; the range of *Fx* is compact and within each speaker's range there are well-defined modes. This type of analysis can be obtained whilst the speaker is talking and, since it depends on the laryngograph wave-form, is unaffected by ambient noise. Two examples of the application of this type of analysis to pathological conditions are given (Wechsler, Neil and Fourcin, 1976).

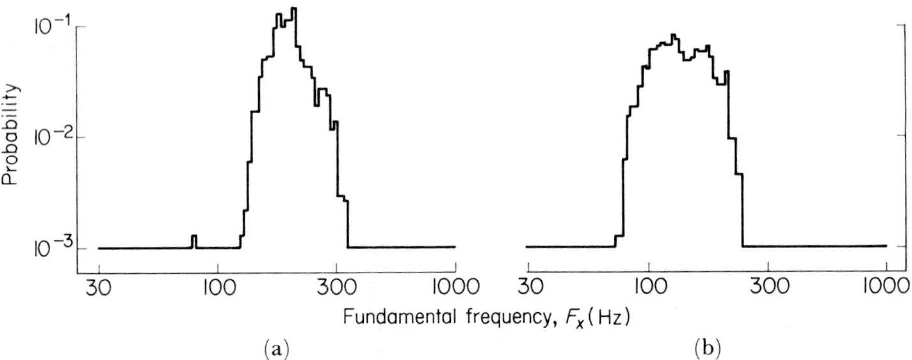

Figure 12.6 Normal voice frequency distributions obtained from long recordings of *Lx* wave-forms. (a) Adult female (50 s voice time); (b) adult male (25 s voice time)

Figure 12.7 (a) relates to a patient who had a fleshy polyp with a large base on one vocal fold; the shape of this voice frequency distribution histogram is markedly different in the low frequencies from the normal analyses shown in *Figure 12.6*. After the surgical removal of the polyp, the patient's voice quality was relatively normal although the range was restricted. This is shown quantitatively in *Figure 12.7 (b)* where it can also be seen that there is a residual low frequency irregularity. This type of information is potentially valuable to the subsequent assessment of the patient's progress. *Figure 12.8* shows the change in voice quality over a period for a patient with

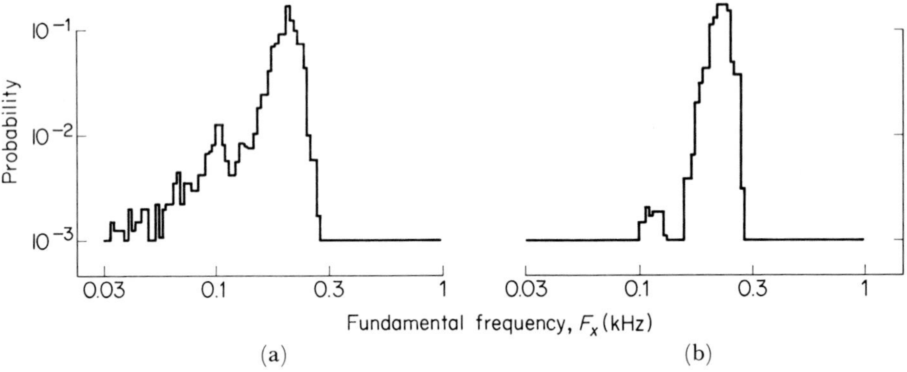

Figure 12.7 Adult female aged 46 years: voice frequency distributions (a) before surgery (35 s voice time); (b) after surgery (44 s voice time)

a left vocal fold palsy, as a result of three months of speech therapy with no surgical intervention. After therapy (*Figure 12.8 (b)*) there was a subjectively evaluated improvement in voice quality and some return of movement in the paralysed vocal fold. Laryngographic tape recordings before therapy and eighteen months later are

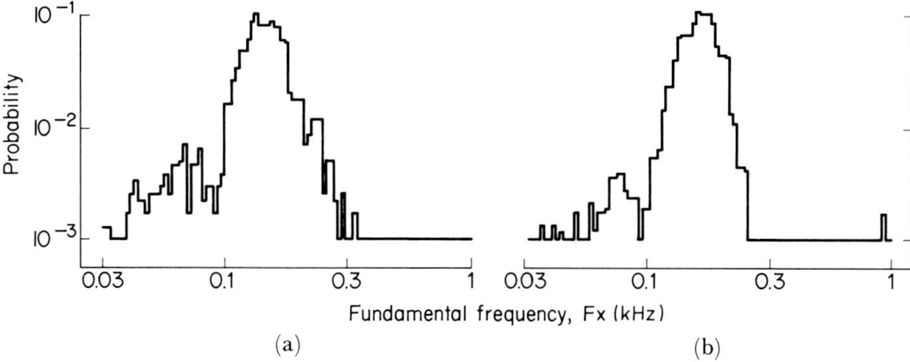

Figure 12.8 Adult male aged 63 years: voice frequency distributions (a) before speech therapy (16 s voice time); (b) after three months' speech therapy (33 s voice time)

basic to the two distributions shown. The later analysis shows a maintenance of improvement with a marked reduction in the abnormal low frequency components of vibration and an essentially normal high frequency tail to the distribution. This correlates well with the auditory evaluation but, additionally, provides a succinct quantitative addition to the case notes which will be useful for later assessment.

The larynx, however, is not the only possible source of sound in speech. It was stated previously that during the production of some sounds the laryngeal mechanism is switched off. At such times another source, a noise generator, comes into action. When the vocal tract is constricted at some point and a considerable volume of air from the lungs is forced past the constriction, turbulence is set up which gives rise to a sound with an irregular, non-repeating wave-form and a more or less extended spectrum. The main difference between this source and the laryngeal source, therefore, is that it generates aperiodic sounds whilst the larynx produces periodic sounds. A second difference is that the laryngeal source is situated at the lower end of the vocal tract whereas the noise source may be placed at various points along the length of the tract; consequently, the effect of the tube upon the noise depends not only on the source-wave but also on its location in the tube.

The noise source may be switched on for an appreciable time in the production of fricative consonants, or for a much shorter time in plosive sounds. It may also be switched on at the same time as the laryngeal source during voiced fricatives and plosives.

The filter system

The vocal tract, from the level of the larynx to the lips, is a tube of irregular shape; the cross-sectional area and the shape of the section vary according to the distance from the larynx and also to the disposition of the articulatory mechanism. The tube acts as an acoustic filter which operates on the source-wave, whether this be coming from the larynx or from a noise-generator at some other point in the tube. The materials which constitute the tube are such as to give the filter a high degree of 'damping' and therefore a considerable part of the energy contained in the source-wave is absorbed as it passes through the vocal tract. The absorption varies greatly with frequency, owing to the resonances of the tube; and the resonances of the tube depend in turn upon the position of the tongue, soft palate and lips. The total length of the tube from glottis to lips is some 15–17 cm; and if we imagined for a moment that this were a straight cylindrical tube of uniform cross-sectional area (of the order of 8 cm^2), there would be three principal resonances in the tube at about 500, 1500 and 2500 Hz. If the glottal source-function were to be applied to such a tube, it would produce at its mouth a vowel-like sound somewhat resembling the vowel in the English word *bird*. The human vocal tract, however, is not such a tube, and resonances occur in it at many different frequencies, mainly because the movement of the tongue introduces narrowing in the tube at several different points. The frequencies of such resonances in the vocal tract are known as formants.

In *Figure 12.9 (a)*, we see the shape assumed by the tube during the vowel of the word 'hid', and the way in which the filter modifies the 'spectrum' of the source-function. For the vowel /i/ the tongue moves forward and high up in the mouth; the space in the pharynx and up to the point of maximum constriction is relatively large.

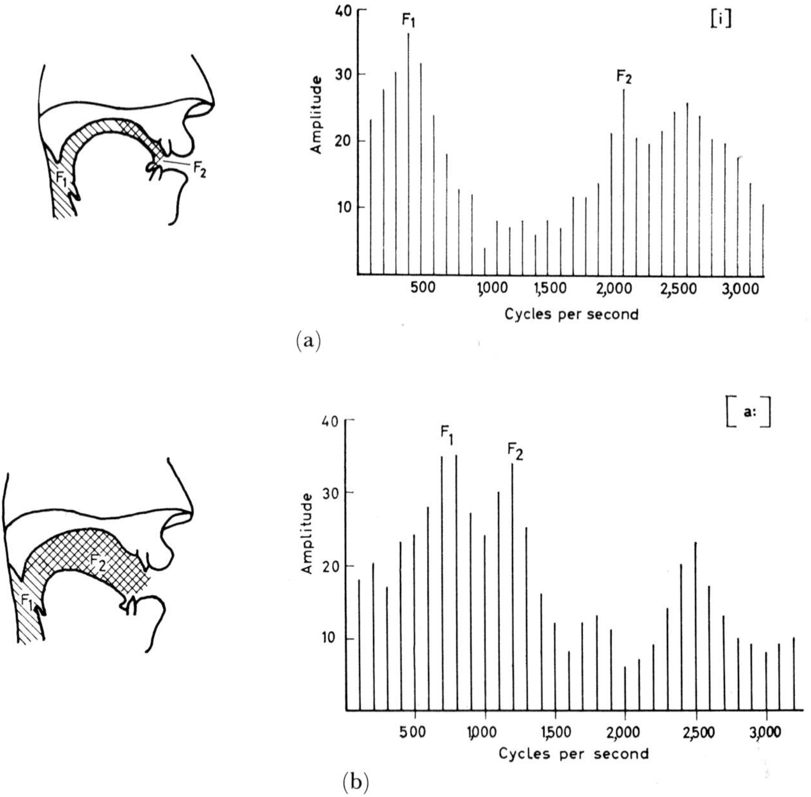

Figure 12.9 (a) Shape of the vocal tract and sound spectrum of the vowel /i/; (b) shape of the vocal tract and sound spectrum of the vowel /a:/

One resonance of the tube is therefore at a low frequency and this produces a peak in the spectrum in the region of 400 Hz. The space in front of the constriction, on the other hand, is small, and this produces a second resonance at a high frequency, in the region of 2100 Hz. A third resonance is to be found at about 2600 Hz.

Figure 12.9 (b) shows the shape of the tract for the vowel /a:/, and the way in which the filter modifies the spectrum of the source-function during this vowel.

The changes in the vocal tract brought about by the movements of articulation introduce continual modifications in the filtering properties of the tract, and hence cause frequent shifts in the position of the spectral peaks. The filter system may also have 'anti-resonances', which produce troughs rather than peaks in the spectrum.

The source and the filter system are together responsible for the sound waves that come from the speaker's mouth. The features of these waves vary continuously with time; there is practically no such thing as a steady state in the acoustics of speech.

The reception of speech

We have seen that the process of speech generation consists essentially of a series of transformations, from the linguistic form of the message in the speaker's brain to the sound waves that issue from the speaker's lips. The task of the receiving mechanism is to perform a series of transformations in the reverse direction, from the sound waves which arrive at the listener's ear to the linguistic form of the message in the listener's brain.

While the movements in speech generation are skilled movements, the movements executed by the hearing mechanism are mechanical – that is to say, they involve no learning. The process of learning to receive speech is carried out by the central cortical mechanisms.

The reception of speech is a two-fold process, consisting first of the 'processing' of information derived from the acoustic input; and secondly, of combining this information with linguistic information drawn from the stock which is already available in the listener's brain.

The acoustic processing of speech

The sound waves which set the listener's drumhead in motion are simply minute changes in air pressure, whose amplitude varies continuously with time. The curve of such pressure changes is identical with an oscillogram of a given utterance, taken in suitable conditions. *Figure 12.10 (a)* shows an oscillogram of one utterance of the sentence: 'She began to read her book'.

The time curve of the pressure variations is transmitted through the middle-ear mechanism to the inner ear, and here they are subject to some form of frequency analysis, so that the oscillogram is no longer an adequate representation of the information that the wave-motions provide. In order to discuss the acoustic aspect of speech, therefore, it is necessary to rely on some transformation of the time–pressure curve which supplies a frequency–intensity analysis at least qualitatively similar to the one carried out by the cochlear mechanism. Such an analysis is usually made with the aid of a spectrograph, a device which measures the spectral distribution of energy in a sound at successive instants and, generally, makes a visible record of changes in the spectrum. A spectrogram of the same utterance: 'She began to read her book' is shown in *Figure 12.10 (b)*.

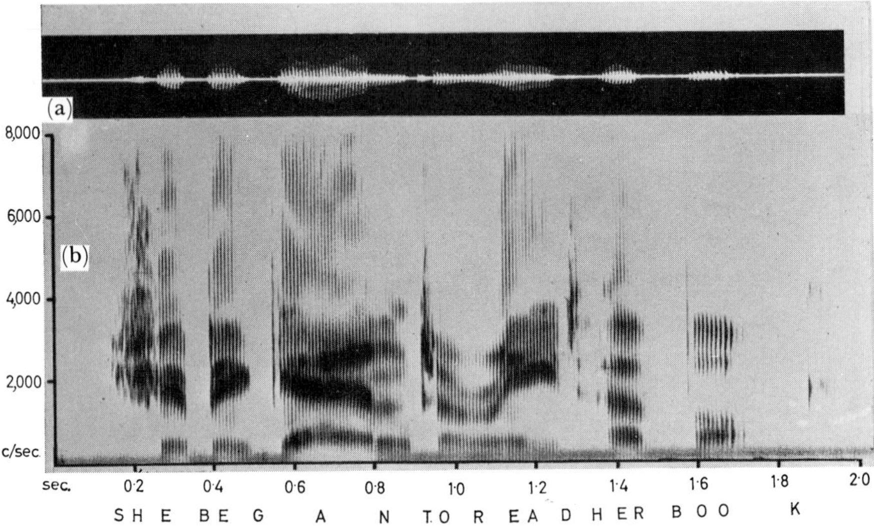

Figure 12.10 (a) Oscillogram of the sentence: 'She began to read her book'; (b) spectrogram of the sentence: 'She began to read her book' (filter bandwidth 300 Hz)

This spectrographic analysis was made by passing the sequence of sounds through a number of filters and registering the amount of acoustic energy in each filter band at succeeding instants throughout the whole utterance. Time is measured on the horizontal axis, frequency on the vertical axis.

It is clear from this spectrogram that speech sounds vary both in their total acoustic energy, and in the way this energy is distributed with frequency. For short spaces of time there is no trace at all (except for the zero line which appears at the bottom of the pattern); this indicates that there is no acoustic output at those moments.

Such silences are to be found at the times which correspond with the complete closure of the vocal tract for plosive sounds. Other sounds show widespread blackness in the pattern, indicating a high level of acoustic intensity. Over a considerable part of the pattern, the trace is broken up by vertical striations; each such stripe represents one cycle of vocal cord action. Thus, wherever these striations occur in the time-pattern, the laryngeal mechanism is switched on and the sound is voiced.

At many places in the pattern, there are broad black bars indicating a high level of acoustic energy in certain frequency regions; these represent the peaks in the spectrum due to the formants of the vocal tract. It is clear from this spectrogram that formant frequencies never remain at the same value for very long; this is due to the fact that the articulators are in almost continuous movement. At many points the change in formant frequency is quite rapid, and these rapid changes are very important for sound recognition. They are known as formant transitions.

At other places, there is a more random black trace which indicates that the noise generator is switched on; there is, for example, an extended one at the beginning of the pattern which corresponds with the occurrence if the fricative /ʃ/.

Acoustic cues in speech recognition

The spectrogram is a means of presenting in a convenient form the information about frequency, intensity and time contained in the sound waves of speech, and it is thus a useful basis for considering the use that is made of such information in the decoding of speech by the brain. In order to do so, however, we must first note some general features of the process of recognition.

The interpretation of a spoken message by a listener is an operation of a very particular kind which has no parallel in human behaviour except the reading of a handwritten message, which is in many ways analogous to the reception of speech.

One important fact about speech recognition is that the listener's brain must be operating on the relations of acoustic values, and not on absolute values; in other words, it must be taking note of the relations of frequency, intensity and time. Another fact which has been established by a whole body of experimental work in recent years is that the listener, in making a single recognition, has a number of acoustic cues at his disposal.

The cues for the recognition of vowels depend mainly on their formant structure; in addition to the formant frequency cues, there are also intensity cues and time cues. The vowel sounds differ from each other not only in total intensity but also in the relative intensity of their formants. From the point of view of the relative duration of the different vowels, those in English divide themselves into two broad classes – long vowels and short vowels; the duration cues are of considerable importance for vowel distinctions when the differences in frequency and intensity are relatively small, a long vowel lasting (on average) one-and-a-half times to twice as long as a short vowel.

The system of acoustic cues for the recognition of consonants is more complex than that used for vowels. The consonant sounds are generally of lower intensity than the vowel sounds, and indeed the distinction between vowels and consonants depends very largely on this intensity difference; even amongst consonants themselves, intensity differences are important cues because, no matter how loud or how soft the speech may be, the intensity relations of the consonant sounds remain fairly constant. *Table 12.4* gives the mean values for the intensity differences in English consonant sounds, expressed in decibels above the level for that consonant sound with the lowest intensity, that is /θ/, as in 'thin'.

Table 12.4 Relative intensity of English consonants*

p	7	dʒ	13	ʃ	19
b	8	f	7	ʒ	13
t	11	v	10	m	17
d	8	θ	0	n	15
k	11	ð	10	ŋ	18
g	11	s	12	l	20
tʃ	16	z	12	r	20

* Intensities are expressed in dB relative to the intensity of /θ/.

In *Table 12.3*, the English consonants were classified according to: (1) the manner of articulation; (2) the place of articulation; (3) the presence or absence of voice. Spectrographic analysis of these consonants shows what acoustic cues are important for dividing the consonants into these categories, but it is not possible to include such a detailed analysis in the present work. Suffice it to say that there is a good deal of evidence that, when the listener recognizes a consonant, he does so in terms of such an articulatory classification rather than directly from its acoustic features.

In the past twenty-five years a considerable body of knowledge concerning the way we hear the difference between speech sounds has been obtained on the basis of experiments with artificially constructed, synthetic, speech. These stimuli have the advantages of: simplicity – so that only one function at a time may be investigated; precision – so that the variability of ordinary speech is not a source of observational error; and range – so that both the full extent and detailed variation of a listener's pattern-processing ability are open to examination.

The following brief examples of synthetic speech pattern forms touch upon the acoustic–auditory nature of these sound differences in regard to intonation, place of articulation, and voice.

Intonation relates to the overall fundamental frequency, intensity and timing of speech and is important to the structure of complete utterances. It is primarily linked to vocal fold vibration and the laryngographic techniques which facilitate this aspect of productive analysis can also provide models for intonation synthesis. In *Figure 12.11* the extreme rising and falling *Fx* curves, 1 and 9, have been obtained from analyses of the speech of a woman saying 'Oh?' and 'Oh!'. The intervening *Fx* contours have been interpolated with reference to the flat stimulus, 5. When these different *Fx* contours are used to synthesize the utterance 'Oh', using formant frequencies appropriate for a woman, the basis is provided for a perceptual experiment in intonation processing. With random presentation of these stimuli at a comfortable listening level to normal subjects, labelling functions of the type shown in the lower half of *Figure 12.11* are typically obtained. Twenty-six presentations of each stimulus in pre-recorded blocks of eighteen were used. Although there are appreciable differences between listeners a consistent labelling ability is apparent and the average curve is a good indication of normal ability. (These results are drawn from experiments by Simon and Fourcin, 1976.)

In *Figure 12.12 (a)* the same stimuli, with stimulus 5 omitted, have been used to assess the perceptual ability of a profoundly deaf child before and after training during one school term with a laryngograph-based display. Before training (by Angela King and Ann Parker: see the figure in the contribution by E. E. Douek) random discriminations were made but at the end of the term a consistent ability to discriminate was found and this is associated with the marked improvement in productive skill which is shown by the central voice frequency distributions. The association of perceptual and productive abilities is important in providing a basis for the continuation of any improvement.

The labelling responses in *Figure 12.11 (b)* have been made by a totally acoustically (post-lingually) deaf patient to electro-cochlear stimuli obtained from the pure *Fx* contours of *Figure 12.11 (a)*. The corresponding electrical wave-forms were low-pass filtered and used to provide a constant current round window stimulation. The extremely well-defined grouping of the resulting stimuli into question and statement response categories gives a striking example both of the way in which an artificially

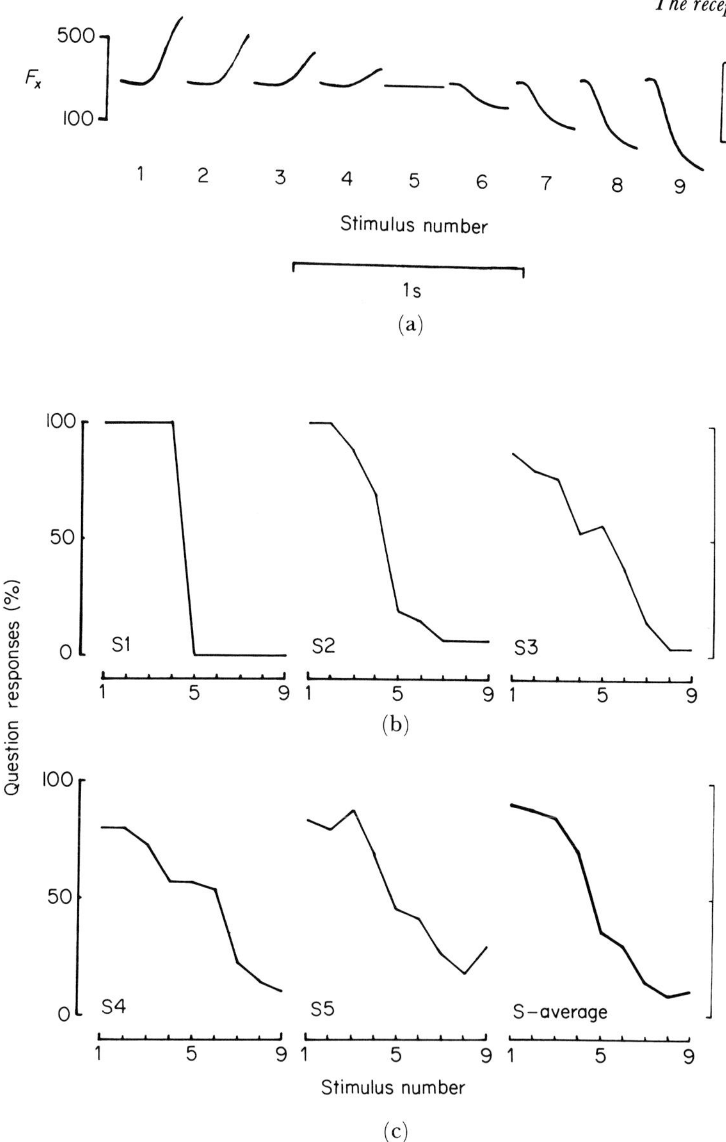

Figure 12.11 A perceptual experiment in intonation processing. (a) *Fx* contours used to synthesize the utterance 'oh'; (b) labelling functions obtained in response to random presentations of the stimuli in (a) from five subjects (S1–S5) and the average response from all Ss

presented speech pattern element is capable of being recognized in a linguistic fashion, and of the potential utility of a single channel electro-cochlear prosthesis, when the auditory nerve has a residual competence for the transmission of temporal information. It is likely that the child, already discussed, is also operating as a result of learning how to process temporal information since with an average pure tone loss of 90 dB between 125 Hz and 500 Hz he is likely to have extremely poor critical band discrimination.

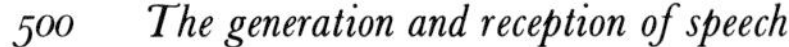

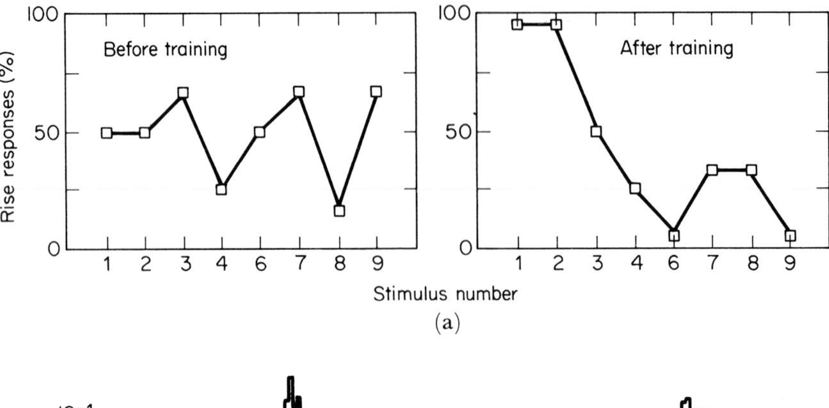

(a)

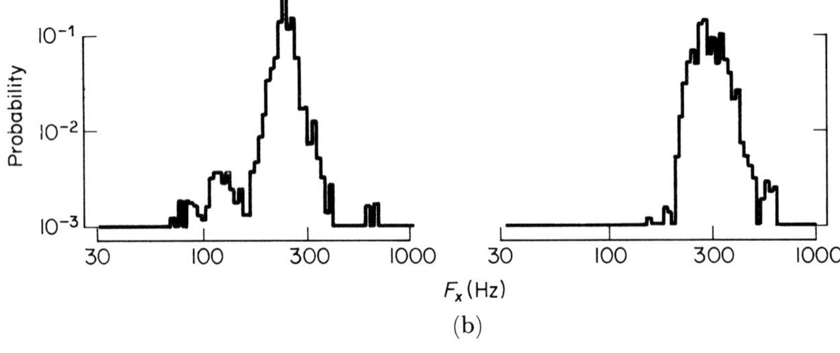

(b)

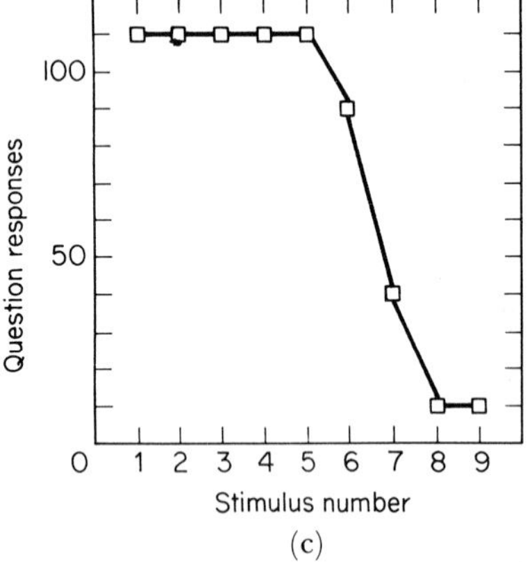

(c)

Figure 12.12 Perceptual response of a profoundly deaf child to random presentations of stimuli 1–4 and 6–9 of Figure 12.11 (a) before and after training; (b) the change in voice characteristics using the analysis of Figure 12.6; (c) *Fx* labelling by a totally, post-lingually, deaf patient for the full range of *Figure 12.11* with electrical presentation of the stimuli

The phonetic feature of place of articulation results in speech sound contrasts which differ in their formant shapings. *Figure 12.13 (a)* gives an example of this for the opposition [ba] on the left versus [da] on the right. All initial formant transitions for [b] rise, whilst only F1 rises for [d] in this vowel environment. By interpolating between these pattern extremes, as in *Figure 12.11* for *Fx*, a set of stimuli can be produced for use in the assessment of labelling ability. These particular stimuli were used (by S. Rosen, 1979), in a study of the influence of range and frequency with normal subjects. These, and related patterns, are beginning to be used in the study of the functional hearing ability of the deaf, when, for example, different hearing aids are compared. *Figure 12.13 (b)* shows an average labelling function for normal listeners responding to a stimulus set derived from this [b–d] contrast. Once more the

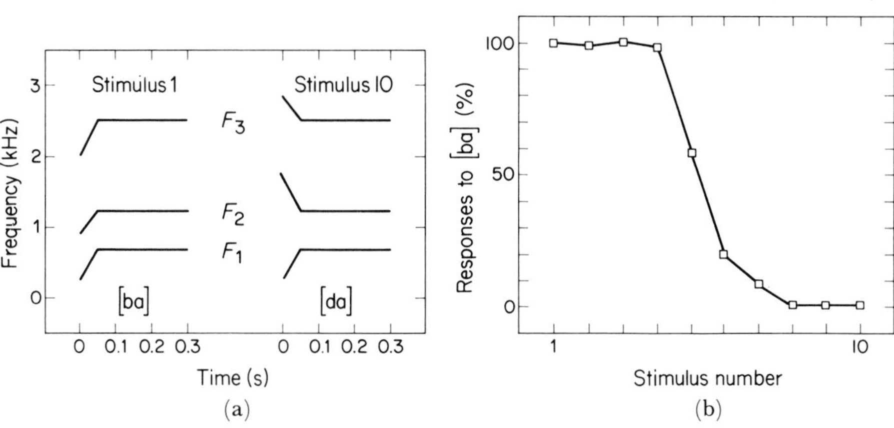

Figure 12.13 (a) Extremes of stimulus range – opposition of [ba] and [da]; (b) average labelling ([ba] responses) for normally hearing listeners

well-defined categorization which is typical of speech perceptual processing is obtained and the function provides a normative reference for the impaired.

Three aspects of initial plosive consonants, in addition to those discussed in the previous example, are introduced in the patterns shown in *Figure 12.14 (a)*. First, this opposition is for the voice contrast. On the left the sound sequence starts immediately with normal voicing; on the right voicing is delayed and there is an initial interval of aspiration. (The total range of larynx vibration onset time, l.o.t., is 70 ms.) Second, the contrast involves velar consonants [g] and [k]. Finally, the burst of noise which ordinarily accompanies the release of an initial plosive has not been omitted, as it has in *Figure 12.13*. Using a stimulus set, produced by interpolating between the pattern extremes which are shown for 'goat' and 'coat', normal listeners label in the way shown in *Figure 12.14 (b)*. A hearing impaired child with very poor hearing above 1 kHz (> 75 dB pure tone loss) has also been able to label these stimuli into two well-defined categories. The possibility that the child's discrimination is based, here, only on the F1 pattern component can be investigated by changing the voiced extreme so that 'goat' now has an unchanging, flat, F1 pattern. This is illustrated in *Figure 12.15 (a)*. Normal listeners are still able to categorize the stimuli from this new range, on the basis of the voice onset time, although they are uncertain about the new extreme 'goat' sounds since the F1 patterning is unnatural. The child's responses to these new stimuli, in *Figure 12.15 (c)*, show that although voicing information is available she cannot use it since the burst and aspiration noises are not available to her. When she is given the same stimuli via a hearing aid characteristic which enhances the importance of high frequency acoustic information, the burst information becomes available and although the F1 pattern shape is not present, labelling, in *Figure 12.15 (d)*, is possible. This example of the interaction between speech pattern, hearing loss and hearing aid is of much more than academic interest and when simple speech pattern audiometers are available to make this type of assessment more generally accessible it may be possible to manage some cases of hearing disability with greater assurance than is possible at present (Fourcin, 1976).

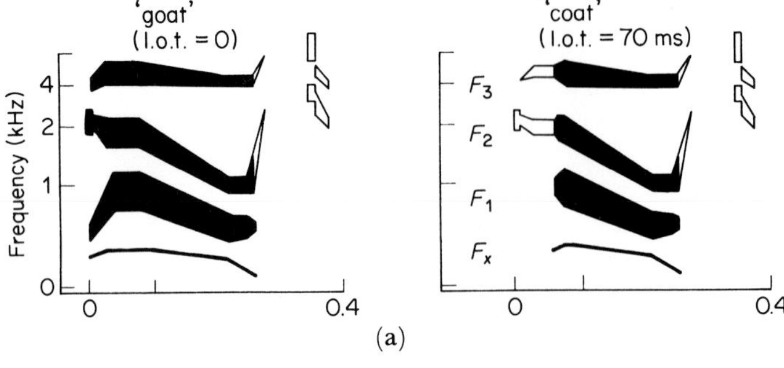

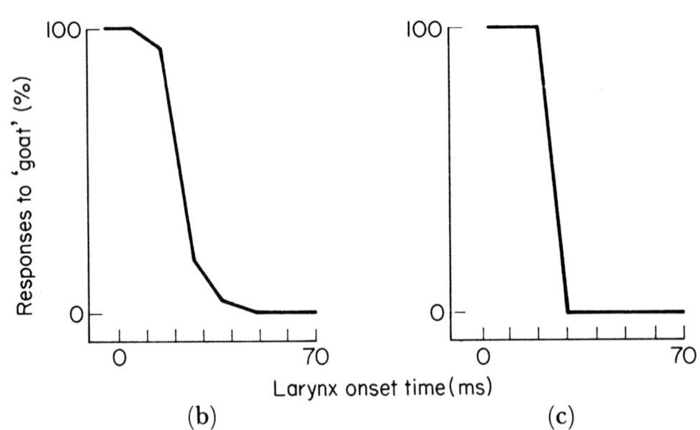

Figure 12.14 (a) Stimulus extremes – the opposition of 'goat' and 'coat'; (b) average response from five normally hearing listeners; (c) responses from a particular child given a flat gain-frequency characteristic hearing aid

The linguistic processing of speech

In considering the function of the brain in the generation of speech, we saw that the speaker must be conversant with a given language; in order to understand the message, the listener equally must have a knowledge of the same language system. Speaker and listener must have a common language.

Much of the decoding of speech depends on knowing what to expect, and on guessing at a solution in accordance with this expectation. Speaker and listener not only share a knowledge of the language system they are using; they also have a profound knowledge of the statistics of the occurrence of phonemes and other units in that language. The weight given to statistical information is very great, and when there are doubts or ambiguities, they are resolved in favour of the solution prompted by statistical evidence. In this way, a mishearing is soon corrected under the pressure of statistical constraints which enforce a correct solution.

The listener reconstructs the morphemes, words and sentences of the message, at each stage relying heavily on his knowledge of linguistic and statistical constraints.

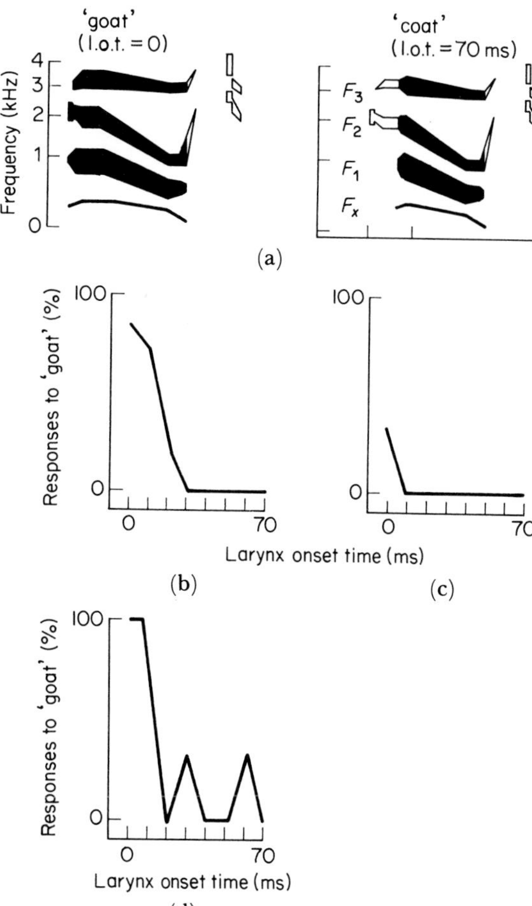

Figure 12.15 (a) Stimulus extremes – the opposition of 'goat' and 'coat' with the voiced extreme of 'goat' changed to have a flat F1 pattern; (b) average response from five normally hearing listeners; (c) responses from the deaf child of Figure 12.14 (c); (d) response from the deaf child of Figure 12.14 (c) given a rising gain-frequency characteristic hearing aid

Although at any time the listener may check back to the sounds he has heard, in order to correct errors or to deal with ambiguities, the actual sounds (in normal working) play little part in the process, once the phoneme sequence has been established.

The rôle of the acoustic processing, therefore, is to provide, as it were, a scaffolding upon which the message can be reconstructed – very largely on the basis of linguistic knowledge already carried in the listener's brain. The reception of speech is thus only partly a matter of hearing; in normal listening conditions we can quite readily take in speech if we hear half the sounds sent to us, for we can fill in the rest from our knowledge of what the sequence must be if the message is to make sense.

Acknowledgement

We are grateful to our colleagues for their contributions and are glad to acknowledge support from the Medical Research Council, Science Research Council, Royal National Institute for the Deaf and the Lady Megany Trust. *Figures 12.4c* and *f* are derived by the use of a computer analysis by Dr M. Hunt of the Joint Speech Research Unit.

References

Delattre, P. C. (1966) *Studies in French and Comparative Phonetics* The Hague; Mouton

Delattre, P. C., Liberman, A. M. and Cooper, F. S. (1955). 'Acoustic loci and transitional cues for consonants' *Journal of the Acoustical Society of America*, **27**, 769

Denes, P. B. and Pinson. E. N. (1963) *The Speech Chain*, New Jersey; Bell Telephone Laboratories

Fant, G. (1960) *Acoustic Theory of Speech Production*, 's-Gravenhage; Mouton

Fletcher, H. (1953) *Speech and Hearing in Communication*. New York; van Nostrand

Fourcin, A. J. (1974) 'Laryngographic examination of vocal fold vibration'. In *Ventilatory and Phonatory Control Systems*, pp. 315–333. (Ed. by B. Wyke). London; Oxford University Press

Fourcin, A. J. (1976) 'Speech pattern test for deaf children', In *Disorders of Auditory Function*. Ed. by S. D. G. Stephens. London and New York; Academic Press

Fourcin, A. J. and Abberton, E. (1976) The laryngograph and voiscope in speech therapy', *Proceedings of XVIth International Congress Logopedics and Phoniatrics*, pp. 116–132 (Ed. by E. Loebell). Basel; Karger

Fry, D. B. (1963) 'Coding and decoding in speech'. In *Signs, Signals and Symbols* (Ed. by S. E. Mason). London; Methuen

Fry, D. B. (1964) 'The correction of errors in the reception of speech', *Phonetica*, **11**, 164

Fry, D. B. (1966) 'The development of the phonological system in the normal and the deaf child'. In *The Genesis of Language* (Ed. by Frank Smith and George A. Miller). Cambridge, Mass. and London; M.I.T. Press *Society of America*, **29**, 117

Fry, D. B. (1966) 'The control of speech and voice'. In *Regulation and Control in Living Systems* (Ed. by H. Kalmus). London; John Wiley

Fry, D. B. (1968) 'Prosodic phenomena'. In *Manual of Phonetics* (Ed. by Bertil Malmberg) Amsterdam; North Holland

Goldman-Eisler, F. (1958) 'The predictability of words in context and the length of pauses in speech', *Language and Speech*, **1**, 226

Goldman-Eisler, F. (1961) 'Continuity of speech utterance its determinants and its significance', *Language and Speech*, **4**, 220

Goldman-Eisler, F. (1961) 'Hesitation and information in speech'. In *Information Theory* (Ed. by C. Cherry). London; Butterworths

Goldman-Eisler, F. (1968) *Psycholinguistics: Experiments in Spontaneous Speech*. London and New York; Academic Press

Gray, G. W. and Wise, C. M. (1959) *The Bases of Speech*. New York; Harper

Lee, B. S. (1950) 'Effects of delayed speech feedback', *Journal of the Acoustical Society of America*, **22**, 824

Liberman, A. M. (1957) 'Some results of research on speech perception', *Journal of the Acoustical Society of America* **29**, 117

Potter, R. K., Kopp, G. A. and Green, H. C. (1947) *Visible Speech*. New York; van Nostrand

Rosen, S. M. (1979) 'Range and frequency effects in consonant categorisation', *Journal of Phonetics*, in press

Simon, C. and Fourcin, A. J. (1976). 'Differences between individual listeners in their comprehension of speech and perception of sound patterns'. In *Speech and Hearing*, pp. 94–125, May. London; University College

Stevens, K. N. and House, A. S. (1955) 'Development of a quantitative description of vowel articulation', *Journal of the Acoustical Society of America*, **27**, 484

Wechsler, E., Neil, W. F. and Fourcin, A. J. (1976) 'Laryngographic analysis of pathological vocal fold vibration', *Proceedings of the Institute of Acoustics*, Edinburgh, 2–16–1/2–16–4

Wells, J. C. (1962) 'A Study of Formants of the Pure Vowels of British English', M. A. Thesis, University of London

Whetnall, E. and Fry, D. B. (1964) *The Deaf Child*. London; Heinemann

Whetnall, E. and Fry, D. B. (1970) *Learning to Hear* (Ed. by R. B. Niven). London; Heinemann

13 Radiographic anatomy of the ear, nose and throat

William B Young and Patricia Hollis

Radiology of the ear, nose and throat

It is almost impossible to have too much clinical information about one's patient provided it can be obtained safely and at a reasonable cost and convenience.

High quality radiography properly interpreted can provide detailed information about anatomy. It can usually determine the extent, and often the degree, of disease. It may at times indicate the likely pathology with fairly high accuracy. It provides a more or less permanent record of all these things, but is, of course, by no means infallible.

It is unrealistic to expect radiological findings always to agree with those found at operation if more than a few days have elapsed between surgery and the x-ray examination; for transitory oedema, and changes due to allergic or short-lived inflammatory states may produce changes on radiographs which are no longer present when the patient comes to operation or proof puncture, even if only a few days later.

Obviously the radiologist should be given a clear indication of the clinical problem if he is to be expected to select the most appropriate positions in which the films should be taken to provide the information required. Equally so, there is need for close consultation between clinician and radiologist when the films are examined and interpreted, for only then can the maximum information be extracted from them.

It is also important to remember that a proportion of patients suffering from diseases of the sinuses and upper respiratory tract, or from obstructive lesions in the oesophagus, suffer from contributory or secondary disease in the lungs, so a routine chest film is often of value, and is in any case a sensible precaution.

In this chapter various standard x-ray procedures and techniques are described and normal radiographic anatomy is illustrated and discussed. As many of the projections to be described involve the head, it is stressed that highest quality results can be consistently obtained only if x-ray apparatus designed specially for skull work is used; and even then only with meticulous technique and attention to detail. It is appreciated, however, that special apparatus is not always available and allowances have been made for this in descriptions in the text.

Current precision equipment

Basic skull table

This equipment developed by Lindgren utilizes both patient and tube angulation. The apparatus has been in use for a number of years and produces high-quality radiographs of the skull with a considerable degree of precision.

Specialized equipment (skull)

Other precision equipment has been developed in the last decade which allows movement of the unit around the patient who is examined always in the supine position. It is a great aid with patients who are unable to cooperate. The technique was developed by Dulac, Delvaux, Ziedses de Plantes and Lindgren and modified by Dulac to simplify the method from its original conception. Three constant reference planes are used, combined with spatial and angle coordinates to achieve exact standard projections and constant magnification of structures demonstrated for any examination area (*see Figure 13.1*).

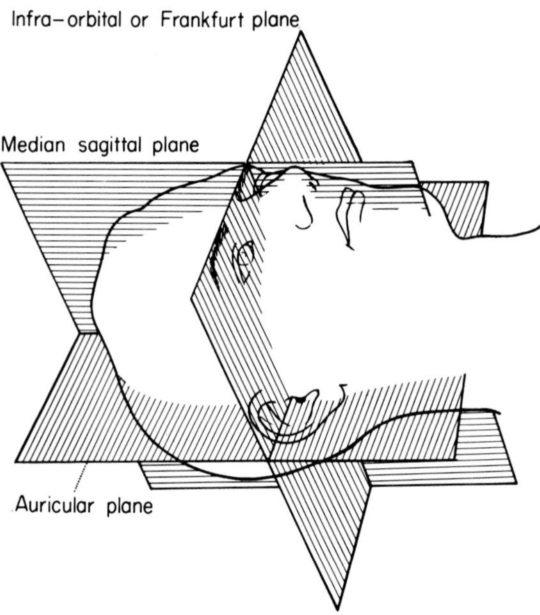

Figure 13.1 Standard projections

Specialized equipment (tomographic apparatus)

There are only a few precision tomographic units on the market which allow a wide combination of tube and film movement such as:

Rectilinear
Elliptical
Circular
Hypocycloidal
Spiral

The minimum selectivity is 0.5 mm, and layer levels may be obtained in minimal increments of 1.0 mm from as little as 0.27 cm above the table top.

The most modern units are ideal for demonstrating small structures as found in the middle ear, using the minimum selectivity. Units should be employed in conjunction with a high output generator which can be used independently of a falling load system for maximum flexibility of mA and time factors. A high-speed rotation tube permits the use of a minimal 0.6 mm focus to obtain optimum resolution.

In any radiological examination of the skull, certain basic steps are taken in the preparation of the patient, and special terminology is used to describe the relative positions of the head and the direction of the x-ray beam. Certain technical points are also important, and a brief mention of all these matters will be made before attempting to give a more detailed description of individual techniques.

Patient preparation

Ear-rings, hair-pins, grips and dentures should be removed. It is also more comfortable for the patient, and eases positioning problems, if shirts, ties, high collars and clothes with zip fastenings are removed.

Lines and planes used

Radiographic base-line – Orbito-meatal base-line

A line drawn from the outer canthus of the eye to the centre of the external auditory meatus. In the neutral position it is regarded as being always perpendicular to the film. It is raised by extending the head and lowered by flexing it. The base-line is always kept at 90 degrees to the film unless stated otherwise.

Interpupillary line
An imaginary horizontal line drawn between the pupils should be at right angles to the film in lateral projections.

Infra-orbital planes and lines

Infra-orbital plane (also known as the Frankfurt plane)
This passes through the lower orbital margins and the roofs of the external auditory canals. An angle of 10 degrees exists between the orbito-meatal base-line and the Frankfurt plane.

Auricular plane

This is at right angles to the infra-orbital plane, and passes through the external auditory canals.

Median sagittal plane

A vertical plane running antero-posteriorly which bisects the skull into two equal halves. It must be aligned at right angles to the film for antero-posterior projections, and parallel to it for lateral projections. Rotation of the head around the vertical axis is referred to as rotation of the sagittal plane – the face being turned to whichever side is indicated.

Coronal plane

A vertical plane at right angles to the median sagittal plane, parallel to the film in antero-posterior projections.

The meatal or auricular plane is a coronal plane passing through the external auditory meatuses.

Tube angulation

This refers to the direction followed by the central ray emerging from the tube.

(a) Cephalically – towards the head.
(b) Caudally – towards the feet.

If fluid levels are being sought a horizontal beam should be used, whether the patient is sitting or recumbent.

Cassette displacement

If the tube is angled the film must be correspondingly displaced approximately 0.5 cm/10 degrees so that the central ray is always directed to its centre.

Radiographic positions

These are named according to the direction of the central ray, the part in contact with the film being put last, e.g. 20 degree occipito-frontal means the central ray is angled 20 degrees caudally, and directed through the occiput to emerge through the frontal bone positioned against the film.

Immobilization

The head must always be carefully immobilized, either by head bands or special clamps and respiration arrested during exposure to reduce unsharpness due to movement.

Film quality

Film definition (a combination of detail and contrast) is improved if:

(a) A Potter–Bucky diaphragm or grid is used, to reduce the amount of scattered radiation reaching the film.
(b) The beam is collimated to include only the structures under examination.
(c) The patient's head is immobilized to prevent movement during exposure.
(d) The smallest focal spot is used compatible with acceptable exposure times, optimum exposure factors, and tube focus loading.
(e) Suitable intensifying screens are used for optimum resolution consistent with the tube or generator output available. Rare earth screens may improve the diagnostic result if exposure factors are limited.

The exposures quoted for radiography relate to the use of a 90 cm focal film distance, medium speed (Fast Detail) intensifying screens, an 8:1 ratio metal grid, and maximum collimation to the area under examination. The exposure factors quoted may be amended to suit departmental requirements, by reducing the mAs factor and increasing the kV.

Grids

The use of specialized skull units permits multiple angulations of the tube around the vertical and horizontal axes, the grid then being rotated precisely to ensure that the incident rays are parallel to the longitudinal plane of the grid slats. If a simple Bucky table is used angulation of the x-ray beam is only possible along the long axis of the grid, so that the head must be rotated or inclined to achieve any angulation other than this.

Area examined

Films taken in the sagittal plane usually include both sides on one film. This has the advantage of allowing close comparison. For other projections, it is advisable to take separate films for each side to allow direct comparison.

Radiological examination of the temporal bone

The degree of pneumatization of the mastoid varies considerably between individuals and is commonly disproportionate on the two sides both in cell distribution and size. Air-cells are absent at birth and the final state of pneumatization is not attained until late adolescence. This process may be interfered with, or modified, by a variety of conditions, not all as yet completely known. In each case an attempt must be made to try to assess the significance of differences in pneumatization of the two sides by noting the presence of bone rarefaction or sclerosis; the overall transradiancy in the middle-ear and mastoid cells; the presence or absence of the ossicles; the thickness and definition of cell walls and the presence of cell destruction.

For general routine purposes three standard projections are recommended for the mastoid areas ($\frac{1}{2}$ axial/2 lateral obliques) or two ($\frac{1}{2}$ axial and full axial) if the internal auditory canals are to be investigated with a view to subsequent tomographic techniques. When both sides are included on the same radiograph, the normal side is available for comparison, unless it too is diseased. When each side is examined separately – as necessitated by certain of the projections to be described – every effort should be made to obtain exactly comparable projections.

When detailed information of small structures such as the facial canal, ossicles, inner ear, or the auditory canals is wanted tomography should be employed. However, for routine examination of the petrous bone it is customary to make a selection from the following projections, bearing in mind that each case presents an individual clinical problem towards the solution of which the examination should be directed.

Standard radiographic projections

(i) Antero-posterior projection through orbits (*see Figure 13.2*) (if AP tomography is not to be undertaken).
(ii) Both 30–35 degree lateral oblique and Stockholm B views.
(iii) Half axial (Slit).
(iv) Full axial (Slit).
(v) Stockholm C or Stenvers.

Antero-posterior projection through orbits *(Figure 13.2)*

This is a projection commonly used during a survey examination when attention is focused on the internal auditory meatus or canal when an eighth nerve tumour is suspected.

The patient lies supine or sits facing the tube. The base-line is depressed 7–10 degrees and the central ray is directed to the median sagittal plane to bisect the interpupillary line, to pass to the centre of the film, the beam being collimated by an eccentric diaphragm or a slit diaphragm 9 × 18 cm maximum to improve definition. Average exposure factors – 70 kV, 120 mAs.

Structures demonstrated

This view projects the internal auditory meatuses through the orbits and allows comparison of the two sides on one film.

30–35 degree lateral oblique – Stockholm B view *(Figure 13.3)*

The two sides are taken separately. The pinna is strapped forward with transradiant tape. The patient sits or lies prone – with the head adjusted to a true lateral position, the side to be examined in contact with the Bucky support. The tube is angled so that the central ray is directed 30–35 degrees caudally to emerge 1.5 cm below and 0.5 cm behind the external auditory meatus under examination and to the centre of the film.

Average exposure factors – 70 kV, 125 mAs.

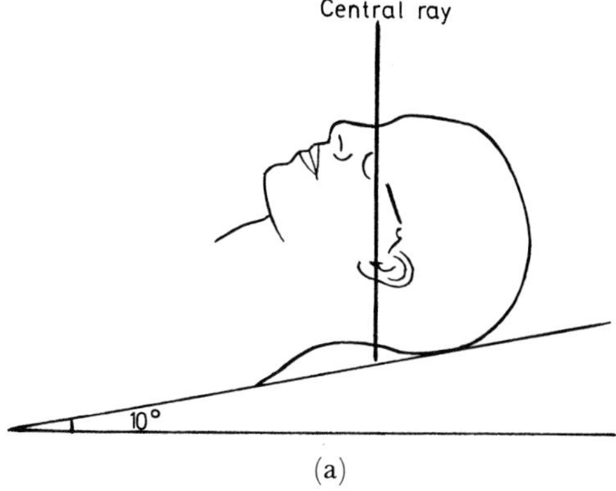

1. Floor of sphenoid sinus
2. Crista galli
3. Cribriform plate
4. Sphenoid sinus
5. Overlap of sphenoids on ethmoids
6. Internal auditory meatus
7. Internal auditory canal
8. Arcuate eminence
9. Superior semicircular canal
10. Maxillary antrum
11. Inferolateral wall of antrum
12. Nasal septum
13. Mandible

(a)

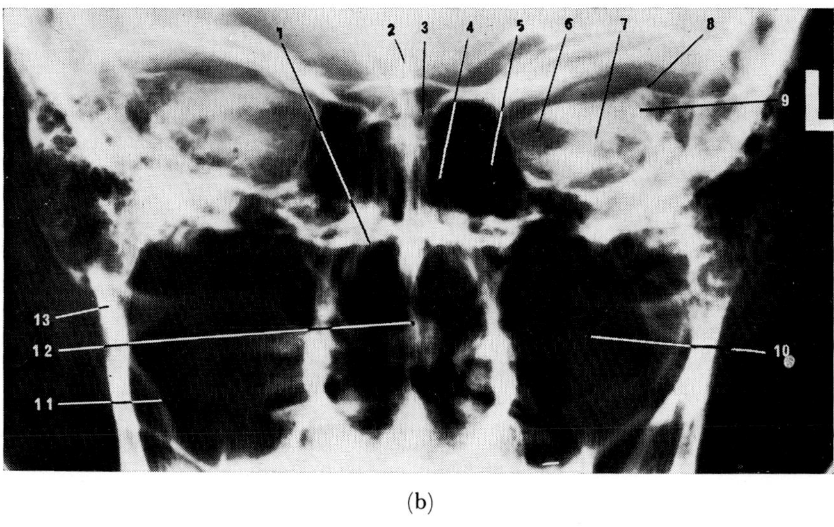

(b)

Figure 13.2 10 degree antero-posterior projection to show internal auditory meatuses through orbits

In this position the central ray strikes the petrous bone obliquely so that it is foreshortened and its apex is projected over the temporo-mandibular joint.

Structures demonstrated

The groove of the lateral sinus is usually well shown and the relationship of cells to it can be determined. Two parallel lines may seemingly mark the anterior wall of the lateral sinus. The anterior of these is the true wall, the other being due to the overhang of the posterior wall of the petrous bone.

The external auditory meatus and the tympanic cavity are largely obscured by the dense bone of the labyrinth. The sinus plate is visible posteriorly, making a triangle with the upper edge of the pyramid. The aditus and attic may be visible, and the antrum too if it is not obscured by smaller overlying cells. A high jugular bulb may present as an area of increased transradiancy close to the lower posterior margin of the external auditory meatus.

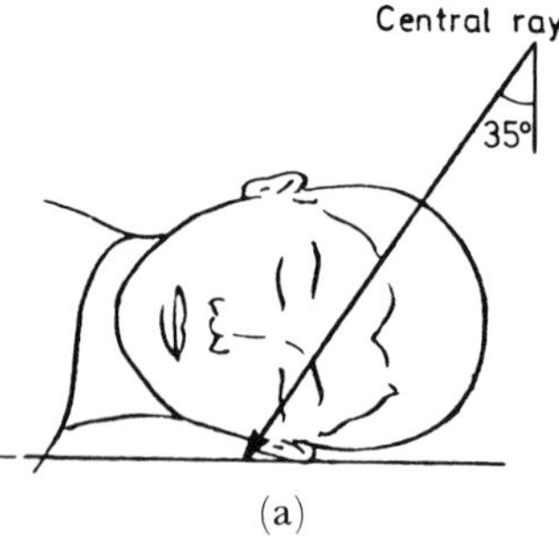

(a)

1. Facial canal cells
2. Peritubal cells
3. Mastoid tip cells
4. Retrosinus (marginal) cells
5. Lateral sinus
6. Sinus plate
7. Cells of sinodural angle
8. Antrum
9. Aditus
10. External auditory meatus (superimposed on middle ear and IAM)
11. Squamous cells
12. Attic
13. Upper anterior wall of petrous bone (middle fossa floor)
14. Zygoma (site of zygomatic cells)
15. Condyle of mandible
16. Dense bone of labyrinth

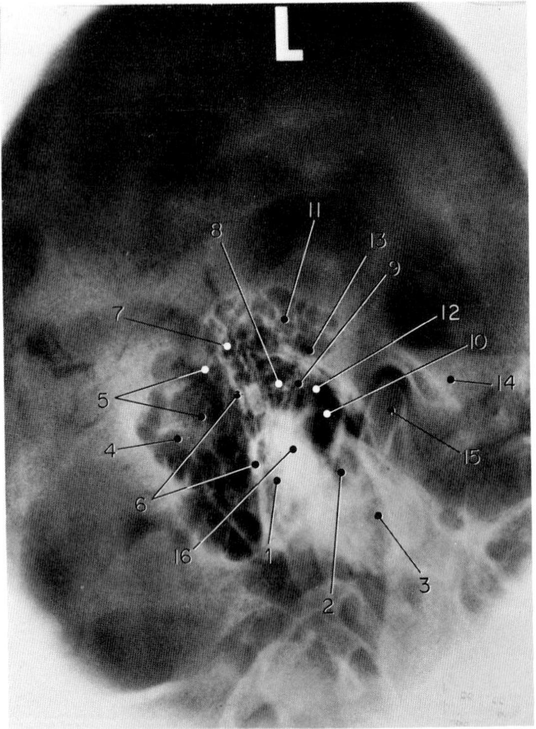

(b)

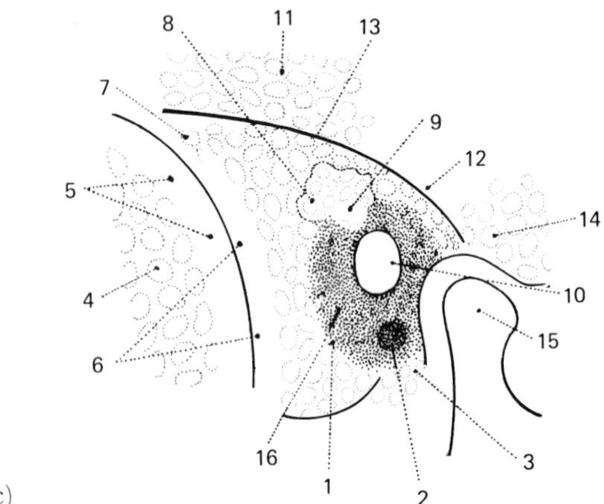

(c)

Figure 13.3 Stockholm B, 30–35 degree lateral oblique view; (a) radiographic technique; (b) 35 degree lateral oblique; (c) diagram of 35 degree oblique

Half axial – 25–35 degree fronto-occipital (Towne's) view. (*Figure 13.4*)

The patient lies supine, or sits, facing the tube with the chin depressed so the orbitomeatal base-line is perpendicular to the film. The central ray is angled 25–35 degrees caudally and directed along the median sagittal plane to pass through the

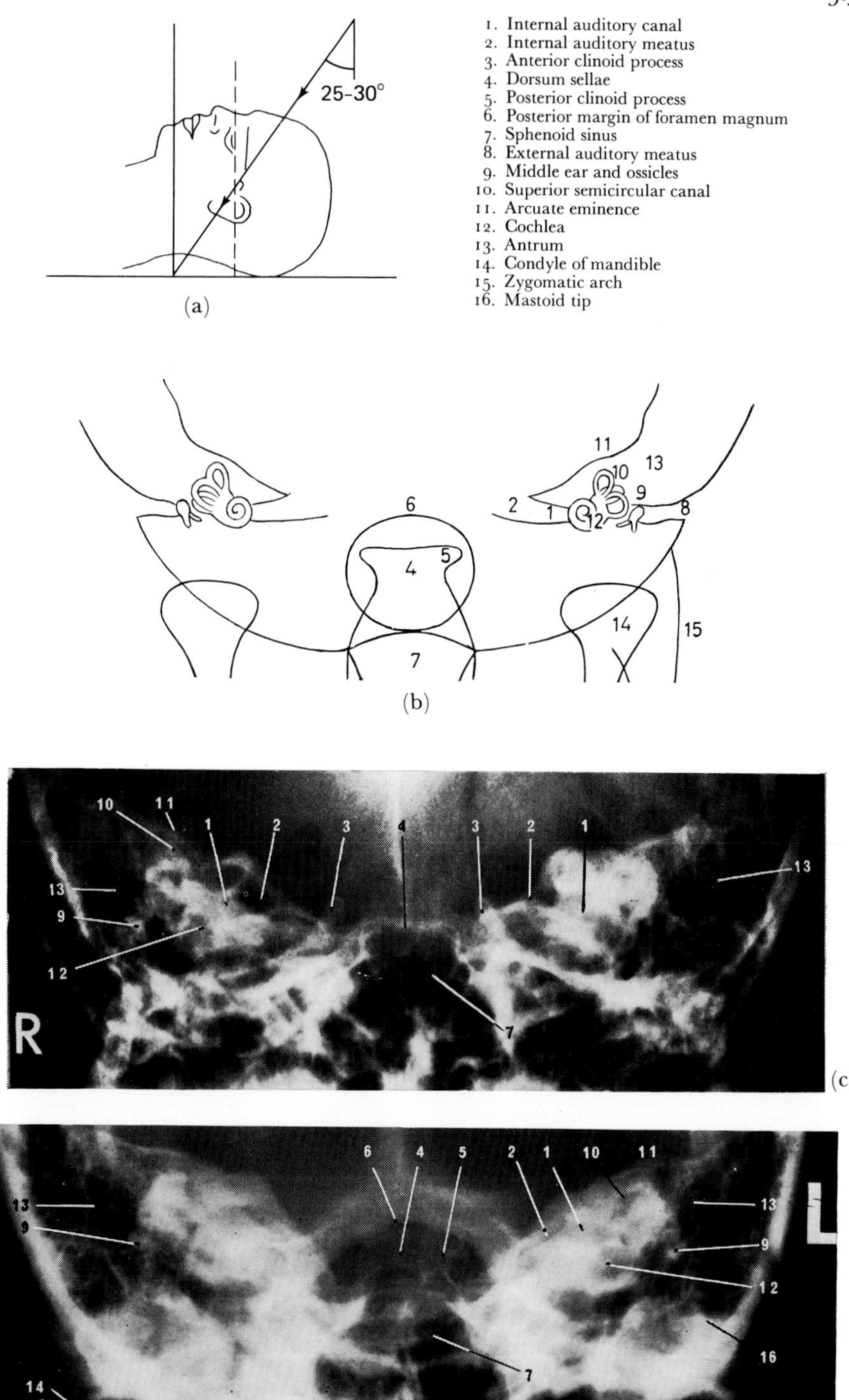

1. Internal auditory canal
2. Internal auditory meatus
3. Anterior clinoid process
4. Dorsum sellae
5. Posterior clinoid process
6. Posterior margin of foramen magnum
7. Sphenoid sinus
8. External auditory meatus
9. Middle ear and ossicles
10. Superior semicircular canal
11. Arcuate eminence
12. Cochlea
13. Antrum
14. Condyle of mandible
15. Zygomatic arch
16. Mastoid tip

Figure 13.4 (a) and (b) 25–35 degree half-axial (Towne's view); (c) 25 degree half-axial view showing anterior clinoid processes; (d) 30 degree half-axial view showing dorsum sellae

intermeatal plane to the centre of the film. The beam is collimated to a slit 9 × 18 cm. Average exposure factors 80–85 kV, 70 mAs.

Both sides are demonstrated on one film and can be directly compared.

Structures demonstrated

The internal auditory meatuses, the mastoid air-cells and antrum, the superior and lateral semicircular canals. With the use of a 25-degree angle the anterior clinoids are shown, whereas with a 30–35 degree angle the dorsum sellae and posterior clinoids are visible. If the *head is over-flexed, the greater part of the foramen magnum and arch of the atlas is visible, and the internal auditory meatuses are projected over the occipital condyles*. If the *head is under-flexed (or the caudal angle is insufficient) the IAMs are obscured by the orbits.*

Full axial – submento-vertical slit view *(Figure 13.5)*

Both sides are demonstrated on one film (*Figure 13.5*). The patient lies supine or sits facing the tube. The head is extended so that the vertex rests against the Bucky support with the base-line parallel to it. The tube is adjusted so that the central ray passes vertically to the median sagittal plane, 0.5 cm in front of the intermeatal plane to cut the base-line at right angles and exit at the centre of the film. Collimation of the beam is limited to 9 × 18 cm and includes only the area of interest. Average exposure factors – 80–85 kV, 150 mAs.

Structures demonstrated

Internal and external auditory canals, the tympanic cavities and ossicles, mastoid air cells, bony eustachian canals, petrous apices, foramina spinosum and ovale. The stylomastoid foramina, the foramina lacera and the carotid canals are also shown. If the head is over-extended the anterior arch of the atlas is projected over the internal auditory meatuses. If the head is under-extended the internal auditory meatuses and middle ear are obscured by the rami of the mandibles.

Samuel (1959) points out that a large jugular foramen should not be mistaken for pathological bone destruction. The foramina may differ considerably in size on the two sides, the right more often being the larger. The petrous apex is pneumatized in about 20 per cent of individuals. Rarely, the tip of the petrous bone is absent.

Lateral oblique – Stockholm C and Stenver's projections

These two projections produce very similar appearances. For the former a skull table with a Bucky grid which can be rotated is required. In both instances less exposure is required to show the mastoid antrum and tip than the internal auditory meatus and canal.

Stockholm C projection (Figure 13.6a, b, c and *d)*

The head is placed in the true lateral position and the central ray angled 28–30 degrees towards the face and 10 degrees cephalically to pass through a point 2 cm in front and 1 cm above the external auditory meatus nearest to the film. The grid is rotated through 72 degrees. Each side is examined separately. A small 9 cm localizing cone is used. Average exposure factors – 75–80 kV, 120 mAs.

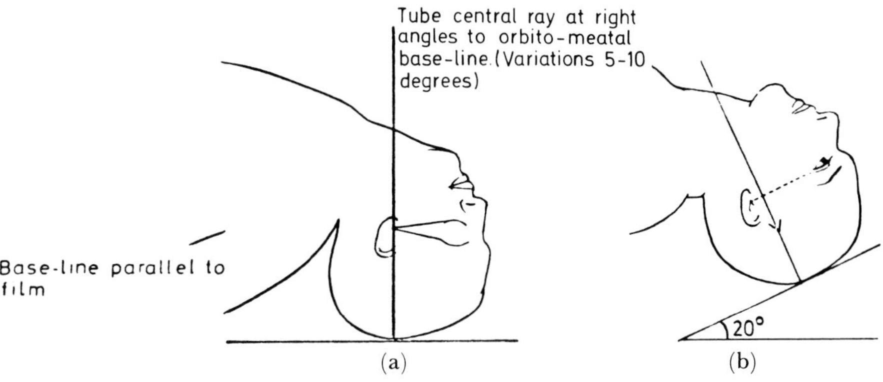

(a) (b)

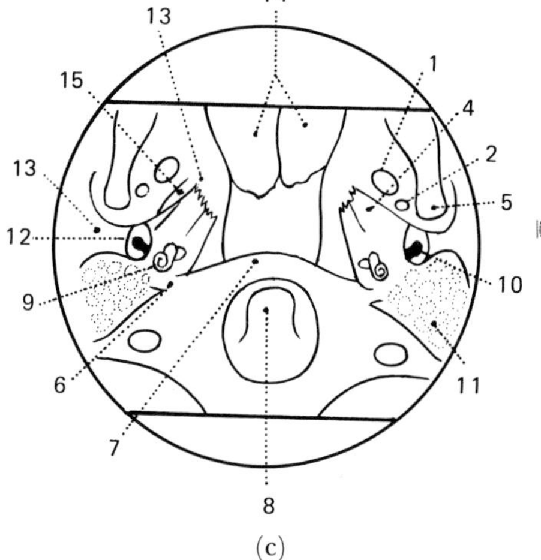

(c)

1. Foramen ovale
2. Foramen spinosum
3. Foramen lacerum
4. Petrous apex
5. Condyle of mandible
6. Internal auditory meatus
7. Anterior arch of atlas
8. Odontoid process of axis
9. Cochlea
10. Middle ear and ossicles
11. Antrum
12. Tympanic ring
13. External auditory meatus
14. Sphenoid sinuses
15. Eustachian tube

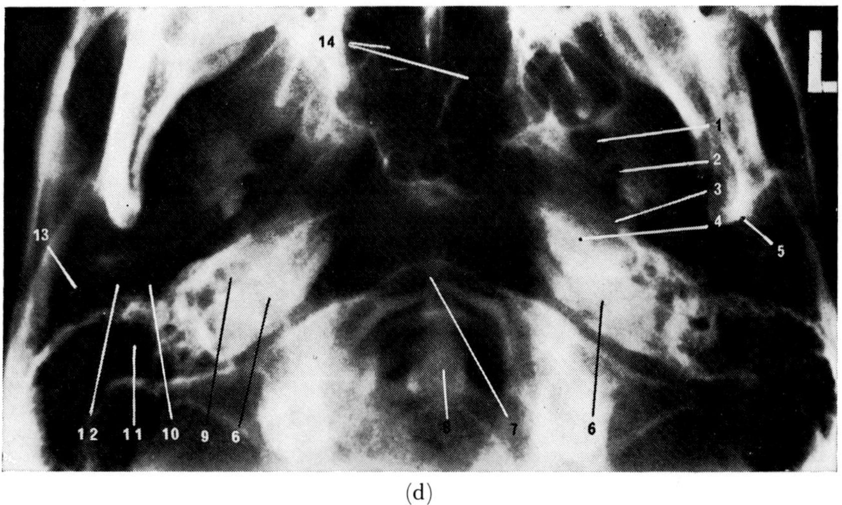

(d)

Figure 13.5 Full axial view

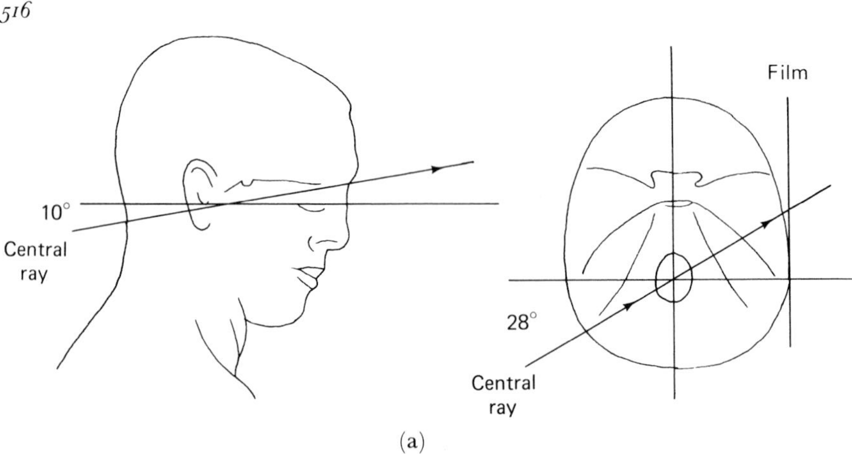

(a)

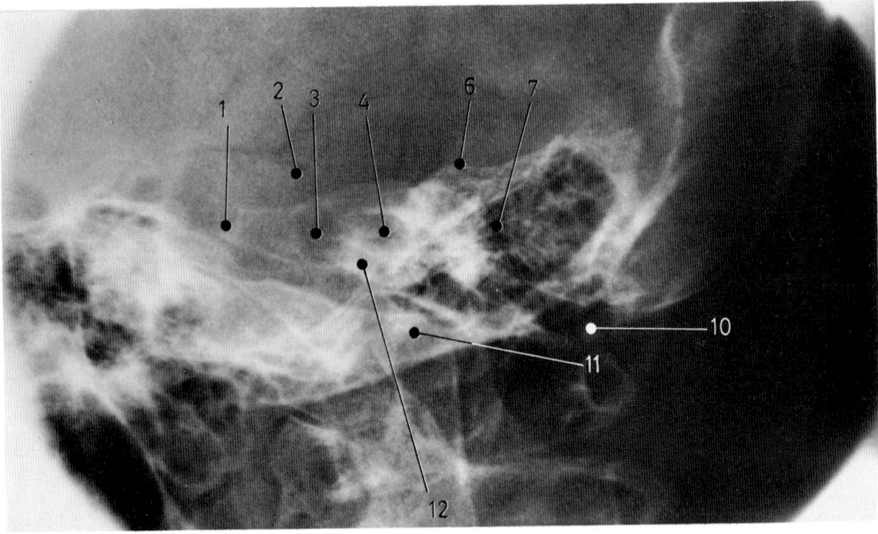

(b)

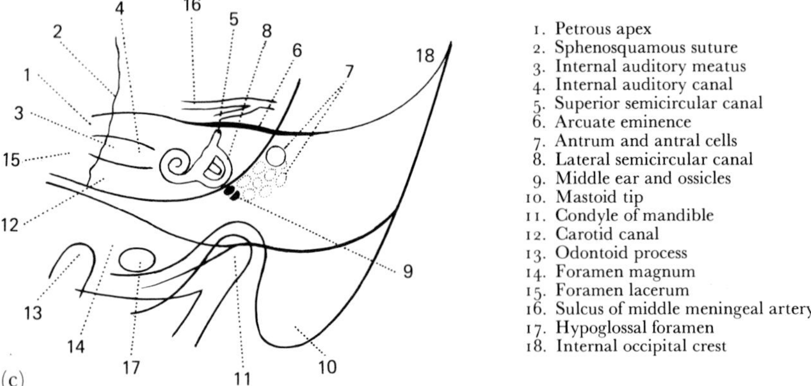

(c)

1. Petrous apex
2. Sphenosquamous suture
3. Internal auditory meatus
4. Internal auditory canal
5. Superior semicircular canal
6. Arcuate eminence
7. Antrum and antral cells
8. Lateral semicircular canal
9. Middle ear and ossicles
10. Mastoid tip
11. Condyle of mandible
12. Carotid canal
13. Odontoid process
14. Foramen magnum
15. Foramen lacerum
16. Sulcus of middle meningeal artery
17. Hypoglossal foramen
18. Internal occipital crest

Figure 13.6 (a) and (b) Stockholm C projection; (c) diagram of Stockholm C and Stenver's projections

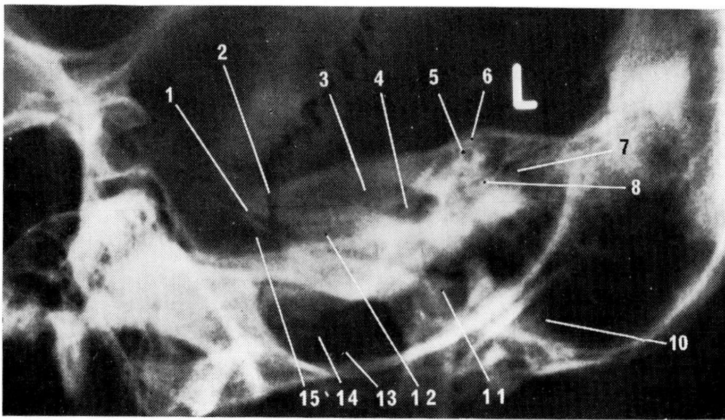

Figure 13.6 (d) Radiograph Stockholm C projection

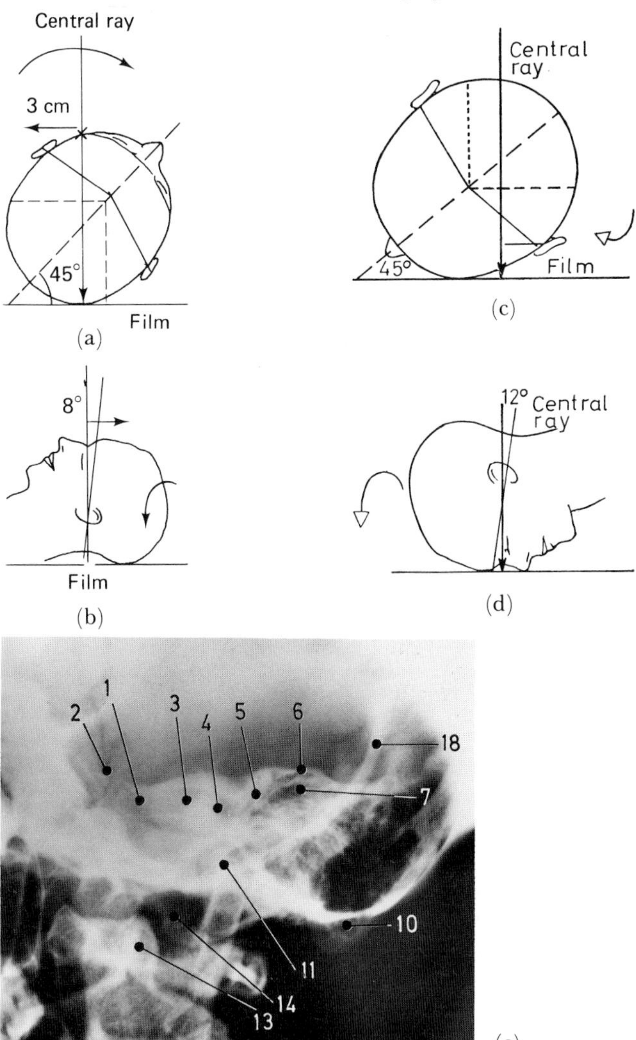

Figure 13.7 (a) and (b) Antero-posterior Stenver's projection; (c) and (d) postero-anterior Stenver's projection (e) Radiograph Stenver's projection

Stenver's projection (*Figure 13.7*)

This technique can be used with an ordinary vertical or horizontal Bucky. The films can be taken either postero-anteriorly or antero-posteriorly sitting or lying down. If postero-anteriorly, the head is inclined laterally 15 degrees away from the side under examination and rotated through 45 degrees, so that the nose, eye and forehead on the side to be examined are in contact with the Bucky support. The central ray is angled 12 degrees cephalically to emerge 2 cm in front, and 1 cm above the external auditory meatus proximal to the film. For the antero-posterior projection the head is rotated 45 degrees away from the side being examined and the base-line is lowered 8 degrees or the central ray angled 8 degrees caudally. The central ray is directed to the zygomatic process 3 cm in front and 2.5 cm above the external auditory meatus remote from the film, to exit to the centre of the film. Each side is taken separately. Average exposure factors – 70–75 kV, 120 mAs.

The antero-posterior projection is more comfortable for the patient, if tomograms are to be taken in this projection.

Structures demonstrated

The undulating line of the upper border of the petrous bone is clearly seen. The lower line of the petrous corresponds to the inferior petrosal sinus.

The superior semicircular canal is usually clearly visible, extending almost to the upper margin of the petrous bone under the arcuate eminence. The horizontal canal may be visible projecting back from its lower end. The angle between these two canals (the so-called 'tractus niche') is often clearly shown. The vestibule may present as a clear area below the superior semicircular canal. The cochlea lies below this towards the apex, being surrounded by dense bone. Cells may be visible above it as a transradiant 'canal' extending towards the apex medial to the superior semicircular canal.

The orifice of the internal auditory meatus is clearly shown as an oval aperture with the canal running back a short distance towards the cochlea. The oblique line crossing the labyrinth from above downwards, and from behind forwards, is produced by the internal occipital crest. By rotating the head a little less than 45 degrees in the postero-anterior Stenver's projection this line can be thrown forwards clear of the petrous apex. This also improves the view of the internal auditory meatus and canal and demonstrates the antrum and labyrinth better. If the angle of rotation is increased above 45 degrees by rotating the head more towards a lateral position the line of the internal occipital crest merges with that of the internal table of the skull and the petrous apex and the tractus niche are shown more clearly. By raising the base-line through 5 degrees a better view of the apex and labyrinth can be attained. The vascular channel running above and parallel to the petrous ridge represents the middle meningeal artery. The spheno-squamous suture runs down more or less vertically over the petrous apex. It usually runs a fairly straight course as it crosses behind the apex and should not be mistaken for a fracture.

Special projections

In the past when chronic attic and mastoid infection was more prevalent, and the more sophisticated types of x-ray tomographic equipment were not available, special

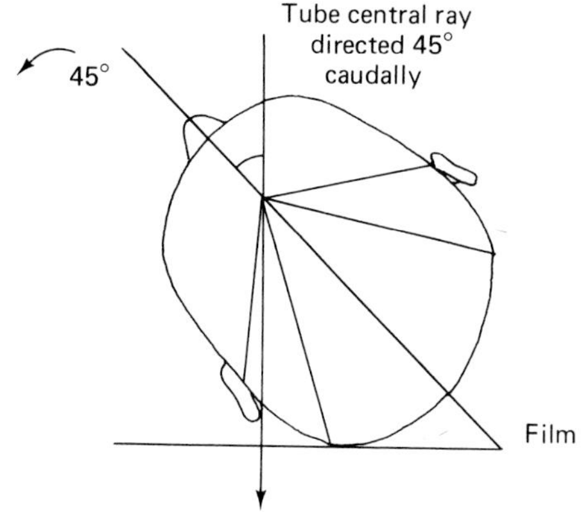

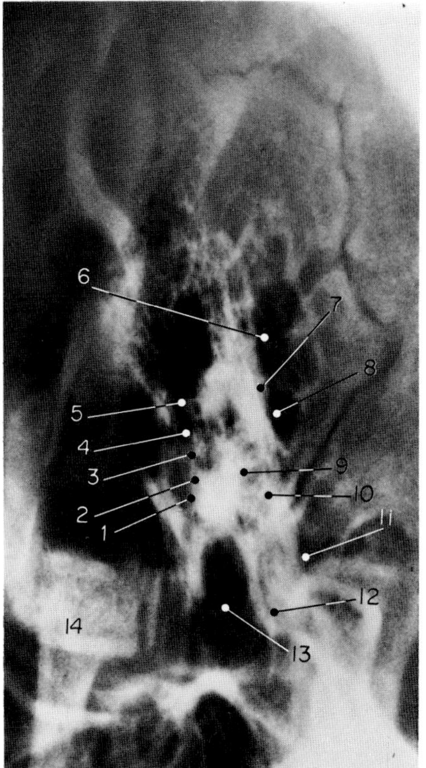

1. Tympanic cavity projected through external auditory meatus
2. Malleus
3. Epitympanic recess
4. Aditus
5. Antrum
6. Squamous cells
7. Posterior wall of pyramid
8. Lateral sinus
9. Cochlea
10. Internal auditory meatus
11. Jugular foramen
12. Petrous apex
13. Carotid canal
14. Condyle of mandible

Figure 13.8 Mayer's projection (modified)

projections were devised in an attempt to show the surgeon the full extent of cell disease or destruction which needed to be extirpated.

Nowadays these projections – apart possibly from Owen's, which is strongly advocated by Compere (1958) – are rarely employed.

Special middle-ear and attic views

Mayer's view (*Figure 13.8*)

Mayer first described an oblique axial view of the petrous bone obtained by placing the patient facing the tube with the base-line raised 10 degrees (modified to 5 degrees) and rotating the sagittal plane through 45 degrees towards the side to be examined. The tube central ray is angled 45 degrees caudally to enter the skull at a point 6 cm above the upper border of the orbit and 6 cm medially from the outer canthus of the eye remote from the film to emerge 5 cm below the tip of the mastoid process nearest to the film and centred to it. A small 13 cm cone is used. Average exposure factors – 80–85 kV, 120 mAs.

Structures demonstrated

This projection shows the middle ear, attic and aditus, but the anatomy is very distorted.

Owen's projection (*Figure 13.9*)

In 1951 Owen described a modification of Mayer's technique which produces far less distortion. More recently Compere has done much to try to popularize this projection which he considers should be a standard one.

The patient faces the tube, the head adjusted to the antero-posterior position. The sagittal plane is rotated through 60 degrees towards the side to be examined. The tube

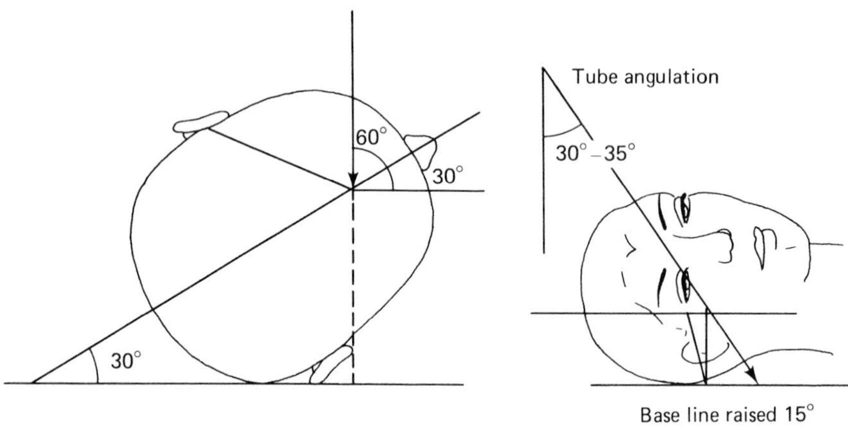

(a)

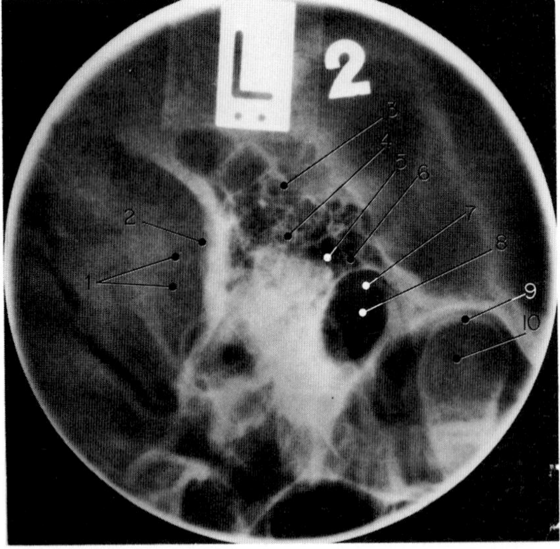

1. Lateral sinus
2. Posterior wall of pyramid
3. Squamous cells
4. Antrum
5. Aditus
6. Epitympanic recess
7. Malleus
8. Middle ear projected through external auditory meatus
9. Temporomandibular joint
10. Condyle of mandible

(b)

Figure 13.9 Owen's view (modified Mayer's): (a) technique; (b) macroradiograph

is angled so that the central ray is directed 30–35 degrees caudally, to a point along the base-line 2.5 cm behind the outer canthus of the eye on the side remote from the film, to exit at a point 1.5 cm below the external auditory meatus proximal to the film. We have found that to prevent the petrous ridge from obscuring the middle ear it helps to raise the base-line from 5–15 degrees depending on individual anatomy. The beam is collimated with a 13 cm diaphragm to the desired area. Average exposure factors – 75 kV, 120 mAs.

Structures demonstrated
The malleus and incus should be projected within the external auditory meatus. The lateral wall of the attic, the aditus and antrum should be clearly visible.

Less common projections

The following two projections were devised to show the middle ear, ossicles and lateral wall of the attic more clearly. They are difficult to interpret and even more difficult to repeat satisfactorily for comparison. It is doubtful if they are worth the time and trouble taken to produce them, for chronic middle-ear and mastoid infection is less common than it used to be and far more satisfactory and exact information can be achieved by modern tomographic techniques.

Guillen's projection (*Figure 13.10*)

The patient lies supine and faces the tube with the base-line 90 degrees to the film. A point just less than 1 cm above the inner canthus is adjusted to lie in the same vertical plane as the tragus of the ear, and the sagittal plane is then rotated 12–15 degrees towards the side being examined. The central ray is directed vertically through the orbit on the same side, to exit through the plane of the external auditory meatus and pass to the centre of the film. Average exposure factors – 65 kV, 120 mAs.

Structures demonstrated
This view is designed to throw the ossicles and middle ear clear of the labyrinth, and to show the lateral semicircular canals and facial canal.

Chausee III view (*Figure 13.11*)

The patient faces the tube with the base-line at 90 degrees to the film. The head is rotated 10–15 degrees away from the side being examined. The central ray is angled 20–30 degrees caudally, to pass midway between the superior lateral orbital margin and the tragus in the plane of the external meatus and to the centre of the film. Average exposure factors – 65 kV, 120 mAs.

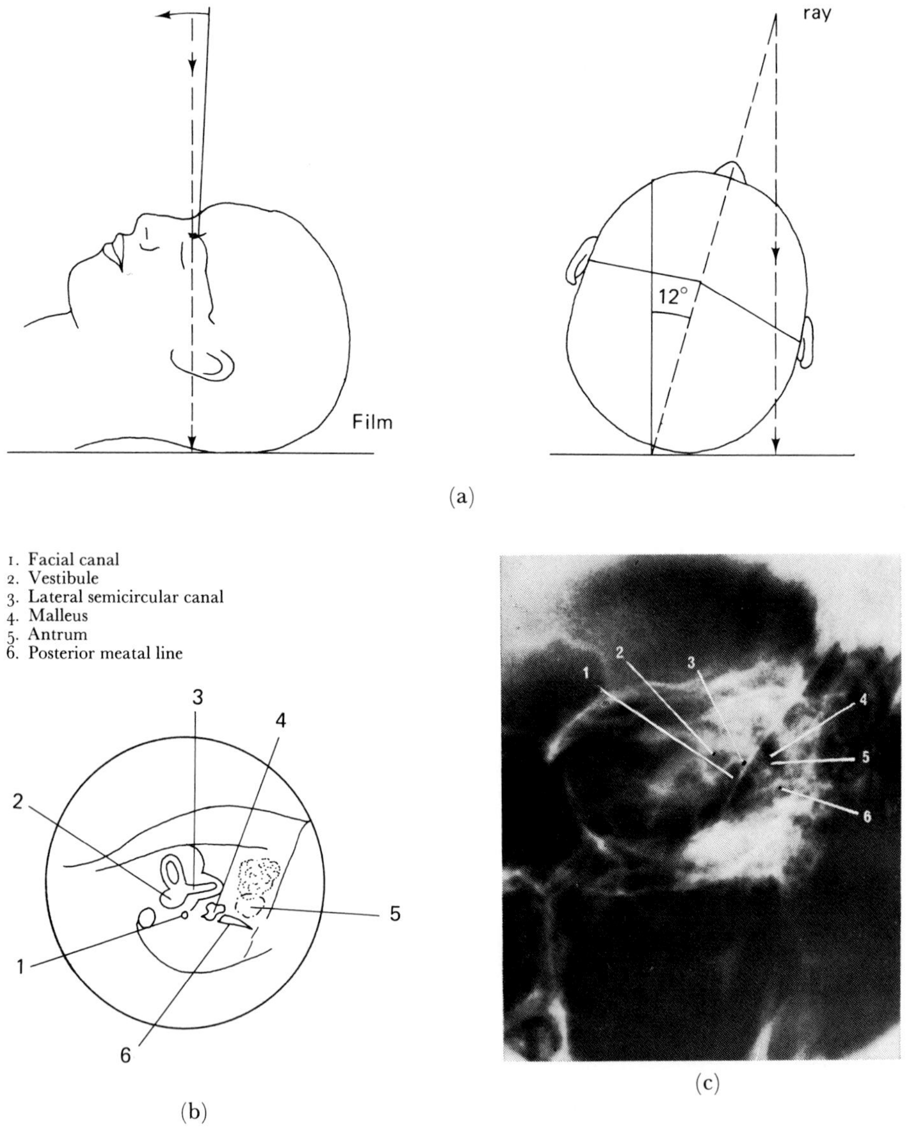

Figure 13.10 Guillen's projection. (a) Technique; (b) structures shown; (c) radiograph

Structures demonstrated

This view is designed to show the attic (epitympanic recess) and its outer wall, which is seen end on, running upwards from the superior margin of the external auditory meatus. The ossicles show a triangular density medial to this, but may be superimposed on the lateral semicircular canal which may be visible just below the transradiancy of the mastoid antrum. This position is very difficult to reproduce satisfactorily and in the case of a cellular or very dense mastoid it may be practically impossible to differentiate structures with any certainty.

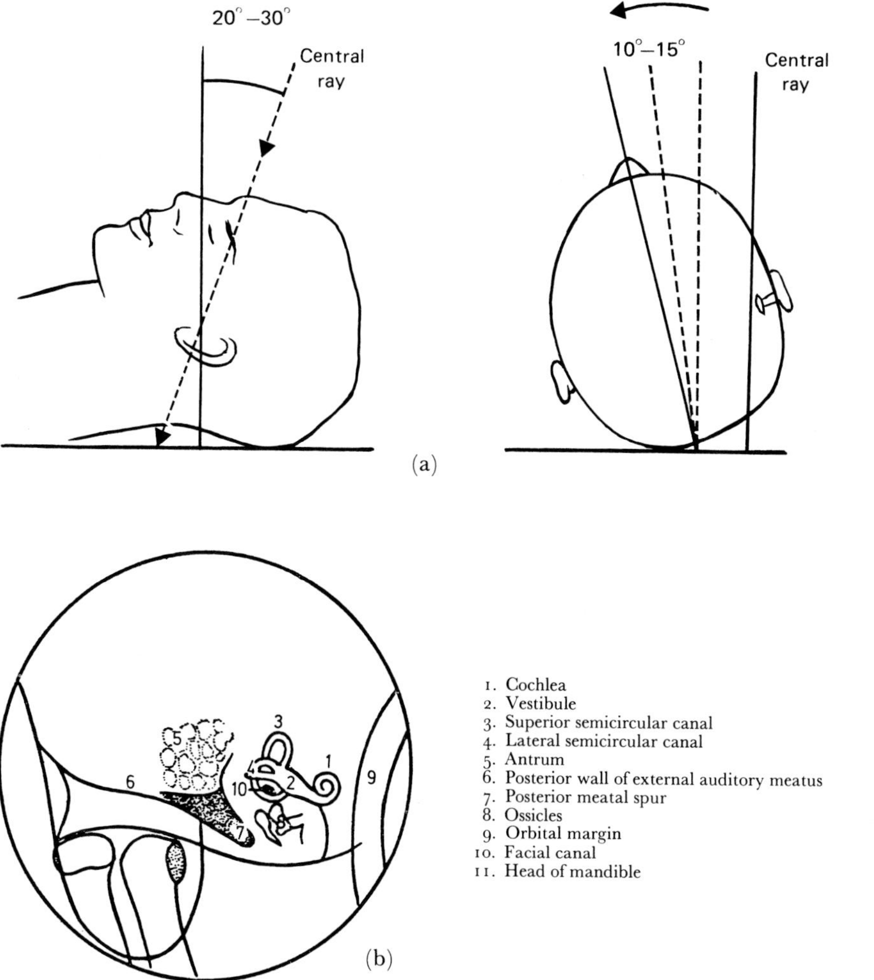

Figure 13.11 Chausee III projection. (a) Technique; (b) structures shown

Special techniques

Macroradiography

Detail can sometimes be enhanced by using a geometric magnifying technique, known as macroradiography. An ultra-fine tube focus is essential (not exceeding 0.3 mm) and the object–film distance is increased – the greater the separation of object and film the greater the geometric magnification providing the ffd remains constant. Electronic magnification using an image intensifier and television linkage is also possible. In practice these techniques seem to have some advantage over the more simple one of using a powerful magnifying glass to look at a conventional film.

Tomography

Tomography is often the only way of assessing anatomical detail in highly cellular or sclerotic mastoids. It provides the best method of demonstrating the extent of destructive processes in the temporal bone and adjacent structures, or of assessing the degree of congenital malformations of the ear. It is often the only reliable way of displaying the facial canal and the labyrinth. Simple tomographic techniques (*Figure 13.12*) utilize longitudinal or transverse tube travel during exposure. If a specialized x-ray unit is available which can achieve a circular, elliptical, hypocycloidal or spiral movement, predominantly longitudinal or transverse structures can be eliminated and fine detail of middle- and inner-ear structures can be obtained. If only linear tomography is available the internal and external auditory meatuses are usually demonstrated more clearly if the direction of tube travel is at right angles to the dominant plane of the structures to be eliminated, and it may be possible to position the patient to effect this.

For any examination in the coronal plane (patient supine) initial survey cuts are usually made at the level of the tragus of the ear and 5 mm above and below it to show

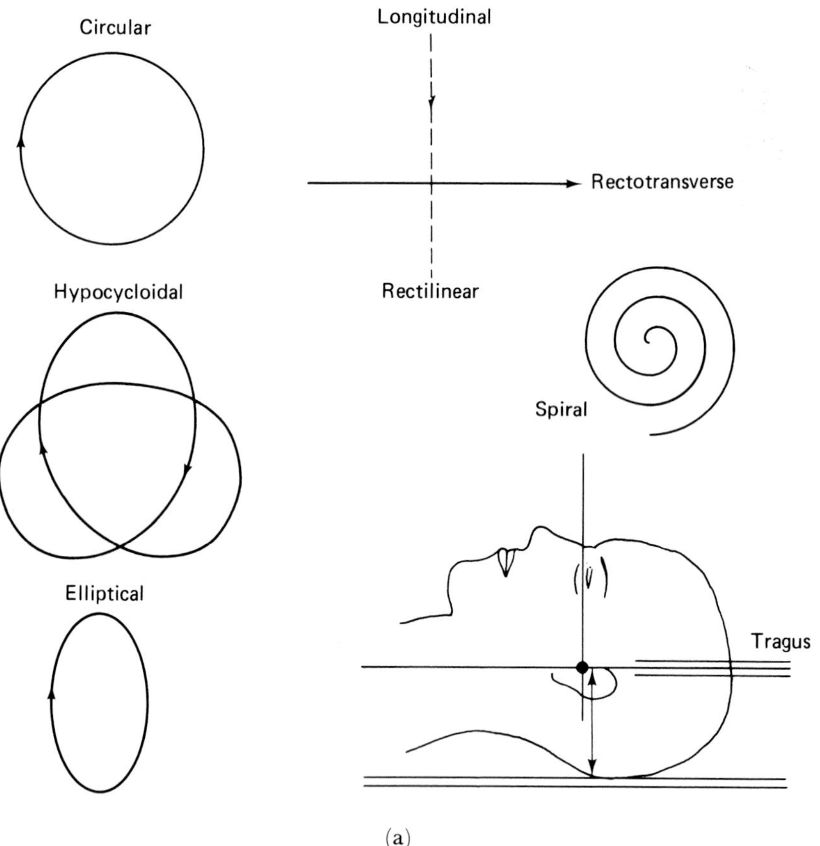

Figure 13.12 (a) Tomography; (b) rectilinear tomogram; (c) rectotransverse tomogram; (d) spiral tomogram

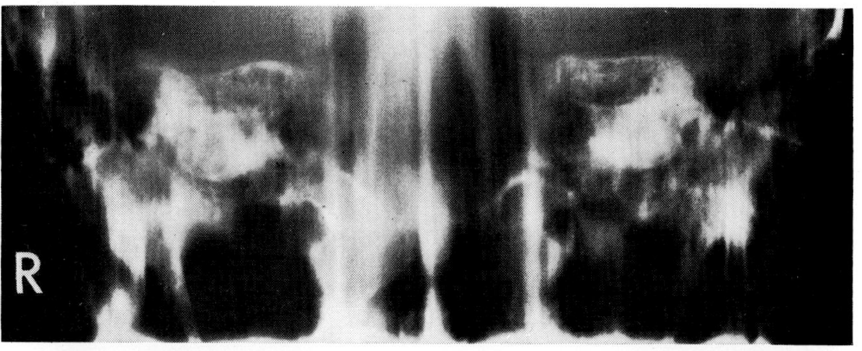

(b)

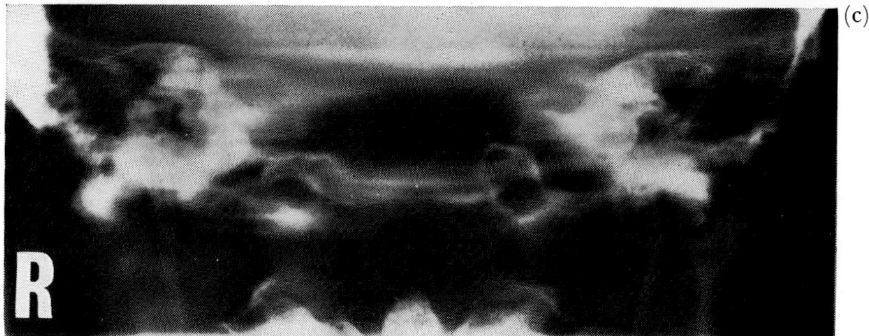

(c)

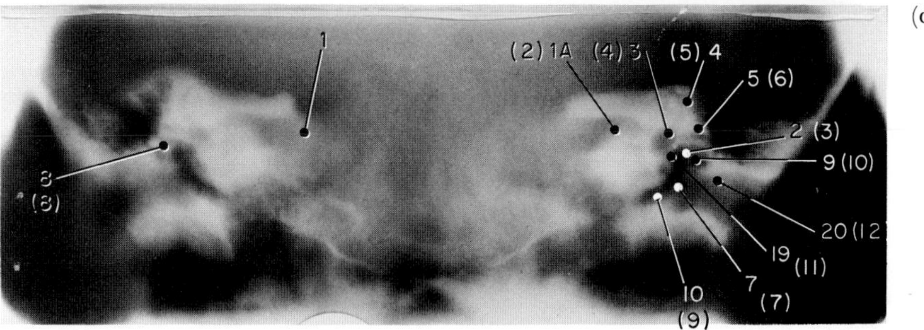

(d)

1. Internal auditory meatus
2. Internal auditory canal
3. Attic
4. Vestibule
5. Superior semicircular canal
6. Lateral semicircular canal
7. Promontory
8. Ossicles
9. Hypotympanum
10. Antrum
11. Oval window
12. Scutum of outer attic wall

the cochlea and canals. When these have been examined, further cuts may be made at appropriate levels, the thickness of and interval between cuts depending on the capability and sophistication of the apparatus. Selectivity depends on the angle or blurring path through which the tube moves and the resolving power of the recording medium. Modern specialized equipment has a maximum selectivity of 0.5–1 mm. It is essential to immobilize the head during the examination and to protect the eyes with lead shields 1 mm thick to reduce the risk of subsequent cataract.

Dosage to the cornea using spiral tomographic movement, fast detail screens, Cronex film, a 1 mm lead shield (double lead foil), 6 × 15 cm collimation and eccentric diaphragm with an exposure of 85 kV/125 mA/3.0 s is 250 mrad.

1. Internal auditory meatus
   1a. Internal auditory canal
2. Facial canal
3. Vestibule
4. Superior semicircular canal
5. Lateral semicircular canal
6. Antrum
7. Middle ear
8. Ossicles
9. Epitympanic recess
10. Hypotympanic recess
11. Cochlea
12. External auditory meatus
13. Tympanic ring
14. Mastoid tip
15. Facial canal (descending limb)
16. Jugular foramen
17. Hypoglossal canal
18. Styloid process
19. Oval window
20. Promontory
21. Round window
22. Spur (lateral wall of attic)

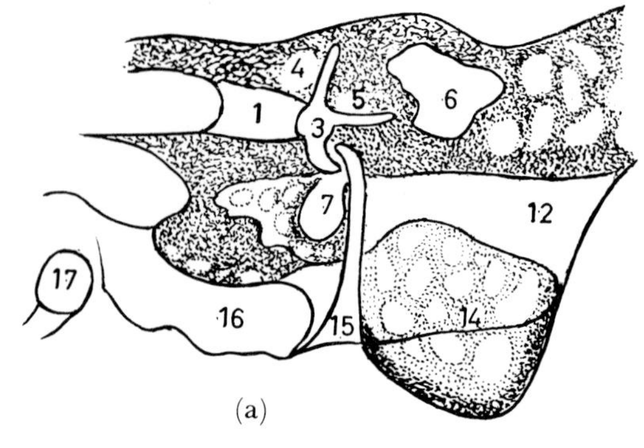

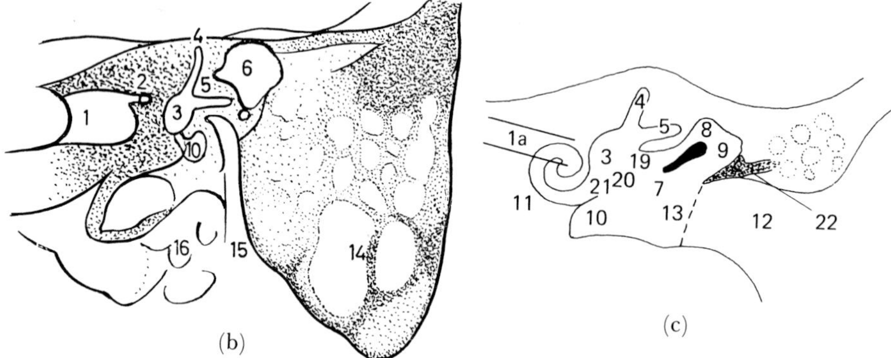

Figure 13.13 Tomography. Antero-posterior projection of left petrous bone: (a) 8.5 cm cut; (b) 9.0 cm cut; (c) 9.5 cm cut

Standard antero-posterior projection (tomography) (*Figure 13.13*)

This is probably the best projection to display the middle and inner ears and the internal and external auditory canals. The two sides are usually projected on the same radiograph but each side may be examined separately. In either case the patient is positioned comfortably in the supine position so that the orbito-meatal base-line is perpendicular to the film. (This position may be modified by depressing the orbito-meatal base-line 7–10 degrees to show the attic and aditus more clearly.) The central ray is directed vertically to the median sagittal plane at the level of the external auditory meatus; or, if each side is being examined separately, to the centre of the orbit at the junction of its middle and inner thirds (2–2.5 cm lateral to the nasion). Initial cuts are taken at the level of the tragus and at 2 mm intervals above and below this point to survey a thickness of 1 cm in total, demonstrating the canals below the level of the tragus and the cochlea above. Average distance from table top 7.5–10 cm without radiolucent pads to support the head, 10–12.5 cm with them.

Middle-ear structures demonstrated: the labyrinth, middle ear, ossicles, fenestra vestibuli and the first and third parts of the facial canal may be seen. The oval window is seen as a gap in the lateral wall of the vestibule. The round window lies a little below this separated from it by the promontory. Occasionally on this projection there seems to be a gap in the lateral wall of the facial canal which should not be mistaken for a true defect. By depressing the base-line 15 degrees (modified Towne's view) a continuous view of the middle ear from the mastoid antrum to the hypotympanic recess can be obtained, but identical positioning at subsequent examinations may be difficult to achieve.

Antero-posterior oblique (Stenvers) projection (tomography) (*Figure 13.14*)

Each side is examined separately. The patient lies supine with the base-line perpendicular to the table. The base-line is depressed through 8 degrees, the head is then rotated through 45 degrees away from the side being examined and the central

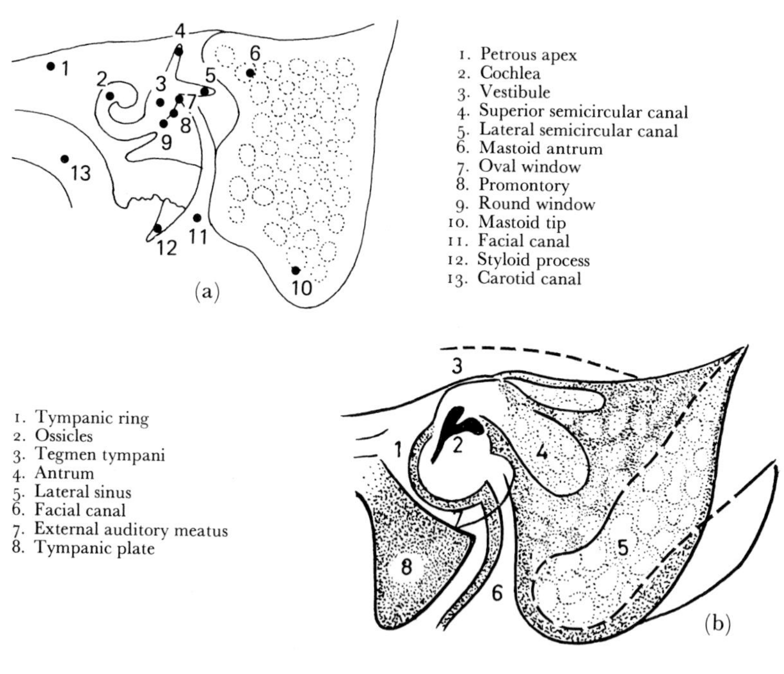

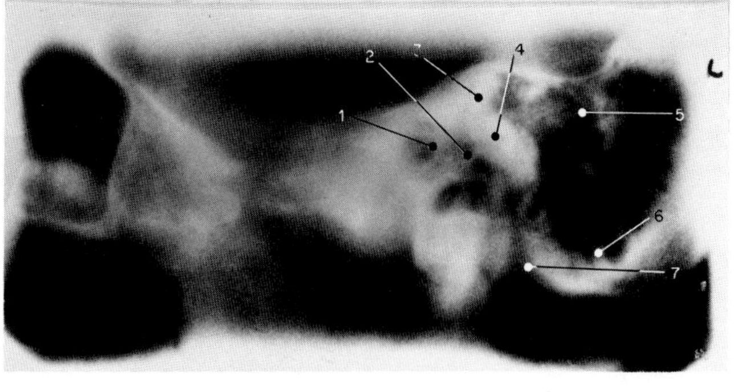

1. Cochlea
2. Vestibule
3. Superior semicircular canal
4. Lateral semicircular canal
5. Antrum
6. Mastoid tip
7. Facial canal

(c)

Figure 13.14 Tomography: antero-posterior oblique projection of left petrous bone. (a) 11 cm cut; (b) 11.5 cm cut; (c) tomogram of 17.3 cm cut

ray is directed to the zygomatic process 4–5 cm in front and 1 cm above the external auditory meatus remote from the film, to exit at the centre of the film. Cuts are taken 2 mm either side of the level of the tragus measured from the table top, average 10.2 cm.

Structures demonstrated: petrous apex, labyrinth and facial canal. The fenestra rotundum may occasionally be visible. The entry of the sigmoid sinus into the jugular foramen is usually clearly demonstrated.

Full axial projection (tomography) (*Figure 13.15*)

Without the use of a specialized skull table incorporating tomographic facilities the patient lies supine with pillows under the waist and upper trunk.

The head is extended so that the vertex comes into contact with the table, with the orbito-meatal base-line aligned parallel to it. With the use of a skull table the film support is lowered and angled forward to allow the patient to be positioned with his neck fully extended and the vertex in contact with the support. The central ray is directed vertically from below the mandible to a point 2.5 cm medial to the tragus if the examination is unilateral; or to a point in the midline bisecting the intermeatal plane if both sides are to be included on the same film. The first cut is taken at the level of the EAM, an average of 10–12 cm from table top, the distance from the table top to the external auditory meatus must be kept constant throughout the examination by immobilizing the head. Subsequent cuts are made 2–4 mm above the EAM (tragus) for the cochlea and 2–4 mm below the EAM for the mastoids and ossicles, and IAMs.

Structures demonstrated: middle ear and its recesses; the auditory canals and meatuses; all the ossicles; petrous apex; bony eustachian tube and the carotid canal. The lateral semicircular canal is shown in its whole length parallel to the film. It is probably the best single view in cases of congenital malformation of the ear.

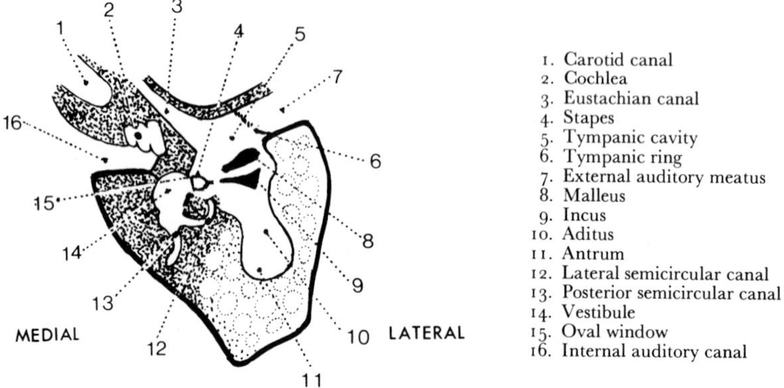

Figure 13.15 Tomography: full axial projection of left petrous bone 11 cm cut

Axial projection of the pyramid (modified Mayer's) (*Figure 13.16*)

Each side is examined separately. The patient lies supine with the base-line depressed to its maximum. The sagittal plane of the head is then rotated 45 degrees towards the

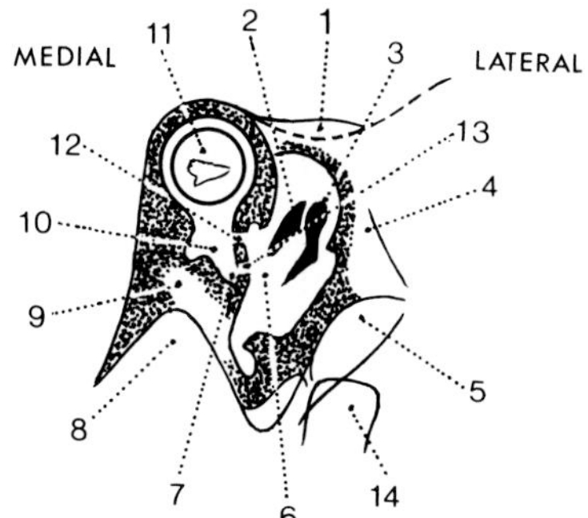

1. Tegmen tympani
2. Incus
3. Malleus
4. Lateral wall of epitympanic recess
5. External auditory meatus
6. Middle ear (tympanic cavity)
7. Basal coil of cochlea
8. Jugular fossa
9. Posterior semicircular canal
10. Vestibule
11. Superior semicircular canal
12. Oval window
13. Round window
14. Condyle of mandible

Figure 13.16 Tomography: axial ('end on') view of the pyramid 6.5 cm cut

side to be examined. The central ray is directed through the prominence of the opposite zygoma 6 cm medially from the external auditory meatus remote from the film to exit 1 cm behind the external auditory meatus nearest to the film. Initial cuts are taken between 4 and 7 cm in the adult.

Structures demonstrated: the whole tympanic cavity with its recesses should be clearly shown. The labyrinth lies medially. All the ossicles can be shown with the vestibule and the oval and round windows. The superior semicircular canal is parallel to the plane.

Lateral projection (*Figure 13.17*)

The patient lies prone, the head supported on a 4 cm transradiant polyfoam block thick enough to support the head in the lateral position, the orbito-meatal base-line parallel and the interpupillary line perpendicular to the table. The central ray is directed vertically 1 cm above the external auditory meatus and to the centre of the film. If attention is focused on the facial canal the centring point is just behind the external meatus. Cuts are taken from approximately 3–6 cm above the table top, the exact level of the middle ear being assessed from the antero-posterior projection.

Structures demonstrated: the bony external meatus, tympanic cavity and descending part of the facial canal should be shown. The malleus lies anterior to the incus and the joint is shown.

Special investigations for suspected eighth nerve or cerebello-pontine tumours

Plain radiography with tomography of the internal auditory meatus will show sufficient enlargement of the meatus or bone erosion to make a diagnosis in only between 65 and 75 per cent of all cases of eighth nerve tumours, as it depends on there being sufficient bone erosion or enlargement of the canal to be detectable by comparing the two sides.

Air-encephalography. After introducing air into the subarachnoid space by lumbar or cisternal puncture, the head is manipulated to manoeuvre it into the cerebello-pontine cisterns. This will demonstrate a tumour, if present, in about 95 per cent of

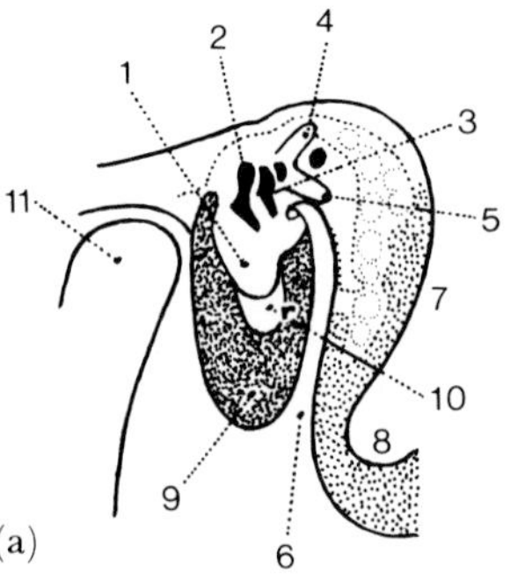

1. Middle ear (tympanic cavity)
2. Ossicles
3. Lateral semicircular canal
4. Superior semicircular canal
5. Facial canal
6. Sigmoid sinus
7. Tympanic plate
8. External auditory meatus superimposed on middle ear
9. Condyle of mandible and temporomandibular joint

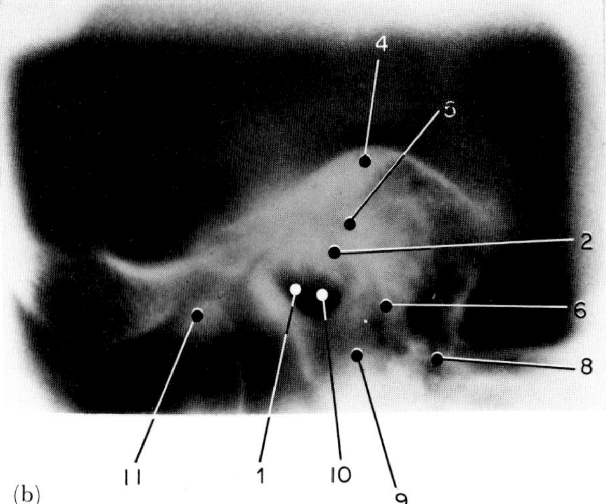

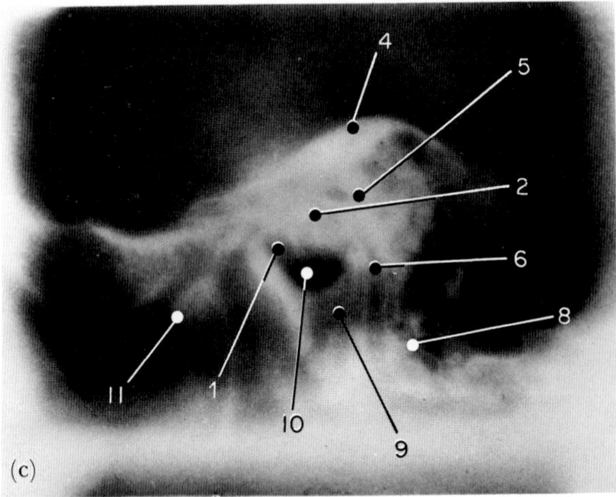

Figure 13.17 Tomography: (a) lateral projection 7.6 cm cut; (b) radiograph 7.6 cm cut; (c) radiograph 7.8 cm cut

cases by silhouetting it against the air in the cistern (*Figure 13.18*). Tomography may be used to show detail more clearly. Both sides are examined and the films compared.

Contrast (internal auditory) meatography. As an alternative to air-encephalography a radio-opaque fluid may be used instead. This is the most effective method of clinching the diagnosis of an eighth nerve tumour when one is suspected and the only method which offers success when the tumour is small or of intracanalicular type. Myodil or metrizamide 6–8 ml, 150 mg per ml saline, which has been advocated recently, is introduced into the subarachnoid space, preferably by cisternal puncture, and the head manipulated under television control to run the opaque medium into each internal auditory meatus in turn. This allows comparison of the two sides and may occasionally reveal an unsuspected lesion on the other side. Obstruction to the flow of opaque medium into the meatus, or a filling defect in the contrast column when the side under examination is dependent, provides the diagnosis (*Figure 13.19*).

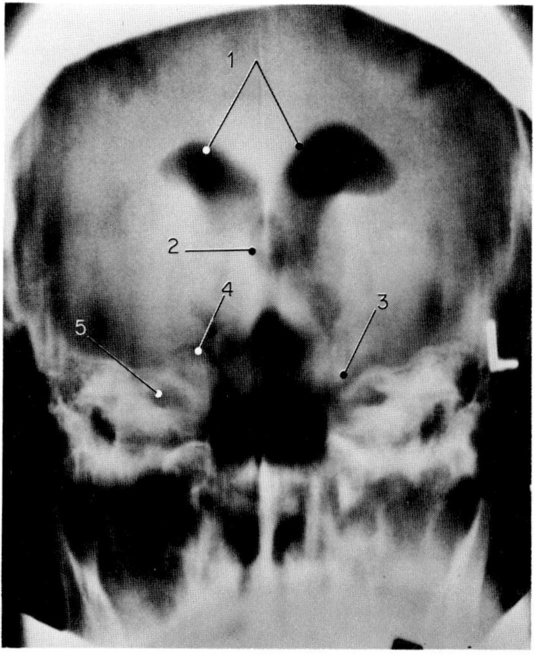

1. Lateral ventricles
2. Third ventricle
3. Air in cerebello-pontine cistern
4. Eighth nerve tumour contrasted by air in cistern
5. Internal auditory meatus

Figure 13.18 Air encephalogram

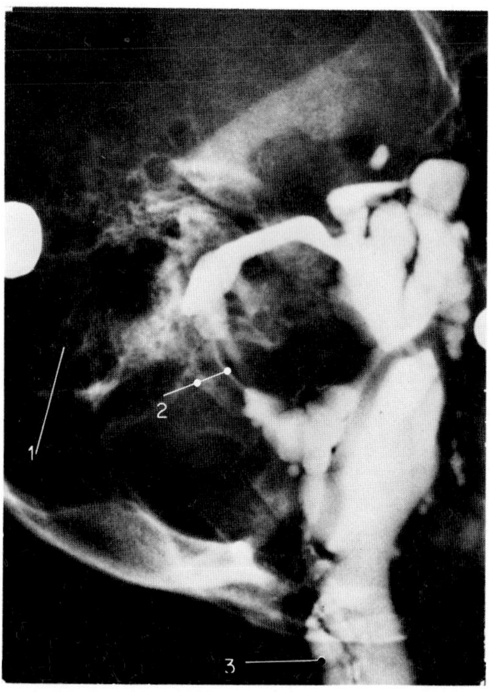

1. Mastoid cells
2. Filling defect due to large eighth nerve tumour
3. Myodil in cervical spinal canal

Figure 13.19 Myodil encephalography (contrast meatography)

Vertebral artery angiography will reveal the cause if due to meningioma in about 90 per cent of cases, by displacement of normal vessels and the demonstration of a tumour blush on the late films.

Computerized axial tomography (CAT) This is a recent technique developed from one devised by Hounsfield whereby two narrow beams of x-rays traverse the head in tandem originally at intervals of 1 degree rotation now increased to 3 degrees as the tubes, which are carried on a gantry, rotate through an arc of 180–240 degrees of a fixed radius around the immobilized head. Each beam is collimated to a band approximately 1 cm wide and the emergent x-rays are picked up and measured by a bank of special detectors which, at a fixed distance, rotate around the head on the side opposite to the source of x-rays. Usually four or five different circuits, 2.5 cm apart, are made, resulting in eight or ten sequential cuts each of 1 cm thickness. The signals from the special detectors are fed to a computer which calculates the sum total of radiation absorbed per unit volume of tissue, during the 180 degree travel of the x-ray source round the head. This information in turn is fed to a minicomputer which records this information either on magnetic tape, from which it can be printed out in numerical format on to paper, or by using additional equipment transferred on to a floppy disc for immediate pictorial display on a screen using a cathode-ray tube system. The latter system not only allows 'reading' during the course of the examination, and therefore control of the examination as it proceeds, but can provide a permanent record, for the image to be photographed, using polaroid or special photographic film which can be inserted in the notes or sent by post to the patient's doctor.

Since the original design, a number of manufacturers have devised equipment using multiple detectors which allows each cut to be completed in under 5 min thereby increasing the scope of the apparatus.

Because different tissues absorb x-rays to different degrees, it is possible to ascribe an absorption coefficient to them according to the degree to which this characteristic effects the transmission of the x-ray beam. Bone has a high absorption coefficient in the neighbourhood of 500 on the EMI scale which arbitrarily scales water as zero and which appears black on the screen. Because of their CSF content the ventricles, cisterns and sulci appear black. Fat has an absorption coefficient less than water whereas oedema – recent haemorrhage and tissue necrosis – brain tissue – congealed blood and calcification, shade progressively through grey to white as the coefficient increases. Bony structures such as the petrous bones stand out almost as on conventional x-rays and an enlargement of the internal auditory meatus or areas of bone destruction can usually be detected unless this is only minimal.

CAT scanning is diagnostically effective in approximately 95 per cent of cases of eighth nerve tumours or meningiomas. This figure is approximately the same as for air-encephalography or arteriography, but the examination is far less unpleasant and considerably less hazardous to the patient than these procedures and, where possible, after routine tomography of the internal auditory meatus, should be the next procedure of choice. In its present state of development CAT scanning is unlikely to demonstrate a tumour of less than 1 cm diameter and even tumours between 1 and 1.5 cm may occasionally be undetectable. This applies especially to intracanalicular tumours which are unlikely to be detected. There is a false positive rate of possibly 2 or 3 per cent. If there is a suspicion of a tumour based on clinical grounds a negative CAT scan should, if possible, be followed by positive contrast meatography (see

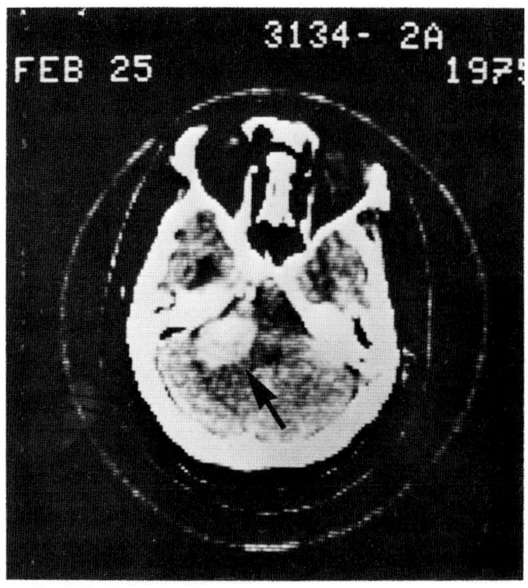

Figure 13.20 Computerized axial tomography (CAT) scan showing intracranial structures, and an acoustic neuroma

above) as this is probably the most effective technique available at present.

Eighth nerve tumours in about one-third of cases appear denser than the neighbouring brain tissue and may distort the surrounding cistern. In about half the cases they have a well-defined darker posterior rim (*Figure 13.20*). Occasionally there is a cystic element in the tumour. They tend to increase in density (or enhance) if a water soluble iodine compound such as that used in arteriography is injected intravenously. Meningiomas tend to be denser than neurinomas and usually enhance even more strongly. *Enhancement* is therefore an essential part of the examination when an eighth nerve tumour is suspected. Large tumours may displace or obliterate the fourth ventricle or be associated with dilation of the third and lateral ventricles. In Von Recklinghausen's disease tumours may be bilateral.

A neurilemmoma of the jugular foramen may present a diagnostic problem as may a metastasis. External carotid arteriography may be necessary to differentiate the former and an x-ray of the chest should be part of the routine work up. Arachnoid cysts may also present a diagnostic problem but do not enhance.

Radioisotope scans. Radionuclides. Recently isotope scanners have been developed along the lines of the brain scanner developed by EMI which greatly enhance the value of this technique. Meningiomas and neurilemmomas tend to take up isotope readily, the former more intensely than the latter, and if over 1 cm in diameter are likely to be demonstrable. This technique which is complementary to rather than competitive with EMI scanning increases the scope of diagnosis when used in conjunction with it.

Radiological examination of the nose

The nasal cartilages are not individually recognizable on routine x-ray films. The paired nasal bones meet medially to form the bridge of the nose. The internasal suture is slightly tortuous and rarely lies exactly in the midline. Sutures separate the nasal bones from the frontal bones above, and the frontal processes of the maxillae inferolaterally. On each side, running down parallel to the naso-maxillary suture is a groove for an anterior ethmoidal nerve.

Usually films are taken after injury to determine fractures or displacements of nasal bone or bones.

Soft tissue lateral view (*Figure 13.21a*)

The patient is examined in the sitting position with the skull adjusted to the lateral position. A non-screen film is used and placed in contact with the lateral aspect of the face. The tube (using a long localizing cone to cover a 7.5 cm circle) is directed horizontally to the root of the nose and to the centre of the film. Alternatively a dental film may be used as it can be held in close contact with the lateral aspect of the nose. Exposure – 50 kV, 32 mAs, 90 cm.

Supero-inferior view (*Figure 13.21b*)

The patient holds an occlusal film lightly between the teeth, so that approximately two-thirds of the film projects forwards. The tube is directed from above so that the central ray passes tangential to the forehead vertically through the root of the nose to the centre of the film. In some subjects a prominent forehead or upper jaw may obscure the nasal bones. Exposure – 65 kV, 32 mAs, 90 cm.

Nasal bones screen type film technique

Lateral (screen film technique) 24 × 18 cm cassette long axis horizontal

The patient sits erect with head in the lateral position (median sagittal plane, parallel interpupillary line perpendicular to the film). Area included on the film from the frontal sinuses above to the upper alveolar margin below.

The tube's central ray is directed horizontally to the root of the nose and to the centre of the film.

Infero-superior (screen film technique)

The patient is seated, the neck hyperextended so that the vertex may be placed in contact with the film support and the orbito-meatal base-line parallel to it.

The TCR is directed horizontally and cephalically towards the median sagittal plane tangential to the upper alveolar margin and the frontal bone in order to demonstrate the nasal bones in plan view (*see Figure 13.21c*)

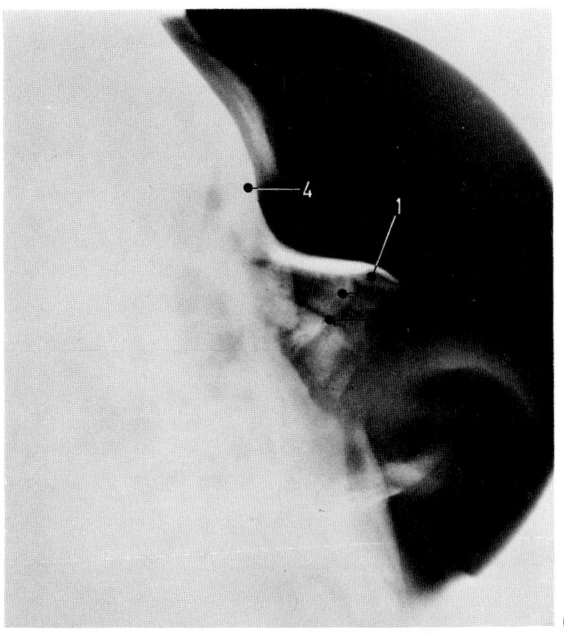

(a)

1. Nasal bones
2. Groove for anterior ethmoidal nerve
3. Nasomaxillary suture
4. Nasal process of frontal bone

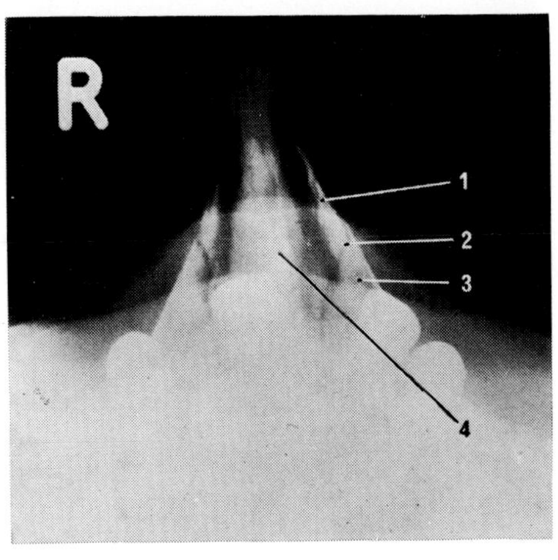

(b)

1. Nasal bones (lateral aspect)
2. Nasomaxillary suture
3. Nasal process of maxilla
4. Septum

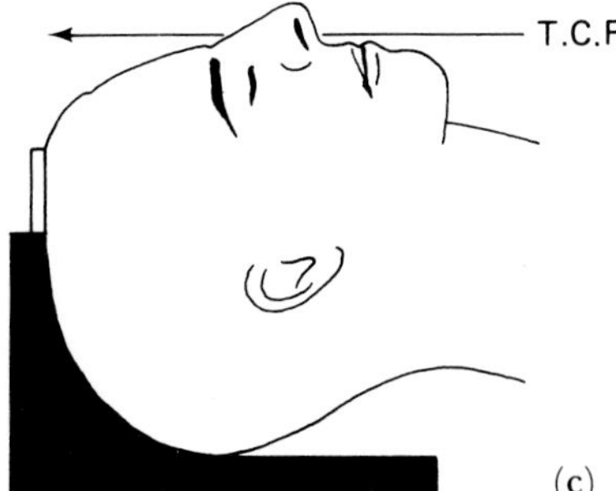

(c)

Figure 13.21 (a) Lateral view of nasal bones. Detail screens film technique 50 kVp/3.2 mAs/100 cm; (b) supero-inferior biew of nasal bones. Detail screens 60 kVp/10 mAs/9 cm diaphragm; (c) cassette technique for nose

Occipito-mental view (*Figure 13.22*)

This view shows the frontal processes of the maxillae and the maxillary processes of the frontal bone. The nasal bones are seen end on.

Paranasal sinuses

If one wishes to try to demonstrate each of the paranasal sinuses free of overlying structures and to obtain more than a single projection of any one sinus it is necessary to take films in five or six different projections. This may be considered unnecessary by practising rhinologists who often ask for a single occipito-mental survey film, but a single film can only help to exclude gross disease for it is impossible to examine all the paranasal sinuses adequately by one projection, and information important to the patient and to the clinician may easily be missed.

As in other radiological examinations it is desirable to have at least two views of any structure, if possible at right angles to each other. With the sinuses this may present practical difficulties because of superimposition and intermediate projections may be necessary. However, in spite of superimposition of the paired sinuses, a lateral view provides information of the sphenoid sinuses and the nasopharynx, and at the same time gives an indication of general sinus topography in depth. If the ethmoids are suspect, special views to show these should be taken.

It may be argued that in all cases a single survey film in the occipito-mental position should be taken first and that other views should be taken only if there is an indication to do so when this is examined. This practice is not always easy to organize in a busy department and it is more practical to carry out a reasonably full examination from the start.

To carry out a thorough examination, at least three, and in most cases four, projections are necessary (occipito-mental, occipto-frontal, lateral and axial). There is little increase in patient's time, no significant hazard from extra radiation, and only small additional cost.

General comments

There is no such thing as a 'normal' sinus from the anatomical point of view because there is no constant pattern of pneumatization and, therefore, there is always individual variation in size and shape. One is therefore discussing average or mean appearances.

Asymmetry of the paired sinuses will usually result in the smaller sinus appearing more opaque because of its thicker bony walls. This should not be mistaken for a pathological state. It is not uncommon for one frontal sinus to be much smaller than its fellow or even to be absent. Less often the antra differ in size though small differences in size are not uncommon. Rarely one maxillary antrum fails to develop and in consequence the maxilla looks uniformly dense on the x-ray film. This is liable to lead to a mistaken diagnosis of infection (*Figure 13.22*). The smaller size of the affected antrum should alert the observer to this possibility.

Hypopneumatization of the frontal sinuses is common in severe erythroblastic anaemia, whether sickle-celled or of mediterranean (Cooley's) type.

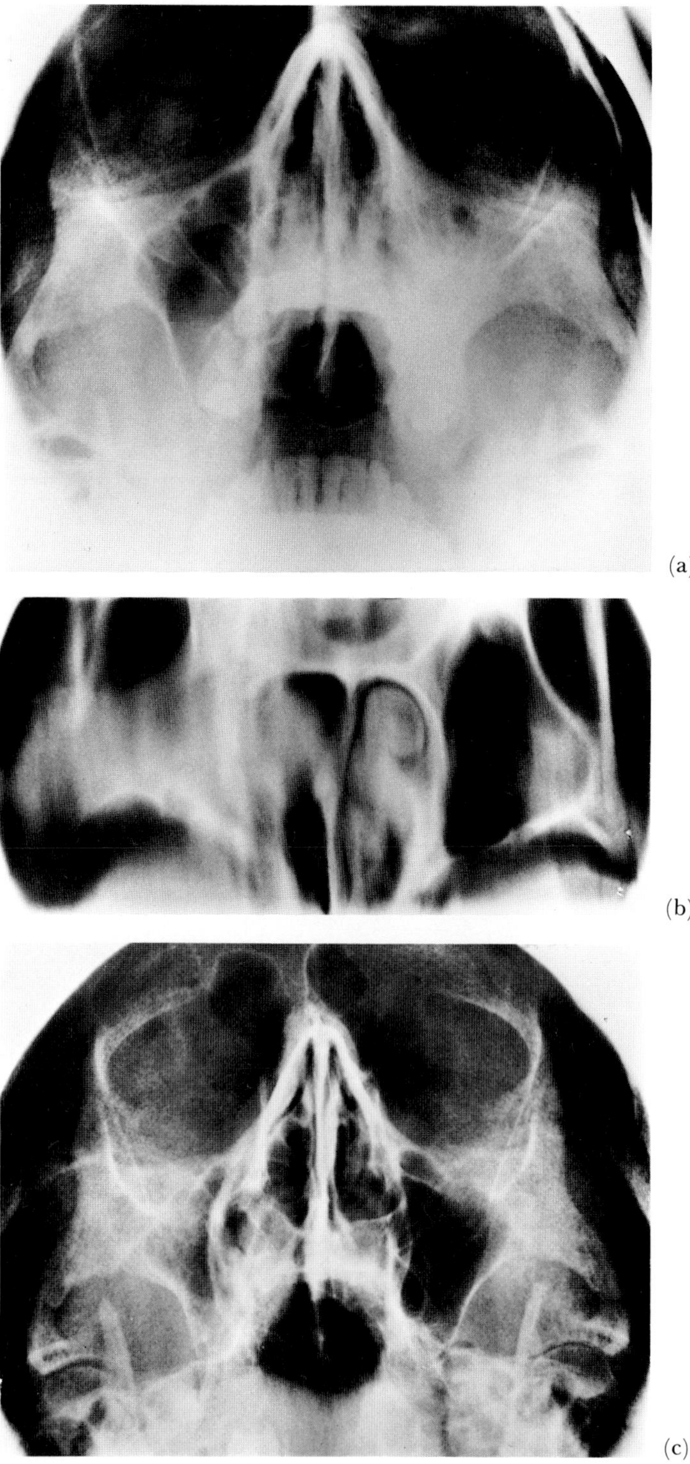

(a)

(b)

(c)

Figure 13.22 (a) Underdeveloped left antrum: occipito-mental view; (b) underdeveloped left antrum as in (a) – the tomograph confirms the diagnosis; (c) underdeveloped right antrum

Hyperpneumatization

Hyperpneumatization of the frontal sinuses is a feature of acromegaly and of Sturge–Weber disease. If unilateral it should suggest a long-standing atrophy of one cerebral hemisphere.

The *maxillary antra* are best shown in the standard occipito-mental and full axial projections though their lower portions are visible on the 15 degree occipito-frontal view. They are superimposed in the lateral view. The antra are not discernible at birth but usually can be made out as small triangular cavities after a few months of life, gradually enlarging towards full development at 16–18 years of age. The alveolar recess is absent in children, being occupied by teeth. It may fail to develop in later life. The roots of the upper pre-molar and first and second molar teeth commonly project into the floor of the antrum. In later life, with loss of teeth, reabsorption of bone may reduce the thickness of the alveolus to a thin bony ridge. Partial bony septa are not uncommon, though complete septa are rare. A zygomatic recess may produce a septate appearance which should not be mistaken for a dental cyst when dental films are taken. On the standard occipito-mental film, the lateral antral wall may present a double contour. This is because it runs backwards and medially. A groove may be seen half-way down this wall caused by the postero-superior dental vessels. Not uncommonly aberrant ethmoidal cells extend into the postero-superior part of the medial antral wall and may even migrate into the orbital plate giving them a double contour. The true origin of these cells usually only becomes obvious when they, or the antrum, are individually infected and become opaque.

The *frontal sinuses* usually show on x-rays from three years of age onwards, reaching their ultimate size at about 18 years. Development and pneumatization tend to be asymmetrical and may be markedly so. Not infrequently one, or both, are absent, and when this occurs there is often persistence of a metopic frontal suture. The septum between the two frontal sinuses is usually thin and commonly deviated to one side. The outlines of the frontal sinuses are normally crenated and ridged with short septa. Loss of this crenated appearance should rouse the suspicion of a mucocele.

Each frontal sinus may consist of one or two components, one extending vertically into the calvarium and the other horizontally into the roof of the orbit. In the postero-anterior projections the two components tend to be superimposed and asymmetry of development may therefore cause marked differences in transradiancy on the two sides. The frontal sinuses are best shown on the 15 degree occipito-frontal projection or the over-tilted full axial view. The latter shows the depth of the frontal sinuses and the thickness of their anterior and posterior walls. They are visible in different degrees of obliquity on other projections described.

The *ethmoid sinuses* are present at birth and reach full development at about 16 years of age. The shape of the labyrinth in life is a flat-sided truncated cone with its base posteriorly. The cells vary considerably in size and number in different individuals, and to some extent on the two sides in the same person. Occasionally cells are so large that only three or four are present.

Migratory (agger) cells may extend forwards to merge with the frontal sinus, or back towards the sphenoids. Occasionally they extend into the greater wing of the sphenoid and the roof of the antrum on one or both sides. The best projection to show the ethmoidal sinuses free of overlying cells is the full axial view (submento-vertical). Oblique views projecting the ethmoids into the orbits show only the posterior and middle cells free from superimposition of cells of the other side (*see Figure 13.27*).

The *sphenoidal sinuses* are not usually visible before four years of age. The two halves usually develop asymmetrically. The septum is usually central anteriorly and deviates to one side as it passes backwards. Accessory septa are fairly common postero-laterally. The degree of pneumatization varies considerably between individuals. Usually the anterior two-thirds of the body of the sphenoid is pneumatized but the sinus may extend back into the dorsum sellae and the posterior clinoid processes, and rarely even into the basi-occiput. At times the sphenoids may extend laterally into the pterygoid plates or greater wings of the sphenoids. If the anterior clinoids are pneumatized each may look like an optic foramen on the oblique views taken for ethmoids or for the optic foramina. The true foramen, however, lies immediately medial to this. More important from the surgical point of view is failure of pneumatization, or partial pneumatization, for the anterior wall of the pituitary fossa may then consist of thick well-corticated bone which may hamper access to the fossa when approached through the nose. The thickness of the anterior wall can nearly always be assessed on the plain lateral film, but tomography provides more exact information.

The sphenoidal sinuses are best shown on the full axial view but may be visible on the standard occipito-mental projection if the mouth is open during exposure. On the lateral film they are superimposed. A decubitus lateral (patient supine, horizontal beam) is the best projection to show fluid levels if present, though these may also be shown if the full axial view is taken with the patient sitting.

Projections for the maxillary sinuses

For general purposes the following four projections allow a good all-round assessment of the paranasal sinuses. It is preferable to take them with the patient seated, and using a horizontal beam wherever possible to show fluid levels if present. The head should be immobilized by a suitable head band or clamp. A specialized skull table gives the best results, but high-quality films can be taken on an upright Bucky stand, or even on a horizontal Bucky table. In the latter case fluid levels will only be shown on projections using a horizontal beam.

Occipito-mental (*Figure 13.23*)

The patient sits facing the Bucky support with the chin resting against it, the median sagittal plane aligned to the midline. The mouth is supported wide open with a transradient perspex 'bite block' and the base-line is adjusted to make an angle of 45 degrees with the film. In older patients it may be necessary to angle the tube central ray caudally to compensate for an inability to extend the head sufficiently, but if a skull table is used with the object table angled through 20 degrees (or more) forwards towards the patient the correct position is consistently maintained, and always allows the use of a horizontal x-ray beam. The tube is adjusted so that the central ray passes horizontally to the midline at the level of the inferior orbital margins and to the centre of the film.

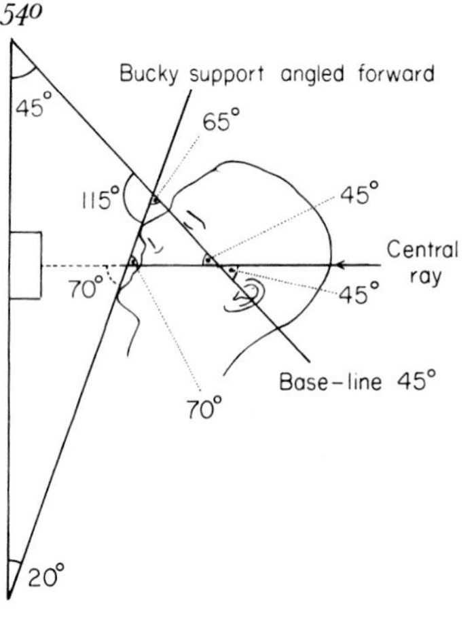

(a)

1. Frontal sinuses
2. Nasal bones
3. Nasal process of maxilla
4. Nasal septum
5. Middle turbinate
6. Postero-lateral wall of antrum
7. Antrum
8. Antero-lateral wall of antrum
9. Inferior turbinate
10. Sphenoid sinus
11. Foramen ovale overlying alveolar recess of antrum
12. Soft tissue shadow cast by lips (dotted lines)
13. Foramen rotundum
14. Infra-orbital foramen
15. Zygoma
16. Superior orbital fissure
17. Innominate line
18. Lamina papyracea of ethmoid
19. Frontozygomatic suture
20. Soft tissue shadow cast by nares (dotted lines)
21. Orbit
22. Ethmoid cells

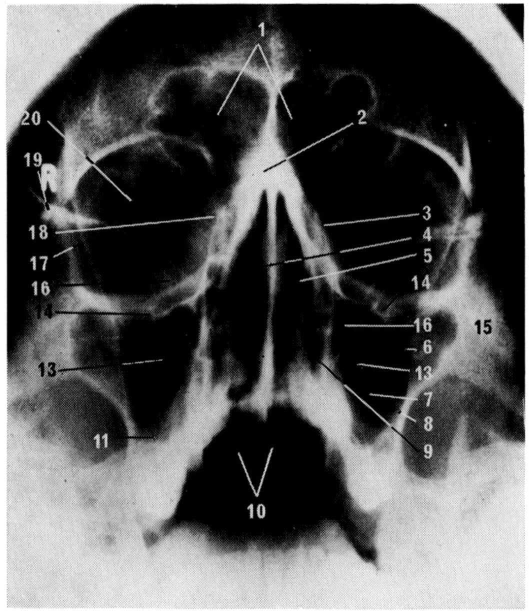

(b)

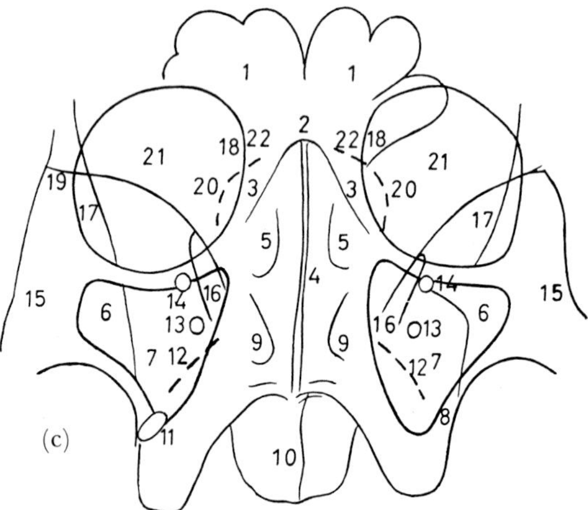

(c)

Figure 13.23 Occipito-mental view of the sinuses: (a) technique; (b) radiograph; (c) line drawing of (b)

Structures demonstrated

The antra are clearly shown. The frontal sinuses are projected obliquely, though their floors are clearly shown. The ethmoid cells are largely obscured, but a few cells may be seen within the nose and medial to the lamina papyracea on the inner wall of the orbit. The sphenoidal sinuses are visible through the open mouth. If, after examining the film a fluid level is suspected, its presence or absence can be confirmed by repeating the view with the sagittal plane of the head tilted 20–40 degrees to the side in question.

15 degree occipito-frontal (*Figure 13.24*)

The patient sits or lies prone with the forehead and part of the nose in contact with the Bucky support. The base-line is adjusted perpendicular to the film and the tube is angled 15 degrees caudally. If a skull table is used the object table is angled 15–20 degrees towards the patient, the central ray is directed horizontally to the nasion, and to the centre of the film.

Structures demonstrated

The frontal sinuses are clearly shown. The upper parts of the antra are obscured by the petrous bones but their lower parts are visible. The floor of the sella turcica, the crista galli, the nasal septum and middle and inferior turbinates can be seen. The ethmoidal and sphenoidal sinuses are superimposed.

Full axial – submento-vertical (*Figure 13.25*)

The patient sits facing the tube. The neck is fully extended, so that the vertex rests against the Bucky support. The base-line should be as near parallel to the film as possible. The central ray is directed 2.5 cm anterior to the intermeatal plane to the midline, from beneath the mandible at an angle of between 90 and 100 degrees to the base-line, and to the centre of the film. Slight over-extension is an advantage as both anterior and posterior walls of the frontal sinuses are then seen ('overshot' axial view, *Figure 13.25 (c)*).

Structures demonstrated

The ethmoidal and sphenoidal sinuses are shown free of superimposed cells. The posterior walls of the antra, petrous apices and base of the anterior and middle fossae of the skull are clearly seen. In elderly patients, or in those with short thick necks, it is often difficult to obtain sufficient extension of the head to bring the base-line parallel to the film. If a skull table is available this can be easily countered by angling the object table forwards towards the patient. If not, the tube central ray must be angled cephalically accordingly, to compensate for lack of head extension.

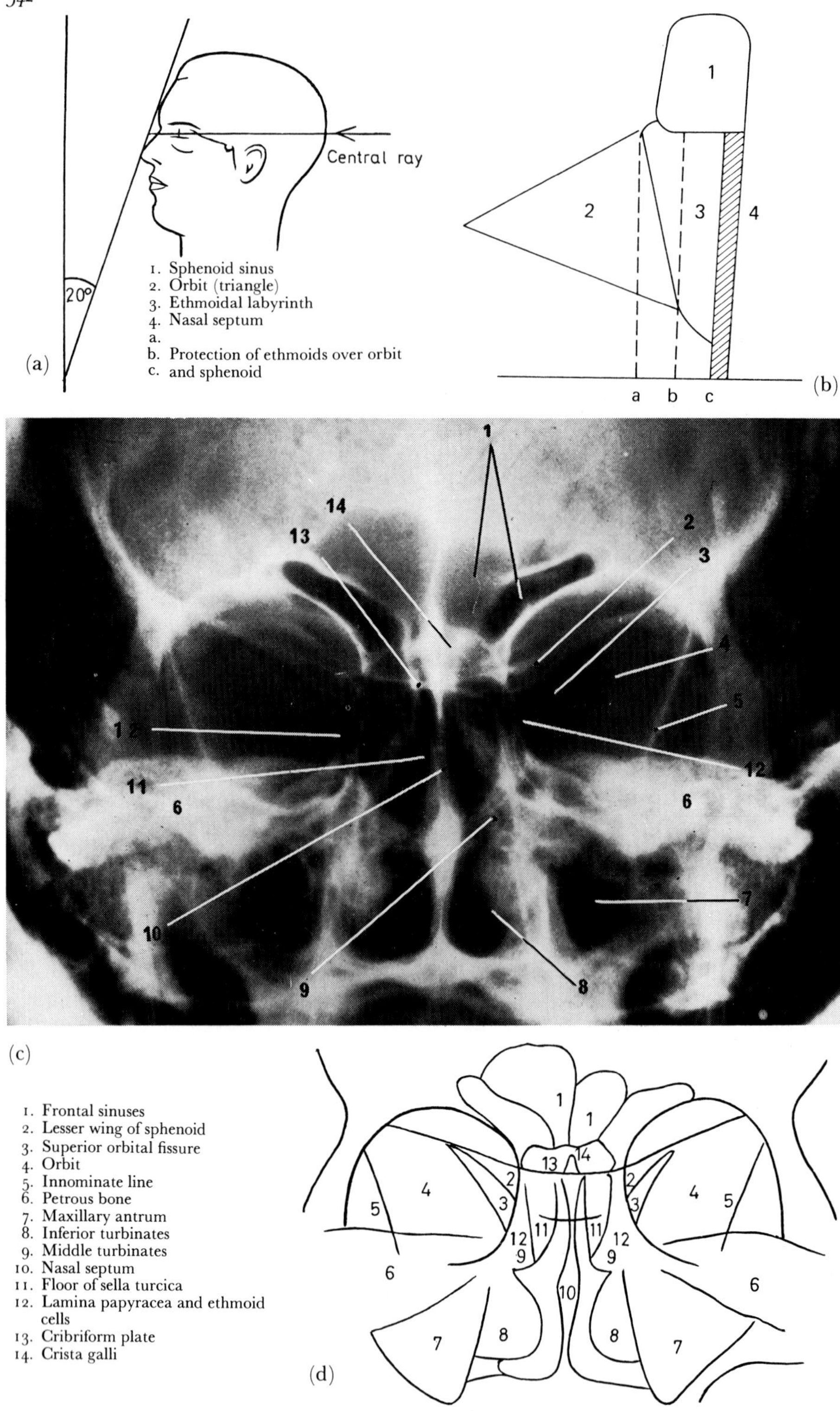

Figure 13.24 15 degree occipito-frontal view of the sinuses; (a) technique; (b) schematic representation of sinuses from above to show overlap (after Hajek); (c) radiograph; (d) line drawing of (c)

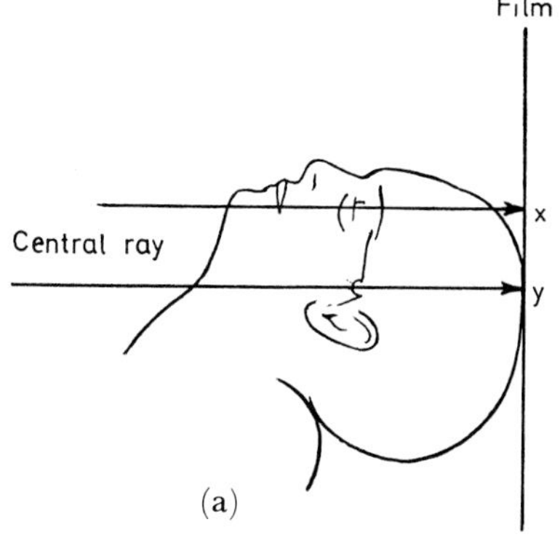

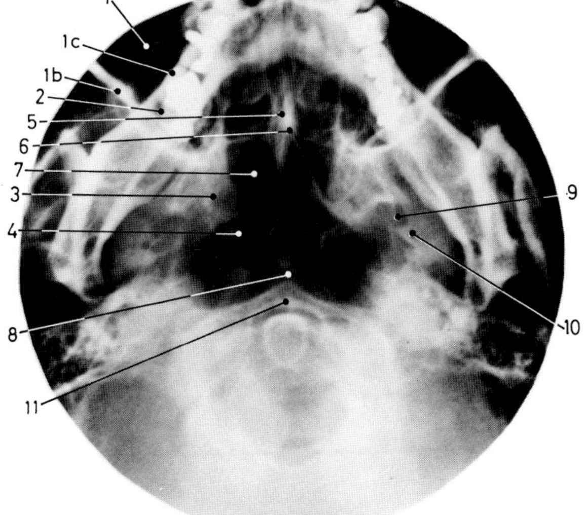

1. Antrum
   b. Posterolateral wall
   c. Medial wall
2. Inferior orbital fissure
3. Great wing of sphenoid
4. Anterior boundary of middle cranial fossa
5. Ethmoid labyrinth
6. Bony nasal septum
7. Sphenoid sinuses
8. Air in pharynx
9. Foramen ovale
10. Foramen spinosum
11. Anterior arch of atlas

(b)

1. Frontal sinus
2. Maxillary antrum
3. Ethmoid labyrinth
4. Nasal septum
5. Paired sphenoid sinuses
6. Air in nasopharynx
7. Foramen ovale
8. F. spinosum
9. Condyle of mandible
10. External auditory meatus
11. Odontoid peg

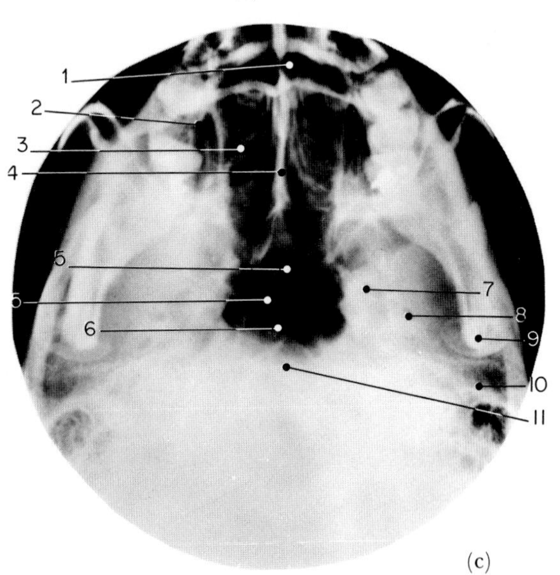

(c)

Figure 13.25 Full axial projection: (a) Centre to x for frontal and ethmoid sinuses. Centre to y for sphenoids. (b) Full axial (submento-vertical – SMV) projection – standard position. (c) 'Overshot' axial view (10 degree cephalic tube angle)

Lateral (*Figure 13.26*)

The patient sits facing the Bucky table and the skull is then rotated into the lateral position. The central ray is directed horizontally to a point behind the outer canthus of the eye and to the centre of the film. When particular interest is directed to the nasopharynx, the patient sits sideways on with the head in the lateral position with the chin protruded. In children under seven the central ray is directed horizontally to a point immediately posterior to the angle of the mandible. In older children or adults the central ray is directed to a point 2.5 cm in front and 3.75 cm below the superimposed external auditory meatuses and to the centre of the film. The focal film distance is increased from the standard 90 cm to 150 cm to reduce magnification. Exposure – 60 kV, 40 mAs, 90 cm (*Figure 13.26*).

Structures demonstrated

On the lateral projection the paired sinuses are superimposed on one another, but the extent of pneumatization of the frontal and sphenoidal sinuses can be gauged, especially in their vertical and horizontal directions. The thickness of the soft tissues in the nasopharynx, the uvula, and the extent of the nasopharyngeal airway can be assessed. Enlarged adenoids can be clearly shown. This view is essential when opaque foreign bodies are being sought, or when surgery on the sphenoid or transnasal implantation of radioactive isotope seeds into the pituitary gland is contemplated.

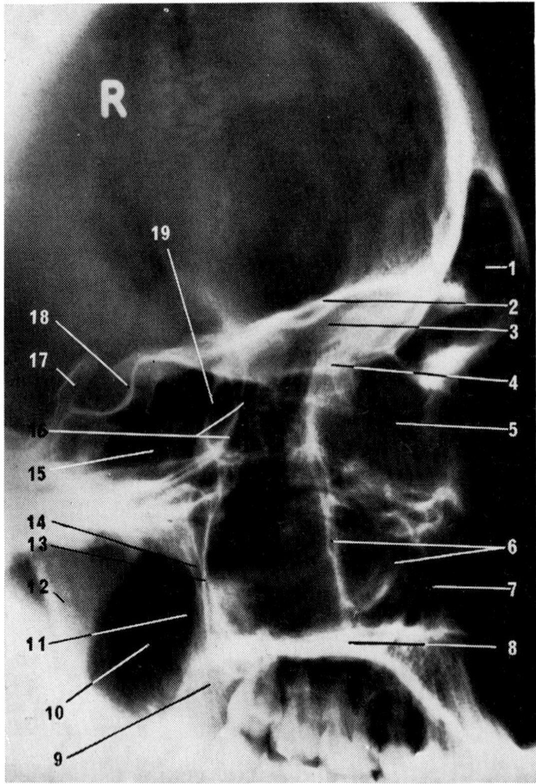

1. Frontal sinuses. Vertical component
2. Floor of anterior cranial fossa
3. Frontal sinuses. Horizontal component
4. Cribriform plate
5. Orbit
6. Zygoma
7. Anterior wall of antrum
8. Floor of antrum
9. Uvula
10. Air in nasopharynx
11. Lateral pterygoid lamina
12. Mandible
13. Posterior wall of antrum
14. Anterior wall of pterygoid process
15. Sphenoid sinus
16. Anterior wall of middle cranial fossa
17. Dorsum sellae
18. Anterior wall of pituitary fossa
19. Anterior wall of sphenoid sinus

Figure 13.26 Lateral view of sinuses; 60 kV, 40 mAs

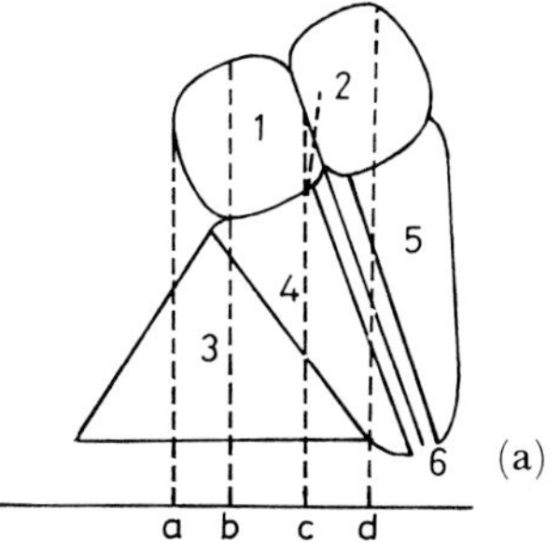

1. Right sphenoid sinus
2. Left sphenoid sinus
3. Orbit
4. Right ethmoid labyrinth
5. Left ethmoid labyrinth
6. Nasal septum

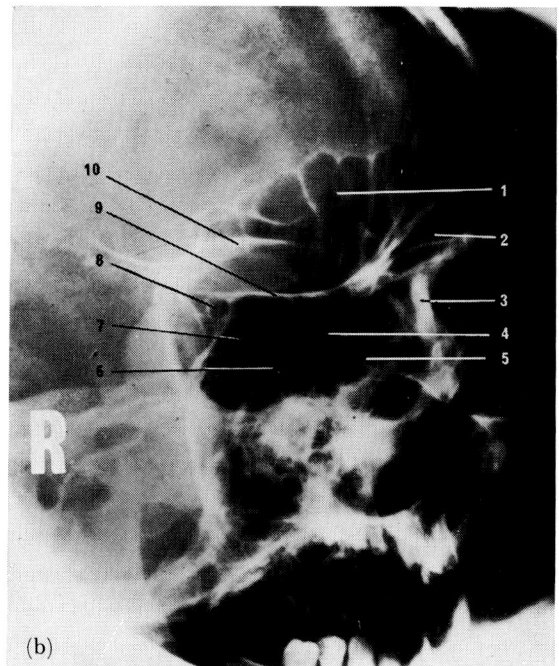

1. Right frontal sinus
2. Left frontal sinus
3. Nasal bones
4. Middle ethmoid cells and left sphenoid sinus
5. Right anterior ethmoid cells
6. Right middle ethmoid cells
7. Right posterior ethmoid cells and right sphenoid sinus
8. Right optic foramen
9. Lesser wing of sphenoid
10. Roof of right orbit

Figure 13.27 40 degree right postero-anterior oblique projection: (a) schematic representation as seen from above (after Hajek); (b) radiograph demonstrating sinuses

Special views for ethmoid cells

35–40 degree postero-anterior oblique (*Figure 13.27*)

The right and left sides are examined separately. The patient is positioned to face the Bucky table and the base-line is adjusted perpendicular to the film, the head is then rotated through 35–40 degrees so that the rim of the orbit, the nose and cheek on the side to be examined, are 'flattened' against the Bucky support. The tube central ray is angled 10–15 degrees caudally (or the base-line raised 10–15 degrees) to prevent the petrous bones obscuring the ethmoids, and directed to pass through the centre of the orbit and the centre of the film.

Structures demonstrated
This view shows the posterior and middle groups of ethmoidal cells with some superimposition of the sphenoidal sinuses on the side to be examined – as well as the optic foramen and floor of the anterior fossa. The frontal sinuses are shown obliquely. Half the sphenoid and a few posterior ethmoid cells of the opposite side are also shown.

Less commonly used projections

30 degree occipito-frontal (*Figure 13.28*)

This is a modified Towne's view. The patient's skull is adjusted to the true antero-posterior position, the tube central ray is angled 30 degrees caudally and directed to the midline at a point 1 cm below the lower border of the orbits and to the centre of the film.

Structures demonstrated

This projection demonstrates the postero-superior and supero-lateral walls of the antra, the superior orbital fissure, the mandibular rami and zygomatic arches.

Vertico-submental (*Figure 13.29*)

The patient faces the Bucky support with the head extended as far as possible and the chin resting on the support. The central ray is angled 40 degrees from the horizontal passes to a point 2.5 cm anterior to the EAM, to the midline and to the centre of the film.

Tomography (*Figure 13.30*)

This is an excellent technique for demonstrating fine detail of the sinuses and is not utilized as much as it should be. It is often the only way to demonstrate fractures or early destruction of sinus walls, and in showing tumours or foreign bodies in the

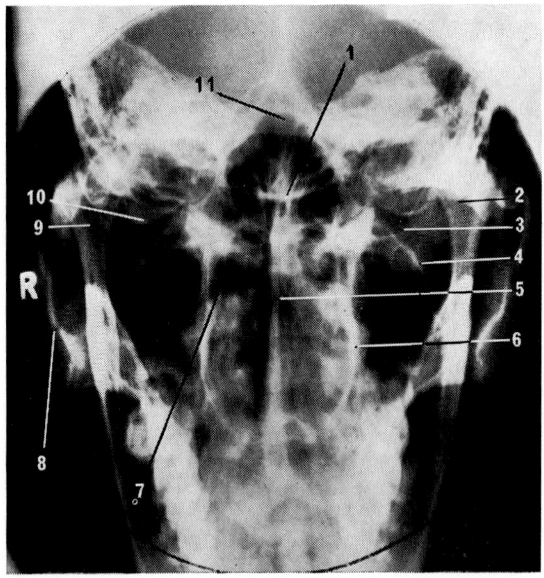

1. Cribriform plate
2. Condyle of mandible
3. Inferior orbital fissure
4. Postero-supero-lateral wall of antrum
5. Nasal septum
6. Nasal process of maxilla
7. Medial wall of antrum
8. Zygomatic arch
9. Condyle of mandible
10. Anterior margin of middle cranial fossa
11. Posterior margin of foramen magnum

Figure 13.28 30 degree occipito-frontal projection of sinuses

1. Antrum
2. Anterior wall of antrum
3. Postero-lateral wall of antrum
4. Lower jaw
5. Bony septum (vomer)
6. Zygomatic arch
7. Anterior boundary of middle cranial fossa
8. Sphenoid sinus
9. Foramen ovale
10. Foramen spinosum

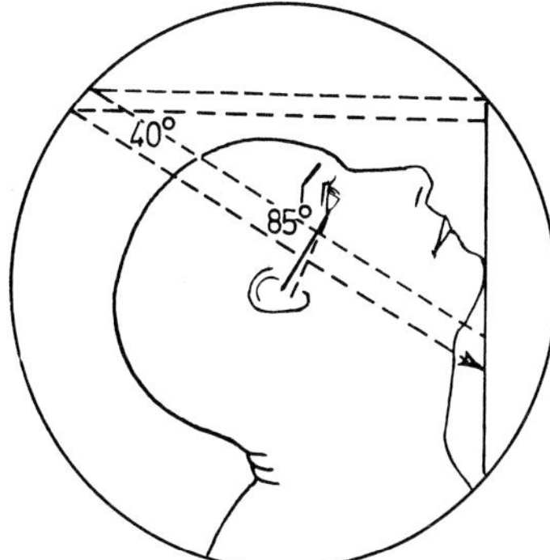

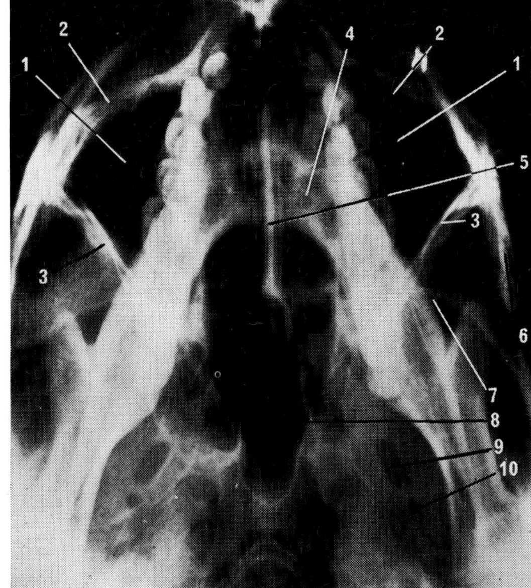

Figure 13.29 Vertico-submental projection

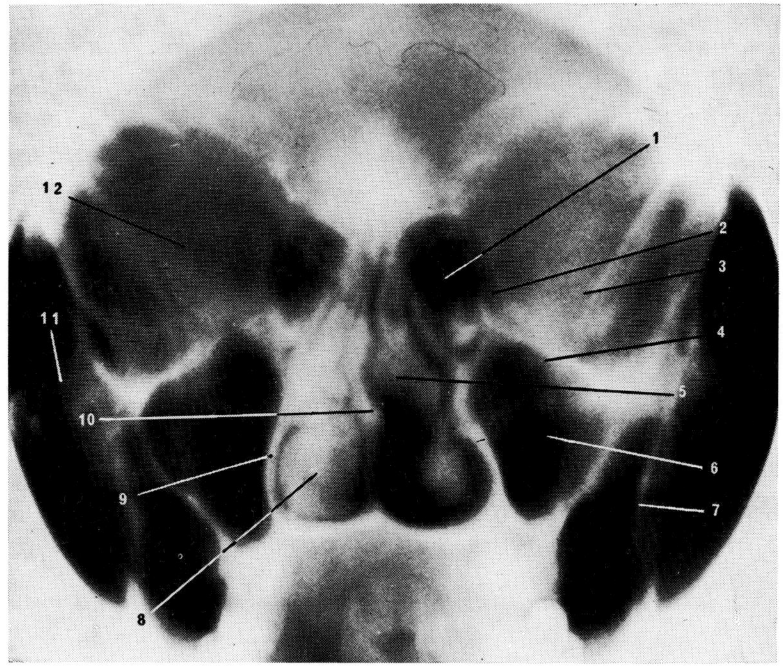

1. Ethmoid labyrinth
2. Medial wall of orbit
3. Innominate line
4. Roof of antrum. Floor of orbit
5. Middle turbinate
6. Antrum
7. Ascending ramus of mandible (blurred)
8. Inferior turbinate
9. Medial wall of antrum
10. Nasal septum
11. Zygoma
12. Orbit

Figure 13.30 Tomography of the sinuses. Section at 18 cm through maxillary sinuses and nose – patient supine

sinuses or nasal passages which not infrequently are invisible, or only poorly shown on conventional films. It should be used routinely in any case of unexplained nasal obstruction, discharge, or bleeding. It may be performed with the head in any of the standard positions to be described though the straight antero-posterior or lateral positions are probably the most satisfactory and most comfortable to the patient. If the apparatus can be used in the erect position so much the better to show fluid levels.

Techniques using opaque media

In some countries attempts are made to demonstrate the confines and contents of the maxillary antra by instilling an opaque medium into them, either by direct puncture or the Proetz manoeuvre. It is claimed that this method also gives some indication of the efficiency of ciliary action, the antra being usually cleared of the medium within 48 h. This may be so with Lipiodol, but if more modern types of water-soluble media are used this does not apply. The method has been little used in this country and it is doubtful whether it provides vital information that cannot be better obtained by other techniques such as tomography.

Radiological examination of the pharynx, larynx and oesophagus

A lateral film of the patient's neck taken at a distance of 1.8 m should be a basic feature of any radiological examination of the nasopharynx, larynx and pharynx, and may be especially helpful to a clinician before he starts his examination of children or nervous individuals when difficulty is expected. A postero-anterior and lateral film of the chest should also be taken as a routine to exclude localized pulmonary or mediastinal disease, such as tumour, aneurysm, pulmonary fibrosis or tuberculosis.

Radiographic technique

The patient sits in a true lateral position with the jaw comfortably protruded, extended and raised. The head is firmly immobilized by a head clamp, the film should include from 3 cm above the upper border of the pinna to the thoracic inlet. The tube central ray is directed horizontally to a point at the level of the thyroid cartilage (C4–5) if interest is centred on the larynx or pharynx. If interest is centred on the nasopharynx or oropharynx the film should include from the pinna to a point 7.5 cm below the angle of the jaw, and the tube central ray directed horizontally to a point 1.25 cm below, and 2.5 cm in front of the external auditory meatus (at the angle of the jaw in the case of a child under five years of age as the facial bones are compressed) and to the centre of the film. In the former case during the exposure, the patient breathes quietly through the open mouth; in the latter he should breathe through the nose with his mouth closed. Average exposure factors (adult) 108 kV, 18 mAs at 1.2 m distance regular screens. Alternatively a high kV technique may be used using 'low dose' film with screens, or a wedge filter to allow visualization of the range of densities from the neck to the thoracic inlet. Exposure factors: 110 kV density 2 + 2 80 mAs, 180 cm ffd using a 100 line 12.8 : 1 grid, and an aluminium wedge filter.

To show the structures low in the neck and upper mediastinum, the central ray is directed to a point below the middle of the clavicle at the level of the thoracic inlet, and to the centre of the film, placed in the Bucky tray. The patient braces the shoulders, clasps the hands behind the back, so that a sandbag may be looped over them to depress the shoulders.

The antero-posterior projection is usually less informative as the air-filled structures of the nasopharynx and larynx are largely obscured by the cervical spine, but it may show tracheal displacement or compression, or a fluid level in a pouch or abscess.

To demonstrate a laryngocele the exposure is made during the Valsalva manoeuvre, but tomography may be necessary.

Long ossified styloid processes are best shown on an antero-posterior film taken through the open mouth.

All examinations should be performed erect if possible to show fluid levels if present, but in young children films may have to be taken recumbent.

Structures demonstrated (*Figure 13.31*)

On the lateral projection air in the upper respiratory passages outlines the valleculae and cavities of the larynx and trachea. Soft tissue structures such as the soft palate, base of tongue, epiglottis and aryepiglottic folds are silhouetted against this air background. Occasionally enlarged tonsils may be seen as oval densities, and the cartilaginous eustachian tube may present as a narrow dark slit when filled with air with a rim around it due to the eustachian cushion. The hyoid bone and, if ossified, the thyroid and cricoid cartilages, can usually be clearly seen. Careful note should be made of the thickness of the soft tissues in the nasopharynx and of the pre-vertebral soft tissues are important, or a bulge or increase in thickness may indicate oedema, abscess, haematoma, cyst or tumour. The state of the cervical vertebrae and discs should also be noted. Surgical emphysema shows as linear streaks of air in the pre-vertebral plane. In adults the soft tissues in the roof of the nasopharynx should measure not more than 1 cm, they should be regular in outline and thickness. In children hypertrophy of adenoids may be so pronounced as to obliterate the air space between the postero-superior wall and the soft palate, and enlarged adenoids may be visible into early adult life.

In infants, especially in the first weeks of life, the pre-vertebral soft tissues normally look thick, especially on full expiration, and this should not be mistaken for a retropharyngeal infection. Films should always be taken on inspiration and if there is any doubt the film should be repeated on inspiration, or a cine run taken with the infant held in an erect lateral position.

The depth of the cervical pre-vertebral soft tissues normally increases slightly from the level of the anterior arch of the atlas down to the lower border of the fifth and sixth cervical vertebrae where it blends with the thicker soft tissue shadow of the cricopharyngeus and upper oesophagus. After the age of two or three it should not measure more than 4 mm in depth. Below the cricoid the soft tissue thickness between the air-filled trachea and the spine should not normally exceed three-quarters of the

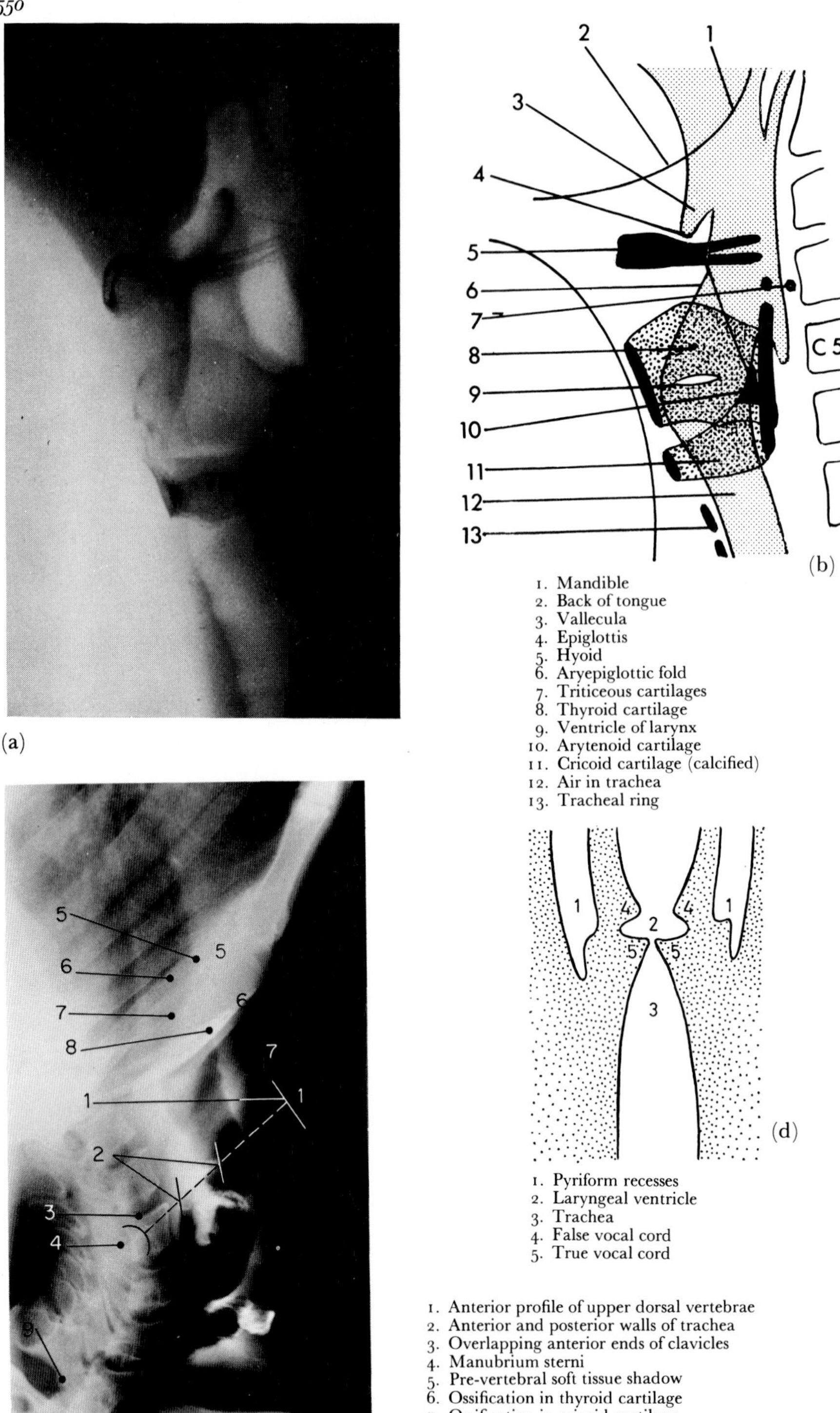

Figure 13.31 (a) Lateral soft tissue film of larynx; (b) schematic drawing; (c) lateral film of thoracic inlet; (d) schematic drawing of AP view of larynx as shown by tomography

diameter of the corresponding cervical vertebra, and should it do so a tumour or inflammation in the post-cricoid region or upper oesophagus should be suspected.

Foreign bodies and growths in the larynx or trachea may be silhouetted against intraluminal air. At the thoracic inlet the trachea usually lies centrally in the antero-posterior projection. On the lateral view (*Figure 13.31d*) it normally lies equidistant between the anterior vertebral border and the posterior profile of the upper manubrium. These relationships may be disturbed by scoliosis or kyphosis, the trachea being displaced towards the concavity of the scoliosis, and forwards with kyphosis. With a straight cervical spine displacement of the air-filled trachea (or barium-filled oesophagus) indicates extrinsic pressure.

Ossification commonly occurs in one or more of the laryngeal cartilages though there is considerable individual variation both in age of onset and extent. It is uncommon before the third decade, and if present earlier, should suggest the possibility of an adrenogenital syndrome. Ossification occurs most commonly in the thyroid cartilage in which it starts posteriorly and inferiorly and slowly extends forwards and upwards. The cricoid tends to ossify from behind forwards. The stylohyoid ligament not infrequently ossifies in its upper part, and occasionally throughout its whole extent. The styloid processes are best shown on an antero-posterior film taken through the open mouth. Rarely ossification occurs in the epiglottis and occasionally the cricothyroid ligament is ossified. Compression of the trachea is usually obvious.

The arytenoids may ossify in the absence of ossification in other laryngeal cartilages and present as dense triangular opacities. If superimposed they should not be mistaken for a swallowed foreign body when the examination has been performed to try to demonstrate one. The same applies to ossified triticeous cartilages. The corniculate and cuneiform cartilages are unlikely to be so mistaken because they lie more anteriorly.

As an alternative, or in addition to the two-film techniques described, the patient can be 'screened' using an image intensifier coupled to a 0.3 mm focus tube. Spot films are exposed in those positions found to show the structures of interest to best advantage. This method has certain advantages. It permits appraisal of dynamic function and allows barium to be given by mouth to show the pharynx and upper oesophagus during the passage of the bolus. Any lack of muscle co-ordination in the act of swallowing such as hesitancy or stasis, or lack of forward propulsion due to ineffectual muscle movement, can be readily seen and recorded on cine film or video tape. The movement of the cords during breathing and phonation can be watched and lack of symmetry is usually obvious. This, too, can be recorded on cine film or tape. After swallowing barium, the soft tissue structures of larynx and pharynx may be sufficiently coated with barium to produce a double contrast effect, and this may be enhanced by the Valsalva manoeuvre. In children, or in adults with language difficulties, the Valsalva effect is best achieved by blowing up a balloon.

Contrast radiography

Larynx and pharynx

This method has proved of value in some hands but a sufficient number of cases must be examined by any single individual to allow him to become expert in the technique and in the interpretation of the results. It is liable to be time-consuming and at times frustrating. Technically the method is often most difficult in patients who have undergone tracheostomy or in those whom the clinician has also had difficulty in examining by conventional methods. On the other hand, when successful the cords and ventricle are clearly outlined and this allows an accurate assessment to be made of paralysis, fixation or displacement of a cord, and will often show the outline, size, and extent of a tumour in the larynx or pharynx.

The throat is sprayed with topical local anaesthetic (2.0 per cent lignocaine) and the larynx can be similarly treated, or the patient can gargle with 2.5 per cent amethocaine mixed with carboxymethyl cellulose. Better still, one or two injections of 1.0 ml, 2.0 per cent lignocaine are made through the cricothyroid membrane into the upper trachea – the needle being withdrawn as the patient coughs. This is quicker, and uses less anaesthetic to produce satisfactory anaesthesia. A viscous contrast medium of the type used for bronchography (Dionosil aqueous) is then injected over the back of the tongue through a fine rubber tube under screen control, the tongue being drawn forwards to make swallowing more difficult. When the larynx and pharynx are satisfactorily coated a cine run is made, or spot films are taken in postero-anterior, lateral, and oblique positions during quiet breathing, phonation, and the Valsalva manoeuvre.

Nasopharynx

The patient lies on his back with the neck hyperextended sufficiently to place the vertex against the Bucky support. Topical local anaesthetic is sprayed through the nostrils into the nasopharynx. After a short interval this is followed by injecting a water-soluble opaque medium such as 45 per cent hypaque, or fluid lipiodol through both nostrils. Films are exposed in the axial and lateral positions after 2 ml have been injected into each side and again after 4 ml. The patient sits up, expectorates excess fluid and two more films are exposed, one axial, one lateral.

Contrast demonstration of the eustachian tube

This is a technique which could well be used more often when tubal obstruction is suspected or is not responding to treatment, or when middle-ear infection persists. It is best performed on a special skull table. The patient lies supine with the neck fully extended as for the full axial (SMV) projection described (page 541, *Figure 13.25*) and 1–2 ml of water soluble contrast – such as 25 per cent Hypaque – is injected into the middle ear to fill it, having instilled 4 per cent topical Amethocaine or Xylocaine into the EAM for a few minutes beforehand. The patient is maintained in the lateral position until it has taken effect. The injection is made through a perforation in the drum when one exists – or directly through the intact drum using a fine needle. In the latter case it is advisable to inject a little local anaesthetic into the middle ear before the opaque medium which tends to be irritant.

Films are exposed in the full axial projection followed by a lateral film using a horizontal beam. The patient is then turned prone and the lateral film is repeated followed by a reversed Towne's ($\frac{1}{2}$ axial) projection.

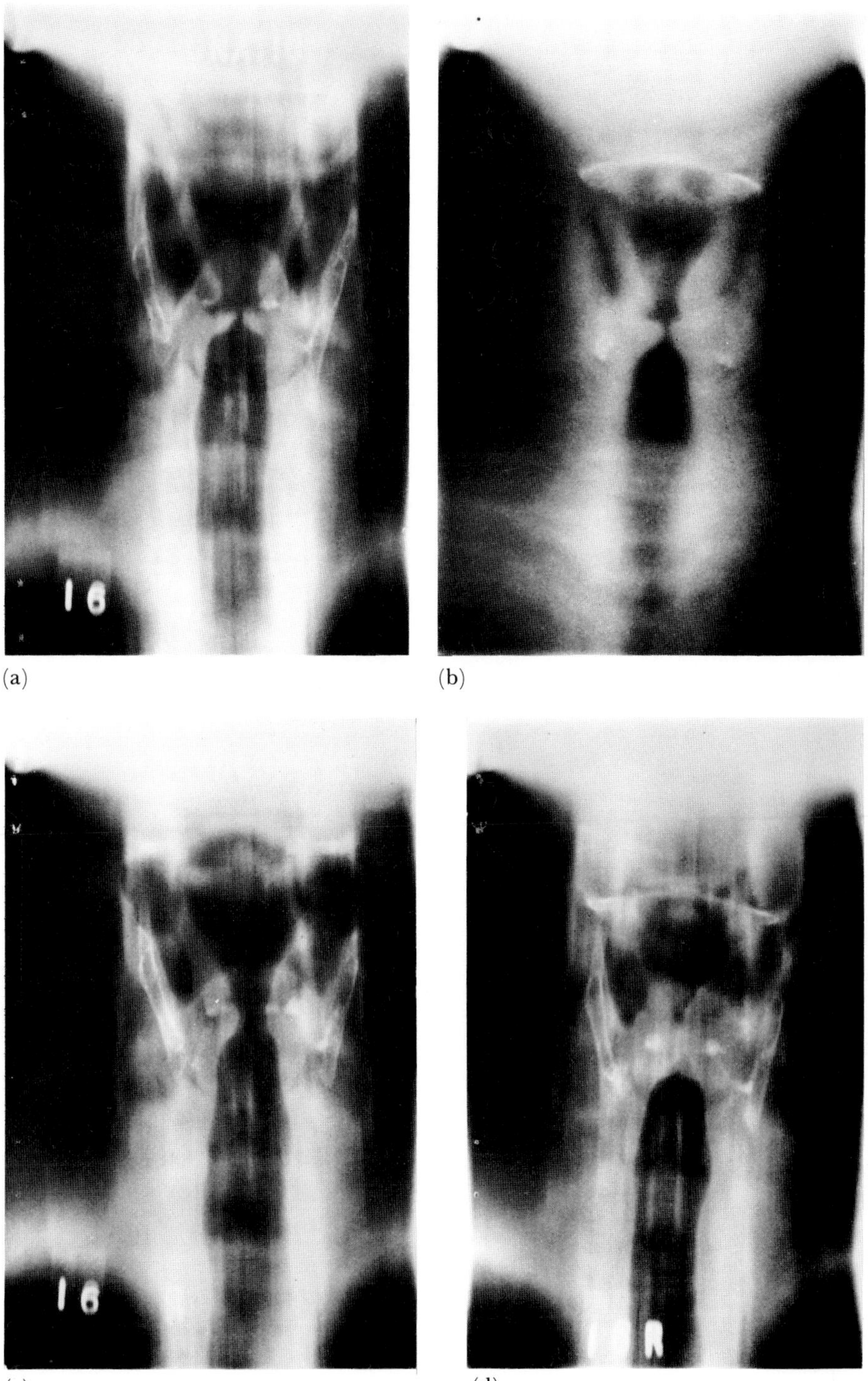

Figure 13.32 Tomography of the larynx (16 cm cut): (a) phonating 'EE' (linear, exposure 80 kV, 0.63 s, 300 mA); (b) phonating 'EE' (spiral, exposure 75 kV, 3 s, 50 mA); (c) Valsalva (linear); (d) quiet breathing (linear)

Tomography (*Figure 13.32*)

This is the most effective method of demonstrating the larynx and subglottic regions. The patient lies supine with the chin raised (and the upper trunk supported, to bring the larynx and trachea parallel to the table top). The tube central ray is directed to the midline over the middle of the thyroid cartilage (C4–5) and cuts are initially made at 2.5 mm intervals, preferably using the linear movement for the initial survey during 'quiet breathing'. The first cut is taken at a level of approximately 2 mm below the anterior skin surface. Further cuts are made if necessary at levels decided upon when the first films are examined. Use of the spiral or hypocycloidal movement on the most useful plane of cut demonstrated on the survey film, and using a selectivity of 0.5 mm will eliminate overlying structures still further. Phonation and the Valsalva manoeuvre may be undertaken either in the initial survey or when further cuts are taken. Further cuts are made if necessary at levels decided on when the first films are examined using a selectivity of 1 mm on the spiral or hypocycloidal movement. Lateral tomographs may also prove valuable, especially if the apparatus can operate with the patient in the erect position.

Oesophagus

This is a tubular organ the diameter of which varies from a potential space to the size needed to accommodate whatever can be swallowed. It normally contains no air though occasionally a small triangular air shadow can be seen on a lateral film just below the level of the cricopharyngeus. Air is almost always visible in this region when there is a foreign body present in the pharynx or upper oesophagus.

The conventional radiological examination is the barium swallow. It is often stated that barium should never be used if it is thought that spillover into the trachea may occur, but provided small amounts only are used there seems to be little danger, especially if postural drainage is used afterwards. Barium is inert and less irritating than most water-soluble contrast media, and usually provides better radiographic detail. In infants, if atresia or a fistula is suspected, it is better to pass a soft rubber tube and to inject a water-soluble opaque fluid, of the kind used for bronchography, only if necessary. Communication between the oesophagus and trachea involves the anterior wall of the oesophagus so that injection of opaque fluid should be made in prone and prone oblique positions under x-ray screen control and films taken as required.

When undertaking a screen examination of the oesophagus the patient is usually given fluid barium to swallow, though occasionally barium paste is used. The radiologist follows the passage of a mouthful of barium from the mouth to the stomach. The situation, extent, and form of physiological and pathological constrictions or filling defects, or any hesitation or hold-up or diversion of the normal flow is noted. Attention is paid to the form and amplitude of peristaltic waves. The lower oesophageal sphincter is tested for competence, by watching the patient swallowing prone while abdominal compression is applied.

Zaino and colleagues (1970) have demonstrated that there is a sphincter 1–2 cm long at the upper end of the oesophagus, below the cricopharyngeus, in which increased pressure can be measured manometrically, and state that this provides the

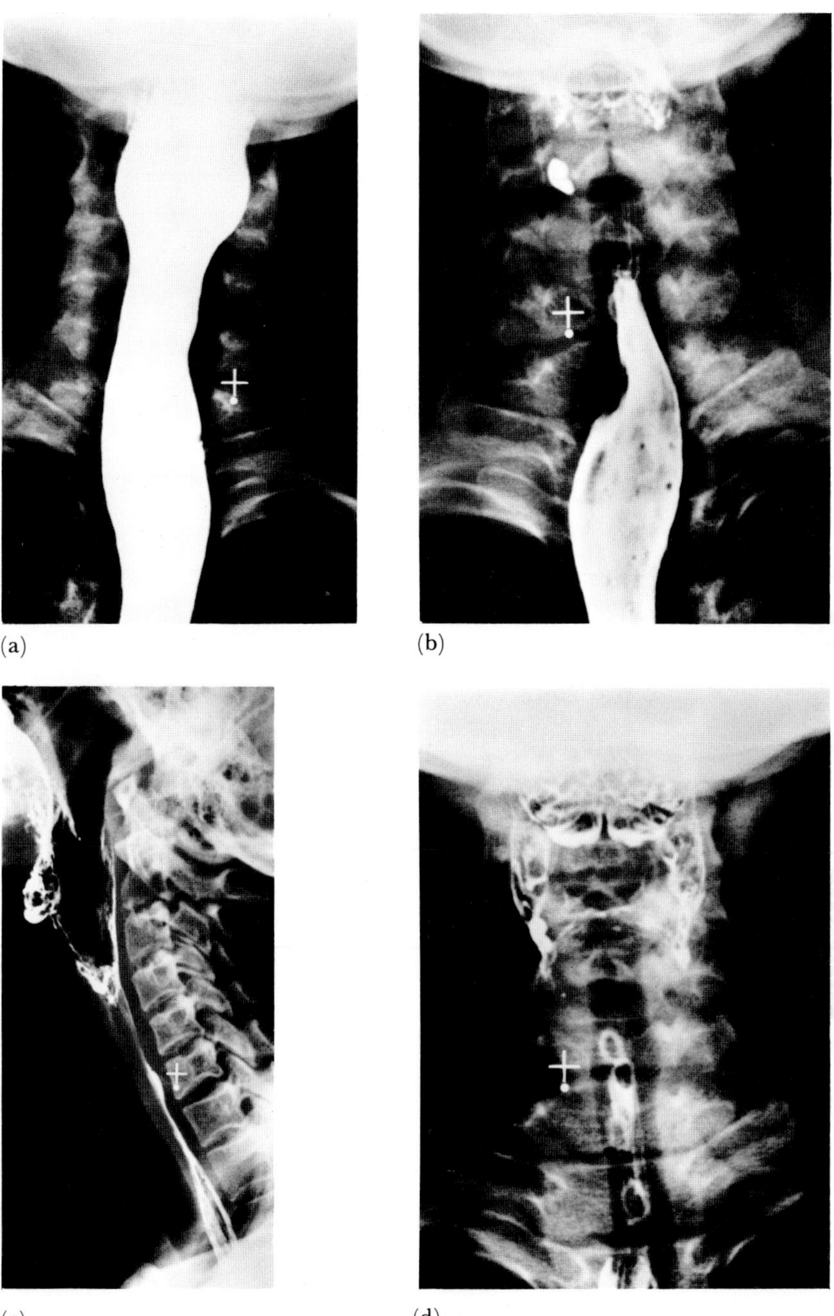

Figure 13.33 Normal barium swallow appearances. (a) Complete filling (antero-posterior; (b) later stage – residue of barium about to descend from pyriform fossa (antero-posterior); (c) lateral view showing valleculae, post-cricoid lumen, and upper oesophagus; (d) antero-posterior view showing valleculae, pyriform fossae and upper oesophageal lumen

true sphincter mechanism for the upper oesophagus and not the circular fibres of the cricopharyngeus.

At times the cricopharyngeus muscle may produce a pronounced indentation of the posterior outline of the filled oesophagus as barium passes through, and this is often especially marked when there is neuromuscular incoordination present, as with bulbar lesions. In about 80 per cent of cases a small thin fold is present anteriorly just below the cricopharyngeus muscle. This should not be mistaken for a web, which is more constant both in presence and size. It has been suggested that it is caused by a submucous vein, but this has not been substantiated.

Image intensification with cine radiography (video-tape), or rapid serial filming using 70 mm or 100 mm film has greatly improved the efficiency of the barium swallow examination and should be used routinely when investigating abnormal patterns of deglutition, whether the result of motor paralysis or incoordination of muscle action. Normally barium flows rapidly through the pharynx and down the oesophagus (*Figure 13.33*). It may coat the sides of the pharynx for a short time and after the first swallow a little may remain in the valleculae and pyriform fossae only to be quickly cleared by a subsequent swallow. Any degree of stasis beyond this should be suspect.

When one attempts to demonstrate or localize a non-opaque swallowed foreign body such as a fish bone, success can sometimes be achieved by persuading the patient to swallow a sandwich of teased out dry cotton wool with a centre of cotton wool soaked in barium. The patient should try and swallow this without mouthing it and saturating it with saliva and, should it be impaled on the fish bone, the site is immediately shown. (*Figure 13.34*).

The upper oesophagus normally deviates a little to the left at the level of the thoracic inlet. It may be indented, compressed or displaced by an enlarged thyroid, or parathyroid gland, or enlarged lymph nodes, as well as by mediastinal tumours or aneurysms of the aortic arch. It is indented anteriorly, and on its left side, by the normal aortic arch and left main bronchus, and when present, the oblique indentation of an anomalous right subclavian artery above the level of the aortic impression is diagnostic. Malformations of the aortic arch, such as a right-sided aorta, or double aorta, may be suspected or diagnosed by the different impressions they produce on the barium-filled oesophagus.

The oesophagus is usually loosely attached to the descending aorta and tends to maintain this relationship throughout life, so that when the aorta becomes elongated and unfolded with atheroma, the oesophagus tends to be displaced with it. An atheromatous aorta may compress the oesophagus at its lower end where it crosses it, and this is particularly liable to happen when the thoracic aorta is tortuous and heavily calcified.

The oesophagus is displaced posteriorly and to the left in its lower third by enlargement of the left atrium in mitral disease. Very occasionally in this condition it may be displaced to the right, and even less commonly it may be mobile and displaced sometimes to the right and sometimes to the left, depending on posture.

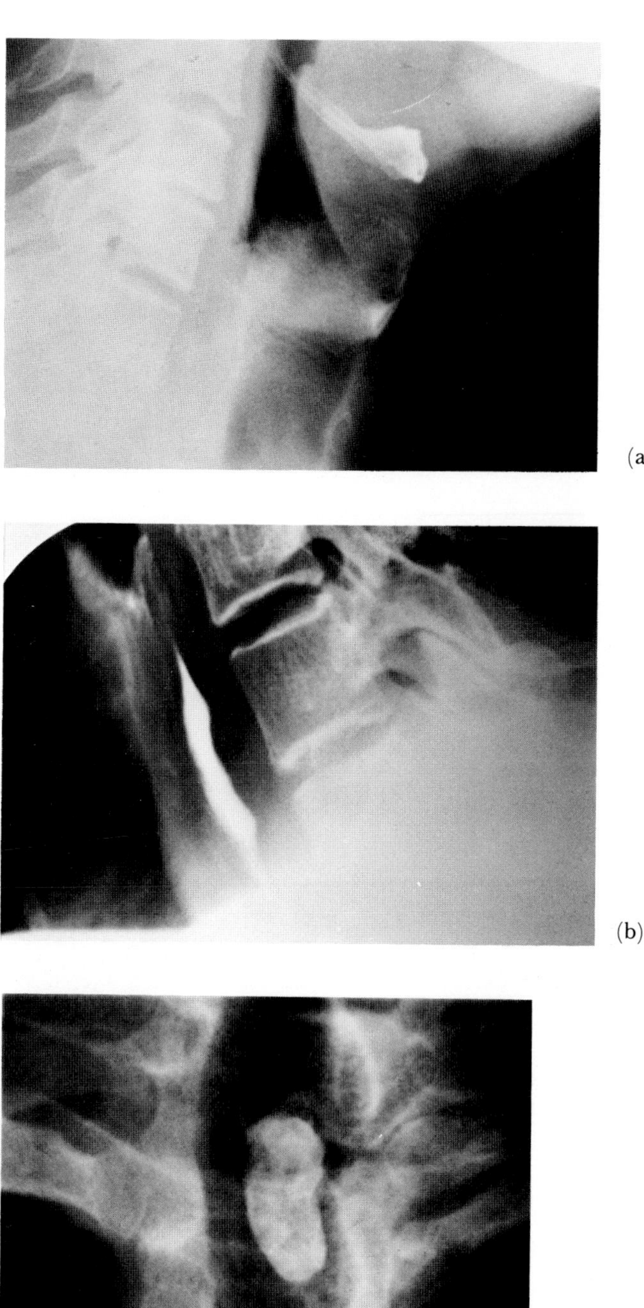
(a)
(b)
(c)

Figure 13.34 Films taken with barium contrast. An impacted dry bay-leaf is disclosed

Acknowledgements

Most of the tomographs were taken by Miss L. Harris to whom we wish to record our thanks. We should also like to thank Dr. Ivan Mosely, Consultant Radiologist, The National Hospital for Nervous Diseases, London for the illustrations of eighth nerve tumours, and Mr. Garfield Davies for the print of the foreign body in the oesophagus.

References

Caldwell, E. W. (1918). 'Skiagraphy of the Accessory Nasal Sinuses,' *American Journal of Roentgenology*, **5**, 569

Chamberlain, W. E. and Young, B. R. (1935). 'Ossification (so-called 'Calcification') of Normal Laryngeal Cartilages Mistaken for Foreign Body, *American Journal of Roentgenology*, **33**, 441

Compere, W. E. Jnr. (1958). *Transactions of the American Academy of Ophthalmology and Otolaryngology*, **62**, 444

Granger, A. (1932). *A Radiological Study of the Paranasal Sinuses and Mastoids*, Philadelphia; Lea and Ribiger

Hartung, A. and Grossman, J. W. (1939). 'Examination of the Larynx and Adjacent Structures with Intrapharyngeal Films,' *American Journal of Roentgenology*, **42**, 481

King T. T. and Ambrose J.A.E. (1977). 'C.A.T. Scanning in Tumours of the cerebello-pontine angle,' *First EMI Scan Seminar-Computerised Axial Tomography in Clinical Practice*, pp. 134–138.

Law, F. M. (1931). 'Interpreting Sinus Roentgenograms,' *Annals of Otology, Rhinology and Laryngology, St Louis*, **40**, 82

Lysholm, E. (1963). *Lysholm Precision Apparatus for Skull and Skeletal Radiography*. (Revised by I. Wickbom.) Stockholm Solma; Elema Schomander

Mayer, E. G. (1930). *Otologische Roentgendiagnostik*. Vienna; Julius Springer

Mayer, E. G. (1962). *Radiology*, **7**, 306

Peele, J. C. and Lejeune, F. E. (1942). 'Roentgenography of Sphenoid Sinus,' *Laryngoscope*, **52**, 522

Proetz, A. W. (1930). 'Displacement Method in Sinus Diagnosis and Treatment; Its Advantages and Limitations,' *Transactions of American Laryngological Association*, **52**, 121

Rees-Jones, G. F. and McGibbon, J. E. G. (1941). 'Radiological Visualisation of Eustachian Tube,' *Lancet*, **2**, 660

Samuel,, E. (1952). *Clinical Radiology of the Ear, Nose and Throat*. London; Lewis

Selander, E. (1946). 'The Roentgen Appearance of the Anterior Wall of the Sulcus Sigmoideus,' *Acta Radiologica*, **27**, 60

Shambaugh, G. E. (1967). *Surgery of the Ear*, p. 112. Philadelphia; Saunders

Spielberg, W. (1927). 'Visualisation of the Eustachian Tube by the Roentgen Ray,' *Archives of Otolaryngology*, **5**, 334

Stenvers, H. W. (1917). 'Roentgenology of Os Petrosum,' *Archives of Radiology and Electrotherapy*, **22**, 97

Walters, C. A. and Waldron, C. W. (1915). *American Journal of Roentgenology*, **2**, 633

Welin, S. (1948). 'The Roentgen Ray Examination of the Paranasal Sinuses with Particular Reference to the Frontal Sinuses,' *British Journal of Radiology*, **21**, 431

Wilson, J. L. and Moseley I. F. (1977). 'A diagnostic approach to cerebellar lesions.' *First EMI Scan Seminar-Computerized Axial Tomography in Clinical Practice*, pp.123–131

Young, B. R. (1940). 'Recent Advances in Roentgen Examination of the Neck,' *American Journal of Roentgenology*, **44**, 519

Zaino, C., Jacobson, H. G., Lepow, H. and Ozturk, C. H. (1970). *The Pharyngo-esophageal Sphincter*. Springfield, Ill.; Thomas

14 Bacteriology in relation to otorhinolaryngology

Paul Noone

Commensal flora of the respiratory tract

The mouth and saliva

Although sterile when secreted and containing some antibacterial properties, the saliva becomes heavily colonized from the mouth with various organisms including:

(1) *Streptococci*. *'Streptococcus viridans'* is a uniform finding in normal subjects. It is not a single species but includes a range of species with differing pathogenic potential. *Str. sanguis*, *Str. mutans* and *Str. mitior* have been implicated in infective endocarditis while *Str. salivarius*, another α-haemolytic organism, is virtually non-pathogenic.

β-haemolytic streptococci are found in at least 5–10 per cent of healthy subjects in the United Kingdom, including Groups A (*Str. pyogenes*), C and G.

Anaerobic streptococci (peptostreptococci) are also easily isolated if strict anaerobic culture is undertaken.

(2) *Staphylococci*. *Staph. epidermidis* (albus) is common in the mouth while *Staph. aureus* is often found too without pathogenic significance.

(3) *Gram-positive rods*. These include Corynebacteria ('diphtheroids'), lactobacilli, which are more common where there are carious teeth, and aerobic sporebearers.

(4) *Gram-negative cocci*. Both Neisseria species and Veillonella (strict anaerobes) are commonly encountered.

(5) *Other anaerobes*. These include fusobacteria (which may be involved in Vincent's angina) and actinomyces species.

(6) *Coliforms (Esch. coli, Klebsiella, Enterobacter and Proteus spp.)* are often present, their numbers increasing in subjects receiving antibiotics. This usually has little pathogenic significance though it may have epidemiological importance in hospital patients.

(7) *Other micro-organisms* are numerous. Many different kinds of *Treponemes* and *Spirillum* species have been described, being frequently isolated from the gums near the dental margin. Vincents' Spirillum is found with fusiforms in synergistic

relationship in Vincents' angina, an anaerobic infection of the gums and mouth.

Mycoplasmata are also present, as are *yeasts* (principally *Candida albicans*). The latter may become the predominant flora when antibiotics suppress the oral bacterial population, and cause thrush.

Nose and nasopharynx

There are marked differences in the microbial flora of these two areas. The flora of the nasopharynx tends to be more varied and abundant. *Str. viridans* and Neisseria species (other than *N. meningitidis*) are the main organisms in the nasopharynx although *Haemophilus influenzae* and *Str. pneumoniae* are frequently present, apparently being more numerous in cold damp weather. Less common are *β*-haemolytic streptococci (especially *Str. pyogenes*) and *N. meningitidis*, though these potential pathogens are by no means uncommon, carrier rates in healthy individuals ranging from 5 to 20 per cent in non-epidemic situations.

By contrast the flora of the *anterior nares* are less abundant. *Staph. aureus* is found in from 20 to 50 per cent of healthy subjects (the numbers may be greater in hospital), *Staph. epidermidis* is present in virtually everyone while diphtheroids and *Str. viridans* are also very common. Less common are Neisseria species, Haemophilus species and *Str. pneumoniae* (though this organism is universally present in infants). *Str. pyogenes* is carried in the anterior nares in less than 1 per cent of healthy subjects – nevertheless its presence in this site is associated with a higher risk of cross infection so that nasal carrier state should be assessed during the investigation of any outbreak of *Str. pyogenes* infection in an at-risk community. Occasionally coliforms and in particular *Proteus mirabilis* are found in the anterior nares of healthy individuals.

Tonsils

The flora are very similar to those of the nasopharynx so that Neisseria species, *H. influenzae* and *Str. pneumoniae* and the organisms encountered in the mouth predominate. *β*-haemolytic streptococci also occur in the tonsils of 5–20 per cent of healthy subjects. The isolation rate from patients with diseased tonsils is higher.

Sinuses, trachea, bronchi and alveoli

These areas are normally thought of as 'sterile'. The organisms inhaled during respiration are largely filtered in the nasal passages and those that pass through the larynx are deposited in the mucosal secretions and removed by cilial action or via the lymphatics. However, *Str. viridans*, Neisseria spp. and Haemophilus spp. may be isolated in small numbers from bronchial specimens of mucus in healthy adults. This may have relevance when assessing the significance of isolates from specimens obtained during bronchial 'washing'.

In patients with tracheostomies, heavy tracheal and bronchial colonization is more readily observed, often without immediate pathogenic significance. Various coliforms, staphylococci, *Ps. aeruginosa* and yeasts may be isolated, the latter two species being selected by antimicrobial chemotherapy.

Ear

The epithelium of the external auditory meatus has very similar flora to the normal skin. *Staph. epidermidis*, *Staph. aureus* and diphtheroids predominate. *Str. viridans*, coliforms (especially Proteus spp.) and *Ps. aeruginosa* are also commonly encountered in healthy individuals. Commensal mycobacterial species may also be detected, apparently being associated with the waxy secretions. This is important to bear in mind if acid-fast stains are being performed.

It is important to know about the commensal flora of the body when attempting to interpret the results of microbiological investigations. The position is made more difficult by the existence of healthy carriers of well-recognized pathogens (e.g. *Str. pyogenes*) and opportunist infections caused by organisms usually of low virulence (e.g. *Ps. aeruginosa* in otitis externa).

Antimicrobial therapy

Furunculosis (boils)

Boils often occur singly or in clusters around the nose, inside the anterior nares, and in the external ear.

This is hardly surprising as *Staph. aureus* is commonly carried in that area. The boil arises when the organism produces a small abscess in a hair follicle.

Antimicrobial therapy

This is not indicated for small boils in otherwise healthy subjects as the condition is self-limiting. It is sensible to treat boils with antistaphylococcal antibiotics in the following circumstances.

(1) *carbuncle* – when drainage (surgical or by use of hygroscopic paste) is also essential;
(2) in patients with debilitating diseases such as diabetes mellitus, leukaemia and 'hard' drug addiction, where complications such as local or metastatic spread of sepsis are a more serious risk;
(3) in otherwise normal subjects who are having repeated episodes.

The antibiotic of choice is currently flucloxacillin 500 mg four times daily or cephradine 500 mg four times daily for 5–7 days usually.

In all these groups as well as in hospital staff such as surgeons and nurses with simple boils, it is advisable to eliminate the carrier state if possible. Obviously the strain of *Staph. aureus* being carried is virulent if boils have been produced and a person with active staphylococcal lesions of the face is a potent disseminator of this virulent organism to hospital patients. Not only will the environment be contaminated by *Staph. aureus* shed on skin particles but there will be gross and repeated contamination of the hands.

Treatment of carriers of *Staph. aureus*

Nasal antiseptic creams such as chlorhexidine applied twice a day for a week will help eradicate carriage in the nose but this will be short-lived if the skin carriage sites are not treated too, especially axillae, umbilicus, perineum and hair-bearing sites including the scalp.

Sore throat, pharyngitis, tonsillitis

More than half the patients seen in general practice with sore throats are probably suffering from viral infections (adenoviruses, para-influenza viruses, etc.) and a sore throat may often be part of the 'common cold' syndrome.

The most common cause of bacterial sore throat is *Streptococcus pyogenes* (i.e. Lancefield Group A β-haemolytic streptococci). The condition usually starts abruptly with sore throat, worse on swallowing, fever and headache. Children and infants may have nausea and vomiting. By contrast with most viruses, nasal stuffiness and discharge is a minor problem if it occurs at all, and involvement of the larynx is rare. Earache is also typical. In susceptible hosts, strains producing erythrogenic toxin will cause 'scarlet fever', the rash coming on 1–5 days after onset of the illness, starting in the chest and neck but rapidly spreading over the abdomen and limbs. The face looks flushed but there is classically circumoral pallor.

The pharynx, tonsils and soft palate appear inflamed though the degree of redness can vary considerably. Typically there is a whitish or yellowish exudate on the tonsils ranging from pinhead lesions to confluent areas. Nevertheless streptococcal pharyngitis may occur without exudates, and exudates may occur in viral infections.

There is marked lymphadenopathy, and the cervical nodes may even suppurate in severe cases; but lymphadenopathy also occurs in viral infections.

The differential diagnosis must also include adenoviruses, para-influenza viruses, primary herpes simplex pharyngitis, herpangina (a Coxsackie A virus infection), Vincents' angina, infectious mononucleosis and diphtheria.

It may thus be difficult to decide whether or not to treat patients with antimicrobial agents. Although most *Str. pyogenes* throat infections are self-limiting the post-infection complications of rheumatic fever, chorea and glomerulonephritis are generally considered too serious to risk and so antibiotic treatment is indicated. It would seem sensible therefore to treat the following groups of patients with sore throats prior to the receipt of bacteriological results once throat swabs have been taken (and sent to the laboratory in transport medium, as *Str. pyogenes* fares badly on dry swabs):

(1) Patients with complications such as quinsy, retropharyngeal abscess, otitis media, or scarlet fever.
(2) Those who have already suffered attacks of rheumatic fever or chorea.
(3) Those with underlying pathology known to compromise host defences such as leukaemia, lymphoma, diabetes mellitus or immunosuppressive therapy.
(4) Where the history and clinical signs indicate the probability of *Str. pyogenes* infection. Thus tonsillar exudates may usually be taken as such a criterion although their presence or absence is by no means conclusive evidence either way.

The drug of choice for streptococcal sore throat is *penicillin*. Penicillin V 250–500 mg orally four times daily taken on an empty stomach for ten days is usually effective. If the condition is serious (e.g. quinsy) then benzylpenicillin 1–2 megaunits 6-hourly should be the initial therapy, oral penicillin only being given when the infection is controlled. The main problem with penicillin V is unreliable absorption (especially if taken with food) and lack of patient compliance. The latter is always a problem in domiciliary patients with drugs needed to be taken four times a day. In such cases, amoxycillin might be useful as it is absorbed well even in the presence of food and only needs to be taken three times a day (500 mg three times daily).

Where the patient is allergic to penicillin, erythromycin (500 mg four times daily) is a useful alternative. Cotrimoxazole is very much a second choice for streptococcal infection.

If a patient has been started on antibiotics and the throat swab comes back as 'negative' for *β*-haemolytic streptococci, the antibiotic can be discontinued as there is no need to 'give a complete course'. Difficulties in interpretation arise when only scanty numbers of *Str. pyogenes* or other *β*-haemolytic streptococci are isolated. This may indicate a coincidental carrier state rather than pathogenic infection. On the other hand, *β*-haemolytic streptococci often survive poorly on throat swabs especially if there are delays in transport to or processing in the laboratory. Thus the numbers isolated may underestimate the numbers in the throat. The sensible course would be to treat all patients yielding *Str. pyogenes* from throat swabs who have symptomatic sore throats.

Other organisms giving pyogenic sore throats include:

(1) Group C and Group G *β*-haemolytic streptococci. The choice of antibiotic treatment is as for Str. pyogenes.
(2) Candida species, especially *C. albicans*.
(3) C. diphtheriae.

Candidiasis (thrush)

Candida species, especially *C. albicans* may cause sore throat and mouth (thrush) and in severe infections may spread the entire length of the oesophagus. The diagnosis is seldom in doubt and it usually occurs as a complication of broad spectrum chemotherapy. Immunosuppressed patients (renal transplant, leukaemia) run an increased risk of being infected and also of having the rare complication of candida pneumonia and/or Candidaemia, both conditions with high mortality.

The treatment consists of stopping broad spectrum antibacterial chemotherapy and commencing local mouth washing (and swallowing) with nystatin suspension or amphotericin suspension. Some patients find nystatin suspension sickly and nauseating.

Between mouth washing, gargling and swallowing, the patients should be encouraged to suck amphotericin lozenges ad libitum.

These antifungal oral preparations are not absorbed from the gastro-intestinal tract.

Systemic antifungal therapy is usually not indicated for oral thrush but in heavily infected immunosuppressed patients or those with suspected pneumonia or candidaemia, one of the following regimens may be followed:

(1) Miconazole 600 mg 8-hourly intravenously. This is a potent new agent still undergoing trial as a systemic preparation although previously widely used as a local vaginal application. It is reliably active against yeasts and preliminary reports are encouraging. It appears so far to be remarkably non-toxic.

(2) Flucytosine 50 mg/kg 6-hourly intravenously/orally. A minority of yeasts are naturally resistant to this agent and resistance apparently developing during treatment has been seen not infrequently. Nevertheless it can be efficacious. Neutropenia, anaemia and thrombocytopenia have been reported rarely.

(3) Amphotericin. Test dose of 1 mg in 10 ml of diluent over 10 min then after 4 h, if no acute toxicity occurs, start at 10 mg/dose and build up to 0.6–1.0 mg/kg intravenously (50 mg maximum) on alternate days, using 5 per cent dextrose as diluent. Hydrocortisone 25–50 mg can help reduce toxic reactions.

This is the broadest spectrum antifungal agent and resistance in yeasts is rare. Nephrotoxicity is the most important manifestation of toxicity and may be the limiting factor in its use.

When treating systemic fungal infection in actively immunosuppressed patients, it is important to reduce the degree of immunosuppression wherever possible or if possible withdraw suppressive therapy completely. This is probably more important than administering antifungal agents.

Diphtheria

Corynebacterium diphtheriae may occur in three subspecies, *mitis*, *intermedius*, and *gravis* (in ascending order of virulence). It usually gains access to the body in temperate climates via the respiratory tract, although in tropical climates cutaneous lesions resembling impetigo may be seen.

The respiratory tract lesions may be *pharyngeal*, with the classic grey membrane firmly attached to the tonsils and fauces; *laryngeal*, sometimes as an extension of the pharyngeal disease which frequently gives rise to the emergency of upper airway obstruction; and the more unusual *nasal* form where there is often a thin bloody nasal discharge.

If in the latter condition the patient has little in the way of constitutional upset he may become an important 'unrecognized' source for dissemination of the disease.

The lethal nature of diphtheria is mainly due to the potent exotoxin produced by the organisms which causes *myocarditis* with tachycardia, cardiac arrhythmias, heart block and heart failure and *peripheral neuritis* which develops 2–6 weeks after the onset of the disease and may affect cranial nerves, the extremities or the muscles of respiration. Motor function is more strikingly affected than sensory.

The most crucial elements of management are therefore early diagnosis and prompt administration of antitoxin. The giving of antibiotics is important in ending the primary disease and eliminating the further elaboration of toxin but is insufficient therapy in itself.

Diagnosis

The classic picture of a patient complaining of sore throat and with a rapid thready pulse and a firmly attached pharyngeal membrane is by no means the common presentation. It may be extremely difficult to differentiate between possible diphtheria, or severe streptococcal pharyngitis, adenovirus infection with exudate, candidiasis, infectious mononucleosis or even severe Vincent's angina. A membrane may not always be present particularly early in the disease. Laboratory confirmation is therefore essential even though it is crucial to start treatment before the diagnosis is confirmed wherever the clinical suspicion is strong.

Throat swabs, including swabs of membranous exudate, are taken for immediate culture and microscopy. Cultural isolation of *C. diphtheriae* is necessary as microscopy, even with Albert's stain, may be misleading except in expert hands. In the United Kingdom few laboratory staff nowadays have a great deal of experience with *C. diphtheriae*. The organism is isolated on special medium such as tellurite blood agar where it produces characteristic colonies in 24–48 h, although up to five days may elapse before growth occurs. It is essential to warn the laboratory of the clinical suspicion of diphtheria as otherwise only routine culture plates will be used and it is difficult to detect *C. diphtheriae* among commensal throat flora on ordinary blood or chocolate agar plates. All isolates of *C. diphtheriae* must be checked for toxin production (usually using the Elek plate) as not all strains are toxigenic and this may have significance when screening for carriers or if the organisms are isolated coincidentally.

Specimens for culture must be taken before antibiotics are administered as the latter may delay or even prevent isolation of *C. diphtheriae*.

Treatment

Patients suspected of having diphtheria should be nursed in isolation with *strict* bed rest. The dose of antitoxin is empirical but in general the more severe the disease and the later the diagnosis the greater the dose. This may range from 10 000 units for mild cases to 100 000 units for severe laryngeal disease. 20 000–40 000 units for moderate pharyngeal disease would seem appropriate. Hypersensitivity is rare but some authorities suggest giving up to half the dose by intramuscular injection and then, providing no adverse reaction occurs, giving the rest by slow intravenous infusion.

Erythromycin is the drug of choice for treating patients with clinically overt disease or in the carrier state, the adult dose being 500 mg orally 6-hourly for seven days. Alternatively, penicillin G 2 megaunits 6-hourly intramuscularly for the disease state or 500 mg orally four times daily for seven days in the carrier state may be used.

Other drugs for the carrier state include clindamycin 300 mg three times daily or rifampicin 600 mg daily, both for seven days.

Tetracyclines, ampicillin and oral cephalosporins may fail to eradicate *C. diphtheriae* from the upper respiratory tract.

Prevention

Routine immunization against diphtheria toxin is to be highly recommended commencing in infancy. 'Booster' doses of the toxoid should be given before primary school entry. Patients with diphtheria should be kept in isolation until at least two cultures of the throat and nose (and other infected sites) taken on successive days, are negative. If the patient has received antibiotics, 48 h should elapse after the ending of therapy, before these check swabs are taken.

Oropharyngeal abscesses

These include *peritonsillar abscess* (quinsy), *retropharyngeal abscess* and *Ludwig's angina* (cellulitis of the floor of the mouth). The former two conditions may occur as complications of streptococcal tonsillitis and are more frequently seen in children.

The essential features of management in all these conditions is securing the airway and draining the pus. Antibiotics serve only as therapeutic adjuncts.

These abscesses are usually caused by mixtures of organisms which may include not only *Str. pyogenes* but also *Str. pneumoniae*, *Staph. aureus* and more frequently obligate anaerobes such as anaerobic streptococci and bacteroides species. Coliforms including *Esch. coli* and *Klebsiella* may also occur.

The initial choice of antibiotic before culture results are available is penicillin G 2 megaunits 6-hourly intramuscularly (adults) although metronidazole may be added to useful effect (1 g suppository or 600 mg orally or 500 mg intravenously, 8-hourly). Alternative choices include cephradine 500 mg 6-hourly and erythromycin 500 mg 6-hourly. Culture results and sensitivity tests may well modify antibiotic treatment, particularly if coliforms predominate.

Laryngitis

This may often be associated with a general upper respiratory tract viral infection such as influenza, adenoviral pharyngitis, para-influenza virus infection ('croup'), rhinoviruses or with measles, or it may be part of a more general bacterial infection such as diphtheria (q.v.).

Primary bacterial infection is rare although secondary bacterial invasion of a viral laryngitis or inflammation caused by noxious fumes occurs more frequently. The usual pathogens include *Haemophilus influenzae* (principally), *Str. pneumoniae*, *β*-haemolytic streptococci and uncommonly *Staph. aureus*.

Swabs should be taken before antimicrobial therapy is started and the initial choice before the results of culture are available should be directed mainly against Haemophilus and streptococci, e.g. ampicillin 500 mg intramuscularly 6-hourly or amoxycillin 500 mg orally 8-hourly. Ampicillin-resistant Haemophilus is still rare in the United Kingdom though occasionally seen.

Alternative therapy includes cotrimoxazole two tablets 12-hourly and erythromycin 500 mg 6-hourly, although resistance to the latter is frequently seen in Haemophilus.

Acute laryngitis, with *tracheobronchitis* and *epiglottitis* is an acute medical emergency more common in children. Rapidly developing respiratory obstruction produced by intense inflammation and oedema may be fatal unless treated promptly and vigorously. The usual cause is infection with capsulated (type b) strains of *Haemophilus influenzae*.

Swabs should be taken of the epiglottis and sent for culture *before antibiotics* are started. Microscopy may reveal many pleomorphic Gram negative cocco-bacilli which are morphologically suggestive of Haemophilus. An overnight culture on chocolate agar (or other suitable Haemophilus medium) can often be confirmed as *H. influenzae* by serological tests so that relatively rapid confirmation is obtained. The patient should be admitted to hospital as the essential management includes securing the airway.

Antibiotic therapy must be started once swabs have been taken and must be aimed primarily against *H. influenzae*. Ampicillin 1 g intramuscularly/intravenously stat. (adult dose) then 6-hourly has been orthodox therapy in later years. Oral therapy can be substituted once the infection has come under control and the emergency situation has passed (e.g. amoxycillin 500 mg three times daily). An alternative is cotrimoxazole 15 ml of intravenous infusion 12-hourly (180 mg trimethoprim, 1.2 g sulphamethoxazole – adult dose). Amoxycillin (and cotrimoxazole) – resistant strains of *Haemophilus influenzae* have been reported with increasing frequency, particularly the capsulated (type b) strains which cause meningitis, septicaemia and epiglottitis. Where resistant strains occur as a local problem, the choice of initial antibiotic therapy rests between chloramphenicol 750 mg intravenously or orally 6-hourly (adult dose) and carbenicillin 5 g intravenously 4-hourly (adult dose).

Paediatric doses:		
	ampicillin	62.5–250 mg four times daily
	amoxycillin	125–500 mg three times daily
	cotrimoxazole	5–10 ml paediatric suspension twice daily
	chloramphenicol	6.25–12.5 mg/kg four times daily (avoid in neonates)
	carbenicillin	100–200 mg/kg intravenously 6-hourly
	erythromycin	125–250 mg kg four times daily

The currently available cephalosporins (except cefuroxime) are not reliably active against Haemophilus; nor are benzyl penicillin, the lincomycins or the aminoglycosides.

Chronic laryngitis

This is not normally an infective condition but is more likely to be attributable to vocal abuse, smoking, inhalation of other irritants, and allergic reactions. Antibiotics therefore serve no useful purpose. Nevertheless rare causes of chronic laryngitis include tuberculosis, syphilis and, it is alleged, sinusitis. It may be wise therefore to perform chest and sinus x-rays; tests for treponemal serology; and take laryngeal swabs for culture, including perhaps mycobacterial culture and microscopy.

Bronchitis

Acute bronchitis may be caused by inhaling irritating gases and fumes but is more often associated with viral infection of the upper respiratory tract generally (q.v.). Bacterial secondary infection is probably much less common than many doctors suppose. Antibiotics are often given without real indication, 'just in case'. This is bad medical practice as it encourages colonization with resistant organisms such as *Staph.*

aureus, coliforms, Pseudomonas and yeasts, and antibiotics are not without their inherent side-effects and risks. When practised on a wide scale this all promotes emergence of resistant strains in the environment.

Among the few groups of patients who probably merit antibiotic treatment to reduce the chances of secondary bacterial infection during an upper respiratory tract viral infection are chronic bronchitics and those with obstructive airways disease.

Sputum and throat swab cultures should be performed to assess the microbial flora. Specific pathogens such as β-haemolytic streptococci or heavy growths of *Haemophilus influenzae* or *Str. pneumoniae* may indicate the need for appropriate antibiotic therapy.

Chronic bronchitis is not primarily an infective disease and antibiotics play little part in improving either long-term prognosis or preventing gradual deterioration of pulmonary function. The underlying pathology results from excessive mucus production and then destruction of ciliated epithelium caused by prolonged irritation by noxious stimuli, in particular tobacco smoking. Bacterial infection usually with *H. influenzae* and *Str. pneumoniae*, occurs secondarily to exacerbations of bronchitis related to irritating inhalations or viral infection.

Antibiotic treatment is therefore directed at curtailing episodes of bacterial infection and preventing bronchopneumonia and further structural damage which infection might produce. The number of exacerbations which occur is not reduced by antibiotics – only their duration and severity. Thus *continuous* antibiotic therapy is usually contraindicated as it merely leads to resistant organisms colonizing the oropharynx, so that bacterial infections during exacerbations are with resistant bacteria. Antibiotics should be given promptly when exacerbations of the underlying disease occur, when upper respiratory tract viral infections occur, or when the sputum becomes purulent-looking. The patient can keep a supply of antibiotic at home which he takes at once in the above situations, before reporting to his general practitioner.

The choice of antibiotic is between amoxycillin, cotrimoxazole and tetracycline. The differences are marginal. Each is active against *H. influenzae* and *Str. pneumoniae*. Resistant strains occur uncommonly. Obviously the particular choice of antibiotic will depend not only on individual resistance patterns but also on patient acceptability and compliance. Side-effects such as diarrhoea are important limiting factors.

Amoxycillin 500 mg three times daily or cotrimoxazole 2 tablets twice daily or doxycycline 200 mg stat. then 100 mg once or twice daily (depending on severity of disease) would seem to be adequate dosage. Oxytetracycline must be given in doses of at least 500 mg four times daily to be effective. Doxycycline is to be preferred not only because of its once (or twice) daily dosage which makes for better compliance but also because it appears to penetrate respiratory tract secretions better and it seems to be non-nephrotoxic. The other tetracyclines are nephrotoxic, especially in the elderly and in those with already impaired renal function.

Sputum culture is not always indicated but should certainly be carried out in the following circumstances.

(1) In all patients with chronic obstructive airways disease admitted to hospital, especially those with acute exacerbations of the underlying disease or those due to receive anaesthesia for elective surgery or other reason.
(2) All chronic bronchitic patients with suspected or confirmed pneumonia,

preferably taking specimens before antibiotic therapy is commenced or at least changed.

(3) In all those with an acute exacerbation and purulent sputum not responding to the usual chemotherapy.

Tracheostomy infections

Tracheostomies do not remain sterile and readily become colonized with a wide range of organisms. The colonization extends into the trachea itself. Providing hygienic maintenance of the tracheal stoma and any indwelling tubes is carried out meticulously each day this should not be of pathogenic consequence.

Nevertheless colonization of the tracheostomy site may be the first step on the way to pneumonia especially in those who are unconscious, receiving assisted ventilation or in intensive care units.

Acceptable colonizing flora include *Str. viridans,* non-haemolytic streptococci, diphtheroids, Neisseria species and *Staph. epidermidis.* Difficulties may arise in interpreting the significance of potential pathogens such as *Staph. aureus,* coliforms (especially klebsiella) and *Ps. aeruginosa.*

On most occasions such colonization signifies very little although in some circumstances (e.g. Intensive Therapy Unit) it may be advisable to apply local antiseptics such as povidone-iodine to reduce infectivity and eliminate the carrier status, particularly with such undesirable organisms as *Ps. aeruginosa.*

Carriage of potential pathogens by asymptomatic patients in their tracheostomy sites can be an important reservoir of infection in specialized units. It is relatively easy for the hands of nurses, physiotherapists and other health workers attending the patient to become contaminated – thus spreading infection. Meticulous handwashing with antiseptic soaps such as povidone-iodine or chlorhexidine must be insisted upon in all those handling tracheostomy sites and tubes.

Pneumonia

In patients with pneumonia it is usually necessary to begin antimicrobial therapy before culture and other microbiological test results are available. The range of pathogens possible is very wide and each demands its own particular optimal therapy. The following scheme suggests a rational approach to initial antibiotic therapy based on a best-guess approach to likely pathogens associated with certain presenting features of the disease. Of course, chemotherapy is only one aspect of treatment and other factors such as physiotherapy, oxygen, assisted ventilation, and isolation (especially important in suspected or established *Staph. aureus* pneumonia) must not be overlooked.

Wherever possible sputum samples should be taken for culture before antimicrobial therapy is started but it is not always easy to obtain sputum (particularly in early lobar pneumonic consolidation) and salivary specimens masquerading as sputum may give misleading results. Intubated patients readily provide useful specimens but in all other patients the specimens are contaminated from the mouth and pharynx. Gram films and semi-quantitative culture of homogenized sputum help discriminate pathogens from upper respiratory tract contaminants, but are by no means totally reliable. In the USA transtracheal aspiration is used in several centres to apparent good effect. The technique has not 'caught on' in the UK. It is unpleasant for the patient and not entirely without hazard. Specimens obtained during fibre-optic bronchoscopy may be useful.

However, in view of these problems, samples of empyema or pleural fluid (if present) may be extremely valuable in yielding pathogens. Blood cultures are very useful too and should always be taken. They are often negative but a positive culture not only reveals the major pathogen(s) but also indicates a worse prognosis.

Choice of initial antibiotic therapy

Pneumonia acquired outside hospital

(1) Classic lobar pneumonia is likely to be caused by *Str. pneumoniae* and the drug of choice is benzyl penicillin 1–2 megaunits 6-hourly intramuscularly. Only after the infection is well controlled should oral therapy be contemplated and then penicillin V should be given on an empty stomach to ensure absorption ($\frac{1}{2}$–1 g 6-hourly).

(2) In patients with chronic obstructive airways disease or chronic heart failure or debilitating illness, mixed bacterial infections occur, often including *Haemophilus influenzae*. Following viral infections (especially during influenza epidemics) these patients often develop *Staphylococcus aureus* bronchopneumonia. An urgent Gram stain of sputum may be helpful in deciding therapy. A safe choice in such cases is probably ampicillin 500 mg intramuscularly 6-hourly *plus* flucloxacillin 500 mg intramuscularly 6-hourly until the results of culture are available. An alternative is chloramphenicol 500–750 mg 6-hourly orally or intravenously.

(3) Friedlander's pneumonia, where the pathogen is *Klebsiella pneumoniae*, is a fulminating acute lobar pneumonia with early cavitation and haemoptysis. It is usually found in alcoholics (following an acute drinking episode) or the malnourished or in the immunosuppressed (renal transplant patients) and the immunologically compromised (leukaemia, Hodgkins' disease). The fatality rate is in excess of 80 per cent in the untreated condition and about 40 per cent when treated. Gram films of sputum may be suggestive. The drug of choice is *gentamicin* intravenously or intramuscularly starting with doses of 2 mg/kg 8-hourly then according to serum values. Peak serum concentrations (1 h post-dose) should be 8 μg/ml or more while trough concentrations (pre-dose) should be $<$ 2 μg/ml to avoid later ototoxic problems. Treatment may have to continue for 2 weeks. Alternative chemotherapeutic choices include chloramphenicol 750 mg 6-hourly intravenously/orally or cephradine 1 g 6-hourly intravenously initially, reducing later to 500 mg 6-hourly.

(4) *Aspiration pneumonia* is usually severe and has a poor prognosis. It is more likely to occur in unconscious or anaesthetized patients, in those with poor cough reflex or with dysphagia. The gastric contents are chemically damaging to the lungs but there is also mixed bacterial infection including anaerobes such as anaerobic streptococci and bacteroides species. Nevertheless coliforms may also occur and antibiotic therapy should be directed against the probable components of the mixed infection. Penicillin G, 1–2 megaunits intravenously (or ampicillin

0.5–1 g intravenously) *plus* gentamicin (1.6–2 mg/kg intravenously or intramuscularly 8-hourly) *plus* metronidazole (500 mg 8-hourly intravenously or 1 g suppository 8-hourly) would seem wise initial therapy to be modified by the results of the culture. The metronidazole is first choice as anti-anaerobic agent.

Alternative therapy includes clindamycin (300–600 mg intramuscularly) instead of metronidazole (and penicillin) or carbenicillin (5 g 6-hourly intravenously) in place of penicillin and gentamicin (although carbenicillin is *not* active against klebsiella species and not as reliable against coliforms and *Staph. aureus* as gentamicin). Chloramphenicol can be used on its own (750 mg intravenously 6-hourly) as it is active against streptococci, haemophilus, most staphylococci, coliforms and anaerobes. It is *not* active against *Pseudomonas aeruginosa*.

(5) Primary atypical pneumonia may be caused by a variety of viral, chlamydial and mycoplasmal agents but the commonest aetiological agent is *Mycoplasma pneumoniae*. There is a wide and varied clinical picture ranging from 'a cold' or 'flu' to a fulminating pneumonia with cyanosis. Usually the onset is less acute than for true bacterial pneumonia and physical findings are often less dramatic than the chest x-rays would suggest. Sputum is scanty and the peripheral white blood count unremarkable. Cold agglutinins may be present but diagnosis is best confirmed by demonstrating a rise in antibody titre during the 2nd week of illness to *M. pneumoniae*. In mild cases antibiotics are not indicated but both tetracycline (0.5 g orally 6-hourly) and erythromycin (0.5 g orally 6-hourly) are effective.

Where the diagnosis is poised between Mycoplasma and *Str. pneumoniae*, erythromycin is the drug of choice because of its activity against both agents.

Psittacosis may give a similar clinical picture to *Mycoplasma pneumoniae* but there is usually a significant history of exposure to psittacine birds. Treatment is with tetracycline (500 mg orally 6-hourly) or chloramphenicol (500 mg orally 6-hourly).

(6) Pneumonia with *Pneumocystis carinii* is an uncommon condition and it is usually seen in children or adult patients who are immunosuppressed. It often develops when the patient has gone into remission from leukaemia following intensive (antileukaemic) chemotherapy. The infecting agent is thought to be a protozoon, normally a commensal in the respiratory tract, which becomes an opportunist pathogen. The development of the condition is usually insidious, the patient being pyrexial and progressively dyspnoeic, distressed and cyanosed.

The chest x-rays are variable but frequently show diffuse and worsening shadowing, classically with 'apical sparing'.

Currently the antimicrobial therapy of choice is high dose cotrimoxazole.

(7) Tuberculosis is not rare and should be considered as a possible cause of pneumonia in the following cases.

(a) Patients with a classic onset of chest infection and a history of weight loss and night sweats.

(b) Patients from areas of high incidence such as the Indian subcontinent, West coast of Ireland, Scottish islands, The Phillipines, etc.

(c) Patients with diseases or treatment suppressing cellular immunity, e.g. Hodgkins' disease, long-term steroids, alcoholics.

(d) Occupations posing special risks, e.g. health workers, such as nurses, doctors, laboratory technicians, post-mortem room attendants.

(e) Patients with haemoptysis.

(f) Those *not* responding to antipyogenic antimicrobial therapy and where there is no evidence of abscess or empyema.

A chest x-ray is essential and microscopy of sputum for acid-fast bacilli can be invaluable – although negative smears do not rule out the diagnosis.

Cultures will not be positive (at the earliest) for two weeks and may take up to eight weeks to yield a confirmatory growth. Treatment must often be started on the basis of the clinical diagnosis where sputum is difficult to obtain; early morning gastric aspirates (i.e. *not* washings and *before* breakfast is eaten) can be useful.

Currently antituberculous therapy is based on rifampicin combined with isoniazid. This is a highly bactericidal combination and has reduced the duration of therapy to nine months, even for severe disease. Normally either ethambutol or streptomycin are given for the first 2–3 months of treatment as triple therapy. Streptomycin should be avoided in the elderly and those with renal disease because of the risk of ototoxicity.

Ethambutol dosage must be reduced after the initial 6–8 weeks high dosage to avoid the risk of optic neuritis.

Isoniazid and rifampicin seem to have a hepatotoxic potential which is greater together than when either is used alone. Nevertheless it is an uncommon occurrence and reversible if recognized early and the treatment is withdrawn.

Resistance to the antituberculous drugs is uncommon (<5 per cent) in the UK. Antituberculous therapy in patients with resistant strains of M. tuberculosis should be guided by physicians with expert knowledge in the field (usually infectious disease or chest physicians).

Pneumonia acquired in hospital

This usually occurs in patients who have received an anaesthetic, have aspirated, are receiving immunosuppressive or cytotoxic therapy, or are having assisted ventilation.

Until culture results are available it must be assumed that infection may have occurred with hospital pathogens including *Staph. aureus*, *Ps. aeruginosa*, Klebsiella and other coliforms.

Sputum cultures, blood cultures and other samples and swabs (such as tracheostomy swab, empyema or pleural fluid) are essential before therapy is commenced. Gram films can be useful.

In patients with chronic obstructive airways disease who have received an anaesthetic, *H. influenzae* and *Str. pneumoniae* are likely pathogens. Nowadays most of these patients receive prophylactic therapy for anaesthetics with ampicillin or cotrimoxazole. A pneumonia developing in such circumstances may well be due to staphylococcus, pseudomonas, klebsiella or other coliform.

Safe initial therapy in such patients (which may be modified as culture results become available) would be ampicillin (1 g intravenously 6-hourly) and gentamicin (1.6–2 mg/kg intravenously or intramuscularly 8-hourly) – adding metronidazole (500 mg intravenously 8-hourly) if aspiration is suspected. In neutropenic patients, carbenicillin (5–7.5 g intravenously 6-hourly) should be substituted for ampicillin.

If the Gram film of sputum strongly suggests staphylococci, flucloxacillin (1 g 6-hourly intravenously/intramuscularly) can be substituted for ampicillin.

Sinusitis

It is particularly common for bacterial infection to supervene during or following viral infections of the upper respiratory tract. The organisms are often *mixed* and are derived from the mouth, the oropharynx and nasopharynx in antral sepsis and from the nasopharynx and anterior nares in frontal sinus infection. This means that there are some differences in infecting flora in the two sites but a good deal of overlap.

Maxillary sinus

The main pathogens in *acute* or *chronic* sinusitis tend to be *Haemophilus influenzae*, *Str. pneumoniae*, other non-haemolytic streptococci, 'commensal' Neisseria species, and (increasingly recognized) obligate anaerobes such as peptostreptococci, bacteroides spp, veillonella, anaerobic corynebacteria and (most difficult to isolate) fusiformis spp. Anaerobes may be present in at least 50 per cent of antral sinus infections referred to hospital specialists. Their presence can be detected clinically whenever foul (faeculent)-smelling pus is evacuated from a sinus, though usually the infections are mixed. Many of these anaerobes will be sensitive to penicillins, cephalosporins and erythromycin although cotrimoxazole will not be as reliably active. Metronidazole and clindamycin will be virtually always active and liable to penetrate the lesions.

Haemophilus influenzae will usually be susceptible to ampicillin, cotrimoxazole, tetracycline and erythromycin, though often resistant to currently available cephalosporins and clindamycin and always resistant to metronidazole.

The streptococci are sensitive to penicillins, cephalosporins, erythromycin and clindamycin though not infrequently less susceptible to cotrimoxazole and (unless obligate-anaerobic strains) resistant to metronidazole.

A suitable choice of antibiotics to be given before culture results of sinus material are available would seem to be:

ampicillin 500 mg intramuscularly 6-hourly or amoxycillin 500 mg orally 8-hourly
plus
metronidazole (600 mg orally 8-hourly or 1 g suppository 8-hourly)

Alternatives are many and include:

cephradine 500 mg 6-hourly + metronidazole
or cotrimoxazole tabs. 2 12-hourly + metronidazole
or erythromycin 500 mg four times daily (alone)
or in acute (non-recurring) situations amoxycillin 500 mg three times daily alone.

Tetracyclines may be useful alternatives, especially in general practice, although resistance is not infrequent in *Str. pneumoniae*, other streptococci and the anaerobes too. Tetracyclines also have a nephrotoxic potential which should be avoided in the elderly and in those with already impaired renal function. Doxycycline is the tetracycline least likely to cause nephrotoxicity. A dose of 200 mg stat. then 100 mg daily may be effective. The once daily dosage certainly encourages patient compliance in a domiciliary setting.

Of course, antibiotics alone are not sufficient therapy, except perhaps in the acute (non-recurring) situation. Drainage of clinically infected antral sinuses is essential.

Specimens are not normally taken in acute sinusitis in general practice. But where the infection does *not* respond to simple antibiotic therapy; where complications occur (v.i.); or where antral drainage is carried out, specimens should be sent to the laboratory for full culture (including anaerobic culture) and sensitivity tests, although antibiotics may be started on a best-guess basis (as outlined above) before results are available.

Two types of specimen are acceptable – direct needle puncture of the antrum, when pure pus may be aspirated without contaminating contact with the upper respiratory tract; or following 'antral washout' when gobs of pus can be recovered. Some contamination inevitably occurs with the washout but semi-quantitative culture can be valuable in distinguishing true pathogens from contaminants. Routine throat or nasopharyngeal swabs are *not* very meaningful.

Frontal sinus

The infecting flora of frontal sinusitis are marginally different. Although *Str. pneumoniae* and anaerobes (anaerobic streptococci, anaerobic diphtheroids, veillonella and fusiforms) are often present, *H. influenzae* is not so predictably present as in antral sepsis. *Staph. aureus* and *Proteus mirabilis* may also be involved and the possibility of the former must always be 'covered' when choosing 'best-guess' therapy for frontal sinusitis (and its complications) before laboratory test results are ready.

Frontal sinus specimens obtained at surgery can be invaluable for reliable microbiological investigation.

A nose swab can be useful but is insufficient on its own. But at least it may reveal *Str. pyogenes*, *Staph. aureus* or *Pr. mirabilis* which may have significance.

The choice of initial antibiotic therapy for frontal sinusitis should cover *Staph. aureus* and one must assume penicillinase production in these organisms till proved otherwise even in domiciliary practice. Resistance to the penicillinase-resistant penicillins such as flucloxacillin, cloxacillin and methicillin or to cephradine, cephalexin, and cefazolin is rare in indigenously acquired *Staph. aureus* infection. One would therefore suggest either:

(1) cephradine 500 mg 6-hourly (intravenously/orally) + metronidazole 600 mg (orally) or 1 g (suppository) 8-hourly

or

(2) ampicillin 500 mg 6-hourly i.m. (or amoxycillin 500 mg 8-hourly orally)
+ flucloxacillin 500 mg 6-hourly i.m. or orally
+ metronidazole 600 mg 8-hourly orally (or 1 g suppository 8-hourly)

Note: this is *not* 'magnapen'

This regimen may well have to be altered in the light of laboratory findings but it is worth remembering that anaerobes may be difficult to isolate even in first class laboratories especially fastidious species such as fusiforms. Not growing them does not always constitute reliable proof of their absence.

Other laboratory studies

Gram film
Pus obtained from any sinus, abscess or collection should always be stained by Gram's method. This can give helpful indications of what to expect on culture. Not only do streptococci and staphylococci show characteristic morphology but so also may the various anaerobes. The presence of micro-organisms in a Gram film may be particularly useful when cultures are 'sterile'. This may occur because of the fastidious nature of the bacteria, as mentioned, or because of antimicrobial therapy already started. This therapy may be sufficient to prevent laboratory culture but inadequate to treat the clinical sepsis effectively.

Gas liquid chromatography (GLC)
Where available this is a useful technique for rapid detection of anaerobes in clinical material – such as pus. An ether extract of the latter is made and injected in nitrogen through a column of activated diatomaceous earth. Volatile fatty acids, the characteristic end products of the metabolism of glucose by the various anaerobic organisms, are then detected by flame-ionization technique. The pattern of fatty acids produced can be so characteristic of a species as to constitute identification, but with mixtures of anaerobes in clinical material it is difficult to do much more than detect their presence. GLC can be carried out within an hour or two of taking the specimen. Nevertheless, a negative finding does not completely rule out the possibility of anaerobes. The equipment is expensive to acquire (though cheap compared with the costly apparatus to be found in most 'ordinary' haematology and biochemistry laboratories nowadays).

It is worth noting that a bedside 'diagnosis' of anaerobic infection can be readily made. Any faeculent or foul-smelling collection of pus or discharging wound – whether antral sinus, subphrenic drainage or brain abscess – is caused by anaerobic organisms (whether or not they are isolated on culture). Of course, not all anaerobic pus smells but it is certainly true that many clinicians wrongly attribute faeculant or foul-smelling pus to 'coliforms', or '*E. coli*'.

Pus produced by coliforms and *E. coli alone* does *not* smell.

Serology
Occasionally it may be useful to attempt detection of *Staph. aureus* or *Str. pyogenes* infections by serological techniques. The *anti-staphylolysin* titre may occasionally be raised in deep seated (and chronic) staphylococcal infection. Thus in osteomyelitis where the microbial diagnosis is in doubt, or it is difficult to obtain specimens for culture, or the picture has been confused by previous antibiotic therapy it is worth undertaking the test, realizing that the usual negative result leaves one in exactly the same dilemma.

For suspected *Str. pyogenes* infections one may attempt to demonstrate a rising (or highly raised) antistreptolysin O (ASO) titre. This may be especially useful in patients with a history of tonsillitis or acute otitis media who have been partially treated with antibiotics and throat swabs are negative. It should also be looked for in cases of osteomyelitis with an unknown pathogen (as above) and of course it is an important test in the investigation of patients with suspected rheumatic fever or chorea.

Complications of sinusitis

The infecting organisms are much the same as those found in sinusitis and usually occur in mixtures. *Staph. aureus, Str. pyogenes, Str. pneumoniae, H. influenzae, Proteus mirabilis* and other coliforms and the various *anaerobes* will have to be considered as likely pathogens. Chemotherapy, once specimens have been taken – including pus (aspirated from the sinus), blood cultures, nose and throat swabs and CSF where appropriate – should be along the lines suggested above for frontal sinusitis, but with bigger dosage, given parenterally initially. Ampicillin 1 g 6-hourly intramuscularly/intravenously + flucloxacillin 1 g 6-hourly intramuscularly/intravenously + metronidazole 500 mg intravenously (or 1 g suppository) 8-hourly.

Cephradine may be given in place of ampicillin and flucloxacillin initially in a dose of 1 g 6-hourly intravenously. It should not be given intramuscularly because of poor absorption from the intramuscular depot. Oral administration gives better blood concentrations. Most cephalosporins penetrate bony and soft tissue lesions relatively well but cross the blood–brain barrier poorly even when there is inflammation. They should therefore be avoided if there is meningitis.

Where the patient is extremely ill and coliforms (*Esch. coli,* Klebsiella, *Pr. mirabilis* or *Ps. aeruginosa*) are isolated on culture or strongly suspected from Gram films of purulent material, then gentamicin is invaluable, given in a dosage initially of 1.6 mg/kg body weight 8-hourly intravenously/intramuscularly (i.e. 120 mg for 70 kg individual or 100 mg for 60 kg person). Dosage should then be monitored according to serum gentamicin concentrations (*see below*) or according to a suitable nomogram based on serum creatinine concentrations (e.g. Mawer *et al.*, 1974). Direct serum assay is more reliable and safer than nomograms used on their own, both from the point of view of giving an adequate dose for efficacy and avoiding toxicity.

Gentamicin should be given together with ampicillin or penicillin G (2 megaunits intravenously/intramuscularly 6-hourly) to cover streptococci, and metronidazole (for anaerobes). Gentamicin should 'cover' *Staph. aureus*, though if the latter has been isolated or is strongly suspected, flucloxacillin may be given with gentamicin.

Like the cephalosporins, gentamicin penetrates even the inflamed blood–brain barrier poorly. Where intracranial sepsis is strongly suspected *chloramphenicol* is highly recommended. It penetrates freely across the blood–brain barrier and has truly broad spectrum activity against streptococci, staphylocci, Haemophilus, coliforms and most anaerobes. (It does not cover *Ps. aeruginosa.*) Because of its restricted use in this country, acquired resistance is rare. So is the dreaded toxicity of agranulocytosis and aplastic anaemia. One must maintain a sense of proportion about the toxic risk and if the risks of sepsis are great, then chloramphenicol offers many advantages, though obviously it is not a drug to be used casually. Like cephradine it gives better blood concentrations after oral rather than intramuscular administration and so should be given by the oral or intravenous routes. An initial dose of 750 mg 6-hourly is indicated for an adult, though this can be cut to 500 mg four times daily when the infection comes under control. Other serious toxic side-effects of chloramphenicol include pseudomembranous colitis and the 'grey baby' syndrome, seen in neonates.

Chloramphenicol should not be used in conjunction with penicillins because of the *in vivo* antagonism, shown classically with *Str. pneumoniae*. It may be combined with metronidazole (to give extra cover against anaerobes). Metronidazole, too, passes the blood–brain barrier easily.

Where there is a chronic or subacute staphylococcal osteomyelitis *not* responding to the therapy outlined above, i.e. flucloxacillin or cephradine (this will probably be due to inadequate dosage or sequestrum formation), then fusidate ('fucidin') 500 mg–1 g 8-hourly (orally/intravenously) plus erythromycin 500 mg–1 g 6-hourly (orally/intravenously) or clindamycin 600 mg 8-hourly (orally/intramuscularly) may be tried. These antibiotics penetrate bone well and are usually active against staphylococci. Occasional resistant strains occur and appropriate laboratory studies should be performed. But note:

(1) If either fusidate or erythromycin is used alone resistance may emerge during therapy. The combination together reduces this risk considerably. Nevertheless the combination given orally causes gastro-intestinal upset in many patients. Enteric coated tablets help reduce this but are even more expensive.
(2) Fusidate should not be combined with cloxacillin or flucloxacillin unless (and until) laboratory studies reveal no antagonism between these antibiotics for the particular strain of *Staph. aureus* involved. This is unpredictable. Fusidate and (flu)cloxacillin may show synergy, antagonism or indifference in their interactions. Where there is antagonism, failure of therapy may occur with serious consequences.
(3) Clindamycin is not only antistaphylococcal but also active against anaerobes and streptococci (it has no activity against coliforms or *Ps. aeruginosa*). This is a useful spectrum for sinus infections and their complications. It certainly should be considered where there is a failure of response to initial therapy. Its reputation for causing pseudomembranous colitis (PMC) restricts its use. Perhaps when the nature and effective treatment (or prevention) of PMC become fully understood, one will be able to use clindamycin more readily with less anxiety.

Finally it must be emphasized that antimicrobial agents alone may not be sufficient to treat the complications of sinusitis. Collections of pus must be drained whether intra- or extracranial, and dead pieces of bone must be excised. Only then can antibiotics deal with the infection effectively.

Otitis externa

This condition occurs relatively frequently and is usually related to underlying allergy or trauma. The superficial infection which may be associated tends to be caused by constituents of the normal flora acting opportunistically.

Staph. aureus, streptococci, Candida, aspergillus, and gram negative bacterial rods, especially *Ps. aeruginosa* and *Pr. mirabilis*, may be implicated but the mere isolation of these organisms from swabs of the external auditory canal means very little since they may be isolated from healthy subjects.

Unfortunately it is all too easy for clinicians to prescribe antibiotic ear drops for patients with a 'sore' or 'discharging' ear. Neomycin, framycetin and gentamicin ear drops are very popular. All too often they serve little therapeutic value and merely promote the emergence of resistant strains of bacteria (gentamicin-resistant *Ps. aeruginosa* is a particularly unwelcome organism) and the development of hypersensitivity to aminoglycosides. The drops are casually applied by the patient with little hope of the agent reaching all or even most of the affected parts of the external canal.

What is usually needed is a thorough cleaning of the external ear and treatment of allergic disorders. Swabs of the affected part should be taken carefully for culture. The results should be treated with reserve. If topical agents are selected then the choice should be of agents *not* used systemically (e.g. framycetin rather than gentamicin) and those to which resistance does not readily emerge (e.g. polymixin or colistin for *Ps. aeruginosa* rather than gentamicin). Of course, topical agents should be used with great caution where there is perforation of the drum. Most popular topical agents are ototoxic, including the aminoglycosides and the polymixins. Finally it is worth noting that 3 per cent acetic acid is highly effective against *Ps. aeruginosa* as well as being cheap. Resistance is not known to occur. It is worth serious consideration as a topical agent for infections caused by this organism.

Systemic antibiotics have no proven place in the treatment of simple otitis externa. Virtually no antibiotic at all will penetrate to the surface of the auditory canal. The only indication for systemic antibiotics is where there is an *invasive* infection of the external ear.

(1) *Severe infection of the pinna*. This is a serious condition as cartilage, once it has become necrotic, is impossible to treat conservatively. The usual pathogens are *Staph. aureus* or *Str. pyogenes* or *Ps. aeruginosa* (see below). It is imperative, once specimens for culture have been taken, to start high-dosage parenteral chemotherapy. Penicillin 2 megaunits 6-hourly intramuscularly plus flucloxacillin 1 g 6-hourly intravenously or intramuscularly would be reasonable initial treatment but if *Ps. aeruginosa* is suspected at all, carbenicillin 5 g 6-hourly intravenously and gentamicin 1.6 mg/kg 8-hourly intravenously or intramuscularly are indicated.

(2) *Furuncles* in the external auditory meatus are nearly always caused by *Staph. aureus*. Swabs of any pus exuding should be sent for culture as well as the usual external auditory canal swabs.

Initial treatment should be with flucloxacillin 500 mg four times daily (orally). If the infecting *Staph. aureus* is shown to be sensitive to penicillin then it should be substituted, penicillin V 500 mg four times daily being up to eight times more active than the same dose of flucloxacillin. If the patient has had much trouble with furuncles then it may be useful to check for any underlying disease (such as diabetes mellitus) and get rid of staphylococcal skin and nares carriage. This can best be achieved by exclusive bathing for a week with anti-staphylococcal soap, chlorhexidine ('Hibiscrub') or povidone-iodine ('betadine', 'steribath') or hexachlorophane, including hair shampoo, combined with twice daily application of chlorhexidine cream to the anterior nares. All clothing should be laundered and dry cleaned during this week and all persons in intimate contact with the patient checked for carriage of the offending *Staph. aureus* (phage typing is necessary). It may prove necessary to 'treat' the household along with the patient.

(3) *Otitis externa malignans.* This uncommon condition is caused by *Ps. aeruginosa* producing an invasive infection of the external auditory canal. Cartilage and soft tissues are destroyed and there may be involvement of the facial nerve and osteomyelitis. A copious, thin bloody discharge is characteristic, sometimes with a greenish tinge and a musty 'Pseudomonas' smell.

Most of the patients have diabetes mellitus or are otherwise debilitated or immunosuppressed. The condition has much morbidity and may be fatal unless treated energetically. This often entailed radical and destructive surgery before effective anti-Pseudomonas antibiotics became available.

The treatment of choice is carbenicillin 5–7.5 g 6-hourly intravenously (or 5 g 4-hourly intravenously) plus gentamicin 1.6 mg/kg intramuscularly or intravenously 8-hourly. Daily local debridement and cleaning and application of colistin or acetic acid should be carried out under microscopy. Serum gentamicin concentrations should be monitored regularly to ensure peak values in the range of 5–10 μg/ml and trough (pre-dose) values of 2 μg/ml or less. Higher trough levels call for longer intervals between doses (e.g. 12 h). Treatment will need to be continued for *at least* 10–14 days and may need to be carried on for longer. Accumulation of gentamicin is more likely to occur in the second week of treatment.

Diabetics are liable to have impaired renal function without any obvious history or symptoms. It is advisable to check renal function early, by creatinine clearance estimation rather than a simple blood urea test. Not only is gentamicin potentially nephrotoxic but carbenicillin administration involves giving a great deal of sodium. Carbenicillin itself comes as a sodium salt, and 30 G means giving 162 mEquivalents of sodium per 24 h. Added to this is the sodium chloride in which the carbenicillin is given (glucose solutions being acidic cause hydrolysis and are to be avoided). Patients with renal impairment (or with cardiac ischaemia) run rapidly into problems of sodium overload and may develop ankle oedema, pulmonary congestion and hypokalaemia. Diuretics (e.g. frusemide or thiazides) and potassium supplements may be necessary additions to the therapy.

Adequately treated in the manner described, otitis externa malignans (*see* Vol. 2) will respond promptly and completely.

Acute otitis media

This is predominantly a disease of young children and is frequently recurrent. It is often part of an upper respiratory tract infection, usually with viruses. Nevertheless bacterial superinfection may readily occur and occasionally may be primary as for example when complicating *Str. pyogenes* tonsillitis.

The usual bacterial pathogens include *Str. pyogenes*, *Str. pneumoniae* and in infants *Haemophilus influenzae*.

It is often difficult to obtain useful specimens. Unless the drum has ruptured and there is a bloody discharge, there is little point in swabbing the external canal as the flora cultured otherwise is totally misleading. In certain special centres it may be possible under microscopic control to aspirate infected fluid from the middle ear through the tympanic membrane. Such specimens should be cultured both aerobically and anaerobically.

Although many episodes of acute otitis media will be self-limiting viral conditions, bacterial superinfection is relatively common and has sufficient morbidity untreated, to warrant a low threshold on the part of the clinician for giving antibiotics. In older children penicillin V 125–250 mg four times daily would be the treatment of choice with erythromycin 125–250 mg four times daily as an alternative for those with penicillin allergy. In infants the added possibility of *H. influenzae* as a pathogen means that penicillin V is not adequate. Amoxycillin 125 mg three times daily should be suitable. Cotrimoxazole 5–10 ml of paediatric suspension twice daily is a suitable alternative, although it is less reliably active against streptococci than the penicillins or erythromycin.

Mastoiditis

This is a condition usually seen in children and most frequently due to *Str. pyogenes*, *Str. pneumoniae* and anaerobes.

Surgical intervention to drain abscesses is essential. Antibiotic treatment initially should be parenteral penicillins, the drug of choice being benzylpenicillin 15–20 mg/kg 6-hourly. When the acute situation is controlled it may become possible to change to penicillin V 125–250 mg 6-hourly (on an empty stomach).

Chronic otitis media

Infection is usually of a secondary, opportunist nature in this condition. The organisms are mixed and tend to be derived from the commensal flora of the external auditory canal or the nasopharynx.

Swabs taken from the distal end of the external auditory canal are of little value (the conventional 'ear swab') but swabs taken (using fine 'pernasal'-type swabs) under microscopic control from the site of infection are more useful.

Cultures should be performed anaerobically as well as aerobically (and in an atmosphere of carbon dioxide).

The organisms isolated include the various streptococci, diphtheroids, *Ps. aeruginosa*, coliforms (such as *E. coli*, Klebsiella, Enterobacter, Proteus spp.) and anaerobes (bacteroides, peptostreptococci, fusiforms, veillonella). Fungi may be involved including candida and aspergillus species.

The crucial feature of management is treating the underlying cause, such as excision of cholesteatoma. The variety of pathogens listed above will probably not be covered by any topical preparation and if underlying causes are not removed the infection will persist. As many of these patients have perforated tympanic membranes, pouring in ototoxic topical agents such as neomycin, framycetin, gentamicin, colistin and the like is not without risk, apart from stimulating the proliferation of resistant organisms. Antibiotics play only a *supplemental* role to surgical measures. There is usually sufficient time to take a fine swab from the site of infection isolating all anaerobes and aerobes and establishing sensitivity and resistance patterns with such a variety of possible pathogens. This is important in the selection of suitable antimicrobial agents which may be administered systemically or locally, depending on the invasiveness of the infection and the penetrating powers of the agent.

Complications of chronic otitis media

The complications of chronic otitis media include subperiosteal abscess, meningitis, sigmoid sinus thrombosis and brain abscess. Abscesses of course necessitate surgical intervention for their drainage. Otogenic abscesses almost always have mixed flora including various streptococci (though *not* Group A usually); *Str. milleri* ('micro-aerophilic streptococci') is common, as well as *Str. pneumoniae* and anaerobic streptococci (peptostreptococci). Other anaerobes occur frequently especially the bacteroides spp. and *B. fragilis* in particular.

This suggests that initial antibiotic cover before culture results of pus are available should be directed against streptococci and anaerobes. Penicillin G in high dosage (3 megaunits 4- or 6-hourly intravenously) and metronidazole (500 mg intravenously or 1 g suppository 8-hourly) would be useful. Clindamycin 300–600 mg intramuscularly 6-hourly is an alternative. (If clindamycin is given by intravenous infusion then it should be given *slowly* over 20–30 min. A quick 'bolus' intravenous injection may cause cardiac arrhythmias.)

Alternatively chloramphenicol 750 mg four times daily intravenously or orally may be given as it covers the major pathogens likely to be involved and penetrates well.

When the neurosurgeon drains a brain abscess it may be useful for him to instil 10–20 megaunits of penicillin G into the abscess cavity.

Tuberculosis of the upper respiratory tract

Nose

Usually the anterior part of the septum and the inferior concha are involved. There may be ulceration and destruction of tissues but involvement of the bone is unusual. In the less acute form the lesions are more fibrotic with the production of warty vegetations.

There is virtually always evidence of tuberculosis elsewhere. Investigations should include chest x-ray, microscopy and culture of scrapings (biopsies) from the lesions and early morning sputum. Syphilis serology should also be checked especially where acid-fast bacilli are not seen on microscopy.

Histological examination of biopsy specimens may also be diagnostic.

Pharynx

Tuberculosis in this area may present as ulcerating or fibrotic ('lupus') lesions. It may also produce a tuberculoma, resembling a malignant mass. This may break down and cause local destruction of soft tissues.

It is almost always secondary to tuberculosis elsewhere (especially pulmonary disease) and the tonsillar glands are usually involved too.

Scrapings of the lesions (or biopsy specimens) are better for mycobacterial microscopy and culture than simple swabs.

Secondary pyogenic infection may occur and routine bacteriological culture should be performed and suitable antipyogenic antimicrobial therapy given in addition to antituberculous therapy.

Larynx

Here tuberculosis is always secondary to pulmonary tuberculosis and may present as ulcers with rapid worsening of the disease, or as more fibrotic lesions ('lupus') with involvement of the surrounding parts including the epiglottis. This usually runs a more chronic course. Direct laryngeal swabs and biopsy specimens may be taken for microscopy and culture. Sometimes a diagnosis is made from histological examination. Where microscopy is negative for acid-fast bacilli, it is important to perform treponemal serology.

A chest x-ray should always be performed. Before effective antituberculous therapy was available, this condition was almost always fatal.

The ear

Tuberculosis of the ear occurs mainly in children with an insidious onset. Often the disease is widespread before there is any outward manifestation. It is secondary to tuberculosis elsewhere and it is postulated that there is spread of mycobacteria up the eustachian tube. Often there is secondary pyogenic bacterial infection too and there may be a dangerous delay in diagnosis of tuberculosis. Sometime labyrinthitis and facial palsy have occurred before the diagnosis is made. Swabs of the lesion may not be sufficient to exclude mycobacterial infection and histology and culture of biopsy specimens is invaluable. Antituberculous therapy may have to be supplemented by mastoid surgery.

Treatment

All forms of upper respiratory tract tuberculosis respond well to standard antituberculous chemotherapy. The treatment is the same for all four conditions listed above:

Isoniazid	300 mg daily (+ pyridoxine 10 mg daily)	for 9 months
Rifampicin	600 mg daily	

Ethambutol 25 mg/kg daily for 6–8 weeks then reduced to 15 mg/kg daily for up to three months.

The above are the most favoured first-line drugs in the United Kingdom at the present time. Very occasionally progressive liver dysfunction occurs which is probably attributable to isoniazid and rifampicin showing synergistic hepatotoxicity. Alternative drugs that may be substituted for one of the above include streptomycin (0.5–1.0 g intramuscularly daily), though this drug should be avoided in elderly patients and those with impaired renal function; para-aminosalicylate (12 g daily); prothionamide (0.5–1.0 g daily) and pyrazinamide (0.5 g three times daily) though the latter three drugs probably cause more toxicity and side-effects than the first-choice agents.

Tuberculous cervical lymph nodes

Although the bovine strain of *Mycobacterium tuberculosis* was the classic cause of this condition before the 1940s, the universal availability of pasteurized milk and tuberculin-testing of dairy herds has virtually eradicated it from Britain.

Tuberculous cervical nodes still occur but more often nowadays are caused by *M. tuberculosis* (human strain), which is chiefly seen in patients with an apparent genetic susceptibility to the disease (e.g. from the Indian subcontinent, Western Ireland); or by so-called 'atypical' species of Mycobacteria, especially *M. avium* and *M. intracellulare* but also occasionally *M. xenopi*. Those organisms are more likely to be seen in the indigenous population.

Treatment is best started with rifampicin 450–900 mg daily (before breakfast) and isoniazid 300 mg daily plus pyridoxine 10 mg daily (to counter some of the side-effects of prolonged isoniazid therapy such as psychosis and peripheral neuropathy). This is continued for 9 months. For the first 3 months a third antituberculous agent is given. Either ethambutol (25 mg/kg daily for 6 weeks, then 15 mg/kg daily for the remaining time), or streptomycin (0.5–1 g intramuscularly daily for 3 weeks then twice weekly for the rest of the period).

Streptomycin should be avoided in elderly patients or those with renal disease. Ethambutol may cause optic neuritis presenting as an inability to read small print and loss of colour vision. It is reversible if detected early and the drug is stopped. This is why it is recommended that the dose is cut after the first 6 weeks of treatment.

Rifampicin causes red tears and red urine which may cause alarm unnecessarily but there is evidence that the combination of rifampicin and isoniazid may be more hepatotoxic than either alone. It is therefore prudent to watch for signs of jaundice, and liver function tests should be performed at the outset as a base-line.

It is essential that a sample of lymph nodes removed for diagnostic histology should be sent for mycobacterial culture and microscopy. A swab is not adequate, and it is important *not* to put the tissue for culture into formalin solutions. This kills the mycobacteria as it fixes the tissues.

Although a diagnosis of mycobacterial infection can be made from histological examination or straightforward microscopy, this in itself may not be sufficient for management. It cannot be simply assumed that acid-fast organisms are *M. tuberculosis*.

Cultural confirmation is needed. It is also important to know antituberculous agent sensitivity patterns and it may be useful epidemiologically to distinguish between human and bovine strains. Culture is also needed to identify the various atypical mycobacteria and to establish their sensitivity and resistance patterns. They may often be naturally resistant to first-line antituberculous drugs and so this may lead to modification of therapy. Choice of drugs must depend on *in vitro* tests although these species are often less virulent and the nodal masses may be successfully treated by simple excision.

Actinomycosis

Cervicofacial actinomycosis accounts for about two-thirds of all cases. It is a chronic suppurating disease with the production of granulomas and the progressive involvement of surrounding tissues including bone. The disease is most often caused by *Actinomyces israelii*, a gram positive, non-acid fast bacterium (*not* a fungus), which can be found in the tonsils and saliva of over a third of normal individuals but especially in those with carious teeth.

It is a strict anaerobe and may take a week or more to grow on anaerobic culture. The infection is endogenous and there is no evidence of cross-infection. The disease can spread and involve the pharynx and larynx, usually with the production of deep ulcers with yellowish pus containing 'sulphur granules' – colonies of the infecting organism. The discharge can be offensive.

Microscopy of the sulphur granules will yield the diagnosis, confirmed by culture.

Treatment

Benzylpenicillin for 6 weeks (2 megaunits four times daily) or tetracycline (500 mg four times daily for 6 weeks). Surgery may be necessary where there is extensive involvement of bony tissue.

Mouth and throat infections in patients with neutropenia, leukaemia, lymphoma

Patients with blood dyscrasias and those who have received anticancer therapy which has led to neutropenia (less than 200 neutrophils/mm^3) become particularly susceptible to various infections including bacteria, fungi and other opportunists such as *Pneumocystis carinii*.

There are large numbers of bacteria in the mouth, pharynx and the alimentary tract. In the neutropenic patient invasion takes place more readily through the oropharynx or intestines and this tendency is increased by the action of cytotoxic agents which not only act on the components of the bone marrow but also damage the pharyngeal and intestinal mucosa.

Many of the pyrexial attacks that these patients suffer are associated with bacteraemia. The lack of neutrophils allows bacterial proliferation and dissemination of sepsis. The outcome if not treated promptly is often fatal. But antibacterial treatment, even with bactericidal drugs, is often not as effective as in patients without neutropenia. Neutrophil infusions appear to be helpful.

Oropharyngeal toilet is important in these patients. As staying in hospital leads to acquisition of hospital opportunist pathogens (especially if antibiotics are given) such as *Klebsiella, Ps. aeruginosa*, Enterobacter spp., etc., it is essential to place such patients in reverse (clean) isolation with sterile food and non-absorbable oral antibiotics designed to suppress such bacteria and also Candida (framycetin, colistin and nystatin form one such regimen).

It is best to give these agents where possible as suspensions which are rinsed round the mouth and throat before swallowing. Otherwise the mouth does not get adequately disinfected.

Throat swabs and gum margin swabs should be taken regularly (e.g. twice a week) to monitor the acquisition of hospital flora. *Ps. aeruginosa* in particular poses a serious threat and every effort must be made to suppress it.

The Gram negative rods and Candida may cause secondary infection of mouth ulcers with invasion. The surrounding tissue becomes swollen and reddened and the ulcer develops a necrotic centre. The patient will probably spike high temperatures but there will be no purulent discharge and little in the way of polymorphs on microscopy even though bacteria are abundant.

Local oral mouth wash is started (if not already being taken) with framycetin 1 g 6-hourly, colistin $\frac{1}{2}$ megaunit 6-hourly and nystatin 6-hourly (or amphotericin 6-hourly) and amphotericin lozenges ad libitum. This must be supplemented with systemic chemotherapy after blood cultures have been taken. The initial choice is carbenicillin 5–7.5 g 6-hourly combined with gentamicin 1.6 mg/kg 8-hourly (at first, then according to serum assay concentrations). This may be modified to other bactericidal drugs as and when the results of cultures and sensitivity tests become available. White cell infusions may also aid resolution of infection and healing.

Some routine precautions to be taken before starting patients on antimicrobial chemotherapy

(1) Allergy and hypersensitivity

(a) Ask the patient for any history of drug allergy or general allergies. If a history of penicillin-allergy is obtained discover whether there is major allergy (anaphylaxis, angioneurotic oedema, serum sickness) or minor allergy (e.g. ampicillin skin rash).

(b) Antimicrobial agents when topically applied are more liable to sensitize than if systemically taken. Penicillins are never used topically in the UK nowadays because of this heightened risk.

(c) Cross-allergenicity exists usually between antibiotics of the same type, e.g. penicillins (a patient allergic to penicillin G should not receive ampicillin, cloxacillin or carbenicillin). Mecillinam also exhibits cross-allergenicity with penicillin. Patients allergic to penicillin show an increased hypersensitivity to cephalosporins compared with the general population. It is a safe rule not to use cephalosporins in patients with a history of major allergy to penicillins.

(d) Cotrimoxazole contains sulphonamide and should not be used in patients allergic to sulphonamide. The Stevens–Johnson syndrome may be precipitated in this way and carries a significant mortality.
(e) Skin-testing is often unreliable for detecting allergic subjects. This is especially true for the penicillins. Skin-testing has been known to precipitate major allergic reactions to the test-substances.
(f) Where there is a life-threatening condition (e.g. endocarditis) for which a penicillin is the drug of choice, it may be possible to give the drug under suitable steroid and antihistamine cover. Advice should be sought from the clinical microbiologist and/or clinical pharmacologist in such circumstances about the choice of antimicrobial agents and appropriate dosage and precautions.

(2) Renal and hepatic dysfunction

It is important to understand the pharmacology of the drugs used and whether or not their metabolism and/or excretion are affected by impaired renal or hepatic function or whether they may cause further damage.

Thus tetracyclines (except doxycycline) may cause further renal damage in the elderly. Nitrofurantoin may also produce further deterioration of renal function in those with pre-existing impairment. Aminoglycosides accumulate excessively in the serum and tissues of patients with impaired renal clearance and may cause further renal damage as well as damage to hearing.

Drugs which are metabolized by the liver and/or excreted via the biliary system should be used at full dosage, even in patients with impaired renal function (e.g. lincomycin, erythromycin, fusidate). Only drugs which are excreted via the kidneys should have their dosage reduced in such circumstances. Drugs which are excreted via the bile or are metabolized by the liver should be used with caution in patients with liver disease.

(3) Pregnancy

Care must be exercised when prescribing for pregnant women or women of child-bearing age who may be pregnant, to avoid any possible damage to the fetus. Many antibiotics cross the placenta. Tetracycline can cause unsightly staining of the teeth and even disorders of bone growth. Cotrimoxazole is best avoided as teratogenic effects have been seen in experimental animals receiving huge doses. It has been suggested that aminoglycosides may cause ototoxic damage in the fetus. Nevertheless untreated sepsis can also produce ill-effects in the fetus and so appropriate antibiotic therapy should be used in pregnant women when indicated (e.g. pyelonephritis, tuberculosis, pneumonia, etc.). It is also worth noting that drugs which act as enzyme-inducers in the liver (e.g. rifampicin) may interfere with the contraceptive effect of the 'mini-pill' and lead to unexpected and unwanted pregnancy.

(4) Young children

Tetracyclines should be avoided in children below 10 years of age because of the staining which occurs in permanent teeth. Erythromycin is usually an effective alternative for most conditions for which tetracycline is used.

Neonates have much poorer renal function than older children and healthy adults, which leads to accumulation of many drugs. Thus penicillins and aminoglycosides are best given 12-hourly in neonates (although neonatal meningitis may call for more frequent dosage of penicillin).

Hepatic function is also poorly developed and this is particularly true of premature neonates. Drugs metabolized by the liver or excreted in the bile are best avoided, e.g. clindamycin and fusidate. Chloramphenicol is particularly dangerous and can produce the 'grey baby syndrome', with significant mortality. Sulphonamides (including cotrimoxazole) are best avoided in neonates as they interfere with the binding of bilirubin to albumin and may cause (or exacerbate) hyperbilirubinaemia.

(5) Interactions with other drugs

Not only may antimicrobial agents react with or interfere with the action of other drugs (e.g. broad-spectrum antibiotics taken orally can heighten the effect of anticoagulants such as warfarin) but they may interfere with one another. Thus penicillin and tetracycline counteract one another against *Str. pneumoniae* in vivo as do penicillin and chloramphenicol. There is also evidence to suggest that ampicillin and chloramphenicol are less effective together than either alone against *H. influenzae* in meningitis.

Cloxacillin and fusidate may interact in synergistic, additive or antagonistic ways against *Staph. aureus* and it is impossible to know which reaction will occur without suitable laboratory tests.

Synergy may be important in clinical situations. Perhaps the best example is the treatment of streptococcal endocarditis (particularly when caused by *Str. faecalis*) by penicillin together with gentamicin.

Combinations of antibiotics may be indicated not only in the treatment of such difficult infections, but also to prevent the emergence of resistant strains of bacteria which may happen when drugs are used singly – as for example in tuberculosis when three drugs are used initially and then two together (when sensitivities are known). Combinations are also used when a single drug does not have sufficient spectrum to cover all the possible bacteria in a mixed infection, for example in faecal peritonitis when an anti-anaerobic agent such as metronidazole or clindamycin is combined with an anticoliform agent such as cotrimoxazole, cephradine or gentamicin.

Nevertheless combinations of antibiotics should not be deployed unless there is a sound clinical or microbiological reason. They are not routinely indicated and there may be harmful effects either because of mutual interference (as described above) or because of 'synergistic' toxicity effects. Thus injected cephalosporins and aminoglycosides combined together produce more nephrotoxicity than when either is used alone. If there are doubts about whether or not a combination of antibiotics should be used, discuss its suitability with the clinical microbiologist.

It should also be noted that drugs may interact chemically when combined in a syringe or in bottles of infusion fluid. The best known example of this is carbenicillin and gentamicin which nullify each other's antimicrobial effect by combining together. The effect is most pronounced when large amounts of drug are mixed in infusion fluid at room temperature; it is less in serum at 37°C in normal serum concentrations. The interaction in serum is only clinically significant in patients with impaired renal function receiving widely-spaced doses of drugs. But, in any event such patients should have their dosage controlled by frequent serum assay.

It is a good rule to avoid mixing antibiotics in syringes or infusion fluid but to give each as an independent 'bolus' intravenously or by intramuscular injection.

(6) Collection of specimens

Specimens for microbiological examination should always be taken where possible, and treatment should be withheld if possible until a microbiological diagnosis is made. Nevertheless it is often necessary to start treatment for a presumed infection before results are available, on a 'best guess' basis, modifying treatment as indicated by clinical developments and laboratory results. It is essential to realize that antibiotics administered before specimens are taken can obscure or prevent diagnosis without treating the clinical condition effectively. This is especially true of serious infections such as endocarditis, septicaemia, meningitis and pneumonia and can be very dangerous.

Blood cultures are particularly valuable as bacteraemia occurs not only in septicaemia but also in many other serious septic conditions, such as pneumonia, osteomyelitis, pyelonephritis, etc. One of the specimen bottles should be suitable for recovering strict anaerobic organisms. It is important to take trouble over obtaining good quality specimens since the bacteriological result can only be as good as the specimen allows. In particular, time spent in collecting satisfactory blood cultures, urine samples, sputum and pus samples is well rewarded. It is, also, very important that samples, especially swabs, should reach the laboratory as quickly as possible after being taken.

Tables 14.1, 14.2 and *14.3* provide a scheme of ready reference and an aid to selection of antibiotics.

Table 14.1 Major pathogens: Gram positive

Organism	*Usually sensitive to*	*Frequently resistant to*
Staph. aureus	Flucolaxacillin*, cephalosporins, erythromycin*, lincomycin*, fusidate*, chloramphenicol*, gentamicin*, amikacin	Penicillin, ampicillin, sulphonamides, tetracyclines
Str. pyogenes (Lancefield Group A)	Penicillin G, penicillin V, erythromycin, lincomycin, chloramphenicol, cephalosporins	Aminoglycosides, tetracycline
Str. pneumoniae	Penicillin G*, penicillin V*, ampicillin*, erythromycin*, lincomycin*, chloramphenicol*, vancomycin	Aminoglycosides, sulphonamides, tetracycline
Anaerobic streptococci	Metronidazole, penicillin G, clindamycin, erythromycin, chloramphenicol	Aminoglycosides, tetracycline, cotrimoxazole

Table 14.1 Major pathogens: Gram positive *(continued)*

Organism	*Usually sensitive to*	*Frequently resistant to*
Clostridium species	Penicillin G, metronidazole, clindamycin*, erythromycin*	Tetracycline, cotrimoxazole, aminoglycosides
Corynebacterium diphtheriae	Erythromycin, penicillin G, fusidate	
Actinomyces spp	Penicillin, tetracycline, metronidazole	Aminoglycosides
Myobacterium tuberculosis	Rifampicin, isoniazid, ethambutol, streptomycin	'Conventional' antibiotics

* This signifies that, although they are relatively rare at present, resistant strains of these bacteria have caused clinical problems. Such resistant organisms are a very unusual problem in patients admitted from domiciliary practice but may pose serious difficulties in particular hospitals or in particular (specialist) units, often those with patients with compromised host defences. In such circumstances advice on appropriate antibacterial chemotherapy should be sought from the clinical microbiologist.

Table 14.2 Major pathogens: Gram negative

Organism	*Usually sensitive to*	*Frequently resistant to*
Neisseria meningitidis	Penicillin G, ampicillin, chloramphenicol, sulphonamide*	
Neisseria gonorrhoeae	Penicillin G*, ampicillin*, tetracycline, cephradine, spectinomycin, kanamycin	Sulphonamide, penicillin V
Haemophilus influenzae	Ampicillin*, tetracycline*, cotrimoxazole*, chloramphenicol, carbenicillin	Penicillin G and V, flucloxacillin, erythromycin, clindamycin
E. coli	Cotrimoxazole*, cephradine*, chloramphenicol, carbenicillin*, gentamicin, amikacin	Ampicillin, tetracycline, sulphonamide
Klebsiella	Cotrimoxazole*, cephradine*, chloramphenicol, gentamicin*, amikacin	Ampicillin, carbenicillin, sulphonamide
Proteus mirabilis	Ampicillin*, cephradine*, cotrimoxazole*, chloramphenicol, carbenicillin, gentamicin, amikacin	Tetracycline, sulphonamide
Other Proteus species ('indole positive')	Cotrimoxazole*, carbenicillin*, gentamicin, amikacin, chloramphenicol*	Sulphonamide, ampicillin, cephradine
Enterobacter spp.	Cotrimoxazole, carbenicillin*, gentamicin, amikacin, chloramphenicol*	Sulphonamide, ampicillin, cephradine
Pseudomonas aeruginosa	Carbenicillin*, gentamicin*, amikacin, colistin	Ampicillin, cephalosporins, cotrimoxazole, chloramphenicol

* This signifies that although they are relatively rare at present, resistant strains of these bacteria have caused clinical problems. Such resistant organisms are a very unusual problem in patients admitted from domiciliary practice but may pose serious difficulties in particular hospitals or in particular (specialist) units, often those with patients with compromised host defences. In such circumstances advice on appropriate antibacterial chemotherapy should be sought from the clinical microbiologist.

Table 14.3 Antibacterial agents

Drug	*Spectrum of activity*	*Route of administration*	*Toxicity and side effects*	*Other points*
Aminoglycosides				
Gentamicin	*Staph. aureus*, *E. coli*, *Klebsiella*, proteus, other coliforms, *Ps. aeruginosa* (not streptococci alone nor anaerobes)	i.v./i.m.	8th nerve (especially vestibular) nephrotoxicity	Toxicity rare with proper monitoring
Tobramycin	Similar; better activity against *Ps. aeruginosa in vitro* not reflected *in vivo*	i.v./i.m.	Similar	Same applies
Kanamycin	Similar to gentamicin but more resistant strains of *Staph. aureus* and coliforms occur. All *Pseudomonas aeruginosa* resistant	i.v./i.m.	8th nerve (cochleotoxic) nephrotoxic	Same applies
Sissomicin	Very similar to gentamicin but possibly more active *in vivo*	i.v./i.m.	8th nerve (vestibular) nephrotoxic	Same applies
Netilmicin	Similar to gentamicin but including some gentamicin-resistant strains	i.v./i.m.	Much less ototoxic than the above compounds. May be less nephrotoxic too	Should still be monitored
Amikacin	Same as gentamicin but active against majority of strains of coliform, *Ps. aeruginosa* resistant to gentamicin and tobramycin. Not active against streptococci nor anaerobes. Useful activity against *M. tuberculosis*	i.v./i.m.	8th nerve (cochleo toxic) nephrotoxic	No more toxic than gentamicin when used in equivalent dosage
Framycetin } Neomycin }	Similar spectrum to kanamycin (i.e. not active against *Ps. aeruginosa*)	Topical or oral (non-absorbed)	Too ototoxic for systemic use	Absorbed from extensive wounds, burns etc. Can cause deafness this way
Streptomycin	Used only for *M. tuberculosis* nowadays although has broad antistaphylococcal and anticoliform activity though not as wide as kanamycin nor gentamicin. Not active against *Ps. aeruginosa*	i.v./i.m.	8th nerve (mixed but mainly vestibular)	–

*Cephalosporins**				
Cephaloridine	Gram positive organisms (including streptococci and staphylococci). Gram negative rods of coliform type although not active against *Ps. aeruginosa*, *Enterobacter*, some species of Proteus and some strains of klebsiella. Some destruction by *Staph. aureus* penicillinase. Little activity against *Bacteroides fragilis*	i.v./i.m.	Nephrotoxicity – although uncommon, potentiated by doses >6 g/24 h; by frusemide and by aminoglycosides	–
Cephalothin	Similar to cephaloridine but slightly wider anticoliform activity; less affected by *Staph.* penicillinase	i.v. (very painful i.m.)	Similar to cephaloridine although slightly less nephrotoxic	Rapidly excreted also metabolized by liver to inactive form
Cephazolin	Similar to cephalothin	i.v./i.m.	Should not be nephrotoxic if <6 g/24 h are used and concurrent administration of frusemide and aminoglycoside avoided	Replacing cephalothin
Cephalexin	Similar to cephaloridine except more active against coliforms and less active against gram positive organisms. Not much useful activity against *H. influenzae*	Oral	Nephrotoxicity very rare	–
Cephadrine	Almost identical with cephalexin. Very stable against *Staph.* penicillinase. Also active against penicillinase-producing *N. gonorrhoeae*	O./i.v./i.m.	Nephrotoxicity rare	Better blood concentrations by oral and i.v. routes than i.m.
Cefuroxime	Similar spectrum to cephradine but slightly wider against coliforms including *Enterobacter*. No activity against *Ps. aeruginosa* or some strains of Proteus. Some activity against strains of *B. fragilis*. Also better activity against *H. influenzae*	i.m./i.v.	Rare nephrotoxicity	Useful for certain resistant bacteria found in hospitals. Otherwise no advantage over existing cephalosporins

* Other cephalosporins and cephamycins (related compounds) are being produced and tested in various countries. They may offer some advantages in particular situations (e.g. cefoxitin has greater activity against *B. fragilis* while cephamandole has good activity against *H. influenzae* – including ampicillin – resistant strains. There is also the possibility of cephalosporins with useful antipseudomonas activity.)

Table 14.3 Antibacterial agents *(continued)*

Drug	*Spectrum of activity*	*Route of administration*	*Toxicity and side effects*	*Other points*
Chloramphenicol	Broad spectrum. Bacteriostatic. Main use – enteric fever (Salmonellae), meningitis (especially *H. influenzae*) local for eye infections; active against rickettsiae, chlamydia, mycoplasma. Can be invaluable as '3rd choice' in severe refractory chest infections. Also active against anaerobes including most strains of *B. fragilis*. Not active against *Ps. aeruginosa*	O./i.m./i.v. topically (eyes)	Agranulocytosis, aplastic anaemia. In neonates, failure of conjugation by liver leads to 'grey baby syndrome'	Diffuses well, even into CSF without inflammation of meninges
Clindamycin Group				
Lincomycin	Similar spectrum to erythromycin (i.e. Gram positive species and some Gram negative cocci and anaerobes but not coliforms or *Ps. aeruginosa*). However less active against *H. influenzae* but more active against *Staph. aureus* and Bacteroides	O./i.v./i.m.	Pseudomembranous colitis	Excreted in bile
Clindamycin	As lincomycin but more active against *B. fragilis*	O./i.v./i.m.	Pseudomembranous colitis	Similar to lincomycin
Colistin	See under 'polymixin'			
Cotrimoxazole	See under 'sulphonamides'			
Erythromycin	Gram positive organisms and strains of *H. influenzae* and Bacteroides. Also active against myoplasma, rickettsiae and chlamydia	O./i.v. (i.m. injection very painful)	Gastric upset. Erythromycin estolate may cause jaundice if given for two or more weeks. Jaundice is not seen with other oral preparations	Excreted in bile. *Staph. aureus* rapidly develops resistance if used alone in such infections
Fusidic acid (Fusidate)	Active mainly against *Staph. aureus* although also active against many anaerobes and corynebacteria	O./i.v. (but not i.m. or s.c.)	Gastric upset	Penetrates bone well. Shows synergy with erythromycin against *Staph. aureus*

Mecillinam	See under 'penicillins'			
Metronidazole	Broad bactericidal activity against strict anaerobes including Bacteroides, fusiforms, clostridia and anaerobic cocci. Also active against amoebae, trichomonas and giardia	O./i.v./suppository	Metallic taste and anorexia-dose related. Antabuse effect if taken with alcohol. Prolonged high dosage may cause reversible peripheral neuropathy. Controversy exists about possible mutagenic properties	Penetrates all tissues and fluids. Has become drug of choice for anaerobic sepsis in UK
Nalidixic acid	Coliforms (E. coli, klebsiella, proteus) Inactive against Gram positive organisms and Pseudomonas	O.	Photosensitivity rarely. Raised intracranial pressure reported in infants. Avoid in pregnant women	Only for urinary tract infection as serum and tissue concentrations are too low
Nitrofurantoin	Coliforms, *Strep. faecalis* and staphylococci. *Not* active against Proteus (*in vivo*) or Pseudomonas	O.	Nausea and vomiting. Contra-indicated in uraemia as it further damages kidneys. Occasional peripheral neuropathy or pneumonitis. Use with caution in G-6-PD deficiency	Only for urinary tract infections as serum and tissue concentrations are too low
Novobiocin	Gram positive organisms (similar to erythromycin). Should not be used alone in *Staph. aureus* infections because of rapid emergence of resistance	O./i.m./i.v.	Rashes, thrombocytopenia. In neonates, interference with bilirubin conjugation	Biliary excretion
Penicillins				
Benzylpenicillin (penicillin G)	Gram positive organisms (especially Streptococci) also Gram negative cocci (*N. meningitidis*; *N. gonorrhoeae*) treponemes and leptospires. Susceptible to *Staph. penicillinase*	i.m./i.v.	Allergic effects. Neurotoxicity with high doses (in renal failure) or with excessive amounts intrathecally (fits, unconsciousness, myoclonic spasms, hallucinations)	
Phenoxmethylpenicillin (penicillin V)	Similar spectrum to penicillin G although markedly less active against *N. gonorrhoeae*	O.	Allergic effects	Variable absorption. Should be taken on empty stomach

Table 14.3 Antibacterial agents *(continued)*

Drug	*Spectrum of activity*	*Route of administration*	*Toxicity and side effects*	*Other points*
Benzathine penicillin	Similar spectrum	i.m.	Allergic effects. Dangerous in allergic subjects	Slow release, sustains low concentrations in patients with rheumatic fever receiving prophylaxis for streptococcal infections
Methicillin	Effective against penicillinase-producing *Staph. aureus*. Much less active than penicillin against sensitive organisms	i.m./i.v.	Allergic effects. Rarely neutropenia and	–
Flucloxacillin Cloxacillin	Effective against penicillinase-producing *Staph. aureus*. Less active against penicillin-sensitive organisms	im./i.v./o.	Allergic effects	Flucloxacillin better absorbed than cloxacillin via the oral route
Ampicillin Amoxycillin	Broader spectrum than penicillin G including also *H. influenzae*, *E. coli*, *Pr. mirabilis*, *Str. faecalis* and Salmonella. Inactive against *Klebsiella*, and Pseudomonas and destroyed by Staphylococcal penicillinase	i.m./i.v./o.	Allergic effects, gut upset, skin rashes (especially in 'glandular fever')	Ampicillin resistance common in *E. coli* and occuring in *H. influenzae* Amoxycillin better absorbed orally even in the presence of food
Carbenicillin	Broader than ampicillin including many strains of *Ps. aeruginosa* and Proteus, *E. coli*, Haemophilus, etc., resistant to ampicillin. Inactive against Klebsiella; and resistant coliforms and Pseudomonas do occur	i.v.	(a) Allergic effects Because of large doses required (20–30 g/24 h), also (b) platelet dysfunction (with bleeding, petechial haemorrhages); (c) sodium and fluid overload and hypokalaemia especially in patients with liver failure, renal failure and congestive heart failure; (d) neurotoxicity with excessive build-up of serum and CSF concentrations	–

Carfecillin	Same as carbenicillin – an ester of carbenicillin. Stable in presence of acid; is well absorbed orally and liberates carbenicillin in blood	O.	Unlikely to have side-effects associated with high dosage. It cannot be used for systemic infections as it is rapidly excreted and only achieves low serum concentrations	
Piperacillin	Similar to carbenicillin but more active. Should become available in UK in near future	i.v.	Allergic effects. Lower dosage needed than for carbenicillin. So should avoid sodium overload and hypokalaemia	–
Mecillinam	Not very active against Gram positive organisms. More active against coliforms (including ampicillin-resistant *E. coli*) and Salmonella species. Inactive against *Ps. aeruginosa* and *H. influenzae*	i.v./i.m./o.	Allergic effects. Cross allergenicity with penicillins	Achieves good concentrations
Polymixins				
Colistin (Polymixin E)	Gram negative organisms except Proteus and Providence. Active against *Ps. aeruginosa*. Not active against Staphylococci nor streptococci nor anaerobes	I.m./i.v.	Systemically – may cause nephrotoxicity and circumoral paraesthesia	Synergy with sulphonamide. Not absorbed when taken orally
Polymixin B	Similar	Too toxic for systemic use. Used orally and topically	–	–
Sulphonamides	Wide spectrum. Bacteriostatic. Sulphadiazine penetrates CSF best but risk of crystalluria. Sulphadimidine, general purpose 'sulpha'. Sulphafurazole is most soluble in urine. Active against Gram positive organisms, coliforms, *N. meningitis*, *N. gonorrhoeae*. Inactive against *Ps. aeruginosa*. Resistant strains not uncommon	O./i.v./i.m.	Rashes, crystalluria, blood, dyscrasia, Steevens-Johnson syndrome rarely. Causes bilirubin to be displaced from albumin in neonates. Never give intrathecal sulphonamide	–

Table 14.3 Antibacterial agents *(continued)*

Drug	*Spectrum of activity*	*Route of administration*	*Toxicity and side effects*	*Other points*
Cotrimoxazole (Trimethoprim and Sulphamethoxazole)	Wider spectrum than sulphonamide including Coliforms, Salmonellae, *Str. faecalis*, *H. influenzae*, Staphylococci, Brucella, and streptococci. Many anaerobes resistant, as is *Ps. aeruginosa*. Resistant strains of klebsiella and *Staph. aureus* a problem in several hospitals	O./i.v./i.m.	As for sulphonamides. Should not be used in patients allergic to sulphonamides. Should be avoided in pregnancy as animal studies have shown teratogenic effects with relatively huge doses. Neutropenia a particular hazard	
Tetracyclines including: Tetracycline, Oxytetracycline, Chlortetracycline, Doxycycline, Minocycline	Bacteriostatic action. Broad spectrum although growing number of resistant organisms including *Staph. aureus*, *Str. pyogenes* (40%), coliforms and now pneumococci. Active against anaerobes although resistance in *B. fragilis* is considerable. Active against mycoplasma, Rickettsia, Chlamydia	O./i.m.	GI upset. Candidiasis. Contra-indicated in renal failure (except doxycycline) as they cause further renal damage and impairment of function. Parenteral (especially IV) administration can cause hepatic damage. Avoid in children and pregnant women because of tooth staining and interference with bone development. Minocycline causes temporary vestibular disturbance in 10% or more of patients	Achieves good concentrations in respiratory secretions
Vancomycin	Bactericidal for Gram positive organisms including staphylococci, streptococci, clostridia, valuable for multiresistant organisms and where there is penicillin hypersensitivity	i.v.	Ototoxic, nephrotoxic. Monitor blood concentrations to achieve peak concentrations of 10–40 μg/ml	

Anti-Tuberculous Drugs				
Isoniazid	Only for *M. tuberculosis*. Very active	O./i.m.	Peripheral neuritis, pellagra, psychosis, drowsiness, agranulocytosis. Hepatitis rarely. Give pyridoxine 10 mg daily concurrently to minimize neurological complications	Resistance rare in UK. Passes into cerebrospinal fluid readily. Mainstay of treating tuberculous meningitis
Rifampicin	Broad spectrum (including Staphylococci, streptococci, bacteroides and coliforms although resistance emerges relatively easily if used alone) but should be reserved for mycobacterial infections, where it is very effective	O.	Red urine, tears and sputum. Rashes, jaundice and gut upset. Intermittent dosage may lead to hypersensitivity reaction ('flu'-like syndrome)	When combined with isoniazid, probably a greater incidence of hepatic dysfunction
Ethambutol	Only for mycobacteria. Very active	O.	Optic neuritis (check visual acuity and colour vision regularly). If caught early, damage virtually always reversible	
Streptomycin	See above under aminoglycosides			(1) Avoid in elderly and those with renal impairment because of increased ototoxic risk
Kanamycin	See above under aminoglycosides			(2) Kanamycin and amikacin may be useful where there is streptomycin-resistance
Amikacin	See above under aminoglycosides			(3) Aminoglycosides are useful (with ethambutol) where there is (severe) liver damage

Table 14.3 Antibacterial agents *(continued)*

Drug	*Spectrum of activity*	*Route of administration*	*Toxicity and side effects*	*Other points*
Paraminosalicylate	Only for tuberculosis (not highly active)	O.	Many toxic effects including hypersensitivity, nausea hypoprothrombinaemia, rashes and (rarely) hepatitis	It is not uncommon for patients to default on treatment because of GI upset, when taking this drug
Prothionamide and (ethionamide)	Bactericidal. Only mycobacteria. Cross-resistance with thiacetazone	O.	Nausea, anorexia. Rarely neurotoxic; Hepatotoxic. Teratogenic (do *not* use in pregnant women)	–
Pyrazinamide	Bactericidal. Very effective with isoniazid. Not active against bovine strains of *M. tuberculosis*	O.	Hepatotoxic. Blood transaminase levels and bilirubin should be regularly checked. May also precipitate attacks of gout	–
Cycloserine	Weakly active against Mycobacteria. In combination helps prevent resistance developing to other (more effective) drugs. 'Broad spectrum' against coliforms	O.	Neurotoxic – including depression, excitability and other disturbances. If this happens stop drug immediately	–
Thiacetazone	Only against mycobacteria. Cross resistance with prothionamide	O.	Rashes, nausea, vomiting, dizziness. (Side effects reported more frequently when used in Indian sub-continent than when used in Africa)	–

References

Garrod, L. P., Lambert, H. P. and O'Grady, F. *Antibiotics and Chemotherapy*, 3rd edn. London; Livingstone

Kucers, A, and Bennett, N, Mck. (1975). *The Use of Antibiotics*, 2nd edn. London; Heinemann

Mawer *et al.* (1974). *British Journal of Pharmacology*, **1**, 45

15 Allergy and rhinitis

L H Capel

> 'The vaccinated person behaves . . . in a different manner from him who has not previously been in contact with such an agent. Yet he is not insensitive to it. We can only say of him that his power to react has undergone a change. For this general concept of *changed reactivity* I propose the term *allergy* . . .'
> Von Pirquet 1906.

Allergy is the specifically altered state of the host after contact with a specific allergen. Further contact with the allergen can have the clinical consequences of *immunity*, which protects from tissue damage, of *hypersensitivity* which is tissue damaging, and of both in the same host. It is possible that these very different clinical consequences may have biological mechanisms which are qualitatively similar.

Rhinitis is a clinically defined condition present if there are one or more of the symptoms of sneezing, running nose and blocked nasal airway. If from clinical or experimental evidence a tissue-damaging allergic hypersensitivity process can be inferred as the cause of the symptoms rhinitis may be qualified as allergic. If no such process can be discovered or inferred as the cause of symptoms it may be qualified as non-allergic. In most patients this distinction can be made. Features typical of a patient with symptoms arising from allergic hypersensitivity are:

(1) a history of symptoms after exposure to a particular substance or season;
(2) a family history of this;
(3) skin prick test positive for one or more of the common allergens.

Common allergens in the United Kingdom are house dust, grass pollens *Aspergillus fumigatus* and cat. It must at once be emphasized that a positive skin prick test reaction draws attention to the patient's constitutional predisposition to react in that way; it does *not* necessarily indicate the symptom-causing allergen. Persons in whom this constitutional predisposition can be demonstrated are more likely to be in the first half of life.

The management of rhinitis is perhaps best indicated by what the patient has to say about the symptoms and by the response to treatment, leading to an empirical and critical use (or omission) of drugs and possibly some change of living habits. An understanding of tissue-damaging allergic reactions is, at the present (1978), perhaps more of academic help in the discussion of causes of disorder and of the successes and failures of management. In the future, however, such an understanding is likely to dictate the management not only of certain forms of rhinitis, asthma and skin disorder, but also of a wide range of human disorder. With the current explosion of knowledge this future seems to approach fast.

This chapter, it is hoped, will be a helpful introduction to the understanding of the nature of allergy, especially its tissue hypersensitivity reactions as they might affect the nose.

Allergy

Allergy is an activity of lymphocytes, their progenitors in the bone marrow and their derivatives in blood and lymphatic and other tissues. These act in association with macrophages, and commonly with polymorphonuclear leucocytes and blood and tissue enzymes including the complement enzyme system. The reaction is set off by a foreign substance entering the body. A first intrusion by a specific foreign substance, an allergen, can set off a non-specific *attack* on the intruder substance and a specific information storage: *memory*. Macrophages take up the foreign material, process it in ways unknown and hand the processed material over to certain lymphocytes with which they come in contact. Thus specifically sensitized, these lymphocytes and their progeny henceforth react to reject subsequent intrusions by the specific allergen.

The clinical consequences of allergy, then, may be immunity, or hypersensitivity or both. From the immune response no symptoms ensue. From the hypersensitivity response ensue symptoms: in the nose these may be sneezing, running and block; in the lungs they may be cough, expectoration and wheeze. The clinical consequences of most hypersensitivity responses in most individuals is transient, for example in hay fever. In some responses in some individuals, however, inflammation may proceed to fibrosis and permanent change, for example in Farmer's lung.

This allergic reaction may be directly by contact of allergen with specifically-sensitized lymphocytes, or indirectly by contact of the allergen with specific immunoglobulins produced by plasma cells in lymph and spleen which are derived from specifically-sensitized lymphocytes. This contact of allergen with specific immunoglobulin can facilitate phagocytosis, for example of bacteria. These specific immunoglobulins are antibodies.

Antibody-mediated tissue damaging reactions can depend on the reaction of allergen with antibody attached to mast cells in the connective tissue of mucous membranes, and the reaction can depend on the formation of complexes of allergen and antibody. These complexes can later involve the complement system and then polymorphonuclear leucocytes. The *complement system* is a series of linked-action enzymes which by chain reaction amplifies the consequences of allergen/antibody complex formation. Different patterns of tissue-damaging allergic hypersensitivity reactions have been modelled, as will be seen.

It is of passing interest to note that the allergy process can be likened to a biological information system in which the processes of memory, reaction, feedback and amplification can be recognized.

Host defence

All living species must successfully defend themselves against virus and bacterial infection and parasite infestation. The defence can be non-specific and it can be allergic. If allergic, the consequence can be immunity and it can be hypersensitivity. In any defence episode all these processes may be at work, but typically one will dominate.

Non-specific host defence

The skin and the mucous membranes with their liquid and usually moving covering provide barrier defence. This barrier is strengthened by commensal organisms which compete with pathogens. In the tissue liquids beyond the barrier are antimicrobial substances and wandering and fixed phagocyte cells of the reticulo-endothelial system.

Allergic defence

Allergic defence is initiated by the intruder, be it virus, bacteria, parasite or chemical, and specific for it. If chemical, it can initiate a specific allergic response only after it has linked to a body protein: such chemicals are called *haptens*. Some chemicals acting in this way, for example, platinum salts, are exceedingly potent causes of hypersensitization.

Specific host defence–allergy

Replenished by the bone marrow, there is a constant traffic of lymphocytes and their derivatives between the blood and the lymphoid tissues – the thymus, the spleen and the lymph nodes. These cells of the lymphatic series move also between the blood and all the tissues of the body.

As the newly formed cells pass from bone marrow they are processed in one of two ways to become:

T lymphocytes – processed in the thymus or by by-products of the thymus;
B lymphocytes – processed (probably) in the gut lymphatic tissue including (probably) tonsils, Peyer's patches and appendix.

In chickens the Bursa of Fabricius, a lymphoid organ near the cloaca, has been identified as a modified organ for this group of lymphocytes, influencing the development of Bursa-dependent lymphocytes or (in other animals by analogy) B lymphocytes.

An appropriate antigen stimulates either T or B lymphocytes to differentiate and proliferate, and in the case of B lymphocytes to synthesize antibodies specific for the allergen. It is a popular hypothesis that this is a specific reaction of clones of cells each of which can respond only to one or a few of all possible antigenic determinants.

An antigen activates B lymphocytes after it is transported to lymph nodes or spleen and T lymphocytes which gather at antigen deposit sites. Antigen can activate lymphocytes only after ingestion and processing by macrophages. Macrophages in contact with lymphocytes then pass on the processed allergenic material via cytoplasmic bridges. Without such macrophage-processing lymphocytes can not be activated. Further, the raw unprocessed allergen can induce tolerance rather than immunity or hypersensitivity.

The response of B cells to allergen which results in their forming antibodies depends on T cells (helper cells) processing or presenting the allergen to the B cells.

Specifically-sensitized T cells can be activated at the site of entry of the allergen. The allergen may, indeed, be tissue-fixed, for example transplant cells and skin or tissue impregnated with bacterial product. Specifically-activated lymphocytes move off to stimulate proliferation of other lymphocytes in the cortical regions of lymph nodes and the white pulp of spleen. These specifically-sensitized T cells act in direct contact with allergens. The instruments of specifically-sensitized T cell action include:

Specific antibody generated by B cells but attached to the T cell. This may be a feature of the Helper mechanism. The B cells make no antibody themselves.

Transfer factor, a low molecular weight extract of T cells which can transfer T cell specific sensitivity to other animals.

Macrophage migration inhibition factor (MIF) inhibits migration of macrophages from the site, presumably increasing the allergic efficiency of T cells at the site when these are exposed to allergen.

Specific macrophage arming factor (SMAF) is released by T cells sensitized by tumour: these give macrophages selective power to kill tumour cells.

Monocyte chemotactic factor induces monocytes to move towards it.

Skin reactive factor increases capillary permeability, which may facilitate the passages of cells and mediators of the allergic process to the tissues.

Other soluble factors also are present. It seems that only a small proportion of cells taking part in a T cell-mediated allergic reaction are specific. These attract other non-sensitized cells to take part in the reaction, and some specifically-sensitized cells thus move off to initiate the generation of more of their kind.

Specifically-sensitized B cells can be activated by soluble allergen and allergen which can be carried to regional lymph nodes or spleen. The allergen is captured by follicular reticular cells and macrophage in the lymph follicles, processed by them and passed on to lymphocytes. These sensitized lymphocytes transform to plasma cells and pass to the medullary cords of lymph nodes and the red pulp of spleen. Here they stay, manufacturing antibody which passes via efferent lymphatics to blood and tissues. Thus the specifically-sensitized B cells act at a distance. Their instruments of action are the immunoglobulins (Ig), complex proteins of molecular weight 150–900 000 which function as antibodies. Antibody immunoglobulins are Y-shaped. Their function is related to domains in their structure: specific antigen binding (the two arms), complement fixation (the stem) and biological activity such as mast cell binding and passage through membranes (the foot). *Figure 15.1* shows this in crude diagrammatic detail. The general outline of the appearance, inferred from biochemical studies, has been confirmed by electron microscopy.

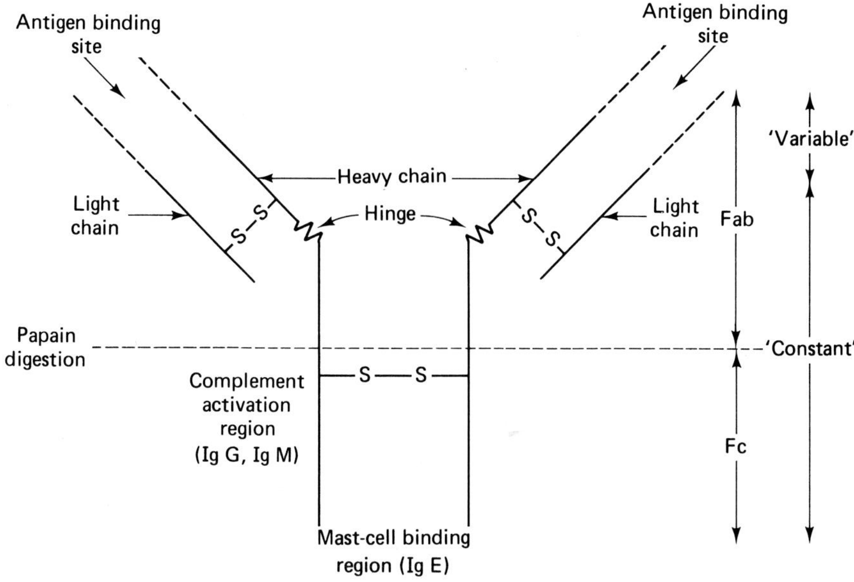

Figure 15.1 The Y-shaped immunoglobulin (Ig) molecule consists of two heavy chains and two light chains. The tips of the arms of the Y (---) are of 'variable' amino-acid structure: they are the antigen binding sites. The rest of the structure is of 'constant' amino-acid sequence structure. Papain digestion (- - -) divides the molecule into two antigen binding fractions (Fab) and one crystallizable fraction (Fc). The Fc portion contains a region responsible for complement activation (IgG and Igm) and a region for mast-cell binding (IgE). When specific antigen binds two adjacent IgE molecules fixed to a mast cell the two Fab portions drop at the hinge, and the mast cell disgorges its granules. This structure can be detected on electron microscopy. – S – S – sulphadryl groups

Classes of immunoglobulins

There are five classes of immunoglobulin, IgG, IgA, IgM, IgD, and IgE in descending order of concentration in serum. Each functions differently in the allergic processes, and they may function in serial and simultaneous cooperation, sometimes one dominating, sometimes another.

Micro-organisms are the common allergens. Each is a minute bundle of antigens. They elicit the typical allergic response. IgM (called a macroglobulin because of its large molecular weight) is produced first. It fixes complement well, facilitating lysis and phagocytosis of cells. IgG is produced second, and in largest quantity; it diffuses more readily than other immunoglobulins into extravascular spaces. It is thus good for neutralizing toxins and it can enhance phagocytosis. IgG can form complexes which precipitate and in certain circumstances it can fix antigens. IgA is concentrated in tears, saliva, sweat and the mucous secretions of the nose, bronchial tree and gut. It seems to be especially important for protecting the gut from micro-organisms, and it is especially efficient at virus neutralization. IgA aided by complement and lysozyme can lyse certain gram-negative bacteria. IgA is produced by plasma cells in the mucous membranes and transported to the lining secretions by association with secretory piece, a component secreted by the lining cells. The IgA-secretory piece combination protects this antibody from digestion in the gut. The function of IgD is unknown. IgE is present in only minute concentration in serum. Its characteristic feature is fixation to mast cells. Its function is unknown, but it has been suggested that it may play a part in resisting helmith infection; the serum IgE level certainly rises on infestation by them.

Recognition of T and B cells

Lymphocytes may be identified as B cells by fluorescent anti-immunoglobulin, and as T cells by spontaneous rosette formation with uncoated sheep erythrocytes. T and B cells can be distinguished morphologically by electron microscopy.

Clinical consequences of allergy

The clinical consequences of allergy are immunity and hypersensitivity. (There can also be immune tolerance which will not be discussed.) On the basis of animal models, Lachman (1975) suggested that there are four Modes of Allergic Reaction resulting clinically in immunity, and four Types of Allergic Reaction resulting clinically in tissue-damaging hypersensitivity. The Modes and Types of reaction may operate serially and simultaneously: characteristically one reaction will predominate, certainly so at a given moment. It is possible also that both immunity and tissue-damaging reaction to the same allergen can co-exist, one predominating.

The components of the Modes and Types of reaction include antigens, macrophages, T and B lymphocytes, non-specific lymphocytes, polymorphs, monocytes, antibodies, active substances released from cells, complement and other enzymes, and the cells of affected tissues.

Though their clinical consequences are so different, there are inevitably close resemblances between the biological models proposed for the modes of immunity reaction and the (more widely accepted) types of tissue-damaging hypersensitivity reaction.

Hypersensitivity

Allergic hypersensitivity predisposes to tissue damage. The processes of allergic hypersensitivity are lymphatic reactions of two sorts: indirect action by sensitized B lymphocytes via antibodies in contact with antigens, and direct action by sensitized T lymphocytes themselves in close contact with antigen. These two sorts of reaction may be called antibody-mediated and sensitized-cell-mediated respectively in terms of the agent apparently in closest contact with antigen, though both are, of course, actions of sensitized (or allergized) cells.

After antigen challenge in sensitized individuals antibody-mediated reactions develop faster than sensitized-cell-mediated reactions. Sensitized-cell-mediated hypersensitivity is therefore called delayed hypersensitivity. On the basis of animal experiments Gell and Coombs (1975) described three types of antibody-dependent tissue-damaging hypersensitivity reactions (Types I, II, and III) and one type of directly-acting sensitized-cell-mediated hypersensitivity (Type IV). In any tissue-damaging allergic hypersensitivity reaction one Type will dominate, but others may take part also, serially or simultaneously, and Modes of immunity may be at work as well. For example, a positive Mantoux test is a Type IV (delayed) tissue-damaging allergic hypersensitivity reaction in an individual likely to have developed a greater immunity to tuberculous infection than one who does not respond in this way.

Types of tissue-damaging allergic hypersensitivity reaction

All forms of allergic reaction depend on processes stemming ultimately from reactions of specific antigens with the products of specifically-sensitized lymphocytes. The processes are of two sorts: those in which the cellular progeny of specifically-sensitized lymphocytes react directly, that is in contact with a specific antigen, and those in which antibodies derived from specifically-sensitized cells react with a specific antigen. If the reaction is tissue-damaging allergic hypersensitivity, then the two processes are respectively cell-mediated hypersensitivity and antibody-mediated hypersensitivity.

Gell and Coombs (1975) have classified the tissue damaging allergic hypersensitivity reaction into four reaction types based on animal models: Types I, II and III are antibody-mediated; Type IV is cell-mediated, as mentioned above.

In the Type I reaction antibody is fixed to certain cells in the connective tissue of mucous membranes (tissue-fixed antibody) and antigen is free in serum and tissue fluids: antigen reacts with cell-fixed antibody on the cell surface. In the Type II reaction antigen is fixed to certain cells (cell-fixed antigen), and antibody is free in serum: antibody acts on cell-fixed antigen on the cell surface. In the Type III reaction both antigen and antibody are free in tissue-fluid or in serum, and these react forming complexes which may be insoluble and precipitate, or soluble and deposit elsewhere in tissues. In the Type IV reaction specific antigen reacts directly with the specifically-sensitized cells, and antibody is not known to take part: typically the reaction is localized to the entry site of the allergen.

The mechanisms of four types of tissue-damaging reactions

(I) Tissue damage is a consequence of enzymes released from the cells to which reacting antibody is fixed.

(II) Tissue damage is a consequence of activation of enzymes free in the tissues adjacent, or of stimulation of phagocytosis.

(III) Tissue damage is a consequence of activation of enzyme systems in the tissues, of release of enzymes from attracted polymorphs and of release of enzymes from involved platelets.

(IV) Tissue damage is a consequence of enzymes and substances released from the sensitized-cell in contact with antigen and of the actions of macrophages stimulated by certain of the released substances.

Usually one of these reactions predominates. More than one can develop serially or coincidentally, however. These reactions will now be discussed in detail.

Type I

The Type I reaction may also be called an *immediate reaction* because of its rapid onset, usually at a maximum within 20 min. Historically it may be called *reagin-dependent*, after the reaginic antibody, the name given before IgE was discovered. The term *anaphylactic* is often used, but sometimes to describe the clinical consequences of the Type I reaction, sometimes to describe the mechanism: historically it has been used to describe certain consequences of Type II and Type III reactions.

The main antibody responsible for the Type I reaction is an immunoglobulin classified as IgE, present only in minute concentration in serum. Its characteristic feature is a tendency to fix to the surface membrane of basophil polymorphonuclear granular leucocytes. These are called basophils in the blood and mast cells in connective tissue. The basophilic granules in the basophils contain enzymes. Basophils in the connective tissue of the mucous membranes of the eyes, nose, bronchial tree, skin and gut are of special clinical importance.

A mast cell has a limited number of receptor sites for the foot-piece of the IgE antibodies: perhaps 100 000. The attached Y-shaped antibodies may be imagined, arms in the air, bristling on the surface of the allergized mast cell. Antigen capture can precipitate a response only if the antigen molecule simultaneously involves the arms of two adjacent antibody molecules. The arms of the antibody molecules then drop to the surface of the mast cell membrane. This initiates a process which results in the liberation of granules from the mast cell. The process involves changes in the cell membrane and the adenylcyclase-cyclic AMP system within the cell and entry of calcium into the cell. The cell is not destroyed in the process. The released granules contain pharmacologically active substances, which are liberated. In man these substances include histamine and probably the slow reacting substance of anaphylaxis (SRS-A).

IgG also can fix to mast cells: it is much less avid for this than IgE, and short-lasting in its attachment. It is of no known clinical importance.

Histamine contracts smooth muscle, including bronchiolar muscle, increases blood vessel permeability, constricts venules (tending to oedema) and increases secretion of lachrymal, nasal, and possibly bronchial glands.

Release of histamine from mast cells may have a physiological function involving dilution of antigen by oedema, attraction of phagocytes and facilitation of tissue repair. Antihistaminic drugs resemble histamine clinically: presumably they block tissue receptor sites preventing histamine action. (Incidentally, antihistamines are also anaesthetic and anticholinergic: this must contribute to any apparent therapeutic effect.) Antihistamines can temporarily reduce the severity of hay fever and the magnitude of the immediate response to skin prick testing through antigen. They have no clinically apparent effect on the severity of allergic asthma. It is suggested that this is because SRS-A is the important pharmacological mediator in asthma. The chemical nature of SRS-A is unknown. Its action is prolonged. No clinically useful SRS-A antagonist has yet been proven (1978). The Type I tissue-damaging allergic hypersensitivity reaction may in theory and sometimes in practice be controlled by:

(1) Counteracting the effects of pharmacological mediators: adrenergic, cholinergic and anti-inflammatory corticosteroid drugs.
(2) Blocking the pharmacological mediators: antihistaminic and, when they are developed, antiSRS-A drugs.
(3) Stabilizing the mast-cell membrane so preventing the release of granules: sodium cromoglycate (and other drugs of similar function now being developed), corticosteroids and adrenergic drugs.
(4) Preventing access of antigen to the mast cell: hyposensitization by injection of increasing doses of antigen. The vaccine is thought to stimulate a development of circulating IgG antibody specific for the antigen and possibly development of specific IgA antibody in mucous membrane. These antibodies, it is thought, would unite with antigens so blocking their access to tissue-fixed IgE antibody on the mast cell: the vaccine is said to stimulate blocking antibody. It has been suggested also that such vaccine might induce tolerance in the T cells which should otherwise be helpers of the antibody-producing B cells. The hopeful use of vaccines in this way is a ritual hallowed by convention rather than conclusive experiment. In the United Kingdom only grass pollen vaccine for hay fever has any proven place in routine clinical practice. Adequately controlled trials of properly standardized vaccines have yet to be made.
(5) Flooding the mast cell receptor sites with non-specific foot-pieces (fc) of the IgE antibody (*see Figure 15.1*).
(6) Avoiding contact with the antigen.

The atopic constitution

The tendency to respond to the common allergens of the environment by the ready production of IgE antibodies specific for one or more of them varies between individuals. About one individual in ten can be identified as a ready producer of specific IgE antibody by use of the skin prick test for one or more of the common allergens: (in the UK) house dust including the house dust mite, grass pollen, cat and the moulds cladosporium and aspergillus. A drop of extract of the material is placed on the forearm and pricked through with a very fine sharp needle by introducing it just sufficiently to enable a gentle lifting of the skin. A weal and flare, with itching, develops within minutes and is at a maximum in about 20 min if the reaction is positive. A positive reaction to one or more of the commonly encountered allergens identifies the subject as a ready producer of specific IgE antibody: such individuals are said to be of atopic constitution. It does not necessarily follow that they suffer symptoms on account of any of the antigens which produce a positive skin test: a positive skin test for grass pollens without hay fever is common, for example.

Where there is, for example, both a positive skin test for grass pollen and symptoms of hay fever, then it is common for blood relatives also to be affected. The atopic constitution tends to run in families. The development of symptoms attributable to the atopic state early in life, eczema in infancy, positive skin tests to a large number of allergens and a tendency to more severe allergic rhinitis or asthma tend to go together.

The earlier in life rhinitis or asthma presents, the more likely it is that the patient will be found to have an atopic constitution: patients in whom these conditions begin in the second half of life are less likely to be of atopic constitution.

The development of specific IgE antibodies in atopic subjects appears to be a consequence of contact of the relevant antigens with the mucous lining of nose, bronchial tree and gut, events which do not lead to the development of IgE antibodies in non-atopic subjects. Injection of the antigen, for example in skin or muscle, affects atopic subjects no differently from non-atopic subjects.

Secretory IgA is the immunoglobulin characteristic of mucous membranes. Since IgA deficiency is commoner in atopic than in non-atopic subjects it has been suggested that atopic subjects might suffer a mucous membrane defect associated with decrease in secretory IgA activity.

Why atopic individuals on exposure to allergen respond some with rhinitis, some with asthma, some with skin and gut symptoms, some sometimes with one symptom and sometimes with another, and some never with any symptoms is unknown. Other features, including disturbances of function of the cell wall and of autonomic nerve transmission, may also be at work.

IgE

Identification of the reaginic antibody, now known as IgE, in serum was achieved from the interpretation of Prausnitz and Kustner's classic and simple experiment in 1921. Kustner was hypersensitive to fish. Prausnitz (incidentally a hay fever sufferer) was not. A small quantity of Kustner's serum was injected into the skin of Prausnitz's forearm. After a delay of a few hours this site was challenged with fish extract; a weal and flare developed, though none developed when the extract was injected elsewhere in the arm. During the waiting period the reaginic antibody became fixed to the skin mast cells (tissue-fixed) and other antibody was neutralized and cleared. For many years this was the only way in which the existence of reaginic tissue-fixing antibodies in serum could be demonstrated. It is an example of that passive transfer of allergic hypersensitivity which is a feature of the Type I and Type III reactions.

IgE is produced in plasma cells found mainly in the lymphoid tissue around the mucous and serous glands of the nose, bronchial tree and gut, including the tonsils and adenoids.

RAST

Specific IgE levels in serum can now be measured in serum by the Radio-Allergo-Sorbent Test (RAST). So measured, these levels variously are related to the history and the results of skin and provocation tests in about three instances in four. For clinical purposes the RAST has no advantage over the history and prick testing. For academic study, and above all for the standardization of antigens for diagnostic and in time therapeutic use, it is of great importance. In serial studies of IgE levels by the RAST it has been found that specific IgE levels wax and wane with the levels of allergen exposure, while total serum IgE levels remain unchanged. Serial measurements could help in demonstrating that exposure to an allergen was responsible for symptoms, for example in an industrial Type I allergy or where it is uncertain whether a substance is both allergenic and the cause of symptoms.

Type II

Type II reactions involve cell-bound antigens. The cell-bound antigen complexing with antibody results in the destruction of the cell. Hence the name cytotoxic hypersensitivity. Commonly the cells are formed elements of the blood (which include platelets). Cell damage results from facilitation of phagocytosis or from activation of part or all of the complement system of enzymes. It has been suggested also that antibody complexed with antigen on the cell surface might attract groups of mononuclear cells of uncertain sort, which cells, Killer cells, then destroy the cell holding the antigen-antibody on its surface. This process, it has been further suggested, might play a part in the rejection of parasites and tumours. Clinical consequences of Type II hypersensitivity include transfusion reactions and Rhesus incompatibility, certain auto-allergic reactions and some drug reactions.

Type III

In the Type III reaction, unlike the Type I and Type II reactions, neither the antigen nor antibody are cell bound: antibody free in blood and tissue fluids awaits antigen free in blood and tissue fluids. IgG is the antibody involved.

The Type III reaction proceeds after a complex of antigen and antibody are deposited in blood-vessel walls. The antigen-antibody complex so deposited then activates components of the complement system of enzymes. This activation of complement attracts polymorphs. Polymorphs accumulate and phagocytize the complexes. These involved polymorphs then liberate proteolytic enzymes which damage the walls of the blood vessels in which the complexes have deposited. Deposition of complexes is facilitated by, and indeed may require, prior increase in vascular permeability. Such increase in vascular permeability can arise, it is suggested, from a Type I reaction which releases vasoactive amines. Thus a Type I reaction may be required to initiate a Type III reaction.

The formation of immune complexes is not necessarily tissue-damaging. If, however, there are relatively high concentrations of antigen and specific IgG antibody, then a Type III tissue-damaging reaction may develop. The reaction can remain local if complexes are developed and remain local, and the reaction can be generalized if complexes develop in the bloodstream where they are carried to the tissues of organs throughout the body.

The animal model of the local Type III reaction is named after Arthus who first described it. Clinical examples of Arthus-like reactions are extrinsic allergic alveolitis arising from inhalation of thermophilic actinomycetes (Farmers' lung), and from inhalation of similar antigens in mouldy sugar cane (bagassosis) and mushrooms (mushroom pickers' lung). Inhalation of serum proteins in the faeces of pigeons and budgerigars can cause illness in their keepers (bird fanciers' lung). The illness may or may not present with wheeze, breathlessness, cough and fever some hours after each exposure. It can proceed to lung fibrosis. Injection of antigen in the skin of the sufferer causes an Arthus-like reaction of oedema and redness some 6 h after injection. In subjects who are atopic as well, a preliminary Type I weal and flare reaction may also be seen.

Soluble antigen-antibody complexes developing within the circulation can be carried throughout the body. They can lodge in any tissue of the body, damaging the structure and functions of organs. Nephritis, arthritis and carditis, for example, can result. Immune complex disorders may be transient or progressive. They can be initiated by drugs and vaccines (serum sickness) and by virus and bacterial infection and parasite infestation. Serum sickness was a dreaded complication of serum therapy before the antibiotic era. The process may also be initiated by some degeneration of the body's own tissues (auto-allergic or auto-immune disorders).

Type IV

The Type IV reaction is set off by the specifically-sensitized cell in contact with its antigen, this contact resulting in changes within the cell and liberation from within it of a number of substances (lymphokines) which are the mediators of the reaction. This specifically-sensitized cell is a circulating lymphocyte. Thus in the Type IV reaction the specifically-sensitized cell mediates the reaction and it may be called the sensitized-cell-mediated hypersensitivity reaction.

Specific sensitized-cell-mediated hypersensitivity may be passively transferred to another non-sensitized animal of the same species by transfer of sensitized cells, but not by transfer of serum. Since the reaction is delayed some 24–72 h it is also called the *delayed hypersensitivity reaction*. Thus the Type IV reaction contrasts with Types I, II, and III in which the sensitized cell is the plasma cell remaining in lymphoid tissue discharging its antibodies into efferent lymphatics. Types I, II and III are antibody-mediated reactions and Type IV is a sensitized-cell-mediated reaction. The antibody-mediated reactions may be passively transferred by serum (Type I – the P.K. reaction) and by antibody-antigen-complement complexes (Type III). Type I is immediate in onset (10–20 min), Type III intermediate (about 6 h) and Type IV delayed (24–72 h).

As with all allergic hypersensitivity and immune reactions the Type IV reaction is initiated by macrophage-processed antigen. The processed antigen combines with specific sites on the surface of the sensitized cell of the T series. Transformation and mitosis follow, with liberation of lymphokines. These lymphokines activate macrophages. The activated (angry) macrophages are responsible for the tissue damage. They are responsible also for killing bacteria and possibly foreign and tumour cells.

A number of lymphokines have been described. The most important is macrophage migration inhibition factor (MIF). This inhibits migration of macrophages from the site and activates them for damage. It can transform macrophages which allow tubercle bacilli to grow within them to macrophages which kill the tubercle. If tumour cells are attacked by T cells sensitized to them a specific macrophage arming factor (SMAF) is invoked. The lymphokines attract mononuclear cells to the lesions, and probably only a minority of the cells involved in the reaction are specifically sensitized lymphocytes.

The clinical consequences of the Type IV reaction include responses to injection, chemical contact, insect bites and homograft rejection.

The typical Type IV infection response is the tuberculin reaction: a perivascular infiltration of monocytes consisting of a majority of lymphocytes and a minority of macrophages developing 24–72 h after intradermal injection of tuberculin. Tuberculous cavitation, caseation and toxaemia and tuberculoid leprosy are other examples. Cell-mediated hypersensitivity is a feature also of certain virus infections (skin lesions in smallpox, measles and herpes simplex), protozoal diseases (Leishmaniasis and schistosomiasis) and fungus diseases (coccidiomycosis, histoplasmosis).

Foreign substances which can bind to body proteins to form antigens can initiate the Type IV hypersensitivity, especially by skin contact. Typical examples include nickel salts (nickel suspenders) neomycin in ointments, the primula plant and poison ivy, picryl chloride and chromates. Thus many examples of industrial contact hypersensitivity are a consequence of Type IV hypersensitivity. Some forms of skin reaction to insect bites are cell-mediated.

In allograft rejection after organ and tissue transplantation it is probable that both cell-mediated and antibody-mediated reactions occur. Whether cancerous tissue is ever controlled by these mechanisms is unknown: immunological surveillance, so-called, has been suggested. Auto-allergic disorder, commonly called auto-immune disorder, is suggested as a consequence of an individual developing damaging hypersensitivity against his *own* tissues. Thyroid and adrenal disorders are examples.

Further study

It will be apparent that the distinctions between allergic immunity and allergic tissue-damaging hypersensitivity are based on models convenient for study and discussion. Immune reactions also are commonly tissue-damaging, but the tissue is commonly bacterial, viral and parasitic invaders and hence foreign to the host. Further, tissue-damage of the host can protect, as in transudations of vascular liquids and cells. It is possible that as more is discovered and understood, then the modes of immunity and the types of tissue-damaging hypersensitivity will come to be described as entities.

At present the management of rhinitis and asthma in the United Kingdom is usually empirical, and most sufferers can be helped by critical use of drugs. In some the drugs have troublesome unwanted effects, and in some their help is inadequate: these sufferers will in future be helped by new knowledge and better understanding of the mechanisms of tissue-damaging hypersensitivity reactions.

References

Gell, P. G. H., Coombes, R. R. A. and Lachman, P.J. (1975). *Clinical Aspects of Immunology*, 3rd edn. London; Blackwell

Mygind, N. (1978). *Nasal Allergy*. Oxford; Blackwell

Roitt, Ivan (1977). *Essential Immunology*, 2nd edn. Oxford; Blackwell

Turk, J. L. (1972). *Immunology in Clinical Medicine*, 2nd edn. London; Heinemann

16 The principles of cancer immunology with particular reference to head and neck cancer

Peter Clifford

'Seek simplicity and distrust it'
Alfred North Whitehead
in *Concepts of Nature* (1920)

Introduction

Interest and the study of cancer immunology developed in the early part of this century, inspired by the therapeutic advances of Pasteur, von Behring, Kitsato and others, in the vaccine treatment of rabies, cholera, tetanus and diphtheria. Paul Ehrlich considered that techniques developed actively to immunize or passively transfer immunity might be developed and used against cancer. Bacteriologists had developed techniques of using pure or attenuated organisms to develop resistance in persons at risk and in those who had acquired infection and were non-resistant; antibacterial sera were used to transfer passive resistance.

The early application of these methods in laboratory animal tumour systems and in human cancer clinics led to confusing and conflicting reports. Ignorance of tissue antigen systems and the rejection of tumour transplants due to *histo-incompatibility* factors led to erroneous claims that the administration of different tumour extracts and indeed bacterial preparations such as Coley's Toxins (Nauts, Fowler and Bogako, 1953) had resulted in the regression of existing cancers in man or the rejection of subsequent tumour transplants in laboratory animals.

The development of pure inbred strains of laboratory animals all genetically identical (syngeneic) enabled tumour rejection due to host and specific tumour factors to be differentiated. The normal tissue cells of these pure-bred animal strains are antigenically similar.

Histocompatibility or transplantation antigens

Antigens are glycoproteins found mainly on the cell membrane but also in the cytoplasm or nucleus. Normally, man or a laboratory animal accepts cells with the same antigen configuration as 'self' and without reaction, but reacts to 'non-self antigens' by the production of an immunoglobulin antibody. Antigens may be defined as molecular structures capable of stimulating the production of a specific antibody, and both usually combine readily. There are a large number of possible glycoprotein combinations (glycoprotein, protein, lipid, lipoprotein, lipopolysaccharide, polypeptide-lipopolysaccharide), but the cellular arrangement of these molecules is governed genetically. Some combinations have been determined, i.e. blood groups; others are referred to as *histocompatibility* or *transplantation* antigens. These are situated on the surface of nucleated cells and determine the antigenic specificity of the individual. It is now known that in man, monkeys, dogs, rats and chickens histocompatibility antigens (HCA) are *genetically determined* by a single major gene locus and a number of minor loci. In man the major locus is referred to as the HLA locus. This system is referred to as the histocompatibility or transplantation antigen system as tissue grafting is most likely to be successful between individuals with similar systems, e.g. identical twins. Similarly normal tissue grafts between highly inbred or syngeneic rodents does not lead to rejection because both donor and recipient have similar histocompatibility or transplantation antigen systems. Since malignant cells develop from normal cells it is not surprising that most of the chemical components of the normal cell are expressed in the malignant cell including HCA. But variations from the normal cell components occur, new antigens may appear, normal antigens may be lost or changed in concentration, and antigens characteristic of normal embryonic or fetal tissue, normally lost or repressed during maturation of the cell, may reappear (*Figure 16.1*).

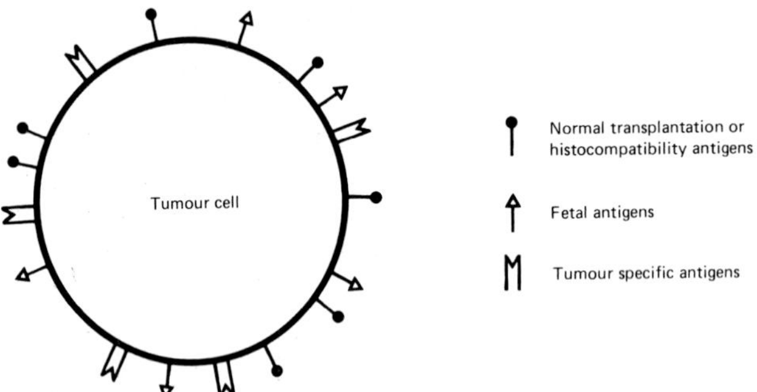

Figure 16.1 Diagrammatic representation of antigen groups which may be represented on tumour cell surface

Tumour-specific transplantation antigens (TSTA)

Some experimental tumours induced in laboratory animals by chemical or viral agents will be rejected by syngeneic recipients because of the presence of additional antigenic components on the cell surface which leads the host to recognize the transplant as 'non-self' or foreign, and may lead to an immune response and rejection. This has led to the conclusion that tumour immunity is probably a special form of transplantation immunity and that the reaction provoked by a tumour inoculation is similar to that responsible for graft rejection (Bach, 1974; Bagshawe,

1974). TSTAs are thought to be glycoprotein molecules, and structural similarities have been found between normal HCAs and TSTAs (Invernizzi and Parmiani, 1975).

Animal laboratory studies have shown very important differences between tumours induced by viral and chemical or physical (irradiation or implantation of multiple filters) carcinogens. Tumour-specific antigens associated with tumours induced by a particular virus are the same for all tumours induced by that virus irrespective of the animal species developing the tumour or the organ system involved. In contrast, tumours induced by chemical or physical agents are specific and different for each particular tumour, so that different tumours induced in the same animal by the same chemical will carry different distinctive tumour antigens (Alexander, 1965). However the TSTA system may be more complex as 'individual' antigens have been identified in virally-induced tumours and some chemically-induced tumours may carry common antigenic properties (Reiner and Southam, 1967).

The histological or morphological appearance does not relate to the TSTA system. Histologically similar tumours may carry entirely different TSTAs and conversely histologically different tumours may carry identical TSTAs, which may indicate a common viral aetiology.

Evidence of immune resistance to cancer in experimental animals

The discovery that many of the early tumour graft rejection experiments resulted, not from a developed host resistance, but from inherited histo-incompatibility differences, led to a disbelief that tumour resistance might have a significant anticancer role. Thomas (1959) was the first to suggest that allograft rejection due to histo-incompatibility might have evolved as a defence against neoplastic disease, and Burnet (1967, 1970) postulated that the immune system has evolved to protect the species against the effects of spontaneous mutagenic cell replication. Such cells would be recognized as 'foreign' and would be killed off so that the species would be preserved from the effects of haphazard abnormal cell reduplication. Burnet applied the term '*immunological surveillance*' to this phenomenon.

Immune reactions operate through the lymphoid system. This system first developed in primitive fishes and all animal species phylogenetically distal to those have a lymphoid system which it is thought conferred a survival advantage. But paradoxically, animal forms with a lymphoid system are highly susceptible to total body irradiation and chemical carcinogens, whereas species lacking a lymphoid system are extremely resistant to irradiation and chemical carcinogens and rarely develop malignancy. It is considered that the higher forms of animal life could only have evolved successfully if their adaptive evolution had been controlled by a developing immune system, for as the capacity for cellular differentiation increased, so did the possibility of mutations induced by environmental factors. The principal function of this immune system was to recognize and destroy these mutant cells whose replication would endanger the orderly development of the species.

Chemically-induced tumours

A new era in tumour immunology began in 1953 following the report by Foley that mice could be immunized against transplanted chemically-induced tumours raised in syngeneic animals following the implantation of methyl cholantrene pellets. The validity of this study was confirmed by Prehn and Main (1957) who showed that while it was possible to immunize syngeneic animals against the growth of transplanted chemically-induced tumours, it was not possible to produce immunity against skin grafts obtained from the original tumour donor host, nor could normal tissue from the donor animal produce immunity against the tumour in the syngeneic recipient. These studies confirmed that *tumour-specific* immunity exists and rejections were not simple allograft rejections (rejections due to HCA differences). The antigenic specificity of each chemically-induced tumour has already been noted, and investigators have established the specificity of immunity to chemically-induced tumours (Review of Alexander, 1965).

Virally-induced tumours

It has been shown that both the DNA (polyoma, SV40, Shape papilloma, Adenovirus 12 and 18) and RNA (Mammary Tumour agent, Gross, Maloney, Rauscher Friend and others) oncogenic viruses produce tumours containing specific antigens capable of inducing rejection responses in syngeneic recipients. Tumours induced by any one virus cross-react antigenically with those of all other tumours induced by the same virus regardless of the histological appearance of the tumour or the animal species developing the tumour (Sjogren, 1967).

Thus it was shown that prior excision of a chemically-induced tumour or prior inoculation of cells from a viral tumour developed in a syngeneic host initiated an immune response which was strong enough to destroy a *limited* number of viable tumour cells given subsequently as a challenge (Klein, 1966; 1968). But it was found that both chemical and viral tumours differ in their antigenic strength, *some being weak and some strong*, and immunological rejection was difficult to establish or demonstrate in weak antigenic systems. Furthermore it was shown that the rejection response was limited in the number of tumour cells that could be eliminated. Resistance to a challenging dose of tumour cells could also be built up in syngeneic animals by inoculation with heavily irradiated viable (but incapable of replication) tumour cells.

Concomitant immunity

Animals with an intact immune system growing an implanted primary tumour may have the capacity to inhibit the growth of a second implant of the same tumour, a phenomenon referred to as *concomitant immunity*. This phenomenon may be relevant to the rate of growth of the primary tumour and to the development of tumour metastases. And it is worth noting that in systems with a weak antitumour response lymphocytes from an immunized syngeneic animal may have a tumour-destructive effect when mixed *in vitro* with viable tumour cells prior to inoculation into a susceptible host.

Spontaneous tumours

The problems associated with demonstrating an immune reaction against an antigenically weak tumour system are well illustrated by the 'spontaneous' mammary carcinoma of the mouse (Mühlbock, 1973). Mice infected with mammary tumour virus (MTV) during nursing, a time when complete immunological competence has not developed, develop a state of immune *tolerance* to a common antigen present in many MTV induced spontaneous mammary tumours. But by safeguarding against the possibility of animals developing '*tolerance*' it has been shown repeatedly that immune resistance against isologous and autochthonous tumours is almost universally demonstrable with proper experimental procedures, and that an important essential relationship exists between the lymphoid system, immunity and malignancy. Thus animals rendered immunologically incompetent by neonatal thymectomy develop malignancies more readily than their intact counterparts.

Evidence of tumour-specific immunity in humans

Though many tumours studied in laboratory animals have been shown to carry tumour-specific antigens capable of eliciting a specific antitumour immune response, the techniques used in laboratory systems are not generally applicable to humans and the search for human tumour antigens has been slow in yielding clear cut and definite positive results. But careful clinical observations and some laboratory data referred to below do support the concept that the immune system may play a very important role in the inception and course of many human cancers (Klein and Oettgen, 1969).

Spontaneous tumour regression

Everson (1967) has reported 176 authentic cases of probable spontaneous regression of cancers. This list includes hypernephroma, neuroblastoma, malignant melanoma, choriocarcinoma and sarcomas of bone and soft tissue. Other workers (Smithers, 1967; Boyd, 1966) have supported this concept, and it is considered that the true incidence of human tumour spontaneous regression is much larger than these reported series indicate. These regressions may have resulted from the effects of immunological factors though the role of other factors such as concurrent infections and pyrexia, hormonal factors and other conditions affecting tumour nutrition may be relevant.

Immunological incompetence and cancer

It has been suggested that the high relative frequencies of tumours and other malignancies in young and old people may relate to relative immuno-incompetence in the early and late (non-reproductive) periods of life. But the exact relationship of ageing to cancer and immune competence is ill-defined. In experimental animals viral and chemical carcinogens are immunosuppressive and this may relate to their effectiveness as oncogenic agents.

In humans a great increase in the rates for malignant disease is known to be associated with inherited immunological deficiency diseases such as congenital agammaglobinanaemia, hereditary ataxia–telangiectasia, the Wiskott–Aldrich and Chedrak–Higashi syndromes.

Corticosteroids have been used for many years in laboratories to depress the immune defence system in animals so that tumours could be transplanted across histocompatibility barriers and also to increase the incidence of metastases. All immunosuppressive agents facilitate malignant adaption, and consequently it is not surprising that spontaneous malignancies have developed in several patients receiving immunosuppressive therapy for renal transplants and in instances where a neoplasm has been inadvertently transplanted with a renal allograft the immunosuppression has facilitated the rapid growth of the allogenic tumour. Regression of both the spontaneous and transplanted malignancies has occurred when the immunosuppression was stopped or became ineffective (Alexander and Good, 1970).

Tumour transplants

A number of experiments in man using autotransplants have shown that patients are usually resistant to subcutaneous transplantation of their own tumour cells (Southam, 1967). It requires the injection of a large number of autochthonous tumour cells to produce tumour growth suggesting that concomitant immunity may play an important role even in patients with advanced cancer. The degree of resistance may be increased by incubation with autologous leucocytes before injection.

Morphological evidence

The observations that some tumours and associated structures show signs of being involved in a 'transplantation' reaction suggests that some tumours may be recognized as 'foreign' or antigenically different by the host and lead to an immunological rejection response. Fisher (1971) refers to a number of early and recent studies in patients with carcinoma of the stomach and breast in whom the degree of lymphocyte and plasma-cell infiltration of the primary tumour and the degree of *sinus histiocytosis* (hallmarks of an immunologically determined rejection response) were co-related with survival.

Though in nearly every animal tumour system which has been fully studied the presence of tumour-specific antigens has been established, the search for human tumour-specific antigens has not been so uniformly conclusive. Serological techniques have been used extensively in attempts to demonstrate antibodies in the sera of patients. This was initially reported by Graham and Graham (1955) in patients with gynaecological cancers. An enormous amount of work has been undertaken since then. In these tests the target antigens were derived from tissue culture lines of human cancer cells (HeLa, J-111 and HEP2) or from tumours prepared from individuals other than the sera donors. In these tests complement fixation (*see below*) and cytotoxicity methods were used to assess a tumour-specific antigen/tumour-specific antibody reaction but in the light of present knowledge of the HLA system it is impossible to consider that any positive results in these studies related to a specific antibody/specific tumour antigen reaction (Review of Fisher, 1971).

Head and neck cancers

There are now strong but not absolute grounds indicating that the Herpes type Epstein Barr Virus (EBV) plays an aetiological role in *Burkitt's Lymphoma* and in *nasopharyngeal carcinoma*, and antibodies specifically related to EBV-determined antigens have been noted in both these conditions (Klein, 1973). The antibody titres vary with the clinical course of these malignancies (Henle and Henle, 1974). The Herpes virus has been strongly implicated in the aetiology of a number of human cancers (Rapp and Duff, 1974; Milnick, Adam and Rawls, 1974). A Herpes Simplex type I antigen (non-viron) leading to the production of specific antibodies has been described in patients suffering with *squamous carcinoma of the head and neck* (Smith *et al.*, 1976), but the constancy and significance of this association requires confirmation.

Gastro-intestinal tract cancers

In 1965 Gold and Freedman demonstrated tumour-specific antigen(s) in adenocarcinomas arising from entodermal epithelium (colon, stomach, oesophagus, liver, pancreas). Similar antigens were found in embryonic and fetal gut, pancreas and liver during the first six months of intra-uterine life. These antigens are now considered to be a normal component of fetal tissue which are repressed during the later stages of gestation. Normally the synthesis of these antigens is repressed in the differentiated tissues of the normal adult, but malignant conversion may re-initiate the synthesis of these constituents by a process of 'de-repressive-de-differentiation' or 'antigenic reversion'. The term carcinoembryonic-antigens (CEA) is applied to this group of reversionary antigens (Gold, 1976). About 85 per cent of patients with carcinoma of some site in the gastrointestinal tract show abnormally high levels of this antigen in the serum. Since the *oral cavity*, *larynx* and *pharynx* are entodermally derived structures, patients with carcinoma of these sites have also been studied but only 55–60 per cent of these patients show abnormal levels of CEA, a percentage nowhere near that which would be clinically useful for diagnosis or management (Berlinger and Good, 1974). Other examples of reversionary tumour antigens include *Alfa Fitoproteins* (AFP) the synthesis of which is re-initiated in hepatocellular carcinoma and in embryonal-cell carcinomas of the ovary and testis, but these have not been demonstrated in head and neck cancers.

Other tumour-specific antigen systems

Antibodies against tumour-specific antigens have been described in three other tumour systems, i.e. Osteosarcoma, Neuroblastoma and malignant Melanoma.

Antibodies against a common *osteosarcoma antigen* have been detected by immunofluorescence in the serum of patients with osteosarcoma (Morton *et al.*, 1969). The same antibody is found in all members of the patient's family, in about 90 per cent of the patient's close contacts, and in 25 per cent of randomly selected blood bank donors. The active sera are immunologically cross-reactive with other sarcomas especially fibrosarcomas, chondrosarcomas and liposarcomas. This cross-reactivity and the fact that family members and personal contacts show a high degree of reactivity suggests a virus-derived antigen.

Hellstrom *et al.* (1968) and Hellstrom and Hellstrom (1974) have demonstrated antibody and lymphocyte toxicity in patients with *neuroblastoma.* The cross-reactivity of lymphocytes from patients with this malignancy and from their mothers, suggests that the neuroblastomas are induced by a common virus that infects both mothers and children, or that mothers are immunized during pregnancy against antigens from the fetal tumour. The fact that there is an unusually high incidence of spontaneous regression reported with these tumours also lends support to the concept of the importance of host-immunological defence mechanisms.

Malignant Melanoma is a tumour that occasionally undergoes spontaneous regression. The primary tumour may remain localized for a long period before dissemination and even in advanced disease some metastases may grow while others regress. Using immunofluorescence and cytotoxicity techniques antibodies have been demonstrated against (a) antigens on the cell membrane, and (b) in the cytoplasm of melanoma cells (Hellstrom and Hellstrom, 1974; Lewis *et al.*, 1969; Lewis and Phillips, 1972; Bodurtha *et al.*, 1975). These two antigen/antibodies differ significantly. The antibody reactive against the cytoplasmic antigen(s) is cross-reactive with melanoma cells other than those from the serum donor which may indicate an antiviral, viral component reaction. In contrast the cell surface reaction is only demonstrable in the autochthonous situation and only in those patients where the disease remains localized. As the disease progresses this latter reaction is no longer demonstrable.

Humoral and cell-mediated immune reactions

As with the immune reaction against 'foreign' transplantation or histocompatibility antigens the reaction to tumour-specific antigens involves a complex interaction of both humoral and cell-mediated factors (Baldwin and Embleton, 1974; Baldwin *et al.*, 1974; Hellstrom and Hellstrom, 1974; Herberman, 1976; Pilch and Golub, 1974). Over the past 30 years a great deal of work has been done, a variety of sophisticated techniques have been evolved, and much has been written, but the effect of the interaction of the humoral and cell-mediated immune reactions upon cancer growth, in patients with localized and in those with metastatic disease, has yet to be defined.

The complex series of biological phenomena which constitute the immune response may be considered under the following headings.

(1) Cells of the immune system.
(2) Antigen recognition.
(3) Humoral immunity.
(4) Cell-mediated immunity.
(5) Genetic control of the immune response.

Basically two classes of mononuclear cells, macrophages and lymphocytes, are responsible for the development of immune responses. The hallmark of such a response is *specificity* which is the unique property of the lymphocytes. The macrophages act as accessory cells playing a non-specific role but may acquire specificity as a result of interaction with a lymphocyte product. Lymphocytes are a highly heterogeneous group of cells and the functions of some subgroups have been identified. The major subclasses are the B (or Bursa) and T (or Thymic) lymphocytes. Miller (1966) described primary lymphoid organs, populated by stem cells from the marrow where lymphoid precursor cells are primed for an immunological function to be discharged at another site in the body (*see Figure 16.2*). Thus the immune system

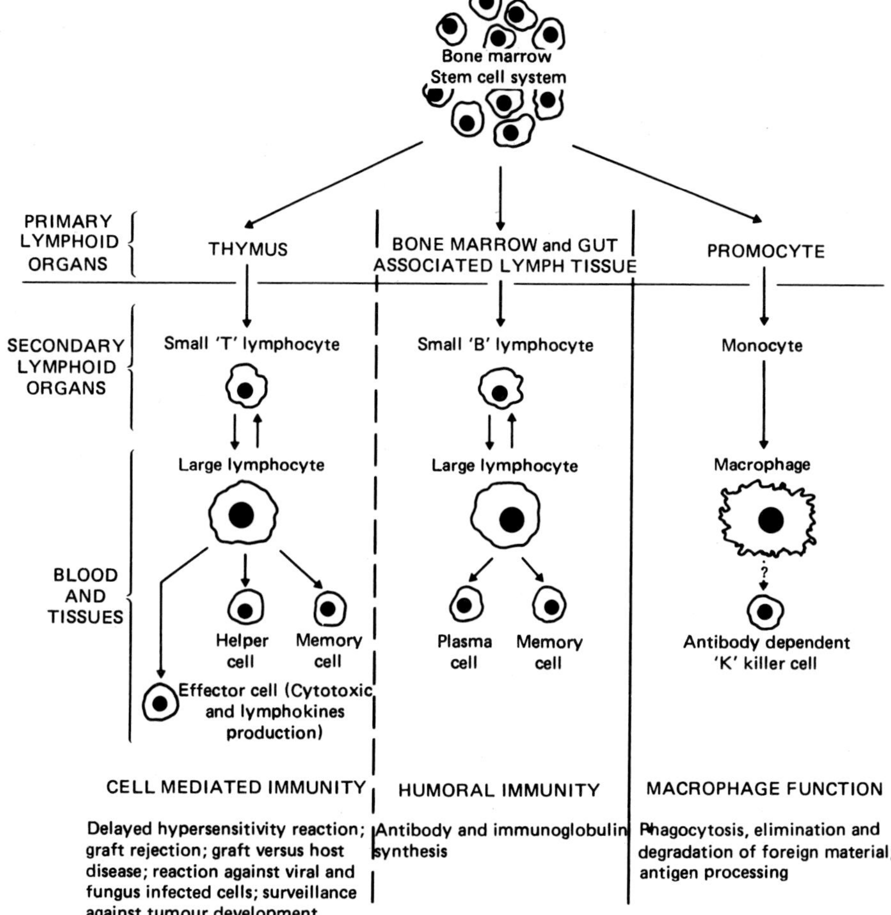

Figure 16.2 The development and differentiation of the organs and cellular components of the immune system

may be divided horizontally into the *primary* (or central) lymphoid organs, Thymus and Bursa or its equivalent, and the *secondary* (or peripheral) lymphoid organs which include lymph nodes, spleen and gut-associated lymphoid tissue (GALT) (Henry and Goldman, 1975).

The T lymphocyte system

The classic experiments of Miller (1961 and 1962) who removed the thymus in neonatal mice, showed that this structure was essential for the development of normal cell-mediated immunity and for some humoral immune responses. Thymectomized animals showed:

(1) A decrease in the number of circulating lymphocytes.
(2) A severe impairment in cell-mediated immunity, i.e. delayed allograft rejection.
(3) A reduced humoral antibody response to some but not all antigens.

Thus it is now known that the thymus is responsible for the production, differentiation and direction of a population of small antigen-reactive lymphocytes concerned with cell-mediated immunity, and a population of memory cells primed by previous contact with antigens. The development and differentiation of the primitive thymic lymphoid precursor cell or thymocyte is induced by a hormonal or humoral substance secreted by the epithelial component of the thymus, isolated and identified as a polypeptide named *thymosin*. It is now thought that the 'self' and 'non-self' recognition is learnt by the T cells through early contact with histocompatibility antigens expressed on the *epithelial tissue of the thymus*.

Thymus-dependent lymphocytes also cooperate with some bone marrow-derived lymphocytes for the production of humoral antibody against some, but not all antigens. The main function of the thymus is to produce and export a population of immunologically competent T lymphocytes to the secondary or peripheral lymphoid organs, i.e. the interfollicular and deep cortical areas in lymph nodes and to the peri-arterial lymphatic sheaths in the spleen. On appropriate antigen stimulation the peripheral T lymphocytes proliferate and these activated cells serve a number of different functions (*see Figures 16.2* and *16.4*).

Effector T cells

These are involved in graft rejection, transplantation and tumour immunity resistance to virus or fungus infected cells, delayed hypersensitivity, auto-immunity and graft versus host reactions. Some authorities classify 'killer' or K cells as specialized T effector lymphocytes (Fakhri and Hobbs, 1972), but others (MacLennon *et al.*, 1973) consider K cells to be a special subpopulation of macrophages which develop independently of the thymus. These cells are non-phagocytic and have no direct action against target cell antigens, but are triggered to kill by antibody bound to the target. K cells have been shown to be tumoricidal *in vitro*.

Regulatory T cells

These may be 'helper' cells enhancing immunoglobulin synthesis or in other situations may exert an inhibitory effect on an immune response and may be referred to as 'suppressor' cells.

Memory T cells

Immunological memory probably resides in T cells taught 'self' by their progenitors. These have a relatively long life span.

It is not known for certain if these different functions are effected through different T cell subpopulations, but some laboratory evidence suggests that this is the case rather than an entirely uniform T cell population having the capacity to serve in a special manner on different occasions.

The B lymphocyte system

The production of humoral antibody is dependent on B lymphocytes including plasma cells. In birds this system is sited in the hind-gut lymphoid organ called the Bursa of Fabricius, hence the term B (bursal) cells. B lymphocytes may be differentiated and counted, as distinct from T lymphocytes, by a process of immunofluorescent tagging. The site of the Bursa equivalent in man is not known but it may be in the gut-associated lymphoid tissue (GALT, *see below*). The precise site is not important but the distinction between B and T lymphocytes (Roitt *et al.*, 1969) is appropriate as the bursa-dependent cells play no part in cell-mediated immunity. It is thought that the non-phagocytic B lymphocytes act in response to stimulus received from mononuclear phagocytic cells. Direct contact between mononuclear macrophages and lymphocytes has been observed (Alexander and Good, 1970). Ingested antigen may be processed in the macrophages and this material or specific RNA may later be transferred to the lymphocyte. Thus 'instructions' following sensitization could be transferred back to the germinal centres and medullary cords so that re-exposure to the stimulus leads to blast transformation and proliferation of B lymphocytes, which differentiate and divide into antibody-forming plasma cells and resting memory cells (*see Figures 16.2* and *16.4*). When suitably stimulated the resting memory cells will re-enter cycle. In some instances B lymphocytes require the cooperation of T 'helper' lymphocytes to recognize certain antigens and proceed to produce antibodies, but this is not necessary for all antigens.

The secondary lymphoid organs

The bone marrow is the original source of the stem cells destined to propagate and develop either as T or B cells; as well it is probable that in adult life the bone marrow retains a role as a source of B lymphocytes (Kongshavn, Hawkins and Shuster, 1976).

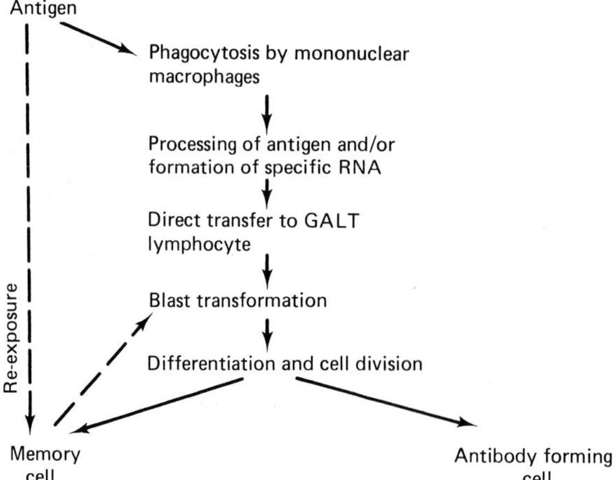

Figure 16.3 Representation of the development of antibody-forming cells and memory cells

Lymph nodes are organized into cortical, paracortical and medullary zones (*see Figure 16.4*) Following appropriate antigenic stimulation lymphoid follicles appear within the cortex indicating that an immune reaction has occurred. The germinal centres are concerned mainly with B cell production but T lymphocytes also develop at these sites (Guttman and Weissman, 1972). Antigens that promote a cell-mediated immune reaction mainly influence the deep cortex or paracortical zone, which is the site of T cell production. Antigens which induce a humoral response result in lymphoid follicle development and the appearance of plasma cells in the medulla. Morphological examination of changes observed in regional lymph nodes can provide information on the immune status of a given individual (Cottier, Turk and Sobin, 1972). The initial maturation of T cells from precursor stem cells and the maintenance and expansion of the T cell population in peripheral lymphoid organs may be controlled by thymic humoral factors. Such a substance, a polypeptide hormone called *thymosin* has been isolated from bovine thymus and the action of this hormone is not species-specific (Thompson, 1976; Goldstein, 1978). Another such substance known as *Transfer Factor* has been described by Lawrence (1969). Transfer factor is a specific mediator of cellular immunity. It is released by sensitized T lymphocytes activated by contact with the sensitizing antigen and it is capable of inducing specific activity in other previously unsensitized lymphocytes. It is capable of transferring in the form of peripheral blood leucocytes, or as a leucocyte extract, a cell-mediated response (i.e. a delayed hypersensitivity response) from a sensitized to a non-sensitized individual and the immunity it induces may persist for months or even for years.

In the spleen T cells are produced in the lymphoid tissues surrounding the follicular arterioles and a proliferative response depends on contact with antigen-reactive lymphocytes which circulate into the spleen through the splenic artery (Henry and Goldman, 1975). The lymphocytes in the primary follicles surrounding the germinal centres serve in the humoral or B cell response.

GALT. In humans this is thought to be the Bursal equivalent and comprises the systemic primary follicles, the lamina propria of the intestinal tract, aggregates of

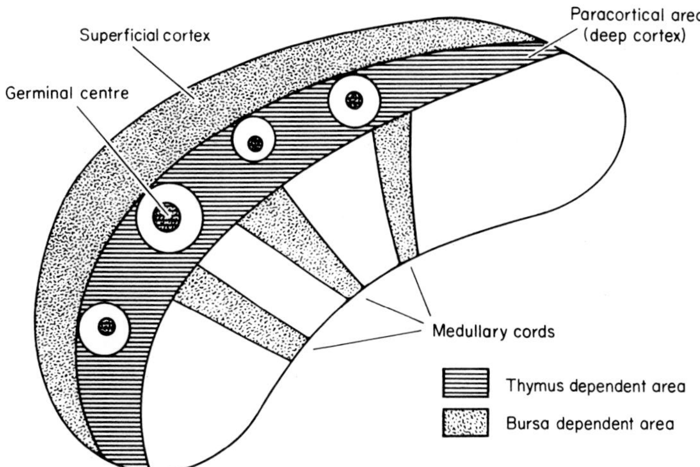

Figure 16.4 Lymph node: diagrammatic representation of the T and B cell areas

primary follicles known as Peyer's patches and the appendiceal lymphoid tissue, but this view is not universally accepted, and some workers consider that in mammals the bone marrow is the real bursal equivalent (Henry and Goldman, 1975).

Circulation of the lymphocytes

Studies (Everett and Taylor, 1967; Ford, 1969; Ford and Gowans, 1969) have shown that lymphocytes circulate from the secondary lymphoid organs (SLO) through lymphatics and thoracic ducts to the bloodstream and back again to the SLO. The great majority of the peripheral blood small lymphocytes are T cells. These pass by efferent vessels from the paracortical area of lymph nodes or the periarteriolar lymphoid tissue in the spleen through the thoracic duct to the bloodstream, later to return to a T cell area by passage through the epithelial cells of the post-capillary venules. The T lymphocyte may remain for some time in the paracortical or similar area in an SLO before returning to the bloodstream via the thoracic duct. The cycle may then be repeated. B lymphocytes circulate from the peripheral bloodstream back to the outer layer of the germinal centres of GALT. The T cell subtype referred to as Memory cells which retain and transmit knowledge of previous contact with a particular antigen also circulate so that thoracic duct lymphocytes transferred from a sensitized to a non-sensitized syngeneic animal will enable the recipient to mount a secondary response on to the antigen to which the donor animal had been sensitized (Gowans and Uhr, 1966). At present cell-mediated immunity working through the T lymphocyte system is considered to be the most significant arm in the host reaction against cancer. Specifically sensitized lymphocytes or lymphocytes armed by Transfer Factor, are capable of destroying tumour cells directly, or of mobilizing macrophages to destroy the tumour cells. Specifically sensitized T cells will on contact with tumour-specific antigens transform to blast cells and divide as well as releasing humoral substances called *lymphokines* which control the macrophages. Several lymphokines have been identified (Krause and Nysather, 1977):

(a) *Blastogenic factor*; causes lymphocytes to increase DNA synthesis and divide.
(b) *Lymphotoxin*; which is thought to have a direct toxic effect on the tumour cell.
(c) *Chemotactic factor*; attracts macrophages to the immediate area.
(d) *Migration Inhibition Factor* (*MIF*); inhibits the migration of macrophages from the area.
(e) *Macrophage Activating Factor* (*MAF*); stimulates macrophages to destroy the tumour cell.

Macrophages and the immune response

These cells are derived from the marrow promonocytes and the blood monocytes. An immune reaction to *some* antigens does necessitate prior processing by macrophages. They can act as phagocytes and process particulate matter, microbacterial and complex antigenic material and convert these substances to forms which are immunogenic. The macrophages constitute a very essential part of the humoral immune response. Possibly by removing antigen complexes from the body fluids these cells may lessen the risk of '*enhancement*'. After exposure to antigen, macrophages release factors that influence *antigen recognition*.

Antigen recognition

In immunologically competent (antigen sensitive, antigen reactive) T and B lymphocytes, the ability to recognize antigens as foreign depends on the pressure of immunoglobulins fixed on the surface of the lymphocyte which functions as an antigen recognition unit. The concept that antibody fixed on the surface of the lymphocyte cell membrane acts as an antigen recognition unit was first proposed by Sell (1967) and was most easily demonstrated in the B lymphocyte (humoral antibody) system. There is now direct evidence that specific antigen receptors exist for the T lymphocyte (cellular immunity) system. Following contact with antigen the lymphocytes undergo transformation into large blast cells which proliferate and differentiate into cells with special roles (*see Figures 16.2* and *16.3*). The ability of an antigen to stimulate an immune response relates to a number of variable factors. The *chemical structure* is a factor which determines whether an antigen is 'weak' or 'strong'. Pure proteins and carbohydrates may be strongly antigenic but lipids are usually weak. Molecules of high molecular weight (500 000 or greater) with a complex polypeptide-carbohydrate or protein structure are among the strongest antigens. The *antigenic density* (the number of antigenic sites on the cell membrane) also determines whether a cell provokes a strong, weak or negligible response.

Humoral immunity

Several classes of antibodies (immunoglobulins) have been identified and it is known that each plasma cell produces only a single particular immunoglobulin, which is synthetized by the ribosomal structures in the cell and is actively secreted. Five classes of immunoglobulins have been described to date, and there are subgroups in each class.

IgG is quantitatively the largest class, forming 80 per cent of the total serum immunoglobulins.
IgM forms 5–10 per cent of the serum immunoglobulin and as with IgG has specific antibacterial, antiviral and antitoxic properties.
IgA is thought to have a role in protecting mucosal membrane from bacterial infection.
IgE. This class of immunoglobulin is involved in allergic and auto-immune states; low levels have been described in cancer patients.
IgD. The biological function of this class is not known at present.

IgM is the first antibody to appear after a primary antigenic stimulus and is very resistant to immunosuppression. *IgG* is formed late in a primary response and appears to have a regulatory role on IgM levels; as the serum level of IgG rises the level of IgM falls. Both these immunoglobulins are synthetized by plasma cells in the medullary and germinal centres of the lymph nodes.

IgM and three of the four subclasses of IgG activate the synthesis of a complex system of serum proteins referred to as *Complement*. It is known that IgA is not concerned with complement synthesis but whether IgE and IgD are involved or not is uncertain. *Complement plays an important role in the humoral system, amplifying the interaction between antigen and specific antibody*. Activation of this arm of the immune system plays an important role in assisting *IgM* and *IgG* to destroy bacteria and *membranolysis* (disrupture of cell membrane) by the binding of tumour-specific antibody to TSA on the tumour cell membrane and *cytolysis* (destruction of the cell) also involves complement. Clinical laboratory tests such as the Wasserman reaction are read as positive or negative depending on whether complement is fixed or not in the interaction. Though cytolysis has been repeatedly demonstrated in *in vitro* studies, it is not known how susceptible human cancer cells *in vivo* are to cytolysis involving complement.

Cell-mediated immunity and tumour cell destruction

It has been postulated that the major and most significant part of a host's reaction against its tumour involves the T cell arm of the immune response. Sensitization by a cell carrying antigens recognized as foreign (tumour, transplantation or histo-incompatibility antigens) leads to the development of specific immunological receptors (immunoglobulins) on the T cell surface which have the capacity of combining with specific antigens on the tumour surface. This specific immune reaction is followed by the synthesis of cytotoxic substances by the lymphocyte which causes swelling of the tumour cell and enzymatic destruction of the cell membrane. This phenomenon occurs within hours of contact but is maximal after 24–48 h, and, in contrast to the humoral reaction, occurs *independently of complement.*

At present it is known that three groups of cell are concerned in the cell-mediated antitumour response. Mainly on evidence from laboratory animals and *in vitro* studies, cancer cells may be destroyed by:

(1) Sensitized Effector T cells which can synthesize ad secrete cytoxic lymphotoxins (Pilch and Golub, 1974). K cells may belong to this group.
(2) Sensitized B lymphocytes either by direct cytotoxic action (Shacks, Chiller and Granger, 1973) or by production of an antibody-like substance which specifically arms macrophages to attack the tumour cell. This effect occurs *independently* of complement.
(3) Cytotoxic macrophages; this may follow activation by sensitized T lymphocytes, lymphokines, or by the production of antibody-like material by sensitized B lymphocytes or by direct action. The macrophages, like the effector T cells can synthetize cytotoxic lymphotoxic type material. The B lymphocytes lack this property. Thus as well as inducing and amplifying antitumour immune response (antigen processing for both B and T lymphocytes) the macrophages may be directly cytotoxic against cells with foreign characteristics (Levy and Wheelock, 1974).

Humoral tumour cell destruction

Destruction of the tumour cell may be by antibody molecule (IgG) and complement causing *cytolysis* (*see Figure 16.5a*) or by T cell mediated enzyme attack (*Figure 16.5b*). The relationship between antigen 'strength', density, specific immunoglobulins and sensitized lymphocytes is biologically very important. If the antigen is strong though the density on the surface is low, immune lymphocytes can react to cause death of the cell. If however, immunoglobulins just bind to the antigen site, the cell will not be recognized as foreign and destruction by an immune-competent lymphocyte will not occur, a phenomenon referred to as *enhancement* (*see Figure 16.5c*). Circulating antibody–antigen complexes (Currie, 1973; Jose and Seshadri, 1974) may also be inhibitory. If antigenic sites on the cell surface are sparse, IgG will not fix sufficient complement to cause cell destruction. In these situations antibody can actually contribute to the prolonged survival of newly neoplastic cells even in a host with fully immunocompetent lymphocytes. Enhancement may thus be a factor of major importance in the survival of cancer cells in immunocompetent patients. In the same way circulating antigen or antibody–antigen complexes can neutralize or 'block' antibody or potentially cancerocidal sites on T lymphocytes (*Figure 16.5c*).

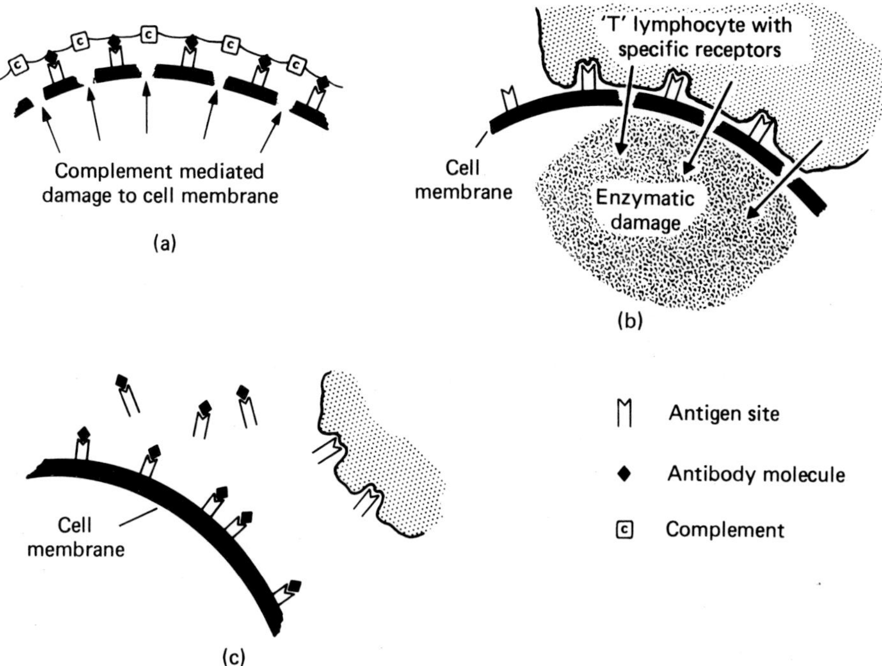

Figure 16.5 (a) Cytolysis: Specific antibody with complement causing cell death by disruption of cell membrane. (b) T cell destruction of target cell by enzymes released by T cell. The sensitized T cell has specific receptors for the specific antigens expressed on the tumour cell's surface. (c) Enhancement: tumour cell 'disguised' by antibody coating distinctive tumour-specific antigens on surface. 'Blocking' of sensitized lymphocyte's specific receptors by soluble antigen or antibody/antigen complexes

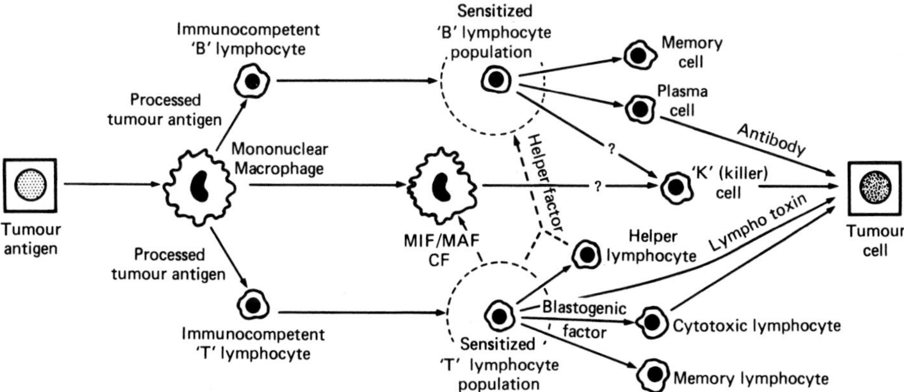

Figure 16.6 The key role of the mononuclear macrophage in initiating a T and B cell response. These cells function maximally in a cooperative, non-independent fashion

T and B cell cooperation

The cell-mediated and humoral arms of the immune response do not function separately (*see Figure 16.6*). In *vitro* studies have demonstrated the existence of T cell factors that regulate B cell response. In general the T cells appear to have a *regulatory* role enhancing and strengthening the B cell response to low doses of antigen and *suppressing* the response to high doses.

Genetic control of the immune response

'Susceptibility to cancer is inherited. The demonstration that some forms of cancer in experimental animals are gene-controlled is not the end of the story; it is merely the beginning' (Law, 1954).

Recently it has become evident that the ability to recognize and respond to a number of antigens as foreign is under genetic control. Genes that specifically control immune responses are termed immune response (Ir) genes. Some, but not all Ir genes are linked to the major histocompatibility gene loci (HLA system) that codes or 'instructs' for the histocompatibility antigens expressed on the cell surface. Though studies are as yet imprecise and not entirely conclusive it has been shown that both the T and B cell systems function under genetically determined control, and it is possible that the antigenicity of a tumour may relate to the capacity of the host to recognize foreign antigens and to initiate an appropriate immune response; so lack of recognition does not equate with lack of antigenicity in all cases. The Ir gene system functions specifically and by controlling specific immune responses to different antigens the resistance or susceptibility to the antigenic components of a particular virus or cancer is determined (Kongshavn, Hawkins and Shuster, 1976; Green, 1974; Klein, 1976). In the past the propensity to develop certain conditions such as allergies have been considered to be influenced by hereditary factors. The studies on the Ir gene system and the concept that resistance and susceptibility to certain diseases including neoplasia is genetically determined has been substantiated in both laboratory animals and in humans. Lilly and Pincus (1973) have described susceptibility genes, Klein (1976) has noted genetically linked resistance factors and Stutman and Dupuy (1972) have described genetic *susceptibility* and *resistance* factors which control the response to Friend leukaemia virus in some animal systems. These workers were able to differentiate between genetically determined absolute and relative resistant states. In the former situation where total resistance related to purely genetic factors immunosuppression failed to make resistant animals susceptible. These studies, albeit conducted in virally induced malignancies in syngeneic laboratory animals lend support to the concept enunciated by Law (1954) that inherited qualities were of fundamental importance in human cancers. Harnden (1976) has reviewed the genetic components in cancer. That susceptibility and resistance to certain cancers is influenced by genetic factors has recently been substantiated by Simons *et al.* (1974, 1975) who have demonstrated an association between the risk of developing nasopharyngeal carcinoma in male Chinese and Tunisians with a certain HLA profile. Oliver (1978) has reviewed the relationship of the HLA system and immunological defences against cancer.

Hormonal influences on the immune system

Manipulation of the endocrine environment is an accepted form of treatment for some endocrine-dependent tumours such as cancers of the prostate and breast (Welbourne and Castro, 1976). In addition to the direct effect on hormone-dependent neoplastic cells hormonal influences have considerable effects on the structure and functioning of the immune system. Orchidectomy and adrenalectomy increase thymus and lymph node size and reactions that depend on the T cells for expression are strengthened. Cortisone, oestrogen, androgens and cyproterone acetate all cause lymphoid tissue atrophy. Testosterone is mildly immunosuppressive and oestrogens depress T cell function (Castro, 1978), but interestingly Magorey and Baum (1971) have noted that the depression of reticulo–endothelial phagocytic activity which follows radiotherapy can be prevented by the simultaneous administration of stilboestrol. It has been noted that cell-mediated immunity was depressed in rats after hypophysectomy (Prentice *et al.*, 1976). Thus the internal hormonal environment may directly influence immunological resistance against cancer.

The afferent and efferent limbs of an immune response

The afferent limb of the immune response

This term is used to describe the transfer of antigenic material leading to the eventual production of specific immunocompetent cells.

Peripheral sensitization describes lymphocytes entering the tumour, reacting with antigen and so becoming sensitized and then passing to the RLN to instruct and stimulate the proliferation of sensitized cells (Brent and Medawar, 1967). But it is now considered that *central sensitization* in the RLN is more likely (Ford and Gowans, 1969) and that antigenic material is either transported by mononuclear macrophages or passes directly to RLN where sensitization takes place.

The efferent limb of the immune response

This relates to the pathways of sensitized cells (macrophages, T and B cells and their subgroups) to the target cells. Anatomical and vascular factors such as the location and blood supply (or lack of it) could affect the access of afferent limb cells to the target tumour cells. The vasculature of tumours is antigenically similar to that of the host so the route of access is not included in an antitumour immunological reaction, as is the case in organ transplantation.

The role of the regional lymph nodes

At present the concept of a proper cancer operation consists of the simultaneous removal of the primary tumour along with the regional lymphatics if an enlarged node is palpable (Stell, 1975; Stell and Green, 1976). In situations where clinical experience indicates a high probability of regional lymph node (RLN) involvement (e.g. supraglottic larynx) a block dissection may be performed in continuity with the primary tumour in the absence of palpable nodes (Bocca, 1976; Stell and Green, 1976). It has been estimated that a node less than 1 cm^3 is not palpable and a metastasis of that size may contain 10^6–10^7 tumour cells. In this view the lymph nodes act as filters and barriers to cancer cells leaving the primary tumour to metastasize, but Fisher and Fisher (1967a,b) have demonstrated that the lymph nodes are not in fact effective barriers and that cancer cells may traverse through the lymph node to leave by efferent lymphatics or through the venous system by way of the nodal lymphatico–venous channels. McKelvie (1976) has studied and described the paths of metastases in head and neck cancers. The spread of the initial metastases is segmental but thereafter 'the slope of spread is steep'. McKelvie has described long range fast paths which may be the route of spread in some tongue and post-cricoid cancers.

In recent years interest in the role of the RLN in the cancer-bearing patient has been stimulated by evidence that the RLN are significantly involved in both afferent and efferent limbs of the immune response to a tumour.

Initiation of tumour immunity

RLN are singularly involved in the initiation of allograft rejection and it is thought that the pattern of reaction against TSA is similar to that against histo-incompatible antigens. The RLN would be similarly involved, but data from human studies to confirm this is slight. Fisher (1971) however, has suggested that the RLN are probably more important for the development of tumour immunity than for the initiation of the transplant or hypersensitivity response.

Maintenance of tumour immunity

Fisher and Fisher (1972) have demonstrated the importance of RLN in the maintenance of tumour immunity, and their work suggests that removal of RLN not involved by tumour may facilitate the outgrowth of residual micrometastases. This concept has also been supported by Crile (1967, 1968). Alexander *et al.* (1969) and Alexander and Hall (1970) have described the cellular changes in RLN in rat sarcomas. Initially the efferent lymphatics carry many large lymphocytes or what Alexander and his colleagues refer to as 'immunoblasts'. As the tumour grows, the afferent antigenic load increases and the efferent output of 'immunoblasts' diminishes. Removal of the primary tumour restores immunoblast production. Black and Speer (1958) described *sinus histocytosis* in RLN draining a primary cancer and related the presence of such a change and the degree of lymphocyte infiltration of the tumour as an indication of the strength of an antitumour immune reaction and so with prognosis. These findings have been confirmed by Hamlin (1968). Thus enlargement of RLN does not necessarily indicate metastatic spread. The margin of error both in 'false positive' and 'false negative' neck RLN examinations is as much as 30 per cent. An enlarged RLN, particularly if it is soft, may represent infection in the drainage field or an immunological reaction (Cutler *et al.*, 1969, 1970). The work of Alexander and his colleagues has shown that the effector immunological reaction of the RLN may be paralysed by antigenic excess. Removal of the antigen source restored immunoblast production. These studies and those of Fisher and Fisher (1972) indicate that RLN not involved by tumour play an important role in the immunological defence system. The problem, of course, still unsolved, is how to detect tumour micrometastases?

Tumour cell destruction

That RLN have the capacity to destroy disseminated living tumour cells is suggested by the work of Hellstrom *et al.* (1968) who demonstrated an *in vitro* inhibition of tumour cell growth by lymphocytes from the host animal's RLN. In humans with nasopharyngeal carcinoma Stjernsward *et al.* (1968) demonstrated tumour-specific increased sensitivity of lymphocytes derived from saphenous lymph nodes which drained the site of infection of an irradiated nasopharyngeal carcinoma cell suspension.

The RLN are now considered to be of *singular significance in the initiation and maintenance of immunity and probably have the capacity to destroy some tumour cells* disseminated by lymphatics. The nodes play a more important role than mere mechanical traps and the absence of tumour cells from the RLN may signify that the host's regional immunological reaction had the capacity to destroy such cells as had metastasized rather than that the tumour cells had not metastasized. It is accepted that the prognosis is better in those cancer patients when lymph nodes are not involved and this may be because this group of patients represents those with a competent antitumour immune system.

RLN in squamous carcinoma of the head and neck

A large tumour can overwhelm or neutralize the host defensive reaction (Fairley, 1969) and there is a limit to the number of tumour cells (10^5–10^6) which can be contained by an effectively functioning immune system. In this context it has been suggested that an 'early' apparently localized primary tumour may contain 2×10^9 cells. Saxon and Parkis (1977) have evaluated the lymphocyte subpopulation in RLN in patients with squamous carcinoma of the head and neck, and compared these subpopulations with that in normal distant lymph nodes and in the peripheral blood. The patients examined had no previous radiotherapy. These investigators noted a relative increase in the B lymphocytes and a relative reduction in the T lymphocyte population, and they failed to identify macrophages in any of the RLN. These authors suggest that the marked preponderance of B lymphocytes may have a prognostic significance. None of these changes were reflected in distant lymph nodes or in the peripheral blood. Berlinger *et al.* (1976) have reported on the value of RLN morphology as an important prognostic parameter in patients with squamous carcinoma of the head and neck. Those whose RLN demonstrated immunological stimulation had five-year survival rates significantly higher than those whose nodes showed no evidence of stimulation.

Some reasons why tumours grow despite host immunity

There is now ample evidence to support the concept that animal and human tumours (carcinoma of the breast, colon, testis, ovary, bladder, endometrium, melanoma, neuroblastoma and various sarcomas) carry tumour-specific antigens (Hellstrom *et al.*, 1971; O'Toole *et al.*, 1973; Hellstrom and Hellstrom, 1974) that are capable of evoking immunological, humoral and cell-mediated responses in the host. Consequently it may be asked why do tumours grow? Possible explanations have been discussed by Fisher (1971), Klein (1972), and Currie (1974). The basic reason why tumours grow apparently in the face of possible immune resistance, may be due to a combination of some of the factors listed below, or because of a biological phenomenon as yet not described. The following list (undoubtedly incomplete) summarizes some of the ways in which a tumour may escape:

(1) Failure or defective recognition (immunodeficiency of the host)
  – genetic
  – environmental.
(2) Immunologic enhancement.
(3) Immune tolerance.
(4) Inadequate antigenic stimulation.
(5) Immunoselection.
(6) Antigenic modulation; shedding and blocking factors.

(1) Immunodeficiency of the host

Reference has been made earlier to the probably profound significance of *genetic factors*; the 'Ir' ('immune responsiveness') gene system. Ir genes do not act by influencing immune responsiveness in general; their action is specific for particular antigens or antigen groups, and may include antigen recognition by T cells, B cell dependent antibody formation and T–B cell cooperation (Katz, Hamaoka and Benacerraf, 1973; Zinkernagel and Doherty, 1974, 1975; Benacerraf and Katz, 1975). The effects of iatrogenic immunosuppression and inherited immunodeficiency states in relation to cancer have been referred to earlier. An example of the significance of these aspects comes from Australia. The strong solar radiation and genetic constitution of a section of the population of that continent makes skin cancer relatively common. The risk is further increased by immunosuppression in renal transplant patients (Marshall, 1973). In instances where an immune recognition deficiency may be responsible for or contributory to tumour growth attempts have been made to promote recognition by linking the tumour antigen with hapten groups or other non-specific immune system stimulants.

(2) Immunologic enhancement

This term describes increased growth of an antigenic tumour under the protection of humoral antibody. The existence of this phenomenon is unquestioned and well-documented (Moller, 1964; Bubenik and Koldovsky, 1965). Several explanations have been advanced; antibody binds with TSA sites on the tumour-cell membrane and so prevents interaction with cytotoxic cells; other suggestions are that antibodies combine with released TSA thus weakening the antigenic stimulus either by interfering with its recognition as foreign by macrophages, or by directing the antigen away from recognition sites (i.e. spleen); the antibody may have a mitogenic effect stimulating tumour growth; the tumour may be rendered less antigenic as the antibody temporarily depletes receptors. This latter was called '*antigenic modulation*' by Boyse and Old (1969). Enhancement was first described by Kaliss (1958) who observed that pre-immunization with lyophilized tumour tissue promoted rather than retarded a subsequent transplant of allogeneic tumour tissue.

The phenomenon has been described in human Burkitt's lymphoma patients (Clifford *et al.*, 1967) and is a real hazard to be remembered in some forms of immunotherapy. In those patients with Burkitt's lymphoma who demonstrated enhancement, the tumour cells were entirely coated with IgG and were entirely resistant to chemotherapy. Splenectomy undertaken to break enhancement had no effect on tumour cells subsequently examined nor on the therapeutic response.

(3) Immune tolerance

In this situation the host fails to recognize the TSA as foreign. Practically all information on this aspect has been derived from virus-induced laboratory tumours. It is optimally produced if the animal first encounters the virus before birth or in the early neonatal period. It may be that cells migrating to the thymus to learn 'self' from the thymic epithelial components encounter the viral antigen and include that moeity in the 'self' complex. Whether tolerance is a factor relating to the growth of human tumours is not known, but Currie (1974) recounts that in all human neoplasms examined specific tolerance could be outruled by the detection of specifically cytotoxic lymphocytes in the peripheral blood. Patients with a variety of tumours react immunologically to immunization with autologous tumour (Currie, 1973). It is unlikely that specific immunological tolerance plays a role in the immunological escape of human tumour cells, but it is conceivable that the two-phase phenomenon 'initiation' and 'promotion' may have significance (Salaman and Roe, 1964). A number of cells affected by the initiating carcinogen may remain dormant for a period, either contained by the immune system or perhaps not evoking a response. Subsequently the co-carcinogen 'promoter' activates a tumour cell population too large to be destroyed by the immune system.

(4) Adequate antigenic stimulation

It is possible that at the inception of a tumour the amount of antigen available may not be adequate to promote an immune response and thus the growth of the tumour outpaces the immune response of the host; an escape mechanism referred to by Old *et al.* (1962) as 'sneaking through'. There is a limit to the number of tumour cells that even a perfectly functioning immune system can destroy and by the time recognition and response have occurred the tumour may have outgrown the cytotoxic capacity of the immune system. Alexander and Hall (1970) have suggested that it is only when the tumour cells outgrow their nutrition and cell death occurs that antigenic release occurs and that an immune response can be initiated. But by then the tumour may have grown beyond control.

(5) Immunoselection

This is a theoretical concept to describe the 'cloning out' of the less antigenic cells. If there are quantitative and qualitative differences in the antigenicity of the cells of a tumour it is conceivable that the host's immune system could most easily destroy the more antigenic cells so that eventually the tumour consists of cells descended from those of least antigenicity. It is not known if this phenomenon occurs in human tumours.

(6) Shedding of antigens: modulation and blocking factors

The glycocalyx (sugar coat) of all nucleated mammalian cells is constantly being shed and re-synthesized. Antigen complexes including HCA and perhaps TSA are not fixed permanently to the cell membrane, and may appear in a soluble form in the serum. It is thought that CEA present in the serum of patients with colonic cancer (Gold and Freedman, 1965) appears as a result of glycocalceal shedding.

The antigen shedding may have a bearing on other phenomena such as *antigenic modulation* and it is conceivable that a tumour cell rendered less vulnerable by shedding antigen is afforded further protection by being surrounded by soluble antigens which may neutralize cell-mediated cytotoxicity, a possible phenomenon which Currie (1974) refers to as an antigen 'smoke screen'.

Currie and Basham (1972) have presented suggestive evidence that tumour-specific antigen complexes are shed from human tumours and leak into the serum and extracellular fluids. Thomson, Steele and Alexander (1973) have demonstrated a similar phenomenon in rats, and Currie and Alexander (1974) have demonstrated the spontaneous shedding of TSA in rat sarcoma cells in culture. These studies elucidated a discouraging and apparently baffling paradox. Hellstrom and Hellstrom (1969, 1970) had described a serum factor which inhibited specific cell-mediated cytotoxicity in Maloney virus-induced sarcoma in mice. This factor was referred to as *blocking antibody* which was thought to react with antigens on the tumour cell surface and were so protected from recognition by specifically sensitized lymphocytes; a type of immunological enhancement (Moller, 1964). *Blocking antibodies* were identified in other laboratory systems and the issue became more confused with the description of a special '*unblocking*' antibody by Bansel and Sjogren (1971). They recognized that tumour cells may continuously shed antigen and that the serum factor which protected tumour cells against specific cell-mediated cytotoxicity is either *free tumour antigen* in soluble form in the serum or *antigen–antibody complexes*. In the latter it is the antigen component which is important (Thomson, 1975). These *blocking* factors operate by neutralizing cell-mediated cytotoxicity, and not by reducing recognition of the tumour cell by antibody coating, to become less vulnerable to a cell-mediated reaction. *Unblocking antibody* represents serum fractions that neutralize the *blocking antigen–antibody complexes* (Baldwin *et al.*, 1974).

Assessment of immune function in the cancer patient

The studies of Mitchison (1955, 1957) indicated that the rejection of histo-incompatible normal and tumour tissue is mediated by lymphocytes, and Klein *et al.* (1960) showed that specific antitumour immunity could be passed from immunized to non-immunized syngeneic animals by the transfer of lymphocytes. Since these initial very significant studies a great deal of scientific work has been done which supports the concept that the major part of the host's immunological response against a tumour is cell mediated and is similar to that leading to allograft rejection (Skamene and Gold, 1976; Calne, 1978). Consequently over the years attempts have been made to assess the capacity of the immune system in patients with cancers to react against their tumours. This is a matter of practical interest because laboratory and clinical studies have shown that the competence of the immune system may relate to *genetic, hormonal and nutritional factors* and determine the response to viral, chemical and radiation carcinogens. The importance of the level of competence of the immune system may determine the course of events after the establishment of a clone of proliferating malignant cells; whether the disease remains localized to a particular anatomical area or metastasizes. The pre-treatment immunological status of patients is important and in particular the ability to demonstrate a strong cell-mediated response is a favourable prognostic sign. Certain hormones and cytotoxic drugs depress immune function. Certain cytotoxic drugs maximally depress B cell function, others T cell function, and there is suggestive evidence that a favourable response to chemotherapy may relate to a synergistic effect in the presence of a strong host immune reaction (Clifford *et al.*, 1967). Furthermore a strong and intact immune system will be less affected by cancer chemotherapy and will recover quicker and more completely than a weak one. Radiotherapy can depress immune reactivity for a considerable period of time after treatment (Stjernsward, 1974, 1977). Major surgery may show depressed immune function for several weeks post-operatively. These two instances indicate the necessity to define pre-treatment immunological capacities. It must be remembered that the presence of a large tumour may in itself cause marked depression of immunological competence (Baldwin and Robins, 1976). It is now recognized that the outgrowth of micrometastases undetected during the period when the primary treatment of the cancer was thought to be complete and successful is the root cause for many failures. A full pre-treatment immune system assessment may be of value in the future in selecting the form of immunotherapy chosen to act against possible micrometastases.

Formerly it was believed that measures which appeared to strengthen cell-mediated immunity against the tumour were all favourable in contrast to those which led to an antibody increase and which were considered to be unfavourable. But it is now thought that the maximal antitumour effect is achieved in situations where the T and B cells function in harmony and that other cell systems such as the mononuclear macrophages play a significant role in tumour-cell cytotoxicity. Attempts to determine the size of the T and B cell counts in the peripheral lymphocyte circulation are now considered inconclusive as the percentage of B and T cells fluctuates, but the absolute peripheral lymphocyte count is of value. Assessment of the functional competence of cell-mediated immunity includes *in vivo* and *in vitro* studies.

Herberman (1976) has reviewed the manner in which the immune status of the cancer patient may be assessed, and such studies have been undertaken on patients with squamous carcinoma of the head and neck by Chretien and Ketcham (1973), Chretien (1975), Parker *et al.* (1975), Tarpley, Potvin and Chretien (1975) and Tanner, Clifford and Carter (1978). These workers have used:

(1) Skin tests for DHR
    Recall antigens.
    DNCB.
(2) Peripheral lymphocyte counts.
    Differential T and B cell estimations.
(3) Lymphocyte function.
    Proliferative response to PHA.
(4) Antibody production.
    Circulating immunoglobulins.
    Antibodies against viral-determined antigens.

In vivo studies of cell-mediated immunity

Skin tests involving the cutaneous injection of antigens to demonstrate a delayed hypersensitivity reaction are widely used as a means of evoking and assessing *cell-mediated immunity.*

(1) *Delayed cutaneous hypersensitivity reaction* (*DHR*)
(a) To tumour cell extracts, autochthonous or allogeneic.
(b) Following primary sensitization to chemicals such as dinitrochlorobenzene (DNCB).
(c) Recall antigens, i.e. mumps, candida, veridase, tuberculin. The majority of adult patients will have previously been exposed to these antigens.

(a) *Tumour cell preparations* Homogenates, cell membrane extracts purified and/or concentrated have been injected intradermally to test for a specific DHR response. Though the aim of this form of testing is clear such factors as possible bacterial contamination and uncertainty regarding the preparation of the test substance causing an alteration in the antigenic substance has led to this form of testing being considered unreliable. But studies such as that reported by Hughes and Lytton (1964), Stewart (1969a, b) and Fass, Herberman and Ziegler (1970) indicated that a positive response could be related to prognosis and with the degree of lymphocyte infiltration of the tumour. Though the methodology and the results of such tests may be questioned, reliable information regarding the patient's capacity to react *specifically* to the tumour may relate to forms of treatment and prognosis.

(b) *DHR to dinitrochlorobenzene (DNCB)* This organic chemical is a potent allergen which is thought to act as a hapten, and by conjugation with a protein becomes immunogenic. It is a substance with which the general population do not normally come in contact and consequently patients and controls may be primarily quantitatively sensitized by applying measured doses to a specified skin area. After an interval to allow sensitization to occur the patient may be challenged by the skin application of controlled amounts of different concentrations of DNCB and the response quantitatively graded. Levin *et al.* (1964) and Eilber and Norton (1970) have described the use of this test in patients with tumours, and Bone and Camplejohn (1973) described response correlated with tumour stage. This test is thought to assess the afferent and efferent limbs of the cell-mediated immune response but it must be stressed that though the test may be a measure of general immune competence it is not a measure of a patient's potential to recognize and mount a *specific* attack against cells carrying TSAs. Bone and Camplejohn used standardized different strengths of DNCB to measure quantitatively the strength of the cell-mediated immune reaction, a method also described by Bleumink *et al.* (1974). Bolton (1975) has described and reviewed the use of this test in oncology and concludes that:

(1) The DNCB response is a safe and useful method of assessing cell-mediated immunity.
(2) Non-specific factors such as the general health and nutritional state may influence the response.
(3) The site of origin of a tumour rather than the disease stage relates to the response, i.e. 'early' breast cancer shows little impairment in contrast to 'early' colon cancer which has marked impairment.
(4) A negative DNCB response is usually associated with a poor prognosis, but the converse does not always apply. DHR to DNCB is one of the best available in clinical oncology, but in evaluating the results it must be stressed that the assessment is *non-specific* and may or may not relate to a possible cell-mediated immune reaction *against* TSA or the tumour cells.

(c) *DHR to recall antigens* The assumption supporting the use of these antigens, derived from bacteria, viruses or fungi is that the subject has had prior exposure and sensitization to the antigens and on testing will demonstrate an established delayed hypersensitivity. The test is simple: a small amount of antigen in a small volume of fluid, usually not more than 0.1 ml, is injected intradermally. A positive DHR may be evident in 4–48 h after testing and appears as an area of hyperaemia and induration measuring at least 5 mm in diameter. Tests are usually read 48 h after testing. Measurements should be made and recorded in two diameters 90 degrees apart. In clinical trials a group of recall antigens are commonly used and a constant concentration and dose of each antigen are used for each trial patient and normal control. Commonly used antigens are:

(1) Purified protein derivative of tuberculin (PPD). This antigen is available in three standard concentrations (Parke, Davis & Co.).
(2) Candida albicans extract.
(3) Mumps antigen.
(4) Varidase (streptokinase–streptodornase).

The use of recall antigens to assess the DHR of cell-mediated immunity may be criticized on the grounds that the degree of previous exposure is quantitatively unknown and a negative response may relate to inadequate prior exposure or to anergy. For this reason testing with an antigen to which prior exposure was unlikely is considered preferable; such a substance is dinitrochlorobenzene (DNCB) a single application of which will sensitize over 90 per cent of the population.

The role of DHR commenced 50 years ago when it was observed that patients with cancer had a decreased incidence of tuberculin-type skin reactions (Renaud, 1926). A failure to respond to a single or even several recall test antigens may have little significance since the degree of prior sensitization is unknown. Even if a response against all recall antigens is obtained this does not give an indication of the capacity to respond specifically to TSA on tumour cells.

(2) *Lymphocyte transfer and allogeneic skin grafting*

These have been used to study cell-mediated immunity. Hattler and Amos (1965) have studied the effects of intradermal transfer of lymphocytes from normal and cancer patients to patients with advanced cancer and noted that the recipients with advanced cancer had a minimal local reaction which suggested to these investigators that patients with advanced cancer have a defective cell-mediated immune response. Similarly as the reaction against TSA has been compared with that against foreign HCAs or transplantation antigens, skin grafts from normal and cancer patients have been exchanged. Several studies have been reported, some suggesting a prolongation of allograft survival in patients with advanced disease. But the results are conflicting (Fisher, 1971). Where there is a general depression of cell-mediated immunity there is also a delay in the rejection of the allograft.

(3) *Laboratory studies*

(a) *Colony inhibition in vitro* This test, originally described by Hellstrom *et al.* (1968), demonstrates that peripheral blood lymphocytes may be capable of inhibiting the formation of miniature colonies when the tumour cells are put in tissue culture. The original study was done on neuroblastoma cells and these workers showed that neuroblastomas carry a common or cross-reacting antigen.

(b) *Lymphocyte reactivity to phytohaemagglutinin (PHA)* Normally when lymphocytes react with a foreign antigen the cells undergo blast-transformation and divide. The same effect occurs when peripheral lymphocytes are cultured with phytohaemagglutinin (PHA), and the response can be monitored by adding tritriated thymidine to the culture. Chretien and Ketcham (1973) have noted impaired reactivity in lymphocytes from patients with squamous carcinoma of the head and neck.

(c) *Lymphocyte cytotoxicity* This test, initially described by Hellstrom *et al.* (1971), tests the direct cytotoxicity of peripheral blood lymphocytes against the donor's tumour grown in microcultures. These workers demonstrated that the majority of cancer patients carry lymphocytes capable of killing their own tumour. This type of test has also been used to elucidate the problem of serum 'blocking' factors which inhibit the cytotoxic effects of the lymphocytes (*Figure 16.6*; Baldwin *et al.*, 1974; Baldwin and Robins, 1976).

The aims and present achievements of clinical studies

In the group of clinical studies noted earlier initial studies were undertaken on pre-treatment cancer patients and controls, and the results subsequently compared with patients' progress usually after two years. It was hoped that the use of these tests would enable patients to be categorized on immunological grounds into groups; those with a favourable prognosis and those with a poor prognosis. The former group could be treated radically and the latter would on humanitarian grounds be treated palliatively. The results of these studies can only be expressed in general and not absolute terms. The ability to demonstrate a DHR to DNCB was prognostically good as were normal lymphocyte counts. The response to recall antigens was unreliable. It may be that these patients had a specific immunodysfunction to their TSA which none of these tests will measure and also that the presence of a large antigenic tumour (if such is the case) will, while present, induce a degree of immunological paralysis. The B and T cell values in the peripheral blood are inconstant and it is now considered that DNCB reactivity and total peripheral lymphocyte count may be reliable indications of *general* immunological competence.

Herpes viruses and head and neck cancer

Humoral antibody responses

Attention of workers in cancer immunology has mainly been focused on the cellular response but the demonstration of antibody is indicative of an immune response (Harris, 1976) and the study of this arm of the immune response may be rewarding as the studies of Klein and his co-workers on the Epstein Barr virus in Burkitt's lymphoma and nasopharyngeal carcinoma (Klein, 1973) indicate. Smith *et al.* (1976) have reviewed previous studies which suggest a relationship between *Herpes simplex virus infection and squamous carcinoma of the head and neck.* Smith and co-workers have described significantly high levels of IgA antibody directed specifically against herpes simplex induced antigens in patients with squamous carcinoma of the head and neck. A high intake of alcohol and tobacco were considered contributary factors but IgA anti-herpes simplex antibodies were less elevated in a comparable control group. The precise significance of these results is not yet clear nor is the role of herpes simplex in relation to head and neck squamous carcinoma fully understood.

Immunotherapy

Because the treatment of head and neck cancers by orthodox radiotherapy, chemotherapy and surgery either as a single modality or in combination therapy is not always successful, it is hoped that immunological manipulations might improve the results of treatment. Laboratory studies have demonstrated that it is possible to immunize animals *specifically* against virus, chemically and physically induced tumours which possess tumour-specific antigens. Such an antigen system has been demonstrated in many human tumours and Morton (1972) believes that adequate and sensitive methods would detect specific antigens in many other human cancers, and that 'the future for immunotherapy in human cancer is bright'. Morton (1972) has reviewed the present status and future potential of the immunotherapy of cancer, and McKhann and Gunnarsson (1974) have described the different forms and optimum requirements of the different forms of immunotherapy at present under clinical trial. Currie (1974) has presented a very factual review of the present state of immunotherapy. The need to define the nature of the *specific* fault in the human immunological defence system, which presumably allows the outgrowth of cells carrying tumour-specific antigens needs to be defined. This information is *not* available. Currie (1974) refers to modern tumour immunology as 'phenomenology', a record of events which we lack the methodology and knowledge to unravel and understand. The host–tumour relationship is complex and attempts to treat patients by *immunological manipulations are associated with hazards such as the enhancement of the tumour growth by antibody, blocking by an excess of soluble antigen and the development of reticuloses*. The situation at present is a doctor's dilemma, and the answer is simply not a matter of stimulating the phagocytes. Three forms of immunotherapy which may be of relevance in the treatment of head and neck cancers will be referred to. Since Mathe *et al.* (1969) described the beneficial effects of using Bacillus Calmette–Guerin (BCG) given with irradiated acute leukaemia tumour cells in the treatment of acute lymphocytic leukaemia, BCG has been a popular agent in immunotherapy. The rationale for its use is that the specific antitumour immunological response may be increased as part of a BCG induced increase in general (non-specific) immunological reactivity. This assumes that the patient has already initiated an immunological response against the tumour-specific antigens of the cancer, which for reasons already referred to, has been ineffectual in controlling tumour growth. Powles (1973) has reported improved results in acute myelogenous leukaemia following treatment with BCG and allogeneic tumour cells. Gutterman *et al.* (1973) have used BCG to treat malignant melanoma following surgical resection for recurrent disease and initial reports indicated benefit for the patient. In *head and neck cancers* Donaldson (1973) reported favourable responses in a group of patients treated with BCG and Methotrexate. Many of the patients included in Donaldson's report had recurrent disease following prior surgery or radiotherapy. This report is of interest and perhaps of significance. Very little is as yet known of the effects of *chemo-immunotherapy* which is the term used by Donaldson to describe the combination of BCG, isoniazid and methotrexate which he used. BCG has been used intradermal, intraplural, intralesion, intravenous, by scarification, multiple puncture, Heaf gun injection and intracavity, but apart from the studies of Mathe and Powles no clear improvement in treatment results has been proven. Apart from the difficulties which may follow uncontrolled manipulation of the immunological system in an imperfectly understood situation, the report by McKhann *et al.* (1975) of two deaths following intralesional injection of BCG due to BCG hypersensitivity, underlines the dangers. *Corynebacterium parvum* (*C. parvum*) has been used in the same way as BCG, as a non-specific reticulo-endothelial stimulant. Fisher *et al.* (1975) have shown that *C. parvum* given with cyclophosphamide produced a more effective tumour inhibition than could be achieved by giving either of these agents separately. Currie and Bagshawe

(1970) had previously studied the effects of this combination and had stressed that the maximal antitumour effect could only be achieved by correctly timing the administration of immunotherapy. These studies suggest that cancer chemotherapy as well as its direct effect against the tumour, corrects some tangle in the immunological system, and as a consequence subsequent immunotherapy is more effective.

Thymosin

The thymus controls the development and maturation of the T cell system by secreting a family of polypeptide hormones collectively known as *thymosin*. Goldstein (1978) has reported that thymosin has the capacity to expand the T cell population above normal levels. This approach is in contrast to the previous use of adjuvants which aimed at activating and focusing the response of an existing lymphoid population. This hormone has been studied in laboratory tumour systems but its use in human clinical trials is still preliminary.

Levamisole

This drug influences cell-mediated immune responses (T lymphocytes) but has little effect on the B lymphocyte system (Symoens and Rosenthal, 1977; Willoughby and Wood, 1977). The effects of this drug are most evident in immunodepressed patients, and trials of its effect on patients who have undergone radiotherapy are in progress. But its precise role in cancer immunotherapy has yet to be decided. More precise knowledge and understanding is required before immunotherapy is brought into general use.

Acknowledgements

The author is grateful to Miss L. Pegus and Mr. Robert Thornton of the Medical Arts Department, and to Mrs. M. Potucek, Photographic Department, Royal Marsden Hospital, who prepared the figures.

Publication of this chapter would have been impossible without the help of my wife, Jayne Clifford, who arranged the text and references.

References

Alexander, J. W. and Good, R.A. (1970). *Immunobiology for Surgeons*, pp. 132–143. Philadelphia, London, Toronto; W. B. Saunders Co.

Alexander, P. (1965). 'Immunological reaction against primary tumours'. In *The Scientific Basis of Surgery* (Ed. by Irvine, W. T.). London; J. and A. Churchill Ltd.

Alexander, P., Bensted, J., Delorme, E. J., Hall, J. G. and Hodgett, J. (1969). *Proceedings of the Royal Society*, **174**, 237

Alexander, P. and Hall, J. G. (1970). *Advances in Cancer Research*, **13**, 1

Bach, F. H. (1974). *American Journal of Clinical Pathology*, **62**, 173

Bagshawe, K. (1974). *British Medical Bulletin*, **30**, 68

Baldwin, R. W., Bowen, J. G., Embleton, M. J., Price, M. R. and Robins, R. A. (1974). *Advances in Biosciences*, **12,** 539

Baldwin, R. W. and Embleton, M. J. (1974). *International Journal of Cancer*, **13,** 433

Baldwin, R. W., Embleton, M. J., Price, M. R. and Robins, A. (1974). *Cancer*, **34,** 1452

Baldwin, R. W. and Robins, R. A. (1976). 'Host immune responses to tumours'. In *Scientific Foundations of Oncology* (Ed. by Symington, T. and Carter, R. L.), pp. 514–520. London; Heinemann Medical Books

Bansel, S. C. and Sjogren, H. O. (1971). *Nature, London*, **233,** 76

Benacerraf, B. and Katz, D. H. (1975). *Advances in Cancer Research*, **21,** 121

Berlinger, N. T. and Good, R. A. (1974). *Otolaryngologic Clinics of North America*, **7,** 859

Berlinger, N. T., Tsakraklides, V., Pollak, K., Adams, G. L., Yang, M. and Good, R. A. (1976). *Laryngology*, **36,** 792

Black, M. M. and Speer, F. D. (1958). *Surgery, Gynaecology and Obstetrics*, **102,** 599

Bleumink, E., Nater, J. P., Koops, S. and The, T. H. (1974). *Cancer*, **33,** 911

Bocca, E. (1976). *Nuovo Archivio Italiano di Otologia, Rinologia e Laringologia*, **4,** 151

Bolton, P. M. (1975). *Clinical Oncology*, **1,** 59

Bone, G. and Camplejohn, R. (1973). *British Journal of Surgery*, **60,** 824

Bordutha, A. J., Chee, D. O., Lancius, J. F., Mistrangelo, M. J. and Prehn, R. T. (1975). *Cancer Research*, **35,** 189

Boyd, W. M. (1966). *The Spontaneous Regression of Cancer*, p. 99. Springfield, Illinois; Charles C. Thomas

Boyse, E. A. and Old, L. J. (1969). *Annual Review of Genetics*, **3,** 269

Brent, L. and Medawar, P. B. (1967). *British Medical Bulletin*, **23,** 55

Bubenik, J. and Koldovsky, P. (1965). *Folia Biologica, Praha*, **11,** 258

Burnet, F. M. (1967). *Lancet*, **1,** 1171

Burnet, F. M. (1970). *Progress in Experimental Tumour Research*, **13,** 1

Calne, R. Y. (1978). *Journal of the Royal Society of Medicine*, **71,** 479

Castro, J. E. (1978). *Journal of the Royal Society of Medicine*, **71,** 123

Chretien, P. B. and Ketcham, A. S. (1973). 'Quantitation of immunologic defects in cancer patients'. In *Proceedings 7th National Cancer Conference*. Philadelphia and Toronto; J. B. Lippincott Company

Chretien, P. B. (1975). *Canadian Journal of Otolaryngology*, **4,** 225

Clifford, P., Singh, S., Stjernsward, J. and Klein, G. (1967). *Cancer Research*, **27,** 2578

Cottier, H., Turk, J. and Sobin, L. (1972). *Bulletin of the World Health Organisation*, **47,** 375

Crile, G., Jr. (1967). *Journal of the American Medical Association*, **199,** 736

Crile, G., Jr., (1968). *Annals of Surgery*, **168,** 330

Currie, G. A. and Bagshawe, K. D. (1970). *British Medical Journal*, **1,** 541

Currie, G. A. and Basham, C. (1972). *British Journal of Cancer*, **26,** 427

Currie, G. A. (1973). *British Journal of Cancer*, **28,** Suppl. 1, 153

Currie, G. A. (1974). 'Immunological escape of tumours'. In *Cancer and the Immune Response*, pp. 56–70. London; Edward Arnold

Currie, G. A. and Alexander, P. (1974). *British Journal of Cancer*, **29,** 72

Cutler, S. J., Zippin, C. and Asire, A. J. (1969). *Cancer*, **23,** 243

Cutler, S. J., Axtell, M. A., Schottenfeld, D. and Farrow, J. H. (1970). *Surgery, Gynaecology and Obstetrics*, **131,** 41

Donaldson, R. C. (1973). *American Journal of Surgery*, **126,** 507

Eilber, F. R. and Morton, D. L. (1970). *Cancer*, **25,** 362

Everett, N. B. and Taylor, R. W. (1967). *International Review of Cytology*, **22,** 205

Everson, T. C. (1967). 'Spontaneous regression of cancer'. In *Progress in Clinical Cancer*, Vol. III, (Ed. by Ariel, I. M.). New York; Greene and Stratton

Fairley, G. H. (1969). *British Medical Journal*, **2,** 467

Fakhri, O. and Hobbs, J. R. (1972). *Lancet*, **2,** 403

Fass, L., Herberman, R. B. and Zeigler, J. (1970). *New England Journal of Medicine*, **282,** 776

Fisher, B. and Fisher, E. R. (1967a). *Cancer*, **20,** 1907

Fisher, B. and Fisher, E. R. (1967b). *Cancer*, **20,** 1914

Fisher, B. (1971). 'The present status of tumour immunology'. In *Advances in Surgery* (Ed. by Welch, Claude E. and Hardy, James D.), Vol. 5, pp. 189–253. Chicago; Year Book Medical Publishing Co.

Fisher, B. and Fisher, E. R. (1972). *Cancer*, **29,** 1496

Fisher, B., Wolmark, N., Saffer, E. and Fisher, E. R. (1975). *Cancer*, **35,** 134

Foley, E. J. (1953). *Cancer Research*, **13,** 835

Ford, W. L. (1969). *British Journal of Experimental Pathology*, **50,** 257

Ford, W. L. and Gowans, J. L. (1969). *Seminars in Hematology*, **6,** 67

Gold, P. and Freedman, S. O. (1965). *Journal of Experimental Medicine*, **122,** 467

Gold, P. (1967). *Cancer*, **20,** 1663

Gold, P., Gold, M. and Freedman, S. O. (1968). *Cancer Research*, **28,** 1331

Gold, P. (1976). 'Cancer immunology'. In *Clinical Immunology* (Ed. by Freedman, S. O. and Gold, P.), pp. 429–437. Hagerstown, Maryland, New York, San Francisco, London; Harper and Row

Goldstein, A. L. (1978). 'Thymosin. Basic properties and clinical potential in the treatment of patients with immuno-deficiency diseases and cancer'. In *Antibiotics and Chemotherapy*, Volume 24, *Application of Cancer Chemotherapy* (Ed. by Schabel, F. M., Jr.), pp. 47–59. Basel, Munich, Paris, London, New York, Sydney; S. Karger

Gowans, J. L. and Uhr, J. W. (1966). *Journal of Experimental Medicine*, **124**, 1017

Gowans, J. L. In *Harvey Lectures*, 1968–1969, p. 87. London; Academic Press

Graham, J. B. and Graham, R. M. (1955). *Cancer*, **8**, 409

Green, I. (1974). *Immunogenetics*, **1**, 4

Gutterman, J. U., Mavligil, G., MacBride, C., Frei, E., Freireich, E. J. and Hersh, E. M. (1973). *Lancet*, **1**, 1208

Guttman, G. A. and Weissman, I. L. (1972). *Immunology*, **23**, 465

Hamlin, I. M. E. (1968). *Cancer*, **22**, 382

Harnden, D. G. (1976). 'The genetic components in malignant disease'. In *Scientific Foundations of Oncology* (Ed. by Symington, T. and Carter, R. L.), pp. 181–189. London; Heinemann Medical Books Ltd.

Harris, J. E. (1976). In *Scientific Foundations of Oncology* (Ed. by Symington, T. and Carter, R. L.), pp. 532–536. London; Heinemann Medical Books Ltd.

Hattler, B. G. and Amos, D. B. (1965). *Journal of the National Cancer Institute*, **35**, 927

Hellstrom, I. E., Hellstrom, K. E. and Pierce, G. E. (1968). *International Journal of Cancer*, **3**, 467

Hellstrom, I., Hellstrom, K. E., Pierce, G. E. and Bill, A. H. (1968). *Proceedings of the United States National Academy of Sciences*, **60**, 1231

Hellstrom, I. and Hellstrom, K. E. (1969). *International Journal of Cancer*, **4**, 587

Hellstrom, I. and Hellstrom, K. E. (1970). *International Journal of Cancer*, **5**, 195

Hellstrom, I., Hellstrom, K. E., Sjogren, H. O. and Warner, G. A. (1971). *International Journal of Cancer*, **7**, 1

Hellstrom, I., Sjogren, H. O. and Warner, G. A. (1971) *International Journal of Cancer*, **7**, 1

Hellstrom, I. and Hellstrom, K. E. (1974). *Cancer*, **34**, 1461

Hellstrom, K. E. and Hellstrom, I. (1974). *Advances in Immunology*, **18**, 209

Henle, W. and Henle, G. (1974). *Cancer*, **34**, 1368

Henry, K. and Goldman, J. M. (1975). 'The lymphocyte'. In *Recent Advances in Pathology No. 9* (Ed. by Harrison, C. V. and Weinbren, K.), pp. 30–72. London; Churchill, Livingstone

Herberman, R. B. (1976). *Cancer*, **37**, 549

Hughes, L. E. and Lytton, B. (1964). *British Medical Journal*, **1**, 209

Invernizzi, G. and Parmiani, G. (1975). *Nature, London*, **254**, 713

Jose, D. G. and Seshadri, R. (1974). *International Journal of Cancer*, **13**, 824

Kaliss, N. (1958). *Cancer Research*, **18**, 992

Katz, D. H., Hamaoka, T. and Benacerraf, B. (1973). *Journal of Experimental Medicine*, **137**, 1405

Klein, E. (1966). 'Tumour Antigens', In *Annual Review of Microbiology*, pp. 233–252. Ed. by C. E. Clifton. Palo Alto, California; Annual Reviews Inc.

Klein, E. (1968). *Cancer Research*, **28**, 625

Klein, E. (1972). *Annals of the Institute of Pasteur* (Paris), **122**, 593

Klein, G., Sjogren, H. O., Klein, E. and Hellstrom, K. E. (1960). *Cancer Research*, **20**, 1561

Klein, G. and Oettgen, H. F. (1969). *Cancer Research*, **29**, 1741

Klein, G. (1973). 'The Epstein Barr Virus'. In *The Herpes Viruses* (Ed. by Kaplan, A. S.). London, New York, San Francisco; Academic Press

Klein, G. (1976). 'Tumour immunology: a general appraisal'. In *Scientific Foundations of Oncology* (Ed. by Symington, T. and Carter, R. L.), pp. 497–504. London; Heinemann Medical Books Ltd.

Klein, G. (1975). 'Immunological surveillance against neoplasia'. Harvey Lecture Series 69, 1973–1974. pp. 71–102. New York, San Francisco, London; Academic Press

Kongshavn, P. A. L., Hawkins, D. and Shuster, J. (1976). 'The biology of the immune response'. In *Clinical Immunology* (Ed. by Freedman, S. O. and Gold, P.), pp. 38–40. Hagerstown, Maryland, New York, San Francisco, London; Harper and Row

Krause, C. J. and Nysather, J. O. (1977). *Annals of Otology, Rhinology and Laryngology*, **86**, 698

Law, L. W. (1954). *Advances in Cancer Research*, **2**, 281

Lawrence, H. (1969). *Advances in Immunology*, **11**, 195

Levin, A. G., McDonough, E. F., Miller, D. G. and Southam, C. M. (1964). *Annals of the New York Academy of Sciences*, **120**, 400

Levy, M. H. and Wheelock, E. F. (1974). *Advances in Cancer Research*, **20**, 131

Lewis, M. G., Ikonopisor, R. L., Nairn, R. C., Phillips, T. M., Fairly, G. H., Bodenham, D. G. and Alexander, P. (1969). *British Medical Journal*, **3**, 547

Lewis, M. G. and Phillips, T. M. (1972). *Journal of the National Cancer Institute*, **49**, 915

Lilly, F. and Pincus, T. (1973). 'Genetic control of murine viral leukemogenesis'. In *Advances in Cancer Research* (Ed. by Klein, G. and Weinhouse, S.), Vol. 17, p. 231. New York and London; Academic Press

MacLennon, I. C. M., Hardy, B., Loewi, G. and Howard, A. (1973). *British Journal of Cancer*, **28**, (Suppl. 1) 7

Magorey, C. J. and Baum, M. (1971). *British Medical Journal*, **1**, 367

Maisel, R. H. and Ogura, J. N. (1976). *Annals of Otology, Rhinology and Laryngology*, **85**, 517

Marshall, V. D. (1973). *Australia and New Zealand Journal of Surgery*, **43**, 214

Mathe, G. *et al.* (1969). *Lancet*, **1**, 967

McKelvie, P. (1976). *Proceedings of the Royal Society of Medicine*, **69**, 409

McKhann, C. F. and Gunnarsson, A. (1974). *Cancer*, **34**, 1521

McKhann, C. F., Hendrickson, C. G., Spitler, L. E., Gunnarsson, A., Banerjee, D. and

Nelson, W. R. (1975). *Cancer*, **35**, 514
Miller, J. F. A. P. (1961). *Lancet*, **2**, 748
Miller, J. F. A. P. (1962). *Nature, London*, **195**, 1318
Miller, J. F. A. P. (1966). *British Medical Bulletin*, **22**, 21
Miller, J. F. A. P. and Mitchell, G. F. (1967). *Nature, London*, **216**, 785
Milnick, J. L., Adam, E. and Rawls, W. E. (1974). *Cancer*, **34**, 1375
Mitchison, N. A. (1955). *Journal of Experimental Medicine*, **102**, 157
Mitchison, N. A. (1957). *Proceedings of the Royal Society*, **B142**, 72
Moller, G. (1964). *Nature, London*, **204**, 846
Morton, D. L., Malmgren, R. A., Hall, W. T. and Schildlovsky, G. (1969). *Surgery*, **66**, 152
Morton, D. L. (1972). *Cancer*, **30**, 1647
Mühlbock, O. (1973). *British Journal of Cancer*, **28**, 96
Nauts, H. C., Fowler, G. A. and Bogardo. F. (1953). *Acta Medica Scandinavica*, **276** (Suppl.), **5**, 103
Old, L. J., Boyse, E. A., Clarke, D. A. and Carswell, E. A. (1962). *Annals of the New York Academy of Sciences*, **101**, 80
Oliver, R. T. D. (1978). *Journal of the Royal Society of Medicine*, **71**, 50
O'Toole, C., Perlmann, P., Unsgaard, B. and Zetterlund, C. G. (1973). *Lancet*, **2**, 1085
Parker, R., Alexander, S., Shaheen, O. H. and Parkes, P. (1975). *Journal of Laryngology*, **89**, 687
Pilch, Y. H. and Golub, S. H. (1974). *American Journal of Clinical Pathology*, **62**, 184
Pointon, R. C. S. and Jelly, G. O. (1976). *Proceedings of the Royal Society of Medicine*, **69**, 414
Powles, R. (1973). *British Journal of Cancer*, **28**, 262
Prehn, R. T. and Main, J. M. (1957). *Journal of the National Cancer Institute*, **18**, 769
Prentice, E. D., Lipscomb, H., Metcalf, W. K. and Sharp, J. G. (1976). *Scandinavian Journal of Immunology*, **5**, 955
Rapp, F. and Duff, F. (1974). *Cancer*, **34**, 1353
Reiner, J. and Southam, C. M. (1967). *Cancer Research*, **27**, 1243
Renaud, M. M. (1926). *Annales de Medecine Interne*, **50**, 1441
Roitt, I. M., Greaves, M. F., Torrigiani, G., Brostoff, J. and Playfair, J. H. L. (1969). *Lancet*, **2**, 367
Salaman, M. H. and Roe, F. J. C. (1964). *British Medical Bulletin*, **20**, 139
Saxon, A. and Parkis, J. (1977). *Cancer Research*, **37**, 1154
Sell, S. (1967). *Journal of Immunology*, **98**, 786
Shacks, S. J., Chiller, J. and Granger, G. A. (1973). *Cell Immunology*, **7**, 313
Simons, M. J., Wee, G. B., Day, N. E., Morris, P. J., Shanmugaratnam, K. and De The, G. (1974). *International Journal of Cancer*, **13**, 122
Simons, M. J., Wee, G. B., Chan, S. H., Shanmugaratnam, K., Day, N. E. and De The, G. (1975). *Lancet*, **1**, 142
Sjogren, H. O. (1967). *Modern Trends in Medical Virology*, **1**, 207
Skamene, E. and Gold, P. (1976). 'Organ transplantation'. In *Clinical Immunology* (Ed. by Freedman, S. O. and Gold, P.), 2nd edn, pp. 449–481. Hagerstown, Maryland, New York, San Francisco, London; Harper and Row
Smith, H. G., Chretien, P. B., Henson, D. E., Silverman, N. A. and Alexander, J. C. (1976). *American Journal of Surgery*, **132**, 541
Smithers, D. W. (1967). *Annals of the Royal College of Surgeons of England*, **41**, 160
Southam, C. M. (1967). *Progress in Experimental Tumour Research*, **9**, 1
Stell, P. M. (1975). *Proceedings of the Royal Society of Medicine*, **68**, 83
Stell, P. M. and Green, J. R. (1976). *Proceedings of the Royal Society of Medicine*, **69**, 411
Stewart, T. H. (1969a). *Cancer*, **23**, 1368
Stewart, T. H. (1969b). *Cancer*, **23**, 1380
Stjernsward, J., Clifford, P., Singh, S. and Svedmyr, E. (1968). *East African Medical Journal*, **45**, 1
Stjernsward, J. and Clifford, P. (1969). 'Tumour distinctive cellular immune reactions against autochthonous cancers'. In *Immunity and Tolerance in Oncogenesis* (Ed. by Severi, L.), pp. 749–758. Proceedings of the IV Perugia Quadrennial International Conference on Cancer, Perugia University
Stjernsward, J. (1974). *Lancet*, **2**, 1285
Stjernsward, J. (1977). *Cancer*, **39**, 2846
Stutman, O. and Dupuy, J. M. (1972). *Journal of the National Cancer Institute*, **49**, 1283
Symoens, J. and Rosenthal, M. (1977). *Journal of the Reticulo-endothelial Society*, **21**, 175
Tanner, N. S. B., Clifford, P. and Carter, R. L. (1978). *Clinical Oncology*, **4**, 99
Tarpley, J. L., Potvin, C. and Chretien, P. B. (1975). *Cancer*, **35**, 638
Thomas, L. (1959). In *Cellular and Humoral Aspects of Hyper-sensitivity States* (Ed. by Lawrence, H. S.). New York; P. B. Hocker
Thompson, D. M. P. (1976). In *Clinical Immunology*, 2nd edn (Ed. by Freedman, S. O. and Gold, P.), pp. 548–550. Maryland, New York, San Francisco and London; Harper and Row
Thomson, D. M. P., Steele, K. and Alexander, P. (1973). *British Journal of Cancer*, **27**, 27
Thomson, D. M. P. (1975). *International Journal of Cancer*, **15**, 1016
Welbourn, R. B. and Castro, J. E. (1976). In *Scientific Foundations of Oncology* (Ed. by Symington, T. and Carter, R. L.), p. 612. London; Heinemann Medical Books Ltd.
Willoughby, D. A. and Wood, C. A. (1977). 'The history and development of levamisole'. In *Forum on Immunotherapy*, Vol. 1. London; Royal Society of Medicine
Zinkernagel, R. M. and Doherty, P. C. (1974). *Nature, London*, **251**, 547
Zinkernagel, R. M. and Doherty, P. C. (1975). *Journal of Experimental Medicine*, **141**, 1427

17 Principles of radiotherapy in head and neck cancer

D B L Skeggs

In the last few decades there have been such immense advances in medicine that interdisciplinary cooperation has become essential to ensure that each patient receives the very best treatment available. Nowhere is this more true than in the management of neoplasms of the ear, nose and throat. As a result of such cooperation, helped by the technical advances both in surgery and radiotherapy, there has been a steady improvement in cure rates. However, an ideal link between surgeon and radiotherapist is not achieved just by the establishment of a 'joint ENT Clinic'. It is essential that there should be mutual respect and understanding by each of the other's capability to deal effectively with each particular problem. The otolaryngologist requires some working knowledge of elementary radiotherapy, in order to appreciate how much his radiotherapeutic colleague is able to do and the nature of the problems that confront him.

What is radiotherapy?

The radiotherapist uses ionizing radiation to destroy tumour cells. His armamentarium of irradiation includes x-rays, electrons, gamma and beta irradiation from natural elements such as radium, or from man-made isotopes such as cobalt 60 and phosphorus 32. More recently, particulate irradiation such as fast neutrons and pi-mesons is being brought into use. Clinicians who do not have close contact with radiotherapists are sometimes under the impression that they are 'scientists' rather than clinicians and that, by the very nature of their work, they must have a profound knowledge of physics. They do have a six-months' intensive course in physics and, having covered this ground, they must retain an understanding of the subject and a feeling for it in relation to the treatment of patients with irradiation. From the otolaryngologist's point of view it is useful to appreciate the following facts.

Penetration

The degree of penetration of all forms of ionizing radiation is related to the energy of the particular beam. X and γ rays behave in an identical manner with respect to their interaction with matter. The absorption is exponential and the higher the energy, the greater will be the percentage dosage received at a particular point. Electrons on the other hand have a finite range and, as a rough guide, one estimates that their range in tissue is approximately 1 cm for every 3 MeV. The intensity of irradiation suddenly drops to 50 per cent, once the electrons have reached their range, with a subsequent, more rapid decrease in intensity of irradiation. This particular characteristic is of great importance when one requires to treat a superficial tumour without causing unacceptable damage to underlying structures (e.g. squamous cell carcinoma of the buccal mucosa.)

Megavoltage irradiation

The term 'megavoltage' is used to describe treatment using x-rays or gamma emission with an energy equivalent to at least 1 million volts. The requirement of the high energy is not only to produce a more penetrating beam in order to treat effectively deep-seated tumours, but at this energy range, two very important features occur.

(1) All tissues regardless of their structure will, weight for weight, absorb the same amount of irradiation (*Figure 17.1*). At lower energy ranges, especially in the 60–140 kV range which is intentionally selected for diagnostic purposes, absorption is proportional to the cube of the atomic number of the material being irradiated and so structures such as bone and cartilage may well receive about eight times as much irradiation as the surrounding soft tissue. Thus, if an attempt is made to cure a tumour in the head and neck with low energy x-rays, bone or cartilage necrosis may occur. This problem confronted earlier generations of radiotherapists, whose highest energy machine was the standard deep x-ray unit working at 250 kV. To overcome this serious disadvantage, high energy x-ray machines and radium teletherapy units started to be built in the late 1930s. The disadvantage of the former machines was that they tended to be unreliable and the radium 'bombs' had a large treatment penumbra and low output, necessitating long treatment times. By the mid 1950s, cobalt teletherapy units with a gamma energy of 1.3 MeV, equivalent to an x-ray beam of 2.6 MeV, were increasingly being brought into use and at the same time, linear accelerators, with an x-ray beam of up to 30 MeV, were being developed.

(2) With beams of an energy up to 1 MeV, the maximum dosage always occurs on the surface. It is for this reason that the early radiotherapists earned a reputation of 'burning' their patients as a deep x-ray beam, by necessity, gave the maximum exposure to the skin rather than to the underlying tumour. With beams of an energy over 1 MeV, the point of maximum intensity gradually increases to come to a peak of 100 per cent at a depth of an increasing number of millimetres below the surface of the skin, the higher the energy of the beam. Thus, the megavoltage beam from a cobalt unit or linear accelerator has the quality known as 'skin-sparing effect' because the maximum intensity is not reached until the beam is well past the surface of the skin. As a result, intense skin reactions are not often seen.

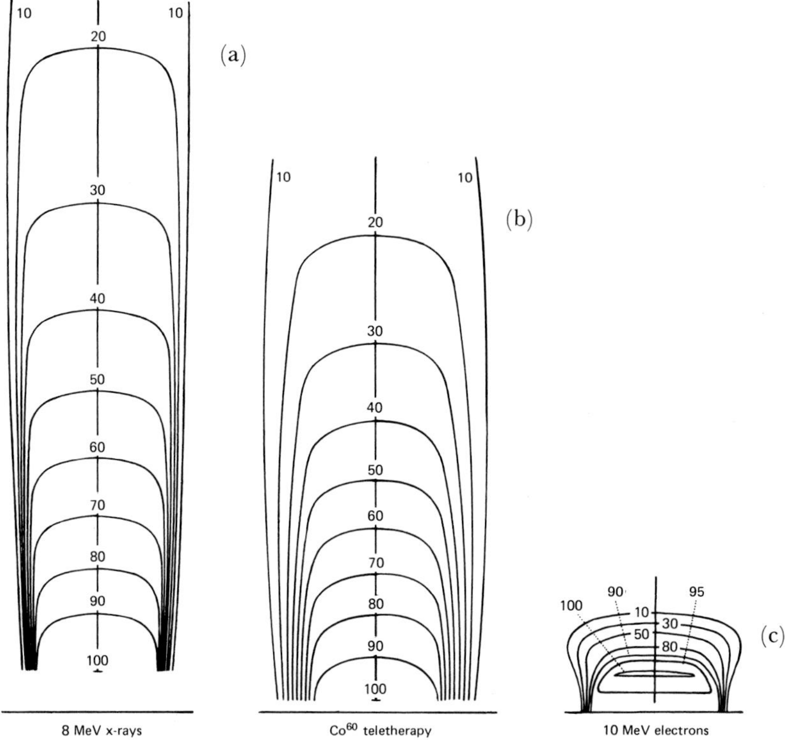

Figure 17.1 The dosage distribution in tissue of: (a) MeV x-rays; (b) cobalt 60 teletherapy beam; (c) 10 MeV electrons. The 8 MeV beam has its maximum dosage at 2 cm depth, has great penetrating power and a 'sharp' edge to its beam. The cobalt teletherapy beam in contrast has a significant penumbra on the edge of the beam, does not have such great penetrating power and its maximum dose is at 4 mm in tissue. The electron beam will be seen to have an effective range of approximately 3 cm in tissue and beyond this there is a very rapid reduction in the amount of irradiation

The inverse square law

All forms of electromagnetic radiation (including ionizing radiation), obey this law, which states that the intensity of irradiation falls off inversely with the square of the distance from the source. Use is made of this physical law when it is required to give a very intense dose of irradiation to a given region, without causing harm to vital adjacent structures. The radiation is applied directly to the tumour either by implantation with radioactive needles or by applying a 'radium' applicator. Conversely, when the intention is to irradiate a deep-seated tumour to a high dose but at the same time, to spare the overlying skin as far as possible, a treatment unit employing a long source-to-patient distance, i.e. a cobalt teletherapy unit or linear accelerator, is used.

The mechanism of radiotherapy

Exactly how ionizing radiation destroys tumours is not fully understood. It is known that irradiation has the power to destroy the reproductive integrity of cells and it probably achieves this partly as the result of the impact of the irradiation on the cell nucleus and partly as a result of chemical changes induced by the ionizing radiation.

Radiosensitivity

The degree of sensitivity to irradiation can, to a large extent, be correlated with the histological structure of the tumour. In practice, tumours are grouped as shown in *Table 17.1*.

Table 17.1

		Dose required
High sensitivity	Tumours of lymphatic origin Embryonic tumours Highly anaplastic tumours	2000–4000 rad
Moderate sensitivity	Reticulum cell sarcoma Squamous cell carcinoma Some adenocarcinomas	5000–6500 rad
Low sensitivity	Tumours of mesodermal origin, such as fibrosarcoma, osteogenic sarcoma	Min. of 7000 rad

In treating a tumour, the aim is to destroy every malignant cell. In practice, it is a well-known fact that the tumours that are most likely to be cured by radiotherapy are those that have been diagnosed at a very early stage. One of the reasons for this is that as a tumour enlarges, the number of malignant cells that it contains increases by a factor of eight each time the tumour doubles in size. Thus, on mathematical grounds the chances of destroying all the malignant cells decreases rapidly as the tumour enlarges. Furthermore, as the tumour enlarges there comes a stage when the cellular proliferation begins to outstrip the vascularity supplying it. The situation then arises when an increasing percentage of the tumour cells are either partially hypoxic or completely anoxic, leading to necrosis. Hypoxia (Gray *et al.*, 1953) protects cells from the destructive effects of radiation and this can be an important factor in a tumour failing to respond to treatment.

Radiocurability

A distinction has to be made between radiosensitivity and radiocurability because the two are not necessarily synonymous. The explanation for this is that many of the more radiosensitive tumours, such as anaplastic carcinomas, although responding locally exceptionally well to the irradiation, may well, by the very nature of their natural history, have disseminated beyond the bounds of the area being treated. Thus, there may be a successful outcome to the treatment locally but the patient succumbs as a result of wider local extension of the disease or possibly distant metastases.

The philosophy of successful radiotherapy

From what has already been said, it is plain that it is essential to obtain a definitive tissue diagnosis for all patients who are to be considered for treatment by radiotherapy. Curative treatment is then based upon the well established axiom, 'small volume – high dose', the corollary of which is, the larger the volume to be irradiated, the smaller the dose it is possible to give. The intention always is to destroy the tumour without causing unacceptable damage to the surrounding normal structures. Fortunately, normal structures will tolerate irradiation rather better than tumour cells, but this differential sensitivity is only marginal and everything possible has to be done to manipulate the treatment in such a way that healthy tissues have the best chance of surviving the onslaught of the radiotherapy. This is achieved partly by limiting the actual volume irradiated (which therefore necessitates very accurate localization of the region to be treated) and also by fractionating the treatment over a sufficient length of time so that the cumulative total dose received by the tumour is sufficient to destroy it, but at the same time will not cause irreparable damage to normal structures. There has also been speculation that the fractionation of dosage makes it more likely that the tumour cells will be treated at different phases of the mitotic cycle and therefore may be more likely to succumb to the treatment. There is a subtle relationship between time and dose and this is calculated in such a way that the normal cells do not receive so much irradiation on each exposure that they are unable to repair the damage that has occurred. At different Centres throughout the world it will be noted that the doses prescribed for tumours vary according to the total overall period of treatment and the number of treatments actually given in that time. When a patient is to be given a radical course of therapy, whenever possible it is desirable to give the treatment five days a week for approximately six and a half weeks, to a total dosage of 6500 rad. This tends to cause the least amount of constitutional disturbance with avoidance of excessive reactions and the lowest incidence of long-term morbidity. Some Centres will give 5500 rad in 20 treatments over four weeks and yet at other Centres, 3600 rad in six fractions over 18 days may be prescribed. As far as the tumour is concerned, all these doses have been calculated to be approximately equal in their lethal effect (Ellis, 1969) but the smaller the number of fractions of treatment and the shorter the period of time, the more likely is one to inflict long-term damage to normal tissues.

When a radiotherapist is planning a treatment, instinctively he thinks not only about the tumour volume that has to be adequately irradiated, but at the same time consideration must be given to the structures that have to be avoided so that there is no long-term disability for the patient.

In the region of the head, the two normal structures that are highly sensitive to irradiation and therefore have always to be considered, are the lens and the spinal cord. A total dose of between 200 and 800 rad may well be sufficient to cause a radiation cataract and a dose in excess of 4000 rad to the cervical spinal cord can result in frank radiation myelitis, which is irreversible and tends to be progressive. Thus, exceptional attention has to be given to accurate localization of the tumour volume to be treated and careful arrangement of the treatment fields, so that adjacent vital structures, such as the eye and spinal cord, do not receive an unacceptable dose. It is thus apparent that exact information with regard to the localization of the tumour from his surgical colleague is all important to the radiotherapist. Special x-ray investigations, and notably the EMI computerized transverse tomography system, can also give vital information for providing the exact details necessary for localizing the tumour volume.

Radiotherapy at special sites

The ear

Tumours on the pinna are usually squamous cell carcinomas though basal cell carcinomas are by no means unknown. The precise pathological diagnosis is important as the basal cell carcinoma requires approximately 4000 rad to ensure its cure, whereas the squamous cell carcinoma must be given a dose in the region of 5000–6000 rad. Generally speaking, for the basal cell carcinoma, successful treatment with no risk of damage to the cartilage, can be given by means of superficial x-ray therapy (130 kV) in approximately 9–10 treatments over 12 days. Epitheliomas on the other hand, cannot be treated to the higher dose level of 6000 rad by means of superficial x-ray therapy without risk of causing necrosis to the underlying cartilage. In these circumstances, a radium mould may be used with the radium conveniently applied in the form of a 'sandwich' (*see Figure 17.2*). The advantage of this system is that radium has a high effective energy equivalent to x-rays of approximately 2.5 MeV, which means that there is no excessive absorption of irradiation in the underlying cartilage; furthermore, on account of the inverse square law, adjacent structures do not receive a high dose.

The external auditory canal

Malignant tumours arising in the external auditory canal are invariably epitheliomas. Although these may appear to be localized and at the time of biopsy may apparently have been virtually completely excised, these tumours have a most unpleasant reputation. The tumour bed must be treated to a radical dose level and subsequently, a very careful watch on the adjacent lymph node drainage for metastatic spread is necessary. Here, electrons of an appropriate energy are ideal as a form of treatment because with a simple straight-on field with the energy specifically selected for the depth of the particular tumour, the full radical dosage of 5000–6000 rad can be given without the underlying or adjacent structures receiving a significantly high dose.

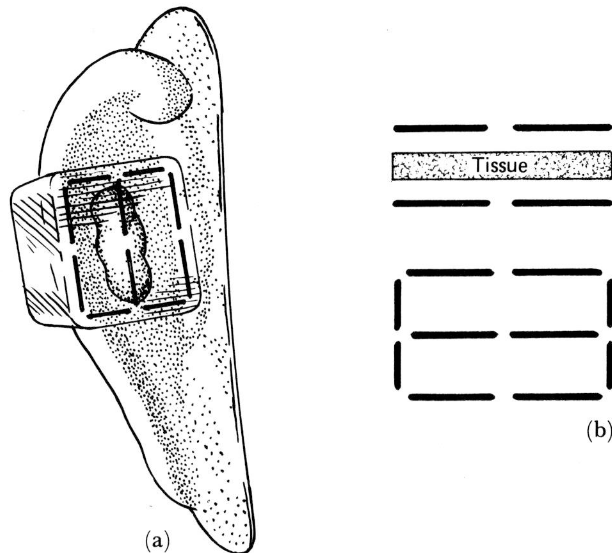

Figure 17.2 (a) Epithelioma of the pinna. This demonstrates an acrylic mould of the pinna expanded into a carrier for radium overlying an epithelioma of the pinna. (b) This diagram illustrates how the radium is loaded for treating an epithelioma of the pinna, with the tumour forming the 'meat' for the sandwich

The middle ear

Tumours of the middle ear are too deep-seated for treatment by electrons of the usual energy available in some departments. Therefore, a technique using two angled fields with cobalt teletherapy or a linear accelerator incorporating a wedge filter in the beam to give homogeneous dosage, is employed (*see Figure 17.3*). The fields are angled so as to confine the dose as far as possible to the tumour volume and to ensure that the brain stem receives a sufficiently low dose. The angle of the wedge is specifically selected to achieve the optimum distribution of irradiation for each particular case. Glomus jugulare tumours are treated in exactly the same way. Prior to the report of Capps (1957) and others, it was accepted that these tumours were not responsive to radiotherapy. However, Capps disproved this and his findings have been subsequently confirmed by radiotherapists throughout the world.

Maxillary antrum

Before starting radiotherapy at any site, histological identification of the tumour is essential. This applies especially to the antrum, where the tumour is most usually a squamous cell carcinoma, though melanomas, lymphomas and sarcomas are known to occur. Usually the diagnosis is established after a 'Caldwell–Luc' has been performed and this approach to the antrum has the added advantage that it allows

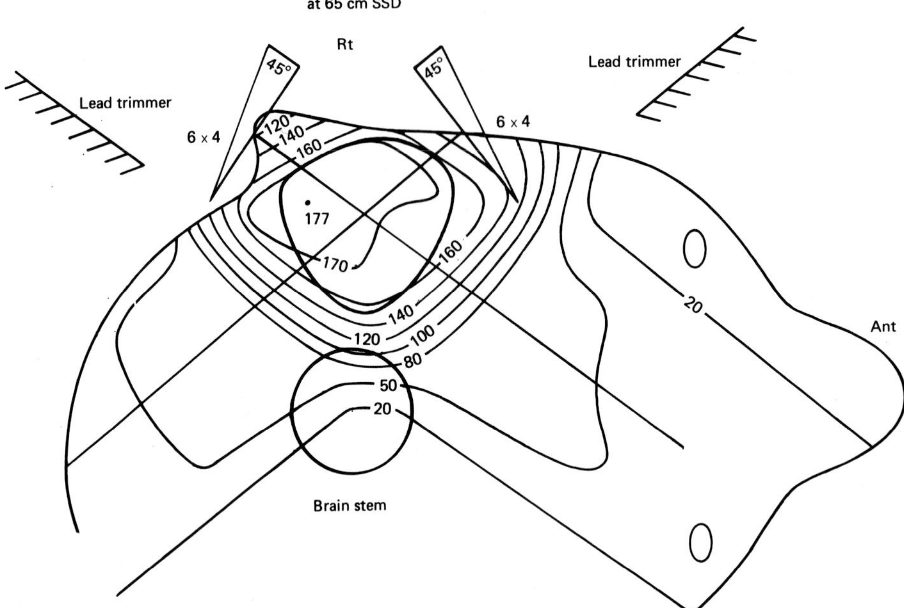

Figure 17.3 Treatment plan for a middle-ear tumour. The treatment dosage is concentrated in the region of the middle ear by directing two angled fields with a special wedge filter in the beam to achieve homogeneity of dosage distribution. It should be noted that this arrangement results in a low dosage being received both by the brain stem and the lens of both eyes. A lead 'trimmer' is positioned on the inner edge of both fields in order to remove the penumbra effect and thereby reduce the dosage received by the brain stem.

drainage of infection that might otherwise cause complications during the radiotherapy. Because of the anatomical relationships of the maxillary antrum, the floor of the orbit has to be included within the treatment volume. Every effort is made to protect the anterior chamber of the eye but the patient must be warned that it is virtually inevitable that sight will be lost on this side and that there is a risk that the eye itself could be destroyed by the treatment. The diagram of the treatment technique (*Figure 17.4*) shows how the two-wedged fields are arranged in such a way that the antrum and its immediate surrounds receive homogeneous dosage, but at the same time the contralateral eye and the brain stem receive the bare minimum. During each treatment, the patient will bite on a special bung between his jaws in order to depress the mandible and with it the tongue so that the tongue, which would otherwise be in apposition with the palate, does not receive the full dose of irradiation. The actual policy with regard to the treatment of antral tumours varies from Centre to Centre concerning the parts that surgery and radiotherapy have to play in the management of the disease. On occasions, palatal fenestration may be performed following radical irradiation and if residual active disease is discovered, it is essential to draw a detailed diagram of the exact area involved. The reason for this is that although radical external irradiation has already been given, it is still possible to give further irradiation in the form of local treatment from a radium mould. An impression is taken of the oro–antral cavity and this is then used to make an acrylic

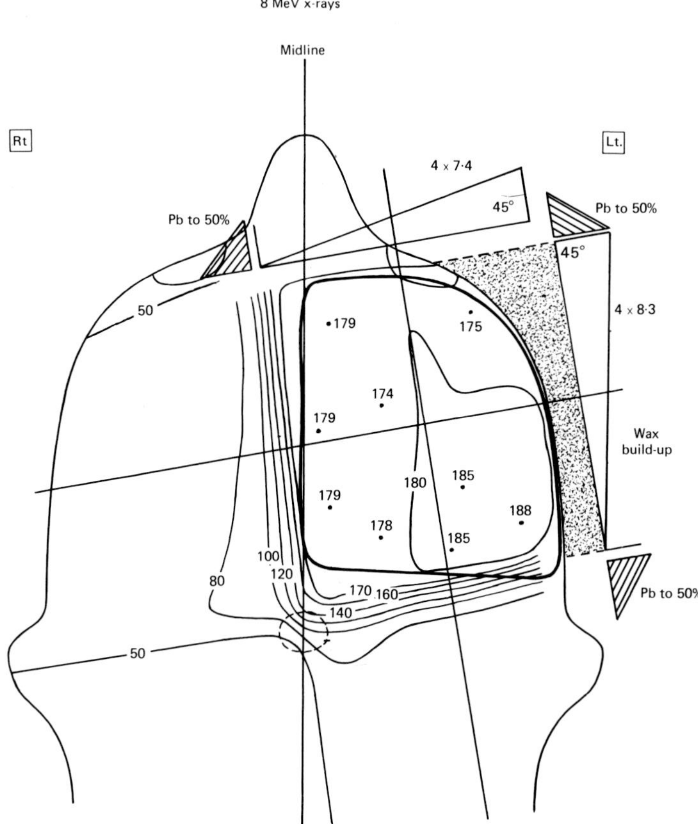

Figure 17.4 Treatment plan for a tumour of the maxillary antrum. Note how the fields are arranged at a slight angle in order to reduce the amount of irradiation being received by the brain stem and the contralateral eye

prosthesis. Then, in cooperation with the surgeon, the radiotherapist will mark on this prosthesis the exact area that he wishes to be loaded with radium. Bearing in mind the inverse square law, this radium applicator may then be inserted to give a very high dose, just where the residual tumour was noted and at the same time the surrounding structures will receive only a minimal amount of irradiation, which will be easily tolerated. The radium applicator is usually worn for 6–8 h a day for eight days, to give a calculated dose of 6000 rad to the site of tumour recurrence.

Ethmoidal sinuses

If an electron beam of sufficient energy to give the necessary penetration is available, a single straight-on field applied to the ethmoids is ideal. Most radiotherapy centres do not have this facility and therefore the treatment has to be given using a combination of two small, parallel opposed, lateral fields together with a small supplementary anterior field. The localization, planning and subsequent treatment has to be very precise in order to spare the eyes from irradiation. Chordomas arising in the region of the basi-sphenoid are treated in a similar manner.

Nose

Within the nasal vestibule and on the septum the tumour most commonly seen is a squamous cell carcinoma. Joint discussion between the surgeon and radiotherapist decides whether surgery or radiotherapy is the treatment of choice. If it is the latter, the standard dose of approximately 6000 rad will be required, which will be delivered by the best means available.

Post-nasal space

Tumours at this site are infrequent in the British Isles. They are most commonly squamous cell carcinomas of varying differentiation or reticulum cell sarcomas. In younger patients, giving a short history, anaplastic lymphomas are most frequently the cause. By contrast, in the Arabian peninsula, post-nasal space carcinomas are frequently seen and most usually are anaplastic carcinomas. At the time of diagnosis, enlarged lymph nodes in the neck are frequently noted, which in the case of anaplastic tumours or lymphomas, may well extend down to the level of the clavicle. Radiotherapy is the only effective treatment available, sometimes supplemented with cytotoxic drugs, and the treatment field has to extend from Reid's baseline downwards. If the tumour is a lymphoma, then all the nodes to the level of the clavicle must be irradiated. If, on the other hand, the tumour is a squamous cell carcinoma, a compromise is usually made in order to reduce the total volume irradiated and thus enable a higher dose to be given. At this site one of the main problems confronting the radiotherapist is the fact that the nodes in the neck may well overlap the spinal cord. The spinal cord in the neck will tolerate little over 4000 rad and this dose must not be exceeded. Usually the primary tumour, together with the lymph nodes in the neck, will be treated initially by cobalt teletherapy or by a linear accelerator, in continuity up to a dose level of 4000 rad. Then, electrons may be applied to the glands in the neck, to bring their total dosage to the required level, whilst the primary tumour area continues to be irradiated by parallel opposed lateral fields with the megavoltage unit. If the tumour is a squamous cell carcinoma and has already produced metastatic lymph nodes, the outlook is indeed bleak. However, if it should be a lymphoma, radiotherapy followed by appropriate cytotoxic drugs may well produce a long-lasting remission.

Tonsil and oro-pharynx

Yet again, establishment of the exact histological diagnosis of the tumour is essential before any decision is made upon how the tumour is going to be treated. If the neoplasm is a well-differentiated squamous cell carcinoma and is entirely confined to the tonsil, one is justified in confining the treatment to the site of the primary tumour together with the adjacent lymphatic drainage. If, on the other hand, the tumour is poorly differentiated, or is a lympho-epithelioma or some variation of the lymphoma family, it is necessary to cover a much larger volume and consideration will have to be given to the advisability of regarding the disease as a midline condition and applying the radiotherapy bilaterally.

Larynx

The results of radical radiotherapy at this site for early tumours arising on the cords are exceptionally good (up to 90 per cent 5-year survival) because the tumour can be very accurately localized and the resultant small volume, which may measure as little as 3 × 5 cm, can be given up to 6500 rad in six and a half weeks, usually with little in the way of side-effects. With such a small field, absolute accuracy of treatment set-up is essential and it is customary to make either a special acrylic cast or a 'jig' of the patient's outline, so that on each occasion the planned treatment may be easily reproduced (*Figure 17.5*). The treatment of more extensive tumours within the larynx is carried out in the same way, but the cure rates are by no means so good. This may be partly due to the fact that the tumour has outgrown its blood supply and may

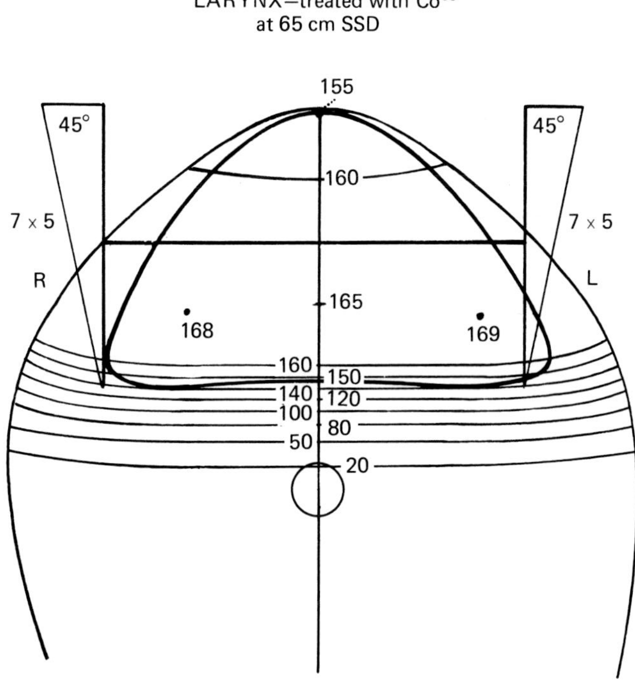

Figure 17.5 Treatment plan for a larynx. The even distribution of dosage within the treatment volume should be noted as well as the fact that the spinal cord is receiving a low dose. The wedge filters are used in this instance to compensate for the curved outline of the neck, thus allowing for the tissue 'deficiency' within the treatment volume and maintaining an even distribution of irradiation

contain a significant percentage of hypoxic cells, and partly because the mathematical probability of destroying such a vastly increased number of tumour cells is small. The experienced radiotherapist usually has a shrewd idea of his chances of curing a particular laryngeal tumour and careful discussion with his surgical colleague is necessary so that each may express his views as to the part that his specialty has to play in the treatment of any particular case.

Tumours of the laryngo–pharynx are treated in exactly the same manner. Generally, they are more advanced and therefore have to be treated by larger fields and do not stand such a good chance of cure. This applies especially to tumours of the pyriform fossa, which tend to present late as the primary tumour may be present for many months before it gives rise to symptoms and by this time may well have given rise to lymph node metastases in the neck.

Post-cricoid carcinoma

These tumours, if not too advanced, may be treated in exactly the same way as laryngeal neoplasms, with reasonably good results.

Carcinoma of the oesophagus

The results of treatment at this site, either by surgery or by radiotherapy, have in the past been far from good. Radiotherapy has failed because in order to ensure that the tumour is fully covered, a margin of 5 cm above and below the limits of the tumour shown on x-ray, has to be covered. Due to the tortuous course of the oesophagus at this site, conventional radiotherapy has to cover a large expanse of normal structures in order to encompass the whole of the tumour volume, thus making it necessary to reduce the overall dose given to the disease. In recent years, promising results have been obtained at the Royal Free Hospital, London, using the system known as the 'Tracking Cobalt', which is able to follow the tumour volume within its distribution in the thorax and at the same time sparing the surrounding normal structures so that they receive the minimum of treatment. Consequently, it is possible to give the oesophageal tumour a radical dose, which is well tolerated by the patient and does not cause unacceptable complications.

Parotid tumours

In general, the primary treatment for parotid tumours is surgery. For the pleomorphic adenoma, there is no indication for radiotherapy, except in a situation where the tumour has been removed on several occasions and the surgeon feels unsure of achieving a satisfactory clearance. After the tumour has been resected, the radiotherapist can implant the tumour bed with radioactive needles such as radium or caesium and these will remain in place for approximately 8 days to give a calculated dose of 6000 rad.

The other indication for radiotherapy for parotid tumours is for the patient who either has an inoperable carcinoma, or has had surgery but in whom complete removal was not possible. In this situation, a straight-on field with electrons is usually ideal as this will ensure that the tumour residuum receives high-dosage irradiation, but the underlying tissues will be spared. If the tumour mass should be so thick that electron therapy is not applicable, then the patient may be planned for treatment with cobalt teletherapy using wedged fields, in a manner rather similar to that used for treating tumours of the middle ear.

Radiation reactions

During his course of radiotherapy, the patient will inevitably develop reactions of the normal tissues. Generally, skin reactions are not severe because with megavoltage irradiation the maximum dosage received occurs at several millimetres below the surface of the skin. When a larynx is being treated, the dose received by the skin from the exit beam is, in fact, greater than the dose received on the side to which the beam is being applied. By the completion of treatment, there will usually be just a moderate erythema with perhaps some dry, spotty desquamation. Any form of trauma, be it due to washing with soap, exposure to sunlight, or even irritation from coarse clothing, will aggravate the normal skin reaction and may even necessitate the suspension of the treatment and thus prejudice its success. Whilst there may be little to see in the way of a reaction on a patient's neck, the mucosal lining on the other hand may show a different picture. Initially, there will be an even erythematous reaction and gradually this will progress to a stage where there is a patchy, fibrinous exudate. This is the ideal stage that should be reached by the completion of treatment and shows that the normal tissues are approaching tolerance. If treatment is allowed to proceed beyond this point, the patchy exudate will progress to a confluent exudate, which signifies that the tissues are being taken beyond tolerance and the end result may be necrosis. The membranous reaction usually starts as an erythema at a dose level of around 4000 rad and a patchy fibrinous exudate starts to develop at around 5500 rad. The underlying mechanism of this effect is that the irradiation causes increased capillary permeability, allowing the fibrin to exude. This reaction will be aggravated by any form of trauma such as smoking, drinking strong alcohol, infection or the use of irritant mouth washes such as salt and water. The patient may complain of dysphagia at this stage and this usually responds well to the use of a soluble aspirin gargle and swallow, just before meals. In order not to prejudice the successful progress of the treatment, it is essential that patients be advised about these complications and their prevention. On occasions, when a patient develops an infection such as monilia, the reaction may temporarily become very brisk and the treatment has to be suspended for a week or so. This is undesirable but it is preferable to do this rather than continue 'regardless', knowing full well that the patient will not complete his treatment successfully. In view of this, it is essential that patients are instructed not to shave using soap and water but to use an electric razor during the treatment. Usually there is some permanent loss of the beard and the patient must be advised not to expose the treated skin to direct sunlight for at least six months following treatment.

Long-term reactions are unusual and may take the form of pallor of the vocal cord or perhaps some localized telangiectasia. From time to time persistent oedema of the laryngeal cartilages occurs and in this situation it is advisable to treat the patient with a suitable broad spectrum antibiotic together with steroids. It may be necessary to give the antibiotic for about a month and for the same time, Prednisolone will be given, starting at a dose of 10 mg thrice daily, which will be gradually tailed off during the same period. In most cases the oedema settles down satisfactorily, though occasionally the patient may be left with some persistent low-grade oedema and a hoarse voice. Fortunately, radiation necrosis of the larynx is virtually unknown in the best Centres. It is important to consider the long-term effect of irradiation upon normal tissues, especially if the necessity for surgery arises at a site that has previously been irradiated. Irradiation causes endarteritis of the smaller vessels and this in its turn will aggravate the tendency for high dosage irradiation to induce fibrosis. In spite of this, laryngectomies following failed radiotherapy seldom run into trouble as a result of modern megavoltage radiotherapy. Electrons, on the other hand, for practical purposes deliver the maximum dosage to the skin and surgery at a site that has received radical electron therapy may well face problems with skin healing.

Some patients complain of dryness following a radical course of irradiation, which is due to the suppression of the normal secretory glands. This symptom may persist but more usually it tends to improve gradually. What the long-term effects to the middle ear are is to some degree a matter of speculation as there is little in the way of reports on human experience or on animal experiments. It would seem likely, however, that high dosage irradiation may induce some degree of fibrotic change in association with the ossicles, which would result in some diminution of acuity of hearing. Perhaps the most serious long-term radiation effect is malignant change but this usually takes in the region of thirty years to manifest itself. Thus, it is seldom seen, but when it does occur it tends to be a sarcoma such as osteogenic sarcoma.

Hyperbaric oxygen

Already it has been stated that hypoxia causes cells to be protected from irradiation. Churchill-Davidson *et al.* (1973) have postulated that a lymph node 1 cm in diameter probably contains 1 per cent of hypoxic cells. The resultant radio-resistance of the tumour cells in that node may well be sufficient for conventional therapy to fail. In such cases, treatment in a hyperbaric oxygen chamber (*Figure 17.6*), with the patient breathing oxygen at a pressure of 30 lb/in^2 (3 atmospheres absolute), has been shown to improve significantly the response of metastatic lymph nodes in the neck and also of extensive tumours of the head and neck that normally do not respond well to conventional radiotherapy. The method of treatment is time-consuming and is undoubtedly a considerable ordeal for some patients, especially if they suffer with claustrophobia. The treatment involves placing the patient in a small pressure chamber and each treatment will require the patient to be in the chamber for at least 1 h. Absolute immobility is essential to ensure accuracy of treatment and this, coupled with barometric problems such as difficulty in clearing the eustachian tubes and variations in temperature within the chamber, make the treatment a considerable trial, especially for the more intelligent patient. In view of this, the course of treatment is carried out in six sessions given twice a week over a period of three weeks, the patient receiving a total dose of 3600 rad, which is approximately equivalent to the standard dose of 6500 rad given in daily fractions over six and a half weeks.

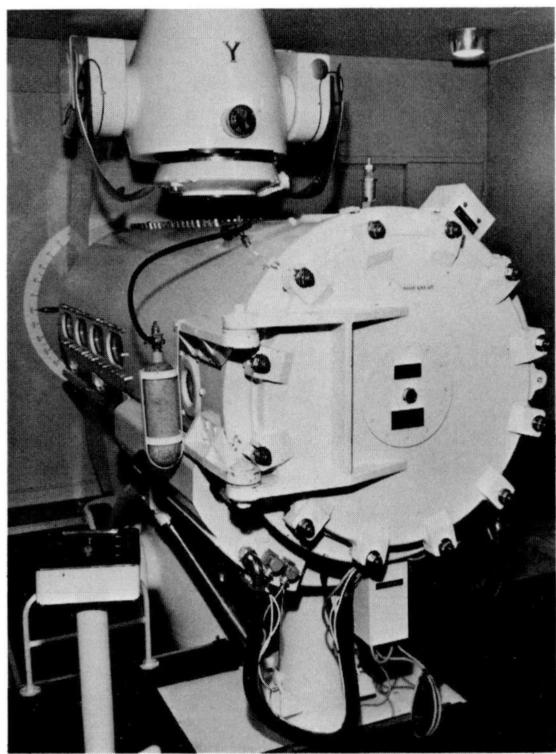

Figure 17.6 Hyperbaric oxygen chamber. This is the chamber in use at St. Thomas's Hospital and it will be noted that the cobalt teletherapy treatment unit associated with it has twin heads in order to reduce the overall treatment time as much as possible. (Permission to use this photograph has kindly been granted by Dr. Ian Churchill-Davidson)

Radiotherapy and cytotoxic drugs in combination

In the treatment of head and neck lymphomas it is usual to treat the primary tumour area, together with the main associated lymph nodes, by means of radiotherapy and then, after an interval, to follow this treatment with the appropriate combination of cytotoxic drugs. Certain cytotoxic drugs, especially Bleomycin and Methotrexate, have been shown to have an adjuvant effect on radiotherapy in the treatment of squamous cell carcinomas. The indication for such treatment would be for a patient who has extensive disease or metastatic lymph node involvement, who is not suitable for treatment by surgery and who would be deemed to have a poor chance of being cured by radiotherapy alone. Bleomycin is most commonly used and 5 mg are given intramuscularly, 30 min before the patient receives his radiotherapy. The potentiation of effect sometimes is remarkable and furthermore, the same increased effect also occurs in the normal tissues. As a result, unless the daily dose of radiotherapy is reduced by about 15 per cent, the patient will develop excessive radiation reactions, which will necessitate the treatment being suspended. In such circumstances, it is advisable to give approximately 850 rad a week, instead of 1000 rad, and to complete the treatment after 6000 rad have been given, instead of 6500 rad. Such combined treatment has undoubtedly improved the otherwise very poor results of treating advanced head and neck epitheliomas. More recently a number of workers, including

Price and Hill, have reported (1978) encouraging results using high dosage combination cytotoxic drug treatment, given preferably before radiotherapy or surgery. On occasions it is given in combination with the radiotherapy, in which case appropriate adjustment of the radiation dosage is necessary.

The general care of the patient receiving radiotherapy

Most patients with cancer have, I believe, a very shrewd suspicion of the nature of their diagnosis, but very few of them are able to discuss it and they do not wish to be told the whole truth. Usually the patient is reaching out for hope and it is essential that the treatment be given in an atmosphere of confidence. From the very start, the patient should realize that the treatment is a team effort and he, the patient, is the most important member of that team. His cooperation throughout the course of treatment is essential and the importance of such precautions as avoiding infections, maintaining oral hygiene, avoiding smoking, drinking strong alcohol and having a good balanced diet, must be stressed. At the very start, when the decision has been made that the patient will receive radiotherapy, it is essential to explain to him exactly what is going to be done for him and what he will experience during that time. Inevitably, on the occasions of the first few treatments, the patient may have a sense of claustrophobia as he will be in the treatment room on his own, but, as it will be explained to him, once he is set up in the correct position and the machine is switched on, the treatment time is only about 2 min and throughout this time he is constantly watched by direct vision through a special window or by means of a closed circuit television system. Many departments have background music which some patients find soothing. Also, in some departments, unusual ceiling designs are painted so that the patient has a subject on which to focus his attention during the treatment, which will help him to keep still and make the treatment time seem less long. During the actual treatment there is no sensation whatsoever; it is as if an x-ray picture has been taken but the exposure is that much longer. As the treatment progresses, so the patient may develop radiation reactions, which have already been described. This will be explained to the patient and he will be told to tell the radiographers of any symptoms that he may develop so that they may be treated promptly. The establishment of a close liaison between the patient and the staff is all-important and at the same time, when possible, the family should also be kept well informed.

References

Capps, F. W. C. (1957). *Journal of the Faculty of Radiology*, **8,** 312

Churchill-Davidson, I. *et al.* (1973). *Clinical Radiology*, **24,** 498

Ellis, F. (1969). *Clinical Radiology*, **20,** 1–7

Gray, L. H. *et al.* (1953). *British Journal of Radiology*, **82,** 638

Price, L. A. and Hill, B. T. (1978). *Scott Brown's Diseases of the Ear, Nose and Throat*, 4th edn. London; Butterworths

18 Principles of chemotherapy in head and neck cancer

L A Price and Bridget T Hill

Introduction

Most head and neck cancers are traditionally treated with some form of surgery, preceded or followed by radiotherapy. Though most of these lesions tend to remain local and spread to a variable degree to regional nodes, cure rates for the advanced lesions, especially those with lymph node involvement, remain poor (Lederman, 1970; Till *et al.*, 1975). The traditional approach to the overall management of head and neck cancer is summarized in *Figure 18.1*. Because the overall disease-free interval

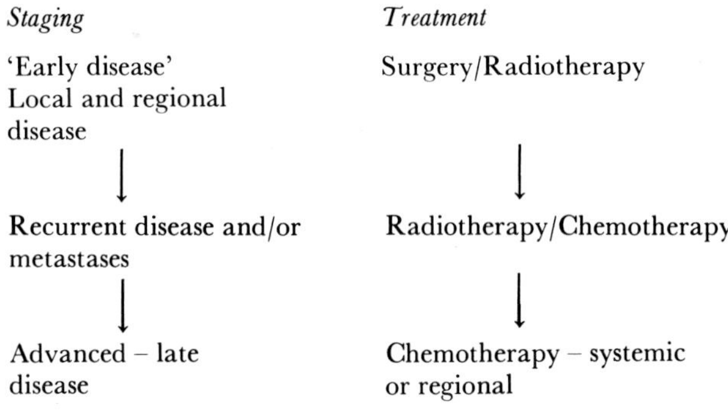

Figure 18.1 The traditional approach to the management of head and neck tumours (adapted from Carter and Soper, 1974)

has not improved for several decades using this approach, this chapter is a discussion of whether the addition of logically designed combination chemotherapy earlier in the disease can improve the prognosis in this group of tumours.

Traditional chemotherapy

Of the 30 'standard agents' given systemically (*see Table 18.1*), 16 drugs have been evaluated against head and neck cancer (all types) of which twelve have consistent activity and four are inactive. These agents and their response rates are listed in *Table 18.2*. Fourteen widely available drugs have never been adequately tested in these cancers. The most effective single agent is methotrexate given by intravenous infusion and followed by folinic acid (Carter and Soper, 1974). Attempts to improve these response rates have involved intra-arterial perfusion and the systemic use of combinations of drugs. Although good results can still be achieved with regional chemotherapy using various combinations of methotrexate, 5-fluorouracil and bleomycin (Espiner and Westbury, 1964; Donegan and Harris, 1976) this approach

Table 18.1 30 'Standard' anti-cancer agents

Actinomycin D; Adriamycin; L-Asparaginase; 5-Azacytidine; BCNU; Bleomycin; Busulfan; CCNU; Chlorambucil; Cyclophosphamide; Cytosine arabinoside; Daunorubicin; Dibromodulcitol; Dibromomannitol; DTIC; 5-Fluorouracil; Hexamethylmelamine; Hydroxyurea; Mechlorethamine; Melphalan; 6-Mercaptopurine; Methotrexate; Methyl-CCNU; Mithramycin; Mitomycin C; Procarbazine; Streptozotocin; 6-Thioguanine; Vinblastine; Vincristine

(After Wasserman *et al.*, 1975.)

Table 18.2 Drug activity in head and neck cancer (all types)

Drug	*Activity*	*Number of evaluated patients*	*Response** (%)
Methotrexate	++	630	47
Bleomycin	++	144	35
Hydroxyurea	+	18	39
Cyclophosphamide	+	77	36
Vinblastine	+	35	29
Adriamycin	+	112	28
Dibromodulcitol	+	50	22
5-Fluorouracil	+	118	15
Chlorambucil	+	34	15
Methyl CCNU	+	40	15
Hexamethylmelamine	+	75	12
6-Mercaptopurine	+	45	12
Procarbazine	–	31	10
Nitrogen Mustard	–	66	8
CCNU	–	50	8
DTIC	–	24	5

Legend: ++, adequate evaluation, drug definitely active.
+, inadequate evaluation, evidence of drug activity but not clearly evaluated.
–, adequate evaluation, drug inactive.
* Response, 50 per cent or greater shrinkage of a measurable lesion.
(After Wasserman *et al.*, 1975 and Bonadonna *et al.*, 1975.)

is no longer widely used for two main reasons: (1) there is a definite morbidity associated with intra-arterial cannulation; (2) similar results can be achieved more safely with properly administered systemic treatment. Attempts at combination therapy have been relatively few, and until 1974 the best response rate for combination chemotherapy was approximately 45 per cent. Some of these results are summarized in *Table 18.3* (after Goldsmith and Carter (1975)). Although good results were obtained by some of these protocols definite toxicity occurred to normal proliferating systems especially bone marrow.

Table 18.3 Combination chemotherapy in head and neck cancer

Drug combination	*Number of evaluated patients*	*Number with > 50% tumour regression*
Bleomycin + methotrexate	4	2
Methotrexate + vincristine	28	15
Bleomycin + adriamycin	8	4
Cyclophosphamide + methotrexate	10	1 CR
Vincristine + 5-fluorouracil		7 PR*
Vinblastine, streptonigrin, thio-phosphoramide, chlorambucil, 6-mercaptopurine, methotrexate, and procarbazine	82	45*

*Definition of response unclear.
(After Goldsmith and Carter, 1975.)

The evidence from the traditional approach suggests that improved therapeutic results may be obtained in squamous tumours at specific sites, notably the oral cavity and maxillary sinuses (Goldsmith and Carter, 1975). Conclusions from these traditional studies are that in spite of occasionally dramatic response rates there has been considerable morbidity, and no dramatic increase in survival. There is a major requirement for a safer and more logically based approach to the chemotherapy of head and neck cancers.

Current concepts

Recently a logical scientific basis for safer and more effective cancer chemotherapy has been proposed involving the application of certain concepts in cell cycle kinetics (Price, 1973; Hill and Baserga, 1975). These ideas now provide an exciting opportunity for a rationale for combining optimal and safe systemic therapy with the best forms of local treatment and suggest reasons why the traditional approach to solid tumour therapy should be re-assessed.

Experimental studies with clinical relevance

In many experimental animal tumours and certain human tumours, where accurate measurements have been possible, there is a constant relationship between increase in tumour cell number and time, and these cells are said to grow exponentially. Exponential growth is especially characteristic of the early period of tumour development, but as the tumour mass increases the growth rate tends to slow. The concept of exponential growth allows a diagrammatic representation of the relationship between tumour cell number and tumour weight, the ability to detect the tumour clinically and the death of the patient (*see Figure 18.2*). Present methods of

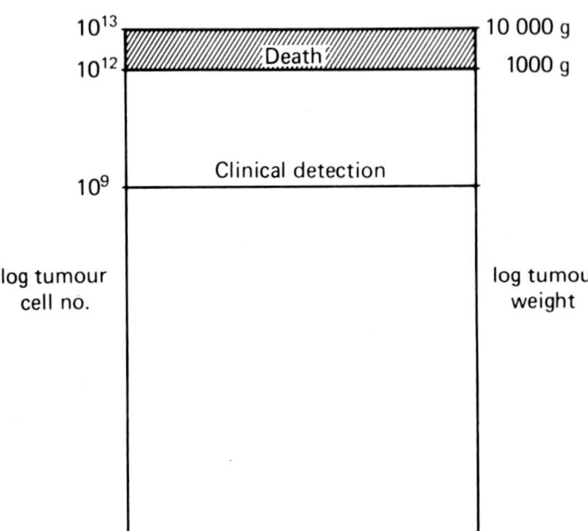

Figure 18.2 The relationship between tumour cell number, tumour weight, clinical detection and the death of the patient (reproduced with the kind permission of Wm. Heinemann Medical Books Ltd., from Hill and Price, 1977)

investigation in man are unable to detect tumours until about 1 g of tumour is present, consisting of approximately 10^9 cells. Since the patient is likely to die when the total tumour burden reaches between 10^{12} and 10^{13} cells (i.e. 1–10 kg tumour weight), it follows that by the time the tumour can be detected it is already at least two-thirds of the way through its lifespan. By definition most tumours are late or advanced at the time of presentation. This same theoretical point applies to the detection of secondary deposits of all cells not removed or destroyed by local therapy. It is therefore possible that the best techniques of surgery and/or radiotherapy will always be unable to cure advanced head and neck cancer since some undetectable malignant cells will be left behind.

In 1965, Skipper and his colleagues showed that chemotherapy is much more likely to be curative if used when the smallest number of malignant cells are present (Skipper, Schabel and Wilcox, 1965; Wilcox *et al.*, 1965). They developed a quantitative assay for estimating the number of tumour cells killed by a given course of drug treatment using a mouse model system. In this way they were able to show that the effect of an antitumour agent on malignant cells follows first order kinetics. This means that for a given treatment, the percentage of the total population (not the absolute number) of tumour cells killed is reasonably constant for cell populations of various sizes. A simplified version of this concept is illustrated in *Figure 18.3*, which shows the relationship between cell number and eradication of the tumour, assuming the same fraction cell kill, the same drug and the same degree of sensitivity of the tumour cells. It is apparent that the same drug, which can be curative when only a small number of tumour cells is present, would be completely useless in treating an animal with a large, advanced tumour. These studies therefore suggest that for chemotherapy to be curative drug treatment should be given immediately after local treatments have removed the bulk of the tumour mass, *provided* that it can be given more safely than it has been in the past.

Effects of a drug which achieves a 6 log cell kill (99·9999%)

'CURE' almost all animals with 10 thousand malignant cells

'CURE' 40 per cent of animals with 1 million malignant cells

'CURE' none of animals with 1 billion malignant cells

Figure 18.3 The relationship between 'cure' rate and tumour cell number (adapted from Skipper *et al.*, 1965). Chemotherapy is most effective when the number of malignant cells present is smallest

A major contribution to chemotherapy, in terms of safety and minimal toxicity to normal bone marrow stem cells, has come from the clinical application of certain concepts of cell cycle kinetics. Stem cells are by definition capable of an infinite number of proliferations. The object of chemotherapy is to do the maximum damage to malignant stem cells with minimal damage to normal stem cells. Bruce and his co-workers developed a technique to measure the effects of 24 h exposure to various chemotherapeutic agents on the survival of the normal bone marrow stem cells and lymphoma stem cells (Bruce, Meeker and Valeriote, 1966). They showed that the drugs could be divided into two categories: those which after an initial reduction in survival do not cause increasing damage to normal bone marrow stem cells with increasing dose (Class II), and those where the bone marrow stem cell kill does increase with increasing dose (Class III). In both classes, there was maximal selective kill of malignant stem cells (*see Figure 18.4*). This selectivity appeared to be based on the fact that in untreated mice most of the normal haematopoietic stem cells were resting, while all the detectable lymphoma stem cells appeared to be cycling. Therefore short courses (i.e. over 24 h) of Class II and Class III agents would cause a much greater kill of malignant as opposed to normal stem cells. If the time of exposure is prolonged, however, this kinetic difference between normal and malignant stem cells is abolished and increasing damage to the normal bone marrow occurs. These initial studies have now been extended to include other agents and have been reviewed by Hill and Baserga (1975) and form the basis for a kinetic classification of antitumour drugs (Hill and Price, 1975). *Table 18.4* classifies the drugs used in the treatment of head and neck cancer in this manner. Bleomycin and hexamethyl-melamine have not been included since data suggest that they have little effect on normal bone marrow stem cells.

In vitro studies with mammalian cells have determined the phase or phases of the cell cycle where anticancer drugs exert their maximal cell killing effects. This means that drugs can be selected for combination chemotherapy which exert their lethal effects primarily in different phases of the cycle. This subject has been reviewed by Hill and Baserga (1975) and *Figure 18.5* indicates where in the cycle the drugs used for treating cancers of the head and neck exert their lethal effects.

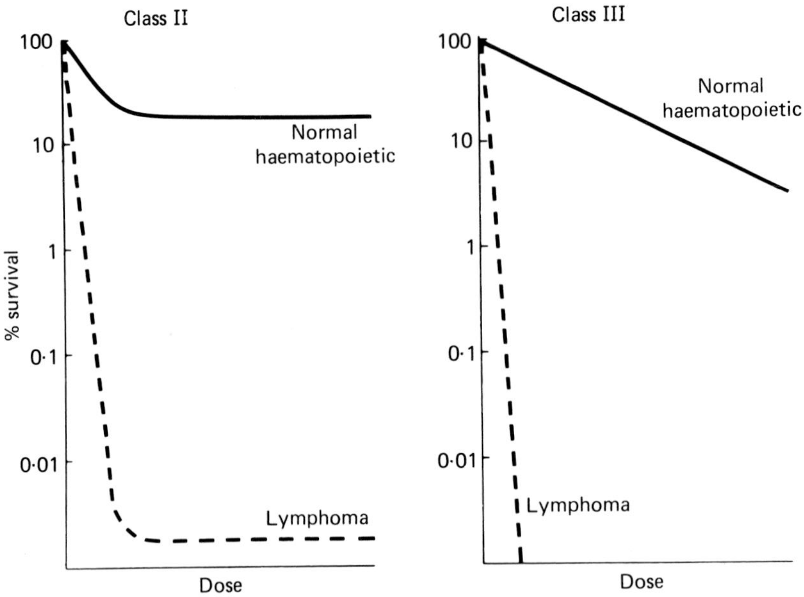

Figure 18.4 The basis of a kinetic classification of antitumour drugs. Dose survival curves for both normal haematopoietic and lymphoma colony-forming units (after Bruce *et al.*, 1966)

Table 18.4 Kinetic classification of antitumour drugs used in the treatment of head and neck cancer

Class II	*Class III*
Hydroxyurea	Adriamycin
6-Mercaptopurine	Chlorambucil
Methotrexate	Cyclophosphamide
Vinblastine	Dibromodulcitol
	5-Fluorouracil
	Methyl CCNU

The experimental findings from these model systems have indicated that the following principles should be applied in the chemotherapy of head and neck cancer: (1) drug treatment should be given when the smallest number of malignant cells is present, i.e. in combination with surgery and/or radiotherapy, (2) chemotherapy should be given over periods of 24–36 h in intermittent courses (approximately 3–4 week intervals, unless methyl-CCNU is included when a 6-week interval should apply to allow marrow recovery between treatments), since this approach would markedly reduce toxicity and lead to safer chemotherapy, (3) a knowledge of the kinetic classification of antitumour agents is essential if chemotherapy is to be given safely. The toxicity of Class II agents to normal stem cells (e.g. bone marrow) is not dose dependent. Class II drugs may therefore be added to combinations without reducing their dose, provided the total treatment time is 24–36 h. Combinations of Class III drugs will be additively toxic to normal bone marrow and therefore doses should be reduced proportionately, (4) the practice of giving small daily doses of

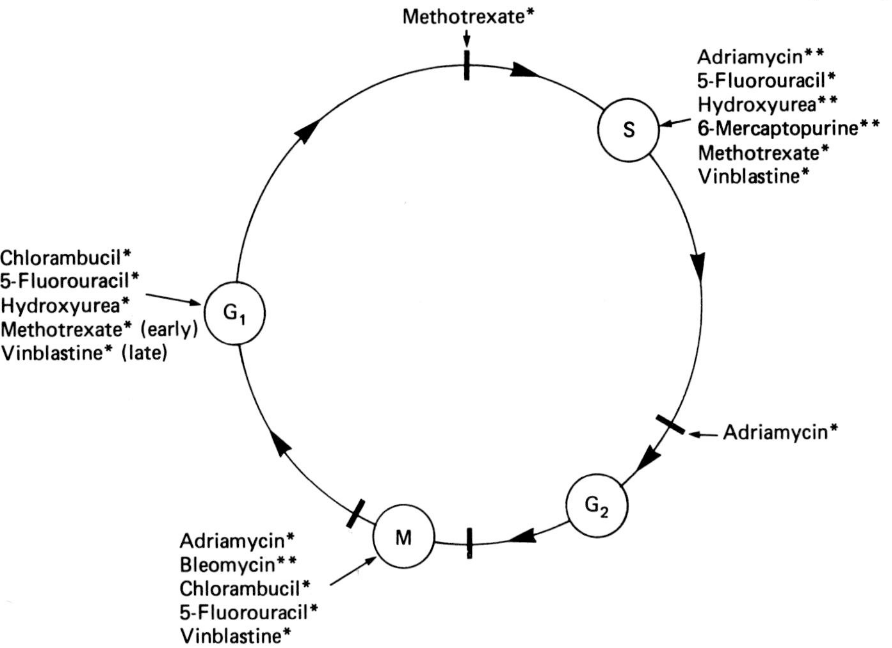

Figure 18.5 The phases of the cell cycle where antitumour agents, used in the treatment of head and neck cancers, exert their cell killing effects. * Indicates more than one site of action of the drug. ** Indicates phase where *maximal* lethal effects of the drug are exerted

drugs from either Class should be avoided, since under these conditions normal bone marrow stem cells will be drawn into cycle and killed. This approach would increase the toxicity to normal bone marrow and may reduce the number of malignant cells that are killed because the treatment has to be postponed or interrupted, (5) when selecting drugs for combination therapy a knowledge of their killing effects in different phases of the cell cycle may be helpful.

Clinical implications of these theoretical concepts

The theoretical points outlined above indicate that chemotherapy can be given much more safely than in the past and also that it should be given early in the disease and as soon as possible after local treatment. Therefore the traditional use of drug therapy in head and neck cancer should be reviewed.

Figure 18.6 shows an ethical and logical way in which the safe integration of chemotherapy into a combined attack with surgery and radiotherapy can be achieved in head and neck cancer.

Logical approach to solid tumour chemotherapy

Test new drugs and combinations in advanced disease

↓

Develop optimum chemotherapy regimen for disseminated disease

↓

Integrate optimum chemotherapy regimen with surgery and radiotherapy in a combined attack in the primary treatment of 'bad-risk' local and regional disease

Figure 18.6 A suggested approach towards the integration of chemotherapy with surgery and/or radiotherapy into a multidisciplinary attack on head and neck cancers (adapted from Carter and Soper, 1974)

Clinical results using this kinetic approach

The principles outlined above have direct clinical application whether head and neck cancer is treated with single drugs or with combination chemotherapy. For example, it is possible to give methotrexate in very high doses with increased therapeutic effect provided certain precautions are rigorously observed. A safe approach is to infuse the drug in 1–2 l of normal saline over periods of 12–30 h in doses of 100–20 000 mg followed by a leucovorin 'rescue' (Goldie, Price and Harrap, 1972). It is essential to maintain a good diuresis during the infusion and to extend the leucovorin 'rescue' appropriately in patients with impaired renal function as judged by low creatinine clearance (Price and Hill, 1977). Similarly, as predicted experimentally, up to 40 g hydroxyurea, a Class II agent, can be given quite safely over 24 h.

The greatest step forward, however, in terms of response rates has been the use of the above concepts in designing combination chemotherapy protocols which are not only safer but also more effective than previous multiple drug treatments given over several days. In 1975 a seven-drug combination not only produced an 80 per cent response rate in advanced squamous cell carcinoma (T_3 T_4 lesions in the TNM classification) but also caused no significant myelosuppression (Price *et al.*, 1975). Forty per cent of the patients in this study survived for at least one year even though they were all considered 'terminal' when treatment started.

Currently the best response rates in the world are being consistently achieved by a simplification of this protocol using a carefully sequenced combination of vincristine, bleomycin, methotrexate, 5-fluorouracil and hydrocortisone given over 24 h with a subsequent leucovorin 'rescue' (Price and Hill, 1977). Apart from a response rate (i.e. a greater than 50 per cent reduction in measurable tumour volume) of over 70 per cent this approach has enormous advantages to the patients, for example (1) they spend only one night out of every three or four weeks in hospital, (2) there is no severe bone marrow depression so that the requirements for intensive supportive therapy using platelets and antisepticaemia regimens is drastically reduced, (3) alopecia occurs only in 6 per cent of patients so treated, and nausea and vomiting are minimal and easily controlled, (4) it is possible to offer intensive chemotherapy without ruining the quality of the patient's life (Price and Hill, 1977; Price *et al.*, 1978). A major implication of these findings is that 'adjuvant' chemotherapy can now ethically be given in an appropriate combination with surgery and/or radiotherapy in an attempt to increase the 'cure' rates in this group of diseases. Although all the lesions in these studies (Price and Hill, 1977; Price *et al.*, 1978) were either undifferentiated carcinomas or various subgroups of squamous cell types histologically, response rates vary at different sites. In general, lesions of the oral cavity responded better than those of the larynx and pyriform fossa. If the patients had had prior radiotherapy the response rate to drug treatment was significantly reduced.

We may conclude that much of the toxicity associated with chemotherapy in the past has been due to the somewhat unscientific way in which the drugs have been administered. Drug treatment using the kinetically-based approach described above is safe and effective (Price and Goldie, 1971; Price *et al.*, 1975; Price and Hill, 1977; Price *et al.*, 1978). Even so there are certain precautions which must *always* be observed if patients with head and neck cancers are submitted to chemotherapy; these are listed in *Table 18.5*.

Table 18.5 Precautions to be observed in all cases receiving chemotherapy

1. Never give another treatment cycle unless the peripheral blood count has returned to its original level
2. Patients with impaired renal function receiving methotrexate must have an extended leucovorin 'rescue', i.e. at least 3 h longer than normal
3. Doses of cyclophosphamide, adriamycin and 5-fluorouracil should be halved in patients who have had thoracic, abdominal or pelvic irradiation
4. Doses of Class III agents should be reduced proportionately if more than one of them is included in a combination
5. Adriamycin should not be given to patients with a history of cardiac failure. The total dose of adriamycin must never exceed 550 mg/m^2. The dose of adriamycin should be halved in patients who have impaired hepatic function
6. Patients receiving drugs which are excreted in the urine, e.g. methotrexate and hydroxyurea, must be adequately hydrated and passing urine while they are having the drug
7. Bleomycin should not be given to any patients with impaired respiratory function

Current trends and future prospects

The necessary requirements now exist for using clinically the logical approach outlined in *Figure 18.6* in the treatment of head and neck cancers. This method offers the brightest hope for an increase in survival times in this group of diseases in the near future. Drug combinations available now if integrated early with surgery and radiation might improve the 'cure' rate at least in certain anatomic sites. In addition new agents presently being screened are showing significant activity; examples are *cis*-diamminedichloroplatinum and possibly porfiromycin. There is already evidence (Clifford *et al.*, 1978) that a multimodality approach produces increased survival compared with historically matched groups. There is a major requirement for prospective controlled studies involving surgery, radiation therapy and chemotherapy to be organized in multidisciplinary clinics. Such studies are already underway in England and The National Cancer Institute in the USA. For the first time for several decades it is permissible to be cautiously optimistic that the overall survival times in head and neck cancers may soon be increased significantly.

References

Bonadonna, G., Beretta, G., Tancin, G., Brambilla, C., Bajetta, E., De Palo, G. M., De Lena, M., Fossati Bellani, F., Gasparini, M., Valagussa, P. and Veronesi, U. (1975). Adriamycin (NSC – 123–127) Studies at the Istituto Nazionale Tumori, Milan, *Cancer Chemotherapy Reports*, **6,** 231

Bruce, W. R., Meeker, B. E. and Valeriote, F. A. (1966). Comparison of the sensitivity of normal hematopoietic and transplanted lymphoma colony-forming cells to chemotherapeutic agents administered *in vivo*, *Journal of the National Cancer Institute*, **37,** 233

Carter, S. K. and Soper, W. T. (1974). Integration of chemotherapy into combined modality treatment of solid tumours, *Cancer Treatment Reviews*, **1,** 1

Clifford, P. T., O'Connor, A. D., Durden-Smith, J., Hollis, B. A. B., Edwards, W. G. and Dalley, V. M. (1978). Synchronous multiple drug chemotherapy and radiotherapy for advanced (Stage III and IV) squamous cell carcinoma of the head and neck. In *Proceedings of the 10th International Conference on Chemotherapy*. Basel; S. Karger AG

Donegan, W. I. and Harris, P. (1976). Regional chemotherapy with combined drugs in cancer of the head and neck, *Cancer*, **38,** 1479

Espiner, H. J. and Westbury, G. H. (1964). Continuous chemotherapy by intra-arterial infusion, *Acta Unio Internationalis Contra Cancer*, **20,** 475

Goldie, J. H., Price, L. A. and Harrap, K. R. (1972). Methotrexate toxicity: correlation with duration of administration, plasma levels, dose and excretion pattern, *European Journal of Cancer*, **8,** 409

Goldsmith, M. A. and Carter, S. K. (1975). The integration of chemotherapy into a combined modality approach to cancer chemotherapy. V. Squamous cell cancer of the head and neck, *Cancer Treatment Reviews*, **2,** 137

Hill, Bridget T. and Baserga, R. (1975). The cell cycle and its significance for cancer treatment, *Cancer Treatment Reviews*, **2,** 159

Hill, Bridget T. and Price, L. A. (1975). Kinetic classification of antitumour drugs, *British Medical Journal*, **3,** 367

Lederman, M. (1970). Radiotherapy of cancer of the larynx, *Journal of Laryngology and Otology*, **84,** 867

Price, L. A. (1973). The application of a kinetic model to clinical cancer chemotherapy. In *Proceedings of the 3rd Eli Lilly Symposium on the Vinca Alkaloids in the Chemotherapy of Malignant Disease* (Ed. by Shedden, W. I. H.), p. 35. Cheshire; SHERRAFF

Price, L. A. and Goldie, J. H. (1971). Multiple drug therapy for disseminated malignant disease, *British Medical Journal*, **4,** 336

Price, L. A. and Hill, Bridget T. (1977). A kinetically-based logical approach to the chemotherapy of head and neck cancer, *Clinical Otolaryngology*, **2,**

Price, L. A., Hill, Bridget T., Calvert, A. H., Shaw, H. J. and Hughes, K. B. (1975). Kinetically-based multiple drug treatment for advanced head and neck cancer, *British Medical Journal*, **3,** 10

Price, L. A., Hill, Bridget T., Calvert, A. H., Dalley, V. M., Levene, A., Busby, E. R., Schachter, M. and Shaw, H. J. (1978). Improved results in combination chemotherapy of head and neck cancer using a kinetically-based approach: a randomised study with and without adriamycin, *Oncology*, in press, to appear in January (1979) issue

Skipper, H. E., Schabel, F. M. Jnr. and Wilcox, W. S. (1965). Experimental evaluation of potential anticancer agents. XIV. Further study of certain basic concepts underlying chemotherapy of leukaemia, *Cancer Chemotherapy Reports*, **45,** 5

Till, J. E., Bruce, W. R., Elwan, A. *et al.* (1975). A preliminary analysis of end results for cancer of the larynx, *Laryngoscope*, **85,** 259

Wasserman, T. H., Comis, R. L., Goldsmith, M., Handelsman, H., Penta, J. S., Slavik, M., Soper, W. T. and Carter, S. K. (1975). Tabular analysis of the chemotherapy of solid tumours, *Cancer Chemotherapy Reports*, **6,** 399

Wilcox, W. S., Griswold, D. P., Laster, W. R. Jnr. *et al.* (1965). 'Experimental evaluation of potential anti-cancer agents, XVII. Kinetics of growth and regression after treatment of certain solid tumours', *Cancer Chemotherapy Reports*, **47,** 27

19 Haematology in relation to otolaryngology

J E Pettit

Haematology is primarily concerned with the structure and function of blood cells and their formative tissues and with the mechanisms of haemostasis. As well as primary blood abnormalities numerous derangements secondary to disease in other organ systems are encountered. Patients with acute leukaemia or chronic lymphocytic leukaemia may develop enlargement of nasopharyngeal lymphoid structures and neutropenic patients commonly have serious infections in the otolaryngologist's area of interest. The otolaryngologist is not infrequently asked to help control persistent bleeding in patients with haemorrhagic diatheses. Some of the drugs used in otolaryngology may have unwanted side-effects which may cause blood cytopenias.

Table 19.1 Normal blood counts

	SI units	*Traditional units*
Haemoglobin	11.5–18.0 g/dl	11.5–18.0 g/100 ml
Red-cell count	$3.9–6.0 \times 10^{12}$/l	$3.9–6.0 \times 10^{6}/\mu l$
PCV or Haematocrit	0.35–0.54	35–54 per cent
Mean cell haemoglobin	27–32 pg	27–32 μg
Mean cell volume	76–96 fl	76–96 μm^3
Mean cell haemoglobin concentration	30–35 g/dl	30–35 per cent
Reticulocytes	0.2–2.0 per cent	0.2–2.0 per cent
	$10–100 \times 10^{9}$/l	10–100 000/μl
White-cell count	$4–11.0 \times 10^{9}$/l	4000–11 000/μl
Platelet count	$150–350 \times 10^{9}$/l	150 000–350 000/μl

Haematological investigation is initiated by haemoglobin estimation, blood cell counting and blood film microscopy. Few surgical patients are denied this basic screening because knowledge of the oxygen-carrying capacity, the leucocyte and platelet levels are essential for correct anaesthetic and surgical management. The normal blood counts in Systeme International d'Unites (SI) and traditional units are shown in *Table 19.1* Appendices to this chapter list the principal abnormalities found during blood film examination and their clinical associations.

Anaemia

Anaemia is present when the haemoglobin or haematocrit is below the lower limit of 'normal' range (*see Table 19.2*). It is important to remember that the mean 'normal' value and the lower limit of 'normal' range (defined by the mean value minus twice the standard deviation) depend on the age and sex of the reference healthy population and their attitude of residence. After puberty the values for males are higher than for females. Although statistical interpretation of normal distribution curves would suggest that 2.5 per cent of a healthy population might have haemoglobin or haematocrit values lower than two standard deviations below the mean, it is essential to exclude disease in patients whose values fall below the limits given.

Table 19.2 Normal variation in haemoglobin and PCV (haematocrit)

	Haemoglobin	*PCV*
Men	13.5–18.0	0.40–0.54
Women	11.5–16.0	0.35–0.47
Full-term infants	13.6–19.6	0.44–0.62
Children : 3 months	9.5–12.5	0.32–0.44
Children : 1 year	11.0–13.0	0.36–0.44
Children : 10–12 years	11.5–14.8	0.37–0.44

The definition of anaemia requires clinical evaluation and haematological study. Enquiry should be made about the patient's symptoms, occupation, diet, drug and chemical exposure and about a family history of blood disorders. Physical signs particularly relevant to the diagnosis of anaemia include pallor, jaundice, glossitis, splenomegaly, liver and lymph node enlargement. With modern automated electronic counters, accurate computed red-cell indices (MCV, MCH and MCHC) readily indicate which morphological class of anaemia is present, e.g. hypochromic, microcytic, macrocytic or normocytic. In many patients blood film microscopy identifies the type of anaemia, e.g. macrocytic anaemia with oval macrocytes and hypersegmented neutrophils suggests a megaloblastic anaemia; red-cell spherocytosis and polychromasia would point to a haemolytic anaemia. The reticulocyte count which reflects the erythropoietic response is also of value in the definition of anaemia.

Anaemia is the result of abnormal red-cell production or excessive loss of red cells. It may be congenital or acquired, primary or secondary to other disease. In many patients the anaemia is not a definitive diagnosis but merely a reflection of an underlying disorder and a final diagnosis must include the pathogenesis of the anaemia, e.g. iron deficiency due to chronic haemorrhage from carcinoma of the stomach. Knowledge of pathogenesis is essential for correct treatment.

Iron deficiency anaemia

Iron deficiency, the most frequent nutritional disorder in Western countries is the commonest single cause of anaemia. It affects mainly women, children and the poor.

The healthy male body contains about 4 g of iron, some 65–70 per cent present as haemoglobin, 25–30 per cent as ferritin and haemosiderin in stores and the remainder present as cellular enzyme iron and circulating iron bound to transferrin. Haemoglobin iron and iron stores are about one third less in females. The daily loss and requirements amount to approximately 1 mg in adult males and children, 1.5–2.0 mg in menstruating females and up to 3 mg or more in a normal pregnancy. Absorption which amounts to 5–10 per cent of the average daily intake of 10–20 mg occurs maximally through the duodenum and jejunum. This amount just balances the daily loss. The important causes of iron deficiency include:

(1) *Blood loss*: Gastrointestinal loss (from oesophageal varices, hiatus hernia, peptic ulceration, aspirin ingestion, gastric or colonic carcinoma, hookworm infestation, ulcerative colitis or haemorrhoids) is particularly important. Haematuria is a less frequent cause. In women excessive uterine bleeding, e.g. from fibroids or menorrhagia, is an additional cause.
(2) *Physiological*: Iron deficiency is common in infancy and adolescence; the expansion of red-cell volume creates increased demands for iron. In women of childbearing age dietary intake may not be adequate to meet the demands created by menstruation, pregnancy, parturition and lactation.
(3) *Nutritional*: Deficient iron in the diet is particularly a problem in the underdeveloped countries, in the elderly and in infants taking unsupplemented milk diets.
(4) *Malabsorption*: Malabsorption is not a common cause. However in untreated coeliac disease iron deficiency is usual and there is associated folate deficiency.

Clinical features

Symptoms include those due to anaemia, e.g. dyspnoea, lassitude and, in many patients, those due to the disorder responsible for iron deficiency, e.g. peptic ulcer. Repeated infections, including those of the upper respiratory tract and middle ear may be a problem in iron deficient infants and children. Pallor is usually present and, in long standing cases, epithelial changes such as angular stomatitis, glossitis and koilonychia occur. There is associated atrophic gastritis and achlorhydria in small numbers of patients and rarely a post-cricoid pharyngeal web may result in dysphagia (Plummer-Vinson/Paterson-Kelly syndrome).

Diagnosis

Iron deficiency anaemia is hypochromic and microcytic with a mean cell volume (MCV) less than 80 fl (femtolitres) mean cell haemoglobin (MCH) less than 27 pg and mean cell haemoglobin concentration (MCHC) less than 30 g/dl. Blood film examination shows red-cell hypochromia, microcytosis, anisocytosis and poikilocytosis. The platelet count may be raised (above 350×10^9/l) particularly if the patient is bleeding. The serum iron is low, e.g. morning samples less than 14 μmol/l (80 μg/100 ml) and the iron-binding capacity is raised, e.g. morning samples above 70 μmol/l (350 μg/100 ml).

Treatment

As well as replacing the iron deficit of circulating haemoglobin and body stores the treatment of iron deficiency includes measures directed towards correcting the underlying cause. Where possible the correction of chronic anaemia should be completed before non-urgent elective surgery.

A six-month course of oral iron therapy is usually sufficient to correct anaemia and replenish iron stores. Ferrous sulphate, succinate, glutamate or fumarate are equally effective. Doses of 60 mg of elemental iron thrice daily are used. Liquid preparations may be used in children.

A course of intramuscular iron (iron dextran or iron sorbitol) is given when the patient is intolerant to oral iron, when bleeding continues or if the patient has a gastrointestinal lesion that may be aggravated by iron. As an alternative a total dose intravenous infusion of iron dextran in saline may be used in selected patients.

Occasionally when the patient's clinical state is severe or when urgent surgery is required a closely monitored delivery of packed red cells is the treatment of choice.

Megaloblastic anaemia

Megaloblastic anaemia is usually the result of vitamin B_{12} or folate deficiency.

Although often suspected on clinical grounds because of pallor, jaundice, glossitis or neurological signs the diagnosis of megaloblastic anaemia depends on the association of red-cell macrocytosis with bone marrow megaloblastic change. The MCV is greater than 100 fl and values of greater than 120 fl are frequent. Oval macrocytes, red-cell anisocytosis and hypersegmented neutrophils are seen in the peripheral blood film. In severe cases there is leucopenia and thrombocytopenia.

The estimation of serum vitamin B_{12}, serum and red-cell folate levels are required to establish which deficiency is responsible for the megaloblastic change. The normal range of serum vitamin B_{12} is 160–925 ng/l (pg/ml). Levels of 0–100 ng/l (pg/ml) are found in severe deficiency. Borderline values of 100–160 ng/l (pg/ml) are found in mild vitamin B_{12} deficiency and in some patients with folate deficiency. The normal serum folate level is 6.0–20 μg/l (ng/ml). While levels of less than 3.0 μg/l (ng/ml) indicate folate deficiency, levels of 3.0–6.0 μg/l (ng/ml) are considered borderline. Normal or raised levels occur in vitamin B_{12} deficiency. The normal red-cell folate level is 160–640 μg/l (ng/ml) packed cells. Low results occur in severe folate deficiency and this test is a good test of tissue folate stores.

Vitamin B_{12} deficiency

The average Western diet contains 7–30 μg of vitamin B_{12} of which 2–5 μg is absorbed. Almost all of the daily intake is in foods of animal origin. The daily requirement is 1–2 μg and the stores in adults amount to 2–3 mg, i.e. enough for 3–4 years if supplies are completely cut off. The absorption of vitamin B_{12} requires intrinsic factor, a gastric glycoprotein which binds the vitamin and transports it to specific receptor sites in the distal ileum where absorption takes place.

The causes of vitamin B_{12} deficiency are listed in *Table 19.3*. Malabsorption of the vitamin is the normal cause and pernicious anaemia is the most important vitamin B_{12} deficiency disorder in most Western countries. Inadequate dietary intake is seen in Vegans, who omit both animal meat and animal products such as milk, eggs and cheese from their diet.

Table 19.3 Causes of vitamin B_{12} deficiency

Malabsorption
Pernicious anaemia
Gastrectomy
Tropical sprue
Ileal resection
Intestinal 'stagnant-loop' syndromes
Nutritional – Vegans

In addition to an anaemia, patients with vitamin B_{12} deficiency may have difficulty in walking, paraesthesias and muscle weakness associated with peripheral neuropathy or degeneration of the lateral and posterior columns of the spinal cord (subacute combined degeneration).

Pernicious anaemia

In pernicious anaemia the megaloblastic change is the result of a severe lack of intrinsic factor due to gastric atrophy. The disease occurs more commonly than by chance in close relations and usually presents over the age of 40. It appears likely that the underlying gastric atrophy is autoimmune in origin since: (1) lymphocytes invade the stomach, (2) transient improvements in the stomach lesion have followed steroid therapy, (3) parietal cell antibodies are found in 90 per cent of patients, (4) there is an association with other possible autoimmune diseases, e.g. autoimmune thyroiditis and myxoedema, Addison's disease and hypoparathyroidism. Radioactive vitamin B_{12} (^{57}Co or ^{58}Co) absorption studies with or without intrinsic factor are useful in confirming that the primary abnormality is gastric rather than intestinal. The urinary excretion method (of Schilling) is most popular. Patients with pernicious anaemia have an increased incidence of gastric carcinoma.

Gastrectomy

The usual body stores of vitamin B_{12} are exhausted 3–4 years following total gastrectomy. Some patients with extensive partial gastric resections also develop megaloblastic anaemia after this period of time. There is often coincident iron deficiency.

Treatment of vitamin B_{12} deficiency

Vitamin B_{12} deficiency, from whatever cause, is corrected and body stores replenished with six intramuscular injections of 1 mg hydroxycobalamin given at intervals over two or three weeks. In pernicious anaemia and most other causes of vitamin B_{12} deficiency, therapy is required for the remainder of the patient's life; 1 mg hydroxycobalamin is given once every three months.

Folate deficiency

The adult daily requirements for folate are about 100 μg. The normal Western diet contains about 600 μg of folate but these compounds may be destroyed by cooking at high temperatures. Maximum absorption occurs through the duodenum and jejunum. The principal causes of folate deficiency are noted in *Table 19.4*.

Table 19.4 Causes of folate deficiency

1. *Nutritional*
2. *Malabsorption*
   Tropical sprue
   Coeliac disease
   Post gastrectomy
3. *Excessive requirement or loss*
   Pregnancy
   Hyperactive haemopoiesis
   Renal dialysis
4. *Antifolate drugs*
   e.g. Methotrexate
   Alcohol

An inadequate diet is the principal cause of folate deficiency and nutritional deficiency is common in countries with 'subsistence agriculture', e.g. India and some parts of Africa, where there is a marked seasonal variation in folate intake. Dietary deficiency also occurs with old age, poverty, in chronic invalids and psychiatric patients.

Malabsorption of folate occurs in coeliac disease and tropical spruce and may also contribute to folate deficiency in some patients following partial gastrectomy.

Pregnancy increases the daily requirements for folate and to prevent the development of anaemia most obstetricians give routine folic acid supplements.

Treatment

Folate deficiency is easily treated; 5–15 mg folic acid daily by mouth for a few days is sufficient to saturate body stores of folate (about 10 mg) in all patients, even those with malabsorption of the vitamin. The dose is usually continued for three months to ensure a complete correction of the anaemia. The decision about maintenance therapy depends on whether the cause of the deficiency can be corrected; such measures as improved diet, a gluten-free diet for coeliac disease or the end of a pregnancy may mean that the deficiency is unlikely to recur.

Secondary anaemias

Anaemias secondary to chronic infections, connective tissue disorders, malignancy, endocrine disorders, liver disease and renal failure form the largest group of anaemias seen in clinical practice. These anaemias respond to the alleviation of the causative disease; standard haematinics such as iron, folic acid or vitamin B_{12} usually have little effect.

Anaemia of chronic disorders

Three components appear to contribute to the pathogenesis of the normochromic or hypochromic normocytic anaemia which occurs in patients with chronic inflammation or malignant disease: (1) reduced iron release from reticuloendothelial stores, (2) an inadequate erythropoietin response to the anaemia, (3) a reduced red-cell survival. Both the serum iron and iron-binding capacity are low, bone marrow iron stores are adequate but siderotic granulation of erythroblasts is reduced. The severity of anaemia is proportional to the activity of the underlying disease and if the haemoglobin is less than 9.0 g/dl there is likely to be an additional cause for the anaemia, e.g. associated haemorrhage, iron or folate deficiency, marrow infiltration or haemolysis.

Anaemia of renal failure

Both acute and chronic renal failure are associated with anaemia which is the result of decreased erythropoietin response and reduced red-cell survival. In many patients blood loss, infection, iron and folate deficiency or microangiopathic haemolytic anaemia complicate the issue.

Anaemia in chronic liver diseases

Many factors may contribute. Blood loss occurs from oesophageal varices or as a result of reduced synthesis of coagulation factors and thrombocytopenia. Folate deficiency, hypersplenism and reduced red-cell survival may also be important in the pathogenesis of the anaemia. Alcohol has a direct toxic action on erythropoiesis.

Anaemia in endocrine disease

Anaemia is present in most patients with hypothyroidism. In hypopituitarism the mild anaemia results from reduced erythropoiesis and responds to replacement hormone therapy. The anaemia found in Addison's disease responds to corticosteroid therapy.

Haemolytic anaemias

Haemolytic anaemias are caused by an increase in the rate of red-cell destruction. Jaundice, splenomegaly, characteristic red-cell changes, e.g. spherocytes or fragmented red cells and an increase in absolute reticulocyte levels above 200 × 10^9/l are findings that suggest active haemolysis. Because of the erythropoietic hyperplasia which accompanies chronic haemolytic anaemia the rate of red-cell destruction may need to be increased several-fold before anaemia develops. Definitive diagnosis of the type of haemolytic anaemia often requires detailed laboratory tests. The life span of the normal red cell is 120 days. In haemolytic anaemia a variable shortening occurs and in severe haemolysis the cells survive only a few days. If serious doubt about haemolysis exists a chromium-51 (^{51}Cr) labelled red-cell survival study may be needed. A classification of the more important haemolytic anaemias is given in *Table 19.5*.

Table 19.5 Haemolytic anaemias

Hereditary red-cell defects	
1. Membrane, e.g.	Hereditary spherocytosis Hereditary elliptocytosis
2. Metabolism, e.g.	Pyruvate kinase deficiency G6PD deficiency
3. Haemoglobin, e.g.	Sickle-cell disease Thalassaemias
Acquired membrane defect	Paroxysmal nocturnal haemoglobinuria
Extracorpuscular abnormality	
1. Immune haemolytic anaemias, e.g.	Autoimmune Drug-induced Haemolytic disease of the newborn Transfusion reaction
2. Red-cell fragmentation syndromes	
3. Hypersplenism	
4. Miscellaneous – drugs, chemicals, infections, toxins	

Haemolytic anaemias comprise only a small fraction of the anaemias seen in clinical practice. However otolaryngologists with patients of African, Mediterranean or Asian origins may not infrequently encounter glucose-6-phosphate dehydrogenase deficiency, Sickle-cell disease or thalassaemia. Haemolytic transfusion reactions are a potential problem for any physician or surgeon.

Glucose-6-phosphate dehydrogenase deficiency

The vital reduction potential of red cells is largely dependent upon metabolic activity of the pentose phosphate shunt. Patients with deficient activity of the enzyme glucose-6-phosphate dehydrogenase (G-6-PD) are particularly prone to drug-induced haemolytic anaemia. Favism (haemolytic sensitivity to the broad bean *Vicia fava*), hereditary non-spherocytic haemolytic anaemia and neonatal jaundice are other manifestations of particular types of G-6-PD deficiency. Numerous variants of G-6-PD have been characterized and many are associated with less activity than the 'normal' Western or type B G-6-PD. The principal racial groups affected are West African, Mediterranean and South East Asian but sporadic G-6-PD deficiency occurs in all populations. The inheritance is sex-linked, affecting mainly males in the hemizygous state.

A large number of drugs have been associated with acute haemolytic anaemia in G6PD deficiency (*Table 19.6*). These drugs or their metabolites are usually oxidant compounds often related to the 8-aminoquinolines or derived from an aniline base.

Table 19.6 Agents which may cause haemolysis in G-6-PD deficient patients

Antimalarials	*Sulphonamides and sulphones*
Primaquine	Sulphanilamide
Pamaquine	Sulphapyridine
Quinacrine	Sulphadimidine
Quinine	Sulphafurazole
Chloroquine	Sulphacetamide
Pyrimethamine	Salazopyrine
	Sulphamethoxazole
Antibacterial agents	Dapsone
	Aldesulphone
Penicillin	Thiazosulphone
Chloramphenicol	Glucosulphone
p-Aminosalicylic acid	
Streptomycin	*Miscellaneous*
Isoniazid	
Nalidixic acid	Stibophen
Nitrofurans – Nitrofurantoin	Probenecid
– Nitrofurazone	Bimercaprol (BAL)
– Furaxolidone	Acetyl phenylhydrazine
	Phenylhydrazine
Analgesics	Quinidine
	Vitamin K (water soluble)
Phenacetin	Naphthalene (moth balls)
Paracetamol	Methylene blue
Aminopyrine	Arsine
Acetanilide	Fava beans

Bacterial or viral infections, diabetic acidosis and other acute illnesses may also trigger haemolysis in G-6-PD deficient subjects. The clinical picture is of rapidly occurring intravascular haemolysis with haemoglobinuria but the severity is partly determined by the nature of the enzyme variant. Negroes with the A-type of deficiency often suffer from less severe anaemia than that observed in the rarer variants found in Northern Europeans. The anaemia rapidly improves on cessation of the offending drug. Patients presenting with symptoms from severe anaemia must be treated with red-cell transfusion. Adequate fluid intake is important as high urine volumes should be maintained during crises of intravascular haemolysis. The diagnosis is made by measuring the G-6-PD activity in the patient's red cells and numerous screening tests are available.

Sickle-cell disease

The abnormal haemoglobin (HbS) in the sickle-cell disorders may be found in association with almost equal amounts of normal adult haemoglobin (HbA) in the heterozygous state designated sickle-cell trait or HbAS. The homozygous state or sickle-cell anaemia (HbSS) is the most hazardous of the disorders. The special characteristic of HbS is its tendency to form tactoid 'crystals' when exposed to low oxygen tensions which convert the normal biconcave discoid red cell into a sickle shape. Aggregations of sickled red cells may block the microcirculation leading to infarctive crises. Their rigid shape confers a short survival.

Any patient of African origins or from the Middle East, Eastern Mediterranean or Indian subcontinent may possess sickle-cell haemoglobin and should be screened for this possibility prior to surgery. If the screening tests for this condition are positive electrophoretic genotyping should be performed.

The homozygous form of HbS disease is characterized by a 'steady state' of chronic haemolysis with periodic crises. In the steady state haemoglobin levels of 6–9 g/dl are usual but patients tolerate this degree of anaemia well because of a lowered oxygen affinity of HbS. The infarctive, haemolytic or aplastic crises require intensive treatment. Precipitating factors include infections, dehydration, exposure to cold, intense muscular activity, hypoxia and acidosis. Rest, analgesics, hydration with 5 per cent glucose and bicarbonate therapy to prevent or treat acidosis are the mainstays of management of the crises. Packed red cells are only necessary if severe anaemia is causing symptoms.

Surgery must be undertaken with reluctance. Emergency operations during crises have a high mortality. The patient should be in a steady state, warm, well hydrated and infection-free before elective operations. For major surgery if the haemoglobin is less than 7–8 g/dl a slow transfusion of packed red cells should be given in order to improve the degree of anaemia in the days before the operation. Fresh blood should be available to replace the blood loss during surgery. Prophylactic broad spectrum antibiotic cover is necessary to minimize post-operative chest infections. The pre-medication should avoid respiratory depression, pre-oxygenation for several minutes should precede the induction of anaesthesia and the anaesthesia should include a technique that gives the best assurance of oxygenation, clear airway and the avoidance of circulatory stasis. Post-anaesthetic oxygen therapy is essential until full clinical recovery has occurred.

Although during normal life most patients with sickle-cell trait (HbAS) usually require no treatment these people may 'sickle' under general anaesthesia. Precautions to ensure optimum oxygenation as outlined above are desirable.

Thalassaemia

The thalassaemias are found mainly in people of the Mediterranean, the Middle East and the Far East. There is a failure to produce normal quantities of either the α-polypeptide chain (α-thalassaemia) or the β-chain (β-thalassaemia) of normal adult haemoglobin (HbA).

In homozygous β-thalassaemia excess free α-chain precipitates to form insoluble red-cell inclusions which lead to a severe haemolytic anaemia. Compensatory marrow hyperplasia produces bone overgrowth and most patients have gross hepatosplenomegaly. The severe anaemia often requires regular transfusion to sustain life. Growth retardation, iron overload and hypersplenism are dominant clinical problems. The peripheral blood film shows marked erythroblastosis, reticulocytosis, red-cell hypochromia, anisocytosis and poikilocytosis. Up to 90 per cent of the haemoglobin is of the fetal type (HbF). Before surgery it is usual to transfuse patients with homozygous β-thalassaemia to a haemoglobin level of 10 g/dl or above.

Patients with the heterozygous form of β-thalassaemia (β-thalassaemia trait) are usually symptomless. They may present with a mild hypochromic anaemia or be detected during studies of relatives of patients suffering from thalassaemia. β-thalassaemia trait may be differentiated from iron deficiency by finding raised haemoglobin F or haemoglobin A_2 levels and normal serum iron and iron-binding capacity.

β-thalassaemia is seen predominantly in South East Asia. The severest form is incompatible with life beyond the late fetal stage and results in stillborn hydropic fetuses. Patients with haemoglobin H disease, a less severe form of α-thalassaemia, commonly present with a moderate haemolytic anaemia. They may also experience severe haemolysis when taking drugs similar to those which cause haemolysis in G6PD deficient subjects.

Haemolytic transfusion reactions

Most severe immediate haemolytic transfusion reactions are the result of ABO blood group incompatibility. Less commonly, IgM antibodies directed against other blood group antigens may be the cause. Severe haemolytic reactions are accompanied by pain along the line of the vein carrying the transfusion, flushing of the face, head throbbing, chest constriction and lumbar pain. These symptoms may be accompanied by tachycardia, hypotension, urticaria, peripheral circulatory collapse, rigors and pyrexia. Obviously many of these reactions are abolished by anaesthesia. Either a fall in blood pressure or an increase in pulse rate may warn the anaesthetist but frequently the first sign of a haemolytic transfusion reaction during surgery is bleeding at a previously dry operation site. The bleeding is caused by decreased coagulation factors and platelets resulting from the disseminated intravascular coagulation which is triggered by the intravascular haemolysis. The clinical presentation of transfusion reactions due to Rhesus blood group incompatibility or other IgG mediated reactions is less severe. The diagnosis of haemolytic reaction is confirmed by finding a positive direct antiglobulin (Coombs) test on samples of blood taken from the patient at the time of the reaction. In severe haemolysis there will be marked haemoglobinaemia with haemoglobinuria.

Apart from stopping the offending transfusion, treatment should be immediately directed towards maintaining the circulating blood volume; plasma volume expanders are given until further compatible blood becomes available. Intravenous corticosteroid and an appropriate antihistamine may diminish the severity of reaction. An infusion of 500 ml of 10 per cent mannitol and the administration of sodium bicarbonate are believed to reduce the risk of anuria following major haemolytic reactions. If *in vitro* haemostasis testing indicates the presence of disseminated intravascular coagulation, heparin therapy and platelet transfusions should be considered. With less severe and delayed haemolytic transfusion reactions urgent treatment is not required. However, many patients will require further transfusion with compatible blood.

Other immediate transfusion reactions

The infusion of *infected blood* results in clinical features similar to those described for ABO incompatibility with profound shock, hypertension, vomiting and often widespread bleeding from disseminated intravascular coagulation; 50–80 per cent of reactions due to infected blood prove fatal. Immediate diagnosis is essential and direct gram staining should be carried out on smears made from the plasma of the infected blood. The responsible organisms are most frequently endotoxin-producing pseudomonas, coliform or achromobacteria capable of growing at low temperatures. Treatment consists of restoring blood volume with compatible fresh blood, intravenous hydrocortisone, careful use of vasocompressor agents, e.g. metaraminol, high doses of appropriate antibiotics, e.g. gentamicin and carbenicillin and platelet concentrates and intravenous heparin if disseminated intravascular coagulation is present. If the patient survives the initial few hours it is likely that management will include the treatment of acute renal failure.

The febrile reactions which were caused by the transfusion of *bacterial pyrogen* are now rare because of the widespread use of disposable sterile plastic transfusion sets. Rises of temperature to 40 °C accompanied by headache may result from *white cell or platelet incompatibility*. White cell and platelet iso-antibodies are generally not formed until the patient has had many transfusions or pregnancies. Although these reactions may be unpleasant they are rarely serious; antihistamine therapy and slowing the drip-rate may allow completion of the transfusion. In sensitized patients the use of washed red cells, or leucocyte filters may diminish such reactions.

Very rarely anaphylactic reactions occur in patients lacking IgA who have a potent anti IgA in their plasma which reacts with donor IgA. Immediate treatment with 1 mg subcutaneous adrenalin, intravenous hydrocortisone and an intramuscular antihistamine is indicated. In such patients, repeatedly washed red cells have still provoked reactions and full protection is provided only by transfusing blood from rare donors lacking IgA.

Aplastic anaemia

In aplastic anaemia there is anaemia, neutropenia and thrombocytopenia which results from reduced haemopoietic bone marrow. The haemoglobin, granulocyte and platelet levels vary from patient to patient but sustained neutrophil counts of less than 0.5×10^9/l and platelet counts of less than 20×10^9/l are associated with a poor prognosis. Patients with aplastic anaemia may present with severe oropharyngeal infection or epistaxis. Infections at other sites, generalized purpura and clinical features of anaemia are common. Splenomegaly, hepatomegaly and lymphadenopathy are unusual.

The blood count reveals a normochromic, normocytic anaemia and the reduced numbers of white cells and platelets seen in the peripheral blood do not include primitive or abnormal forms. The reticulocyte count is low. Bone marrow examination is essential to differentiate aplastic anaemia from other causes of pancytopenia, e.g. aleukaemic leukaemia, megaloblastic anaemia, hypersplenism, infiltration of the marrow with carcinoma or myeloma.

In about half the patients, aplastic anaemia follows exposure to a toxic agent such as a drug, chemical or virus (*see Table 19.7*). Chloramphenicol and phenylbutazone

Table 19.7 Toxic agents associated with bone marrow depression

Agents whose effect is regular and dose dependent		
1. Ionizing radiation		
2. Cytotoxic drugs		
3. Benzene		
4. Arsenic		
Agents whose effect depends on idiosyncrasy		
Anti-inflammatory type drugs	:	Phenylbutazone*, Indomethacin, Colchicine, Gold salts**
Antibiotics	:	Chloramphenicol, Streptomycin, Sulphonamides, Amphotericin B, Isoniazid
Anticonvulsants	:	Mephenytoin*, Trimethadione*, Paramethadione*, Phenytoin, Primidone
Antithyroids	:	Carbimazole*, Thiamazole*, Thiourea, $KClO_4$
Hypoglycaemic drugs	:	Tolbutamide, Chlorpropamide
Pyschotrophic drugs	:	Chlorpromazine*, Promazine*, Meprobamate*, Pecazine*, Amitriptyline
Miscellaneous drugs	:	Chlorothiazides**, Organic arsenicals**, Hair dyes, Acetazolamine, Quinidine, CCl_4, Trinitrotoluene
Insecticides	:	DDT, Lindane, Parathione
Viruses	:	Hepatitis, congenital rubella, infectious mononucleosis

* Selective neutropenia usual toxic effect.
** Selective thrombocytopenia usual toxic effect.

are the two most frequently associated drugs in Europe and North America. Aplastic anaemia may also follow cytotoxic therapy for disseminated malignancy or leukaemia. A group of congenital aplastic anaemias occurs in childhood. In *Fanconi's anaemia* there are often associated abnormalities of skin, bone, genital development, spleen and kidneys.

Treatment

Current management of aplastic anaemia includes intensive supportive therapy, the use of androgens and bone marrow transplantation.

Red-cell transfusions are given to raise the patient's haemoglobin to a symptom-free level, e.g. 9–11 g/dl. Patients with massive haemorrhage require *fresh whole blood* supplemented by *platelet concentrates*. Platelets are also indicated for continuing haemorrhage. The use of prophylactic platelet transfusion is controversial. Many patients with aplastic anaemia are continuously at risk from severe thrombocytopenia for months or years. As catastrophic haemorrhage is a frequent cause of death soon after presentation, there is a definite place for regular platelet transfusions in the early management of patients with repeated minor haemorrhages or purpura.

Because of severe neutropenia infections are the other principal causes of death. In febrile patients blood cultures should be taken and vigorous attempts made to identify the responsible organism by direct examination of potentially infected material as well as by culture methods. Many lethal infections arise from the patient's own microbial flora, e.g. pseudomonas, anaerobes, *E. coli*, *Staphylococcus aureus*. Persistent unexplained pyrexia should be treated with empirical broad-spectrum bacteriocidal antibiotics, e.g. gentamicin and carbenicillin. When the infective agent and its sensitivities are known appropriate changes in antibiotic therapy should be made. If cell separator facilities are available *leucocytes* from normal donors or patients with chronic granulocytic leukaemia frequently improve patients with life-threatening infections. HL-A matched leucocytes are preferable but it is not often possible to obtain them.

Anabolic androgens have occasionally been successful in initiating a regeneration of erythropoiesis and, less frequently, granulopoiesis and thrombopoiesis. *Bone marrow transplantation* is currently under trial. The best results have been obtained when HLA matched, mixed lymphocyte culture compatible siblings are available as donors.

Neutropenia

Neutropenia may be part of a general bone marrow failure, as in aplastic anaemia or acute leukaemia, or due to hypersplenism. In other patients with neutropenia there is no anaemia or thrombocytopenia. Some of the causes of selective neutropenia are listed in *Table 19.8*. A variety of congenital neutropenic syndromes have been

Table 19.8 Causes of neutropenia

1. *Selective neutropenia*
   Drug-induced
   Idiopathic
   Familial syndromes
   Cyclical
2. *Bone marrow failure*
   e.g. aplastic anaemia, leukaemia,
   malignant infiltration, myeloma
3. *Splenomegaly*
4. *Severe megaloblastic anaemia*
5. *Miscellaneous*
   Viral infections, e.g. hepatitis, influenza
   Fulminant bacterial infections, e.g. typhoid
   Hypersensitivity and anaphylaxis
   Felty's syndrome
   Systemic lupus erythematosis

described and a mild asymptomatic reduction in neutrophil levels are found in many people of West African ancestry. Neutropenia may be the earliest sign of drug-induced marrow damage and if the drug is stopped further generalized bone marrow suppression may be prevented. Drugs which may cause selective neutropenia include the phenothiazides, antithyroids, anticonvulsants, sulphonamides, phenindione and phenylbutazone (*see Table 19.7*). Although a drug-hapten antibody mechanism was responsible for the agranulocytosis which occurred with aminopyrine and dipyrone therapy (*see below*) drug-dependent antibodies have rarely been identified in neutropenias associated with other drugs which probably have a more direct myelotoxic action. Bone marrow examination is essential to determine whether the neutropenia is the result of depressed granulopoiesis or of accelerated removal of neutrophils from the blood; it may also reveal evidence of leukaemia, megaloblastic change or marrow infiltration.

Patients with acute severe neutropenia (absolute neutrophil counts $<0.2 \times 10^9$/l usually present with fever and infection). They should be admitted to hospital and nursed in separate rooms with 'reverse barrier' isolation techniques or placed in 'laminar flow' rooms or plastic isolators if these intensive care facilities are available. The infective organisms should be isolated and vigorously treated and leucocyte concentrates judiciously used as already described.

Although many drug-induced neutropenias are reversible and recovery occurs one to two weeks after stopping the drug, in other patients the bone marrow damage is permanent. Infection remains the dominant problem in patients with chronic neutropenia. Early recognition of infection is essential and antibiotic and supportive therapy must be initiated without delay. Chronic infections of the skin and nasopharynx are frequently encountered in these patients. Vulnerability to infection occurs when the neutrophil count is below 0.5×10^9/l. An exception to this rule is the patient with the familial condition of 'idiopathic benign neutropenia' in which a reduction in neutrophil count results from a permanent increase in the marginating fraction of blood neutrophils; such individuals have few infections, normal granulopoiesis and adequate numbers of neutrophils in inflammatory exudates; and they require no therapy.

Acute agranulocytosis (Schultz' syndrome, agranulocytic angina)

Between 1922 and 1934 there were many reported cases of acute agranulocytosis in patients taking the analgesic aminopyrine. Seven to ten days after the onset of therapy, or immediately if the drug had previously been taken, susceptible individuals suddenly developed a chill, with high fever, tachycardia and headache. If the drug was continued the number of neutrophils in the peripheral blood fell to zero or very low levels and the patient developed a painful gangrenous ulceration of the soft palate, tonsils, pharynx, gums and tongue. Septicaemia, profound shock and death followed in many cases. It has now been established that the neutropenia which occurred in about 1 per cent of patients taking the drug was the result of a hypersensitivity reaction. After 1934 aminopyrone was no longer widely prescribed and the incidence of associated severe neutropenia rapidly increased. However a few years later further cases of agranulocytosis and death followed the introduction of the drug dipyrone which was a derivative of aminopyrone.

A similar drug-activated antibody reaction has rarely been demonstrated with other drugs causing neutropenia. Single case reports have included patients taking sulphapyridine and phenylbutazone.

The leukaemias

The leukaemias are a group of disorders of unknown aetiology characterized by an accumulation of abnormal white cells in the bone marrow. Common but not essential features include abnormal white cells in the peripheral blood, a raised white-cell count, evidence of bone marrow failure: anaemia, neutropenia, thrombocytopenia, and involvement of organs other than marrow, e.g. liver, spleen, lymph nodes, skin, gums, brain.

The acute leukaemias

The acute leukaemias are generally associated with a predominance of undifferentiated cells. 'Lymphoblastic leukaemia' is thought to originate from cells of the lymphoid series in the marrow and the acute myeloid leukaemias are classified into various subclasses depending upon the dominant cell type present, e.g. myeloblastic, promyelocytic, myelomonocytic, monocytic and erythroleukaemia.

The common presenting features of the acute leukaemias are symptoms of anaemia, fever, infections and haemorrhage. Blood counting reveals progressive anaemia, neutropenia and thrombocytopenia; total white-cell levels are frequently elevated to 100×10^9/l.

Cytotoxic drugs, e.g. vincristine, rubidomycin, cytosine arabinoside, mercaptopurine, methotrexate, are used to achieve clinical and haematological remission. In an attempt to reduce continually the 'hidden' leukaemic cell population rotating cycles of different cytotoxic drugs are given for up to two years if an initial remission has been achieved. The benefit of prophylactic central nervous system irradiation, intrathecal methotrexate, immunotherapy and bone marrow transplantation are currently under investigation. Supportive measures such as isolation procedures, intensive antibiotics, red-cell transfusion and the use of leucocyte and platelet concentrates are of great importance and are similar to those already described for aplastic anaemia and neutropenia.

Recent trials have indicated that the median survival of children with lymphoblastic leukaemia treated with intensive chemotherapy and prophylactic nervous system irradiation is greater than five years. In acute myeloid leukaemia remissions are more difficult to achieve and shorter, the value of cyclical therapy is less obvious and the median survival of treated patients is less than six months.

Chronic granulocytic leukaemia

Chronic granulocytic leukaemia comprises 20 per cent of the leukaemias and is most frequently seen in middle age. In most patients there is a replacement of normal bone marrow by cells with an abnormal G group chromosome (the Philadelphia or Ph^1 chromosome). A great increase in total granulocyte mass occurs with high blood white-cell counts, e.g. $50–600 \times 10^9$/l, massive splenomegaly and symptoms of hypermetabolism such as weight loss, lassitude, night sweats, anorexia and fever. There is often failure of red-cell and platelet production with anaemia and thrombocytopenia but the platelet count is sometimes elevated. The differential count reveals a predominance of neutrophils and myelocytes.

Chronic granulocytic leukaemia has a surprisingly stable clinical course with a predictable response to palliative therapy with busulphan in the chronic phase of the disease. Other forms of therapy include the drugs dibromomannitol and hydroxyurea and splenectomy. There is a high rate of 'metamorphosis' to a more acute disorder often referred to as the 'blastic crisis'. Associated features of this change include the patient becoming refractory to therapy, anaemia, thrombocytopenia or thrombocytosis, leucocytosis on leucopenia, an increase in blast cells in the blood and marrow and blast cell infiltrations of lymph nodes, other organs and soft tissues and new chromosome changes. The median survival is 3–4 years. Death usually occurs from 'metamorphosis' or from haemorrhage or infection.

Chronic lymphocytic leukaemia

Chronic lymphocytic leukaemia comprises 25 per cent of the leukaemias and occurs chiefly in the elderly. Large numbers of apparently mature lymphocytes accumulate in the blood, bone marrow, spleen and liver. In advanced disease there is often generalized lymphadenopathy and bone marrow failure with anaemia, neutropenia and thrombocytopenia. Associated hypogammaglobulinaemia results in an increased susceptibility to infections. However, many patients with early disease are asymptomatic with no abnormal physical findings.

Although most patients with chronic lymphocytic leukaemia have a leucocytosis of $30–300 \times 10^9/l$ (70–99 per cent lymphocytes) the diagnosis should be suspected if there is a persistent lymphocytosis of more than $5.0 \times 10^9/l$. Lymphocytes comprise more than 30 per cent of the marrow cell total. About 15 per cent of patients develop a secondary autoimmune haemolytic anaemia.

Patients in bone marrow failure or with troublesome organomegaly and lymph node enlargement are treated with prednisone, chlorambucil and cyclophosphamide. No improvement of immunological capacity occurs with this therapy and attention must be directed towards the prophylaxis and treatment of infections. Irradiation is useful for treating lymph nodes or local tissue deposits causing pressure symptoms.

Multiple myeloma

In multiple myeloma a neoplastic proliferation of plasma cells in the bone marrow causes lytic bone lesions, bone marrow failure and a monoclonal protein in the serum, urine or both. Eighty per cent of patients present after the age of 40. Presenting features include back pain, pathological fractures, normocytic anaemia, neutropenia and thrombocytopenia. Deposition of Bence-Jones protein in the kidney, amyloidosis, hypercalcaemia and pyelonephritis may all contribute to renal failure. Associated amyloid disease may also cause macroglossia. Interference of coagulation factor activity by the myeloma protein and thrombocytopenia may produce a haemorrhagic diathesis. Rarely polymerization of myeloma IgG or IgA causes a 'hyperviscosity syndrome' with heart failure, nervous system manifestations or purpura. This syndrome is more frequently seen in the related monoclonal IgM gammopathy, Waldenstrom's macroglobulinaemia. Management of myeloma includes palliative therapy with melphalan and prednisone and supportive measures, e.g. blood transfusion for anaemia, irradiation for painful skeletal lesions and plasmapheresis for hyperviscosity syndrome or bleeding due to paraprotein interference with coagulation.

Polycythaemia

The term polycythaemia or its synonym erythrocytosis refers to a pattern of red-cell change that usually includes an increase in haemoglobin above 18 g/dl, a red-cell count above 6×10^9/l and a haematocrit above 0.55. The causes of polycythaemia are listed in *Table 19.9*. Initial blood volume studies are required to establish whether

Table 19.9 Causes of polycythaemia

Primary
- Polycythaemia vera

Secondary
- Due to compensatory erythropoietin increase in:
  - High altitudes
  - Cardiovascular disease
  - Pulmonary disease
  - Increased affinity haemoglobins
- Due to inappropriate erythropoietin increase in:
  - Renal disease – carcinoma, cysts, vascular impairment
  - Hepatocellular carcinoma
  - Cerebellar haemangioblastoma
  - Adrenal tumours

Relative
- 'Stress' polycythaemia
- Dehydration : vomiting, water deprivation
- Plasma loss : burns

the polycythaemia is 'real' where there is an increase in total red-cell volume or 'relative' where there is no increase in total red-cell volume. The red-cell volume may be determined by ^{51}Cr or ^{99m}Tc labelled red-cell methods and the plasma volume should be independently measured with the ^{125}I-albumin dilution method. The normal results using these methods are:

Total red-cell volume,	men	: 26–33 ml/kg
	women	: 22–29 ml/kg
Plasma volume		: 40–50 ml/kg.

Polycythaemia vera

In polycythaemia vera the increase in red-cell volume is the result of endogenous myeloproliferation. The underlying defect is probably of the marrow stem cell as in most patients there is accompanying leucocytosis and thrombocytosis. Clinical symptoms are due to hypervolaemia and hyperviscosity: headaches, plethora, pruritus, dyspnoea, blurring of vision, thrombosis and haemorrhage; and to hypermetabolism: night sweats and weight loss. Some patients suffer from gout and there is associated hypertension in about one third of patients. Supportive findings that suggest polycythaemia vera rather than a secondary polycythaemia include; leucocytosis and thrombocytosis, marrow hyperplasia involving granulopoiesis and megakaryocytes as well as erythropoiesis, splenomegaly, raised levels of serum uric acid, leucocyte alkaline phosphatase, serum vitamin B_{12} and B_{12} binding capacity. Radiological studies, measurement of arterial oxygen concentration and haemoglobin studies may be required to exclude a cause of secondary polycythaemia.

Treatment of polycythaemia is directed at reducing the red-cell volume and consequently the blood viscosity. This is achieved by repeated venesection, administration of radioactive phosphorus (^{32}P) or by myelosuppressive drugs, e.g. busulphan or chlorambucil. Transition to myelofibrosis occurs in 20 per cent of patients and a smaller fraction of patients develop acute leukaemia.

Surgery in patients with uncontrolled polycythaemia vera carries with it a 75 per cent incidence of major haemorrhage or thrombosis with an associated mortality of about 30 per cent. Patients effectively controlled at the time of surgery have a low incidence of complications. When major elective surgery is indicated patients should be treated with ^{32}P or myelosuppressive drugs until a near normal blood count has been achieved. In the case of an emergency procedure a rapid haemodilution should be accomplished by venesection accompanied by an infusion of equivalent amounts of an electrolytic solution or low molecular weight dextran. Blood lost by surgical bleeding should be replaced with fresh blood.

Haemorrhagic disorders

Normal haemostasis depends on interaction between circulating platelets, blood vessel wall and clotting factors. Platelet and coagulation factor deficiency and, more rarely, defects of the microcirculation result in prolonged bleeding.

The diagnostic approach to a bleeding disorder requires thorough clinical and laboratory assessment. Enquiry must be made whether the bleeding disorder has been lifelong and whether there is a family history of bleeding. While purpura, excessive bleeding from superficial cuts or abrasions and mucosal haemorrhage suggest a platelet disorder, deep haematomas, haemarthroses, haematuria and delayed wound healing are more characteristic of coagulation factor deficiency. Bruising occurs with both types of defect. A number of screening tests are used in the diagnosis of a bleeding disorder. The bleeding time and platelet count are essential to detect quantitative and qualitative platelet defects. The prothrombin time is sensitive to deficiencies of coagulation factors II, V, VII and X and is typically prolonged in liver disease, vitamin K deficiency and during oral anticoagulation. The activated partial thromboplastin time is sensitive to deficiencies of factors V, VIII, IX and X and thus is able to detect the most important hereditary coagulation disorders, haemophilia (deficiency of factor VIII) and Christmas disease (deficiency of factor IX). This latter test is also sensitive to the presence of heparin. In disseminated intravascular coagulation low fibrinogen levels and fibrin degradation products can be detected by the fibrinogen titre, the thrombin time and one of the screening tests for serum fibrin degradation products; thrombocytopenia should be confirmed by platelet counting and prolongation of prothrombin time and activated partial thromboplastin times indicate reduced levels of coagulation factors. The results of haemostasis screening tests in the vascular purpuras are usually normal.

The vascular purpuras

Hereditary telangiectasia

The dilated microvascular lesions of this condition appear during childhood and become more numerous with age. In addition to extensive involvement of mucous membranes and skin, A–V fistula may be found in the liver, spleen and lungs. Recurrent epistaxis, chronic gastrointestinal bleeding and haemoptysis produce a state of severe iron deficiency which requires extensive iron replacement therapy. Ethinyloestradiol has diminished bleeding in some patients.

Ehlers Danlos syndrome

In this rare hereditary condition defective perivascular connective tissue results in recurrent ecchymoses, epistaxis, muscle haematomas, gastrointestinal bleeding and haematuria. There is no effective treatment.

Henoch–Shonlein purpura

This hypersensitivity reaction is usually seen in childhood. The purpuric rash which typically involves the buttocks and limbs is often accompanied by localized subcutaneous oedema and there may be painful joint swelling, haematuria and abdominal pain. In most cases the disorder is self-limiting but occasional patients develop renal failure.

Scurvy

Gingival bleeding and perifollicular haemorrhages on the flexor surfaces of the legs and buttocks are a characteristic sign in vitamin C deficiency. With severe scurvy there is more widespread bruising and painful periosteal haemorrhage occurs in children.

Thrombocytopenia

The main causes of thrombocytopenia are listed in *Table 19.10*.

Table 19.10 Causes of thrombocytopenia

A. *Platelet production failure*
(i) *Selective megakaryocyte depression*
Drugs, chemicals, viruses
(ii) *General bone marrow failure*
Aplastic anaemia, leukaemia, myeloma, myelosclerosis, marrow infiltrations
B. *Abnormal platelet destruction*
(i) *Immune*
Acute and chronic idiopathic thrombocytopenias; Secondary, e.g. CLL, SLE-lymphomas, drug-induced, post transfusion
(ii) *Disseminated intravascular coagulation*
C. *Abnormal platelet distribution*
Splenomegaly
D. *Dilutional loss*
Massive transfusion of old blood to bleeding patients

Acute thrombocytopenic purpura

Acute thrombocytopenic purpura is more common in children. It usually follows vaccination or an infection, e.g. chicken pox, measles, rubella or infectious mononucleosis. An allergic reaction is presumed but not often proven. In typical cases, petechiae develop rapidly and bleeding may occur from the nose, gums, vagina, gastrointestinal or urinary tracts. Usually there is spontaneous recovery. Occasionally the disease passes into a chronic form and very rarely death occurs from intracranial haemorrhage. Treatment consists of blood transfusion, platelet concentrates and short-term prednisone therapy.

Chronic idiopathic thrombocytopenic purpura

Chronic idiopathic thrombocytopenic purpura (ITP) has an immune origin; sensitivity tests are able to show an antiplatelet IgC in the serum of most patients. It occurs predominantly in adults, particularly in women between 20 and 50 years. The onset is insidious with petechial haemorrhage, easy bruising and menorrhagia. Epistaxis and mucous membrane bleeding occur in some cases but intracranial haemorrhage is rare. Usually the platelet count is 10 to 50 $\times$ 10^9/l and the platelets in the peripheral blood film appear large. Increased numbers of megakaryocytes are seen in marrow aspirates.

It is important to exclude a drug as the cause of the thrombocytopenia. Secondary immune thrombocytopenia occurs sporadically with systemic lupus erythematosis, sarcoidosis, tuberculosis, carcinoma, lymphoma and with autoimmune haemolytic anaemia.

Less than 10 per cent of adult patients with chronic ITP recover spontaneously. The initial treatment of choice is high dose prednisone. Splenectomy or immunosuppressive drugs are recommended in patients who do not respond to steroids. Platelet concentrates should be given to patients with major haemorrhage.

Drug-induced thrombocytopenia

Drug-induced thrombocytopenia may result from generalized toxic marrow depression (*see* p. 687), or with some drugs such as chlorothiazide, tolbutamide, from a selective megakaryocyte depression. However, it is now believed that most drug-induced thrombocytopenias are caused by an allergic mechanism. The most frequently reported drugs have been quinine, sedormid, paraminosalicylate, sulphonamides, chloroquine, digitoxin, stibophen, rifampicin and the gold salts.

The onset may be gradual or the patient may present with an acute syndrome heralded by a chill, headache and flushing. In severe cases in addition to purpura there is epistaxis, oropharyngeal mucosal haemorrhage and bleeding into the gastrointestinal, urinary, and female reproductive tracts. Recovery occurs after a few hours or days with rapidly metabolized drugs but may take months in gold sensitivity. The platelet count on presentation is frequently less than 10×10^9/l, normal or increased megakaryocytes are found in marrow aspirates and drug dependent antibodies against platelets may be detected by *in vitro* techniques. Negative *in vitro* results may arise because an active metabolite, rather than the drug itself, is involved in the *in vivo* allergic reaction.

All suspect drugs should be stopped. Short-term corticosteroids may be helpful and platelet concentrates are given to patients with severe bleeding. The patient must avoid the offending drug and any structurally related drugs.

Hereditary thrombasthenia

In this rare condition there is recurrent epistaxis, bruising, gastrointestinal bleeding and menorrhagia. Although the platelet count is normal, the bleeding time is prolonged, there is capillary fragility, clot retraction is abnormal and the platelets do not aggregate with APP or thrombin. Severe bleeding episodes should be treated with platelet concentrates.

Acquired qualitative platelet defects

Functionally defective platelets contribute to the bleeding tendency in uraemia. This dysfunction is decreased by dialysis. Abnormal platelet function has also been demonstrated in the myeloproliferative disorders, polycythaemia vera, essential thrombocythaemia and myelosclerosis, in patients with macroglobulinaemia and in liver disease.

Aspirin therapy produces an irreversible inhibitory effect on the platelet 'release reaction' and this may contribute to the associated gastrointestinal bleeding. Occasionally there is mild purpura, abnormal surgical bleeding occurs, the bleeding time is prolonged and *in vitro* platelet aggregation tests are abnormal. Aspirin therapy accentuates bleeding in patients with other haemorrhagic disorders.

Coagulation factor deficiency

There are ten plasma factors necessary for normal blood coagulation. Deficiencies may be inherited, usually of a single factor, or acquired, when several factors may be reduced. Haemophilia, Christmas disease and von Willebrand's disease are the most frequently encountered hereditary disorders. Liver disease, anticoagulant overdosage and disseminated intravascular coagulation are the most commonly acquired coagulopathies.

Haemophilia

Although a sex-linked inheritance pattern is well established, 25 per cent of haemophiliacs have no family history of the disease. The defect is an absence or low plasma level of functional coagulation factor VIII. Immunological studies are able to identify an inactive factor VIII related protein in the plasma.

The clinical problems associated with haemophilia correlate well with the plasma factor VIII activity; patients with less than 1 per cent factor VIII usually have severe disease. Painful joint haemorrhages and subsequent deformity dominate the clinical problems. Muscle haematomas may cause nerve and blood vessel compression; haematuria is often a problem. Operative and post-traumatic haemorrhages are life threatening in both severely and mildly affected cases.

The activated partial thromboplastin time is usually prolonged. However this test may fail to detect a mild deficiency and factor VIII assays must be performed in all suspected haemophiliacs.

Bleeding episodes are treated with fresh plasma, fresh frozen plasma, cryoprecipitate and factor VIII concentrates. The circulating level required to initiate and maintain haemostasis varies with the type of bleeding. Spontaneous minor bleeding and early haemarthroses respond to fresh plasma or cryoprecipitate and the factor VIII level should be elevated to 5–20 per cent of normal. To treat dangerous muscle or soft tissue haematomas or to cover dental extraction, the level of factor VIII should be elevated above 20 per cent. For major surgery and serious accidents it is essential to maintain a level of factor VIII above 40 per cent for 6–10 days after the operation or following the trauma. To achieve these higher plasma levels of activity it is necessary to use large amounts of cryoprecipitate or factor VIII concentrates.

Antibodies to isologous factor VIII develop in about 5 per cent of haemophiliacs. These may sometimes be overcome by massive replacement therapy. Plasmaphoresis has also been used to treat severe bleeding in patients with factor VIII inhibitors.

Christmas disease

The inheritance and clinical features of Christmas disease are identical to those of haemophilia. The activated partial thromboplastin time is usually prolonged but the factor VIII clotting activity is normal. Diagnosis is established by demonstrating low or absent plasma factor IX activity.

The principles of management are similar to those in haemophilia. Bleeding episodes are treated with fresh plasma, fresh frozen plasma or factor IX concentrates. The activity levels required to maintain haemostasis under variable haemostatic stress are similar to those described for haemophilia.

Von Willebrand's disease

This bleeding disorder has an autosomal dominant pattern of inheritance and affects both sexes. Operative and post-operative haemorrhage, epistaxis and excessive bleeding from superficial cuts and abrasions are characteristic. Haemarthroses and muscle haematomas are rare.

In severely affected patients the bleeding time is prolonged, the capillary fragility test is positive and there is a variable deficiency of factor VIII activity. Most patients show greatly reduced factor VIII related protein by immunoelectrophoresis, an absence of Ristocetin-induced platelet aggregation and poor retention of platelets in glass bead columns. The laboratory results in mildly affected patients are somewhat variable. The defect in patients with this syndrome is not established but it appears likely that the deficient protein has relevance both to plasma factor VIII activity and to certain platelet functions.

Treatment consists of fresh-frozen plasma, cryoprecipitate or factor VIII concentrates. Single infusions are associated with sustained and often delayed increases of factor VIII activity.

Liver disease

Biliary obstruction results in impaired absorption of vitamin K with a consequent decreased synthesis of factor II, VII, IX and X by the liver parenchymal cells. With severe liver disease there is a deficiency of these factors and, in addition, reduced levels of factor V and fibrinogen. Hypersplenism associated with portal hypertension may produce thrombocytopenia. These multiple abnormalities contribute to increased surgical bleeding in patients with liver disease. The degree of haemostatic defect is best judged by prolongation of prothrombin and bleeding times.

Patients with liver disease should receive 20–50 mg vitamin K_1 daily for three days prior to liver biopsy or surgery. Fresh frozen plasma will replace the deficient clotting factors. Surgical blood loss is best replaced by fresh whole blood which provides platelets in addition to coagulation factors.

Anticoagulant overdosage

The coumarin and indandione anticoagulants are vitamin K antagonists and produce anticoagulation by decreasing the liver synthesis of factors II, VII, IX and X. Haemorrhage is the main side effect and epistaxis is often the first indication of overdosage. Alcohol may increase the effect of anticoagulants by inhibiting the oxidative process concerned with their elimination, and other drugs, e.g. phenylbutazone, chloral hydrate and clofibrate may potentiate anticoagulant action by displacing them from their plasma protein binding sites. Overdosage is confirmed by finding excessive prolongation of prothrombin time or a thrombotest result of less than 5 per cent.

If the bleeding is severe vitamin K_1 20–50 mg intravenously and fresh frozen plasma or fresh blood should be given.

Disseminated intravascular coagulation

Widespread intravascular deposition of fibrin with consumption of coagulation factors and platelets occurs as a consequence of many disorders and may be associated with a fulminant bleeding syndrome. This process may be initiated by the entry of procoagulant material into the circulation, e.g. in patients with premature separation of the placenta, amniotic fluid embolism, haemolytic transfusion reactions, widespread mucin-secreting adenocarcinomas, promyelocytic leukaemia or it may result from generalized endothelial damage and collagen exposure, e.g. during shock, viraemia, acidosis or hypothermia. Septicaemia with Gram-negative organisms is a frequent cause.

In acute syndromes the blood may fail to clot because of gross fibrinogen depletion. The thrombin time and fibrinogen titre are abnormal and there are high levels of serum fibrin degradation products. Thrombocytopenia is usual and fragmented red cells may be seen on blood film microscopy. Although screening tests for coagulation factor deficiency, e.g. prothrombin time, activated partial thromboplastin time, are prolonged in the acute syndrome, with more chronic forms an increased synthesis may result in normal levels of coagulation factors and normal screening test results. Fibrinogen assays will document the severity of fibrinogen depletion.

Treatment in disseminated intravascular coagulation is primarily directed towards correcting the causative disorder. In acute syndromes supportive therapy with fresh blood, fibrinogen and platelet concentrates are often required. The use of heparin is controversial.

Appendix 19.1: Red-cell abnormalities and associated conditions

Red-cell abnormality	*Associated conditions*
Hypochromia	Iron deficiency, thalassaemia, sideroblastic anaemia

Anisocytosis and Poikilocytosis	Non-specific finding in many blood disorders, iron deficiency, vitamin B_{12} or folate deficiency, myelosclerosis and marrow infiltration
Microcytosis	Iron deficiency, thalassaemia
Macrocytosis	Vitamin B_{12} or folate deficiency, liver disease, during a reticulocytosis
Polychromasia	During reticulocytosis, myelosclerosis and marrow infiltration
Spherocytosis	Hereditary spherocytosis, other haemolytic anaemias
Target cells	Iron deficiency, liver disease, thalassaemia, haemoglobinopathy, post-splenectomy
Acanthocytes	Liver disease, post-splenectomy
Red-cell fragmentation	Drug-induced haemolytic anaemia, disseminated intravascular coagulation or microangiopathic haemolytic anaemia
Erythroblasts	Myelosclerosis, marrow infiltrations, leukaemia, in severe or rapidly developing anaemia

Appendix 19.2: Normal leucocyte counts, variations, and associated conditions

Neutrophils	Normal count : 2.5–7.5 × 10^9/litre
Neutrophilia	Bacterial infection, haemorrhage, trauma, connective tissue disorders, infarcts, malignancy, polycythaemia vera, chronic granulocytic leukaemia
Neutropenia	Marrow hypoplasias, drug induced, splenomegaly, vitamin B_{12} or folate deficiency, marrow infiltration
Eosinophils	Normal count : 0.04–0.44 × 10^9/litre
Eosinophilia	Allergy, parasitic infection, skin disorders, Hodgkin's disease, chronic granulocytic leukaemia
Basophils	Normal count : 0.00–0.10 × 10^9/litre
Basophilia	Myeloproliferative disorders, chronic granulocytic leukaemia, mast cell disease

Monocytes	Normal count : 0.2–0.8 × 10^9/litre
Monocytosis	Chronic bacterial infection, protozoal and rickettsial infections. Monocytic or myelomonocytic leukaemia
Lymphocytes	Normal count : 1.5–3.5 × 10^9/litre
Lymphocytosis	Viral infections, particularly rubella and other exanthemata, hepatitis, infectious mononucleosis pertussis, lymphocytic leukaemia and some lymphomas. Normal infants and children have higher levels than adults
Lymphopenia	Irradiation, steroid or immunosuppressive therapy
Atypical reactive forms	Infectious mononucleosis, hepatitis, viral infections

20 Anaesthesia for otolaryngology

R A Green

Introduction

Anaesthesia for otolaryngology is often said to be the most demanding of all types of anaesthesia because both surgeon and anaesthetist require access to the same area of the body. Whether or not this claim is justified, it is certainly true to say that in this field of surgery the closest cooperation between surgeon and anaesthetist is required. The objective of this chapter is not to teach anaesthesiology to the surgeon nor to teach the anaesthetist anaesthetic techniques for otolaryngological surgery. It is rather to help the ENT surgeon to understand some of the anaesthetists' problems in this field and to provide information on pre-operative and post-operative management whenever this may be influenced directly and indirectly by the anaesthesia required.

Assessment and preparation of patient for general anaesthesia

One cannot over-emphasize the importance of careful preparation of patients for operation, be it a minor or major procedure. In addition to a careful physical examination the surgeon and anaesthetist must remember that for him it is a routine procedure, but for the patient it is probably once in a lifetime, unfamiliar and frightening. Therefore great care should be taken to give simple but comprehensive explanations, and to provide suitable pre-operative sedation. With regard to the latter the approach to children is essentially different from that of the adult and will be considered separately.

Pre-operative assessment

A careful general history is the most important aspect of pre-operative assessment so far as the anaesthetic is concerned and is best carried out in a routine methodical manner. The use of a procedure sheet as shown in *Table 20.1* is helpful and avoids omissions.

Table 20.1 Procedure sheet

General history		
Physical fitness:		
Fit and active normally.		
CVS	Chest pain	
	Palpitations	
	Oedema	
	Shortness of breath at rest	
	Exercise tolerance (ability to climb stairs)	
RS	Cough	
	Haemoptysis	
	Smokes	
	Bronchitis or asthma	
CNS	Fits	
	Faints	
	Blackouts	
	Headaches	
GIS	Appetite	
	Weight	
	Abdominal pain	
	Bowel function	
General questions		
When did you last have an anaesthetic?		
Are you attending your family doctor for anything?		
Are you, or have you recently taken any medicine, tablets, drugs or injections?		
Drugs:	1.	
	2.	
	3.	
	4.	
Have you had any serious illnesses in the past?		Yes/No
Illnesses:	1.	
	2.	
	3.	
	4.	
Have you any allergies?		
	Iodine	Strapping
	Antibiotics	Other
Have you any history of abnormal bleeding?		
Do you wear dentures or contact lenses?		
Examination		
CVS	Pulse	
	Blood pressure	
	Apex sounds	
	Heart sounds	Added sounds
RS	Trachea	
	Expansion	
	Percussion note	
	Breath sounds	
GIS	Liver	
	Kidney	
	Spleen	
CNS	Reflexes	
	Muscle tone	

Routine investigations
Haemoglobin – sickle cell test where applicable
Nose and throat swab
Urine examination – sugar, protein
Chest x-ray – where indicated
ECG when indicated

Pre-operative preparation

Children up to seven years old

Young children should, whenever possible, be admitted to hospital with a parent or guardian. When this is not possible visiting hours should be unrestricted so as to allow the mother access to the child at all times should this be considered desirable. A careful explanation of the routine procedure prior to operation should be given to both mother and child, preferably by the anaesthetist, before the child is settled down for the night.

Night sedation
Children rarely require night sedation but with the nervous child it is frequently advantageous. This should be given by mouth in a palatable form. Many excellent preparations are available.

Elixir chloral (100–200 mg/year of age). This is a safe and well-tried preparation but due to its bitter taste which is difficult to mask, it has been widely replaced by dichloralphenazine (Welldorm) 20 mg/kg or triclofos sodium (Tricloryl) 25 mg/kg. All three compounds have a duration of action of 6–8 h with very little hangover, and act by the release of trichlorethanol after absorption from the stomach and small intestine. Welldorm has the advantage of containing phenazone which is a mild analgesic. (It has been known, very rarely, to cause blood dyscrasias when used over a long period of time.)

Promethazine hydrochloride (Phenergan Elixir) This can be made up in a reasonably palatable syrup (5 mg in 5 ml) for night sedation, a dose of 0.3 mg/kg is adequate. As it is claimed to have anti-analgesic properties it is more useful before than after operation.

The benzodiazepines These compounds are used as night sedatives mainly in adults, but may also be effective for the very anxious child. The mode of action is by its depressant effect on the limbic system, particularly the amygdala which is that part of the system which relays 'emotional' responses. The two drugs in this group most commonly used for children are diazepam (Valium) 0.2 mg/kg and nitrazepam (Mogadon) 0.2 mg/kg. Valium syrup (2 mg in 5 ml) is a convenient preparation for children.

Food and drink

Some food and drink restriction is necessary pre-operatively, but many hours of starvation and fluid restriction can be very harmful in the very young and should be avoided. Studies involving children routinely starved prior to surgery, show that 20–30 per cent are both hypoglycaemic and acidotic by the time premedication is given (Thomas, 1947). Perhaps even more important is the dehydration which may occur due to fluid restriction in hot weather. It is unnecessary and unwise to restrict fluid intake for longer than 4 h. The administration of fruit juice or other sugar-containing fluids (10 ml/kg) 4 h before operation is recommended. There is no evidence to suggest that this is unsafe. The patients most likely to suffer are those for morning operation, starved overnight.

Premedication

It is generally agreed that small infants, less than 10 kg, do not need premedication. With the older child the most important preparation still remains a satisfactory rapport between nursing staff, anaesthetist and the patient, but in practice under the conditions usually prevailing in the average hospital surgical ward, some pre-operative sedation is required. The first decision to be made in young children is whether this should be given by injection or by mouth. The parenteral premedicants, usually based on morphine with or without an additional sedative, are unquestionably the most predictable in their effect, but are not always so readily accepted by the patient. The final decision must depend upon the individual case.

Intramuscular premedication Intramuscular injections are never painless, no matter how experienced the nurse administering them may be. In addition many children have an almost pathological fear of injections. It is for these reasons that, despite the obvious advantages of this route of administration, it should not be undertaken without careful thought and explanation to the patient. The doctor ordering the premedication rarely sees its administration, and is therefore often unaware of the problems involved.

Morphine or pethidine remains the most useful drug for this purpose and is usually accompanied by atropine, although with modern anaesthetic techniques atropine is not always necessary. This should be given 1 h before operation. In the nervous child it is often helpful to precede this injection by a sedative such as trimeprazine or diazepam, by mouth, 4 h before operation. Thus the routine could be:

Trimeprazine (2 mg/kg) or diazepam (0.2 mg/kg), 4 h pre-operatively, followed by pethidine (1 mg/kg) or morphine (0.2 mg/kg), with or without atropine (0.01 mg/kg) 1 h pre-operatively.

For the very excitable child this regime may prove ineffective and a more potent form of intramuscular premedication may be required. For this purpose ketamine hydrochloride (Ketalar) may prove invaluable.

Ketamine is prepared in vials containing 10, 50 and 100 mg/ml. The 100 mg/ml is recommended for intramuscular injection in small children because of the small bulk required. A dose of 5–7 mg/kg will produce a quiet child within 15 min. Unlike the barbiturates and most other sedative drugs, it does not have a normal sedative and hypnotic action, but is primarily a cataleptic, with analgesic and anaesthetic properties. The recovery period may be fairly prolonged – a full 2 h required for full ambulation. In adults this recovery period is frequently characterized by vivid dreaming with a certain amount of psychomotor activity and confusion making it unsuitable for their use, but these disturbances are uncommon in children if they are allowed to recover undisturbed.

Oral premedication Oral premedication is usually preferred by children, but has the disadvantage of an irregular absorption rate which makes its action slightly unpredictable. However, it would appear to be the method of choice in this age group. The following drugs are recommended:

Trimeprazine (Vallergan), diazepam (Valium) and triclofos sodium (Tricloryl).

Trimeprazine is one of the most useful of the phenothiazine group of drugs for oral premedication since it has both sedative and antihistaminic properties; however, its anti-adrenergic activity may occasionally cause some cardiovascular depression when a relatively large dose is accompanied by an unusually rapid rate of absorption. Careful observation of the child is therefore necessary after its use. The recommended dose for premedication is 3–5 mg/kg with a maximum dose of 120 mg given 2 h prior to operation.

Diazepam is a useful drug for premedication, but the degree of sedation seems less consistent than with trimeprazine. However, the minimal effect it has on the cardiovascular and respiratory systems makes it useful for the poor risk child. The drug can be given in tablet form, 2, 5 and 10 mg tablets being available, or as a pleasant valium syrup containing 2 mg of diazepam in 5 ml of syrup. A dose of 0.4–0.8 mg/kg will be required to achieve basal narcosis and this should be given at least 2 h pre-operatively.

Triclofos is described under night sedatives but may also be used for premedication in children (Boyd and Manfold, 1973). Elixir tricloryl (100 mg/ml) given in a dose 65–75 mg/kg will usually achieve good results and is particularly useful for the poor risk child.

Rectal premedication From time to time both the oral and intramuscular routes for premedication prove unsatisfactory for one reason or another in which case the rectal administration may be a useful alternative. The two drugs most commonly used for this purpose are thiopentone and methohexitone.

Thiopentone (Pentothal) can be prepared in tap water as a 2 per cent solution or more conveniently given as a specially prepared rectal suspension which contains 2 mg of thiopentone in a 10 ml Abbosert syringe; 44 mg/kg (200 mg/ml) is given 15 min prior to operation.

Methohexitone (Brietal Sodium) is prepared as a 10 per cent solution in warm tap water and given in a dose of 22 mg/kg body weight. Absorption is rapid and sleep occurs within 5 min.

N.B. With both these rectal preparations careful and constant nursing care with the child on his side is essential from the time of administration until the patient is placed in the care of the anaesthetist.

Children over seven years and adults

A careful explanation of the procedure involved in the anaesthetic and surgery should be given the night before the operation. For example, the patient should be told whether or not he will wake up with a sore throat, a gastric tube or tracheostomy in position, or an intravenous drip running. It is waking up to the unexpected which frightens many patients.

Night sedation

The requirement for night sedation prior to operation will vary considerably from patient to patient, and therefore they must be treated individually. With the very anxious patient, sedation should ideally begin a few days before admission to hospital; a small dose of diazepam 2–5 mg thrice daily is useful for this purpose.

A good sleep on the night before operation is essential. Patients who are accustomed to night sedation should be allowed to take the drug of their choice in a slightly increased dose. Nitrazepam 5–10 mg (Mogadon) is a useful night sedative. If the operation is planned for the afternoon an additional morning sedative, such as lorazepam or diazepam, might be required for the anxious patient. Barbiturate sedatives are not usually recommended prior to operation owing to their anti-analgesic properties.

Premedication

In the older age group premedication is usually given intramuscularly owing to its greater reliability. However, oral premedication may be perfectly satisfactory for the patients who show a marked preference for this route. Pethidine, morphine and papaveretum (Omnopon) are the most popular premedicant drugs as they produce both euphoria and sedation, but in some patients they may initiate nausea and vomiting, making the addition of an anti-emetic a wise precaution. The phenothiazines are useful for this purpose as they have both sedative and anti-emetic properties in addition to a mild antisialogogue activity. Pethidine 1.5 mg/kg, morphine 0.2 mg/kg or papaveretum 0.3 mg/kg with promethazine 0.5 mg/kg make a good combination of drugs.

When irritant inhalational anaesthetic agents are to be used antisialogogue drugs such as hyoscine or atropine must be included in the premedication, but with the less irritant agents this is not always necessary. Indeed, in ENT surgery, where the respiratory tract is involved and intubation is usually essential, a moist respiratory mucosa will often reduce post-operative discomfort. If the anaesthetist uses suxamethonium for intubation, he may regard the inclusion of atropine in the premedication as mandatory.

Special considerations regarding pre-operative and post-operative drugs

Special consideration must be given to the preparation and premedication of patients who are suffering from chronic disease, or who are under treatment for conditions unrelated to the proposed operation.

Cardiovascular disease

Pre-existing cardiovascular disease is seldom a contraindication to anaesthesia and surgery provided all efforts are made, with the cooperation of the physicians, to see that the patient has reached his optimal fitness, before undertaking 'cold' surgery. The choice between local and general anaesthesia often has to be considered, and this choice may be a difficult one, requiring considerable experience. Given the services of an experienced anaesthetist, general anaesthesia has much to be recommended in the cardiac patient. The avoidance of fear and tension is very important in these patients and good premedication followed by a smooth, careful induction and maintenance of anaesthesia with constant monitoring is frequently the best way of achieving this aim. Under certain circumstances however, local anaesthesia may be the safer option; for example, patients with fixed cardiac output disease such as constrictive pericarditis, severe vascular disease and certain cardiomyopathies present a special hazard during the induction of general anaesthesia. These patients can usually be managed satisfactorily under local anaesthesia whilst being carefully sedated with intravenous diazepam.

Heart block

This constitutes a serious anaesthetic hazard and merits full consultation with a cardiologist regarding the advisability of pre-anaesthetic treatment with drugs such as ephedrine before surgery is contemplated. These cases should only be anaesthetized by an experienced anaesthetist, but with careful management general anaesthesia is not contraindicated. An external pacemaker may be indicated.

Hypertension

This is no contraindication to general anaesthesia but a special word should be said about patients on hypotensive drug therapy, as they are put at a slightly increased risk under general anaesthesia because the drugs used potentiate the hypotensive effect of many anaesthetic agents. This instability of blood pressure has led some anaesthetists to insist that specific hypotensive therapy is discontinued well in advance of the administration of a general anaesthetic, the period of time being dependent upon the normal length of action of the drug. With this view others will disagree. If the symptoms and risks associated with the untreated hypertension are sufficient to warrant active treatment, then it would appear unwise to expose the patient to these risks prior to the stress of an operative procedure. In addition, successful hypotensive therapy is often extremely difficult to establish in terms of dose adjustment, and to interrupt a satisfactory maintenance regime for any reason requires most careful consideration. This is not to suggest that the administration of an anaesthetic to a patient receiving hypotensive therapy is devoid of special risk, but this risk can be reduced to a minimum by careful attention to the anaesthetic agents used. If, despite these considerations the anaesthetist feels that hypotensive treatment should be discontinued, this decision should not be finalized until he has discussed the specific problems involved with the physician in charge of the case.

Coronary artery disease and aortic insufficiency

A clear history of coronary infarction within the previous 6 months or a history of severe aortic valve insufficiency is normally taken to indicate that general anaesthesia should be avoided whenever possible.

The presence of *anginal pain* always constitutes a special hazard as all anaesthetic techniques tend to produce vasodilatation and if the coronary arteries are prevented by disease from participating in this dilatation, uncompensated hypotension will inevitably lead to coronary insufficiency. It is therefore those patients whose anginal pain is not normally adequately relieved by vasodilator drugs such as glyceryl trinitrite who are at special risk, and for whom it is important to avoid general anaesthesia whenever possible. The patient who obtains ready relief from anginal pain can be expected to tolerate carefully administered general anaesthesia, for his coronary arteries are likely to participate in the overall vasodilatation produced by anaesthesia, cardiac perfusion thus being maintained. Premedication may, with benefit, include the patient's usual coronary dilator drug.

Respiratory disease

Acute upper respiratory infections are always a contraindication to ear, nose and throat surgery under general anaesthesia, and whenever possible the acute condition must be treated before surgery is contemplated.

Ludwig's angina is a condition characterized by the spread of inflammatory oedema throughout the neck, pharynx and larynx, and is particularly hazardous where general anaesthesia is concerned. Tracheostomy may be required to relieve respiratory obstruction in this condition and should be carried out, if possible, under local anaesthesia. If general anaesthesia is necessary, it should be assigned to an experienced anaesthetist and under no circumstances should an intravenous anaesthetic be given. It is essential that the surgeon is scrubbed up and ready to perform emergency tracheostomy or laryngotomy before the induction of anaesthesia is started (*see also* 'Upper Respiratory Obstruction').

Chronic bronchitis and emphysema

These, if severe, may present problems to the anaesthetist and local anaesthesia should be used whenever possible, but general anaesthesia is not always contra-indicated. Every effort should be made to get the patient to optimal fitness by the use of physiotherapy, antibiotics and bronchodilators before surgery under general anaesthesia is contemplated. Premedication with promethazine will serve both to reduce respiratory secretions and to minimize the likelihood of bronchospasm. Atropine should be avoided as its excessive drying effect may result in the production of highly viscous secretions which are difficult to eliminate.

Tuberculosis

With a positive sputum, this carries the risk of spread of the disease, and contamination of the anaesthetic apparatus, so local anaesthesia should be used when possible. Rigorous antituberculous treatment is essential before general anaesthesia is contemplated.

Asthma

This is no contraindication to general anaesthesia. The premedication should contain bronchodilator rather than bronchoconstrictor drugs therefore pethidine should be used in preference to morphine, and the phenothiazines in preference to the barbiturates. The patient should be allowed to continue his routine bronchodilator treatment prior to operation, whether it be ephedrine, salbutamol, isoprenaline or hydrocortisone. If steroids have been used over many months, then the dose should be increased immediately before and for a while after the operation. An aminophylline suppository given with the premedication is often helpful.

Blood disorders

Anaemia

In simple iron deficiency anaemia, general anaesthesia is not contraindicated, but whenever possible the anaemia should be corrected prior to operation. Anaemic patients generally require lower doses of all drugs as compared with normal patients, and of course special care to provide adequate oxygenation during and after anaesthesia is essential. The same principles apply to patients with hyperchromic pernicious anaemia.

Sickle-cell anaemia

Sickle-cell disease is a chronic, familial, haemolytic anaemia which is usually found in African and West Indian patients, and is due to the presence of haemoglobin S in the patient's blood. Two forms of the disease exist. The heterozygous (AS) disease (sickle-cell trait), in which general anaesthesia is not contraindicated and the homozygous (SS) disease in which general anaesthesia is best avoided.

Patients suffering from homozygous (SS) disease run a very high risk of haemolysis and multiple infarction if they are exposed to minor degrees of central or peripheral hypoxaemia, hypercarbia and hypothermia (Searle, 1973). Should general anaesthesia prove unavoidable in these patients the following precautions must be taken.

(1) The patient must be admitted to hospital.
(2) A period of pre-oxygenation before the induction of anaesthesia is advisable.
(3) Pre-anaesthetic administration of sodium bicarbonate to establish a base excess may be considered necessary. This may be given by intravenous infusion of 50–100 ml of an 8.4 per cent solution.
(4) Hypoxia, acidosis and hypotension during anaesthesia must be scrupulously avoided. Adequate temperature control to avoid hypothermia is also important.
(5) Oxygen therapy should be continued post-operatively until recovery is complete.

Routine screening All African and West Indian patients should be screened for sickle-cell anaemia as part of the pre-operative preparation. This may be carried out initially by using a commercial macroscopic test; 0.02 ml of blood is added to 2 ml of a buffered solution containing saponin (red-cell lytic agent) and sodium hypochlorite (reducing agent). If haemoglobin S is present a turbid suspension develops in 3–5 min. In the absence of haemoglobin S the solution remains clear. If the test proves positive and the haemoglobin is less than 11 g per cent, on no account should a general anaesthetic be administered until further examination by electrophoresis has eliminated the possibility of both SS (homozygous) or SC disease being present.

Treatment of sickle-cell crisis Should a sickle-cell crisis occur post-operatively, as indicated by pain in joints or abdomen, haematuria, disturbance of vision, circulatory collapse or prolonged unconsciousness, the following measures should be taken:

(1) Continuous oxygen therapy and the administration of bicarbonate to maintain a base excess.
(2) Haemolysis may lead to severe anaemia which should be treated with transfusion of packed cells if the haemoglobin level falls below 8 g per cent. Unnecessary transfusion is harmful as it may result in an increase in blood viscosity (Howells *et al.*, 1972).
(3) Infarction will be heralded by pain in the limbs, chest and abdomen. This should be treated with analgesics and the intravenous infusion of Macrodex 40 to reduce blood viscosity. It has also been suggested that magnesium sulphate, 2 ml of a 50 per cent solution, should be administered every 4 h.

One of the common causes of death in these patients is pulmonary embolism, and it is therefore suggested that all patients who complain of limb or abdominal pain should be immediately heparinized (Howells *et al.*, 1972).

Thalassaemia

The management of patients suffering from this rare type of anaemia is similar to that described under hypochromic anaemia, but there are two additional problems. First, anaemia may prove difficult to treat. Secondly, these patients develop an abnormal hypertrophy of the bone marrow, which leads to a characteristic overgrowth of the maxilla. This may make laryngoscopy very difficult and sometimes impossible.

Bleeding diatheses

A history of abnormal bleeding in patients who are to undergo ENT surgery must always be taken seriously and a correct diagnosis made before surgery is contemplated. Frequently, a careful history will reveal no suspicion of disease, but, if in doubt, the cause of the bleeding must be established. The following laboratory tests should be ordered:

Full blood count, including platelets.
Bleeding time.
Clotting time.
Prothrombin time.

Should an abnormality be revealed, special tests will be carried out by the haematologist to identify the precise nature of the defect.

Disorders of clotting

(a) *Haemophilia* Haemophilia is an inherited sex-linked disease manifest only in the male and is due to the absence or deficiency of antihaemolytic globulin (AHG – Factor VIII). Clinically the patients may be separated into three groups according to the AHG levels.

(1) AHG Plasma levels over 25 per cent.
These patients seldom present problems to either surgeon or anaesthetist.
(2) AHG Plasma levels 5–25 per cent.
These patients must always be treated by the haematologist before ear, nose and throat surgery is contemplated.
(3) AHG Plasma levels below 5 per cent.
These patients are usually severely handicapped and only essential surgery should be contemplated and then only after careful control by the haematologist.

In all haemophiliacs undergoing surgery general anaesthesia is preferred. Local infiltration or nerve blocks should not be used. Pre-operative and post-operative drugs should be given intravenously or by mouth. Intramuscular drugs should be avoided. Aspirin, with its tendency to produce gastric haemorrhage should not be used. For operations on the nose or pharynx careful intubation is essential, but the nasal route should be avoided. Extubation should be delayed until satisfactory haemostasis has been established and careful observation in the post-operative period should be provided.

(b) *Von Willebrand's disease* This disease affects both sexes and although the bleeding diathesis is associated with the presence of large, tortuous, fragile capillaries, patients frequently have a low plasma AHG and therefore exhibit many of the characteristics of haemophilia.

(c) *Christmas disease* This disease is characterized by a deficiency in Factor IX and clinically resembles haemophilia. Its correction requires the administration of Factor IX rather than AHG. Unlike haemophilia, the female carrier has a tendency to bleed.

Capillary and platelet disorders
This group of diseases include hereditary haemorrhagic telangiectasia and the thrombocytopoenic purpuras. The problems which confront the anaesthetist are those associated with the very low haemoglobin so often present in these patients. The surgeon and anaesthetist must always bear in mind that the preservation of the patient's veins for the purpose of transfusion may be life saving.

Diabetes
There is no single scheme in the management of these patients for surgery which will cover all cases. Generally speaking, it is wiser to aim at a high blood sugar rather than risk hypoglycaemia.

(a) *Minor surgery of short duration* General anaesthesia for minor surgery in the controlled diabetic presents no problems, provided the following precautions are taken.

(1) Anaesthesia is administered approximately 4 h after the last meal, which should preferably be a light breakfast of normal calorie content.
(2) Premedication, other than atropine if required, is omitted.
(3) Anaesthesia is maintained at a light level, so as to obtain rapid recovery.

(b) *Major surgery of long duration* Alteration of pre-operative diet and antidiabetic drugs may prove unnecessary but some physicians prefer to reduce both the calorie intake and equivalent insulin dose by about one third. If prolonged feeding difficulties are anticipated an intravenous drip is essential during the post-operative period.

The following intravenous routine may be used. One litre of 5 per cent dextrose followed by 500 ml normal saline every 12 h. This should be accompanied by 4-hourly urine tests and the administration of insulin as follows:

If urine is blue or green to Benedict's Test	No insulin
If urine is yellow	10 units sol. insulin
If urine is orange	15 units sol. insulin
If urine is red	20 units sol. insulin

Blood sugar estimations should be carried out at regular intervals as a check.

(c) *Emergency surgery* If the diabetic patient is uncontrolled and urgent surgery is necessary, local anaesthesia should be used whenever possible. If general anaesthesia is contemplated 50 g of dextrose accompanied by 24 units of soluble insulin may be given pre-operatively and a 5 per cent dextrose drip containing 12 units of insulin per litre should be given during the operation and over a period of 6 h. Further treatment should be controlled by frequent blood sugar estimations. Whenever possible the advice of a diabetes specialist should be sought.

Patients on drug therapy

Antidepressants

Patients on antidepressant drugs require special pre-operative and post-operative management. Two groups of antidepressants require special mention because of their interaction with drugs commonly used before, during and after surgery.

(1) *Monoamine oxidase inhibitors* (*MAOI drugs*) These drugs are used in the treatment of exogenous and reactive depression, and patients receiving treatment, although often uncommunicative, will usually admit to having been forbidden to eat cheese and other thiamine-containing foods. Such information will help the surgeon to identify the recipient of this large group of drugs, the most common of which are shown in *Table 20.2*.

Table 20.2 Monoamine oxidase inhibitor drugs

Approved or chemical name	*Trade name*
Etryptamine	Monase (Upjohn)
Iproniazid	Marsilid (Roche)
Isocarboxazid	Marplan (Roche)
Mebanazine	Actomol (ICI)
Nialamide	Niamid (Pfizer)
Pargyline	Eutonyl (Abbott)
Pivazin, Pivazide	Tersavid (Roche)
Phenelzine	Nardil (Warner)
Pheniprazine	Catron, Cavodil (Benger)
Tranylcypromine	Parnate (SKF)
Tranylcypromine, Trifluoperazine	Parsteline (SKF)

Certain drugs are absolutely contraindicated when the patients are taking MAOIs.

(a) Pressor amines such as amphetamines and mephenteramine.
(b) Nasal decongestants, such as ephedrine and phenylephedrine.
(c) Ephedrine by injection which may be indicated for the treatment of bronchospasm or asthma.

In the presence of MAOIs these drugs may produce dangerous hypertension which will require immediate treatment with an alpha-adrenergic blocking agent. Phentolamine Mesylate (Rogitine) 5 mg intravenously is the drug of choice.

Other drugs should be used with caution.

(a) Pethidine, especially when given intravenously, may cause excessive respiratory depression, hypo- or hypertension, excitation, sweating, nausea and coma. This is due to inhibition of the liver enzyme which metabolizes pethidine.
(b) Morphine, codeine and other narcotic analgesics have been claimed to cause interaction, but the evidence is less convincing.
(c) All drugs metabolized in the liver, such as barbiturates, phenothiazines and the benzodiazepines may be potentiated and therefore should be used in reduced dosage.

Whenever possible, patients on MAOI drugs who are on the waiting list for surgery should be taken off the drugs at least three weeks before the operation. If this is not possible, local anaesthesia would be preferred. There is no contraindication to the inclusion of adrenaline and noradrenaline in the local anaesthetic, since these substances are destroyed in the body, not by monoamine oxidase but by catechol-*o*-methyl transferase.

(2) *Tricyclic antidepressants* These drugs are used for the treatment of endogenous depression, the two most commonly used compounds being amitriptyline (Triptizol) and imipramine (Tofranil). They do not interact with the sedative and analgesic drugs used before and after surgery, but the additional use of such drugs as diazepam, chlorpromazine and perphenazine have been shown to increase the serum levels and therapeutic effects of the tricyclics. The most important effects of the tricyclics as far as

surgery is concerned, is that they appreciably increase the patients' sensitivity to adrenaline and noradrenaline (*see* section on 'Local Anaesthesia').

Steroid therapy

Prolonged steroid therapy may result in suprarenal depression giving rise to inability to tolerate 'stress'. Operative procedures, whether undertaken under general or local anaesthesia, provide such a stress stimulus. When performed upon patients not receiving steroids, but who have received them during the past two months, the patient should be covered by an appropriate course of steroid treatment. If the patients are still on steroid therapy the dose should be increased before and for a few days after the operation.

The 'pill'

There is some justification for discontinuing the contraceptive pill prior to surgery on two accounts. First because it may increase the likelihood of post-operative thrombosis, particularly if hypotensive anaesthesia is used. Secondly, because it interferes with plasma cholinesterase levels and may in consequence lead to a sensitivity to the muscle relaxant, suxamethonium (Scoline).

Pregnancy

All surgical procedures should be avoided in the first 12 weeks of pregnancy. The risk of abortion during this period as a consequence of operative stimulation may be theoretical rather than real, but should such an abortion occur spontaneously and fortuitously, the operative stimulus will almost certainly be cited as having been causative. Also, during these early weeks it is not permissible to administer any drug, unless it has been established that it is free from ill-effects on the fetus; particular care should be taken in respect of the tranquillizing agents.

In the final weeks of pregnancy the increased intra-abdominal pressure predisposes to respiratory embarrassment and gastric regurgitation, so that general anaesthesia should be undertaken with care. There is also some risk – possibly only theoretical – of inducing premature labour.

Between 12 and 30 weeks, there is no contraindication to general anaesthesia. However, the patient may require some increase in dosage of all anaesthetic and pre-anaesthetic drugs, owing to their increased blood volume. Liberal oxygenation during anaesthesia is indicated.

Recent general anaesthesia

All anaesthetists will agree that, ideally, general anaesthesia should not be repeated at less than 6-week intervals. If repeated anaesthesia cannot be avoided, harm seldom occurs provided the anaesthetist is aware of the nature of the previous anaesthetic.

The main concern arising from repeated general anaesthesia at short intervals is that the patient may become sensitized to one of the anaesthetic drugs. Two drugs in particular are liable to cause trouble, althesin and halothane.

Althesin Anaphylactic reactions have been reported with althesin when the drug is repeated at short intervals. There is some evidence to suggest that this is due to a sensitization to the solubilizing agent used in the preparation of the drug (Watt, 1975).

Halothane Fatal jaundice following the repeated administration of halothane, although very rare, has been reported and has become the subject of very considerable controversy (Strunin and Simpson, 1972).

There is no evidence that halothane is more hepatotoxic than any other halogen-containing anaesthetic agent; but there is a possibility that repeated administration, at less than 6-week intervals, may cause a sensitivity type of hepatitis or that the halothane may change the immune response to a dormant hepatic virus. The fact that the histological change in the livers of these patients is indistinguishable from that seen in infective hepatitis, may give some support to the latter theory, but a sensitivity response seems a more likely explanation.

A pyrexia of unknown origin on the third or fourth day after operation is a feature of this condition and may suggest a sub-icteric hepatitis. Unexplained jaundice after halothane anaesthesia will contraindicate its subsequent use within 6 weeks.

Mode of action of anaesthetic drugs

It is perhaps enough for both anaesthetist and surgeon to know that anaesthetics work, in that they render the patient unconscious – immobile and free from pain – thus allowing surgery to proceed with the minimum of discomfort for all involved. But for the more enquiring mind it may be helpful to discuss how and why they work.

Faced with one group of compounds with one specific action on the nervous system the answer to these questions could possibly be simple, but this is not the case – indeed, many books have been written on the subject. One can therefore only scratch the surface of the problem and whet the appetite of the reader.

Anaesthesia can be produced by large molecular structures such as steroids and by simple hydrocarbons such as cyclopropane C_3H_6 and even inert mono-atomic agents such as xenon. This would suggest that there are many mechanisms involved; but our knowledge of nerve conduction with its obvious simplicity does not make this likely. We must therefore find some common theory of action which will accommodate the widely variable structure of known anaesthetic drugs.

The early pioneer work of Myer and Overton (1899–1901) found that the potency of most anaesthetic agents was closely related to the water to oil (olive oil) partition coefficient. These early conclusions fit in well with the results of more recent experiments by Hong and Hubell (1972) who, using artificial model systems containing phospholipid bi-layers, were able to demonstrate that the lipid region is the primary site of action of inhalational anaesthetics. As a consequence of this action the protein configuration of the membrane surrounding the nerve axon is altered, thus increasing its permeability to various ions.

It is well established that local anaesthetics produce their effect by altering the permeability of the axonal cell membranes to Ca^{++} and Na^{+} ions and thus altering the action potential of the nerve impulse. It seems likely that general anaesthetics might act in a similar way, although the concentration of a general anaesthetic required to block conduction locally is considerably greater than that required to produce general anaesthesia. This perhaps can be explained by postulating that the smaller diameter neurons in the CNS require a much smaller disturbance in protein configuration to interrupt conduction. The actual site of action may be at the synapses which are very sensitive to some agents, but the diversity of structure of anaesthetic agents makes this unlikely. Evidence seems to suggest that a CNS (brain) blockade at the reticular formation is the likely site, but there is still much to learn (Miller, Paton and Smith, 1972).

To sum up, it would seem probable that anaesthetic agents expand the lipid part of the cell membrane – all being lipid soluble – and thus increase the activity of the lipid molecule. This in turn disturbs the protein configuration and in so doing changes the permeability of the membrane to sodium and calcium ions, thus interfering with the conduction to the brain. This process has been shown to be readily reversible.

Local anaesthesia

Local versus general anaesthesia

With modern improvements in general anaesthetic techniques there is a very limited place for local anaesthesia in ENT surgery but it must be admitted that under certain circumstances local anaesthesia provides a safer and more satisfactory form of pain relief than general anaesthesia. Also there are patients who have a genuine fear of general anaesthesia and to whom local anaesthesia should be offered as an alternative. It is therefore important that both surgeons and anaesthetists involved in ENT surgery should be familiar with the pharmacology of local anaesthetics and the relevant blocking techniques.

Local anaesthetics in combination with general anaesthesia also play an important role as a method of providing haemostasis, particularly in operations involving mucous membranes.

Pharmacology of local anaesthetic solutions

Local anaesthetics produce a reversible block of conduction in nerve endings and axons by altering the permeability of the axon membrane and thus interfering with the passage of Na^+ ions across that membrane. This transfer of ions is responsible for the action potential. The site of action of the local anaesthetic is at the node of Ranvier where the myelin sheath is thin or absent, thus allowing easy access to the 'local'. The electrical impulse is capable of jumping one or two nodes, so at least 6–10 cm of nerve should be covered by the local in order to guarantee a successful block. This is an important fact when considering the minimal dose required. The speed at which local anaesthetics penetrate the nerve axon is inversely proportional to the fibre diameter. This is of practical significance, since the smaller sensory fibres are more rapidly affected than the larger motor fibres. The sequence of sensory blockade is pain, followed by temperature, light touch and pressure.

The rate of absorption and distribution of the local anaesthetic will depend upon a number of factors including the chemical structure of the drug used and its concentration, the state of ionization of the solution relative to the pH of the tissues injected and the vascularity of the tissues.

Local anaesthetic solutions are in two forms, the uncharged free base and the ionized form, the degree of ionization depending upon the pH of the prepared solution and the buffering effect of the tissue fluid at the injection site. It is the uncharged form of free base that penetrates the lipid barrier of the nerve sheath as only this form is lipid-soluble. Thus the quality of anaesthesia is governed to some extent by these factors. Two examples support this phenomenon. Benzocaine which is insoluble in water does not exist in the ionized form and therefore cannot be used by injection, but owing to its high lipid solubility is an excellent topical anaesthetic. On the other hand, injections of local anaesthetics into inflamed tissues which have a low pH, produce poor anaesthesia. This is because the proportion of free uncharged base will be reduced by the acid pH of the tissue and delay the penetration of the drug into the nerve axon. The same problem may occur with some commercially prepared solutions containing adrenaline, as these preparations have a low pH. It is often more satisfactory to add adrenaline immediately before use.

Toxic action of local anaesthetics

The toxicity of local anaesthetics is very variable and will be described under the specific agent. Because of this wide range in toxicity it is important that the operator makes himself thoroughly familiar with one or two drugs which he will use exclusively.

The rate of absorption of the drug and the ultimate blood level achieved will depend upon the concentration of that drug and the vascularity of the tissue into which it is injected. These factors must always be taken into consideration when determining the dose to be used, and the need to add a vasoconstrictor. Because of the variability in the rate of absorption, the possibility of an inadvertent intravenous injection and the serious consequences of a toxic reaction, it is always wise to have an open vein (intravenous drip or butterfly needle) whenever local anaesthetics are being used, so that immediate treatment can be given.

Stimulation of CNS

Local anaesthetic agents are essentially central depressants, but despite this the first signs of overdose are central excitation and convulsions, because the inhibitory cells in the brain are affected before the excitatory cells, thus causing over-stimulation. Such stimulation will occur with lignocaine when the blood level reaches about 8 μg/ml of blood, and will, not infrequently, cause death from asphyxia if the convulsions are not treated immediately. Simple twitching and other mild excitatory phenomena may be controlled with small doses of thiopentone and diazepam intravenously but to control major fits it is necessary to give a paralysing dose of muscle relaxant followed by intubation and controlled respiration.

Cardiovascular depression

Moderate blood levels of a local anaesthetic will depress the heart and its conductive tissue, frequently producing bradycardia and occasionally a reduction in cardiac output. It must be remembered that patients in cardiac failure are often acidotic and therefore local anaesthetics become more ionized in the tissues, increasing their toxicity.

Respiratory depression

Following central stimulation, toxic doses of local anaesthetic will lead to profound respiratory depression.

Allergic reactions

Allergic reactions to local anaesthetics are very rare but when they do occur they may cause oedema, bronchospasm and circulatory collapse. Treatment should be based on antihistamines and corticosteroids, followed by adrenergic drugs and full circulatory support.

Methaemoglobinaemia

This occurs with a number of local anaesthetics, but most commonly with prilocaine. One of the breakdown products of prilocaine, *o*-toluidine, causes oxidation of haemoglobin to methaemoglobin. Following the administration of 500 mg or more of prilocaine, the methaemoglobin level may rise to as much as 5 per cent producing a distinct cyanotic tinge to the patient within 4–6 h. Although this is of little clinical significance it may present problems of diagnosis and is therefore best reversed. The methaemoglobin is readily reduced back to haemoglobin by giving, intravenously, 1 per cent methylene blue in a dose of 1–2 mg/kg.

Vasoconstrictors

The addition of a vasoconstrictor to local anaesthetics has three important functions:

(1) It reduces the toxicity of the 'local' by delaying absorption.
(2) It prolongs the action by retaining the drug at the site of injection.
(3) It provides a degree of tissue ischaemia, which is particularly important in microsurgery and intranasal operations.

Adrenaline

Adrenaline is the vasoconstrictor most commonly used in combination with local anaesthetics. In fact, many commercial preparations of lignocaine, prilocaine, bupivacaine and others have adrenaline already added. Although these preparations are convenient, they have some disadvantages. For example, the amount of adrenaline is frequently too high – some containing up to 1:80 000 adrenaline, where 1:200 000 would be perfectly adequate; also some commercial preparations containing adrenaline have a low pH which will increase ionization of the local and thus delay penetration into the nerve axon. It is always more satisfactory to add the adrenaline just before use. Finally because adrenaline is a toxic substance, a total dose of 0.5 mg (0.01 mg/kg) should not be exceeded and it must be used with special care in many circumstances, for example:

(1) In patients suffering from ischaemic heart disease, hypertension or thyrotoxicosis.
(2) When the patient is under general anaesthesia and halothane, trichlorethylene or cyclopropane are being administered.
(3) In patients who are receiving tricyclic drugs. These drugs inhibit the destruction of catecholamines and may in consequence considerably potentiate the cardiovascular effects of the adrenaline. If it is considered necessary to use adrenaline, the tricyclic antidepressants must be withdrawn for at least three days beforehand. One must not confuse the tricyclic antidepressants with the monoamine oxidase inhibitors which have no effect on adrenaline toxicity since they are destroyed in the body, not by monoamine oxidase, but by catechol-*o*-methyl transferase.

Felypressin (PLV.2 Octapressin)

This synthetic vasoconstrictor is a useful alternative to adrenaline as a vasoconstrictor agent where that drug is contraindicated. It has a very low systemic toxicity and does not affect coronary circulation or cause myocardial irritation. Its hypertensive effect is also slight (Katz, 1965).

Felypressin may be used in patients receiving tricyclic drugs without ill effect and also in patients under general anaesthesia with halothane, cyclopropane or trichlorethylene (Trilene). It has the disadvantage that the optimal vasopressor effect is not reached for 1–15 min after injection, but unlike adrenaline it does not produce a secondary dilatation (Green and Coplans, 1973). It is most effective in combination with prilocaine. It is available in a 3 per cent solution of prilocaine containing 0.005 mg of felypressin in 1 ml and is prepared in dental cartridges for easy administration.

Phenylephedrine

This compound has a weaker vasoconstrictor activity than adrenaline and should be used in a concentration of 1:2500. It is however, more stable than adrenaline and has a much longer action as a vasoconstrictor. It has less action on the heart than adrenaline and is less likely to produce dysrhythmias should it be given intravenously by mistake. It is therefore often the drug of choice.

Cocaine

May be used primarily as a surface vasoconstrictor for mucous membranes (*see below*).

The properties of specific local anaesthetic drugs

Local anaesthetics given in the wrong dose and in the wrong circumstances may be dangerous. It is therefore a good principle to be thoroughly familiar with one good drug for each situation and confine one's use to those drugs. Four drugs should cover all the needs for regional and topical anaesthesia of the ear, nose and throat, as follows.

Cocaine

Cocaine was the first drug to be described as a local anaesthetic in 1884 and today its use is almost exclusively confined to surface anaesthesia of the eye, nose and throat. It is extremely toxic when injected. The safety of this drug as a surface anaesthetic is dependent upon the marked vasoconstrictor action it has on small vessels, a property not found in any other local anaesthetic. It is this property of vasoconstriction which is responsible for maintaining the place of cocaine in nasal surgery. If surface anaesthesia alone is required, one of the alternative, safer topical anaesthetics should be employed. For topical anaesthesia and vasoconstriction of the nose, throat and larynx cocaine should be used in a 4–10 per cent solution of the hydrochloride or as a 25 per cent paste. The stronger solutions are possibly less toxic than the weaker solutions on mucous membranes because they are more slowly absorbed but the total dose should not exceed 3 mg/kg, with a maximum of 200 mg in a fit adult.

The toxic effects of cocaine are related to its intense sympatheticomimetic activity as it potentiates the action of noradrenaline and catecholamines; for this reason the addition of adrenaline to cocaine solutions and paste is by some regarded as unnecessary and dangerous, although the combination has been used by many nasal surgeons without mishaps (Lee and Bryce Smith, 1976). The main features of toxicity are an increase in blood pressure and respiratory rate, frequently with intense pallor. This may progress to coma or convulsions. Pyrexia may also be a prominent symptom of cocaine poisoning.

Amethocaine (Pentocaine, Decicaine, Tetracaine)

For the ENT surgeon, amethocaine has its primary use as an alternative to cocaine for surface anaesthesia. Only this aspect of the drug will be discussed here. Unlike cocaine, amethocaine lacks the intense vasoconstrictive activity of cocaine, indeed it has a direct action on blood vessels to cause dilatation, but owing to its very high potency it proves to be a very useful surface anaesthetic for the larynx, pharynx and trachea. For preference it should be used in a fine spray in 0.5–1 per cent solution, the maximum dose being 1 mg/kg; about 4 ml of a 1 per cent solution in the average adult. It should be remembered that the absorption from the bronchial mucous membrane is very rapid – almost as rapid as in intravenous injection – and the rate of hydrolysis slow. It is therefore wise to spray in divided doses giving 5 min between each dose. Particular care should be taken with children.

Like procaine, the drug is broken down in the body by plasma cholinesterase to para-amino benzoic acid which inhibits the action of sulphonamides. The solutions may be sterilized by autoclaving once or twice, but repeated autoclaving may destroy its activity.

Amethocaine (Decicaine) is also prepared as a 65 mg lozenge, which may be sucked over a period of 20 min prior to endoscopy (see below).

Lignocaine (Xylocaine – lidocaine, USP)

Lignocaine is probably the best all-round local anaesthetic to use in ENT surgery for both topical and regional anaesthesia, as it has a rapid onset of action and provides intense analgesia of short duration. It does not produce vasoconstriction but unlike amethocaine vasodilatation is not evident. It is stable in solution, and may be repeatedly autoclaved, but should not be left in copper or nickel containers as ions are liberated which are irritant to the tissues (Lee and Bryce Smith, 1976).

Following absorption, the drug may produce considerable drowsiness and amnesia from its central action, a fact frequently welcome during surgery under local anaesthesia.

The drug is metabolized in the liver and excreted by the kidney. Metabolism may occasionally give rise to cyanosis due to the formation of methaemoglobin, but this is rare and far less common than with prilocaine. The methaemoglobinaemia is seldom incapacitating and may be readily reversed by the administration of 1 per cent methylene blue – 1–2 mg/kg intravenously. The rate of metabolism is increased by premedication with phenobarbitone (Di Fazio and Brown, 1972).

Topical use

Many preparations of lignocaine are available for topical anaesthesia. All are very effective but their duration of action is short, 15–20 min.

Lignocaine Spray is the commonest preparation used in the UK. It is prepared as a pink or green solution, and should be administered by a spray or ultrasonic nebulizer, in a metered dose. Maximum dose is about 240 mg (6 ml) for the average adult.

Xylocaine Viscous is a preparation which contains 2 per cent lignocaine in a mucilage base. It is particularly useful for anaesthesia prior to oesophagoscopy; if 5 ml is moved around the mouth and swallowed, up to 20 min anaesthesia may be achieved, making a good alternative to the decicaine lozenge.

Regional anaesthesia

The justified popularity of lignocaine for regional anaesthesia is based on three factors: its relatively low toxicity, its excellent spreading properties and its good penetration powers into nerve tissue. The short duration of its action may sometimes be a disadvantage, but the addition of adrenaline (1:200 000) will frequently prolong its analgesic effect for as much as 2 h. A 0.5 per cent solution is all that is required for infiltration anaesthesia; and the total dose of 500 mg (100 ml) should not be exceeded (7 mg/kg body weight). If no vasoconstrictor is used the dose should be limited to 3 mg/kg. For nerve blocking procedures a 1 per cent solution of lignocaine is usually adequate and it is never necessary to exceed 1.5 per cent.

Prilocaine hydrochloride (Citanest)

This local anaesthetic has similar properties to lignocaine and can be used as an alternative in comparable concentrations. The maximum safe dose of the plain solution is 400 mg. It is less toxic than lignocaine and has a slightly longer action, but is much more likely to produce methaemoglobinaemia. It has vasoconstrictor activity so that the addition of a vasopressor will only slightly increase the length of its action; it is therefore often the drug of choice for infiltration analgesia into highly vascular areas such as the head and neck and when adrenaline is contraindicated (e.g. for patients with thyrotoxicosis, hypertension or on tricyclic antidepressant drugs). A 3 per cent prilocaine solution with felypressin is marketed for use in a dental syringe; a dose of 7 mg/kg (15 ml) should not be exceeded.

Bupivacaine (Marcain)

Bupivacaine is derived from mepivacaine and was first used clinically in 1963. It has a potency of approximately four times that of lignocaine and has three times the length of action, but the onset is much slower. Bupivacaine is more protein-bound than lignocaine and is therefore less toxic and cumulative. Its use in ENT surgery would appear to be limited as it is less suitable than lignocaine and prilocaine for infiltration anaesthesia and is not very effective as a topical anaesthetic. However, for nerve blocking procedures such as stellate block and regional block for maxillo-facial surgery, where a prolonged action is required, it may prove useful. Little advantage is gained by adding adrenaline to the solution. The drug is marketed as a 0.25 per cent and 0.5 per cent solution with or without adrenaline. Unless muscle relaxation is required 0.25–0.375 per cent solutions provide adequate conditions. The total dose given at one time should be limited to 2 mg/kg body weight (25 ml of 0.5 per cent solution in the average adult).

Etidocaine hydrochloride (Duranest)

This recently introduced, local anaesthetic drug is related to lignocaine, but has a considerably longer action similar to bupivacaine and is more toxic. It may prove a useful alternative topical anaesthetic agent to lignocaine.

Preparation for local anaesthesia

Adequate preparation and premedication, prior to local anaesthesia for major surgery in any region of the body, is essential. It is of particular importance in ear, nose and throat surgery, when communication with the patient during surgery may be difficult or impossible. The lack of effective sedation may wreck an otherwise correct technical procedure, as an anxious patient is likely to anticipate pain with every sensation and react accordingly.

The preparation should begin well in advance of the operation, with a full explanation of the procedure and a warning that local anaesthesia may not always completely abolish the sensation of touch, but will always prevent pain.

Premedication should be designed to suit the individual case. Morphine or papaveretum with hyoscine is often used, because of the euphoria and amnesia which these drugs produce. The drying effect of the hyoscine may be a disadvantage in head and neck surgery, as the patient will be unable to get any relief by wetting his mouth or lips. The phenothiazines are probably a better choice. Promethazine or trimeprazine in a dose of 25–50 mg intramuscularly, given 1 h prior to surgery, are useful drugs for this purpose, and may be combined with an opiate.

If the patient arrives in the theatre in an anxious state of mind, despite the premedication, he should be helped further by intravenous doses of a suitable sedative. One of the soluble benzodiazepines will probably be the drug of choice.

Diazepam (Valium) is the most popular drug in this group, as it gives good sedation and a remarkable degree of amnesia. It should be given slowly, intravenously, in a dose of 5–30 mg, particular care being exercised in the elderly who are very sensitive to its central depressant effect and may not tolerate more than 5 mg. The drug should never be injected into a small vein, i.e. back of hand or wrist, unless it is diluted at least ten times. The consequence of such an injection will be a painful venous thrombosis occurring up to a week after the injection and taking many months to clear completely.

Lorazepam (Ativan) is a less well-tried drug for this purpose, but would appear to be a useful alternative. There is evidence to suggest that the incidence of venous thrombosis when injected into small veins, although not inconsiderable, is less than with diazepam. The drug should be given intravenously in a dose of 2–6 mg about 15–30 min before surgery. A fairly long period of sedation can be expected.

Anaesthesia for adenotonsillectomy (children)

The operation of adenotonsillectomy carries a low mortality but is not without its risks. The figures for 1957–1961 show a mortality rate of 1:10 000 and there is no reason to believe that this has changed in recent years. Although haemorrhage is, without question, the commonest cause of death, general anaesthesia comes a close second. The greatest risk is in the re-anaesthetizing of the child for post-operative haemorrhage (Tate, 1963).

Preparation of the patient

Apart from the problems of premedication which are discussed earlier, the child must have a careful medical examination to eliminate recent infection and intercurrent disease, and to evaluate whether or not antibiotic cover is required. Blood examination, with grouping and the saving of serum for cross-matching, is essential at some stage, but unless the child appears clinically anaemic or has a bleeding tendency it seems unnecessary to subject a fretful nervous child to blood-letting prior to anaesthesia. This will frequently make the anaesthetist's job more difficult and the child's visit to hospital more 'traumatic'. The collection of blood after the child is anaesthetized is time enough, and is usually much simpler for all concerned. Blood loss during adenotonsillectomy is seldom sufficient to require replacement, but Shalom (1964) in a controlled series found that two out of five children, mostly in the very young, came close to needing fluid replacement. Provided that the total loss is less than 10 per cent of the patient's blood volume (80 ml/kg body weight) replacement with Hartmann's Ringer lactate is quite adequate, but with a greater loss than this whole blood replacement will be necessary.

Methods of anaesthesia

In recent years it has been established practice to intubate children of all ages for adenotonsillectomy and tonsillectomy, using the method originally described by Doughty in 1957. The correct tubes and connections must be used to facilitate the insertion of the specially designed split gag; and to prevent obstruction of the tube by the tongue plate (*Figure 20.1*). This method has its obvious advantages, particularly in

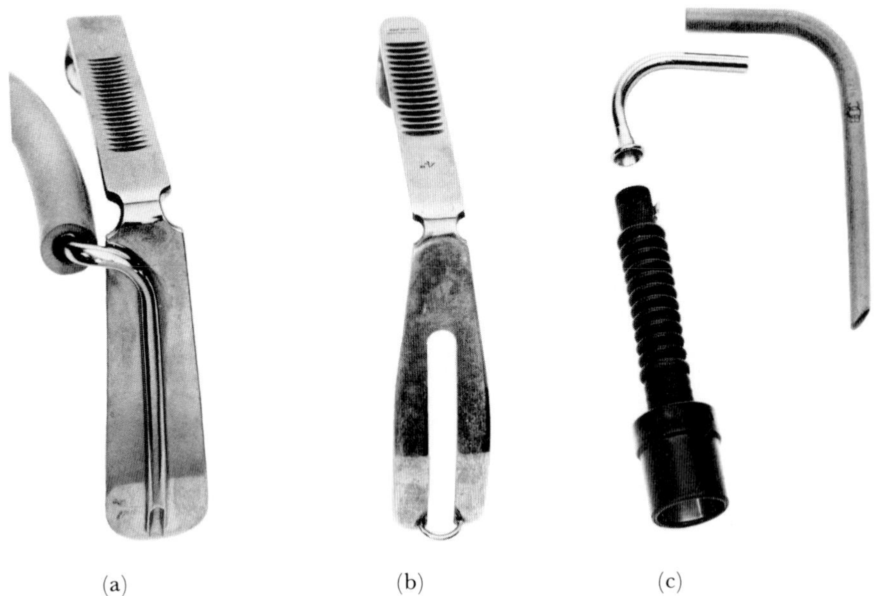

Figure 20.1 Gags and tubes used in tonsillectomy. (a) Boyle–Davis gag; (b) split gag: note groove in tongue plate to accommodate endotracheal tube; (c) tube and connection used with split gag

the older child, as lighter anaesthesia can be used and stridor due to laryngeal stimulation is prevented. However, particularly in the smaller child, many surgeons and anaesthetists still prefer the older, open method of anaesthesia using the Boyle–Davis gag. It is simple, avoids the possible trauma of intubation, the laryngeal spasm which occasionally occurs on extubation and the extra bulk of equipment in a small mouth. The choice of method should be a joint decision between the surgeon and anaesthetist. All ENT anaesthetists must be familiar with both techniques.

The maintenance of anaesthesia is usually by nitrous oxide and oxygen supplemented with ether or halothane, halothane being the most commonly used supplement at the present time. Ether in inexperienced hands is the safer of the two drugs and provides prolonged post-operative analgesia, but it has the disadvantage of being explosive, more irritant, more nauseating and more slowly eliminated than halothane. Halothane is easier to manage than ether, but owing to its high potency and cardiovascular depressing effect, considerably more care and minute-to-minute observation is required. Recovery is very rapid with halothane, but unlike ether it provides no post-operative analgesia. As a consequence the child may be very restless and noisy. This restlessness can be avoided by giving an intramuscular analgesic immediately before the cessation of the anaesthetic. The dose of analgesic should be adequate but not sufficient to produce respiratory depression. Pethidine 1.2 mg/kg or morphine 0.2 mg/kg for a child who has not had a narcotic in the premedication and about 60 per cent of the pre-operative dose if he has, is adequate and safe. No further post-operative narcotic analgesic should be required after these doses.

Recovery

Skilled supervision of the patient after tonsillectomy is probably the most important single factor in maintaining a low morbidity and mortality rate. The patient must be nursed in the lateral position (*Figure 20.2*). This position should be initiated immediately after discontinuing the anaesthetic and before extubation, and maintained until full consciousness has been established. Careful observations of pulse and blood pressure are essential for the first 24 h and signs of bleeding such as swallowing, tachycardia and vomiting recorded. If persistent bleeding is observed narcotic analgesics should be used with caution in adults and never in children. Failure to control the bleeding must be treated with intravenous fluid replacement and early return to theatre.

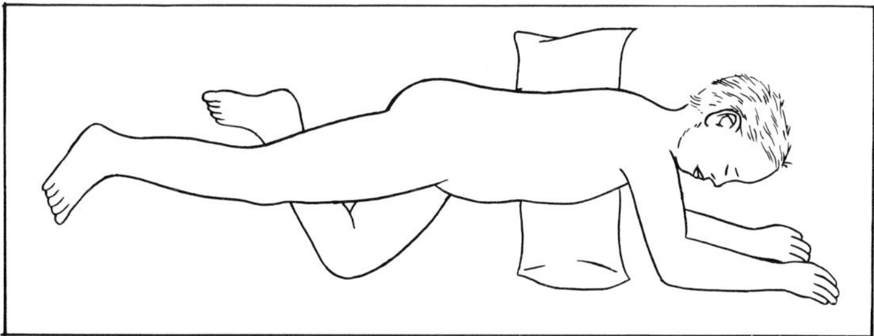

Figure 20.2 Recovery position after naso-pharyngeal operations. Note (1) Extended upper leg and flexed lower leg; (2) pillow placed under thorax which should be used for children, but is unnecessary for adults

Anaesthesia for tonsillectomy in adults

General anaesthesia

Provided there are no adenoids or other contraindications a nasotracheal tube is usually convenient, but oral intubation can be employed using a split gag and a cuffed Oxford tube. Quiet anaesthesia without coughing and straining is essential for good operative conditions. On completion of the operation extubation should be carried out with the patient in the left lateral position.

Local anaesthesia

Local anaesthesia for tonsillectomy is rarely performed when skilled general anaesthesia is available, but this unpleasant procedure may occasionally be necessary.

Technique

The patient is seated in a chair with the head well supported, but adequate facilities for lowering the head should be available in the not uncommon event of fainting.

An Amethocaine lozenge is sucked half an hour before spraying the pharynx with 10 per cent cocaine. Injections are then made, using 5 ml of 1 per cent lignocaine and adrenaline into the following sites:

(1) Upper pole of posterior pillar.
(2) Upper part of the anterior pillar.
(3) The triangular fold, near the lower pole.
(4) The supratonsillar fossa.

Anaesthesia for post-tonsillectomy bleeding

Anaesthesia for post-tonsillectomy bleeding is one of the most hazardous of all anaesthetic procedures in ENT surgery, and the emergency most likely to give junior and senior anaesthetists alike a nightmare. The patient, frequently a small child, is often shocked from hypovolaemia. Vasoconstriction makes venipuncture difficult, and regurgitation after induction of anaesthesia is likely, due to a stomach full of blood. In addition, blood in the mouth may restrict vision during intubation.

The safe management of these patients must depend upon a close cooperation between surgeon and anaesthetist. The following considerations are vital.

(1) The patient must be brought to theatre as soon as it is considered that bleeding is not going to stop with conservative treatment.
(2) Central depressants should not be used in an attempt to quieten a bleeding, restless child, unless continuous uninterrupted supervision is available.
(3) Whenever possible an intravenous drip should be set up and blood taken for

cross-matching before induction of anaesthesia is started. It is however frequently preferable to get on with the operation rather than wait for cross-matched blood to be available.

(4) Anaesthesia should not be started until the patient is on an adjustable operating table and an efficient suction apparatus available and working.

(5) If the oropharynx is fairly clear of blood and clots, anaesthesia may be induced in a head-up supine position using halothane with or without a curare-like muscle relaxant for oral intubation. Nasal intubation is best avoided in these patients. The use of suxamethonium to provide relaxation may lead to trouble, as it has a tendency to produce an increase in intragastric pressure with the consequent risk of gastric regurgitation.

(6) If bleeding is still brisk and large clots, which cannot be removed, are still present in the pharynx, anaesthesia should be induced with the patient in the right lateral, head-down position, and the staff prepared to cope with large quantities of regurgitated blood from the stomach as soon as anaesthesia has been established. In skilled hands intubation should be possible but is more difficult in this position. Alternatively, particularly in the small child, the Boyle–Davis gag can be inserted under deep anaesthesia while the patient is still in the lateral position, and after sucking the pharynx clear he can be turned into the tonsillar position, intubation thus being avoided. Vomiting of blood on recovery must be expected and care taken to prevent pulmonary aspiration. Some anaesthetists like to attempt aspiration of the stomach before the patient leaves the theatre, by passing a wide bore gastric tube.

Anaesthesia for endoscopy and endoscopic surgery

Most endoscopic procedures can be carried out successfully and safely under local anaesthesia, but in children and the majority of adults greater comfort for both patient and surgeon, as well as improved operating conditions, can be better achieved by a combination of local and general anaesthesia.

General anaesthesia for oesophagoscopy, gastroscopy and pharyngoscopy has never presented any problems for the anaesthetist, as tracheal intubation provides safety for the patient and good access for the surgeon, but with bronchoscopy and laryngoscopy a very different problem arises; that of airway sharing. There must of necessity be a compromise between ideal operating conditions and perfect safety for the patient. A close cooperation between the anaesthetist and surgeon with full understanding of each other's problems and a willingness for the surgeon to abandon the operation at any stage, if requested by the anaesthetist, are essential for perfect safety. In recent years, with the advancement of new endoscopic operative techniques requiring greater relaxation and longer surgical procedures, the problems of anaesthesia have increased and in consequence new techniques have been devised.

General anaesthesia in bronchoscopy

Three separate principles are used in general anaesthesia for bronchoscopy, and each has its place according to circumstances.

(1) Anaesthesia with spontaneous respiration

The maintenance of spontaneous respiration during bronchoscopy is essential for safety under a number of circumstances, which include patients with copious secretions, inhaled foreign bodies, bronchial-pleural fistulae and lung cysts. It is also very reassuring in small children in whom even short periods of apnoea may lead to severe hypoxaemia. Halothane without a muscle relaxant will provide adequate conditions for the surgeon under most circumstances, particularly if it is accompanied by good topical anaesthesia. The major disadvantage with this procedure is that sufficient relaxation may be difficult to achieve in the healthy adult patient.

(2) Anaesthesia with apnoea and oxygen insufflation

For short bronchoscopic procedures, up to 20 min anaesthesia and complete relaxation can be maintained by intermittent doses of an intravenous anaesthetic and suxamethonium. Oxygenation is adequately maintained by insufflating oxygen at a rate of 6–10 l/min into the trachea through a small nasal-tracheal catheter (5 mm diameter), placed with its tip close to the carina. There are two disadvantages of this technique: a progressive rise in alveolar carbon dioxide tension (3 mmHg/min) which limits the time available for operating; and the frequent development of severe muscle pains resulting from the use of suxamethonium. In addition one must not ignore the fact that intermittent suxamethonium may occasionally lead to a rise in serum potassium with its consequent cardiac effects (Vaughan and Lunn, 1973).

(3) Anaesthesia with apnoea using a Venturi-type injector for positive pressure ventilation

This method of anaesthesia is similar to the insufflation technique except that instead of supplying O_2 through a nasal-tracheal catheter, a small injector unit (*Figure 20.3*) is attached to the bronchoscope. Oxygen under high pressure is injected intermittently through this unit, producing a Venturi effect which, with entrained air will effectively inflate the patient's lungs (Sanders, 1967).

Adequate ventilation can be maintained for an almost unlimited time in the apnoeic, relaxed patient by this method, providing good conditions for bronchoscopy, without a rise in P_{CO_2} or fall in oxygen tension (Bali, Dundee and Stevenson, 1973).

The main disadvantage is that the surgeon is exposed to intermittent blasts of expired air which may represent a potential hazard in the transmission of infection from the patient to the operator, as well as proving unpleasant (Bethune, 1976). However, for the procedure likely to last more than 15–20 min and where there is no cross-infection risk, this may well be the method of choice.

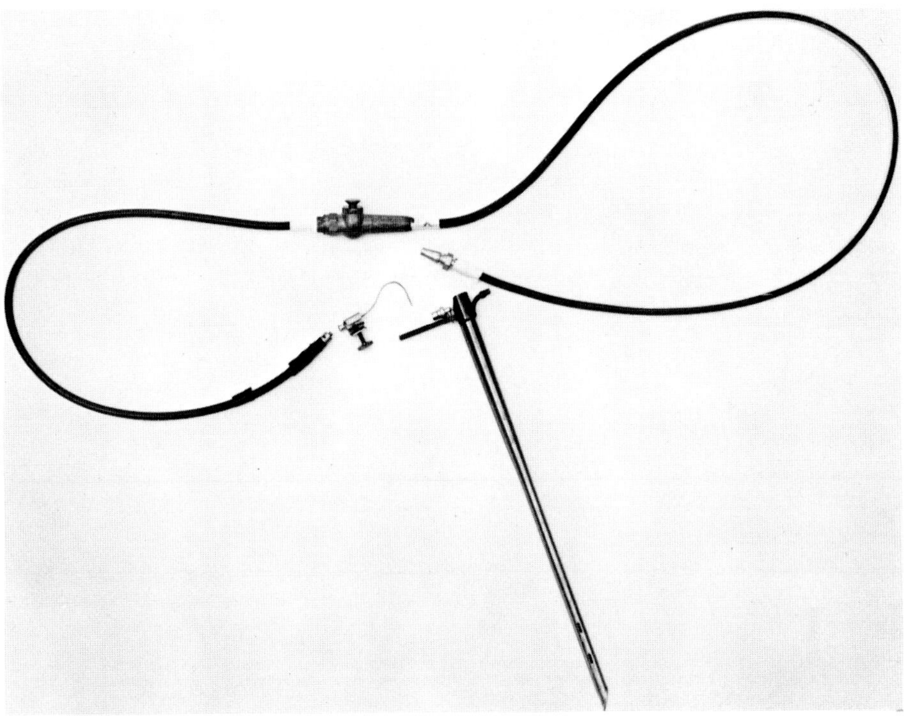

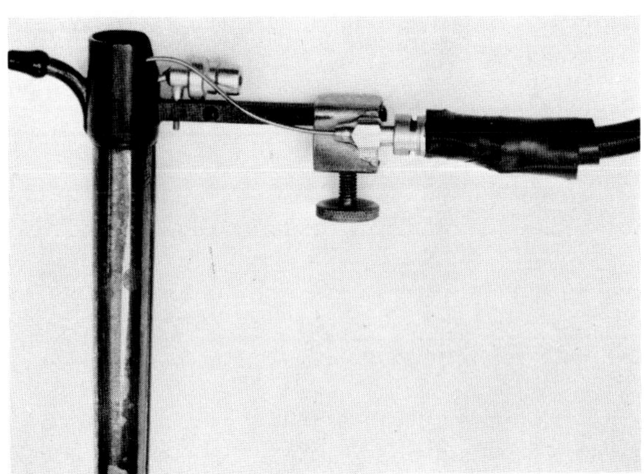

Figure 20.3 Injector unit for use in bronchoscopy. (a) Complete unit showing release button; (b) unit attached to bronchoscope

General anaesthesia for microlaryngoscopy

Anaesthesia for microlaryngeal surgery presents the anaesthetist with problems not described for bronchoscopy. The surgery is often prolonged and the surgeon may be hampered by any reasonable-sized tube passed between the cords for the purpose of maintaining respiration. As in other endoscopic procedures under general anaesthesia close cooperation between the surgeon and anaesthetist is essential. Three separate techniques will be described, each having its merit according to circumstances.

General anaesthesia with spontaneous respiration

The patient is anaesthetized with an intravenous agent, nitrous oxide, oxygen and halothane and taken down to a depth of anaesthesia to provide relaxation. The larynx, pharynx and trachea are then sprayed thoroughly using a metered volume of 2 per cent amethocaine (1 mg/kg) or 4 per cent lignocaine (2 mg/kg). A 3 mm plastic tube or a Foley catheter (Lewis, 1977) is then passed through the larynx, via the nose, and adjusted to lie in the trachea just short of the carina. The laryngoscope is passed and secured in position by the surgeon under deep halothane anaesthesia (Gordon and Sellars, 1971). Continued anaesthesia and quiet respiration are maintained by using intravenous fentanyl in sufficient dose to depress respiration to about 8/min (0.005 mg/kg). Oxygen is blown through the naso-tracheal catheter at 12–15 l/min. This ensures adequate oxygenation and effectively prevents blood and debris entering the trachea during the operative procedure. If the Foley catheter is used and should respiration become too depressed with evidence of respiratory insufficiency the lungs can be ventilated by inflating the balloon at the end of the catheter at a rate of about 10/min. It is seldom necessary to use this device.

This technique, favoured by the author, provides good conditions for prolonged microlaryngeal surgery, and leaves an unobstructive view for the surgeon (*Figure 20.4*). The fentanyl is readily reversed by naloxone at the end of surgery and recovery from anaesthesia is rapid. The disadvantages of not having the profound relaxation

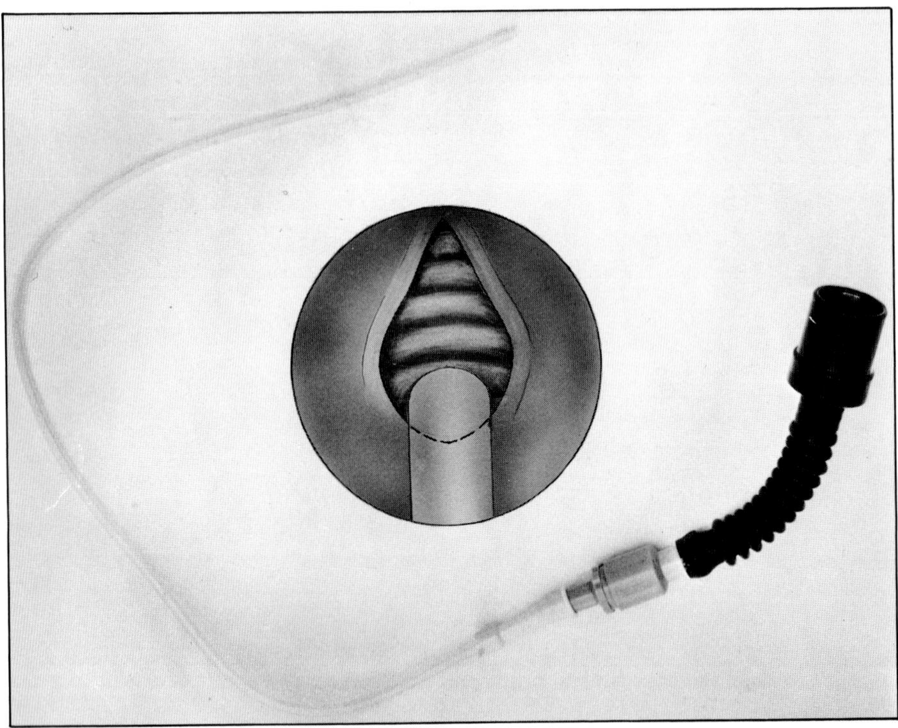

Figure 20.4 View of larynx with 3 mm tube *in situ*. (a) Note unobstructed view of larynx; (b) 3 mm plastic tube

provided by the use of suxamethonium are not insurmountable. Post-operative nausea may be encountered but this is usually avoided by giving an anti-emetic.

General anaesthesia with intubation

There are unquestionable advantages in having a cuffed endotracheal tube *in situ* during microlaryngoscopy when faultless airway protection is considered of paramount importance, but such tubes must be of sufficient size to allow adequate respiratory exchange and may therefore limit surgical access. The original Pollard tube (Pollard, 1968) has a wide oral portion and a narrow cuffed tracheal portion in an attempt to cut down respiratory resistance to a minimum. Many surgeons find this tube inconveniently bulky (*Figure 20.5*). More recently, Coplans (1976) described the use of a long 5 mm cuffed nasotracheal tube. This tube gives perfect airway protection and, provided hand ventilation through a circle absorber is used, adequate respiratory exchange for up to 45 min. The tube allows adequate access to $\frac{4}{5}$ of the larynx (*Figure 20.6*) and in no way hampers laryngoscopy.

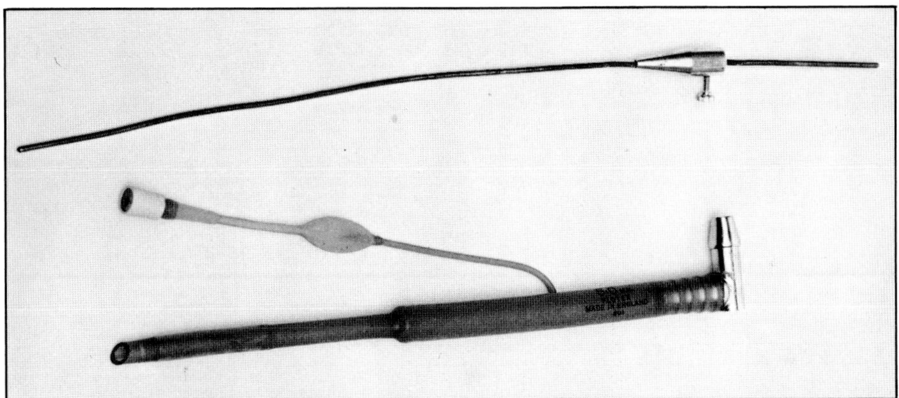

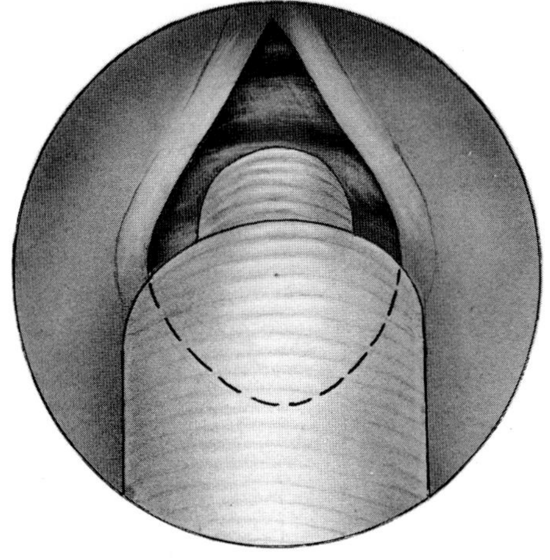

Figure 20.5 View of larynx with Pollard tube *in situ*. (a) Note restricted view of posterior part of larynx; (b) Pollard tube

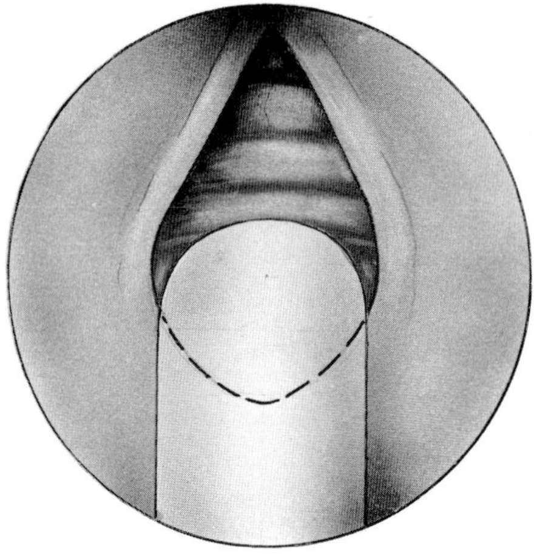

Figure 20.6 View of larynx with Coplans' tube *in situ*. Note good view of four-fifths of larynx

General anaesthesia with apnoea using a Venturi-type injector for positive pressure ventilation through a Carden endoscopy tube

The Carden laryngoscopy tube which was first described in 1975 (Carden, 1975) consists of a 2½-in cuffed silicone rubber tube into which a narrow delivery tube has been fixed (*Figure 20.7*). The tube is placed beyond the glottis with a pair of Magill forceps so that it lies in the trachea just short of the carina. The cuff is inflated and the delivery tube is attached to a Venturi-type injector which can provide adequate inflation of the lungs and an unobstructive view for the surgeon.

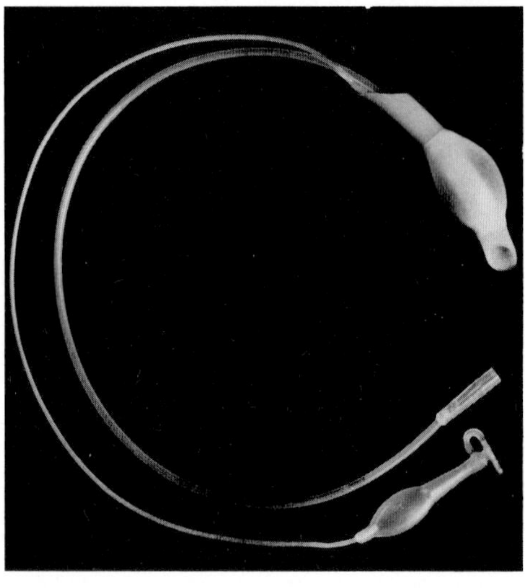

Figure 20.7 Carden endoscopy tube

Anaesthesia for upper respiratory obstruction

Upper respiratory obstruction, whatever its aetiology, will always present a hazard to general anaesthesia, and that hazard will be considerably increased if the obstruction is associated with inflammatory oedema of the pharynx and glottis.

Oral obstruction

Oral obstruction may present itself in many ways and always leads to problems for the anaesthetist. Congenital abnormalities limiting the oral airway include microstoma, macroglossia and hypoplasia of the mandible with prolapse of the tongue. Tumours of the jaw and tongue may encroach on the oral airway and inflammatory conditions of the jaw and teeth may lead to severe trismus. Ludwig's angina, being an inflammatory condition of the submaxillary space, may obstruct the oral airway with oedema of the soft tissues of pharynx and glottis, and also cause trismus. Mouth opening may be severely restricted by temporo-mandibular arthritis or the wiring together of the jaws for the treatment of mandibular fracture. The problems of anaesthesia in these patients are two-fold.

(1) The basic problems, which occur in all patients with upper respiratory obstruction in terms of pre-operative preparation and choice between local or general anaesthesia, are discussed under emergency tracheostomy (*see* p. 736).
(2) The problem of maintaining an airway without free access to the oral cavity.

Two options are open to the anaesthetist, nasal intubation or tracheostomy.

Nasal intubation should be attempted whenever possible. This can frequently be achieved blind and is safest when performed under local anaesthesia. The nose is thoroughly prepared with a 10 per cent cocaine spray and, using a soft long-bevel tube, tracheal intubation is performed through the nose during deep inspiration. This technique is not difficult to master (Verrill, 1963). In the absence of inflammation and with an unobstructed nasal airway, it is justified to perform this procedure under light general anaesthesia, provided muscle relaxants are not used.

If blind nasal intubation is not possible *tracheostomy* should be performed under local anaesthesia.

Pharyngeal obstruction

Severe pharyngeal obstruction may be due to cystic lesions of the pharynx and larynx or to inflammation such as peritonsillar and retropharyngeal abscesses. These lesions always run the risk of rupture due to instrumentation required for intubation, with the consequent hazard of inhalation of infected material if general anaesthesia is used. For this reason preliminary aspiration should ideally be carried out under local anaesthesia.

Ludwig's angina

Ludwig's angina, in addition to producing oral obstruction, may lead to gross pharyngeal oedema, the management of which is discussed under emergency tracheostomy, but the dangers of general anaesthesia cannot be over-emphasized particularly if intravenous agents are used for induction.

Laryngeal obstruction

The problems of anaesthesia for laryngeal obstruction in the adult are discussed in this chapter under 'Laryngectomy' and 'Tracheostomy'. Any operation involving the obstructed infant larynx should be preceded by tracheostomy, because an airway which is just adequate pre-operatively will almost certainly become obstructed by oedema post-operatively. The pre-operative tracheostomy will always be greatly assisted by intubation under general (inhalational) anaesthesia without the use of muscle relaxants. In the very young, under a week old, intubation may usually be performed without anaesthesia. If the obstruction is severe enough to bring the accessory muscles of respiration into use then the tracheostomy should be performed under local anaesthesia.

Laryngotracheobronchitis

This dramatic condition may necessitate tracheostomy in the very young and the question of using local or general anaesthesia will always arise. In experienced hands general anaesthesia with orotracheal intubation may be justified as it will greatly assist the surgeon. An inhalational technique must always be used, with facilities for performing an emergency tracheostomy immediately at hand (Seward and Fraser, 1961). When in doubt the operation should be performed under local anaesthesia using an oral sedative such as trimeprazine (0.3 mg/kg).

Tracheal obstruction

Tracheal obstruction may present many problems for both surgeon and anaesthetist particularly if the lower part of the trachea is involved. The problems are discussed in this chapter under 'Tracheal Stenosis'.

Anaesthesia for emergency tracheostomy

Whenever possible, tracheostomy should be carried out as a planned unhurried procedure under general anaesthesia using a cuffed endotracheal tube to prevent contamination of the airway during the initial stages of the operation. The operative procedure and indications are fully covered elsewhere in this book (Vol. 4).

In the emergency situation where there is some degree of respiratory insufficiency and tracheostomy has been considered necessary, the method of anaesthesia to be adopted must always be carefully and fully discussed between the surgeon and anaesthetist before the operation is contemplated. The anaesthetist must never be placed in a position in which he is persuaded to carry out a general anaesthetic against his better judgement, as he and he alone will fully appreciate the difficulties he may encounter, and the limitations of his capabilities of overcoming these difficulties, in terms of help, equipment and experience. If the risks of general anaesthesia are considered too great, then the procedure must be performed under local anaesthesia despite its many difficulties and disadvantages.

General anaesthesia

The advantages of general anaesthesia with intubation, for tracheostomy in the partially obstructed patient, are obvious. It should always be considered, but only performed if the necessary skills and facilities are available. The worst that can then happen is that a planned tracheostomy may have to be replaced by an emergency tracheostomy or laryngotomy. It is important to remember that, merely by rendering the patient unconscious, a partial obstruction can be rapidly converted into a complete obstruction, impossible to relieve by intubation and requiring instant surgery to save life.

The following preparations are essential before undertaking general anaesthesia in these patients.

The patients should not receive narcotics prior to induction of anaesthesia. Atropine should be used with caution, as it not only stimulates the cerebral cortex, thus raising oxygen requirements, but also increases the viscosity of the secretions making complete obstruction of the diminished airway more likely. Premedication with the phenothiazine derivatives, in carefully assessed doses, will often produce effective sedation without serious respiratory depression. The surgeon and his assistant should be gloved and ready for an emergency should it occur. Induction of anaesthesia must be performed in the operating theatre, after an attempt to obtain full oxygenation and CO_2 elimination. This can often be achieved by a helium–oxygen mixture for 10–15 min before induction (Green and Day, 1954). In the absence of severe respiratory obstruction and hypoxaemia, anaesthesia can be induced with an intravenous barbiturate and muscle relaxant, but if significant signs of obstruction are present at this time then an inhalational induction should be employed, and anaesthesia taken to a depth of good relaxation. The anaesthetist must then attempt intubation having available a range of endotracheal tube sizes. Should attempts to intubate lead to total obstruction and make location of the larynx impossible, the surgeon must instantly perform laryngotomy or tracheostomy at the anaesthetist's request. Anaesthesia can then be continued through the tracheostomy tube.

Tragedies with these patients are practically always due to a casual approach to the problem by both surgeon and anaesthetist and failure to appreciate the suddenness with which serious problems can arise and cardiac arrest ensue.

Anaesthesia for laryngectomy and pharyngolaryngectomy

Major resection surgery of the larynx and pharynx is very often carried out as a combined operation, involving both ENT and general surgeons. Many of these patients are elderly and suffering from advanced carcinoma which has been previously treated with radiotherapy. They therefore tend to be anaemic and generally in poor condition and prone to bleeding, so that the safety of anaesthesia, haemorrhage control and fluid replacement are major problems.

Laryngectomy

Pre-operative assessment

The majority of patients who come to surgery are those in whom radiotherapy has failed to control the disease. Chronic bronchitis and emphysema are common in such patients and these conditions should be vigorously treated with physiotherapy, antibiotics and antispasmodics to obtain optimal fitness before surgery. A variable degree of chronic respiratory obstruction is inevitable, and it is important that this should be carefully assessed by the surgeon and anaesthetist before the form of the operation and anaesthetic is planned. It is very helpful if the same anaesthetist gives the anaesthetic for both the pre-operative biopsy and the laryngectomy. This will enable the anaesthetist to assess how best to achieve control of the airway during the major operation.

Control of the airway

(1) Intubation under general anaesthesia is possible in the majority of cases and is certainly the least unpleasant procedure for the patient, but it should not be attempted in the presence of severe obstruction without careful thought and experience. However confident of success the anaesthetist may be, the surgeon must be immediately at hand should an emergency tracheostomy be required.
(2) In the severely obstructed patient awake intubation can usually be performed under sedation with intravenous diazepam (0.15 mg/kg) and careful preparation with local anaesthetic, without undue discomfort to the patient.
(3) Elective tracheostomy under local anaesthesia is probably the safest method of establishing an airway through which the general anaesthetic can be administered, if severe obstruction is present. This method, however, is unpleasant for the patient and there is some evidence that a tracheostomy performed in this way increases the rate of local recurrence of the carcinoma.

Anaesthetic technique

Premedication
If respiratory obstruction is present it is often prudent to omit respiratory depressant drugs from the premedication and to rely upon tranquillizers such as the diazepines. Atropine may be used but if controlled hypotension is anticipated atropine is best avoided, as the tachycardia induced may make control of blood pressure more difficult.

The maintenance of anaesthesia
Anaesthesia presents few problems once the airway has been established. Controlled hypotension may be helpful if block dissection is to be performed. When the trachea is severed the endotracheal tube is removed after thoroughly pre-oxygenating the patient and a sterile tube is inserted by the surgeon into the tracheostome. This change-over should be performed as quickly and smoothly as possible. The surgeon who does not appreciate the need for speed in this manoeuvre may cause his anaesthetist considerable anxiety.

Pharyngolaryngectomy

Surgery for pharyngeal carcinoma is major and mutilating and the operative mortality is high, but if it is required to alleviate the patient's desperate symptoms such hazards must be faced. 'Diseases desperate grown, by desperate appliances are relieved or not at all' (Shakespeare, Hamlet IV iii 9). Success must depend upon the combined efforts of the whole surgical team.

Pre-operative assessment

In contrast to the patients requiring laryngectomy, these patients rarely present any respiratory or cardiovascular difficulties. The main problems are those of malnutrition and electrolyte imbalance so it is important to see that the electrolyte balance, anaemia and nutritional deficiencies are all corrected as far as possible. An electrocardiogram should be recorded prior to surgery.

It is very important to explain carefully and fully to the patient, the extent and consequences of the operation and be sure that he fully understands.

Premedication

Premedication should be adequate using a sedative and narcotic agent. Pethidine and promethazine make a suitable combination. If hypotensive anaesthesia is to be used atropine is best avoided.

Anaesthetic management

Three main problems confront the anaesthetist in this type of surgery:

(1) The control and replacement of blood loss.
(2) The control of heat loss.
(3) Access to the patient.

The control of blood loss
The use of hypotensive anaesthesia to control blood loss is very helpful in this type of surgery but not accepted by all. Gorham, Baskett and Clements (1965) concluded

that a low blood pressure might prejudice the viability of the colon and therefore should be avoided. Condon (1971) also avoided the use of hypotension as he felt that a normal blood pressure was necessary for adequate perfusion of the graft. However, Campkin (1970) maintained a systolic blood pressure between 40 and 65 mmHg during the neck dissection and brought it back to normal levels prior to transposition of the colon, a technique which would seem to satisfy all requirements.

Whether or not hypotensive anaesthesia is used, accurate fluid replacement is essential and requires careful monitoring.

Monitoring

Continuous monitoring of blood pressure and a record of the electrocardiogram are essential. When hypotension is used, invasive methods of recording arterial blood pressure are justified with an intra-arterial line whenever possible. Sophisticated pressure recording equipment using transducers is advantageous, but expensive and not always available. A simple device described by Zorab *et al.* (1969) using a length of tubing and an aneroid pressure gauge should be found in any department and serves the purpose well (*Figure 20.8*).

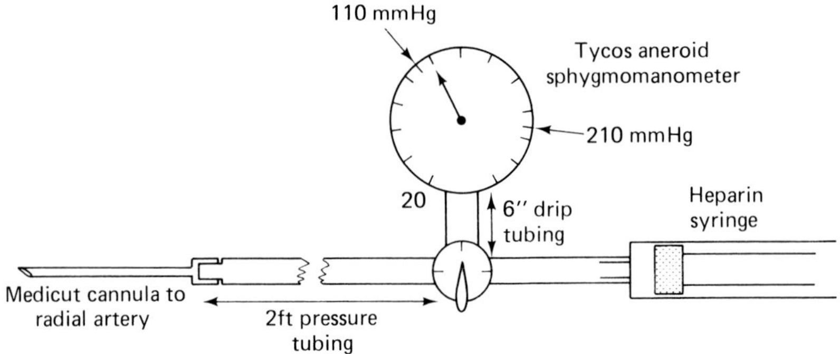

Figure 20.8 Simple apparatus for recording arterial pressure. Note 3-way tap for flushing cannula with heparin solution

Although a continuous central venous pressure record would prove very useful for accurate fluid replacement, most anaesthetists working in this field have found that accurate recordings during the operation are difficult because of surgical manipulation in the neck.

Cardiac dysrhythmias are common during the mobilization of the oesophagus and the transference of the stomach or colon to the neck. This makes continuous electrocardiogram recording essential in order that the anaesthetist can assess cardiac function accurately. It may be necessary to ask the surgeon to stop surgical manipulation from time to time to allow recovery of heart function.

Control of body temperature

Loss of body heat may be considerable during these long operative procedures and many anaesthetists have found a marked improvement in the patient's general postoperative condition by using a heating blanket during the operation to maintain body temperature. A continuous recording of rectal temperature should be made.

Access to the patient
A major problem confronting the anaesthetist when two surgical teams are busy, is that of physical access (Simpson, 1960). Monitoring equipment, although valuable, cannot be a substitute for direct contact. Each surgeon should have a limited number of assistants, and visitors should not be allowed to push their way in at the expense of the anaesthetist's control over his patient. 'Muscling in' may also lead to the dangerous consequences of apparatus becoming disconnected.

Maintenance of anaesthesia

The problems of maintaining anaesthesia are similar to those of laryngectomy. If hypotension is used, normal blood pressure must be re-established for the abdominal part of the operation so as to avoid ischaemia at the anastomoses. The flexibility of sodium nitroprusside is useful for this purpose (*see* 'Hypotensive Anaesthesia'). Rupture of the trachea has been known to occur at the site of the tracheal cuff, when it becomes unsupported after mobilization of the oesophagus, making inflation of the lungs impossible. A short-cuffed endotracheal tube should therefore always be available, so that it may be passed beyond the split in order to re-establish respiration, and allow access for tracheal repair.

Tracheal stenosis

Tracheal stenosis may occur as the result of direct injury, but the increasing use of tracheostomy and intermittent positive pressure ventilation (IPPV) (with cuffed tubes) in intensive therapy, has become the most common cause of tracheal stenosis in recent times. The frequency of stenosis following such therapy is uncertain, reports varying from 1 to 20 per cent (Grillo, 1969; Andrews and Pearson, 1971). The site of the stenosis is likely to be at one of three locations.

(1) The most common site is at the level of the stoma itself, where infection has caused fibrosis or where the surgical method of fashioning the stoma has been faulty.
(2) At the site of the cuff where pressure has been applied to the trachea. The likelihood of stenosis occurring at this level will depend upon a number of factors including the cuff pressure used and the circulatory state of the patient during the early stages of therapy. There would appear to have been a decrease in the incidence of stenosis at this level in recent years since the introduction of the low-pressure cuff, and the practice of deflating the cuff for short periods in every hour. There is good evidence to suggest that the relationship between the cuff pressure and the capillary blood flow in the tracheal mucosa also plays a vital part in this injury (Crawley and Cross, 1975).
(3) Least commonly, stenosis occurs at the level of the tip of the tube where there has been trauma from movement associated with prolonged IPPV and persistent coughing, particularly if the tube is too rigid and incorrectly angled (Bassett, 1971).

The diameter of the trachea has to be reduced by more than 60 per cent before symptoms become evident and the exercise tolerance is reduced. Respiratory distress and stridor may not occur until the diameter has been reduced to less than 6 mm. In these severe cases tracheal dilatation may afford temporary relief, but resection will be required to effect a permanent cure.

Anaesthesia for tracheal resection

This type of surgery presents the surgeon and anaesthetist with problems of respiratory control similar to those for laryngeal surgery, with the exception that, following tracheal section, an endotracheal tube in the distal tracheal segment can considerably hamper access to the anastomosis. Therefore, many leading chest surgeons resort to cardiopulmonary bypass as a means of maintaining oxygenation. The following method of anaesthesia may be a useful alternative for the ENT surgeon.

Method of anaesthesia

Following induction of anaesthesia, an uncuffed endotracheal tube is passed through the stricture into the trachea beyond, and anaesthesia maintained with positive

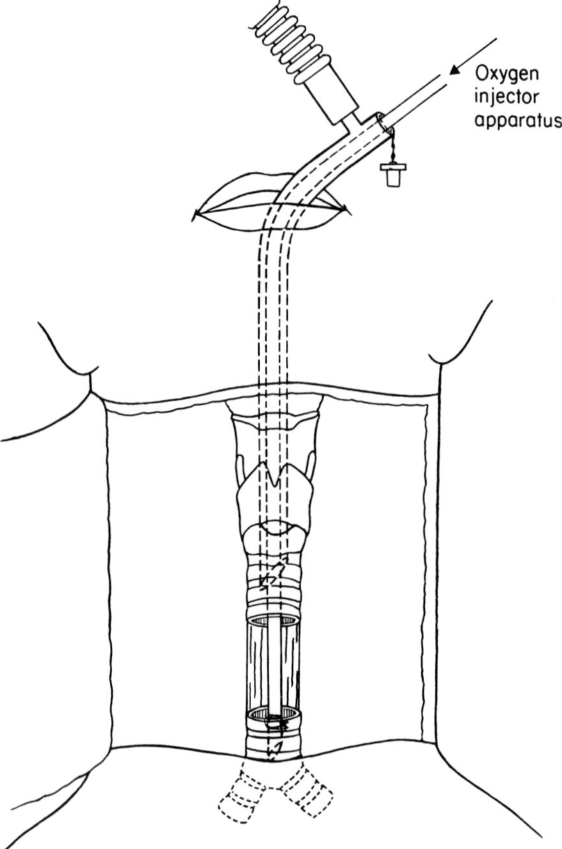

Figure 20.9 Position of endotracheal tube and catheter prior to tracheal anastomosis. Note stitch to anchor plastic tube to distal portion of trachea

pressure respiration. When there is a deviation of the trachea it is important that the bevel of the tube is cut in such a way to avoid the opening lying against the wall of the deviated trachea. As soon as the resection has been completed a long plastic tube, 1.5 mm internal diameter, is passed down the endotracheal tube into the distal portion of the trachea (*Figure 20.9*). If the stenosis is very low two tubes may be passed, one down each bronchus. The polythene tube is secured with a stitch to the wall of the distal tracheal segment and the endotracheal tube is withdrawn into the proximal tracheal segment. The lungs are inflated by attaching an injector to the polythene tube and opening the valve for approximately one second, twelve times a minute (Bethune, Collis, Forster and Burbridge, 1972).

As soon as the anastomosis has been completed the polythene tube is withdrawn and ventilation continued through the endotracheal tube. This technique may avoid the necessity to use the cardiopulmonary bypass in an attempt to maintain oxygenation during this operation (Harley, 1971).

The bloodless field in ENT surgery

The control of haemorrhage in surgery is primarily the responsibility of the surgeon. However, in certain surgical techniques a relatively dry field is so crucial that the anaesthetist may be asked to change the circulatory state of the patient, in order to assist the maintenance of haemostasis. The surgeon should understand the limitations within which this can safely be achieved. Variation in the amount of bleeding during any particular surgical technique depends upon:

(1) The venous pressure at the site of operation.
(2) The state of the peripheral arteriolar circulation.

These two parameters must be carefully and safely controlled.

Venous pressure

Provided the patient's circulatory function is normal the control that the anaesthetist can exercise on venous bleeding will depend upon three main factors: correct posture, a careful induction technique without coughing and straining and an adequate airway throughout. Whether these conditions are achieved with spontaneous breathing or controlled ventilation is a matter of personal choice (Deacock, 1971). Careful avoidance of venous congestion will go a long way to obtaining good haemostasis, but on its own will not be sufficient in all situations.

Peripheral blood flow

Reduction of peripheral arteriolar circulation may be achieved by the use of local vasoconstriction or by induced hypotension. The decision to use induced hypotension needs special experience and careful consideration of surgical requirements and the patient's safety. The decision must follow thorough pre-operative assessment of the patient's fitness for such a procedure, and clear indications for its use. After the decision it is important that anaesthesia is conducted only by an anaesthetist with specific training and experience.

Pre-operative assessment

A careful cardiovascular examination and drug history are essential, with electrocardiogram, chest x-ray, full blood count, and sickle-cell test when indicated. Evidence of myocardial ischaemia or cerebrovascular insufficiency must be regarded as an absolute contraindication to any hypotensive technique. In some other conditions, hypotension is probably best avoided:

(1) Hypertensive patients who are being controlled with drug therapy.
(2) Diabetic patients who may become unstable when treated with ganglionic blocking agents.
(3) Pregnancy at any stage.
(4) Patients suffering from severe anaemia or other blood dyscrasias.
(5) Hypo- and hyper-thyroid states.
(6) Patients taking a contraceptive pill.

Techniques of controlled hypotension

From experience it has been established that provided venous return from the site of operation to the heart is in no way impaired, a relatively dry operating field can be achieved with a systolic blood pressure between 65 and 55 mmHg in the majority of subjects. Pressures below 55 mmHg at arm level run the risk of cerebral ischaemia particularly with a head-raised position. The anaesthetist attempts to obtain these pressures by a balance between lowering the cardiac output and decreasing the peripheral resistance but at the same time maintaining tissue perfusion at a level consistent with metabolic needs. In head and neck surgery a reduced cardiac output is usually achieved by pooling blood in the lower limbs and splanchnic area with posture and muscle relaxation, while at the same time reducing the contractile force of the myocardium and heart rate with halothane and a β-blocking agent such as practolol or a combined alpha and beta blocker – Labetalol (Trandate). The state of peripheral resistance may be regulated in three ways:

(1) Central depression of the vasomotor centre – usually with halothane.
(2) Ganglionic Blockade. The drugs normally used are hexamethonium, with an action of about 1 h, pentolinium tartrate which has a somewhat longer action than hexamethonium, and trimetraphan camsylate (Arfonad) (given by continuous perfusion) which has a very short action.
(3) Peripheral Vasodilatation. This may be achieved by using sodium nitroprusside – a powerful and very short-acting peripheral vasodilator first introduced into anaesthetic practice in 1955 (Page, 1955; Taylor, Sykes and Lamming, 1955). It is used in a very dilute solution as a fast intravenous drip. Although this drug itself is non-toxic it is broken down in the body into thiocyanide and cyanide which

may be toxic in large doses particularly in patients with Vitamin B_{12} deficiency and malnutrition. The drug should be administered with caution and avoided in patients with impaired liver function. In anaesthetic practice however the maximum thiocyanate levels attained have proved to be well below the toxic level (Jones and Cole, 1968). It is unquestionably the drug of choice when a minute-to-minute control of blood pressure is required. A maximum dose of 1.5 mg/kg should not be exceeded.

Monitoring during hypotensive surgery

Careful monitoring of the patient during this type of anaesthesia is an important part of the safety requirement and must be continuous and uninterrupted. The type of monitoring required will depend upon the operative procedure. Apart from adjusting the blood pressure to maintain an adequate circulation to the vital organs, careful monitoring of blood loss is essential, as the patient's ability to compensate for a reduction in blood volume is lost.

(1) *Blood pressure monitoring* For microsurgery and for minor operative procedures where normally blood loss is likely to be less than 500 ml, non-invasive methods should be used. An oscillotonometer or a sphygmomanometer cuff with doppler sensor are perfectly adequate.

For major surgery where despite the use of hypotension considerable blood loss is inevitable (*see* 'Laryngopharyngectomy') continuous monitoring using an intra-arterial line should be considered. If the knowledge and equipment are available such a procedure will add to the safety of the patient.

(2) *Electrocardiogram* Although the information provided by an electrocardiogram during surgery is often not as specific as one would like, it is always of assistance in assessing the patient during hypotensive anaesthesia. A pre-operative electrocardiogram should always be available for comparison.

(3) *Central venous pressure (CVP)* It is vital that the blood loss should be replaced immediately and accurately during hypotensive anaesthesia, making central venous pressure measurement important in major surgery. As with intra-arterial blood pressure reading and other invasive monitoring techniques, CVP monitoring carries a small morbidity in its own right, and therefore should not be used for minor surgery unless the indications for it are very strong.

(4) *Temperature recording* Prolonged major surgery under hypotension, because of the interference with normal temperature-regulating mechanisms, carries a high risk of excessive body-cooling. Therefore the accurate recording and controlling of body temperature may greatly assist the well-being of the patient.

(5) *Electro-encephalography* At the present state of our knowledge the useful information obtained from an EEG Monitor does not warrant the extra trouble involved. This is not to say that in the future it will not have its place.

Post-operative care

The rate of recovery of patients after hypotensive anaesthesia will always vary with the technique of anaesthesia used and therefore experienced recovery-care is essential. When the longer-acting hypotensive agents are employed the return to a normal blood pressure may be gradual. It is important that the patient should be kept flat until he appears to be fully conscious and alert, and the blood pressure has risen above 90 mmHg systolic. The patient can then be gradually elevated to the head-up position. Failure of the blood pressure to rise satisfactorily may be due to a number of factors.

Low cardiac output Failure of cardiac output to increase after minor surgery where beta blockers and halothane have been used is often associated with a bradycardia and is readily corrected with intravenous atropine. The use of a vasopressor may be indicated but is seldom necessary. If a reasonable diastolic pressure is not maintained and the coronary blood flow is at risk then the controlled and short-term use of isoprenaline (a β stimulant) may be indicated. It should be administered at a rate of 2–4 mg/min using an intravenous drip containing 2–4 mg/500 ml of dextrose saline or in a 'bolus' of 1–2 mg.

Hypovolaemia After major surgery continued careful attention to fluid replacement is essential – and CVP recording must be maintained. Dextran 70 may be used to maintain blood volume in an emergency if cross-matched blood is not immediately available.

Cyanide toxicity With the increasing use of sodium nitroprusside, toxicity may be encountered. In assessing the post-operative condition of patients after hypotensive anaesthesia using sodium nitroprusside it must be remembered that, although this method of producing controlled hypotension during surgery is safe and very valuable in experienced hands, both for adults and children, doses in excess of 10 mg/kg/min can produce serious toxic effects (Vasey *et al.*, 1974). Should toxicity occur, as indicated by metabolic acidosis and persistent hypotension, treatment should be instituted immediately by one or more of the following methods.

(1) An adequate quantity of sodium bicarbonate should be given intravenously to correct acidosis; 200–500 mmol may be required (MacRae and Owen, 1974).
(2) The intravenous infusion of vitamin B_{12a} (hydroxocobalamin) may be required to reduce the cyanide toxicity (Posner, Rodkey and Tobey, 1976). It is recommended that 22.5 mg of B_{12a} is given for every 1 mg of sodium nitroprusside used – this may be administered prophylactically.
(3) Sodium nitrite may be given intravenously in a dose of 0.1 mg/kg injected over a period of 4 min. This induces methaemoglobinaemia which has an increased affinity for cyanide. Alternatively, the inhalation of amyl nitrite may be effective for the same reason.
(4) The addition of calcium gluconate to matched ACD blood, in a dose of 1 mg/ml.
(5) The intravenous infusion of sodium thiosulphate in a dose of 150 mg/kg in 50 ml of water given over 15 min.

Middle-ear and mastoid surgery

General considerations

Anaesthesia for surgery of the middle ear has in the past required no special skills that are not necessary for other operations on the head and neck. With the recent advancement of this type of surgery and the almost universal use of the microscope, it has become incumbent on the anaesthetist to provide an operation field that is almost bloodless. Failure to produce such conditions may result in the necessity to abandon the operation, as blood obscuring the operative field can make surgery impossible. Also the continuous use of suction within the middle ear may cause physiological damage and therefore seriously affect the outcome of the operation. To achieve ideal conditions for minor surgery such as suction clearance and myringotomy, with or without the insertion of grommets, presents few problems, but in major surgery, including stapedectomy, tympanoplasty and labyrinthectomy, a combination of induced hypotension and the topical use of vasoconstrictors is frequently necessary. The depth to which the anaesthetist is willing to lower an individual patient's blood pressure must depend upon circumstances but, provided anaesthesia is smooth throughout, it is seldom necessary or wise to lower the systolic blood pressure below 60 mmHg.

Minor surgery

Examination of ears under a microscope and myringotomy are simple procedures which form a considerable part of ear surgery under general anaesthesia and are frequently carried out as a day-stay procedure. The anaesthesia should, therefore, be simple and whenever possible conducted without tracheal intubation. Anaesthesia with nitrous oxide, oxygen and halothane using a naso-pharyngeal tube or an airway clip (*Figure 20.10*) will prove perfectly adequate for most patients.

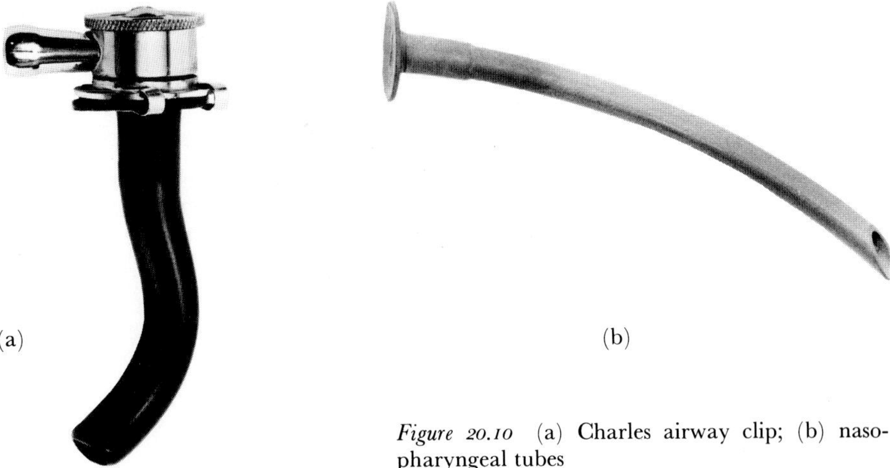

Figure 20.10 (a) Charles airway clip; (b) naso-pharyngeal tubes

Major surgery

Because major ear surgery under general anaesthesia often requires the use of hypotensive techniques, special care is necessary with the pre-operative assessment of these patients.

Pre-operative assessment
In addition to the routine examination required for any patient undergoing an operation, a specially careful history should be obtained from those patients who are going to be subjected to hypotensive anaesthesia.

An enquiry into past illnesses such as heart disease, thromboses and thrombo-embolic phenomena are very important as patients with a history of such illnesses should not be exposed to hypotension during anaesthesia. Special attention should also be paid to past and present drug therapy, particularly drugs which affect the cardiovascular system such as hypotensive agent, β-blockers and mono-amine oxidase inhibitors. These problems are discussed under controlled hypotension (p. 744).

Premedication

There are no particular rules concerning premedication for ear surgery, but it is prudent to include an anti-emetic in the regimen and many anaesthetists prefer the exclusion of atropine if hypotension is contemplated.

Induction of anaesthesia

As discussed under hypotensive techniques a smooth induction is absolutely essential for successful haemostasis. Most anaesthetists prefer to intubate and control respiration for these procedures. The muscle-relaxant used should not increase blood pressure, pulse rate or cardiac output – thus curare is preferable to suxamethonium, parcuronium or gallamine. The larynx and trachea should be thoroughly sprayed with local anaesthetic to avoid coughing following intubation. It is essential to use a non-kinkable or armoured tube of adequate size (*Figure 20.11*). Following induction the patient is placed on the operating table in a 10–15° head-up tip.

Maintenance of anaesthesia

The control of the blood pressure and monitoring devices required are described fully under 'Bloodless Field Surgery' (p. 743). For middle-ear surgery, because of the small blood loss, invasive methods of blood pressure monitoring are seldom considered necessary. Before the end of the operation the anaesthetist will frequently be requested to turn off the nitrous oxide so as to prevent the increased middle-ear pressure created by nitrous oxide from dislodging the drum.

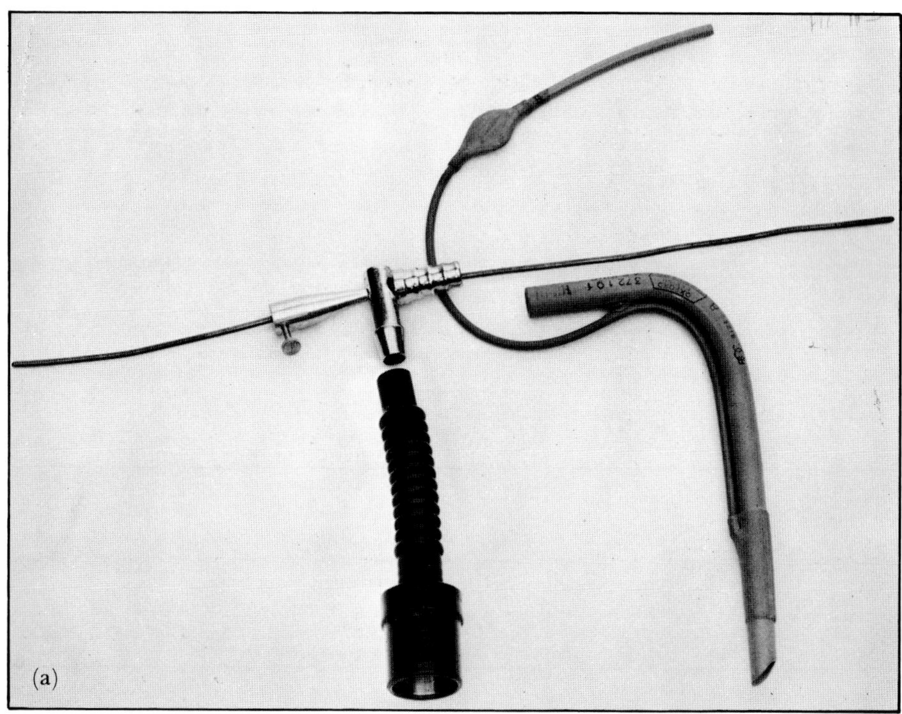

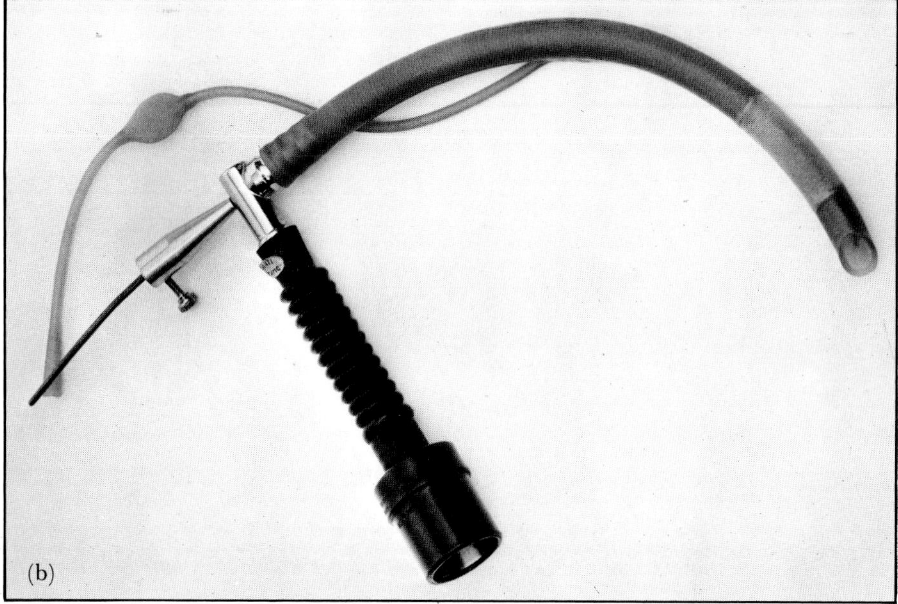

Figure 20.11 Non-kinkable endotracheal tubes. (a) Cuffed armoured tube with stilette in position for easy introduction; (b) Oxford tube. A stilette is needed to introduce the tube in adult patients

Recovery

Recovery is frequently slow after this type of anaesthesia and therefore good recovery care is essential. If hypotension has been used the blood pressure should be allowed to rise slowly, but should be within 20–30 mmHg of its original level before the patient is allowed to remain unsupervised. Nausea is not an uncommon feature after middle-ear operations due to disturbance of labyrinthine function. Therefore the routine use of prochlorperazine (Stemetil) 12.5 mg, perphenazine (Fentazin) 2.5 mg, cyclizine (Valoid) 50 mg is recommended.

Anaesthesia for nasal operations

No matter what operation is performed on the nose and adjoining structures, from major nasal reconstruction to submucous diathermy, the principles of anaesthesia must remain the same. They are faultless maintenance and protection of airway, and minimal bleeding at the site of operation. The first is the absolute responsibility of the anaesthetist and the second can be considerably aided by the anaesthetic technique used.

Maintenance and protection of airway

The surgeon must appreciate that the flexed position of the head and its frequent movement required during these operations may make the anaesthetist's task in maintaining a safe airway difficult. Nevertheless, the careful preparation of the respiratory tract with a short-acting local anaesthetic and the use of non-kinkable cuffed orotracheal tubes will considerably reduce the risks of coughing and tube obstruction. However it is helpful as well as being courteous if the anaesthetist is warned before major changes in position of the head are made. This will avoid the occasionally embarrassing and sometimes dangerous disconnection and kinking of the breathing apparatus.

Control of bleeding

Although the control of bleeding during nasal surgery must primarily be the concern of the surgeon, the anaesthetic technique used can influence considerably the ease by which he can gain this control. The general principles involved are described in detail under the heading 'Hypotensive Anaesthesia' (p. 744). The author feels that for the bulk of nasal surgery, except for the occasional difficult rhinoplasty and extensive cancer surgery, the additional hazards of providing controlled hypotension are not justified, as careful local preparation of the nose and skilled general anaesthesia will provide excellent conditions.

After careful induction of anaesthesia and intubation, a throat pack must be inserted. The pack should be moistened with water or a water-soluble grease such as polyethylene glycol. Paraffin and other insoluble lubricants should be avoided as these may cause a lipoid pneumonia if they enter the lungs.

Local preparation of the nose may be started prior to induction of anaesthesia by the use of adrenaline packs or cocaine spray, but equally good results can be obtained by carrying out the preparation after induction of anaesthesia and thus avoiding additional discomfort for the patient, provided time is allowed for full vasoconstriction before surgery is commenced. This preparation is frequently performed by the surgeon using a mixture of cocaine crystals and adrenaline, or a specially prepared cocaine paste containing 25 per cent cocaine in a soft paraffin. Alternatively it may be more conveniently carried out by the anaesthetist using a modified Moffett technique described by Curtiss in 1952, for nasal operations under local anaesthesia.

Moffett technique

The solution is made up as follows: 2 ml 8–10 per cent cocaine, 1 ml 1:1000 adrenaline and 2 ml 1 per cent sodium bicarbonate are mixed in a container and drawn up in a 5 ml syringe. The patient is placed with the head extended over a pillow. 1.5 ml of the mixture is then instilled into each nostril. This will pool in the roof of the nose. The head is then rotated first to one side and then to the other, over a period of 10 min. Finally the remaining 2 ml of solution is sprayed into the nose on both sides to cover the mucous membranes in the anterior compartment of the nose. Good vasoconstriction is achieved in this way (*Figure 20.12*).

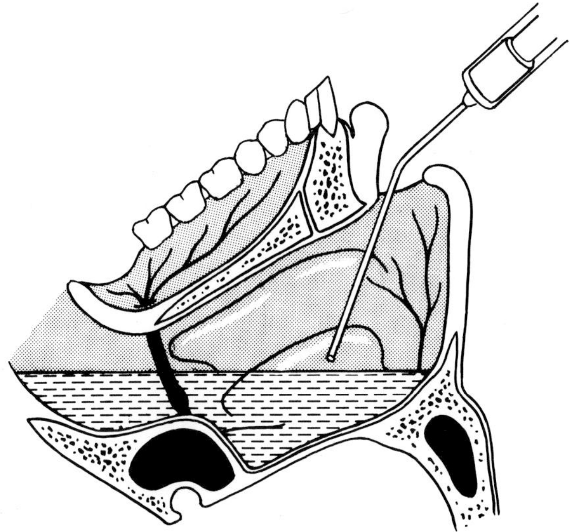

Figure 20.12 Moffett technique

In addition to the topical preparation of the nasal mucosa, adrenaline (1:200 000) may be injected submucosally by the surgeon. It is important that the anaesthetist is warned well in advance before this is carried out, as serious cardiac irregularities may arise if the injection is made before he has time to adjust his anaesthetic drugs accordingly (*see* section on 'Local Anaesthesia', p. 718).

On completion of surgery, it is the anaesthetist's responsibility to see that his pack is removed and that the pharynx is clear of blood. The patient should then be placed on his side before extubation, and an airway inserted. The lateral position must be maintained until all reflexes are active and the patient is awake. He may then be sat up to reduce venous congestion and bleeding. Pain is not usually a feature following these operations but mild analgesics may be required. For the adult an injection of pethidine 75 mg and phenergan 25 mg will usually settle the patient satisfactorily for the first night.

Injuries to the nose and face

Severe trauma to the nose and face is perhaps more the realm of the dental and maxillofacial surgeons than the ENT surgeon, although each may have to deal with the problems in an emergency. Whoever conducts the surgery, the anaesthetist's problems remain the same. These are the maintenance and protection of the airway, which may involve correcting the patients' posture, a difficult intubation or an emergency tracheostomy.

Early management

The immediate necessity after severe facial injury, particularly if unstable fractures are present, is to establish and maintain a good airway. This may be achieved in a number of ways:

(1) The patient must be nursed on his side in the 'recovering-tonsil' position.
(2) The tongue must be held forward, particularly in the unconscious patient, either by an artificial airway or by pulling the tongue forward with a clip or stitch.
(3) If the nose is not fractured or bleeding, a naso-pharyngeal tube passed blind down one nostril may prove helpful. Several types of tube are available, but a naso-tracheal tube cut to the appropriate length to give maximum air entry, and fastened with a pin, is usually the most satisfactory (*Figure 20.13*).
(4) In the deeply unconscious patient a naso- or orotracheal tube may be passed.
(5) If these methods prove unsuccessful an emergency tracheostomy may prove necessary.

Once a stable airway has been established further treatment can be contemplated.

Anaesthesia for corrective surgery

Anaesthesia should be induced carefully on the operating table, bearing in mind the possibility that the regurgitation of a large quantity of blood from the stomach may occur at any time. Naso-tracheal intubation should be performed whenever possible, but if gross nasal injury is present an orotracheal tube may be necessary for the first stage of the operation. At the end of the operation when fixation of the fracture has been completed it is often helpful to pass a naso-pharyngeal tube down the free nostril and to shorten the naso-tracheal tube so that two naso-pharyngeal tubes ensure a good airway post-operatively.

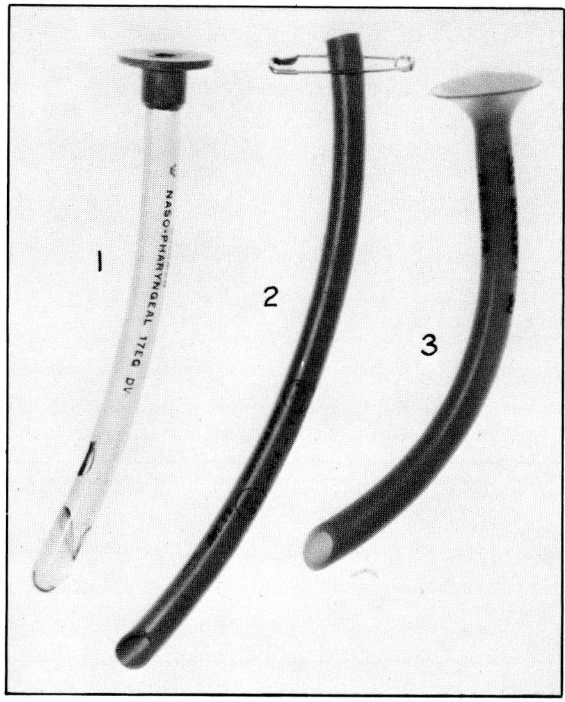

Figure 20.13 Naso-pharyngeal tubes. (2) shows method of adjusting length of tube with a pin

The difficult intubation

All anaesthetists and surgeons are faced from time to time with the necessity to intubate a patient on whom attempts at intubation using standard equipment have proved impossible, and other methods have been sought. This problem may be tackled in a variety of ways.

Blind nasal intubation When there is a relatively normal larynx, but owing to anatomical peculiarities the larynx cannot be visualized, blind intubation will often succeed.

Bronchoscopic intubation By threading a suitable size of naso-tracheal tube over a fibre-optic bronchoscope, the two instruments together may be passed through the nose and directed under vision towards the larynx. As soon as the tube is between the cords the bronchoscope is removed. This can be performed under local or general anaesthesia (Taylor and Towey, 1972).

Guided, blind intubation This method described originally by Waters (1963) was used for patients with severe trismus as the result of cancrum oris. The technique involves threading a length of vinyl plastic tubing through a Tuohy needle which has been inserted into the glottis via the cricothyroid membrane. The tubing is then directed up through the larynx and into the pharynx. A special hook passed down the nose is made to engage the tubing and to pull it out through the nose. This tubing may then act as a guide down which a naso-tracheal tube can be inserted.

Control of intractable pain from malignant disease in ENT

Pain arising from the ear, nose and throat, when associated with neoplasm, is frequently alleviated by operation, radiotherapy or treatment with cytotoxic drugs. In the minority of patients, however, the pain remains unremitting despite these measures, and is then classified as intractable pain requiring other methods of alleviation.

When chronic pain involves the face, it would appear to be less well tolerated than pain elsewhere in the body and to have some special psychological significance leading to a higher incidence of suicide than other types of chronic pain. If no clear cause for the pain is apparent it is only too easy to regard it as psychogenic in origin, only to find a neoplasm a few months later.

The management of such pain must be the primary responsibility of the surgical team looking after the patient, but undoubtedly the best results are obtained by a multidisciplinary approach involving surgeons, physicians, oncologists, anaesthetists and nursing staff. These patients are, generally speaking, inadequately dealt with in the average busy general hospital. There is a tendency for the specialist to be slightly embarrassed by his inability to help the patient further and so to quickly pass by on his ward rounds. The day-to-day management may therefore be left, in the first place, to the house surgeon who frequently has no special experience of analgesics and how to administer them and in the second place to the ward sister who can only administer drugs under instruction and is therefore limited in her ability to deal with the problem effectively. There is much to be said for the setting up of special pain-relief clinics and terminal care units to which these unfortunate patients can be sent. Such units can acquire the extensive knowledge and experience required for their management. Three main approaches are involved in the care of these patients:

(1) The treatment of the malignant process itself (discussed elsewhere in relevant chapters).
(2) The symptomatic management of the pain.
(3) Terminal care.

Symptomatic management

The symptomatic management will involve either the interruption of various pain pathways or the careful administration of analgesic and psychotrophic drugs. The methods chosen will often be influenced by the limited prognosis of the sufferer.

Interruption of pain-conducting pathways

This direct approach to the pain problem should be considered as early as possible in the progress of the patient's disease, as soon as the cancer therapy has been completed and before the patient has become demoralized by useless suffering. If the pain can be controlled in this way, it is unquestionably preferable in the early stages to the use of analgesic and narcotic drugs. The nerves of the head, neck and pharynx are usually accessible to peripheral block or section.

Trigeminal nerve

Chemical destruction of the trigeminal nerve may be necessary in advanced malignancy involving all three branches of the nerve. The block should be performed under x-ray control using an image intensifier and either phenol or alcohol injected into the Gasserian ganglion as it lies in the cave of Meckel. Alcohol gives a more long-lasting effect than phenol, but is more likely to give corneal anaesthesia. The results using alcohol are good and the complications few in expert hands (Penman, 1953), but spill-over to other cranial roots can occur with unfortunate results. The use of 5 per cent phenol in glycerine is far less hazardous as the solution is not so diffusible and is heavier than cerebrospinal fluid. Good results can often be achieved. A more selective analgesia can be obtained by radio-frequency coagulation to the sensory roots involved, by inserting a probe through the foramen ovale into the root sheath. The results can be repeatedly checked by using methohexitone anaesthesia and allowing the patient to wake, from time to time, or with the use of sophisticated impedance recording under continuous anaesthesia (Sweet and Wepsic, 1974). If the equipment for selective treatment by radio-frequency is not available then the individual divisions of the fifth nerve can be treated (*Figure 20.14*).

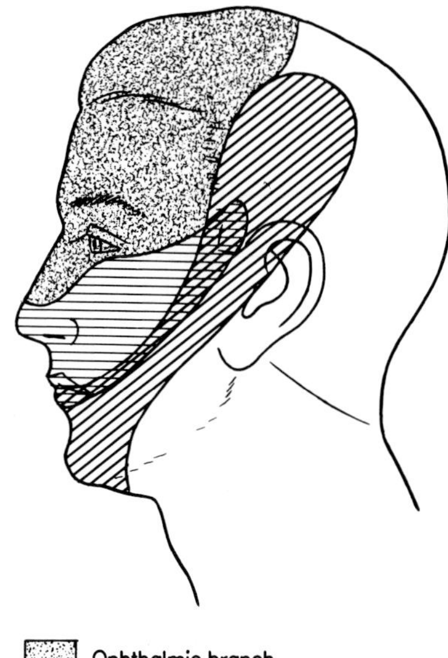

Figure 20.14 Sensory distribution of trigeminal nerve

Ophthalmic division It is usually the ethmoidal branch of the ophthalmic fifth division which is painfully involved in advanced malignant tumours of the maxilla. Unfortunately owing to the close proximity of this nerve to the optic nerve itself, it is unwise to attempt a permanent block using a neurolytic agent for fear of causing visual disturbances. Some relief, however, may be achieved by blocking the supra-orbital nerve as it runs over the orbital ridge. Five per cent phenol in water will frequently give prolonged relief.

Maxillary division After emerging from the foramen rotundum this nerve lies in the pterygopalatine fossa where it is most easily reached with a needle. The successful block of this nerve results in cessation of painful impulses coming from maxillary antrum, tonsils, gums and lower part of nose and is therefore particularly useful for pain from carcinoma of maxillary antrum and tonsil. The simplest technique for blocking this division is the anterior approach from in front of the neck of the mandible and this is also the least disturbing to the conscious patient. The patient lies supine looking directly forward. The mandibular notch is located by asking the patient to open his mouth. The condyle of the mandible is felt to ride forward, in which position it lies over the mandibular notch and a mark can be made on the skin (*Figure 20.15*). With the mouth closed, a skin weal is made over this mark and an 8 cm

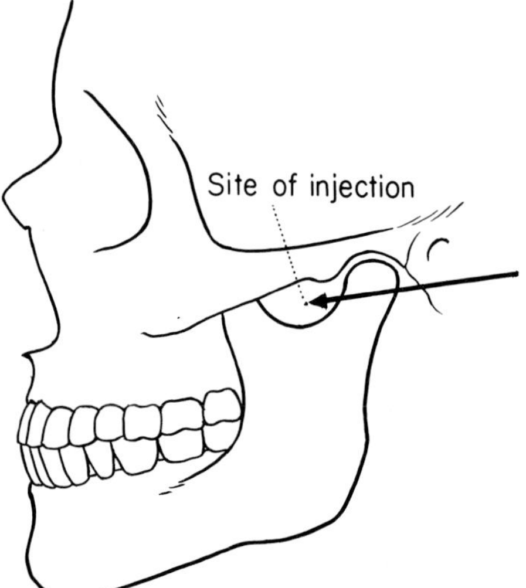

Figure 20.15 Site of injection for block of maxillary and mandibular divisions of trigeminal nerve

needle with marker is inserted and directed towards the back of the eyeball. At a depth of approximately 5 cm the needle will strike the lateral pterygoid plate. The marker is then set 1 cm from skin and the needle re-inserted slightly more anteriorly to pass beyond the plate. Paraesthesia may be felt in the distribution of the nerve. If a special insulated needle is used further confirmation of its position can be gained by electrical stimulation (Greenblatt and Dennerson, 1962). Approximately 3 ml of 6 per cent aqueous phenol may be injected.

Mandibular division Intractable pain resulting from carcinoma of tongue and lower jaw may be alleviated by injecting the mandibular nerve with a neurolytic agent.

The technique is similar to that described for the maxillary division through the mandibular notch. The nerve is blocked in the pterygoid fossa as it emerges from the foramen ovale. When the needle reaches the pterygoid plate it is re-inserted slightly posteriorly to reach the mandibular division and 3 ml of 6 per cent phenol may be injected.

Glossopharyngeal nerve

Malignant disease of the oropharynx can be associated with very severe pain either as a result of the disease process or as a direct result of radiotherapy. Unfortunately blocking of the glossopharyngeal nerve with either local anaesthetic or a neurolytic agent can be a hazardous procedure owing to the close proximity of the vagus and hypoglossal nerves. Nevertheless the risks may be justified if other methods of pain relief prove inadequate.

Technique A narrow gauge 5 cm needle is introduced at right angles to the skin just below the external auditory meatus through a point midway between angle of jaw and tip of mastoid process. With the aid of an image intensifier, lateral and submental views, the needle is directed posterior to the styloid process with its tip lying close to the jugular foramen. A preliminary block should be carried out with local anaesthetic to assess its effect, before a neurolytic agent is used. Owing to the risk of pharyngeal paralysis this block should never be performed on both sides (Montgomery and Cousins, 1972).

Glossopharyngeal neuralgia

The use of cryotherapy has been described for the treatment of glossopharyngeal neuralgia by Brain (1975). Its application in the treatment of chronic pain due to neoplasm has received some attention; unfortunately, the pain relief is frequently short. However, it compares favourably with the effect of phenol and alcohol (Lloyd, Barnard and Glynn, 1976).

Vagus nerve

Tuberculosis or malignant disease of the larynx may cause pain, severe enough to warrant some neurolytic procedure. Blocking of the vagus nerve itself is never justified but a block of its superior laryngeal branch may be very rewarding.

Technique The patient lies supine and a skin weal is made over the notch of the thyroid cartilage. A 5 cm needle is inserted through the skin weal and directed towards the greater cornu of the hyoid bone. The neurolytic agent is deposited just below the greater cornu. Both nerves may be injected through the same puncture.

Upper cervical nerves

In malignant disease of the larynx pain may extend beyond the larynx itself, necessitating injection of the second and third cervical nerves, in addition to the superior laryngeal branch of the vagus.

Technique The patient lies supine with the head rotated away from the side to be treated, and extended over a pillow. A skin weal is made 1.5 cm below the mastoid process. This should lie over the transverse process of the second cervical vertebra. The third and fourth cervical processes lie below at 1.5 cm intervals. The needles are advanced through these points until they reach the transverse processes. The transverse processes lie quite superficially and care must be taken that the needles do not pass through the paravertebral foramina and enter the subarachnoid space. Careful aspiration is necessary before injection of any neurolytic agent. Destruction of the upper cervical nerves in conjunction with the superior laryngeal nerve, can be a very valuable procedure in controlling intractable pain from malignant disease of the larynx.

Analgesic and psychotrophic drugs

Analgesic drugs must inevitably play a major part in the treatment of chronic pain of malignant origin and generally speaking they should be given orally unless there is some special contraindication. The mild analgesics should always be given in adequate dosage in the early stages. Their use frequently fails because they are not given often enough. The objective must be to control pain and not merely to alleviate it and therefore the analgesic should be repeated before the previous dose has worn off. The length of action of each drug will vary from individual to individual, but remains fairly consistent in each individual, so the dose regime can soon be determined. Good pain control can usually be achieved in this way in most patients without greatly increasing the dose required. The overwhelming range of drugs available may cause much confusion, but generally speaking there is very little to choose between them. The analgesic chosen to maintain pain relief should be that drug which produces the fewest side effects in an effective dose. Many patients with chronic pain become agitated and depressed, making the combination of an analgesic and tranquillizer or psychotrophic drug very helpful. Small doses of a phenothiazine such as promethazine 10 mg, chlordiazepoxide (Librium) 10 mg or diazepam (Valium) 5 mg given three times a day will help the agitated patient. For the depressed patient amitriptylline 10 mg or imipramine (Tofranil) 25 mg given two or three times a day makes a good combination with the analgesic drug.

When the disease has progressed to its terminal stage, it is then time to resort to the more powerful narcotic drugs. The same principles discussed for the mild analgesics apply, i.e. to give an effective dose as frequently as necessary and by mouth whenever possible. Pain relief should be achieved and the fear of causing addiction should not detract from this objective. In fact, drug addiction is not a common feature in cancer pain. The patients are only too willing to come off their drugs if other methods of relief can be achieved. Pethidine 50–200 mg, methadone 50–150 mg and Diconal (dipipanone 10 mg with cyclazine 30 mg) by mouth are good drugs with which to start. It may be necessary to progress to morphine and heroin at a later stage. Nausea and constipation are common side effects of these drugs and should be controlled with anti-emetics and aperients.

Terminal care

The care of the terminal patient, as already mentioned, is best carried out in a special unit, or if adequate special attention is available, in the patient's own home. Above all, the patient requires our constant concern, and assurance that they are not being abandoned, or allowed to suffer unnecessary pain (Saunders, 1967). Narcotic analgesics should be supplied on demand and it has been suggested by Schofield, Saunders and others that they should be left by the bedside and the patient allowed to regulate his own dose frequency (Schofield, 1971). Experience has shown that this 'privilege' is not abused by the patients.

The 'Brompton Mixture' containing 10 mg morphine, 10 mg diacetyl morphine and 10 mg of cocaine in a palatable mixture containing gin or brandy or similar mixtures are invaluable in terminal care. Although these mixtures do lead to dependence this is unimportant and probably over-emphasized (Twycross, 1972). The cocaine is often omitted from this mixture as its stimulant effect can lead to considerable restlessness.

Nausea and vomiting may make oral administration impossible, in which case rectal or intramuscular administration may be necessary. Rectal oxycodone (Proladone) or other rectal preparations of analgesics may prove useful. Repeated intramuscular injections of large volumes of fluid into the emaciated patient may cause considerable distress. This can be overcome to some extent by taking advantage of the very high solubility of diamorphine. The appropriate dose may be dissolved in a very small volume of an anti-emetic to make a low volume injection.

The effect of pollution by anaesthetic agents

Apart from the well-known explosive hazards of certain anaesthetic agents such as ether, ethyl chloride and cyclopropane the possible harmful effect of anaesthetic vapours on the personnel in the operating theatres has drawn little attention until recent years.

Although the exposure to anaesthetic vapours is probably about 50 per cent greater for the anaesthetist than for the surgeon, except perhaps during tonsillectomy, all members of the surgical team are exposed to some extent.

The possibility that exposure to these vapours may be harmful was first considered in 1967 as the result of a questionnaire to 300 Russian anaesthetists in which the majority complained of fatigue and other symptoms. The significant revelation in this series was that 18 out of 31 pregnancies among these anaesthetists terminated in spontaneous abortion and only 7 pregnancies were without complications. A more recent survey in 1974 on a range of operating theatre personnel, in the USA and Glasgow compared with a control group show no very conclusive results (Cohen, 1975) but there was evidence that carcinoma and infective diseases of the liver and kidney are more common, particularly among females. The results of many surveys relating to reproduction following the original Russian findings are slightly more significant in favour of some adverse influence of the polluted theatre environment upon the progress of pregnancy, both when the woman herself is exposed and when the husband alone is exposed. However, the ASA (American Society of Anaesthesia) sum up the problem saying: 'The conclusion that operating room personnel are subject to a health hazard and that such a hazard is the result of anaesthetic gases in the ambient air of the operating theatre, must be advanced with caution'.

There is a tendency to implicate halothane rather than any other of the pollutants in the operating theatre in the present argument, probably because halothane is the most commonly used of the recently introduced inhalational anaesthetic agents. However, recent experiments by Corbett *et al.* (1973) and Bruce (1974) in pregnant rats have shown a greater embryotoxic effect with N_2O than with halothane. There is evidence that anaesthetic agents affect the immune response to infection, although the result of this is more likely to be in the patient than in the theatre personnel; it may be of significance in the cause of so-called halothane hepatitis and the increased incidence of infections which occur in theatre personnel.

In conclusion it must be stressed that there would appear to be some relation between working in operating theatres and a raised morbidity among such personnel especially in relation to reproduction. This evidence must not be ignored.

The prevention of operation theatre pollution is obviously more the concern of the anaesthetist than the surgeon as he is more at risk, but it is the eye and ENT surgeon more than any other surgeon whose risk, if there is indeed a risk, will approach that of the anaesthetist. Effective antipollution methods are expensive, but 'clean' technique and good general control of the theatre environment by adequate air-conditioning must always be sought.

References

Andrews, M. J. and Pearson, F. G. (1971). *Annals of Surgery*, **173**, 249

Bali, I. M., Dundee, J. W. and Stevenson, H. M. (1973). *British Journal of Anaesthesia*, **45**, 1063

Bassett, H. F. M. (1971). *Proceedings of the Royal Society of Medicine*, **64**, 890

Bearman, A. J. (1962). *Anesthesiology*, **23**, 130

Bethune, D. W. (1976). *Proceedings of the Royal Society of Medicine*, **69**, 672

Bethune, D. W., Collis, J. M., Forster, D. M. and Burbridge, N. J. (1972). *Anaesthesia*, **27**, 81

Boyd, J. D. and Manfold, M. L. M. (1973). *British Journal of Anaesthesia*, **45**, 501

Brain, D. J. (1975. *Practical Cryosurgery*, 69

Bruce, D. L. (1974). *Anesthesiology*, **41**, 71

Campkin, T. V. (1970). *British Journal of Anaesthesia*, **41**, 1073

Carden, E. and Crutchfield, W. (1973). *Canadian Anaesthetic Society Journal*, **20**, 378

Cohen, E. N. (1975). *Anesthesiology*, **41**, 321

Condon, H. A. (1971). *British Journal of Anaesthesia*, **43**, 1061

Coplans, M. P. (1976). *Anaesthesia*, **31**, 430

Corbett, T. H., Cornell, R. G. and Lieding, K. (1973). *Anesthesiology*, **38**, 260

Crawley, B. E. and Cross, D. E. (1975). *Anaesthesia*, **30**, 4

Curtiss, E. S. (1952). *Lancet*, **1**, 989

Deacock, de C. A. R. (1971). *Proceedings of the Royal Society of Medicine*, **64**, 1226

Di Fazio, C. A. and Brown, R. E. (1972). *Anaesthesiology*, **36**, 238

Doughty, A. G. (1957). *Lancet*, **i**, 1074

Gordon, M. and Sellars, S. (1971). *Anaesthesia*, **26**, 199

Gorham, A. P., Baskett, P. J. and Clement, J. A. (1965). *Anaesthesia*, **20**, 279

Green, R. A. and Coplans, M. P. (1973). *Anaesthesia and Analgesia in Dentistry*, p. 306. London; Lewis

Green, R. A. and Day, B. L. (1954). *Lancet*, **i**, 602

Greenblatt, G. H. and Dennerson, J. S. (1962). *Anaesthesia and Analgesia*, **41**, 599

Grillo, H. C. (1969). *Journal of Thoracic and Cardiovascular Surgery*, **57**, 52

Harley, H. R. S. (1971). *Thorax*, **26**, 493

Hong, K. and Hubell, W. L. (1972). *Proceedings of the National Academy of Science, U.S.A.*, **69**, 2617

Howells, T. H., Huntsman, R. G., Boys, J. E. and Mahmood, A. (1972). *British Journal of Anaesthesia*, **44**, 975

Jones, G. O. M. and Cole, P. (1968). *British Journal of Anaesthesia*, **40**, 804

Katz, R. L. (1965). *Anesthesiology*, **26**, 619

Lee, J. A. and Bryce Smith, R. (1976). *Practical Redional Analgesia*, p. 12. Amsterdam; Excerpta Medica

Lee, J. A. and Bryce Smith, R. (1976). *Practical Regional Analgesia*, p. 17. Amsterdam; Excerpta Medica

Lewis, R. B. (1977). *Anaesthesia*, **32**, 366

Lloyd, J. W., Barnard, J. D. W. and Glynn, C. J. (1976). *Lancet*, Oct. 30, 932

MacRae, W. R. and Owen, M. (1974). *British Journal of Anaesthesia*, **46**, 795

Miller, K. W., Paton, W. D. and Smith, E. B. (1972). *Anaesthesiology*, **36**, 339

Montgomery, W. and Cousins, M. T. (1972). *British Journal of Anaesthesia*, **44**, 383

Page, I. H. (1955). *Circulation*, **11**, 188

Penman, J. (1953). *Lancet*, **i**, 760

Pollard, B. J. (1968). *Anaesthesia*, **23**, 534

Posner, M. A., Rodkey, F. L. and Tobey, R. E. (1976). *Anesthesiology*, **44**, 330

Sanders, R. D. (1967). *Delaware State Medical Journal*, **39**, 170

Saunders, C. M. S. (1967). *Annals of the Royal College of Surgeons*, **41**, 162

Schofield, P. B. (1971). *British Journal of Medicine*, **3**, 773

Searle, J. F. (1973). *Anaesthesia*, **28**, 48

Seward, E. H. and Fraser, R. A. (1961). *British Medical Journal*, **2**, 987

Shalom, A. S. (1964). *Journal of Laryngology and Otology*, **78**, 734

Simpson, K. (1960). *Proceedings of the Royal Society of Medicine*, **53**, 843
Strunin, L. and Simpson, B. R. (1972). *British Journal of Anaesthesia*, **44**, 919
Sweet, W. H. and Wepsic, J. C. (1974). *Journal of Neurosurgery*, **40**, 143
Tate, N. (1963). *Lancet*, **ii**, 1090
Taylor, P. A. and Towey, R. M. (1972). *British Journal of Anaesthesia*, **44**, 611
Taylor, T. H., Sykes, M. and Lamming, J. (1955). *British Journal of Anaesthesia*, **42**, 859
Thomas, D. K. (1974). *British Journal of Anaesthesia*, **46**, 66
Tobias, M. A. (1977). *Anaesthesia*, **32**, 359
Twycross, K. (1972). Personal communication
Vasey, C. J., Cole, P. V., Linnell, J. C. and Watson, J. (1974). *British Journal of Medicine*, **ii**, 140
Vaughan, R. S. and Lunn, J. N. (1973). *Anaesthesia*, **28**, 118
Verrill, P. (1963). *British Journal of Anaesthesia*, **35**, 237
Waters, D. J. (1973). *Anaesthesia*, **18**, 158
Watt, J. M. (1975). *British Medical Journal*, **3**, 205
Zorab, J. S. (1969). *Anaesthesia*, **24**, 431

Index